THE ENCYCLOPEDIA OF NUTRITION & GOOD HEALTH

ROBERT A. RONZIO
PH.D., C.N.S., F.A.I.C.

Facts On File, Inc.

The Encyclopedia of Nutrition and Good Health reports information and opinions of medical literature which may be of general interest to the reader. Although the author has made every effort to assure that all the information in this book is correct at the time of printing, the reader is advised that medical knowledge is constantly changing, and this book should not be relied upon without the consultation and advice of a physician. In addition, in any book of this scope, some errors may occur. The author and Facts On File, Inc. disclaim any responsibility for any consequences that may result from any use or reliance thereon by the reader.

The Encyclopedia of Nutrition and Good Health

Copyright © 1997 by Robert A. Ronzio, Ph.D., C.N.S., F.A.I.C.

Facts On File, Inc.
11 Penn Plaza
New York, NY 10001

Library of Congress Cataloging-in-Publication Data

Ronzio, Robert A.
The encyclopedia of nutrition and good health / Robert A. Ronzio.
p.   cm.
Includes bibliographical references.
ISBN 0-8160-2665-3 (hc : alk. paper)
ISBN 0-8160-3755-8 (pb : alk. paper)
1. Nutrition—Encyclopedias.   I. Title.
RA784.R646   1997
613.-2′03—dc20   96-17868

Facts On File books are available at special discounts when purchased in bulk quantities for businesses, associations, institutions or sales promotions. Please call our Special Sales Department in New York at (212) 967-8800 or (800) 322-8755.

You can find Facts On File on the World Wide Web at http://www.factsonfile.com

Text design by Cathy Rincon
Cover design by Dorothy Wachtenheim

Printed in the United States of America

VB INNO 10 9 8 7 6 5 4 3
(pb) 10 9 8 7 6 5 4 3 2

This book is printed on acid-free paper.

Contents

Acknowledgments

To complete this encyclopedia, I drew on the support of many friends, colleagues, students and family. The concept for the book originated from stimulating early morning conversations with Jeff Kelly, Ph.D. Lendon Smith, M.D., and Lisa Meserole, N.D., R.D., provided valuable suggestions in the early stages of this work. Denny Hannem, Loren Freeman, Amy Nystrom, Kathlyn Swann, L.Ac., Gary Buhr, N.D., Ralph Golan, M.D., Nass Ordoubadi, M.D., and John Hibbs, N.D., provided me with unwavering support. Jonathan Wright, M.D., generously offered the use of his extensive collection of reprints on nutritional medicine. Elizabeth Wales's advice during the evolution of this work proved to be invaluable. Patricia Ronzio, M.Ed., provided clear insights, and she has been a constant source of inspiration throughout. Her constant faith helped bring this long-term project to fruition.

Foreword

Health care reform has already occurred, and almost the only major part of society trying very hard not to notice is the health care industry itself . . . including most medical doctors, dentists, hospitals and insurance companies! Urged by literally millions of their constituents, politicians are beginning to enact health care reform legislation, although for now in bits and pieces.

Perhaps you thought that health care reform was defeated in the 1994 U.S. Congress. It wasn't, although your congressmen and senators thought so, and the newspapers, radio and television all told us so. Our Congress defeated a radical program of "insurance coverage reform," but who (except for politicians) thinks insurance coverage is the same as health care? It takes very little reflection to understand that it isn't!

Real health care reform has happened regardless of the actions of health care professionals, the health care industry and politicians because so many of us have decided to take back primary responsibility for our own health. Millions started this process with jogging and other forms of exercise, began to feel better, and started looking at improved diet, along with vitamins and minerals. More recently, herbal remedies and homeopathy have surged in popularity. Meditation, visualization, acupuncture, massage, chiropractic, naturopathy, and many other natural health care practices have moved from the fringes to the mainstream of public awareness. While medical doctors (particularly our own) are still viewed with respect, they're no longer the only health care authorities, but just one voice among many. More and more of us have decided to stay healthy using our own resources, consulting professionals only when our own efforts have failed, or when we can't find important information.

There are many reasons for this *real* health care reform, including the limited effectiveness and multiple side effects of drugs, chemotherapy and radiation. Over 100,000 of us die every year from side effects of prescription drugs, while many more die of chemotherapy and radiation. The incredible cost of modern high-tech medicine has forced many of us to examine self-care and other more natural alternatives, while driving health care insurance premiums sky-high and government insurance programs into near-bankruptcy.

The explosion of both interest in and information about health and illness prevention (as well as slowing the aging process) has been another major force behind real health care reform. Public demand for access to self-care information led to over two million letters and phone calls to our Congress in 1994—not to support or defeat insurance coverage reform, but to successfully support a baby step toward real health care reform, the [(Dietary Supplement Health and Education Act)] which prevented the FDA from further choking off information about the use of vitamins, minerals and herbs, and even made this information a little more available in natural food stores. Legislation before Congress in 1996 (the Access to Medical Treatment Act) would truly reform health care by making access to any type of health care available, restoring a freedom lost approximately a century ago.

Since so many of us are asking for information, we're getting it! In the 1990s hardly a day goes by without a newspaper or broadcast report about health and diet, health and exercise, or health and a vitamin, a mineral, an herb. The majority of these reports originate in research literally pouring out of our universities, a situation unimaginable in the 1960s and 1970s. Information about taking care of our own health seems to be everywhere! The first and largest question for many of us is "Where do I find reliable information about my body, health and nutrition?" And almost as importantly, where can it be found in one place, without taking too much time?

Which brings me to the *Encyclopedia of Nutrition and Good Health* and Professor Bob Ronzio, a colleague and friend. While a professor at Bastyr University in Seattle, he was recognized as a master teacher. His discussions and guidance were always comprehensive and well-organized and, just as importantly, interesting and understandable. While Dr. Ronzio has retired from his professorship, he hasn't quit teaching, but this time he's broadened his efforts to reach all of us interested in taking care of our own health with this *Encyclopedia.*

There are many nutrition encyclopedias, but none combine detailed explanations of all the individual nutrients from A to zinc with so many other aspects of health. Dr. Ronzio explains, in understandable terms, nearly all major and minor organs, and the functions of many organ systems. He even discusses many individual types of cells and molecules! He includes descriptions and explanations of nearly every hormone,

whether well-known or obscure. There are entries for a variety of body functions, such as exercise, aging, absorption, metabolism and many more.

And "nutrition" doesn't just mean vitamins and minerals: He discusses foods both major and minor, from meat, wheat and milk to tapioca and tangerines. He doesn't forget non-foods in what we're eating this century, including food chemicals, colorings, artificial preservatives and other things that really shouldn't be in our food supply.

Herbal remedies aren't neglected either. You'll find here all the "major" ones as well as many lesser-known. Since he had the time (Dr. Ronzio says the encyclopedia took six years), he's included discussions of most common health problems, and a number of uncommon ones, too.

I'll stop the listing here, as you can find all of this and more for yourself in the pages that follow. As you do, you'll be one of the tens of millions of real health care reformers, taking an active, informed role in guiding your life-long program of good health. And that is what *real* health care reform is all about!

—Jonathan V. Wright, M.D.

Introduction

The average American consumes an estimated 50 tons of food during a lifetime in order to grow, to replace wear and tear, and to operate the body's elaborate machinery. This staggering amount of food represents the sum of daily choices regarding the type, quality and quantity of foods. These crucial choices reflect a complex interplay of factors including family upbringing, the availability and cost of food, and religious or philosophical beliefs. Increasingly people select foods for health reasons. A "health revolution" is in progress that dramatically increases available information as well as how we think about health. New discoveries about how the body uses nutrients and the long-term benefits of a healthy diet are announced almost weekly.

This revolution has changed our thinking about how the body functions. All organ systems are closely linked. Extensive studies have documented this mutual interdependence, especially among the brain (the nervous system), hormones (the endocrine system) and the immune system. For example, we cannot understand digestion without considering the effects of hormones, immune tissue and nerves on the digestive tract. To put it another way, by examining the digestive system, we gain a deeper understanding of how the nervous system and immune system work.

In addition, the health revolution is changing the way physicians view nutrition. The perspective of simply treating disease is gradually shifting to disease prevention through lifestyle modification, emphasizing the importance of diet for optimal health. Inadequate nutrition is linked to some of the most profound diseases of the last half century. These were once believed to be the inevitable consequences of aging—arthritis, senility, diabetes, obesity, cardiovascular disease and osteoporosis. Now, manipulating specific nutrients can help treat certain conditions, and eating appropriate foods can reduce the risk of cancer and chronic degenerative diseases. As a further benefit, nutrition functions as a bridge between traditional and complementary medical disciplines, and nutritionists and medical professionals more frequently work in partnership with their clients and patients in order to achieve their health goals.

Americans face many challenges and opportunities for improving health, and there are pragmatic reasons for exploring nutrition options. The explosive growth in medical costs emphasizes the cost effectiveness of prevention and the importance of nutrition in providing optimal health. Although *under-nutrition* is the overriding concern among many societies, *over-nutrition* with excess calories along with *under-consumption* of key nutrients is far more prevalent in the United States. We now realize that prolonged physical and emotional stress from living in an industrial society like ours can deplete critical protective nutrients. Chronic exposure to potentially damaging chemicals in food, water and air lowers the body's ability to fend off infections and cancer.

Given the broad impact of nutrition on health, it is not surprising that interest in maintaining health has never been stronger. Patients and consumers are increasingly more knowledgeable and more willing to ask questions. They want to become more informed, and they feel empowered as they take greater responsibility for their own health. Life-style choices, including a commitment to exercising and eating wisely, help achieve a more productive, healthier and more satisfying life in order to reach a genetically determined potential. One of my clients put it this way: "I can't change my job, I can't change my kids and I can't change my spouse, but I can change the way I eat." It is often difficult to change environmental factors over which we have limited control, nor can we change our genetic makeup. However, making informed choices about diet can help level the playing field when it comes to feeling better, looking good and being more active.

The amount of nutrition-related information now available can be overwhelming. Popular sources about foods, diets and nutrients include a vast assortment of books, magazine and newspaper articles, talk shows, food advertisements, personal experience of friends and family members, and guidance by knowledgeable professionals. The fundamental issue lies in deciphering this mountain of information without becoming lost. The often expressed sentiment, "Since everything causes cancer (or is fattening), why bother?" is an example of consumer frustration.

In working with clients and teaching nutrition for many years in settings ranging from family programs to graduate school courses, I saw the need for a basic source book that could serve as a one-stop introduction to the world of nutrition and foods. This *Encyclopedia of Nutrition and Good Health* can provide the key to unlock nutrition facts. I have attempted to demystify scientific concepts by simplifying them, so the reader can grasp the essential ideas quickly and easily. The encyclopedia is accurate and understandable. My goal has been clarity without sacrificing accuracy. I have eliminated the scientific jargon that can hinder understanding of the fundamentals. The encyclopedia is objective; it does not advocate a particular diet or vitamin. It does not promote "cure-alls"; indeed, no single food or nutrient can guarantee health or prevent disease.

The Encyclopedia of Nutrition and Good Health is up to date and comprehensive. I have sifted through many thousands of scientific papers and have carefully evaluated recent advances in nutrition, food technology and medicine. My analysis and synthesis of this information is based upon 30 years of experience as a biochemist with a keen interest in human metabolism, nutrition and clinical laboratory practice, and as a biomedical researcher and a professor. The encyclopedia describes the nutrition and food-related terms and concepts you are likely to encounter. It provides current information on foods and food technology, food labels, vita-

mins, minerals, and major nutrients such as fats, carbohydrates and proteins. I describe what each nutrient is and how it works in the body, as well as its impact on health.

The encyclopedia is more than a supplement guide. You will find a discussion of food-related conditions, including eating disorders, obesity, addiction, dieting and weight loss, food sensitivities and chronic degenerative diseases. The ramifications of global issues such as world hunger are discussed. As a practical aid to consumers, I have included summaries of food labels and dietary guidelines. For those who wish to explore key topics further, I have provided over 400 up-to-date references.

Nutrition is an expanding branch of science, and it holds much promise as additional details become understood. However, we still do not have a totally complete picture of the roles played in human health by specific nutrients and other substances in food. Sometimes there are differences of opinion among experts when various hypotheses are presented to explain observations. This is natural and inevitable. Experimental data can be interpreted in different ways: Results from animal studies do not always translate to humans. There can be other experimental limitations. For example, only a small population of white, middle-aged males may have been studied. How do these results apply to women, elderly persons or different ethnic groups?

Nutritionists and health care providers of many disciplines do agree that diet and individual nutrients are mainstays of health, although opinion is still divided regarding the optimal amounts needed. Such controversy can be confusing and frustrating. Where there is disagreement in the scientific literature, I have taken a middle ground in describing the pros and cons. The history of science teaches us that with continued research and clinical studies, even the most perplexing questions will eventually be answered, and that some of the ideas now considered visionary will evolve to become universally accepted facts.

Please consult your physician for any medical problem you may have, rather than relying on self-diagnosis or self-medication. Armed with information, you will be able to ask more questions and become better informed about your individual situation, whether your focus is lowering elevated cholesterol, protecting yourself against disease, combating the effects of pollutants, losing weight, or boosting your immunity. Consider *The Encyclopedia of Nutrition and Good Health* a nutrition translator, a stepping-stone on your path to wellness. This encyclopedia prepares you for the 21st century.

In Health,
Robert A. Ronzio, Ph.D., C.N.S., F.A.I.C.
Houston, Texas

To my family, Patricia, Lora
and Cynthia, for their love;

To Henry and William, who represent the next generation;

To the memory of Anthony R. and Roberta B. Ronzio;

And to people everywhere
who want to learn more about their health
and the fascinating world of nutrition.

absorption Generally, the passage of liquids into solid materials and of gases into liquids and solids. In terms of nutrition, absorption refers to the passage of substances into body fluids and tissues. Digestion is only the first step in the assimilation of nutrients. This chemical breakdown of food particles releases AMINO ACIDS, GLUCOSE, FATTY ACIDS, VITAMINS and MINERALS, which must then be absorbed by the intestine in order to be used by the body. Nutrients enter cells lining the intestine (the intestinal mucosa) and then are drawn into underlying cells, where they may enter either the lymph or bloodstream for distribution to tissues throughout the body. Tissues absorb nutrients from blood via capillaries, the smallest blood vessels. Gases, too, are absorbed. Blood becomes oxygenated in the lungs by absorbing oxygen from inhaled air and releasing carbon dioxide that was absorbed from tissues.

Absorption requires a disproportionately large surface area to meet the body's needs. Consider the total area of the small intestine, which is a highly specialized absorptive organ. Though this tube is only about 20 feet long, it has a highly convoluted surface. Furthermore, the cells lining the surface, VILLI, are covered with microscopic, hairlike projections (MICROVILLI) that dramatically increase the absorptive area to a quarter the size of a football field. The microvilli move constantly, to trap nutrients and partially digested food, which is further digested. The upper regions of the small intestine, the lower DUODENUM and upper ILEUM, are most active in absorbing nutrients. Other regions of the gastrointestinal tract carry out limited absorption: The stomach absorbs some ALCOHOL, glucose, ions and water, and the colon absorbs primarily water and minerals. (See also DIGESTIVE TRACT; MALABSORPTION.)

Accent The trade name for MONOSODIUM GLUTAMATE (MSG). MSG, a common FOOD ADDITIVE, is used as a FLAVOR ENHANCER.

Accutane The trade name for isotretinoin, an oral prescription drug. This derivative of VITAMIN A is used to treat cystic ACNE, a severe and persistent form characterized by pitting and scarring. Cystic acne accounts for less than 5% of acne patients. Accutane can cause severe BIRTH DEFECTS and must be avoided during pregnancy. Taking Accutane with ALCOHOL or with VITAMIN A supplements can cause toxicity. Vitamin A has not proven effective for cases of severe acne.

acerola (acerola cherry, acerola berry) Acerola fruit is a product from the Caribbean and is one of the richest natural sources of VITAMIN C. Acerola juice contains nearly 40 times more vitamin C than orange juice. Acerola extract is sometimes added to natural vitamin C supplements. Because of its very limited availability, the amount added to supplements is usually very small; an acerola-enriched vitamin C preparation may contain as little as a tablespoon of acerola extract per barrel of vitamin C powder.

acesulfame-K (acesulfame potassium; Sunette) This non-caloric, ARTIFICIAL SWEETENER tastes approximately 200 times sweeter than table sugar (SUCROSE) and lacks the bitter aftertaste of SACCHARIN. The United Nations Food and Agriculture Organization endorsed acesulfame-K as a satisfactory artificial sweetener in 1983. Acesulfame-K was approved in 1988 by the U.S. FDA as a sugar substitute to be used in packets or as tablets and now is approved for use in chewing gum and in powdered drink mixes. Unlike ASPARTAME, acesulfame-K can be used in cooking because it does not break down at oven temperatures. Its use in baked goods and in soft drinks is pending approval.

Questions have been raised regarding the safety of acesulfame-K. Theoretically, it would not be expected to be absorbed by the body. Nonetheless, some studies suggest that large doses raise blood CHOLESTEROL levels in diabetic laboratory animals and increase the number of lung and mammary tumors in other animals.

acetaminophen   See ALCOHOL-DRUG INTERACTIONS.

acetic acid   A fermentation product of wine. During fermentation certain bacteria produce acetic acid by oxidizing alcohol when exposed to air. VINEGAR contains 4 to 6% acetic acid, which gives vinegar its characteristic sour taste. As vinegar, acetic acid is a common ingredient in food preparation.

One of the simplest organic acids, acetic acid contains only two carbon atoms. It is classified as a weak acid because it is only partially ionized, unlike strong mineral acids, such as hydrochloric acid.

Acetic acid plays a pivotal role in metabolism. To be metabolized, acetic acid must be activated as acetyl CoA, in which acetic acid is bound to a carrier molecule, COENZYME A, which is in turn derived from the B vitamin PANTOTHENIC ACID. Metabolic pathways that oxidize fatty acids, carbohydrate and amino acids for energy, all yield acetyl CoA, the common intermediate by which carbons from these fuels enter the KREB'S CYCLE to be oxidized to carbon dioxide. Alternatively, acetyl CoA can be used as a building block. It forms saturated fatty acids, cholesterol and ketone bodies. Nerve cells can use it to form the NEUROTRANSMITTER, ACETYLCHOLINE. Tissues combine acetic acid with amino sugars to form a family of sugar derivatives like N-acetylglucosamine and N-acetylgalactosamine that help define recognition sites on the surface of cells and blood group specificities, such as the A, B, O and Lewis blood groups used in blood typing.

acetoacetic acid (acetoacetate)   The most prevalent of the KETONE BODIES, which are acids produced by the liver. Acetoacetic acid is a useful fuel; it is readily oxidized by the heart and brain for the production of ATP, the energy currency of cells. Though small amounts of ketone bodies are normally produced by liver metabolism, an excessive buildup of acetoacetic acid and its derivative, BETA HYDROXYBUTYRIC ACID, in the blood (ketonemia) can occur during excessive fat breakdown, when the liver cannot completely oxidize massive amounts of fatty acids released from fat (ADIPOSE TISSUE). Conditions conducive to excessive acetoacetic acid production include STARVATION (prolonged FASTING), crash DIETING, uncontrolled DIABETES MELLITUS and chronic ALCOHOLISM.

Ketone body production serves an important role in the physiologic adaptation to starvation. With prolonged starvation, the blood levels of ketone bodies rise, and more of them cross the BLOOD-BRAIN BARRIER to be taken up by nerve tissue, where they are burned for energy. Consequently, the brain requires less blood glucose (blood sugar) for energy at a time when this fuel is at a premium. The sustained build-up of acetoacetic acid in the blood (KETOSIS) can acidify the blood, leading to metabolic ACIDOSIS, and alter the acid-base balance of the body, a potentially dangerous condition. (See also ELECTROLYTES; FAT METABOLISM.)

acetone   The simplest ketone. Ketones are an important class of organic compounds. Acetone is a volatile compound that forms spontaneously by the breakdown of the KETONE BODY, ACETOACETIC ACID. Unlike its parent compound, acetone is a metabolic dead end and cannot be metabolized for energy production. Its occurrence is a sign of severe and prolonged imbalanced carbohydrate and fat metabolism. Acetone has a characteristic sweet, ether-like odor, which accounts for the characteristic breath of individuals with uncontrolled DIABETES MELLITUS. Acetone and ketone bodies are excreted in urine under conditions promoting extensive mobilization of fat stores, as STARVATION and metabolic disorders. (See also ACETOACETIC ACID; FAT METABOLISM; KETOSIS.)

acetylcholine   One of the best characterized NEUROTRANSMITTERS. This family of brain chemicals carries nerve impulses between individual nerve cells (neurons) and between neurons and muscle cells. Acetylcholine is involved in memory, in processes associated with thinking, in muscle coordination and in many other functions. Nerves that secrete acetylcholine are called cholinergic neurons. An electrical impulse traveling down such a neuron liberates acetylcholine, which then floods across the gap (synapse) separating the neuron from an adjacent cell, where it binds to its neighbor. A bound neurotransmitter in turn triggers an electrical impulse or other reaction in the receiving cell. Acetylcholine is destroyed by the enzyme cholinesterase, which clears it from the synapse and prepares it for the next impulse.

The brain synthesizes acetylcholine from CHOLINE, a nitrogen-containing ethanol derivative, and acetyl CoA, an activated form of acetic acid. Therefore, administering choline, or the phospholipid LECITHIN, a dietary source of choline, might be expected to increase brain acetylcholine levels. This strategy has been used in clinical trials to treat TARDIVE DYSKINESIA. Up to 50% of patients in mental hospitals suffer from this condition, characterized by uncontrolled twitches of muscles of the face and upper body. Apparently this is a side effect of certain tranquilizers and antipsychotic drugs, which may cause a deficiency of acetylcholine in critical regions of the brain. (See also SENILITY.)

acetylsalicylic acid   The chemical name for ASPIRIN.

achlorhydria   A condition resulting from the lack of STOMACH ACID production. DIARRHEA, stomach discomfort and bloating are common symptoms of achlorhydria. Achlorhydria has serious ramifications. It can lead to MALNUTRITION, even when the diet is well balanced, because achlorhydria drastically reduces the efficiency of DIGESTION. A chronic MALABSORPTION syndrome leads to deficiencies of VITAMIN B$_{12}$, CALCIUM, IRON and other nutrients and sets the stage for chronic FATIGUE, OSTEOPOROSIS, ANEMIA and serious infections. The causes of achlorhydria remain unknown. However, lowered stomach acid production is associated with anemia, stomach inflammation, CELIAC DISEASE, diabetes, lupus, myasthenia gravis, rheumatoid ARTHRITIS and some forms of cancer.

Limited stomach acid production, not the absence of stomach acid, is termed HYPOCHLORHYDRIA. It is not as severe a condition as achlorhydria, though unless corrected, the ensuing malabsorption syndrome can have similar, detrimental long-range effects on health. In either situation patients may be advised to take supplemental hydrochloric acid in the form of BETAINE HYDROCHLORIDE or glutamic acid hydrochloride with meals to enhance digestion. These supplements should be used with medical supervision because of the danger of overdosing with these strong acids. (See also ACID; GASTRIC JUICE.)

acid A large family of compounds that taste sour and can neutralize bases to create salts. Strong acids like hydrochloric acid (STOMACH ACID) and sulfuric acid (battery acid) give up all of their protons in water and lower the pH, the effective hydrogen ion concentration. A pH of 7.0 is neutral, that is, neither acidic nor basic, while pH values less than 7.0 are considered acidic. Exposure to strong acids tends to damage cells and tissues. The stomach is the only organ normally exposed to strong acids, but it is protected from injury by a heavy mucous layer.

In contrast to strong acids, organic acids are classified as weak acids because they donate only a portion of their hydrogen ions, lower the pH to a lesser degree, and are less dangerous to tissues. Many compounds in foods are weak acids, including CITRIC ACID, ACETIC ACID and TARTARIC ACID. Several weak acids are used as FOOD ADDITIVES, including benzoic acid, CARBONIC ACID and alginic acid. As food additives and recipe ingredients, weak acids add tartness to foods. Weak acids are common intermediates, products of cellular processes that sustain life, including: LACTIC ACID, KETONE BODIES, PYRUVIC ACID, acetic acid, FATTY ACIDS, SUCCINIC ACID, citric acid, even the nucleic acids DNA and RNA. GLUTAMIC ACID and ASPARTIC ACID (two common AMINO ACIDS) are classified as acidic amino acids, and are more acid than most.

In the body, weak acids characteristically have lost all their hydrogen ions and exist as a family of anions (negatively charged ions) classified as "conjugate bases" because they have been completely neutralized by the buffer systems of blood. In the blood, lactic acid exists as its anion, lactate; acetoacetic acid (a ketone body) as acetoacetate; citric acid as citrate, and so on. Often the names of acids and their anions are interchanged in nutrition literature. (See also ELECTROLYTES.)

acidemia The condition in which blood becomes acidic. (see also ACIDOSIS.)

acid-forming foods Foods that create acidic residues after they have been broken down by the body. Protein-rich food, such as EGGS, MEAT and poultry, produce acidic residues when oxidized for energy. The combustion of sulfur-containing amino acids tends to acidify the body (acidic residue). In contrast, fruits and vegetables make the body more alkaline or basic. They contain magnesium, calcium and potassium salts of organic acids, which yield an alkaline residue when oxidized. Fruits are accordingly classified as alkali-forming foods, even though juices and fruit taste acidic (sour). Excretion of organic acids (potential renal acid load) can be calculated for various foods based on their content of sodium, potassium, calcium, magnesium, chloride, phosphorus and sulfur. Choosing more alkaline foods may ameliorate osteoporosis, autoimmune conditions such as rheumatoid arthritis, and chronic inflammation. (See also ACID.)

Remer, T. and Manz, F., "Potential renal acid load of foods and its influence on urine pH," *Journal of the American Dietetic Association*, 95:7 (July 1995), pp. 791–97.

acidifiers Common additives that increase the acidity (lower the pH) of foods and beverages. Acidifiers provide tartness and enhance flavors of processed foods. The increased acidity inhibits the growth of microorganisms; thus acidifiers act as preservatives. Certain acidifiers can also retard spoilage by acting as antioxidants, preventing chemical changes due to oxygen. This group of additives includes ADIPIC ACID (adipate), TARTARIC ACID (tartrate), benzoic acid (benzoate) and CITRIC ACID (citrate). (See also ACID; FOOD ADDITIVES.)

acid indigestion (heartburn, esophageal reflux, gastric reflux) A condition characterized by a burning pain near the stomach. Typically this occurs an hour or so after a heavy (fatty) meal and is often relieved by taking ANTACIDS or by drinking MILK. Acid indigestion is the most common gastrointestinal complaint in the United States. One in ten persons suffer daily attacks. The pain associated with acid indigestion is caused by STOMACH ACID backing up into the ESOPHAGUS, the region of the throat connecting the mouth with the stomach.

What causes acid indigestion? Air gulped when swallowing large bites of food can keep the passageway open. Some food allergies and food sensitivities may trigger acid indigestion by relaxing the sphincter muscles that normally seal off the stomach juices from the esophagus after eating. Though the stomach lining is protected from acid by mucus, the unprotected esophagus is irritated by repeated exposure to acid.

To prevent acid indigestion, eat slowly and chew food thoroughly. Avoid those foods and beverages that cause adverse reactions. Common examples include fatty foods, CHOCOLATE, COFFEE, CITRUS FRUIT and alcoholic beverages. Consult a physician for any chronic stomach pain. What feels like acid indigestion may actually be inadequate stomach acid (hypochlorhydria). Seek immediate medical attention if experiencing a crushing pain in the middle of the chest that extends to the left arm. These symptoms could indicate a heart attack.

acidophilus (*Lactobacillus acidophilus*) A species of the bacterium *Lactobacillus* that produces lactic acid by fermenting LACTOSE (milk sugar). This organism in the upper intestinal tract forms a symbiotic relationship with its human host. Other acid-producing bacteria, including *bifidobacteria*, are predominant in the lower intestine. Acidophilus is a member of the normal intestinal microflora, the so-called "friendly bacteria," which produce nutrients like BIOTIN and VITAMIN K. Acidophilus and other Lactobacillus species help balance the digestive system by maintaining conditions that inhibit the growth of yeasts like candida, as well as potentially dangerous bacterial species. Without beneficial bacteria to control them, such opportunistic microorganisms can multiply rapidly, leading to a full-blown infection.

A variety of conditions can drastically lower or eliminate the intestinal acidophilus population. Treatment with broad-spectrum antibiotics, such as tetracycline, imbalances gut microecology because these antibiotics destroy benign as well as disease-producing bacteria. More generally, an unhealthful life-style and a diet high in SUGAR and PROCESSED FOODS also adversely affect beneficial intestinal bacteria.

Acidophilus is a common food supplement that may help repopulate the gut with beneficial bacteria to prevent hard-to-control yeast infections; to break down milk sugar for those with LACTASE DEFICIENCY; to control travelers' DIARRHEA; to relieve CONSTIPATION; to treat vaginitis (when administered as acidophilus douches); and to decrease the production of potential CARCINOGENS by certain bacteria populating the gut. (See also CANCER.)

Chaitow, Leon and Trenev, Natasha. *Pro Biotics*. Northampton, England: Thorsons, 1990.

acidophilus milk (sweet acidophilus milk)   ACIDOPHILUS bacteria are sometimes added to low-fat MILK by the producer. Consumption of acidophilus milk and of yogurt may help lower blood cholesterol levels. Milk and yogurt labels should specify viable (active) acidophilus cultures, since PASTEURIZATION destroys acidophilus bacteria.

acidosis   The acidification of the blood and other body fluids. This condition can be due to acid accumulation or to the loss of bicarbonate buffering capacity from kidney disease. The pH of blood is tightly regulated; the normal range is between pH 7.3 and 7.4. A drop in blood pH below pH 7.3, which corresponds to increased hydrogen ion concentration, could signal excessive acidity of the blood (ACIDEMIA). Homeostatic mechanisms (the body's regulatory system of checks and balances) help prevent acidosis. Bicarbonate and serum proteins take up hydrogen ions to neutralize excessive acid rapidly, while the kidneys more slowly compensate for acid production by excreting surplus hydrogen ions. Prolonged acidosis requires medical attention because it slows down many vital functions, including nerve transmission and heart muscle contraction. Symptoms of acidosis include nausea, vomiting, DIARRHEA, headache, rapid breathing and, eventually, convulsions.

Two forms of acidosis are recognized: metabolic and respiratory. Metabolic acidosis can occur when metabolic acids accumulate excessively. For example, when the body burns FAT at a high rate, the liver converts FATTY ACIDS to KETONE BODIES, acidic substances. This condition may occur during crash DIETING, FASTING, uncontrolled DIABETES MELLITUS or chronic ALCOHOLISM. Excessive ingestion of acids, such as in aspirin poisoning, also causes acidosis. Metabolic acidosis can also result from vomiting or diarrhea, which cause excessive loss of electrolytes like bicarbonate and upset the acid/base balance. Renal disease may prevent the kidneys from adequately correcting acid production.

Respiratory acidosis can occur when breathing does not adequately remove carbon dioxide. Shallow breathing, associated with respiratory disease, can cause excessive CARBON DIOXIDE in the lungs, in turn causing carbon dioxide blood levels to rise and upset the bicarbonate buffer system of the blood. (See also BUFFER; FAT METABOLISM; KETOSIS; STARVATION.)

Lownstein, Jerome. *Acids and Bases*. New York: Oxford University Press, 1993.

acidulant   A food additive that acidifies prepared foods and beverages. Citric acid and sodium dihydrogen phosphate are examples. (See also ACIDIFIERS.)

acne   An inflammation of the skin, especially around hair follicles and oil-secreting glands (sebaceous glands) of the skin. Acne is the most common skin ailment. It affects the face and, less frequently, the back, shoulders and chest. This distribution follows the body distribution of sebaceous (oil-secreting) glands. Acne is more common in males and affects an estimated 80% of Americans between the ages of 12 and 24. Acne occurs in two forms. In acne vulgaris blockage of the oil from the skin's sebaceous glands can lead to bacterial growth and inflammation, manifesting as blackheads and pustules. The second form, acne conglobata or cystic acne, is more severe, with cyst formation and scarring.

The causes of acne are unknown, though heredity plays a role. Other factors are oily skin, emotional stress, production of androgens (male hormones), use of oral contraceptives and oil-based cosmetics, food allergies and reliance on highly processed convenience foods. Exposure to steroids, machine oils, coal tar derivatives and chlorinated hydrocarbons (such as certain solvents and pesticides) can cause acne-like lesions. Vitamin A (retinol) reduces the activity of sebaceous glands and skin thickening around follicles, and is required for healthy skin. It has been used to treat acne; however, the massive doses effective in cystic acne are also likely to produce toxicity because vitamin A, unlike the B complex, accumulates with extended use. Vitamin A derivatives, ACCUTANE and Retin-A, have been used to treat forms of acne and psoriasis. These drugs seem to inhibit inflammation.

Other nutritional factors affect skin health and thus may play a role in treating acne. For example, the trace mineral chromium may help with glucose (blood sugar) utilization by the skin and improve skin metabolism. ZINC, which is involved in wound healing, tissue regeneration and inflammation control, may also be important for the skin. Zinc supplementation for several months may be efficacious for some acne patients. Vitamin E is implicated because it helps reduce oxidative damage. Simple sugars suppress the immune system, and their consumption should be restricted, along with high-fat foods.

ACTH   See ADRENOCORTICOTROPIC HORMONE.

activated charcoal   An effective absorbent used in medicine. Pharmaceutical-grade charcoal is highly absorbable, unlike charcoal used for cooking purposes. Activated charcoal is a pourable black slurry that can be purchased from drug stores. It reduces bilirubin (BILE PIGMENT) in cases of JAUNDICE of newborns, and it has been used to help treat nausea, vomiting and travelers' DIARRHEA and to help control FLATULENCE, because it absorbs ingested toxic chemicals when administered orally. Preliminary studies suggest that oral doses of activated charcoal also help lower LOW-DENSITY LIPOPROTEIN (LDL), the undesirable form of blood CHOLESTEROL. Consult a health care professional before taking activated charcoal, and obtain immediate medical attention for poisoning (any toxin-induced interference with normal body functions). A local phone directory will list poison control centers.

acute Pertaining to any new condition or disease that has a relatively short duration. In contrast, a chronic condition is a recurrent phenomena of long duration that could last months or years.

addiction A chemical dependency. The compulsive use of a substance and denial of the problem characterize addictions. CRAVINGS occur when an addictive substance is withdrawn, and unfulfilled cravings are associated with the pain and DEPRESSION of withdrawal.

Addicted persons are often malnourished, and may be overweight or underweight. Individuals addicted to narcotics and stimulants are often in poor health due to their disinterest in food and in their personal well-being. Intravenous drug users tend to consume inadequate diets—low in protein, vitamins and minerals, and high in refined carbohydrates. They generally have a loss of appetite; they may suffer from maldigestion (incomplete digestion), leading to malnutrition syndromes.

Medical supervision is recommended before abstaining from ALCOHOL, narcotics, tranquilizers or sleeping pills. Regardless of the form of chemical dependency, nutrition offers a powerful adjunct to recovery and to restoring the body's biochemical balance. This approach typically involves several steps:

- Establish new eating patterns. Frequent meals are recommended to stabilize blood sugar and prevent hypoglycemia (low BLOOD SUGAR): breakfast, a mid-morning snack, lunch, an afternoon snack, dinner and a late snack. Avoid eating huge meals or skipping meals.
- Avoid sugary, refined foods such as pastry, candy, soft drinks, ice cream and ice cream substitutes. Avoiding sugar can help stabilize blood sugar levels.
- Eat a varied, balanced diet to provide less saturated FAT and more NUTRIENTS. Making healthful food choices is simplified with EXCHANGE LISTS, available in standard nutrition texts. To make up for decreased consumption of sugary foods, emphasize VEGETABLES. For dark-green leafy vegetables besides spinach, consider CHARD, KALE and COLLARD greens. In the cabbage family, consider BROCCOLI, BRUSSELS SPROUTS, CAULIFLOWER and Chinese cabbage. For orange-colored vegetables besides CARROTS, consider winter squash. Among whole GRAINS, include MILLET, RICE, TRITICALE, RYE and BUCKWHEAT. LEGUMES are also important. Experiment with various kinds of BEANS and PEAS, such as CHICKPEAS and LENTILS. Include a variety of FRUITS, dairy products, nuts, lean MEAT, poultry, FISH and SHELLFISH.
- Avoid foods to which you are sensitive. For assistance consult a specialist who treats food and chemical sensitivities. Eliminating COFFEE and cigarettes facilitates the body chemistry's return to normal.

- Work out a supervised nutritional treatment program to meet individual needs. Supplements may help remedy deficiencies and diminish withdrawal symptoms. In addition to the B complex vitamins and MINERALS, the list of supplements may include GLUTAMINE, VITAMIN C and NIACINAMIDE. (See also ALCOHOLISM; ADDICTION AND SUGAR; APPETITE.)

Kalvinas, P.W. and Samson, H.H., eds. "The Neurobiology of Alcohol and Drug Addiction," *Annals of the New York Academy of Sciences* 654 (1992).

Phelps, J.K. and Nourse, A.E. *The Hidden Addiction and How to Get Free.* Boston: Little, Brown, 1986.

addiction and sugar Addiction to refined CARBOHYDRATES in general and to sucrose (table sugar) specifically is a controversial topic. On the one hand is the belief that sugar has no effect on behavior, and that it has little effect on health other than promoting tooth decay. A U.S. FDA task force concluded in 1986 that typical sugar consumption does not generally pose a health hazard. The opposite view contends that sugar addiction is a common phenomenon. Preferring sugar and sweets seems to be programmed at infancy. A craving for sweets often develops later in life, and in this sense sugar may be psychologically addicting. Compounding the problem of defining sugar addiction is the general observation that related symptoms are rather vague, including a change in mood or feeling shaky when abstaining from sugary foods.

One hypothesis proposes that addicted persons have a drive to achieve a sense of well-being and to overcome depression. Some addicted persons seem to have an abnormal metabolism of NEUROTRANSMITTERS, chemicals that carry signals from one nerve cell to another cell. A primary example is the linkage between low serotonin (the brain chemical) and depression, and the correlation between high sugar, high-fat diets and increased brain serotonin levels. Evidence suggests that eating certain sugary foods stimulates the production of brain peptides (ENDORPHINS), which trigger pleasant feelings. It has been hypothesized that the formation of endorphins may be abnormal in some individuals, possibly leading them to compulsive eating behavior like BULIMIA NERVOSA. (See also APPETITE; BLOOD SUGAR; NATURAL SWEETENERS.)

additives See FOOD ADDITIVES.

adenine A building block of DNA, the genetic blueprint of the cell, and of RNA, the cell's messenger that directs protein synthesis. Adenine is also used to manufacture ATP (adenosine triphosphate), the energy currency of the cell, as well as several enzyme helpers (COENZYMES) required to produce energy. These include coenzyme A, derived from the B vitamin pantothenic acid; FAD (FLAVIN ADENINE DINUCLEOTIDE) from riboflavin; and NAD (NICOTINAMIDE ADENINE DINUCLEOTIDE) from niacin.

In DNA adenine constitutes one of the four bases that make up the alphabet of the genetic code, and it stabilizes the unique double helix based on the attraction and complementary bonding between two parallel DNA chains.

Chemically, adenine is a cyclic structure belonging to the family of purines. Adenine is synthesized in the body from three amino acids (ASPARTIC ACID, GLUTAMINE and GLYCINE).

Therefore, adenine is not an essential dietary nutrient. (See also GOUT; GUANINE.)

adenosine triphosphate   See ATP.

adipic acid (hexapedioc acid)   A common food additive in vegetable oils, adipic acid prevents their oxidation and retards rancidity, thus acting as an ANTIOXIDANT. As an acidifier, adipic acid adds tartness to soft drinks, throat lozenges, gelatin desserts and powdered, fruit-flavored beverages. Adipic acid is readily metabolized and is considered a safe food additive. (See also CHELATE).

adipocyte   Fat storage cell. The adipocyte is like a balloon; it expands in size when fat is added and it shrinks when FAT is depleted. Adipocytes form ADIPOSE TISSUE, specialized for fat storage. The number of adipocytes increases during early childhood and adolescence as the amount of adipose tissue increases. At other stages in life, fat is deposited in, or released from, existing adipocytes. Stored fat comes from the diet or the liver adipocytes take up fatty acids from chylomicrons, which transport dietary fat in the blood, and from VLDL (very low-density lipoprotein), which transports fat synthesized by the liver. Adipocytes also synthesize fat from blood glucose in response to the hormone insulin. Conversely many hormones initiate fat breakdown in adipocytes: epinephrine, glucagon, growth hormone and androgens, among others. (See also LIPOGENESIS; LIPOLYSIS.)

adipose tissue (body fat, depot fat)   Fat storage is a specialized function of adipose tissue. As such, it represents the major fuel depot of the body and is as essential to normal function as any other tissue. Body fat serves other important functions: It insulates the body against low environmental temperatures and serves as a shock absorber. Typically, fat stored in adipose tissue represents 15 to 20% of men's weight and 20 to 25% of women's average weight. Women usually have more fat than men because fat is an important energy reserve during pregnancy and lactation.

Adipose tissue synthesizes fat after a high carbohydrate meal in response to the hormone INSULIN. During FASTING, STARVATION or stress, a second hormone EPINEPHRINE (adrenaline) signals adipocytes (fat cells) to break down stored fat into FATTY ACIDS, which are released into the bloodstream. They are rapidly absorbed and oxidized for energy by muscles. In contrast the brain relies on blood sugar to meet its energy needs.

The fact that an adult can consume approximately 2 pounds of food a day or 700 pounds of food a year with only small changes in body fat indicates how well the body regulates weight when the calorie intake matches the total body requirements.

Of course, common experience suggests that body fat can increase. For example, fat accumulation often accounts for the weight gain of middle-aged Americans. Older people tend to EXERCISE less and the metabolic rate slows with aging. An individual's optimal body fat at any age depends upon many factors, including inheritance, body build, sex and age. Standard HEIGHT/WEIGHT TABLES or the BODY MASS INDEX can be used to estimate an appropriate body weight for an individual.

Excessive body fat is not healthy for many reasons. OBESITY carries with it the increased risk of cardiovascular disease, hypertension and some forms of cancer. It is interesting to note that the distribution of body fat plays a role in defining the risk for heart disease. Abdominal fat (the "spare tire" profile) carries a greater risk for CARDIOVASCULAR DISEASE than fat accumulated around hips and thighs (the "pear" profile).

The general approach to losing fat stored in adipose tissue is exercising and eating nutritious meals, while decreasing caloric intake. Dieting without exercise decreases muscle mass (not desirable) as well as the fat in adipose tissue, and the weight regained after a crash diet is mostly fat (also not desired). Cycles of dieting and not dieting also cause loss of muscle mass. Since muscle burns more ENERGY per pound than fat, DIET cycling may increase the difficulty of losing weight permanently. The number of fat cells in adipose tissue—the storage bags themselves—cannot be lost by dieting or exercise. The only way to lose fat cells of adipose tissue is by LIPOSUCTION, a surgical procedure. (See also FAT METABOLISM.)

ad lib   From the Latin phrase, *ad libitum*, meaning freely available, to be consumed as desired. In nutrition, this term usually refers to animal feeding studies in which caged animals have free access to food and water. Animal studies examining the effects of changes in fat or fiber content in the diet could be ad lib. Other experiments restrict access to food, such as studies to examine the effects of caloric restriction on longevity.

adrenal glands   Triangular-shaped glands, attached to the kidneys, which secrete two types of hormones that regulate tissue metabolism and blood composition. There are two adrenal glands, and each gland is divided in two parts. The outer cortex secretes three classes of steroid hormones (adrenocorticosteroids), each with a different primary function. The GLUCOCORTICOIDS consist of CORTISOL and corticosterone. Their function is to develop a sustained response to stress. They increase blood GLUCOSE; stimulate the synthesis of liver GLYCOGEN; mobilize amino acids from protein; and stimulate ADIPOSE TISSUE to break down stored FAT and release free fatty acids into the bloodstream. MINERALOCORTICOIDS (mainly ALDOSTERONE) direct the kidney to conserve SODIUM and water, and therefore they play a key role in electrolyte and water balance. ANDROGENS (such as testosterone) are anabolic hormones that stimulate muscle protein synthesis and decrease the rate of protein breakdown, leading to an increase in growth rate. Androgens develop and maintain male secondary characteristics, such as genitalia, enlarged larynx, hair growth and muscular development. Testosterone maintains the prostate gland, seminal vesicles and sperm production of the testes.

The inner region of the adrenal gland, the medulla, is a major source of stress hormones. It functions independently of the cortex (outer layer). The medulla synthesizes a family of hormones (CATECHOLAMINES) that are derived from tyrosine: EPINEPHRINE (adrenaline) and norepinephrine. Epinephrine is released when a threatening situation is perceived. The medulla increases the heart rate and the rate of breathing, constricts blood vessels and relaxes bronchioles (the small air passageways of the lungs). It stimulates the release of free FATTY ACIDS from fat stored in adipose tissue, and the release of glucose from glycogen. The effects of norepinephrine resemble those of epinephrine, described above, though it is less active. It, too, increases the liberation of free fatty acids, stimulates the central nervous system and increases heat production. Norepinephrine increases blood pressure by constricting blood vessels in most organs.

The function of the adrenal glands is severely affected by sustained, long-term stress, leading to the GENERAL ADAPTATION SYNDROME. In earlier stages of adaptation to chronic stress, the adrenal cortex produces large amounts of cortisol. This creates a highly catabolic state, in which muscle, fat and glycogen are degraded, leading to chronic FATIGUE. Stressed adrenal glands may be linked to abnormal blood sugar regulation, to muscle protein breakdown and to suppression of the immune system. In later, extreme stages of adaptation to chronic stress, cortisol production is depressed when the adrenal cortex can no longer be activated by signals from the pituitary gland. Inadequate cortisol in turn can lead to hypoglycemia (low blood sugar) and to chronic fatigue. (See also ENDOCRINE SYSTEM; HORMONE; HYPOGLYCEMIA, POSTPRANDIAL.)

adrenaline   The British term for EPINEPHRINE. In the United States, it is used in a nonmedical connotation to indicate heightened emotion due to stress-induced release of the hormone.

adrenocorticotropic hormone (ACTH)   A polypeptide HORMONE produced by the anterior lobe of the PITUITARY GLAND and secreted to activate and sustain the ADRENAL GLANDS. ACTH release from the pituitary gland is regulated by the hypothalamus via a hormone, corticotropin releasing factor (CRH). ACTH stimulates the production of all steroid hormones of the adrenal gland, where it stimulates the conversion of cholesterol to steroid hormone precursors. ACTH also acts on ADIPOSE TISSUE to mobilize FAT and to increase blood levels of FATTY ACIDS. Inadequate ACTH leads to atrophy of the adrenal cortex, while excessive ACTH causes hyperplasia, the excessive growth of adrenal tissue. (See also CORTISOL; ENDOCRINE SYSTEM; FAT METABOLISM.)

adulterated food   A food is classified as adulterated if it contains extraneous material, dangerous amounts of poisons or filth, or if it has been processed or stored under unsanitary conditions. In terms of food for interstate commerce, the U.S. FDA monitors environmental contaminants, toxins from microorganisms, bacterial levels, and potentially harmful substances. Since it is impossible for food to be 100% pure, tolerances have been set for each type of contaminant. Very hazardous materials can be ruled so dangerous that no amount should be detected (a "zero tolerance"). (See also RISK.)

adult onset diabetes   See DIABETES MELLITUS.

advertising   Billions of dollars are spent each year on advertising food, and much of this is focused on specific markets. Food ads for breakfast cereals and junk food, for example, focus largely on the children's market. Toys, comic books, giveaways and polished commercials can hinder young people from making independent judgments on how to eat a balanced diet. Instead, their choices may rely on the direction of advertisers. TV advertising plays a prominent role, where cartoons featuring food commercials dominate children's programming. Young people may see 11,000 junk food ads on TV annually. Most of these emphasize PROCESSED FOODS—low in nutrients and high in CALORIES, SUGAR, SALT and FAT. The American Academy of Pediatrics concluded that less than 3% of advertising during children's programs focuses on healthful food, such as fruit and milk. Excessive TV watching increases the risk of childhood obesity. The AAP concluded that there is a direct link between commercials promoting high-calorie food and health problems, and in 1991 recommended a ban on food commercials geared toward children.

The Better Business Bureau's Children's Advertising Review Unit was founded in 1972. It is composed of representatives from the media, ad agencies and others, and its goal is to monitor truth in advertising in radio, TV and the printed word for children up to the age of 12, according to self-regulating guidelines. It will review material before it is publicized upon request. The group provides a forum for information exchange and relies on a panel of academic professionals to provide expertise on the impact of images on children. (See also CONVENIENCE FOOD; EATING PATTERNS; FOOD ADDITIVES; OBESITY.)

Taras, Howard L. and Gage, Miriam, "Advertised Foods on Children's Television," *Archives of Pediatric and Adolescent Medicine* 149:6 (June 1995), pp. 649–52.

aerobic   Refers to a physiologic or cellular process requiring oxygen. Cellular RESPIRATION is the aerobic process by which oxygen diffuses into cells and is used in the oxidation of fuel to produce ENERGY. The waste product of respiration is carbon dioxide. Aerobic also refers to the ability to function only in the presence of oxygen. For example, aerobic bacteria that are potential pathogens (disease producers) do not flourish in the intestine when the availability of oxygen is limited. (See also ELECTRON TRANSPORT CHAIN; OXIDATIVE PHOSPHORYLATION.)

aerobic exercise   Sustained physical EXERCISE involving moderate to high levels of exertion and characterized by increased heart rate and accelerated breathing. Vigorous activity associated with hard work and athletic sports can raise the pulse rate sufficiently to strengthen the cardiovascular system. Conditioning refers to increased physical endurance due to increased muscle mass and a strengthened oxygen delivery system, including heart, arteries and lungs, as a result of aerobic exercise. (See also FITNESS.)

aerobic respiration   See RESPIRATION, CELLULAR.

aflatoxin   A mycotoxin, a family of toxic compounds derived from filamentous fungi (molds) growing on foods and on grains used for animal feed. Aflatoxin is produced by ASPERGILLUS, a storage mold that often infests damp grains and nuts. Nuts such as pistachios, ALMONDS, WALNUTS, pecans and PEANUTS are susceptible to MOLD. Very low levels of aflatoxin often contaminate peanut butter. Spot checks have shown that this contamination is usually below the U.S. FDA limit. In the 1970s and again in the 1980s hot drought conditions caused outbreaks of mold in corn in the United States and, consequently, widespread aflatoxin contamination.

Concern has focused on aflatoxin because it is a potent liver CARCINOGEN. The amount of aflatoxin permitted by the U.S. FDA is 15 parts per billion, though levels as low as one part per billion can cause liver cancer in certain species of experimental animals. As yet there is no compelling evidence that aflatoxin consumption in the low amounts usually encountered in Western nations causes cancer. In regions of Africa where peanut consumption and consequently aflatoxin intake is very high, population studies suggest a correlation with liver cancer in humans. Recent research suggests that aflatoxin B-1 and hepatitis may contribute to liver cancer in China and Africa.

The recommendation is to avoid moldy, discolored or off-flavor nuts. Molds and fungi send out microscopic filaments beyond the immediate, visibly moldy area and cannot be easily removed. Furthermore, aflatoxin is not completely destroyed by cooking. Therefore moldy food, except cheese, should be discarded, rather than cutting out the mold. (See also CANCER PREVENTION DIET; FOOD TOXINS; FUNGUS.)

Ibeh, I.N. et al. "Dietary Exposure to Aflatoxin in Male Human Infertility in Benin City, Nigeria," *International Journal of Infertility* 39:4, (1994), pp. 208–14.

agar An organic FOOD ADDITIVE that forms non-digestible gels. This extract from seaweed has no odor or flavor. It is used occasionally as a THICKENING AGENT in the manufacture of whipped cream, ice cream, jelly, jam and MAYONNAISE. It prevents the drying out of frosting on baked goods. In microbiology, agar gels in petri dishes are used extensively to culture microorganisms for identification purposes.

aging The progressive decline over time in physiologic function, including reflexes, vision, hearing, short-term memory and learning, physical strength and endurance, DIGESTION, cardiovascular function and immunity. Though these changes often begin in the mid-twenties, heart functioning, memory and reasoning need not drop significantly until very late in life.

Aging is commonly associated with chronic diseases. These include CANCER, diabetes, OSTEOPOROSIS, PERIODONTAL DISEASE, OBESITY, SENILITY, CARDIOVASCULAR DISEASE (STROKE, HEART ATTACK, ATHEROSCLEROSIS, etc.) and AUTOIMMUNE DISEASES (such as RHEUMATOID ARTHRITIS and SPRUE). A growing body of evidence indicates that chronic diseases are not inevitable, but are related to many controllable factors, including diet. The common expectation that decreased physical ability will accompany aging often leads to diminished exercise at mid-life or later, setting the stage for narrowed arteries, elevated blood CHOLESTEROL, and heart and kidney disease.

Possible Causes of Aging

Cellular-molecular theories of aging are currently popular. According to these theories, genes may limit a person's life span, and there may be genes for longevity and predisposition to ALZHEIMER'S DISEASE, cancer and schizophrenia. The longevity determinant gene hypothesis predicts that a few key genes regulate the rate of aging of an organism. Aging may be the result of the improper readout of genes occurring during aging. Accumulated oxidative damage is another molecular explanation of tissue aging; it is hypothesized that the body gradually loses the ability to repair damage caused by oxidation to genetic material, as well as to cellular machinery. The damaging agent is believed to be FREE RADICALS, highly reactive fragmented chemicals, including extremely dangerous forms of oxygen that contain an impaired electron, which bombard tissues and attack DNA, proteins and cell walls.

Senescence could be linked to the structure of chromosomes. The tips of chromosomes are protected by telomeres, structures formed of DNA and protein. With successive cell divisions, telomeres become progressively shorter, reaching a point at which they can no longer protect the chromosome and cell division ceases. Because senescent cells are no longer able to protect organs and blood vessels, they possibly contribute to aging.

An alternate theory states that aging is regulated by the brain, the IMMUNE SYSTEM and HORMONES—the "neuroendocrine immune system." This complex system integrates all body functions, and the brain and the hypothalamus, the pituitary gland, the thymus gland and the pineal gland are implicated in the aging process. Evidence suggests that during aging, these organs gradually lose the ability to maintain the HOMEOSTASIS (the internal equilibrium) of the body. Brain pain-killer substances (enkephalins) no longer adequately balance the neuroendocrine immune system, leading to a decline in the ability to regulate homeostasis. With declining hormone production, tissue protein synthesis, immunity and reproduction decrease markedly. It is well established that the immune system gradually loses its ability to kill cancer cells with aging. Because it fails to discriminate "self" from "non-self," the immune system can begin to attack the body it is supposed to protect, causing the autoimmune and chronic diseases of aging.

Drastically limiting caloric intake may slow the age-related physiologic decline in experimental animals and increase their longevity dramatically. While this approach is a useful research tool, this is an impractical approach to slowing aging in humans. Few adults would volunteer to restrict their CALORIES by 20% or more for a lifetime.

On the other hand, prevention seems a much more feasible approach to counteract aging. It is estimated that only about 30 percent of aging characteristics are genetically based. Consequently how a person lives is the major key to a healthy old age. Staying active physically and socially contributes to successful aging. Regular physical activity, continued social relationships, the ability to recover from losses, and a feeling of control over one's life are predictors of successful aging.

Aging and Memory

Short-term memory functions and the speed of recall often decline with aging. Though annoying, forgetfulness need not be debilitating. Memory serves as the basis of learning. Because memory is selective, it will usually serve the learning process throughout life: Though perhaps slower to learn, an older person can be more accurate. It seems clear that the mental faculties of most older people remain functioning when exercised and challenged by a commitment to life-long learning and activity. Furthermore, research suggests that people may be trained to partially recover their mental function apparently lost during aging.

Forgetfulness can be caused by depression, by the use of alcohol, tranquilizers and sleeping pills, by certain drug interactions and by any factor that decreases the supply of oxygen to the brain. Malnutrition can also cause mental deterioration. In this regard, antioxidants may be particularly important because free radical damage may play a role in mental aging. Older experimental animals fed antioxidants dramatically can improve their mental performance with a concomitant decline in oxidized brain proteins. Such experiments suggest the buildup of oxidized protein, the result of free-radical attack, may cause brain cells to age.

Preventive medicine proposes that making wise life-style choices sets the stage for health later in life. The following life-style choices increase the odds of living longer:

- Avoid cigarettes. Smoking can lead to cancer, cardiovasular disease and emphysema.
- Take care of all emotional needs to reduce the stress of daily living and thus strengthen the immune system. Chronic stress leads to elevated cortisol, which suppresses the immune system.
- Keep mentally active; individuals who use their reasoning power retain it longer.
- Exercise regularly to slow deterioration of sensory and physical abilities. AEROBIC EXERCISE can increase fitness and endurance throughout a lifespan.
- Eat wisely. A varied, balanced diet with minimally processed food is the foundation for lasting good health.

Nutrient Needs During Aging

Elderly persons are prone to MALNUTRITION for several reasons. They are more likely to eat alone and so take less interest in meal preparation; and they are more often disabled and immobile; thus they are less likely to eat properly. More than 30% of homebound older individuals may have difficulty in preparing their own meals. Low-fiber, high carbohydrate meals typify the diets of many elderly persons. They use more laxatives and medications for long periods. Furthermore, many elderly persons have periodontal disease and poor teeth. Their senses of smell, taste and sight decline, making eating less appealing and STOMACH ACID production gradually drops, decreasing nutrient uptake even with an adequate diet.

Evidence indicates that superior nutrition may prevent unnecessary illness and disability from shortening a productive life. Therefore, the following health decisions are recommended:

- Avoid excess calories and alcohol. Surplus calories regardless of their source are converted to fat. Excessive body fat contributes to the risk of heart disease, hypertension and some forms of cancer. Besides the risk of addiction, excessive alcohol can damage the liver, pancreas and brain, in addition to depleting the body of nutrients.
- Your physician may check your stomach acid production. Low stomach acid production sets the stage for inadequate digestion of nutrients like vitamins and minerals and for malabsorption and subclinical deficiencies.
- Make informed choices regarding nutritional supplements. They can affect the quality of health of those who are nutrient deficient, though eating wisely.

- Choose a diet based on dietary guidelines for Americans as a foundation. A BALANCED DIET, one that provides adequate amounts of all nutrients and fiber from varied, minimally processed foods without excessive calories and fat, is of paramount importance.

Relatively little is known regarding specific nutritional needs of people over the age of 65, although more research is being done in this area. Attention has focused on three classes of nutrients as being especially important in aging: minerals, vitamins and antioxidants.

Minerals   Diminished digestion and ABSORPTION can lead to deficiencies of MAGNESIUM, IRON, ZINC, COPPER and CALCIUM. Older persons probably need more than the current calcium RDA of 800 mg because the ability of the intestine to absorb adequate calcium declines progressively with age. The common experience is that the bodies of elderly women and men remove calcium from their bones to meet their calcium needs. Supplementation with calcium and vitamin D, or calcium with low-dose estrogen for postmenopausal women, seems to be more effective in slowing bone losses than supplementation with calcium alone. Normally iron stores increase throughout adult life in men and in women after menopause. However, blood loss due to chronic aspirin use and bleeding ulcers can cause iron deficiency; 5% of elderly men are iron deficient in the United States. CHROMIUM stores in the body decline steadily with age and this may contribute to the decline in the regulation of blood sugar. Chromium assists in insulin action and helps blood sugar regulation in some diabetics. Low chromium is correlated with elevated blood cholesterol levels.

Vitamins   There are indications of increased vitamin needs in elderly people; however, no definite proof that vitamin supplements increase the life span has been offered. Many elderly Americans obtain less than 50% of the RDA of VITAMIN B6. Medications, such as penicillin, estrogens and antihypertensive drugs, interfere with this vitamin. Folic acid and vitamin B12 are less well absorbed in elderly persons and the RDAs should be higher. Inadequate diet and decreased uptake of fat-soluble vitamins probably account for the increased need for VITAMIN A and VITAMIN E with aging, and extra vitamin E may boost immunity, thus helping elderly persons resist disease. VITAMIN D requirements may increase during aging because the skin gradually loses its ability to manufacture the vitamin. Patients with hip fractures may be deficient in vitamin D.

Another problematic nutrient for elderly people is VITAMIN C, a versatile antioxidant. Consumption may be low with diets relying on processed, over-cooked foods and lacking adequate fruits and vegetables. Vitamin C may protect against cataracts and atherosclerosis. The RDA for RIBOFLAVIN is believed to be too low for elderly people. Geriatric outpatients can exhibit low-THIAMIN levels and evidence suggests that RDA of this critical nutrient is greater for older people than for middle aged individuals.

Antioxidants   Several nutrients seem to protect the body throughout life against damage by free radicals, highly reactive forms of oxygen that can attack cells. Trace minerals like copper, SELENIUM and zinc, as well as vitamins C and E plus BETA CAROTENE, function as antioxidants. Together with vitamin A they also help keep the immune system balanced. The immune system protects the body against bacterial and viral diseases and defends against cancer.

Other ingredients in foods, especially fruits and vegetables act as ANTIOXIDANTS. They strengthen the body's defenses and protect against cancer. These include FLAVONOIDS, PHYTO-ESTROGENS (ISOFLAVONES), indoles, coumarins, terpenes, organosulfur compounds including diallyl disulfide and others, lignans, saponins, ISOTHIOCYANATES and CAROTENOIDS. Certainly many more remain to be identified. From hundreds of studies, it is clear that diets that provide ample fruits, legumes and vegetables protect against many of the degenerative diseases that commonly occur with aging. As an example, middle-aged men and women who eat plenty of fruits and vegetables are significantly less likely to experience cardiovascular disease and strokes.

More research is required to determine the optimal intake of anti-aging nutrients. Foods with anti-aging nutrients include orange-colored vegetables (CARROTS, squash) and dark-green leafy vegetable (CHARD, KALE, SPINACH) for vitamin A and beta carotene. Fresh fruit like ORANGES, frozen citrus juices, and BROCCOLI provide VITAMIN C. Vegetable oil, WHEAT germ and nuts supply vitamin E while whole GRAINS, SEAFOOD, cabbage, onions and garlic provide selenium. (See also DEGENERATIVE DISEASES; DHEA; SENILITY.)

Gutteridge, John M., "Hydroxyl radicals, iron, oxidative stress, and neurodegeneration, *Annals of the New York Academy of Sciences*, 738 (November 1994), pp. 201–13.

Johnson, Kathleen and Kligman, E.W., "Preventive Nutrition: Disease-specific Dietary Interventions for Older Adults," *Geriatrics*, 47: 11 (November 1992), pp. 39–49.

agricultural chemicals   See PESTICIDES.

AIDS (Acquired Immune Deficiency Syndrome)   A modern, global epidemic involving the destruction of white cells (lymphocytes) required for immunity. Ultimately, the immune system fails due to infection by the Human Immunodeficiency Virus (HIV). A number of life-style factors have been implicated in increased physiologic susceptibility to HIV infection: overconsumption of refined foods; intestinal leakiness to foreign materials due to alcohol or pain medications (NSAIDS); inadequate diet and malnutrition; malabsorption; use of recreational drugs; repeated infections, including sexually transmitted diseases; use of medications that weaken the immune system; blood transfusions; as well as stress and smoking. Relatively few carefully designed and controlled clinical studies of nutrition and HIV infections have been carried out to permit general conclusions.

As a result of increased susceptibility to disease due to lowered immunity, AIDS patients may develop pneumonia, Karposi sarcoma, a cancer of the connective tissue, and diseases due to infectious agents, including the yeast CANDIDA ALBICANS, Epstein-Barr virus and herpes simplex virus. Low nutritional status contributes to these diseases.

HIV-infected persons are more susceptible to parasites, such as CRYPTOSPORIDIUM, a common contaminant in municipal water supplies. The recommendation is to avoid all public tap water and to drink water that has been boiled or filtered.

Weight loss characterizes HIV infection, but the causes remain ill-defined. In AIDS patients this may be due to MALNUTRITION or it may be due to the lack of appetite (anorexia) associated with the subsequent severe infections or cancer. Anorexia is worsened by depression. Oral and throat yeast infections, early symptoms of depressed immunity, can also compromise food intake.

There is no definitive proof so far that nutrients and proper nutrition alone can cure AIDS or destroy HIV viruses. However, there is a growing belief that they can strengthen the body's defenses. This is reflected by the interest of HIV-positive patients and patients with AIDS in nutrient-dense diets more in accord with published dietary guidelines.

There is no cure for AIDS; however, several nutrients, food-related materials and enzyme preparations boost the immune system and may offer protection against the risk of CANCER and infection in some individuals with AIDS.

Trace nutrients   ZINC deficiency is common in patients with AIDS and may indicate trace mineral malnutrition or malabsorption. Zinc plays an important role in maintaining the immune system. Zinc inhibits an enzyme needed for HIV production. Selenium deficiency may be part of the malnutrition seen in AIDS patients. It is a COFACTOR for enzymes that serve as antioxidants. Selenium helps protect against liver and colon cancer in experimental animals, and clinical studies of the effects of selenium supplementation on cancer prevention are being carried out. Other vitamins and minerals, such as vitamin A, folic acid, vitamin B_{12} and potassium, may be deficient in some AIDS patients.

Enzymes   Megadoses of a variety of ENZYMES, including SUPEROXIDE DISMUTASE, are being used as antioxidants. There is no clear evidence that their use diminishes or prevents symptoms.

Antioxidants   Evidence suggests that HIV-infected patients undergo chronic oxidative stress, with decreased antioxidants: vitamin C, CAROTENOIDS, COENZYME Q, GLUTATHIONE and selenium. Oxidative stress can promote HIV replication and decrease immunity. Antioxidant nutrients may lower the risk of cancer in the general population, and the same may be true for HIV-infected patients. BETA CAROTENE and carotenoids may lower the risk of many cancers, including those of the lung, bladder, stomach, esophagus and prostate. Beta carotene can increase the numbers of T-helper cells. Significantly, the standard American diet is deficient in beta carotene. VITAMIN C boosts immunity, helps protect against viral and bacterial infections, and may decrease the risk of stomach, esophageal and cervical cancer. It increases serum antibody levels and supports the function of the thymus gland and lymphocytes. Furthermore, vitamin C supports healthy connective tissue and assists in wound healing. FLAVONOIDS are associated with vitamin C in plants and enhance vitamin C therapy. Many flavonoids function as antioxidants and several types may stimulate the immune system. Glutathione supports the immune system and functions as a major antioxidant. N-acetylcysteine, a derivative of the sulfur amino acid CYSTEINE, can enhance glutathione levels.

Egg lipids   Mixtures of LECITHIN and other fatty materials from eggs have been used with some positive results in small clinical studies. Although there is a lack of strong evidence of its effectiveness, these mixtures are still being used. They are apparently non-toxic, though long-term effects are unknown.

Herbs Several herbs, such as GOLDENSEAL (*Hydrastis canadensis*), have been shown to enhance several aspects of immune function. The most active component of goldenseal is berberine, a broad-spectrum antimicrobial agent effective in treating the severe diarrhea that is typically seen in AIDS patients. Herbal treatment based on Chinese medicine is also being studied. Certain formulations inhibit viruses and boost the immune system. Garlic seems to enhance immunity and to combat opportunistic organisms associated with AIDS, including Candida albicans, cryptococcus, herpes virus and mycobacteria.

Gramlich, L.M. and Mascioli, E.A., "Nutrition and HIV Infection," *Nutritional Biochemistry*, 6 (1995), pp. 2–11.

Watson, Ronald R., ed. *Nutrition and AIDS*. Boca Raton, Fla.: CRC Press, 1994.

airline meals Over the years, airlines have revised the meals they serve in order to meet consumer expectations for more healthful choices. Changes include more chicken and less beef and fewer saturated fats, like coconut and palm oil.

Special airline meals fall into several categories. Religious meals include Kosher, Hindu and Muslim. For medical conditions, bland, diabetic, gluten-free, low-calorie, low-carbohydrate, low-cholesterol, low-fat and low-sodium meals may be offered. Other options include a fruit plate, seafood, strict vegetarian, ovolactovegetarian, and infant, toddler and child meals. First-class meals follow the same nutritional standards.

Beverages are important, especially on long flights. The healthiest options are mineral water or fruit and vegetable juices, compared to coffee, tea and soft drinks.

A brown-bag, carry-on meal is always an option for those with special dietary needs or with food sensitivities.

alanine (Ala, L-alanine) One of the simplest amino acids used to build PROTEINS. Alanine is readily formed in the body from PYRUVIC ACID, a direct product of glucose utilization; hence, it is classified as a non-dietary, essential amino acid.

In addition to serving as a protein building block, alanine plays an important role in transporting the toxic waste product, ammonia, out of muscle. Ammonia is produced when muscle cells break down amino acids for energy. Cells couple ammonia with a simple acid called pyruvic acid to form alanine, which is then released into the bloodstream. The liver next absorbs alanine and removes ammonia, which it rapidly converts to UREA, the ultimate nitrogenous waste of the body. The liver converts pyruvic acid back to glucose, which is released into the bloodstream. Blood glucose is taken up by the muscle, where it is broken down to pyruvic acid, which is then ready to accept ammonia and thus completes the cycle.

Alar (daminozide) A chemical used until recently to improve the color, yield and storage qualities of APPLES. It is not a pesticide. Until the late 1980s, Alar was used on an estimated 5 to 10% of the American apple crop. It was also used on cherries and peanuts. Alar is a systemic pollutant, meaning it is distributed throughout the plant and cannot be washed off. Alar has caused cancer in experimental animals,

and concern was raised that, because young children drink more apple juice for their body weight than do adults, they are more susceptible to the potential risk.

In 1989 Alar was withdrawn by the manufacturer, Uniroyal Chemical Company. The following year it was formally banned by the EPA. Alar is still sold abroad, however. About 50% of apple concentrates for apple juice comes from foreign countries where Alar is widely used, and imports may be contaminated by Alar. (See also PESTICIDES.)

albacore (*Thunnis [germo] alalunga*) A type of tuna with white meat. Albacore is a small tuna characterized by a large pectoral (side) fin. One of the smallest tuna, albacore usually weigh less than 40 lbs. (18 kg). They are found near the surface of warm or temperate seas throughout the world, where they feed on anchovies, sardines and other small fish. Albacore have been called the "chicken of the sea" because their white meat is comparable to chicken in flavor. Albacore is the highest quality canned tuna and is an excellent protein source. The food value of 3 oz. (85 g) (packed in water): calories, 135; protein, 30 g; fat, 1 g; cholesterol, 48 mg; calcium, 17 mg; iron, 0.6 mg; sodium, 468 mg; zinc, 0.94 mg; vitamin A, 32 retinol equivalents; thiamin, 10.03 mg; riboflavin, 0.1 mg; and niacin, 13.2 mg (See also FISH OIL.)

albumin A class of water-soluble proteins. Albumins are soluble in dilute salt solutions but are insoluble in pure water. Important members of this class are serum albumin and ovalbumin. The liver produces serum albumin, the most plentiful protein in serum. Serum albumin transports ions like CALCIUM, free FATTY ACIDS, and lipophilic (fat-soluble) materials like BILIRUBIN through the blood. Serum albumin also helps buffer the blood. It is a highly charged molecule (polyelectrolyte) that cannot pass through cell membranes and thus helps maintain the electrolyte balance of body fluids.

Ovalbumin is one of the most abundant proteins of egg white. The Roman author Pliny recorded the name of egg white as albumen. Ovalbumin is an excellent source of sulfur-containing amino acids, such as CYSTEINE, and this accounts in part for the excellent food value of egg protein. (See also ELECTROLYTES; LIVER.)

alcohol (ethanol, grain alcohol, ethyl alcohol) A class of organic compounds containing a hydroxyl group (–OH). Alcohol is also a common term for the simple alcohol ETHANOL, the product of FERMENTATION. As a constituent of alcoholic beverages, ethanol is the most common, and longest used, sedative. To produce alcohol, special strains of yeast are incubated with CARBOHYDRATES of FRUIT juices and GRAINS together with other nutrients. Under anaerobic conditions (in the absence of oxygen), these microorganisms ferment sugar to ethanol and CARBON DIOXIDE to obtain energy. The immediate product of the fermentation of grapes is WINE. When malted grains and hops are fermented, the product is BEER. Distillation, a process introduced in the Middle Ages, produces alcoholic beverages with a higher alcohol content. These include rum, whiskey, liqueurs and the like. Beer and wine are perhaps the most popular beverages among moderate drinkers. A mug of beer (11 oz., 4.5%), a glass of table wine (4 oz.) and a shot (jigger; 1.5 fl. oz.) of liquor (80 proof) contain about the same amount of alcohol (9 to 13 grams.)

Excessive consumption of alcoholic beverages is a major factor in subclinical and severe MALNUTRITION because alcoholic beverages contain little else besides CALORIES. A glass of red wine contains 88 calories; a bottle of regular beer, 146; and a shot (1.5 fl. oz.) of whiskey (90 proof), 110 calories. VITAMIN, PROTEIN and MINERAL content of alcohol is exceedingly low, though wine may contain a significant amount of iron. For this reason, alcoholic beverages are classified as low nutrient density or EMPTY CALORIES. To the extent they are consumed, they displace nutrient-dense foods.

ALCOHOLISM leads to disturbances of the GASTROINTESTINAL TRACT: Excessive ethanol directly or indirectly increases chronic intestinal inflammation associated with MALABSORPTION, compromised digestion and "leaky gut," in which the intestine more readily absorbs toxins and potentially harmful substances from food and microorganisms that the body recognizes as foreign (antigens). This can set the stage for FOOD INTOLERANCE and systemic effects. Alcohol affects the liver, where altered glucose and glycogen METABOLISM, fat formation and fat export can lead to fatty deposits (FATTY LIVER). The ability of the liver to detoxify other potentially damaging materials can also be compromised.

The blood alcohol level is affected by the amount of alcohol ingested. Water and juice slow the absorption of alcohol, while carbonation increases the rate of uptake into the bloodstream. Alcohol with food is less intoxicating. How alcohol is metabolized is another factor. A portion of the ingested alcohol is destroyed by enzymes in the stomach that are more active in men than in women; consequently, women generally have a lower tolerance to alcohol. The liver's capacity to destroy alcohol in the blood is limited, and when the liver's metabolic system is saturated, a fraction of ethanol in the blood is destroyed each hour. The remaining alcohol readily penetrates the blood-brain barrier and interacts with the central nervous system. Alcohol can pass from maternal blood into breast milk; therefore, lactating mothers may wish to abstain from drinking.

Some studies suggest that a single alcoholic drink a day may slightly reduce the risk of heart attack and stroke in some individuals. Moderate alcohol consumption increases the level of HDL, the beneficial form of cholesterol that tends to protect against heart disease. Alcohol also inhibits platelet formation, which is required to form blood clots. Moderate alcohol use may also help prevent age-related decline in reasoning and problem-solving. The apparent benefits decline after more than one or two drinks, however. The American Heart Association does not recommend drinking alcoholic beverages to prevent heart disease because of the hazards of alcohol abuse.

Possible consequences of excessive alcohol consumption include the following:

Mental retardation in infants Drinking during pregnancy can lead to FETAL ALCOHOL SYNDROME.

Addiction Alcoholism is one of the most common addictions.

Intoxication Excessive alcohol can lead to a progressive deterioration of mental functioning. Alcohol is a depressant and slows down the nervous system, especially the brain. While moderate drinking can be relaxing, being intoxicated means the control centers are blocked, which can lead to memory lapses, decreased coordination, loss of inhibitions, confusion, mood swings and depression. Most individuals will be adversely affected when the alcohol content of the blood rises above a threshold value. Legal intoxication in the United States is often defined as having a blood alcohol content ranging from 0.01 to 0.02%, depending upon the state. (Normally, the alcohol content of the blood is negligible.) Drunk drivers contribute significantly to traffic fatalities in the United States. Do not drink and drive.

Aggravated high blood pressure Excessive alcohol consumption can worsen hypertension.

Increased risk of disease Alcohol injures the liver (CIRRHOSIS), the pancreas (PANCREATITIS) and the brain. It causes intestinal inflammation, interferes with nutrient uptake and may increase uptake of toxins. Heavy drinkers have increased risk of heart failure, and alcohol causes a dangerous enlargement of the heart. For this reason some researchers do not recommend that anyone past the age of 50 drink alcoholic beverages. Alcohol increases the risk of cancer of the esophagus, mouth and breast. A drink a day may slightly increase the risk of breast cancer in women.

Surplus calories One gram of ethanol provides seven CALORIES, almost as much as FAT. One beer is equivalent to 150 calories. One shot (1.5 fl. oz.) of 80 proof gin, vodka or rye whiskey contributes about 110 calories that supply no other nutritional value. Alcohol even increases the body's need for vitamins.

Exposure to sulfites Wine contains SULFITE, which can cause reactions in sensitive people. (See also ALCOHOL-DRUG INTERACTIONS.)

Menzano E. and Carlen P.L. "Zinc Deficiency and Corticosteroids in the Pathogenesis of Alcoholic Brain Dysfunction: A Review," *Alcoholism, Clinical and Experimental Research*, 18:4 (July/August 1994), pp. 895–901.

alcohol-drug interactions Alcohol interacts with many medications. Drinking ALCOHOL can alter the way the body metabolizes drugs. As an example, the liver adapts to alcohol consumption by increasing its battery of drug-destroying ENZYMES. Because a heavy drinker may metabolize a sedative rapidly, its effects could wear off sooner than in a non-drinker, leaving the heavy drinker undersedated. Read prescription labels carefully before drinking, and inform dentists, physicians, pharmacists and other health care providers if you drink.

Interactions include:

Analgesics Non-prescription pain killers, such as Tylenol, that contain acetaminophen can damage the liver of those who consume several drinks a day. ASPIRIN together with alcohol increases stomach bleeding.

Antidepressants Monoamine oxidase inhibitors, AMPHETAMINES and tricyclic antidepressants like Imipramine cause severe reactions, such as increased sedation, if taken with alcohol.

Antihistamines Drinking after taking drugs like benadryl can lead to excessive drowsiness.

Arthritis medications Indocin and other drugs prescribed for arthritis taken with alcohol can irritate the gastrointestinal tract and may cause dizziness.

Barbiturates Never combine alcohol with drugs like amytal or phenobarbital, which is the most hazardous combination. The additive effects of taking the depressants can lead to respiratory failure and coma.

Diabetic medications Individuals taking Diabinese, Orinase and other sulfonureas to treat diabetes will probably not be able to tolerate alcohol because these drugs can make the user ill after drinking alcoholic beverages.

Niacin Large doses of niacin taken with alcohol can reduce blood pressure excessively.

Prescription pain killers Codeine and narcotics combined with alcohol cause increased sedation. Do not drive in this condition.

Sedatives and tranquilizers Combining alcohol and tranquilizers like Valium, and Thorazine can lead to oversedation and extreme drowsiness.

alcoholism Estimated to be the most common untreated illness and the most serious drug problem in the United States, alcoholism is characterized by an uncontrollable urge to drink, a tolerance to increasing quantities of ALCOHOL, blackout episodes and withdrawal symptoms during abstinence. Alcoholics frequently deny that they have a problem.

The costs of alcoholism to society are enormous. Excessive alcohol is involved in one out of ten deaths in America and typically shortens the life span by 10 to 12 years. Alcoholism contributes to accidental death, crime, violence and abuse. According to the National Highway Traffic Safety Administration, half of all fatalities due to automobile accidents have occurred in crashes in which the driver or pedestrian had been drinking. Estimates of the total cost of alcoholism to society range from $65 billion to $117 billion. Alcohol abuse occurs among young people as well as the elderly, encompasses people of all social and economic backgrounds, and women as well as men. Children of alcoholics are more likely to abuse alcohol and drugs. Individuals may be born susceptible to alcoholism due to imbalanced body chemistry; however, the social environment obviously plays an important role.

The alcoholic individual faces profound health consequences in terms of MALNUTRITION, heart failure, high blood pressure, damage to pancreas, liver, stomach and brain, and increased risk of cancer of the mouth and esophagus. Even moderate alcohol intake can cause birth defects if the mother drinks during pregnancy.

Alcoholism is treatable; however, recovery depends upon the person's willingness to accept help. Individualized recovery programs work best and may incorporate family counseling, psychotherapy, support groups, rehabilitation programs, education, behavior modification, vocational guidance and exercise. Nutritional and medical treatment is often recommended to remedy nutritional deficiencies, alcohol-related disorders and to speed detoxification. A number of clinics treat alcoholism by incorporating life-style changes affecting DIET and EXERCISE, while eliminating CAFFEINE and nicotine. Alcoholics Anonymous (AA) can provide a very strong support system for recovery. (See also ADDICTION.)

aldicarb (Temik) A very toxic insecticide widely used on POTATOES, SOYBEANS, PEANUTS and citrus crops. Aldicarb was assumed to break down rapidly after application. However, tests show that it can persist in soil for years and contaminate crops planted in the same soil later. Several instances of aldicarb poisoning indicate the potential hazard of using this pesticide. Aldicarb-contaminated watermelons caused serious illness to thousands of persons in 1985. In 1988 aldicarb-contaminated vegetables, such as hot-house cucumbers, lead to sporadic outbreaks of illness.

Symptoms of aldicarb toxicity include seizures, disorientation, blurred vision and gastrointestinal disorders. The EPA recently limited the use of aldicarb and directed states to determine areas susceptible to contamination and then to monitor them, to assure concentrations do not exceed the limits set by the EPA. Activated charcoal filters can remove aldicarb from drinking water. (See also PESTICIDES.)

aldosterone A hormone of the adrenal glands responsible for regulating sodium in the blood. It is classified as a corticosteroid, a group of hormones synthesized by the adrenal cortex. Aldosterone is the principal MINERALOCORTICOID, which directs the kidney to conserve SODIUM by reabsorbing sodium and water from urine. In the kidney, aldosterone stimulates the renal tubules to release potassium and hydrogen ions in place of sodium, thus increasing urine acidity. Mineralocorticoids also increase sodium reabsorption from sweat, saliva and gastric juices. Other steroid hormones, deoxycorticosterone, corticosterone and progesterone, can also cause sodium retention, though they are much less active.

Stimuli that increase aldosterone secretion include surgery, anxiety, physical trauma, high potassium intake, low sodium intake, and diseases of the heart, liver and kidney. The pituitary hormone ACTH stimulates steroid hormone release from the adrenal glands. Aldosterone is also regulated by the kidneys in response to low serum sodium levels. The kidneys produce an enzyme, RENIN, which forms the hormone ANGIOTENSIN in the blood that stimulates aldosterone release. (See also ADRENAL GLANDS; ANTIDIURETIC HORMONE; FLUID BALANCE.)

ale An alcoholic beverage resembling BEER. Like beer, ale is brewed from hops, CEREAL GRAINS and MALT. Ale is "heavier" than beer, with a stronger flavor and deeper color. FERMENTATION conditions for ale production differ from those of beer production. In ale production fermentation occurs at higher temperatures. Yeast rises to the top of the fermentation vat, resulting in a pronounced hops flavor. The ALCOHOL in beer and ale supplies 146 calories per 12 oz. Other nutrients are present only in trace amounts. The term EMPTY CALORIES applies to the low nutrient value of all alcoholic beverages.

alfalfa (*Medicago sativa*) A LEGUME used primarily for fodder throughout the world. As a nutritional supplement, this plant is a rich source of TRACE MINERALS, BETA

CAROTENE, ESSENTIAL FATTY ACIDS, VITAMIN K and the B complex vitamins. Alfalfa contains significant FIBER and is a rich source of PROTEIN (25% by weight). In Asia alfalfa leaves are used in the form of greens as a vegetable.

Claims that alfalfa boosts the immune system may relate to its trace mineral content. It also has antibacterial activity, and there is some evidence that alfalfa can induce liver detoxifying enzymes that destroy toxins and pollutants. Alfalfa contains several classes of compounds, including saponins, sterols, flavonoids and coumarins, which can affect the body. For example, alfalfa saponins decrease blood cholesterol levels in lab animals. Alfalfa may reduce damage due to radiation, perhaps due to the antioxidants it contains. Individuals who have heart disease, who are pregnant, who have a tendency to clot easily or take anticoagulants should avoid alfalfa supplements because their vitamin K content may promote blood clotting.

Alfalfa sprouts are a healthful alternative to lettuce, containing beta carotene, VITAMIN C and trace minerals at levels higher than found in iceberg lettuce. In contrast with most lettuce, alfalfa sprouts are not treated with pesticides. Alfalfa sprouts (100 g) provide 54 calories; protein, 6 g; carbohydrate, 9.5 g; fiber, 3.1 g; fat, 0.4 g; calcium, 215 mg; iron, 2.3 mg; thiamin, 0.13 mg; riboflavin, 0.14 mg; niacin, 0.5 mg.

algae Simple plants found in fresh water and oceans throughout the world. Algae are largely undifferentiated and, unlike terrestrial plants, algal leaves and stems are composed of the same tissue. Some are edible and have been consumed throughout history. In this context, seaweed or marine algae are particularly important. Brown algae represent most of the edible seaweed harvested. Seaweed species are either cultivated or collected along coastal intertidal zones. In Japan, six types are consumed, and together they account for an estimated 10% of the country's total food production.

Edible brown algae, which represent most of the edible seaweed harvested worldwide, include arame, hiziki, kelp and kombu. Edible red algae include CARRAGEENAN (Irish moss), dulse and nori. These "sea vegetables" are rich sources of magnesium, iron, iodine and calcium, and some are as rich in vitamins such as vitamin C, beta carotene, vitamin E and the B complex as the best cultivated sources. In addition, various algae are used commercially as sources of gums (agar, carrageenan and ALGINATE). Carrageenan has the ability to form salt gels in milk products and is used to keep fats from separating, and to thicken ice cream. Alginic acid (alginate) in brown seaweed can bind toxic metals in the body and speed their removal. These algae can be added to soups, vegetables, salads, bean dishes and grains to add zest and boost nutritional value. Their flavor is neither fishy nor salty.

There is little information on toxic metal contamination of any domestic or imported seaweed. One study found very low amounts of arsenic, cadmium, lead and mercury in common imported varieties; the levels were well below limits set by the Food Chemicals Codex of the Food and Nutrition Board. Mercury levels were far below the limits set for fish.

alginate (ammonium, calcium, potassium and sodium salts of alginic acid) A food additive obtained from the giant kelp, a brown algae commercially harvested off the coast of California. Alginate is a major constituent of the cell wall and consists of polymers of acidic sugars. Alginate is used by the food industry as a thickening and stabilizing agent because calcium alginate forms very stable gels in water. It prevents jelly in pastries from melting during baking and provides smooth textures to ice cream, YOGURT and CHEESE, candy, whipped cream in pressurized cans and canned frosting. Alginate also helps keep cocoa butter dispersed in chocolate milk. The red pimento stuffed in green olives contains the most alginate (6%) of any food source. Alginate is not used in acidic foods and beverages, such as salad dressings and soft drinks, because it forms a sediment under these conditions.

Alginate is on the GRAS (GENERALLY RECOGNIZED AS SAFE) list of the U.S. FDA. Short-term animal testing indicates that alginate is not absorbed by the body and is not toxic. Because alginate forms highly charged gels in water, it remains to be determined whether it can limit the absorption of minerals and other nutrients by the body. (See also FOOD ADDITIVES.)

alimentary canal See DIGESTIVE TRACT.

alimentation The physiologic processes by which food nurtures and maintains the body. These include chewing (mastication), swallowing and digesting food. Alimentation also encompasses the ABSORPTION of NUTRIENTS (vitamins, minerals, amino acids, fat, carbohydrates) by the intestine and their use in CATABOLISM (energy production) and in ANABOLISM (building cellular constituents). The term alimentary canal refers to the digestive cavity running from the mouth to the anus.

Artificial alimentation refers to feeding a patient artificially either by intravenous procedures or by a nasal tube. Forced alimentation is feeding a patient who is unwilling to eat. (See also DIGESTION; HYPERALIMENTATION.)

alitame A non-caloric ARTIFICIAL SWEETENER pending approval by the U.S. FDA. This sweetener was developed to be safer than ASPARTAME. Unlike aspartame, alitame does not contain PHENYLALANINE and consequently would likely be safe for individuals with PHENYLKETONURIA (PKU), a genetic intolerance for this amino acid.

alkalemia A blood condition characterized by excessively alkaline (excessively high pH). A blood pH greater than 7.4 is considered alkaline and represents an accumulation of hydroxide ions and depletion of hydrogen ions, CARBON DIOXIDE and CARBONIC ACID. The body is exquisitely buffered to keep blood pH slightly alkaline, within a very narrow range, 7.35–7.45. However, this equilibrium can be shifted by loss of STOMACH ACID through vomiting; by the consumption of alkaline medications such as those used to treat ulcers; and by rapid breathing (hyperventilation), which rapidly decreases the body's stores of carbon dioxide.

The body compensates for alkalemia and reestablishes normal blood pH by slowing the respiration rate (breathing); this increases the level of carbon dioxide in the blood, which spontaneously forms more carbonic acid. The kidneys can compensate for elevated pH by excreting alkaline urine. (See also ALKALOSIS; BUFFER; ELECTROLYTES.)

Lownstein, Jerome. *Acids and Bases.* New York: Oxford University Press, 1993.

alkali-forming foods   See ACID-FORMING FOODS.

alkaline   A solution with a pH greater than 7.0, which is considered neutral. Alkaline solutions are also called "basic," as opposed to "acidic." Milk, blood, egg yolk and milk of magnesia are examples of slightly alkaline solutions. Solutions of baking soda (sodium bicarbonate) and ammonia form mildly alkaline solutions. In contrast, the corrosive metallic hydroxides such as sodium hydroxide (lye, caustic soda) are very strong bases and are very alkaline. They destroy tissue, create burns and are considered toxic substances.

alkaline tide   The slight rise in blood pH following a meal, when the blood temporarily becomes more alkaline. When the stomach produces hydrochloric acid (stomach acid) for use in digestion, it removes a fraction of negatively charged CHLORIDE ion from circulation. Chloride is then replaced by BICARBONATE in the blood, which tends to raise blood pH. As the meal is digested, chloride ions are reabsorbed by the intestine and again enter the bloodstream. In turn, bicarbonate is reabsorbed and the pH returns to normal. The urine may become more alkaline during gastric digestion as the body compensates for the change in blood pH.

alkaloid   A large, diverse class of organic compounds prevalent in the plant kingdom. They contain nitrogen and function as bases. Often alkaloids profoundly affect the body's physiology, and purified alkaloids are even more active. Examples of potent alkaloids include morphine, cocaine, quinine, strychnine, nicotine, CAFFEINE (COFFEE) and theobromine (CHOCOLATE). Depending upon the application and the dose, alkaloids may be used in therapy or they may cause toxicity. Socrates was killed by the alkaloid coniine that occurs in hemlock. Eating quail that have eaten poison hemlock can cause food poisoning. Alkaloids such as nicotine and caffeine are addictive substances. Morphine and cocaine are controlled substances due to their addictive properties.

alkalosis   Excessive alkalinity (elevated pH) of body fluids caused by either an accumulation of alkaline substances or a reduction in ACIDS. Alkalosis is thus more general than ALKALEMIA (alkaline blood). Respiratory alkalosis occurs with hyperventilation, aspirin poisoning, abnormal brain function, or inadequate oxygen supply, as may occur during exertion at high altitudes. Metabolic alkalosis occurs with severe vomiting due to losses of hydrogen ions and chloride ions (stomach acid); losses of potassium due to diuretic therapy; and ingestion of sodium bicarbonate (or other alkaline substances). Symptoms of both types of alkalosis include shallow breathing, a tingling sensation at fingertips and toes, muscular cramps and convulsions. Like prolonged ACIDOSIS, alkalosis requires medical intervention. (See also BUFFER; ELECTROLYTES.)

allergen   A substance or agent that causes an allergic reaction. Allergens provoke the IMMUNE SYSTEM when it senses an allergen as a foreign or "non-self" substance and overreacts. This "hypersensitivity" may be immediate, when symptoms appear within minutes to several hours after exposure, or it can be delayed, when symptoms appear hours after exposure or longer.

Allergens are very common. Inhaled materials that are potential allergens include dust, pollen, animal dander, perfume and pollutants such as smoke and volatile chemicals. At the top of the list of food allergens are dairy products, nuts (e.g., PEANUTS, filberts, CASHEWS), GRAINS (especially WHEAT and CORN), SOYBEAN products, CITRUS FRUITS and SHELLFISH. The binders and other ingredients of vitamin supplements, as well as HERBS and SPICES, can cause allergies in susceptible individuals. Prescription drugs (including penicillin), antisera and constituents of infectious agents (including pathogenic bacteria and viruses, yeast and parasites) can be allergens. Physical agents, including radiation, heat and pressure may also provoke inflammation, an aspect of the immune response. In provoking an immune response, allergens typically react with ANTIBODIES, protective proteins formed by specialized cells of the immune system. (See also ALLERGY, FOOD.)

allergic rhinitis   This condition refers to allergy symptoms associated with the chronic inflammation typical of hay fever: a perpetually stuffy, runny nose, sneezing, puffy bags and dark circles under the eyes, and a puffy face. Allergic rhinitis can lead to chronic earaches, especially in children, and to inflamed sinuses (sinusitis). It is more common among children, but can occur at any age. Allergic rhinitis is the result of a specific type of antibody, IgE, which binds to mast cells, defensive cells of the immune system, to stimulate inflammation. Therefore allergic rhinitis can be measured by a skin test. Nasal symptoms occur immediately after exposure to common allergens, including pollen, animal dander, house dust, mites, insects, mold and foods. Perfumes, deodorants and pesticides are not uncommon agents. Identification of the offending substance and reduced exposure are important; complete avoidance may be curative. Antihistamines are sometimes used to relieve initial symptoms. H_1-antihistamines such as terfenadine are the most frequently used medications to relieve symptoms; they have little effect on congestion, however. Cromolyn sodium is frequently used to stabilize mast cells and decrease symptoms. This drug has the fewest adverse effects of any anti-allergic medication. (See also HISTAMINE).

Bernstein, Jonathan, "Allergic Rhinitis: Helping Patients Lead an Unrestricted Life," *Postgraduate Medicine*, 93:6 (May 1, 1993), pp. 124–132.

allergy, food   An abnormal reaction of the immune system to normally harmless foods. An allergic response involves two aspects of the immune system: circulating ANTIBODIES and specialized attack cells. Each branch of the immune system can react to foods as though they were foreign invaders. In contrast, other types of FOOD SENSITIVITY such as LACTOSE INTOLERANCE do not depend on antibody reactions, nor do they involve other aspects of the immune system.

Allergy patterns may change during a lifetime; old sensitivities may vanish, and new ones may appear according to the health of the immune system and to the amount of allergen exposure. Introducing solid foods before an infant's DIGESTIVE TRACT is fully developed carries an increased risk of the development of food allergies. Children are more likely to suffer from allergies than adults, though they often outgrow them. Individuals who have relatives with allergies are more prone to develop food allergies themselves. Food allergies are more likely to occur with inadequate nutrition, infections, and physical and emotional stress. Faulty DIGESTION and intestinal inflammation can allow food ALLERGENS to penetrate intestinal barriers and enter the bloodstream.

Depending upon how food allergy is defined, estimates of the prevalence of food allergies range from 2% to 25% of the U.S. population. Opinion is also divided regarding the predominant form of food allergies. Those who consider food allergy an uncommon phenomenon focus on the readily observable, rapid systemic reactions to foods. These generate hay fever–like symptoms (immediate hypersensitivity). Other research indicates that typical food allergies are complex immune reactions resulting in delayed hypersensitivity. They frequently involve antibodies in the blood (IgG type), and symptoms develop over hours or days after consuming the problem food. This delay increases the difficulty in relating a specific food to sometimes vague symptoms.

The most common symptom of food allergy is FATIGUE. Other symptoms range from those typical of PREMENSTRUAL SYNDROME to hypoglycemia, eczema, irritability, achy joints, puffy eyes with dark circles, or postnasal drip. Food allergies may produce asthma in the respiratory tract; in the brain, insomnia, mood changes, confusion or fatigue; in the gastrointestinal tract, INDIGESTION, irritable colon, CONSTIPATION or DIARRHEA.

A simple, proven method of coping with food allergies is abstinence. To help identify troublesome foods, keep a diet diary for a week or two, carefully recording all that you eat and any symptoms you experience. Avoiding the offending food for several days to several weeks may allow the immune system to return to normal. If symptoms recur when the questionable food is eaten again, that food is probably the culprit. ROTATION DIETS have been devised to minimize exposure to allergenic foods. Because allergy-restricted diets can be difficult to balance nutritionally, those who have multiple food allergies may wish to consult both a physician and a nutritionist. Individuals with food allergies often need to find substitutes for common foods. A wide variety of food allergy cookbooks are now available to help plan delicious, nutritious meals. The U.S. Government Printing Office publishes *Cooking for People with Food Allergies*. (See also ALLERGY, IMMEDIATE; ALLERGIC RHINITIS; CHALLENGE TESTING).

Crook, William G. *Detecting Your Hidden Allergies.* Jackson, Tenn.: Professional Books, 1988.
Rapp, Doris J. *Is This Your Child?* New York: William Morrow, 1991.

allergy, immediate (immediate hypersensitivity) An inflammatory reaction responsible for the familiar hay fever, asthma and hives due to exposure to an ALLERGEN. These symptoms seldom leave any doubt as to their cause; the watery eyes, asthma, hives and swelling result from a very rapid over-reaction after exposure to an allergen. The key lies within mast cells, defending cells embedded in tissues, which carry a bound ANTIBODY (IgE) on their surfaces. Upon contact with an invader, mast cells release inflammatory agents such as histamine and leukotrienes that evoke swelling, itchiness, copious mucous secretion, and the spasm of muscles of the intestinal tract and of air passageways (bronchioles).

Common materials often trigger fast-developing reactions: dust, pollen, animal dander, medications, disease-producing microorganisms and pollutants. Seafood, milk, sulfites, peanuts, nuts and strawberries are a few of the food-related causes of immediate hypersensitivity. It may come as a surprise that immediate allergic reactions account for a small fraction of food allergies. Most food allergies are of the slow-reacting type.

Anaphylactic shock is the condition resulting from allergic reaction and affects the whole body quickly. It produces labored breathing, fever, erratic heartbeat, violent coughing, hives and edema, even convulsions. This severe response can be life-threatening. Individuals who are susceptible to severe allergy attacks may be advised to carry injectable medications ("bee sting" kits containing adrenalin or other drugs). See also ALLERGY, FOOD; ALLERGIC RHINITIS.)

allspice (*Pimenta officinals*; Jamaican pepper) A spice prepared from ground, unripened, reddish-brown berries of an evergreen tree found in the Caribbean, Central America and Mexico. Its name derives from the observation that its aroma resembles a blend of cloves, cinnamon, nutmeg and juniper berries. This versatile spice can be used singly or in combination with other seasoning. Fresh-ground allspice has more flavor. Allspice is used to season sausage, salt beef, pickle sauces and marinades.

almond (*Prunus amygdalus*) A cultivated, elongated nut with white meat and a brown skin. The almond tree resembles the peach, to which it is related. The almond originated in Asia and was known to the Romans as the "Greek nut." There are two varieties: the sweet almond and the bitter almond, which has a stronger flavor. Almond extracts are used to flavor cakes and pastries, and slivered or flaked sweet almonds are used in cakes, cookies and pastry. Dried almonds are served raw or roasted and salted. Nuts roasted with coconut or palm oil dramatically increase their caloric content and increase their saturated fat content. Almonds are also used as ingredients of stuffings and couscous, and they can accompany fish or poultry dishes (the garnish is known as amandine). Almonds are a good source of calcium and they are also rich in oil. Most of the oil is monounsaturated and more closely resembles olive oil than typical vegetable oils like safflower oil, which are high in polyunsaturates. One ounce (28 g) of raw, sweet almonds provides 167 calories; carbohydrate, 5.7 g; fiber, 3 g; fat, 14.8 g; protein, 5.9 g; calcium, 75 mg; iron, 1.0 mg; niacin, 0.95 mg; thiamin, 0.06 mg; riboflavin, 0.22 mg.

aloe vera A succulent plant with long pointed leaves that produces a juice with medicinal properties. There are hundreds of different aloe species. Aloe extracts are a folk remedy, long used to treat mild burns including sunburn, insect bites, abrasions, minor cuts and chafing, fever blisters, poison ivy, and to relieve joint inflammation and allergic reactions. Research has yielded mixed results. Most human studies have been uncontrolled. Evidence suggests that aloe vera may help heal ulcers and gastrointestinal inflammation and fight infections by boosting the immune system. Although a 1985 U.S. FDA study group concluded that aloe vera did not heal burns, recent clinical studies indicate burn healing is speeded up by aloe, possibly by improving collagen formation and by improving blood flow to damaged areas. There is preliminary evidence that aloe may help prevent severe conditions such as cancer. Very rarely, aloe vera may cause a rash in sensitive people, and pregnant women should not take aloe internally. Aloe does have its limitations. Adding aloe vera skin gel may slow the healing of infected surgical incisions compared to standard postoperative treatment.

alpha linolenic acid   Chemically speaking this fatty acid has 18 carbons and a pair of double bonds. It cannot be synthesized by the body and must be obtained from the diet. A POLYUNSATURATED FATTY ACID, it is classified as an essential dietary nutrient. Alpha linolenic acid is the smallest of the omega-3 family of polyunsaturated FATTY ACIDS, distinguished by subtle structural differences in which the double bonds begin at the third carbon from the end. It is the building block of larger omega-3 acids, including EICOSOPENTAENOIC ACID and docosohexaenoic acid (DHA), which in turn form the PG$_3$ class of PROSTAGLANDINS, hormone-like substances that decreases inflammation, decreases blood clotting and lowers blood cholesterol. PG$_3$ prostaglandins help return the body to equilibrium after physical stress or injury.

Omega-3 fatty acids are deficient in the standard American diet, and this deficiency may be linked to an increased risk of heart attacks and inflammation associated with degenerative disease. Chronic, severe deficiencies impair vision, increase inflammation, and diminish learning curves in experimental animals. The utilization of alpha linolenic acid may be limited in some disease states. The nervous system and brain contain high levels of the omega-3 fatty acids, and there is a positive relationship between the content of these fatty acids in the diet and vision and brain function. Pre-term babies need DHA because their livers are not mature enough to synthesize it from alpha linolenic acid.

Good dietary sources of the omega-3 fatty acids are limited. Breast milk contains omega-3 fatty acids, suggesting their importance in the infant's growth and development. Food processing destroys or removes the omega-3s, and there are none present in fast foods like pizza, fried fish sandwiches, fried chicken or hamburgers. The most common sources are FISH and FISH OILS, FLAXSEED OIL and pumpkin seeds; fish oil and flaxseed oil are sold as supplements. The American Heart Association recommends eating several servings of fish weekly. Because oils containing essential fatty acids readily oxidize and become rancid they need to be protected from oxygen and heat. They are usually packaged with ANTIOXIDANTS such as VITAMIN E. Buying small quantities of these oils and refrigerating them in sealed containers after opening reduces the risk of rancidity. These oils should not be used for cooking.

Kinsella, John E., "Alpha Linolenic Acid: Recent Overview," *Nutrition*, 8:3 (1992), pp. 195–96.

alpha tocopherol   See VITAMIN E.

aluminum (alum, aluminum silicate, sodium potassium aluminate)   A metallic ion that is widely distributed in water and soil. Drinking water often contains aluminum beyond levels leached from soil and clay because aluminum hydroxide is often added to municipal water supplies to clarify drinking water.

Aluminum is often added to food. Aluminum compounds make PROCESSED FOOD more creamy and pourable. They are quite versatile and are found in INFANT FORMULA, pickles, relishes, beer, cream of tartar, grated cheese, canned foods, BAKING POWDER and self-rising FLOUR. Aluminum is also found in the medicine chest: A major source of aluminum is ANTACIDS (such as Maalox), which have a high aluminum hydroxide content. Antiperspirants, over-the-counter analgesics (pain relievers, like buffered aspirin for arthritis) and other pain medications all contain aluminum. The average daily intake from all sources ranges from 10 to 100 mg. Most of this is not absorbed; of the fraction of aluminum that is absorbed by the body, most is subsequently excreted.

Although aluminum is not a heavy metal, accumulated evidence suggests that this substance may be harmful. Aluminum causes dialysis dementia, SENILITY and brain damage in young patients undergoing hemodialysis for kidney failure. Their increased aluminum intake is due to the use of antacids containing aluminum and to the elevated aluminum content of water used for dialysis. More generally, high levels of aluminum may inhibit phosphate uptake by the intestine and may increase calcium losses by excretion by the kidneys. The imbalance may cause brittle bones and may disturb bone formation. Other evidence suggests that excessive aluminum impairs the body's immunity.

Aluminum seems to accumulate in the brain with age, and high levels of aluminum are found in the brains of victims of ALZHEIMER'S DISEASE. Whether this is a cause or an effect of senility is not known, but a controversial report from Great Britain correlated the occurrence of Alzheimer's disease with the increased levels of aluminum in drinking water.

Patients with kidney disease and anyone regularly consuming antacids that contain aluminum compounds should be aware of the risks. Avoid taking medications (like buffered aspirin) containing aluminum with orange juice (CITRIC ACID); this combination can dramatically increase aluminum uptake in the body. Avoid placing acidic foods like tomato sauce, apple sauce and SAUERKRAUT in aluminum foil or in uncoated aluminum cookware because these foods dissolve aluminum, which can be absorbed. Avoid aerosol antiperspirants because the aluminum they contain is more readily absorbed through nasal passages.

Duggan John M. et al., "Aluminum Beverage Cans as a Dietary Source of Aluminum," *Medical Journal of Australia*, 156:9 (May 4, 1992), pp. 604–05.

Alzheimer's disease   A progressive, degenerative disease of the brain and the leading cause of SENILITY in the United States. It affects millions Americans and 15% of the U.S. population over the age of 65. This condition is characterized by an irreversible memory loss and the inability to think logically. There is no cure, and little can be done to delay the progress of the disease. Alzheimer's disease results from the death of nerves that represent main links between two regions of the brain responsible for thought processes and memory, the forebrain and the hippocampus. These nerves become embedded with protein (beta amyloid) deposits and become ineffective, tangled masses. The clinical aspects of this disease are associated with a deficiency of ACETYLCHOLINE, a NEUROTRANSMITTER chemical made by neurons that helps carry nerve impulses between cells. Currently, diagnosis of Alzheimer's disease is very difficult, yet a comprehensive diagnosis is critical in treating the senile patient.

Alzheimer's disease may affect as many as four million Americans. Most victims are over 65, but the disease can strike adults in their forties or fifties. This disorder affects almost half of those who are 85 or older. Symptoms occurring before the age of 65 are designated presenile dementia, Alzheimer's type (PDAT); after 65, it is senile dementia, Alzheimer's type (SDAT).

Despite intensive research over the last decade, it is not known whether Alzheimer's disease is a function of AGING, or whether it is the result of a specific disease process. Alzheimer's seems to be a multifaceted disease, with environmental and genetic factors contributing. One form seems to run in families, involving an inherited defect in mitochondria, the cell's energy-producing machinery. There is an association with Down's syndrome and thyroid disease. Smoking a pack of cigarettes a day increases the odds of developing Alzheimer's disease.

Another hypothesis for Alzheimer's links chronic CALCIUM deficiency to increased uptake of ALUMINUM and silicon by the brain. Aluminum concentrates in the brains of patients with the disease; whether this is a cause or an effect is unknown. In postmenopausal women, estrogen (hormone) replacement therapy may help prevent Alzheimer's. The importance of estrogen in brain health is gradually being recognized. Alternatively, there may be alterations in nerve cell membranes. Other evidence links immune system activation with the disease process.

Research points to the following possible causes of senility: exposure to toxins, oxidative damage due to FREE RADICALS, abnormal protein metabolism, slow viruses, the narrowing by cholesterol deposits of arteries feeding the brain, ZINC and VITAMIN B_{12} deficiencies, head trauma, and adverse drug reactions that decrease blood and oxygen supply to the brain.

Nutritional approaches to treatment employ CHOLINE and lecithin (phosphatidylcholine) supplements. The rationale for their use is based on the fact that the brains of diseased patients do not make enough acetylcholine, and supplying this building block could boost acetylcholine production. Results of clinical studies have not shown consistent improvements. Researchers have used drugs that help maintain acetylcholine levels with mixed results. A growth promoter called nerve growth factor may enhance brain function in aged experimental animals. However, no treatment so far developed changes the ultimate course of Alzheimer's disease (See also CARNITINE; SENILITY.)

Flieger, Ken, "Despite New Clues, Alzheimer's Mystery Remains Unsolved," *FDA Consumer*, 26:2 (1992), pp. 17–21.
Harman, Denham, "Free Radical Theory of Aging: a Hypothesis on Pathogenesis of Senile Dementia of the Alzheimer's Type," *Age*, 16 (1993), pp. 23–30.

amalgam fillings   Mixtures of heavy metals, primarily silver and mercury, used to fill cavities in teeth. Silver amalgam fillings release traces of MERCURY and minute amounts enter the bloodstream after chewing. The American Dental Association's position is that the silver amalgam used to fill cavities has a safe track record and that few people (perhaps one in a million) are sensitive to mercury. On the other hand, a number of dentists and preventative medicine physicians argue that the small amount of mercury released from amalgam fillings can lead to a wide range of conditions such as memory loss, insomnia, chronic headaches, high blood pressure and tinnitus (ringing ears). The Swedish Dental Association no longer recommends mercury fillings, and the Swedish government plans a phaseout of amalgam fillings.

Several plastic materials can be used to fill teeth in place of amalgams. However, removal of amalgam fillings and substituting composite fillings has had mixed results in patients. Faulty dental fillings are a common cause of periodontal disease. The mercury from silver amalgam fillings could exacerbate this condition because mercury depletes important anti-oxidant enzymes—CATALASE, GLUTATHIONE and glutathione peroxidase—in gum tissue.

Drasch G. et al., "Mercury Burden of Human Fetal and Infant Tissues," *European Journal of Pediatrics*, 153:8 (1994), pp. 607–10.

amanita   A genus of mushroom that includes many poisonous species, along with a few edible ones. Amanita species can be confused with the edible champignon, leading to mushroom poisoning. The most common cause of mushroom poisoning is the ingestion of *A. phalloides* (death cap) and *A. virosa* (destroying angel). These species produce specific toxins called amatoxins and phallotoxins, compounds with cyclic amino acid structures. A single mushroom may contain enough of these poisons to kill an adult. Eating the mushroom can cause liver, heart, kidney or cardiac damage as well as symptoms of common shock and delirium.

amaranth (*Amaranthus cruentus*; grain amaranth)   A nutritious alternative to WHEAT. The tiny spherical seeds are the size of poppy seeds. Originally grown in Mexico as a staple food of the Aztecs, it was eaten in rituals of Native Americans until the Spanish conquest of Mexico, when its cultivation was outlawed. Amaranth is now cultivated in the United States, and its excellent nutritional qualities account for its present popularity. Amaranth possesses a higher protein content than most cereal grains; the nutritional value of amaranth PROTEIN approaches that of milk. Its protein contains a high percentage of the essential AMINO ACID lysine, which is low in other grain protein like wheat. Amaranth does not contain typical wheat ALLERGENS, nor does it contain GLUTEN; therefore, people allergic to wheat can often eat amaranth because it belongs to an unrelated plant family. Amaranth is available in health food stores as a whole grain, a flour and as crackers and breakfast cereals. Amaranth flour has a nutty flavor and can be used to supplement wheat flour. Popped amaranth seed is mixed with honey to make a Mexican confection known as alegria. Amaranth species have also been cultivated in Asia as a source of greens (een choi in China, hiyu in Japan and chaulai in India). One hundred grams of amaranth provides protein, 15 g; carbohydrate, 66 g; fiber, 4.5 g; fat, 5.7 g; and fiber, 4.5 g.

amine   A very large family of basic organic compounds that contain nitrogen. Amines become positively charged ions (cations) in the blood. Physiologically important amines include the hormones EPINEPHRINE (adrenaline) and norepinephrine, and neurotransmitters such as ACETYLCHOLINE and

SEROTONIN, chemicals released by activated nerve cells. CHOLINE serves as a raw material for both acetylcholine and LECITHIN, a common lipid of cell membranes. All amino acids used to build proteins have properties of amines. Tyramine found in fermented foods is an amine that can cause headache and food sensitivities. A variety of amines in food can react with the food additive nitrite to produce cancer-causing substances (nitrosoamines).

amino acid metabolism   Chemical processes by which amino acids are either synthesized or are broken down and are used for energy in the body. Amino acid synthesis is important because approximately half of the different amino acids used as protein building blocks can be made from carbohydrates. Amino acids such as alanine, glutamic acid and glutamine made by the brain and muscle help transport nitrogen waste products via the bloodstream to the liver for disposal. When amino acids are degraded, the first step (transamination) releases nitrogen with the help of vitamin B_6. The final nitrogen-containing waste product is urea.

The second step of amino acid degradation requires the oxidation of the carbon atoms of amino acids to produce ATP, the energy currency of cells. The waste product is carbon dioxide. An alternative route permits the liver to convert most amino acids to blood sugar (glucose) when the diet does not provide adequate carbohydrates that can be digested to glucose to fuel the brain. This process is called GLUCONEOGENESIS. Heme (the pigment of red blood cells), neurotransmitters (brain chemicals that carry nerve impulses), purines (building blocks of RNA and DNA) and hormones represent important amino acid derivatives. (See also UREA CYCLE.)

amino acids (alpha amino acids)   Small organic acids that serve as raw materials of PROTEINS. The 50,000 to 100,000 different proteins in the body are combinations of just 20 different types of amino acids. During protein synthesis, amino acids are linked together like beads on a string to form long chains (polypeptides). Each type of protein possesses a unique amino acid sequence, specified by the cell's genes.

As the name implies, each amino acid possesses an amino group and a carboxylic acid functional group, and therefore amino acids behave as both acids and bases. They also possess side chains with different properties. For example, certain amino acids, like ASPARTIC ACID and GLUTAMIC ACID, are acidic; others like ARGININE and LYSINE are basic; METHIONINE and CYSTEINE contain sulfur. Another group repels water and has the branched chains: VALINE, LEUCINE and ISOLEUCINE.

Just as hands and feet are mirror images of each other, amino acids occur as mirror image forms (optical isomers). The left-hand forms are designated as "L," and the right-handed opposites are designated as "D." Only L-amino acids are supplied by food and synthesized in the body, and only the "L" forms occur in proteins. Therefore, unless indicated otherwise, an amino acid can be assumed to be the "L-" form when mentioned in nutrition literature. The only common amino acid that does not exist as optical isomers is glycine, the simplest of amino acids.

DIGESTION of food proteins releases amino acids, which are absorbed in the intestine. Depending on the person's body size and the type of protein that is consumed, 55 g to 65 g of protein a day supplies adequate amino acids for an adult. Few Americans are likely to be protein-deficient, because the typical U.S. diet generally supplies twice as much protein as needed. With a varied diet, neither a meat eater nor a knowledgeable VEGETARIAN needs extra protein to obtain adequate amino acids.

MEAT, FISH, POULTRY and dairy products like EGGS are the best sources of essential amino acids. Proteins that provide ample amounts of essential amino acids are said to be COMPLETE PROTEINS. Several plant proteins approach the quality of animal protein: soy, AMARANTH and QUINOA are examples. However, most plant proteins are deficient in at least one essential amino acid. For example, LEGUMES are low in methionine; CORN is low in lysine. These foods can be balanced during the day by eating "complementary" protein foods that provide ample amounts of those amino acids deficient in another food.

Surplus dietary amino acids may be used for energy, and amino acids from the breakdown of cellular protein can be important fuel sources when food intake is inadequate. After 12 to 24 hours without food, muscle protein breaks down rapidly, releasing amino acids into the bloodstream and processing them in the LIVER. The liver removes nitrogen and converts it to urea, while converting the amino acids to GLUCOSE and releasing it into the bloodstream to maintain blood sugar levels. In this way, most amino acids can contribute to blood glucose; consequently, muscle protein can help fuel the brain during starvation when the glucose supply becomes critical.

Ten amino acids are designated as dietary "non-essential" amino acids because they are synthesized by the body and do not need to be supplied in food. On the other hand, the diet must provide the other eight amino acids to prevent malnutrition. These dietary "essential" amino acids are LYSINE, valine PHENYLALANINE, TRYPTOPHAN, ISOLEUCINE, LEUCINE, METHIONINE, and THREONINE. Two other amino acids may be conditionally essential. HISTIDINE may not be formed in adequate amounts by infants and growing children, and ARGININE may be inadequately synthesized by adults with liver disease and by breastfeeding mothers.

Amino acids like phenylalanine and arginine, thought to stimulate growth hormone release and thus promote fat loss, are neither safe nor effective methods for weight control. Large amounts (several grams per day) of single amino acids used as supplements or additives, can drastically affect the body and damage the kidneys. The therapeutic use of amino acids is still in experimental stages. The U.S. FDA removed amino acids from the GENERALLY RECOGNIZED AS SAFE list of FOOD ADDITIVES, and it is prudent to consult a health care provider before supplementing with individual amino acids. (See also BIOLOGICAL VALUE; CHEMICAL SCORE; FOOD COMPLEMENTING.)

Fuller, M.F., Garlick P.J., "Human Amino Acid Requirements. Can the Controversy Be Resolved?" *Annual Review of Nutrition*, 14 (1994), pp. 217–41.

amino sugars   A family of nitrogen-containing sugars. Cells attach nitrogen to the simple sugars GLUCOSE and GALACTOSE to produce GLUCOSAMINE and galactosamine, respectively. These and similar amino sugars are used to produce carbohydrate-containing proteins (GLYCOPROTEINS) that coat cell surfaces, and for structural materials (MUCOPOLYSAC-CHARIDES) that help form the matrix of cartilage for ligaments and joints.

ammonia (NH_3)   The nitrogen waste produced primarily from AMINO ACID metabolism. Ammonia is highly toxic to the nervous system and the brain. It may interfere with metabolic processes required for energy production in the brain. Normally the brain transforms ammonia into glutamine, a safe, neutral amino acid released into the bloodstream. Next, glutamine is absorbed by the intestine, which releases the ammonia for disposal by the liver. Normally the liver very efficiently metabolizes ammonia to UREA, the ultimate non-toxic waste product, via the UREA CYCLE to keep the level of ammonia in the blood at very low levels. Urea is excreted safely in urine. Ammonia is also produced in the intestinal tract by bacteria. Ammonia is absorbed by the intestine and transported directly via the portal vein to the liver for disposal.

Liver disease, such as CIRRHOSIS, reduces urea production and leads to elevated blood levels of ammonia (ammonemia), which causes neurological abnormalities. Genetic defects in the ammonia disposal mechanism of the urea cycle generally lead to brain damage.

ammoniated glycyrrhizin   See GLYCYRRHIZIN.

amphetamines   Prescription drugs that stimulate the central nervous system. Benzedrine sulfate, Amphaplex 10, Bexidrine and Biphetamine are examples of amphetamines which temporarily suppress APPETITE and were once prescribed for weight loss. Amphetamines are now used to control hyperactivity in children and to control bouts of uncontrollable sleepiness (narcolepsy). Amphetamine abuse can cause exhaustion, ADDICTION, suicidal depression during withdrawal, cardiac problems, insomnia, HYPERTENSION and MALNUTRITION. (See also ALCOHOL-DRUG INTERACTIONS; APPETITE SUPPRESSANTS; DIETING.)

amygdalin   See LAETRILE.

amylase (alpha amylase)   The enzyme produced in the body that breaks down starch. Starch digestion begins in the mouth with amylase secreted in saliva, as saliva is mixed with food during chewing. Starch digestion is completed in the intestine by amylase secreted by the pancreas.

Amylase converts starch to a two-sugar fragment called maltose, which is too large to be absorbed. Therefore the intestinal enzyme MALTASE degrades maltose to glucose, which is readily taken up by the intestine and transported as blood glucose. (See also CARBOHYDRATE; DIGESTIVE TRACT.)

amylopectin   The water-insoluble form of STARCH. Plants synthesize this very long chain of glucose units as a storage form of energy, often to nurture the future embryo, seedling or sprout. It is often the major form of starch and it possesses a highly branched, bushy structure resembling liver GLYCOGEN (animal starch). In contrast, AMYLOSE is made up of single straight chains of glucose units. Amylopectin forms a paste in hot water. Starch occurs in seeds, tubers and root vegetables as both amylopectin and amylose, though the ratio of the two forms varies with the source. Cooking softens starch granules, making them available to DIGESTION by AMYLASE. The ultimate product of amylopectin digestion is GLUCOSE. Commercial processing converts starch to glucose, then to high FRUCTOSE CORN SYRUP, a major sweetener. (See also COMPLEX CARBOHYDRATE; FRUCTOSE; POLYSACCHARIDE.)

amylose   A water-soluble form of STARCH found in seeds, tubers and root vegetables. It is made up of long chains of glucose units, and often contains a thousand or more glucose units. Amylose differs from the other prevalent form of starch, AMYLOPECTIN, which is highly branched. Amylose forms large spiral configurations when dissolved in water and can react with iodide to form a characteristic blue-purple pigment. Amylopectin and amylose occur together in starch, and the relative amounts vary depending on the plant sources. During digestion, AMYLASE breaks down amylose to maltose, a disaccharide composed of two glucose units. An intestinal enzyme, MALTASE, then hydrolyzes maltose to the simple sugar glucose, the ultimate product of starch digestion.

anabolic steroids   A family of steroids, related to the male sex hormone TESTOSTERONE. These are classified as prescription drugs used to make up for hormone imbalance and deficiencies. However, synthetic analogs of testosterone have been obtained illegally by athletes and by teenage males to build muscles, and the U.S. FDA has described steroid abuse as a drug epidemic. While testosterone stimulates growth during adolescence, the synthetic derivatives can cause many side effects. Athletes compound this unsafe practice by "stacking" anabolic steroids—taking a combination of brands at 10 to 100 times the recommended doses for weeks at a time.

In men the side effects of anabolic steroids use include: lowered sperm count, enlarged prostate gland, shrinking testicles, balding and enlarged breasts. If taken before puberty, anabolic steroids can stunt growth. These effects seem to be reversible if anabolic steroids have been used for a short time. Some women body builders also use steroids to build muscle. Side effects in women do not seem to be reversible: masculinization, including increased muscles, increased size of clitoris, growth of facial hair, a deepening voice, shrinkage of breast size, uterine atrophy and menstrual irregularities. Severe cases of acne and bouts of rage are signs of anabolic steroid use especially in males. Anabolic steroid use can have more subtle, long-term detrimental effects; damage may show up years later as a HEART ATTACK, high blood pressure, CANCER and liver damage in both men and women.

anabolism (biosynthesis)   Processes involved in synthesizing the molecules needed for cellular growth and maintenance. Thus the formation of PROTEIN, DNA, RNA, LIPID, CARBOHYDRATE, FAT and GLYCOGEN are anabolic processes. Anabolism consumes chemical energy in the form of ATP and NADPH (a reducing agent), which are supplied by CATABOLISM, the energy-yielding oxidative processes involved in degradation. Optimal function and health rely upon a balance of anabolic and catabolic processes (homeostasis). These two branches of metabolism are controlled by the endocrine (hormonal) system, which in turn responds to external influences such as diet. Anabolic processes require small building blocks supplied by breaking down starch, protein and fat in foods to build larger molecules. Glycerol and fatty acids are the subunits of fat; amino acids yield proteins; and glucose yields glycogen. Fat and carbohydrate degradation provides an energized form of ACETIC ACID (acetyl CoA) to synthesize fatty acids and cholesterol. Other specialized products are also assembled from several different types of smaller precursors. For example, heme, the iron-containing pigment of the oxygen transport protein hemoglobin, is synthesized from an amino acid (GLYCINE) and succinic acid, a common intermediate in energy-producing pathways.

Growth and an anabolic state, seen as an increase in body mass and muscle mass, occur during childhood, adolescence, pregnancy and strenuous physical activity, such as body building. The weight gained in these situations represents increased protein, bone or fat, not fluids. Increased fat stores and accumulated body fat represent stored surplus energy in adults and can result from too little exercise, the over-consumption of FOOD, heredity or a combination of the above factors. (See also ADIPOSE TISSUE; ANABOLIC STEROIDS.)

anaerobic   Cellular processes that do not require oxygen. Energy can be produced in cells without oxygen. Anaerobic GLYCOLYSIS refers to an (energy yielding) process by which ATP, the energy currency of the cell, is produced from GLUCOSE without the participation of oxygen. As an example, skeletal muscle produces LACTIC ACID and ATP from glucose when oxygen supplied to muscle is inadequate to meet energy needs during strenuous physical exertion. Accumulated lactic acid is then converted back to glucose during the recovery period following EXERCISE when the oxygen supply is again adequate. Anaerobic processes are important for certain bacteria as well. Anaerobic bacteria in the intestine grow without oxygen and block the growth of potential disease-producing microorganisms. Anaerobic fermentation of sugar by yeast yields alcohol-containing products such as wine and beer. (See also AEROBIC; CATABOLISM.)

analgesics   A family of pain killers that excludes narcotics. ASPIRIN, phenacetin and ibuprofen are over-the-counter medications and among the most widely used over-the-counter drugs. Analgesics also lower body temperature when administered for fever, and usually lower inflammation and pain. Analgesics such as salicylates, pyrazolones, acetaminophen, indomethacin and ibuprofen are commonly referred to as "non-steroidal anti-inflammatory drugs" (NSAIDs).

Aspirin is the most widely used of the salicylate drugs. Besides relieving pain, aspirin also relieves fever (antipyretic) and reduces inflammation (anti-inflammatory). Aspirin blocks the synthesis of prostaglandins of the PG2 family. These hormone-like lipids are believed to stimulate inflammation and sensitize nerves to pain. Aspirin seems to specifically block cyclooxygenase, the first enzyme directly involved in prostaglandin synthesis.

The nonsalicylate analgesics include derivatives of ACETIC ACID (indomethacin); of PROPIONIC ACID (ibuprofen [Advil, Motrin], naproxen [Anaprox]); of fenamic acid (mefenamic acid [Ponstan, Ponstel]); of enolic acids (phenylbutazone [Alkabutazone, Nadazone]). They are believed to block the synthesis of prostaglandins as does aspirin. A number of NSAIDs also block lipooxygenase, the enzyme that metabo-lizes the complex fatty acid ARACHIDONIC ACID to LEUKOTRIENES, which promote inflammation. Others also inhibit the action of neutrophils, invading cells actively engaged in attacking foreign substances and invading cells. Some may unmask suppressor T cells (lymphocytes), which weakens the immune response. Acetaminophen does not block prostaglandin synthesis, and therefore it is suitable for mild pain but not tissue inflammation or joint stiffness. The other NSAIDs are suitable for treating inflammation as well as pain and swelling.

NSAID use carries certain risks. As an example, phenylbutazone (mentioned above) can interact with alcohol to cause ulcers and bleeding. It may cause sedation and it is passed through breast milk to the nursing child. This drug is not recommended for use by children under age 15. Similar precautions apply to ibuprofen and indomethacin. Prolonged use can cause weight gain, eye damage and reduced hearing. Acetaminophen can damage the liver. (See also ALCOHOL-DRUG INTERACTIONS.)

anaphylaxis   An extreme reaction of the immune system in response to exposure to foreign substances. Insect bites, drugs, injected serum and certain foods can create anaphylaxis. This abnormal response or immediate hypersensitivity is usually very rapid in susceptible individuals who may have been sensitized by previous exposure, and may produce shock ("anaphylactic shock"). The massive release of histamines and other inflammatory agents leads to spasming of smooth muscles, especially those of the air passageways, and to widespread EDEMA due to the increased water leaking out of capillaries. Symptoms range from asthma to fever, itching, hives and flushed skin in mild cases, to chest constriction, irregular pulse, painful, labored breathing and convulsions in severe cases. Anaphylaxis can be life-threatening and may require emergency room care. (See also ALLERGIC RHINITIS; ALLERGY, FOOD; ALLERGY, IMMEDIATE.)

androgen   A class of steroid hormones that promotes secondary male characteristics (masculinization). Androgens function in the body to stimulate anabolic processes such as deposition of muscle protein. Examples include TESTOSTERONE and androsterone, produced by gonads.

The synthetic ANABOLIC STEROIDS resemble testosterone. These drugs have been obtained illegally by male and female athletes and by those who wish to speed up or increase muscle mass and decrease body fat beyond the rate obtainable by training. The use of anabolic steroids causes physical and mental changes that may be irreversible and increase the risk of disease. (See also ANABOLISM.)

anemia   A condition characterized by subnormal levels of HEMOGLOBIN, the oxygen-binding protein in blood. Half a million Americans are at risk for anemia, including 40% of pregnant women, pre-menopausal women, vegans (those who eat no animal products), adolescents relying on junk food diets, infants and children with inadequate diets. Anemia may result from either an inadequate number of RED BLOOD CELLS (erythrocytes) or an abnormally low hemoglobin content of red blood cells. With deficient functional red blood cells, the oxygen supply to tissues is inadequate for optimal RESPIRATION, causing shortness of breath, FATIGUE, weakness, pallor, headache and lowered resistance to infection. There are two general types of anemia based on red blood cell size. Megaloblastic anemia is characterized by large red blood cells; their shortened life span results in a decreased number of cells. Microcytic anemia is characterized by small red blood cells with reduced hemoglobin content.

Many nutritional deficiencies lead to anemia. Inadequate dietary IRON, COPPER, FOLIC ACID, PROTEIN, VITAMIN B_6, VITAMIN B_12, VITAMIN C, VITAMIN A, VITAMIN E and RIBOFLAVIN can cause this condition. Each of these nutrients is required for the production of red blood cells (ERYTHROPOIESIS). Iron deficiency anemia is the most common diet-related anemia in the United States and it represents the last stage of iron deficiency. It is characterized by small, pale red blood cells (microcytic anemia), due to chronic blood loss or inadequate iron intake. Symptoms include FATIGUE, pallor and shortness of breath. Studies of the nutritional status of developed nations have routinely found up to 30% of a population with iron deficiency. Groups that are at highest risk are children under the age of two years, teenage women, pregnant women and the elderly. Pregnancy drastically increases the requirement of iron. In terms of blood loss the most common causes of iron deficiency are excessive bleeding during menstruation and intestinal bleeding due to parasites, ulcers or malignancy. Iron deficiency can be caused by impaired iron uptake by the intestine, due to a lack of stomach acid (ACHLORHYDRIA) or from chronic diarrhea. With iron deficiency, the resulting anemia can be treated by iron supplementation.

Deficiencies of either folacin or vitamin B_12 can cause anemia because each is essential for DNA synthesis and deficiencies impair erythrocyte production. Folic acid deficiency is much more common because folic acid stores in the body are small, yet folic acid participates in many biosynthetic reactions. On the other hand, vitamin B_12 is stored in the liver, and only trace amounts are required daily for a few specific functions. Anemia due to inadequate folic acid and vitamin B_12 produces large (macrocytic) cells with a short life span. This form of anemia can occur when intake of fresh vegetables is very limited, or when the need for folic acid outstrips intake, as may occur during pregnancy or in ALCOHOLISM. Treatment with folic acid can ameliorate megaloblastic anemia, yet mask an underlying vitamin B_12 deficiency. This point emphasizes that treatment of anemia requires expert medical supervision.

Anemia can also indicate a serious condition unrelated to diet. Non-nutritional causes of anemia include chronic blood loss and congenital defects in red blood cell formation, such as thalassemia or sickle cell anemia, due to mutant hemoglobins, and spherocytosis (spherical red blood cells). Hemolytic anemia is the result of excessive hemolysis (destruction of red blood cells) in susceptible people exposed to bacterial toxins, toxic chemicals, or drugs that may produce JAUNDICE. Anemia also may result from reduced nutrient uptake due to the presence of parasites and chronic infections, gastrointestinal disease or bowel resection. (See also HEAVY METALS; HEMATOCRIT; LEAD; MALNUTRITION.)

Pruthi, R.K., Tefferi, A., "Pernicious Anemia Revisited," *Mayo Clinic Proceedings*, 69:2 (1994), pp. 144–50.

anemia, aplastic   A form of ANEMIA in which the numbers of RED BLOOD CELLS as well as white cells are reduced. This type of anemia is caused by exposure to chemicals (such as solvents), toxic heavy metals, some drugs like chloramphenicol, or ionizing radiation (like X rays). Radiation therapy, chemotherapy and lead poisoning can damage bone marrow, thus reducing red blood cell production. Both the blood platelet count and immunity decline, with a concomitant increased susceptibility to infection. Destruction of the bone marrow is potentially life-threatening.

anemia, pernicious   A form of ANEMIA caused either by a dietary deficiency of VITAMIN B_12 or by inadequate B_12 absorption. It is characterized by quite large red blood cells (macrocytic) that are overloaded in the hemoglobin (hyperchromic). Low vitamin B_12 consumption is a concern for strict VEGETARIANS who avoid meat and meat products. Pernicious anemia is also caused by inadequate vitamin B_12 uptake. Normally, the gastric lining secretes a protein called INTRINSIC FACTOR that's needed to specifically bind vitamin B_12. Because this protein is required for vitamin B_12 absorption by the intestine, inadequate intrinsic factor production, even with adequate dietary B_12, can cause pernicious anemia.

Pernicious anemia affects the nervous system as well as the blood. Symptoms include memory loss, weakness, personality and mood swings, and numbness and tingling in the hands and feet. If this anemia continues unchecked, nerve damage may be irreversible. Pernicious anemia is most common in males between the ages of 40 and 65 years who have a family history of the condition. Treatment for intrinsic factor defect involves vitamin B_12 injections. Oral doses of vitamin B_12 can remedy dietary deficiencies when intrinsic factor production is normal. (See also FOLIC ACID.)

angiotensin   A protein-like hormone formed in the blood that raises blood pressure. Angiotensin contracts the muscles of CAPILLARIES and ARTERIES (vasopressor), which increases resistance for blood flow. Angiotensin is liberated by the action of RENIN, an ENZYME formed by the kidneys, on a serum protein (angiotensinogen) produced by the liver. The release of renin by the kidneys is triggered when they experience lowered blood flow, for example, due to dehydration. Angiotensin also plays an important role in the regulation of blood pressure by stimulating the ADRENAL GLANDS to secrete ALDOSTERONE. Aldosterone, in turn, promotes sodium retention and water retention by the kidneys, to help regulate water balance. (See also ANTIDIURETIC HORMONE; HYPERTENSION.)

animal drugs in meat   See MEAT CONTAMINANTS.

anion   A negatively charged ion. Anions are the opposite of CATIONS, which carry positive charges. Important anions are formed when weak acids ionize. Anions, together with their cation counterparts, occur in blood and are called electrolytes. They are required to maintain the appropriate effective concentration of ions and proteins in the blood. Key anions in blood are chloride (Cl^-), phosphate ($H_2PO_4^-$ and bicarbonate (HCO_3^-). Chloride (Cl^-) is the predominant anion in body fluids. Neither chloride nor phosphate can be made by the body; they are essential nutrients to be supplied by the diet. Phosphate and bicarbonate ions help buffer blood at nearly a constant pH. These anions are examples of "conjugate bases," formed when weak acids ionize. (See also ELECTROLYTES.)

anise (*Pimpinella anisum*)   An HERB belonging to the parsley family. Anise originated in India and was cultivated in ancient China and Egypt. The fruit, aniseed, is dried and used as a seasoning. The distinctive, licorice-like flavor of anise extract adds to the taste of shortbread cakes, such as pizella (Italy) and pains a l'anis (France). Anise is used in certain candies. Crushed aniseed together with cinnamon and coriander is used to make a liqueur (anisette). Chopped anise leaves have been used in pickled vegetables and soups.

annatto (*Bixa orellara*)   A yellow-red, natural, vegetable food-coloring agent obtained from a small tropical tree that is native to Central America. Annatto is prepared from the pulp of the fruit and from the waxy layer around the seeds, and is used to give a yellow or orange color to several cheeses (Cheddar, Cheshire, Edam) and to smoked haddock, butter and a variety of pastries and sweets.

anorexia   Loss or lack of appetite. Many conditions cause anorexia: DEPRESSION; drug ADDICTION, especially to cocaine; alcoholism; fever; and stomach disorders. Medical procedures such as radiation therapy and the use of chemotherapy in cancer treatment may also cause anorexia. This is a major concern because the resulting malnourished state retards healing and recovery and increases the risk of infection in patients. (See also ANOREXIA NERVOSA.)

anorexia nervosa   An EATING DISORDER involving compulsive STARVATION, resulting in a loss of 25% or more of the body weight. Like BULIMIA NERVOSA, it has become much more common in America during the last 15 years and has reached epidemic proportions. Anorexia is characterized by a sudden or severe weight loss, a continued effort to lose weight, a refusal to maintain normal body weight, a failure to grow during adolescence, missed consecutive menstrual periods (amenorrhea), plus nausea, bloating or constipation. Starvation symptoms include ACIDOSIS, KETOSIS and ELEC-TROLYTE imbalance. Behavioral aspects include food hoarding, food phobia, ritualization of food preparation while eating very little, eating alone, phobia of being obese, and feeling fat when actually underweight. Anorexics seem to prefer protein over carbohydrate. A ZINC deficiency may be involved in the disease because zinc supplements (25 mg/day) have helped some patients gain weight.

Although boys and men can be anorectic, 90 to 95% of patients are girls and women. Anorexia and bulimia together affect 5% of young women in developed nations, although the disorder is absent from less developed nations. Anorexia usually begins with a desire to lose weight or to prevent weight gain. Extreme social pressure to be trim, an abnormal family environment, an imbalanced ENDOCRINE SYSTEM or nervous system can trigger this behavior. The typical patient is a white, female adolescent who is a bright overachiever, attempting to meet high parental expectations and wanting more control over her life. Low self-esteem may be an issue.

Anorexia is a multi-faceted disorder and a broad-based treatment approach has been most successful. Therapeutic programs use nutrition counseling, individual psychotherapy, behavior modification, family counseling and medications when required. Such a multidisciplinary approach involves nutritionists and dietitians, nurses, physicians, social workers and counselors, and self-help groups. Their goals are to establish and maintain a desired body weight while resolving emotional issues and improving the home environment. Fundamental to nutritional care is a counseling program to help patients change their attitudes about food. Depending upon the patient's nutritional status, a nutritional program might entail nutritionally balanced meals, adjusted for patient preferences, vitamin and mineral supplements to remedy deficiencies, slow refeeding with progressive increments in total daily calories to reach the desired level of calories; and ongoing nutritional counseling. Anorexics will be managed by an outpatient treatment program or by hospitalization, when weight loss has been severe, when there are serious metabolic problems, when the family is in crisis, or where the patient is suicidal. Nutritional rehabilitation programs vary according to the severity of the condition, but less restrictive approaches seem to have better results for weight gain. Psychotherapy usually focuses on feelings about body image, self-esteem, food, control of one's life and choices, and gaining independence from harmful family influences. Long illnesses, severe weight gain, a dysfunctional family background, late age of onset of the illness and late occurring treatment make recovery more difficult.

The mortality rate is about 6–10% due to mineral imbalances. The National Association of Anorexia and Associated Disorders and the American Anorexia/Bulimia Association are among the resources available to anorexics. (See also DIET; MALNUTRITION.)

Woodside, D.B., "A Review of Anorexia and Bulimia Nervosa," *Current Problems in Pediatrics*, 25:2 (1995), pp. 67–89.

anorexigenic   Capable of diminishing the APPETITE. Disease influences (diabetes, obesity, cancer) and pharmacological agents (anorectic drugs, naloxone) can diminish appetite. Certain substances produced by the body also modulate appetite, and hormones are likely to be involved. Somatostatin and corticotrophin releasing factor (produced by the hypothalamus to control secretions by the pituitary gland) and hormones of the gastrointestinal tract (vasoactive intestinal peptide) decreased feeding in experimental animals when trace (picomolar) quantities were administered directly to the brain.

anosmia   A loss of the sense of smell. The lining of the nasal passage contains 3 cm. by 5 cm. patches of specialized cells that have receptors for volatile (gaseous) compounds. Binding of aromas to the receptors stimulates nerves that carry impulses to the brain via the first cranial nerve. The smelling apparatus loses its effectiveness if an odor persists; the nerves apparently become fatigued and cannot be effectively stimulated repeatedly. They do not lose the ability to discriminate other odors, however. The loss of the sense of smell is age-related. Aging is associated with a permanent decline in the ability to identify the quality of an odor. Individuals who experience difficulties with olfactory sensitivity are likely to experience difficulties with respect to taste. Colds, infections and injury can alter one's sense of smell.

antacid   A substance that neutralizes STOMACH ACID. Antacids are frequently used to relieve ACID INDIGESTION (heartburn), which manifests itself as a pain in the upper abdomen. Acid indigestion is very prevalent; it affects one-third of Americans. Medications to relieve this condition are some of the most widely used over-the-counter drugs. Antacids are also used therapeutically to treat peptic ulcers. Stomach pain can be due to stress or emotion, and not simply the result of excess stomach acid. However, a severe pain could point to a more serious condition, such as a heart attack. Therefore, seek medical attention for any severe chest pain accompanied by short breath, weakness and sweating.

Antacid use poses potential problems, and antacids should be used only occasionally. They work best when taken one-half to two hours after a meal. Antacids may block the action of medications, such as tetracycline, digitalis and anticonvulsants. Protracted use of antacids interferes with calcium METABOLISM and bone formation. Constipation or diarrhea are the two most common adverse reactions to antacid use. In particular, antacids that contain ALUMINUM hydroxide or calcium carbonate can lead to constipation. Regarding aluminum-containing antacids, there are indications that aluminum intake should be minimized because aluminum may cause calcium and phosphorus depletion. Aluminum hydroxide seems to have minimal complications when combined with magnesium hydroxide.

Calcium carbonate is a common antacid. Although it neutralizes acids effectively, it may cause acid overproduction later (rebound effect). Calcium carbonate can also block iron uptake. Another option is sodium bicarbonate, a major ingredient of several popular antacids. However, it should be noted that the typical American diet provides excessive sodium, and sodium bicarbonate antacids could increase the burden for sodium-sensitive people. A further reservation: Bicarbonate-based antacids may promote alkaline blood (alkalosis) or they may alter kidney or heart function.

Calcium carbonate is the major ingredient of several antacids. They have been recommended because they are inexpensive and calcium carbonate has a high content of calcium (40% of the weight). However, taking antacids as a calcium supplement can seriously lower stomach acidity and decrease the efficiency of digestion. Under normal conditions most forms of calcium supplements (calcium aspartate, calcium carbonate, calcium gluconate and calcium orotate) are absorbed about as well as the calcium in whole milk. Remember that calcium uptake requires an adequate intake of VITAMIN D, magnesium, COPPER and ZINC, while adequate physical EXERCISE promotes calcium deposition in bones. (See also BONE; OSTEOPOROSIS.)

anthocyanins   A family of plant pigments responsible for red to blue-red colors in BLACKBERRIES, RASPBERRIES, BLUEBERRIES, CHERRIES and the like. They belong to the family of FLAVONOIDS, plant substances that are non-nutrients but have beneficial effects. When eaten, these materials bind to connective TISSUE, where they crosslink and strengthen COLLAGEN, the primary structural protein of the body. Liberal consump-

tion of flavonoid-rich foods may be appropriate for individuals subjected to oxidative stress and chronic inflammation. Flavonoids generally function as antioxidants to prevent tissue damage by free radicals, highly reactive molecules that can attack cells. They help counter inflammation and associated pain by blocking the production of proinflammatory agents including prostaglandins and leukotrienes. (See also PHYTOCHEMICALS.)

anti-aging nutrients   See AGING.

antiarchitic   Refers to compounds related to vitamin D that are capable of preventing RICKETS, the disease that results from a severe deficiency of VITAMIN D. Vitamin D is a family of 11 closely related sterols with similar activity; however, only two account for most of the vitamin D activity in foods. Ergocalciferol (vitamin D_2) is the commercial, supplemental form, and cholecalciferol (vitamin D_3) occurs in animal tissues and is the major form in fish oils. The precursor of vitamin D_3, dehydrocholesterol, occurs in the skin where it is activated by sunlight to vitamin D_3. The body converts vitamin D to the active form, calcitriol, which is a hormone.

antibiotic-resistant bacteria in food   If disease-producing bacteria become drug resistant, medicine could lose its most powerful weapon against disease. Although antibiotic use could theoretically destroy a given bacterial population, mutation frequently produces strains that are drug-resistant. Bacteria are very adaptable to selective environmental pressures. Furthermore, genetic mechanisms of bacteria permit drug-resistant genes to spontaneously transfer between bacterial strains. Bacteria multiply rapidly and a drug-resistant strain can quickly replace a drug-sensitive bacteria. There is ample evidence that widespread drug resistance has already occurred worldwide. Most bacterial strains are resistant to at least one antibiotic, and some disease-producing bacteria are resistant to all known ANTIBIOTICS.

Because half of the U.S.-produced antibiotics are used in feed for poultry, cattle and pigs, consumer groups have expressed concern that massive use of antibiotics may lead to drug-resistant bacteria, which could then be passed on to humans. Investigations have concluded that dairy cattle fed antibiotics were probably the source of the drug-resistant strain of SALMONELLA that caused the largest outbreak of FOOD POISONING in the United States in 1985 when contaminated low-fat milk affected 190,000 people in six midwestern states, as judged by Centers for Disease Control.

There are other warning signs of drug-resistant pathogenic bacteria. For example, individuals who eat chicken and Cornish game hens treated with tetracycline are twice as likely to contract bacterial gastroenteritis (inflammation of stomach and intestines) as those who do not eat these POULTRY. Presently 80% of the bacteria causing strep infections resist tetracycline; 25% of the bacteria causing meningitis resist penicillin; 25% of salmonella causing diarrhea resist ampicillin and tetracycline. (See also MEAT CONTAMINANTS.)

antibiotics   Chemicals that destroy or prevent growth of microorganisms including bacteria, molds and FUNGI. Natural or synthetic compounds are used extensively as antibiotics to treat infectious diseases in animals and plants as well as in humans. Sulfanilamides, penicillins and erythromycins are examples of major families of these drugs. Antibiotics impact human health in several ways. The prolonged use of broad-spectrum antibiotics in treating disease drastically alters the intestinal microflora by destroying beneficial bacteria. The loss of beneficial bacteria can permit less desirable, opportunistic microorganisms like yeast to flourish, cause intestinal inflammation, and decrease production of nutrients important in maintaining health of the colon.

Antibiotics can affect specific vitamin requirements; chloramphenicol blocks RIBOFLAVIN and vitamins B$_6$ and B$_{12}$, for example. Penicillin increases potassium requirements. Antibiotics can decrease nutrient absorption in general by altering the intestinal lining. Neomycin interferes with the uptake of FAT, AMINO ACIDS, CARBOHYDRATE, water-soluble and fat-soluble VITAMINS, CALCIUM, IRON and VITAMIN K. Tetracycline decreases absorption of fat, amino acids, calcium, iron, MAGNESIUM and ZINC, while increasing the rate of urinary excretion of riboflavin, FOLIC ACID and VITAMIN C.

Antibiotics can have a direct impact on the food supply. Half the antibiotics produced in the United States are applied to livestock. The benefits are more rapid growth and healthier animals. On the other hand the potential exists for generating drug-resistant pathogenic bacteria and persistent antibiotic residues in meat and dairy products. The application of antibiotics in animal husbandry and the permissible levels of antibiotic residues in animal products are regulated by the U.S. FDA. The following examples illustrate the dimensions of this food safety issue.

Chloramphenicol This drug can cause ANEMIA in humans due to damage to bone marrow. Though banned from use with food-producing animals, periodic spot inspections showed it was widely used in cattle and hogs in the 1980s. The degree to which chloramphenicol continues to contaminate meat through illegal application, and the degree to which such a contamination affects health, are unknown.

Penicillin This common antibiotic is used to treat dairy herds, among others. The allowable penicillin level in milk is 0.01 units per milliliter (about 20 drops) of MILK, but spot checks have found 10 times this level in commercial milk. Such high levels can cause allergic reactions in susceptible individuals.

Sulfamethazine This sulfa drug is a widespread contaminant in meat, POULTRY and milk. One-fourth of milk sampled in the late 1980s was contaminated, despite the U.S. FDA ban on this drug in milk. Sulfamethazine is suspected of being a CARCINOGEN. (See also ACIDOPHILUS; ANTIBIOTIC-RESISTANT BACTERIA IN FOOD; MEAT CONTAMINANTS; PESTICIDES.)

antibodies A class of PROTEINS produced by the IMMUNE SYSTEM to combat viruses, bacteria and FUNGI and to neutralize foreign substances. Antibodies are made in response to foreign substances by B cells, a type of lymphocyte or white cell found in bone marrow or the lymphatic system. The progeny of B cells are called plasma cells and are responsible for antibodies appearing in body fluids in COLOSTRUM and on mucosal surfaces. The body produces millions of different antibodies and each type of antibody attacks a different foreign material (ANTIGEN).

Antibodies represent a huge diversity because the body is subjected to so many different antigens. The basis of this diversity lies in antibody structure, which allows a close fit with the antigen, much like a lock fitting in a keyhole. Antigen-antibody binding then enables scavenger cells to engulf and degrade antigens. Long after exposure to the antigen, information for synthesizing it remains embedded in special lymphocytes called memory cells that enable the body to produce antibodies rapidly when again threatened by the foreign invaders.

Antibodies reacting to normally harmless materials may trigger overreactions of the immune system and may cause autoimmune disease, in which the body attacks its own tissues. Insulin-dependent DIABETES MELLITUS and rheumatoid ARTHRITIS are examples. Allergic reactions are another example of an overreaction of the immune system.

In nutrition the most important classes of antibodies are IgE, IgG and IgA. IgE antibodies are responsible for rapid allergic symptoms (immediate hypersensitivity) related to HISTAMINE release: red, runny nose, hives, asthma, swelling, itching or, in extreme situations, extreme shock (ANAPHYLAXIS). This class of antibody is important in tissues and is less prominent in the blood.

IgG (gamma globulin) is the major class of antibodies found in the blood. Elevated IgG is implicated in slow-developing food allergies (delayed hypersensitivity). After avoiding foods that cause such allergies, the immune system can return to normal as allergen-specific IgG gradually disappears from the blood. It may then be possible to tolerate allergenic foods if eaten infrequently.

Secretory IgA is the major antibody released by mucosal surfaces such as the mouth and the intestinal tract, where it binds potentially dangerous microorganisms and prevents their sticking to tissue and initiating infections. Secreted IgA is also an important antibody in colostrum and breastmilk that helps protect the nursing infant from infection until its own immune system is able to mount a vigorous defense. (See also ALLERGEN; ALLERGY, FOOD; ALLERGY, IMMEDIATE; BREASTFEEDING; IMMUNE SYSTEM; ROTATION DIET.)

anticaking agents A class of FOOD ADDITIVES used to maintain free-flowing powdered and granular materials. These useful additives are added to table salt, powdered sugar, malted milk powders, garlic and onion powders, powdered coffee whiteners, vanilla powder, BAKING POWDER, dried egg yolk and seasoning salts. Examples include DEXTROSE and silicates (aluminum silicate, magnesium silicate, sodium calcium aluminosilicate, calcium silicate and silicon dioxide). These agents are judged to be safe food additives. (See also ALUMINUM; SODIUM.)

anticancer diet See CANCER-PREVENTION DIET.

anticancer nutrients See CANCER.

antidepressants Prescription drugs used to treat DEPRESSION. These drugs cause severe reactions when taken with ALCOHOL or when different antidepressants are taken simultaneously.

Tricyclic antidepressants (like imipramine) seem to block brain messages relating to depression. About 50% of those who take mood elevating drugs also crave food, including sweets, tend to gain weight, and experience insomnia and FATIGUE. These drugs are not habit forming, but should not be taken with alcohol. In combination with monoamine oxidase inhibitors (see below) they can cause convulsions. When taken at the same time as cocaine, tricyclic antidepressants cause severe intoxication.

Monoamine oxidase (MAO) inhibitors (e.g., Nardil, Parnate) also block signals in the brain relating to depression. These drugs often cause a dry mouth and painful, slow urination. Patients with high blood pressure or with heart, liver or kidney problems should avoid them. MAO inhibitors are dangerous when combined with alcohol and are deadly when combined with tricyclic antidepressants and AMPHETAMINES. MAO inhibitors can also interact with TYRAMINE, a substance in WINE, aged CHEESE and other foods, to produce severe high blood pressure.

Amphetamines are stimulants, and unlike the other two classes of antidepressants they increase alertness and decrease fatigue. They have been prescribed as short-term APPETITE SUPPRESSANTS. Amphetamines can be deadly if taken with MAO inhibitors or cocaine.

antidiuretic hormone (ADH, vasopressin) A pituitary HORMONE that decreases urine output and conserves water in the kidney. ADH represents the body's primary water-conserving mechanism. The anterior pituitary gland releases ADH into the bloodstream in response to physiologic stress, dehydration, diminished blood volume, or high sodium concentration in the blood. The mechanism involves these steps. First, receptors located in the HYPOTHALAMUS detect increased osmolarity (ion concentration) of blood, then the hypothalamus stimulates the pituitary gland to release ADH. (See also ENDOCRINE SYSTEM; HOMEOSTASIS.)

antigen A foreign material recognized by the IMMUNE SYSTEM. Antigens stimulate the formation of specific antibodies, which bind the provoking antigens to neutralize them. Generally, a single type of antibody recognizes one type of antigen. Antigens may be PROTEINS, glycolipids, POLYSACCHARIDES, microorganisms or cells. The body has the ability to neutralize a huge number of antigens because it can synthesize an immense variety of antibodies. Since some antigens may share common structural features, antibodies may cross-react. Thus antibodies against cow's milk may cross-react with goat's milk, and antibodies against wheat protein (gluten) can cross-react with similar proteins in other grains. (See also ALLERGEN; ALLERGY, FOOD.)

antihistamine See HISTAMINE.

antimetabolite A drug that interferes with cell division. By mimicking an enzyme's usual nutrient reactant, an antimetabolite tricks the cell's machinery and prevents normal growth. Sulfa drugs are bacterial antimetabolites that block the bacterial synthesis of the B vitamin folic acid, required for bacterial growth. Because animal cells depend on folic acid in the diet and cannot synthesize it, they are immune to sulfa drugs. A somewhat different strategy underlies the use of the anticancer drug methotrexate. Methotrexate attacks cancer cells that have a high rate of growth, by blocking the activation of folic acid to its biologically active form (coenzyme). Without a ready supply of the coenzyme form, cancer cells stop growing rapidly.

antimycotic agents FOOD ADDITIVES used to prevent SPOILAGE. These PRESERVATIVES retard growth of YEASTS and molds. Examples are sorbates, sodium benzoate and calcium propionate. Sorbic acid and potassium and sodium sorbates retard spoilage in CHEESE, syrup, jelly, cake, MAYONNAISE, soft drinks, WINE, dried fruit, MARGARINE and soft candy. Sorbates are readily broken down in the body and are considered safe additives. SODIUM BENZOATE, which occurs naturally in FRUIT and VEGETABLES, prevents the growth of most microorganisms but requires acidic conditions for its antimicrobial action. CALCIUM PROPIONATE prevents the growth of mold and several bacteria and is a common additive in bread to be stored at room temperature. These too are safe food additives.

antineuritic An agent that is capable of relieving damaged nerve inflammations (neuritis). The inflammation of peripheral nerves of the whole body may be due to nutritional deficiency, toxic exposure or metabolic imbalance. Neuropathy or nerve damage may result from long-term deficiencies of the B vitamins thiamin, niacin, vitamin B_6, vitamin B_{12} or pantothenic acid due to dietary deficiencies or to chronically poor absorption by the intestine. As an example, THIAMIN counteracts neuritis, a typical symptom of severe thiamin deficiency. Alcoholics are prone to thiamin deficiency and neuritis because alcohol rapidly depletes the body's thiamin stores. (See also MALNUTRITION.)

antioxidant A compound that prevents or retards the oxidation of sensitive molecules found in the body or in foods. Antioxidants occur in many foods naturally as nutrients or non-nutrients, or as synthetic additives. Antioxidants typically block oxidation by preventing damage caused by FREE RADICALS, extremely reactive forms of oxygen and other molecules that lack an electron and tear electrons from molecules they meet. In the body likely targets are DNA, proteins and lipids (unsaturated fatty acids). Free radicals form in the body by normal cellular processes. These include phagocytosis (engulfing viruses and bacteria) by immune cells; incomplete reduction of oxygen as mitochondria burn fuels; production of hydrogen peroxide by the breakdown of fatty acids and the generation of NITRIC OXIDE, a free radical that functions as a localized vasodilator, a defensive chemical, and as neurotransmitter. Free radicals and reactive forms of oxygen occur by chemical modification of pollutants and toxic substances within the liver. Free radical damage may contribute to CANCER, CARDIOVASCULAR DISEASE and AGING; consequently, antioxidants are a current focus of extensive medical research. It is intriguing that certain antioxidants are both anticancer nutrients and antiaging nutrients. Because there is such a large variety of reactive molecules and free radicals, the body requires a wide range of antioxidant defenses. A "pecking order" exists among antioxidants; some are more readily oxidized than others and will be consumed rapidly unless replenished or recycled in the body. Certain antioxidants are "preventive inhibitors," that is, they block the initiation of free radical attack. Preventive inhibitors include defensive enzymes like CATALASE and GLU-

TATHIONE PEROXIDASE (destroy hydrogen peroxide and lipid peroxides) and SUPEROXIDE DISMUTASE (destroys superoxide), chelating agents like CITRIC ACID that lock up metal ions, proteins that bind metal ions, including ALBUMIN, transferrin and FERRITIN. Other antioxidants, "chain breakers," convert free radicals to stable (safe) products. VITAMIN E and VITAMIN C are essential chain-breaking antioxidants. It is worth remembering that under certain conditions an antioxidant may become an oxidant (prooxidant activity). If the antioxidant becomes a free radical, then it, too, must be disarmed and regenerated.

Antioxidants as Nutrients

VITAMIN A, BETA CAROTENE, VITAMIN C and VITAMIN E, and SELENIUM are key antioxidant nutrients.

CAROTENOIDS, including beta carotene trap free radicals, while vitamin A helps guide normal tissue development. Inadequate carotenoid intake increases the risk of cancers of the lung, bladder, esophagus, stomach, colon, rectum, prostate and skin. Three large-scale randomized clinical trials designed to examine the preventive effects of beta carotene over many years have now been completed. These studies indicate that when used alone, beta carotene does not prevent cancer or heart disease in high-risk people (for example, heavy smokers, drinkers or those exposed to asbestos) or in low-risk people (Physicians' Health Study). Indeed, there are hints that unless beta carotene is protected by another antioxidant, such as vitamin E, it may actually increase damage. A multitude of studies indicates that the consumption of foods rich in carotenoids—including lutein, LYCOPENE, zeazanthin, as well as beta carotene—protect against cancer, cataracts and cardiovascular diseases.

Vitamin C destroys water-soluble free radicals and protects against cancer. It is needed for a healthy immune system and it also speeds wound healing. Vitamin C also protects LDL from oxidation.

Vitamin E acts as a fat-soluble, free radical trap that seems to protect the brain from free radical damage and to partially reverse age-related decline of the immune system in experimental animals. Clinical studies indicate that vitamin E can protect against cardiovascular disease. Vitamin E is believed to block the oxidation of LOW-DENSITY LIPOPROTEIN (LDL) cholesterol. Oxidized LDL damages arterial walls and triggers the build-up of fatty deposits that can eventually cause heart attacks.

Selenium works together with vitamin E by helping an enzyme system (GLUTATHIONE PEROXIDASE) block free radical attack and to disarm reactive lipids. Selenium is also required for a healthy immune system. Selenium deficiency increases the risk of cancer of the esophagus, stomach and rectum.

Antioxidants as Non-nutrients in Food

In addition to vitamins, trace minerals, fiber and carotenoids, vegetables and fruits provide many other ingredients important for long-term health. Vegetables and fruits contain orange-red and yellow pigments called carotenoids. They include carotenes such as beta carotene and LYCOPENE (from tomatoes) and xanthophylls, oxygen-containing derivatives such as zeazanthin and lutein. Xanthophylls occur at high levels in dark green leafy vegetables. Though relatively few carotenoids serve as sources of vitamin A, they help protect the body as versatile antioxidants and they enhance the immune system, complementing the actions of beta carotene. Fruits, vegetables, seasoning, spices and herbs (tea), possess a wide range of complex-molecules called polyphenols (FLAVONOIDS) and phenolic acids that are complex ring structures. Flavonoids include ISOFLAVONES (soybean), flavones (such as QUERCETIN from tea, berries, fruits) and flavonones (such as naringenin and HESPERIDIN from citrus), flavanonols (such as catechins, condensed and hydrolyzable TANNINS), anthocyanins (purple, red and blue pigments of fruits and berries), coumarins (from citrus), ellagic acid (from grapes), and others. In general flavonoids possess multiple properties; thus they can quench free radicals, inhibit inflammation, strengthen capillary walls and reduce oxidative damage to serum cholesterol. The optimal intake of flavonoids and carotenoids is not known and the long-term effects of supplementation with large amounts of phytochemicals has not been studied. It should be pointed out that beta carotene, vitamin C and even vitamin E under the appropriate conditions can become oxidants (prooxidants). Certain flavonoids also exhibit prooxidant properties. Chelated (complexed) iron in the presence of vitamin C can generate free radicals spontaneously in the test tube and this could be a potential problem in the body with iron overload diseases. Finally, certain flavonoids can specifically block the thyroid-hormone generating enzyme in thyroid cells. As with many dietary constituents, a little may be beneficial, while a lot could be harmful.

Foods rich in vitamin A and beta carotene and related carotenoids include orange-colored vegetables like carrots and squash plus dark-green leafy vegetables like CHARD, kale and spinach. Fresh fruit, frozen juice concentrate, and vegetables like green pepper and BROCCOLI supply vitamin C. Vegetable oil, wheat germ and nuts provide vitamin E. Selenium occurs in whole grains, seafood, CABBAGE, onions and GARLIC. Fruits and vegetables also provide flavonoids.

Antioxidants Made by the Body

GLUTATHIONE is a sulfur-containing antioxidant present in very large amounts in the cytoplasm. Besides helping to keep proteins reduced, it assists amino acid transport, helps regulate the internal oxidation state of the cell, maintains vitamin E in a reduced state and detoxifies potentially harmful substances.

COENZYME Q assists mitochondria to burn fat and carbohydrate for energy and it functions as a lipid soluble membrane antioxidant together with vitamin E, which it protects. Coenzyme Q production declines with age and the heart may become deficient in this nutrient.

URIC ACID is found in the blood. It is a nitrogen-containing waste product from the breakdown of DNA and RNA.

CITRIC ACID, succinic acid and other complex organic acids generated by metabolism can bind iron and copper, preventing them from catalyzing of free radical-generating reactions.

MELATONIN, a hormone produced by the pineal gland, possesses strong antioxidant properties.

BILIRUBIN, a breakdown product of HEMOGLOBIN, acts as an antioxidant in blood.

Antioxidants as Food Additives

Antioxidants are extensively utilized to prevent or retard deterioration that produces off-flavors or color changes in foods, making them less appetizing or less nutritious. Oxidation can also be promoted by enzymes in foods when exposed to air. This explains why apples, bananas, pears, peaches and potatoes darken after being sliced. The food industry often employs synthetic antioxidants, particularly butylated hydroxyanisole (BHA), butylated hydroxytoluene (BHT), ethylene diaminetetracetic acid (EDTA), and PROPYL GALLATE, as well as vitamin C, as preservatives to extend the shelf life of processed foods by preventing free radical damage.

Spontaneous oxidation of fats and oils in the presence of oxygen, sunlight and metal ions causes rancidity unless blocked by antioxidants. BHA and BHT are used to prevent rancidity in fats and oils, particularly in baked goods like crackers and cookies. Their safety has been questioned. EDTA is a common additive in salad dressings, MARGARINE, MAYONNAISE, sandwich spreads, pureed fruits and vegetables, as well as cured shellfish, BEER and soft drinks. EDTA is judged to be a safe food additive. Propyl gallate retards spoilage of fats and oils and is often used with BHA and BHT to maximize their antioxidant effects. Several studies with experimental animals suggest that propyl gallate may cause tumors. A close relative of vitamin C, erythroboric acid, is a common antioxidant used in the preservation of processed meats such as bologna, frankfurters and BACON. SULFITES are used as antioxidants to prevent discoloration of fruit and vegetables. Spices and herbs, including thyme, rosemary and sage, are sometimes used as food additives to retard spoilage. (See also ATHEROSCLEROSIS.)

Frei, Balz, ed. *Natural Antioxidants in Human Health and Disease.* New York: Academic Press, 1994.

Singh, Ram B. et al., "Effect of Antioxidant Rich Foods on Plasma Ascorbic Acid, Cardiac Enzyme and Lipid Peroxide Levels in Patients Hospitalized with Acute Myocardial Infarction," *Journal of the American Dietetic Association*, 95:7 (July 1995), pp. 775–80.

antipasto   Cold hors d'oeuvres (from the Italian *ante*, meaning before, and *pasto*, for main course of the meal). A wide variety of foods is suitable for antipasto: marinated vegetables and fish; olives; hard sausages like salami; anchovies; sardines; pickled onion, beets, peppers, artichoke hearts, garbanzo beans; and hard cheeses and soft cheeses like ricotta, along with a crunchy bread like breadsticks.

antiscorbutic   Capable of preventing SCURVY, the disease caused by chronic vitamin C deficiency. Sources of VITAMIN C (ascorbic acid), usually fresh fruit and vegetables, relieve the symptoms of scurvy. Although scurvy has been known since the time of the ancient Egyptians, the antiscorbutic effect of limes and other fruit was not discovered in Europe until late in the 18th century, after experiments involving diets of British seamen. It was not until 1907 that scurvy was discovered to be caused by a nutritional deficiency. Though still prevalent in developing nations, scurvy in developed countries is usually associated with alcoholism and poverty. Sodium erythroborate, an antioxidant used with vitamin C in processed meats, has no antiscorbutic effects.

antivitamin (vitamin antagonist)   A compound that diminishes the effect of a vitamin by specific mechanisms rather than by a general effect. The following examples illustrate the diversity of antivitamins. Drugs can act as antivitamins, thus the anticancer drug methotrexate is a FOLIC ACID antivitamin. The drug prevents tumor cells from making tetrahydrofolate, the coenzyme or activated form of folic acid required for DNA synthesis. Another case is isoniazid, a drug employed to treat tuberculosis, which is an antagonist of VITAMIN B_6. This drug blocks the utilization of vitamin B_6 by the bacteria causing the disease. Dicumarol, a drug that prevents blood clots (anticoagulant), is an antagonist of vitamin K. Antivitamins occur in foods. For example, AVIDIN, a heat-sensitive protein in raw egg white, binds biotin and prevents its uptake in the intestine. The viscera of raw fish contain a thiamin antagonist, thiaminase, which breaks down this vitamin in the intestine. The ackee plum of Jamaica contains a riboflavin antagonist and has caused an illness related to riboflavin deficiency. A vitamin or nutrient can become an antivitamin of another. For example, very high levels of vitamin A block the effects of vitamin K. (See also ANTIMETABOLITE.)

apoenzyme   An inactive form of an enzyme, lacking the appropriate small helper molecule (cofactor or coenzyme) required for activity. Apoenzyme thus refers to only the protein (polypeptide) portion of an enzyme. Enzymes that require coenzymes or metal ions to assist them in catalyzing reactions are entirely inactive unless they are combined with their non-protein helpers. Cellular protein-synthesizing machinery produces apoenzymes, and coenzymes and metal ion cofactors are added later to create a holoenzyme, which is active because it contains the required helper group.

apoferritin   The iron-free protein required for iron storage in tissues. Apoferritin must be first synthesized in cells before their iron atoms combine with apoferritin to form FERRITIN, the iron-storage protein. Ferritin, a large rust-red protein, contains a mixture of iron hydroxide and iron phosphate and accounts for most stored iron, especially in the intestinal lining, LIVER, spleen and bone marrow. Apoferritin can be contrasted with another apoprotein of iron metabolism, transferrin. Transferrin transports iron in the bloodstream to sites in the body that require iron, especially the bone marrow. Generally, transferrin is about 30% bound up with iron. Because 70% of its binding capacity is available for more iron, this apoprotein offers a reserve of iron transport capacity in the blood.

apolipoprotein   A family of proteins that are ingredients of serum LIPOPROTEINS, the lipid-protein complexes that transport FAT and cholesterol in the lymphatic system and bloodstream. There are at least nine different apoproteins associated with different lipoproteins, including Apo A, Apo B, Apo C, Apo D and Apo E. Apo A is located on HDL (high-density lipoprotein), the desirable form of blood cholesterol, and serves as an analytical marker for this lipoprotein. Apo B and Apo E occur as LDL (LOW-DENSITY LIPOPROTEIN), the undesirable form of blood cholesterol. They guide LDL binding to tissues like muscle so that cholesterol can be taken up. Apo C is a constituent of both VERY-LOW-DENSITY LIPOPROTEIN

(VLDL) and CHYLOMICRONS, which transport fat in the blood. Apo C activates an enzyme (lipase) in blood vessels that liberates FATTY ACIDS from these carriers to be absorbed by tissues. Apo D helps transfer CHOLESTEROL between lipoproteins in the blood.

appestat The hypothetical center in the brain that may regulate APPETITE and food intake. While the exact site of regulation of appetite is not yet defined, it probably involves the HYPOTHALAMUS, a part of the brain that regulates HUNGER and thirst. Hunger may be regulated much like a thermostat to balance the body's energy requirements. Possibly one mechanism stimulates feeding and a second suppresses intake. Current research implicates ENDORPHINS and enkephalins, substances that function as endogenous painkillers of the brain, in determining what and how much is eaten and when it is eaten. Other implicated brain chemicals include the neurotransmitter SEROTONIN, which promotes a sense of well-being and quiets the body; GALANIN, a brain protein that increases appetite for fat; and LEPTIN, a protein that decreases appetite. Leptin is released into the bloodstream by fat cells that signal the brain (hypothalamus) to stop sending signals that trigger eating fat and carbohydrate while increasing the metabolic rate of fat tissue.

appetite The learned desire to eat, often a specific food, for taste and enjoyment. Appetite is a pleasant feeling based on previous experiences with foods. Appetite can be triggered by association with aromas, meal time, memories and certain food advertisements. In contrast, HUNGER relates to the innate need to eat and is associated with an unpleasant sensation coupled with a physiological need. A variety of foods may satisfy hunger.

Appetite is determined by many factors, including social influences (religion, philosophy, cultural taboos); taste and palatability; state of health (diabetes, cancer); effect of medications; preferences and aversions learned by experience; environmental factors such as climate; and metabolic factors (hormone levels, caloric requirements).

The physiologic basis of appetite and hunger is not well understood. The hypothalamus of the brain seems to be the interpretative center and clearing house for hunger signals. Anxiety, stress and psychological disturbances may cause the release of appetite-stimulating chemical signals from different regions of the brain.

Multiple chemical messengers including as many as 25 neuropeptides affect food intake. Neuropeptide Y is a brain protein that induces lab animals to consume more fat and carbohydrate. It is produced by the hypothalamus and other regions of the brain. The levels of neuropeptide Y are modulated by hormones and by blood glucose levels. Another brain protein called GALANIN stimulates an appetite for fat. CHOLECYSTOKININ, a gut protein hormone that is also produced in the brain, is believed to stimulate feeding behavior also.

Appetite and exercise

After beginning an EXERCISE program, appetite may increase during the first few weeks then return to normal, while moderate exercise (15 miles per week of jogging or walking) may suppress appetite. Research suggests that exercise increases the intake of CALORIES by normal-weight men by an average of 200 calories, even when they burn an additional 600 calories. On the other hand, exercise does not seem to increase normal-weight women's caloric intake above the levels needed to make up for those burned by exercising. Regular exercise may not increase appetite or excessive eating in overweight women. (See also CRAVING.)

appetite suppressants A variety of drugs and plant products are used to curb appetite. PHENYLPROPANOLAMINE is the major ingredient of non-prescription diet pills. This drug temporarily curbs appetite but can cause important side effects. Individuals with diabetes, kidney disease, thyroid disease, DEPRESSION and high blood pressure should avoid phenylpropanolamine. Amphetamines (Dexedrine, Benadrine) are prescription drugs used to temporarily curb appetite, although appetite generally returns within two weeks. Bulking agents are forms of plant fiber that swell in water, filling the stomach and creating satiety. PSYLLIUM, GUAR GUM and GLUCOMANNAN fall into this category. These bulking agents are often included in protein powders used in weight loss protocols to help satisfy hunger. Serotonin and endorphin levels in the brain induce a sense of well-being, and a new generation of appetite suppressants based on new discoveries has been designed or is on the drawing boards. For example, dexfenfluramine has been designed to increase the levels of serotonin in the brain. This drug has recently been approved by the FDA, although it remains controversial. By FDA standards the effects on weight reduction are modest and there are potential side effects. Prozac, another drug that alters brain serotonin levels, can cause mood imbalances and there is a concern that dexfenfluramine may similarly affect mood. (See also DIETING; FIBER.)

Silverstone, T., "Appetite Suppressants: a Review," *Drugs*, 43:6 (1992), pp. 820–36.

apple (*Malus pumila*) The rounded fruit of the apple tree; originated in Asia Minor. It has been cultivated for thousands of years and today is the most widely cultivated fruit tree in the world. Apples are one of the most popular fruits in North America and in Europe. Though there are an estimated 7,000 varieties, only 20 are available in the United States and just eight account for 80% of apple sales: Red Delicious, McIntosh, Golden Delicious, York, Rome Beauty, Stayman, Granny Smith and Jonathan. Apples are typically 2.5 to 3.5 inches in diameter and range in color from russet red to yellow. The flesh can be white (Cortland) or yellow (Golden Delicious). The flavor may be tart (Winesap) or sweet (Grimes).

Apples are available year round because they store well when refrigerated, although this decreases the content of VITAMIN C. Certain varieties like Delicious, McIntosh and Rome Beauty store better than others. On the other hand, apples stored at room temperature become mealy and will turn mushy. Apples are used in a wide variety of desserts (turnovers, fritters, tarts, puddings, compotes, pies, strudels) and in jams, jellies and apple butter. A significant percentage of the European and U.S. apple crop is used to produce apple juice and CIDER.

Goals of North American apple breeding programs include developing apples that will ripen before early

August, when the first traditional red apples, the Jonathans, ripen. Another has been to develop apples that ripen in November. Eventually apples should be available that will extend the apple season (fresh picked apples) from early August to late October.

A typical unpeeled apple with only 80 to 125 calories can be served as a low-calorie, low-fat dessert or snack and can provide one of the recommended two to four servings of fruit per day. Unpeeled apples are an important source of FIBER; an apple can supply about 20% of the minimum of fiber recommended for daily consumption. Most of the fiber is soluble fiber (PECTIN). The sweeter the apple the greater the sugar (FRUCTOSE) content. Commercial applesauce may contain added sugar. For comparison a half cup of apple butter provides 186 calories; a half cup of sweetened apple sauce, provides 92 calories; a half cup of unsweetened apple sauce, 50 calories. A typical 3.25-inch-diameter apple (212 g) provides calories, 125; protein, 0.4 g; carbohydrate, 32 g; fiber, 6.6 g; potassium, 244 mg; vitamin C, 12 mg; and traces of other vitamins.

apricot (*Prunus armeniaca*)   The oval FRUIT of a tree belonging to a member of the peach family. The ripened, fragrant fruit is golden yellow and has little juice, unlike the plum to which it is related. Apricots originated in China, where wild apricots were harvested 7,000 years ago. Apricots were later cultivated in India and were introduced into the Mediterranean after the Greek conquest under Alexander the Great. The name is derived from the Latin term for early ripening. Apricots are best picked when ripe. They do not store well and can become grainy and soft; consequently, canned apricots maintain their texture and are frequently used in desserts and fruit salads. Apricots are also used in jams, pastries and cakes. Dried apricots are exported by California, Iran, Australia and Turkey. Apricots are a rich source of POTASSIUM, BETA CAROTENE and FIBER. Three apricots (106 g) provide calories, 51; protein, 1.15 g; carbohydrate, 11.2 g; fiber, 2.23 g; potassium, 361 mg; vitamin A, 317 retinol equivalents; vitamin C, 8 mg; and small amounts of other vitamins.

arachidonic acid   A long chain POLYUNSATURATED FATTY ACID that is the parent of important hormone-like agents called PROSTAGLANDINS and LEUKOTRIENES. It is a complex fatty acid, with 20 carbons and four double bonds. Arachidonic acid belongs to the Omega-6 family of unsaturated fatty acids, which are derived from the ESSENTIAL FATTY ACID, LINOLEIC ACID. Because arachidonic acid can be made in the body, it is not classified as one of the essential nutrients. MEAT and dairy products are rich sources and they contribute to the body's supply.

Arachidonic acid is processed by the "cyclooxygenase pathway," a series of enzymes that yield prostaglandins and related compounds. Prostaglandin PGE_2 and its relatives can increase BLOOD PRESSURE, induce BLOOD CLOTTING and cause pain and inflammation. ASPIRIN and non-steroidal anti-inflammatory drugs are effective pain relievers because they specifically block the cyclooxygenase enzyme. Another prostaglandin from arachidonic acid, PGI_2, helps to counterbalance blood clotting, while still another derivative of arachidonic acid, prostacyclin, blocks blood clotting. Therefore, aspirin use carries the added risk of increased bleeding.

A second chain of reactions, the "lipooxygenase pathway," converts arachidonic acid to leukotrienes, extremely powerful inflammatory agents linked to the allergic response including swelling and pain. Fish oils are rich in the omega-3 family of unsaturated fatty acids, rather than the omega-6 fatty acids. Because they block leukotriene production from arachidonic acid, fish oils can reduce excessive chronic inflammation.

arginine (Arg, L-arginine)   A basic amino acid. Arginine helps form the nitrogenous waste product UREA, as part of the chain of reactions called the UREA CYCLE, which disposes of the toxic waste ammonia in the LIVER. More generally arginine helps build PROTEINS. Arginine and LYSINE are classified as basic rather than acidic amino acids. Arginine is often considered a non-essential amino acid because of the capacity of the body to synthesize it. However, endogenous arginine formation may be inadequate in newborn infants and in adults with liver disease. Arginine also participates directly in the urea cycle of the liver. Arginine is also converted to NITRIC OXIDE to regulate blood pressure.

Good dietary sources of arginine are nuts, raw cereals, MEAT, FISH and POULTRY. Arginine supplements have been used by athletes to increase growth hormone production and increase muscle mass. Whether growth hormone levels can be manipulated by diet is controversial. Oral doses of arginine can stimulate the production of anabolic hormones such as INSULIN and prolactin.

Animal studies of arginine supplementation have produced intriguing results. Arginine speeds up wound healing in lab animals, and in patients. Arginine-rich diets also increase T-cell function in patients with traumatic injury or surgery. In experimental animals arginine activates the thymus gland and lymphocytes. It may enhance the release of growth hormone and prolactin, which indirectly stimulate the immune system. The estimated doses of arginine required to bolster immunity (up to 30 g daily) may cause bone disorders in children and adolescents. High doses of arginine may cause nausea and DIARRHEA. The use of large doses of individual amino acids is considered experimental and long-term effects on health are being worked out; therefore, their use therapeutically should be under the guidance of a physician.

Brittenden, J.M.B. et al, "L-arginine Stimulates Host Defenses in Patients with Breast Cancer," *Surgery*, 115:2 (1994), pp. 205–12.

ariboflavinosis   A disease arising from a chronic deficiency of the B vitamin RIBOFLAVIN. Symptoms characterizing this condition include sores on the tongue (bald tongue), sores at the corners of the mouth, dermatitis, and blood vessel formation in the cornea. Oral doses of riboflavin rectify this deficiency. Typically malnutrition produces a general deficiency of most B complex vitamins, rather than of a single vitamin like riboflavin because they occur together in foods. Furthermore, riboflavin is one of the enrichments of BREAD and cereals in the United States and deficiency is uncommon. However, the dietary requirement for riboflavin increases under certain conditions. For example, riboflavin in MILK is destroyed by sunlight, thyroxine (thyroid medication) decreases riboflavin absorption in the intestine, and boric acid increases urinary loss of this vitamin. There may be populations in America for whom riboflavin intake is a problem. A nutritional survey of the U.S. population (NHANES I) revealed that nearly 22% of African Americans could be riboflavin deficient.

aromatic compounds   A family of organic compounds related to benzene. Typically their ring or cyclic structures are composed of alternating single and double bonds. Benzene (one ring, an industrial solvent), naphthalene (two rings, an ingredient of moth balls) and BENZOPYRENE (four rings) are all carcinogens. Benzopyrene is a product of charcoal grilled or BARBECUED MEAT.

Aromatic rings are constituents of a wide range of physiologically important compounds. For instance, the amino acids PHENYLALANINE, TYROSINE, HISTIDINE and TRYPTOPHAN contain aromatic ring structures. Important body regulators like epinephrine (adrenaline), norepinephrine and serotonin (nerve chemical neurotransmitters) and histamine (an inflammatory agent) are aromatic compounds, as are estrogens (female hormones).

Aromatic compounds are made more water-soluble, hence excretable by the kidneys, through ring oxidations carried out by liver "detoxifying" enzymes (oxidases). Unfortunately, these enzymes can transform the aromatic compounds into highly reactive ones during oxidation, and they can become carcinogens (cancer-causing agents). (See also CYTOCHROME P450.)

arrowroot (*Maranta arundinacea*)   The starch or flour from the underground stems or rhizomes of several Central American tropical plants. The name refers to its former use by Indians to treat wounds inflicted by poisoned arrows. As a food, pulped tubers produce a white fluid that is dried, powdered and milled. Arrowroot flour can be used in wheat-free dishes. This thickening agent can replace CORNSTARCH in recipes for soups, cream sauces, pie fillings, puddings, and glazes that need to remain clear after cooking. Arrowroot thickens at a lower temperature than wheat flour and cornstarch. Sauces prepared with arrowroot should be served soon after thickening, because the consistency will not hold. Arrowroot has a neutral flavor and does not need to be cooked to remove residual taste. It is ideal for sauces that should not boil.

arsenic   A toxic, heavy metal. Arsenic as a pollutant occurs in smog and cigarette smoke. High doses are thought to interfere with neurological development in children and to increase the risk of some types of CANCER. As an ingredient in some pesticides, it can contaminate produce.

Arsenic may be an essential trace nutrient. In very low amounts it is a growth promoter in POULTRY and pigs. It plays an as yet unknown function in METABOLISM in animals and perhaps in humans as well. Traces of arsenic occur in common foods: FISH, SHELLFISH, poultry and cereals. (See also HEAVY METALS.)

arteriosclerosis   A group of pathological conditions characterized by thickened, stiffened arteries. Alterations in the intima or the media (the innermost or outermost vessel layers) can cause arteries to lose their elasticity. Arteriosclerosis alters the function of tissues and organs, including the brain, where it can cause major pathological changes. ATHEROSCLEROSIS is a type of arteriosclerosis in which arteries accumulate waxy deposits called PLAQUE.

The cause of arteriosclerosis is unknown, though AGING, altered fat metabolism and family history have been implicated. DIABETES MELLITUS, HYPERTENSION, increased blood FAT and blood CHOLESTEROL levels, cigarette smoking, OBESITY, being male, an inability to cope with STRESS, and physical inactivity increase the risk of this disease. A typical treatment program entails regular exercise; stress management; abstinence from smoking; control of diabetes, high blood pressure and weight; and lowering dietary cholesterol and saturated fat. (See also CARDIOVASCULAR DISEASE.)

artery   A vessel transporting oxygenated blood away from the heart. Most arteries carry oxygenated blood and nutrients to peripheral tissues like muscle. Arteries lead to arterioles (minute arteries), which in turn lead to capillaries, the smallest vessels. In the capillaries oxygen, glucose and other nutrients are delivered to cells. In exchange, blood acquires waste products like ammonia and carbon dioxide. Because the vascular or blood circulatory system is a closed system (that is, blood returns to its starting point, the heart), blood flows out of capillaries to veins (vessels that lead blood back to the heart). Blood is pumped to the lungs to release carbon dioxide in exchange for oxygen. The pulmonary artery, carrying blood from the heart to the lungs, is the only artery that does not carry oxygenated blood. Several arteries are prone to plaque accumulation. The arteries feeding the heart (coronary arteries) are prime candidates for disease in men. (See also CARDIOVASCULAR DISEASE.)

arthritis   A family of inflammatory diseases of the joints, including chronic degenerative joint diseases. Thirty-seven million Americans suffer from various forms of arthritis; two-thirds of them are women. Many conditions are predisposing factors for joint inflammation, including viral infection (Lyme disease); some types of FOOD POISONING; disruption of the body's chemistry (GOUT); a disruption of the IMMUNE SYSTEM (AUTOIMMUNE DISEASE); certain bacterial infections (pneumococcus, staphylococcus and streptococcus); certain parasitic infections (Giardia); physical injury; OBESITY; and physical and emotional STRESS. Arthritis is associated with AGING and heredity also plays a role.

Osteoarthritis is the most common form of joint degeneration. It affects weight-bearing joints, especially the hips and the knees. In this type of degeneration the affected joint may exhibit worn cartilage, with bone overgrowth and bone spurs. Osteoarthritis is related to abnormal calcium metabolism and stress or injury to the joint. Symptoms include morning stiffness, pain that worsens with joint function, localized tenderness, creaking, cracking of joints during movement and restricted mobility. In primary osteoarthritis, degenerative wear and tear often occurs after the age of 50, without trauma or previous inflammatory disease, because with aging there is a decreased ability to restore normal collagen and cartilage. Secondary osteoarthritis refers to a disease caused by a factor in the patient's medical history, such as a prior injury.

Nutritional Considerations in Osteoarthritis

VITAMIN E and VITAMIN C seem to enhance the stability of cartilage constituents (chondroitin sulfate). The essential amino acid methionine and manganese are also needed to produce chondroitin sulfate. VITAMIN A and vitamin B_6, as well as ZINC and COPPER are needed for collagen, the structural protein that helps form cartilage. A deficiency of these nutrients can accelerate joint deterioration.

Rheumatoid arthritis refers to inflamed joints with overgrowth of joint tissue and swollen and stiff joints that often cripple the patient. Symptoms include fatigue, low-grade fever, joint stiffness and pain, in addition to painful, swollen joints. Generally, small joints are first affected. Unlike osteoarthritis, rheumatoid arthritis is an autoimmune condition, in which the body attacks itself. Specifically, antibodies are launched against joint tissue. Investigation has centered on possible factors including foods that trigger this reaction. Though some medical opinion disclaims the effects of food on arthritis, accumulated clinical evidence indicates that certain foods can aggravate arthritis in susceptible individuals and that food allergies can increase joint pain. Common foods in this category are nuts, dairy products like MILK and CHEESE, grains like CORN and WHEAT, and BEEF. Vegetables of the NIGHTSHADE FAMILY may be implicated. Individuals who are sensitive to tomatoes, pepper or eggplant may experience less joint pain when abstaining from these foods. Vegetarian diets may be beneficial in rheumatoid arthritis perhaps due to the decreased consumption of ARACHIDONIC ACID. This polyunsaturated fatty acid, found primarily in MEAT and dairy products, contributes to inflammation through its conversion to certain prostaglandins and leukotrienes, hormone-like compounds that stimulate the inflammatory process. Fish and fish oil benefit some patients. Fish oil also reduces the formation of these inflammatory substances, hence the overall effect of eating cold-water ocean fish is to reduce inflammation. (See also ALLERGY, FOOD; DEGENERATIVE DISEASES.)

Boris, M. and Mandel, F. S., "Foods and Additives are Common Causes of the Attention Deficit Hyperactive Disorder in Children," *Annals of Allergy,* 72:5 (May 1994), pp. 462–68.

artichoke (*Cynara scolymus*)   The leafy, edible buds of a perennial plant resembling the thistle; the fleshy base is surrounded by scale-like leaves. The artichoke originated in Sicily and is now widely cultivated in other warm climates. In the United States, globe artichokes are cultivated in mid-coastal regions of California. The artichoke has diuretic properties and has a long folk history in treatment of liver complaints. Research supports its therapeutic effects. Artichokes contain cynarin, a substance that has significant regenerating effects and stimulates bile flow from the LIVER.

The heart of the artichoke and its scaly leaves are edible after cooking. Artichokes are used as a filling in omelettes and as fritters. Artichoke hearts can be stuffed, used as a garnish or served cold with sauce. Canned artichokes are prepared from the hearts and leaves of young buds. When packed in oil, canned artichokes should be drained and rinsed to lower the calorie content. Artichokes supply fiber and minerals. A medium-sized artichoke (120 g) contains 53 calories; protein, 2.8 g; carbohydrate, 12.4 g; fiber, 4.0 g; fat, 0.2 g; calcium, 47 mg; iron, 1.6 mg; potassium, 316 mg; niacin, 0.71 mg; and small amounts of other vitamins.

artificial flavors (flavoring agents)   These flavors represent the largest group of FOOD ADDITIVES and are used to replace more expensive natural flavors and to improve the taste of manufactured or synthetic foods. Although approximately two-thirds of all food additives are flavorings and flavoring agents, they are used in very small amounts. Common examples include FUMARIC ACID, HYDROLYZED VEGETABLE PROTEIN, vanillin and cinnamaldehyde. MONOSODIUM GLUTAMATE (MSG) is classified as a FLAVOR ENHANCER rather than a flavor.

The U.S. FDA does not require specific flavoring agents to be listed on the food label because they are consumed in small amounts. Consumption averages no more than several ounces a year per person. Substituting an artificial flavor for the natural food or flavor lowers the price; however, the consumer needs to be made aware that artificial ingredients have been used. The U.S. FDA permits the general term "artificial flavoring" to be used. Though nonspecific, this designation is still helpful to consumers because foods that list artificial flavorings on their food labels will probably contain little of the natural food that would normally provide that flavor.

The long-term safety of many synthetic or natural flavors has not been rigorously studied, although the review process has weeded out several natural and synthetic flavorings. Natural root beer flavoring (safrole) was shown to cause CANCER in animals and was withdrawn in 1960. The safety of cinnamon flavor, natural or synthetic, has been questioned. It is similar to cinnamyl anthranilate, which was used in grape and cherry flavors in ice cream and beverages until the U.S. FDA proposed in 1982 that it be banned because it causes cancer in lab animals. Benzylacetate, an artificial flavoring used in chewing gum, puddings and candy, was found to cause cancer in rats and mice by the National Toxicology Program. On the other hand, many flavors, for example caramel, are safe. A major stumbling block in moving forward with assessing the safety of artificial flavors is that the most prevalent artificial flavors, which might pose a health threat, have not been prioritized for toxicological studies. (See also CONVENIENCE FOOD; FOOD LABELING; PROCESSED FOOD.)

Jacobson, M.F., *The Complete Eater's Digest and Nutrition Scoreboard.* Garden City, N.Y.: Anchor Press/Doubleday, 1985.

artificial food colors (food dyes, certified food colors, synthetic food dyes, FD&C colors, coal tar dyes) Synthetic colors account for 80% of food coloring agents used in the food industry, and these synthetic additives pose a greater health risk than any other class of food additive. Because manufactured and processed foods often lack the fresh colors of whole foods, synthetic dyes have been used for years to make such foods look more appetizing or more wholesome. They provide no nutritional benefits.

Certification of artificial food colors (indicated by the FD&C designation) implies the dyes meet standards of purity, but does not assure safety. The D&C designation stands for dyes permitted only in drugs and cosmetics, not foods. Most dyes need not be specified on food labels, and instead they can be grouped under the heading "artificial coloring." Consequently the consumer may not be able to identify the dyes used in a processed food or beverage. Six dyes can be used in any food: FD&C Blue No. 1 and No. 2, Green No. 3, Red No. 40 and Yellows No. 5 and No. 6. They are common additives in candy, soft drinks, desserts like ice cream, baked goods and SAUSAGES. Citrus Red 2 is used only to color orange skins.

How safe are artificial food colors? Many studies with experimental animals suggest that artificial food dyes cause cancer. Few safety studies were carried out before the DELANEY CLAUSE, forbidding the addition of cancer-causing agents to any food, became law in 1962. Examination of the safety of synthetic dyes in use before 1960 has been gradual. Debate centers around the issue of whether additives that slightly increase the risk of CANCER represent a tolerable risk and can be used in food.

Safety concerns about approved synthetic dyes can be summarized as follows. FD&C Red No. 40 is a suspected cause of lymph tumors in experimental animals. It is widely used in soft drinks, sausage, gelatin desserts, other desserts and candy. A long controversy surrounds FD&C Red No. 3. It causes thyroid and lymph tumors in experimental animals. FD&C Yellow No. 5 (TARTRAZINE) is the only dye that must be specifically listed on food labels. Some asthmatics and individuals allergic to ASPIRIN are also allergic to this dye, which is used in soft drinks, sausage, baked goods, candy and gelatin desserts. FD&C Blue No. 1 causes chromosomal damage, and FD&C Blue No. 2 may cause brain tumors in experimental animals. Both are used in candy and soft drinks. FD&C Yellow No. 6 has been placed on permanent approval by the U.S. FDA, although it may cause adrenal kidney tumors in rats. FD&C Green No. 3 causes bladder tumors in experimental animals. (See also ALLERGY, FOOD; CARCINOGEN; CONVENIENCE FOOD; FOOD LABELING.)

Jacobson, M.F. *The Complete Eater's Digest and Nutrition Scoreboard.* Garden City, N.Y.: Anchor Press/Doubleday, 1985.

artificial sweeteners   Very common FOOD ADDITIVES used in processed foods and low-calorie beverages. To satisfy consumers' desire for sweets without the surplus CALORIES of sugary, fat-laden foods, food and beverage producers rely on artificial sweeteners. Only three artificial sweeteners are currently approved in the United States: ASPARTAME, SACCHARIN and ACESULFAME-K. These additives contribute few or no calories. CYCLAMATE, the first artificial sweetener, has been banned. Nutrasweet (aspartame) accounts for nearly 75% of the $1 billion artificial sweetener market. However, its instability to heat has restricted its use to powdered mixes, soft drinks, gum and a sweetener for coffee. Saccharin is heat stable and contains no calories, but when used alone some users find a metallic aftertaste. Acesulfame-K is the newest of the approved artificial sweeteners. It, too, is heat stable, and may find use in baked goods.

Several lines of evidence suggest that artificial sweeteners probably do not assist with weight loss. Artificial sweetener consumption tripled in the 1980s, but natural sweetener consumption also increased rather than declining. The use of artificial sweeteners has not lowered the incidence of OBESITY in the United States; just the opposite may be true. Obesity is a major health problem for many Americans. Women saccharin users were found to be more likely to gain, not lose, weight than non-users. No study suggests that artificial sweeteners diminish APPETITE. Artificial sweeteners may actually trigger a CRAVING for carbohydrates, increase appetite, especially after eating, and thus contribute to a craving for high-calorie desserts.

Several companies are developing new heat-stable sweeteners to replace aspartame. Sweeteners that are 10,000 times sweeter than sugar, but supply no calories and can be used in baked goods, are being developed. Pending FDA approval are SUCRULOSE, 600 times sweeter than sucrose (table sugar), and ALITAME, 2,000 times sweeter than sucrose. Thus artificial sweeteners seem destined to remain an important class of food additive. (See also CONVENIENCE FOOD; DIET; NATURAL SWEETENERS.)

Boris, M. and Mandel, F.S., "Foods and Additives Are Common Causes of the Attention Deficit Hyperactive Disorder in Children," *Annals of Allergy,* 72:5 (May 1994). pp. 462–68.

ascorbic acid   See VITAMIN C.

ascorbyl palmitate   A fat-soluble antioxidant FOOD ADDITIVE, derived from VITAMIN C (ascorbic acid). Ascorbyl palmitate helps retard rancidity in VEGETABLE SHORTENING by preventing the oxidation of unsaturated fatty acids. It is used to add vitamin C to fortified foods and to vitamin supplements as well. Palmitic acid, a common fatty acid, is linked to ascorbic acid to make it fat-soluble. (See also ANTIOXIDANTS.)

asparagine (Asn, L-asparagine)   One of the 20 AMINO ACIDS employed as a building block for PROTEINS. It was the first amino acid to be isolated (from asparagus juice in 1806). Asparagine is formed in the body from the amino acid ASPARTIC ACID and thus is classified as a non-essential amino acid. Cells convert aspartic acid to asparagine by the enzymatic addition of ammonia. This process creates a neutral (uncharged) amino acid from an acidic one.

asparagus (*Asparagus officinalis*)   A vegetable with succulent shoots and scale-like leaves, belonging to the lily of the valley family. Asparagus was known to the ancient civilizations of Egypt and Rome. Though it still grows wild in Europe, it is widely cultivated. Asparagus is a perennial and its underground stem produces white, purple or green shoots or spears. Asparagus root has been used as a mild diuretic in folk medicine. Martha Washington and Mary Washington are the principal varieties grown in the United States.

Asparagus deteriorates quickly, unless refrigerated after harvesting. When kept at room temperature for two days, spears lose half their vitamin C content and they become tougher. Asparagus should be steamed or cooked before use in omelettes and scrambled eggs, in salads, served AU GRATIN or plain, hot or cold, with a sauce or pureed. Asparagus shoots supply vitamins and minerals and are quite low in calories. Four medium-sized spears (cooked, 60 g) contain 315 calories; protein, 1.6 g; carbohydrate, 2.6 g; fiber, 1.1 g; iron, 0.4 mg; potassium, 186 mg; vitamin A, 50 retinol equivalents; niacin, 0.63 mg; vitamin C, 16 mg; and small amounts of other vitamins.

aspartame   By far the most popular ARTIFICIAL SWEET-ENER in America, aspartame is nearly 200 times sweeter than sucrose. The patent for this sweetener expired in 1992 and several versions of aspartame are now marketed. Aspartame contains two amino acids, ASPARTIC ACID and PHENYLALA-NINE, plus methanol (wood alcohol). Though a caloric sweetener, fewer aspartame calories are needed to obtain a degree of sweetness comparable to that of table sugar. Aspartame does not have a bitter aftertaste, nor does it contribute to tooth decay. It has been approved by the U.S. FDA for use in fruit juice-based drinks, malt beverages with less than 3% alcohol, baking mixes and flavored beverages.

Aspartame was approved by the U.S. FDA as a safe substitute for table sugar for healthy people consuming up to 23 mg per pound of body weight. For reference, a can of diet soft drink typically contains 180 to 200 mg of aspartame. Aspartame is not safe for everyone. It can be unsafe for genetic reasons; people with the inherited disease of phenylalanine metabolism, PHENYLKETONURIA, cannot metabolize high levels of phenylalanine, and they must avoid aspartame because its digestion produces phenylalanine. Food labels must warn individuals with phenylketonuria that the product contains phenylalanine, though products do not list the amounts of aspartame they contain.

Certain individuals may be sensitive to aspartame. There have been occasional reports of migraines, disorientation, ringing ears and confusion after eating foods containing aspartame. Reactions occur in women three times more frequently than in men. Although an adult may tolerate the aspartame in six cans of diet soda, this might be too much for a child, because of the child's smaller body weight. Aspartame is not recommended for pregnant and nursing women or for infants less than six months.

Wein, Debra, "Are artificial sweeteners safe? EN updates a sticky issue," *Environmental Nutrition*, 18:2 (February 1995), pp. 1, 4.

aspartic acid   (Asp, L-aspartic acid)   An acidic amino acid and one of the 20 amino acids incorporated into proteins. Aspartic acid possesses an extra acidic functional group. Aspartic acid is readily formed from OXALOACETIC ACID, a KREB'S CYCLE intermediate that is produced during the conversion of carbohydrate to energy. Hence it is a non-essential amino acid.

In addition to serving as a protein building block, aspartic acid is the precursor of the amino acid ASPARAGINE. It also donates nitrogen atoms to create UREA, the main nitrogenous waste product of the body, and to synthesize PURINES, the raw materials of ATP, DNA and RNA. During starvation, oxaloacetic acid can be converted to blood sugar (glucose) by the liver, and therefore aspartic acid is classified as a glycogenic amino acid.

aspergillus   (*Aspergillus flavus*)   A common mold known to produce AFLATOXIN B, the most potent, naturally-occurring CARCINOGEN for liver cancer. Aflatoxin was discovered in the early 1960s in England when thousands of turkeys consumed moldy groundnut meal and developed severe liver lesions. This mold is widespread and occurs in soil, air and forage throughout the world. Different strains produce varying amounts of mycotoxins (mold toxins). As "storage fungus," it develops when foods are stored. Aspergillus has long been studied by food technologists. Foods often contaminated with aspergillus after storage include PEANUTS, CORN, BARLEY, CASSAVA, cottonseed meal, peanut meal, rice, soybeans and wheat. In addition, aspergilli can contaminate fruits, several meats, spices, cheddar cheese and various prepared foods. Improper drying and storage, high humidity and mechanical damage to grains or nuts favor mold growth and widespread contamination. Food contaminated by mold should be discarded. Its toxins cannot be washed off. (See also FUNGUS.)

aspic   A gelatin-based salad with a clear body. Aspic jelly is prepared from the clarified broth of boiled meat, fish or poultry. Shellfish, vegetables or fruit can also be set in a molded jelly. Powdered gelatin can be dissolved to prepare gels for desserts and entrees. Aspics can be colored and flavored with wine or sherry. Fresh pineapple juice contains a very powerful degradative enzyme that will break down gelatin. Therefore, cooked rather than fresh pineapple should be used.

aspirin   (acetylsalicylic acid)   One of the most widely used analgesics (pain relievers). More than 20 million pounds of this over-the-counter medication are sold in the United States each year. In addition to reducing pain aspirin reduces fever and swelling associated with inflammation. Several grams daily are often prescribed to treat the symptoms of ARTHRITIS. At the cellular level, aspirin blocks the formation of PROSTAGLANDINS and thromboxanes, hormone-like compounds that promote pain, fever, swelling and tissue reddening, from ARACHIDONIC ACID, their immediate fatty acid precursor.

Moderate aspirin use may combat a variety of diseases. Previous studies had indicated that aspirin can reduce deaths from heart attack when given soon after the attack. Long-term population studies further demonstrated that daily aspirin use lowers the risk of HEART ATTACKS in men and women by reduced blood clotting. These observations are explained by aspirin's blocking prostaglandins that promote the clumping of small blood cell fragments called platelets. This is a critical step in the formation of blood clots that could be life threatening. Aspirin may be recommended for men over 50 who have one or more risk factors for CARDIOVASCULAR DISEASE, such as hypertension, cigarette smoking, diabetes, obesity or family history of heart disease. A nutritional approach to lowering the risk of cardiovascular disease would be to reduce saturated FAT consumption.

Other potential benefits of aspirin include preventing dangerous high blood pressure during pregnancy; helping victims suffering from dementia due to minor strokes; and reducing the risk of cancers of the esophagus, stomach and colon, according to studies by the American Cancer Society. Most of these benefits are evident with low dosage—the equivalent of one tablet daily or every other day. Aspirin's long history of use has defined potential risks. Aspirin can cause water retention, decrease kidney function, and promote allergic-like reactions in susceptible people. Asthmatics are more likely to react to aspirin. For the person with food allergies, aspirin can accentuate allergy symptoms. Some effects of aspirin can be observed after short-term usage. For example, aspirin use increases VITAMIN C loss after only four to five days.

Because aspirin thins the blood, it may cause bleeding in individuals who are prone to stomach irritation or ULCERS; who have a history of hemophilia, hemorrhagic stroke, uncontrollable high blood pressure, eye problems due to diabetes, liver or kidney disease; who are facing surgery; or who are in the last trimester of pregnancy. Aspirin increases gastric bleeding, especially in the elderly who drink alcoholic beverages. Aspirin should not be used by people taking other nonsteroidal anti-inflammatory drugs or drugs to thin the blood. Children and teenagers up to the age of 18 should not be given aspirin for viral infections because it increases the risk of Reye's syndrome (a serious condition affecting the central nervous system, liver and heart). (See also ALCOHOL-DRUG INTERACTIONS; ALLERGY, FOOD.)

The Dutch TIA Trial Study Group, "A Comparison of Two Doses of Aspirin (30 mg vs. 283 mg) in Patients after a Transient Ischemic Attack or Minor Ischemic Stroke," *New England Journal of Medicine*, 325:18 (1991), pp. 1261–66.

as purchased (A. P.)   Refers to untrimmed foods with inedible portions (bone, husk, rind) intact. This term describes food available from retail outlets. The term "as purchased" appears in tables describing the nutrient composition of foods, where it is important to indicate the form of a specific food that was analyzed.

assessment, nutritional status   The use of objective data to determine an individual's nutritional status. Dietitians and nutritionists collect data from clients in order to develop appropriate individualized plans that assure that nutritional goals will be met. Typically an in-depth nutrition assessment includes four components: anthropometric measurements, laboratory tests, physical exam and clinical evaluation and diet analysis. Anthropometric measurements provide basic data like height and weight. Commonly these measurements are used to calculate a BODY MASS INDEX (BMI) which is the weight in kg divided by height in meters. Body fat is often estimated from measurement of tricep skinfold thickness or midarm circumference. The major problem with interpreting anthropometric values is that there are no universally agreed upon standards for comparison. Additionally, human error can result in inconsistent measurements. Other means of assessing body fat and lean body mass such as measuring electrical conductivity of a region of the body (BIOELECTRIC IMPEDENCE ANALYSIS) are common in clinics.

Chemical laboratory tests can aid in detecting marginal nutritional deficiencies. However, interpretation depends upon the clinician's understanding of the many factors that may affect a given parameter. Typical markers include serum albumin, the most prevalent non-cellular protein in blood, which has been used to assess the adequacy of dietary protein. Serum transferrin, a blood protein that transports iron, is affected by iron deficiency anemia, pregnancy and by serum iron overload. Urinary creatinine, a waste product from muscles, can help determine muscle protein stores, since the amount of creatinine excreted in the urine is proportional to a person's muscle mass. However, creatinine excretion decreases with age. Health of the immune system is compromised by nutrient deficiencies, and total lymphocytes (white cell) count is often used to assess the status of the immune system. Infections and steroid therapy can invalidate this as a nutrition parameter.

Physical Exam and Clinical Evaluation

Although clinicians can usually identify patients with moderate to severe malnutrition, they may be less experienced at identifying patients with mild nutritional depletion. A medical history evaluates health status and uncovers underlying health issues and factors that can affect nutrition, such as alcohol and drug use, chronic disease, disabilities, or use of medications. While some signs relate directly to nutritional deficiencies as noted above, further investigation may be needed to define the underlying cause. For example, a fatty stool may indicate pancreatic insufficiency or inadequate bile production, or impaired absorption as in celiac disease. Conditions such as shortness of breath, diarrhea, constipation, nausea, gingivitis, physical pain, poor-fitting dentures, and medications may interfere with food intake and digestion. Emotional stress can lead to anorexia or depression and dramatically affect nutrient consumption. Many life-style factors influence food intake, including income, family structures, eating habits, physical activity, accessibility to food, use of alcohol and drugs, and philosophical or religious beliefs.

Dietary history is an essential part of nutrition assessment. The simplest form is the 24-hour recall. An interview or a questionnaire is used to determine all foods eaten in the preceding 24 hours and to estimate the quantities by using plastic food models of typical serving sizes. Alternatively, food consumption frequency can be estimated using a food checklist (food frequency questionnaire), for weekly or monthly intake of 40 to 80 of the most frequently used foods. This is a descriptive, qualitative approach. In contrast, food records and diet diaries describe the individual's current food intake, recorded daily in terms of common household measures. To involve the client in behavior modification, she or he may also be required to record eating patterns, including locations, times, events and feelings associated with a given meal. For evaluation, intake data are translated into nutrient intake. Food composition tables form the basis of detailed nutrient intake calculations, and extensive computer software is available to aid in dietary analysis. Food scoring systems can be based on identifying foods that are the main contributors to the elevation of blood cholesterol, that contribute saturated fat or that compose a major food group.

In the final analysis, dietary nutrient intake is compared to a standard for evaluation. Typically this is the Recommended Dietary Allowance (RDA). Since the RDAs are derived for large populations, an individual's calculated nutrient intake that is somewhat lower than the RDA need not indicate a deficiency. Nutrient intake values less than two-thirds of the RDA are best interpreted as placing the individual at risk for under-nutrition.

Lipkin, Edward W. and Bell, Stacey, "Assessment of Nutritional Status, The Clinician's Perspectives," *Clinics in Laboratory Medicine*, 113:2 (June 1993), pp. 329–52.

assimilation   The process by which nutrients are incorporated into cells and tissues of the body. Assimilation is the culmination of digestion and absorption. Food entering the body can be thought of as raw materials that first must be broken down to individual nutrients by digestion. The nutrients must then be taken up into the bloodstream by absorption, and then used by cells for growth and maintenance through a complex array of chemical reactions controlled by enzymes and categorized as METABOLISM. Therefore, interference at any stage—digestion, absorption, assimilation—can lead to malnutrition regardless of whether the individual is consuming a balanced diet.

asthma   An inflammatory respiratory disorder with labored breathing, chest constriction, wheezing and coughing. Asthma affects an estimated 10 million Americans of all ages. This respiratory condition occurs when muscles surrounding small air passageways spasm, thus restricting air flow in and out of the lungs. The inflammation of mucous membranes and overproduction of mucus further obstruct air flow. It is the resistance to air flow that produces the wheezing sound so characteristic of asthma.

Asthma is an aspect of an allergy attack called immediate hypersensitivity because the effects appear within hours of an allergic reaction. A wide range of external factors can cause asthma, including inhaled allergens (pollen, mold spores, animal dander, dust); foods (EGGS, nuts, CHOCOLATE, shellfish); and some drugs. Alternatively, internal causes like upper respiratory tract infections can cause persistent asthma.

There are five classes of medications used for chronic inflammation. For treatment of acute asthma attacks, EPINEPHRINE and bronchodilators, cromolyn sodium or glucocorticoids (anti-inflammatory steroids), can be used. However, steroids have been linked to bone loss and other problems. Antihistamines are often prescribed for the wheezing, sneezing and itching associated with allergy attacks. Eliminating the offending allergens is a direct way of avoiding further distress when the allergens occur in the home or workplace. Many asthmatic patients respond to nutritional approaches. Food allergies are related to an estimated 75% of childhood cases and to approximately 40% of adult asthmatics. ELIMINATION DIETS, in which allergenic foods are avoided for one to four weeks, may alleviate symptoms. Corn, wheat, citrus fruits, dairy products, fish and chocolate are often implicated. Certain additives can cause symptoms. FD&C yellow No. 5 (tartrazine) can trigger asthma. SULFITES, which are common preservatives, trigger asthmatic attacks in susceptible people. Sulfites appear in wine and certain salad-bar vegetables that have been pickled or canned and in other processed foods.

Certain nutrient deficiencies are also associated with asthma, vitamin B_6 and magnesium are noteworthy. Vitamin C serves as an antiinflammatory agent and may be helpful. Sulfite sensitive people may benefit from vitamin B_{12} and molybdenum. In some asthmatics with low stomach acid, supplemented hydrochloric acid may help reduce symptoms. (See also ALLERGIC RHINITIS; ALLERGY, IMMEDIATE; HISTAMINE.)

atherosclerosis (hardening of the arteries)   A progressive, chronic CARDIOVASCULAR DISEASE characterized by thickening of arterial walls and deposits called atherosclerotic PLAQUE. Atherosclerosis is the major cause of heart disease, a widespread condition in the United States where an estimated 65 million people have a form of heart or blood vessel disease. Atherosclerosis occurring in arteries supplying oxygen to the heart causes coronary heart disease and contributes to HEART ATTACKS. Medical progress and changes in diet and life-style have significantly reduced the number of deaths from atherosclerosis in the last decade.

There are multiple causes for clogged arteries; some, like heredity, age and gender, are risk factors that cannot be controlled. In an estimated 5% of cases, a genetic defect in the transportation and utilization of CHOLESTEROL is implicated. On the other hand, many factors can be controlled to reduce an individual's probability of developing atherosclerosis. HYPERTENSION (high blood pressure) and OBESITY contribute to atherosclerosis. Family history often accompanies these conditions, yet life-style choices can limit their impact. For example, the failure to cope adequately with stress can affect the course of hypertension and obesity, while excessive consumption of alcohol or calories contributes to obesity. A sedentary life-style contributes to obesity and elevated blood cholesterol. As other examples of personal choice and disease risk, cigarette smoking can cause hypertension and high dietary saturated fat often leads to high blood cholesterol.

The roots of atherosclerosis generally go back to childhood, when the inner surfaces of arteries first become rough; then "fatty streaks" develop as deposits of lipids, fibrous tissue, calcium and blood components accumulate. During adolescence and early adulthood further deterioration of the wall can lead to further accumulation of calcium and cholesterol in arterial walls. The body can respond to fatty streaks by forming tough and fibrous deposits called plaque. One form of plaque consists of proliferated cells and a second type consists primarily of accumulated lipids, especially of cholesterol and cholesterol linked to fatty acids. Thickening and hardening of plaque with calcium can progress throughout a lifetime and can ultimately narrow arteries sufficiently to restrict blood flow and cause clot formation. Often the blood clot blocks the already obstructed artery, preventing oxygen and nutrients from reaching tissues it would normally feed.

The initial events in plaque formation are not completely understood. However, a growing body of clinical evidence implicates an oxidized form of cholesterol called LOW-DENSITY LIPOPROTEIN (LDL). LDL transports cholesterol from the liver to all other tissues, and LDL is the most prevalent cholesterol carrier in blood. LDL cholesterol can be a target of FREE RADICALS, highly reactive and damaging forms of oxygen; in the process, LDL cholesterol becomes oxidized. Possibly an early event in atherosclerosis, phagocytic cells that patrol artery walls (macrophages and neutrophils among others) ingest oxidized LDL at damaged arterial sites and in the process become transformed into "foam" cells that accumulate lipids. Muscle cells may migrate into the developing mass as it develops into a fatty streak.

Atherosclerosis has also been proposed to be the result of the tumor-like growth of arterial cells injured by oxidized cholesterol, carcinogens or other agents such as HOMOCYSTEINE, a degradation product of the amino acid methionine. Alternatively, mechanical injury to the arterial wall may induce clumping of platelets, cell fragments required in blood clot formation. Still others propose that localized overproduction of growth factors (platelet-derived growth factor) could stimulate underlying smooth muscle to proliferate. The detailed involvement of platelets, oxidized blood lipids, circulating carcinogens, antioxidants, macrophages and white blood cells in plaque formation and abnormal lipid metabolism is still being actively investigated.

Laboratory blood tests to measure an individual's risk of developing atherosclerosis have become increasingly sophisticated. Elevated blood lipids have often been regarded as a risk factor for atherosclerosis. However, elevated serum triglycerides (FAT) and elevated serum cholesterol levels are at best only crude indicators of risk of cardiovascular disease. A ratio of total serum cholesterol to HDL-cholesterol is more useful. HDL (HIGH-DENSITY LIPOPROTEIN) helps remove cholesterol from tissues and returns it to the liver for disposal or redistribution, thus HDL serves a quite different role from LDL.

An even more accurate assessment of risk of atherosclerosis can be obtained from a determination of the ratio of specific marker proteins, apoprotein B, a marker for LDL-cholesterol, to apoprotein A, a marker for HDL-cholesterol. Another cholesterol carrier called Lipoprotein (a), a close cousin of LDL, may be useful as a predictor of heart disease for children, especially for those whose parents or parent had suffered a heart attack before the age of 42. Elevated homocysteine is considered an independent risk factor.

Recent evidence suggests that atherosclerosis may be reversed. One protocol prescribes a near-vegetarian diet supplying only 10% of total CALORIES from fat and 5 mg of cholesterol a day; abstinence from smoking and alcohol; 30 minutes of exercise daily at least six times per week; at least an hour daily of stress-reduction exercises, including yoga and meditation, with twice weekly meetings in a support group. The mental as well as the physical aspects of this program seem essential for its success in opening arteries partially blocked through disease. (See also HYPERCHOLES-TEROLEMIA; VEGETARIAN.)

Ornish, Dean, Brown, S.E., Scherwitz, L.W., "Can Lifestyle Changes Reverse Coronary Heart Disease?" Lancet, 336 (1990), pp. 129–33.

Witztum, Joseph L., "The Oxidation Hypothesis of Atherosclerosis," Lancet, 344 (September 17, 1994), pp. 793–98.

atopic dermatitis See DERMATITIS.

ATP (adenosine triphosphate)   A compound containing "high energy" phosphate bonds that function as the energy currency of cells. ATP contains chemical ENERGY and must be constantly replenished and recycled within cells. It is used for all energy-requiring processes including synthesis of all cellular constituents (proteins, fat, lipids, polysaccharides, DNA) and cell division, movement and muscle contraction, nerve impulses and even the maintenance of ELECTROLYTE balance in cells. ATP is not stored and it cannot be eaten to increase its level in the body.

ATP is produced by CATABOLISM, the summation of all chemical processes in the cell that convert energy stored in fat and carbohydrate to ATP. MITOCHONDRIA, subcellular structures that function as the cell's powerhouses, produce most of the ATP in many types of cells, except red blood cells, by the oxidation of fat and carbohydrate. The cellular mechanism coupling this oxidation with the trapping of about 40% of the released energy as ATP is called OXIDATIVE PHOSPHORYLATION. In this process, electrons obtained from fuel oxidation pass through a sequence of electron carrier proteins (CYTOCHROMES), which operate like a bucket brigade. Simultaneously, inorganic phosphate ions attach to

ADP (adenosine diphosphate) to form ATP, while oxygen is reduced to WATER.

VITAMINS of the B complex assist the enzymic machinery of the mitochondrial engine in its energy conversions. Without B vitamins, fuel is not burned efficiently, curtailing ATP output. They do not create ATP nor are they burned as fuel, however. (See also CARBOHYDRATE METABOLISM; FAT METABOLISM; KREB'S CYCLE.)

atrophy (tissue wasting)   A reduction in size and function of a tissue, organ or structural element of the body. MALNUTRITION, decreased physical activity, a change in hormone balance, reduced cell proliferation and diminished oxygen supply can cause atrophy of tissues. Emaciation characterizes extreme starvation, ANOREXIA or disease processes preventing nutrient assimilation.

attention deficit-hyperactivity syndrome   See HYPERACTIVITY.

au gratin   From the French term for a golden crust on the surface of a prepared dish. In the United States this term usually refers to a food coated with grated, strongly flavored cheeses or bread crumbs and melted butter, therefore higher in calories than baked or steamed foods. A scalloped or sauce dish can be lightly coated with bread crumbs, crushed corn flakes, ground nuts or cracker crumbs and heated to form a golden brown crust. More generally, vegetables, fish and pasta dishes can be cooked so that a layer forms on the surface, thus protecting underlying food from drying out.

autoimmune diseases   Disorders of the IMMUNE SYSTEM in which the body attacks itself. Normally, the body employs the immune system to discriminate very carefully between foreign invaders, which are attacked, and its own tissues. In autoimmune diseases, the immune system mistakenly produces ANTIBODIES against specific tissues. Such an attack can lead to crippling damage. Studies to define underlying causes suggest there is a major breakdown in the way the body discriminates between foreign cells (non-self) and its own tissues (self). Monitoring self-recognition is a complex process involving many components of the immune system that are currently being studied:

- Normal controls (T helper cells) that regulate B cells responsible for forming "self-directed" antibodies may be bypassed. T cells and B cells are the two major types of lymphocytes (white blood cells).
- "Rheumatoid factor," antibodies present in 50% to 95% of patients.
- Defects in the production of cells regulating antibody production (T helper cells or T suppressor cells) due to genetic defects or defects caused by viruses.
- Specific antibody binding sites. HLA antigens on cell surfaces are linked to a susceptibility to several autoimmune diseases, like insulin-independent diabetes and lupus erythematosus.
- FOOD SENSITIVITY and ALLERGY are implicated in some cases.

Examples of different autoimmune diseases include the following: rheumatoid ARTHRITIS, insulin-dependent DIABETES MELLITUS, multiple sclerosis and lupus. Myasthenia gravis (a muscle disease), scleroderma (hardening of the skin) and inflammatory bowel disease (colitis) are also likely candidates.

Rheumatoid arthritis A disease progressing from inflammation of the joint to a deterioration of cartilage. It is characterized by special antibodies, "rheumatoid factors" in the blood that can be measured clinically. Patients with rheumatoid arthritis have increased amounts of a specific type of "histocompatibility" (HLA) antigen. These antigens control transplantation reactions. In some cases food allergies are implicated.

Insulin-dependent diabetes Glucose accumulation in the blood due to the destruction of insulin-producing cells of the pancreas. With the loss of the ability to make INSULIN, there is an absolute requirement for the hormone. This disease is also characterized by the presence of a specific kind of antibody recognition site (histocompatibility or HLA antigen). The best early marker of this disease appears to be an antibody against the insulin-producing tissue (beta cells of the pancreas).

Lupus erythematosus (systemic) A chronic inflammatory disease that can attack many organs, especially their connective tissues. It is much less common than rheumatoid arthritis and occurs most frequently in women between the ages of 20 and 40. The rate of occurrence has steadily increased in the last 30 years, though its cause is unknown.

Multiple sclerosis (MS) Characterized by blurred vision and a gradual loss of control of movement as nerve tissue is damaged. There is also spotty damage to the motor and sensory nerves. This disease apparently begins early in life. Early stages are characterized by feeling clumsy and heavy, with "pins and needles" sensations and feeling light-headed. Living in northern states increases the risk of getting MS. One or two people per thousand Americans have the disease. The cause of MS is unknown, nor is there a proven cure. Abnormalities in the immune response have been detected in patients with MS, possibly triggered by a prior viral infection. Most nutrition research has focused on decreased dietary FAT and increased ESSENTIAL FATTY ACIDS. (See also NIGHTSHADE FAMILY.)

Granholm N.A., Cavallo, T., "Autoimmunity, Polyclonal B-cell Activation and Infection," *Lupus*, 1:2 (1992), pp. 63–74.

avidin A protein in egg white that binds to BIOTIN, making this B vitamin unavailable for intestinal absorption. Avidin is one of several nutrient binding proteins in egg-white that help prevent bacterial growth, which could threaten the fertilized egg. Avidin binds biotin so tightly and selectively that it has been used to experimentally induce biotin deficiency in animals, which otherwise is difficult to study. There is no risk of biotin deficiency due to avidin when consuming cooked eggs because avidin is inactivated by heat. (See also ANTIVITAMIN.)

avitaminosis A vitamin deficiency disease. Such diseases can be caused by a dietary deficiency, by maldigestion or by the MALABSORPTION of a vitamin. Though rare in industrialized nations, acute vitamin deficiency diseases are all too common throughout developing nations, especially among children and elderly populations. Preclinical signs and symptoms usually precede the appearance of a full-blown deficiency disease such as SCURVY (VITAMIN C); PELLAGRA (NIACIN); BERIBERI (THIAMIN); RICKETS (VITAMIN D); and ANEMIA (various vitamins such as FOLIC ACID and VITAMIN B_{12}, among others). The minimal daily requirement was a standard operationally defined by the minimal amount of a nutrient that must be supplied to prevent deficiency disease. (See also MALNUTRITION.)

avocado (*Persea Americana*) A fruit native to Central and South America, and cultivated in the United States in California and Florida. Avocados vary from bell-shaped and green to pear-shaped with a coarse, shell-like skin, depending on the variety. This fruit is unusually high in fat, ranging from 5% to 20% by weight, though most of it is monounsaturated. A monounsaturated oil derived from the avocado is rather expensive and resembles OLIVE OIL in fatty acid composition. Avocado oil contains 69% monounsaturated FATTY ACIDS and 14% POLYUNSATURATED FATTY ACIDS. The corresponding values for olive oil are 72% and 9% respectively. These monounsaturated oils are more healthful than saturated oils and polyunsaturates because they lower LDL cholesterol while maintaining HDL cholesterol levels with typical high fat consumption.

The flesh has a buttery consistency and a mild flavor. Fresh avocados may be used as hors d'oeuvres or in salads, mousses and souffles. Sliced avocados darken rapidly when exposed to air and room temperature. The enzyme-catalyzed darkening can be reduced by refrigeration, by lemon juice or vinegar. One half of an avocado, 4 inches long (100 g) provides calories, 160; protein, 2.0; fat, 15 g; carbohydrate, 7 g; potassium, 600 mg; iron, 1.0 mg; vitamin A, 60 retinol equivalents; vitamin C, 8 mg; niacin, 1.9 mg; thiamin, 0.1 mg; riboflavin, 0.1 mg.

azodicarbonamide A FOOD ADDITIVE used to age (condition) wheat flour. Aging is an oxidation process. During aging flour constituents, including protein, are chemically altered to yield an elastic dough that is lighter and easier to manage. Elastic doughs can rise more readily with the carbon dioxide released by leavening agents. Before the use of food additives, wheat flour was stored for several months in order to alter the properties of gluten. Flour conditioning agents now accomplish the same result in a matter of days. (See also FLOUR.)

baby food   Foods other than milk and formula fed to infants during their first year. Commercially prepared baby foods in jars (cooked or pureed food) and in packets (as dehydrated food) offer a large variety of wholesome and nutritious food, including meats, cereals, vegetables, fruits, desserts and combination foods. Food consistency varies from strained to chunky according to the developmental age of the child.

No ARTIFICIAL FOOD COLORS or ARTIFICIAL FLAVORS are added. However, FOOD ADDITIVES may be included to inhibit molds, increase texture or soften foods. Until the 1980s, most bottled baby foods contained MODIFIED CORNSTARCH as a thickener. This questionable food additive is now seldom used in baby foods.

Salt and SUGAR have been traditional additives to manufactured baby foods. Ironically, these were often added to satisfy the parent's taste. Baby foods are now either unsweetened or contain lower amounts of sugar than previously, and manufacturers have eliminated salt. There is no health reason for adding SODIUM, SUCROSE, MONOSODIUM GLUTAMATE (MSG) or PRESERVATIVES to baby foods. Furthermore, tastes for salty and sugary foods can be acquired, which suggests a potential risk of establishing a child's preference for processed food at an early age. Although all ingredients are listed on baby food labels, the labels can be misleading. For example, "high meat" dinners need be only 26% meat in baby food, and "chicken and rice" for babies need be only 5% chicken according to regulations. (See also BREASTFEEDING; FOOD LABELING.)

Dusdieker L.B., Getchell, J.P., Liarakos, T.M., Hausler, W.J., Dungy, C.I., "Nitrate in Baby Foods, Adding to the Nitrate Mosaic," *Archives of Pediatric and Adolescent Medicine*, 148:5 (1994), pp. 490–94.

Kurtzweil, Paula, "Labelling Rules for Young Children's Food," *FDA Consumer*, 29:2 (March 1995), pp. 14–18.

Bacillus cereus   A bacterium capable of causing food poisoning. There are two forms of *B. cereus* food poisoning: In the diarrheal form, infection is associated with vegetables, sauces, puddings, pastry and meat dishes that have been improperly refrigerated after cooking, permitting bacterial spores to begin growing. The bacteria produce toxins (enterotoxin) in the intestine that cause symptoms including severe diarrhea and abdominal pain and, occasionally, associated nausea. Symptoms generally appear 10 to 12 hours after consuming contaminated food and usually diminish within 24 hours.

A second food poisoning syndrome (emetic syndrome) is due to the production of a different toxin, which is produced in the food itself. Fried rice is often a culprit in Asian restaurants. In the typical scenario, boiled rice is allowed to dry; then it may be stored overnight or longer before it is fried. Bacterial spores that are heat-resistant may form. Symptoms generally appear within one to five hours and include nausea, vomiting and malaise.

To minimize this source of food poisoning, freshly cooked food is best eaten hot. Food allowed to cool slightly and kept warm for extended periods may promote bacterial growth. Cooked food should be kept hot or cooled rapidly and refrigerated.

bacon Smoked and cured cuts from the back, rib area of the hog. Bacon is a high-fat food that is usually thinly sliced, fried or grilled. Bacon burns easily, and old bacon burns twice as fast as fresh. Bacon, 100 g or about 3 oz, cooked and drained of FAT, still represents 573 calories, and most of this is due to SATURATED FAT. Canadian-style bacon resembles HAM and comes from a muscle in the eye of a pork loin; it should be cooked more like ham. It is a leaner meat than U.S. bacon; 100 g equals 183 calories.

NITRITES are added to bacon and other cured meats to retard bacterial growth and to maintain a brighter color. The legal limit of nitrite in bacon was set at 100 ppm (parts per million) in 1985. Cancer researchers are concerned that nitrite can react with nitrogen-containing compounds (AMINES) in foods to form a potent carcinogen (cancer-causing agent) called nitrosoamine. Among cured MEATS, levels of nitrosoamines were found to be highest in bacon because it is fried at high temperatures, which promotes nitrosoamine formation. The U.S. Department of Agriculture requires that VITAMIN C (ascorbic acid) or another ANTIOXIDANT be added to minimize the formation of nitrosoamine when the meat is cooked. (See also MEAT.)

bacteria, intestinal Microorganisms that normally grow in the human INTESTINE. In adults the intestine contains more bacteria than there are cells in the body. The colon contains most of the intestinal bacteria, weighing typically 4 to 6 pounds and including non-spore-forming anaerobic bacteria, anaerobic streptococci and acid-forming bacteria. In this regard, lactobacillus species and bifidobacter species are most important. In a healthy person the bacterial flora are relatively constant. This is remarkable, considering the many pounds of food ingested daily and the huge number of microorganisms in the environment.

"Friendly" gut bacteria are important in maintaining a healthy intestinal flora that benefit the body. Lactobacillus species occupy the lower portions of the small intestine, where they adhere to the intestinal wall and prevent potential pathogens (disease-producing microorganisms) from growing on the intestinal wall. The exclusion of potential pathogens from attachment sites on the intestinal wall where they might colonize in the presence of normal bacteria is referred to as microbial interference. Lactobacillus and bifidobacteria break down carbohydrate to produce LACTIC ACID, which helps create an acidic environment that is unfavorable for many potential pathogenic microorganisms. These bacteria also produce substances that limit the growth of undesirable organisms, including yeasts.

Intestinal bacteria ferment much of the FIBER and undigested carbohydrate, which are further metabolized by bacteria to short-chain fatty acids (ACETIC ACID, PROPIONIC ACID and BUTYRIC ACID) and methane and hydrogen. The short-chain fatty acids may supply more than 10% of the body's energy needs, and butyric acid specifically promotes the health of the colon. Other useful bacterial products include VITAMIN K and BIOTIN in quantities usually adequate to meet most daily requirements.

A state of imbalanced intestinal bacteria is called dysbiosis, which is characterized by low levels of desirable bacteria and the appearance of harmful, opportunistic organisms. Many factors can cause dysbiosis. The most common cause is the chronic use of broad-spectrum antibiotics that destroy many types of bacteria, including the beneficial ones. A Western-style diet, characterized by high meat, high fat and low fiber consumption, favors dysbiosis. Stress, inadequate stomach acid to sterilize food in the stomach, and aging can imbalance gut bacteria.

Pancreatic insufficiency can lead to carbohydrate maldigestion and inflammation or other alteration of the intestine, which can limit carbohydrate digestion and uptake. Excessive undigested carbohydrate resulting from maldigestion and MALABSORPTION can promote bacterial proliferation leading to DIARRHEA, FLATULENCE and bloating. LACTOSE INTOLERANCE, which is due to the inability to digest milk sugar, leads to intestinal discomfort when bacteria are able to ferment undigested lactose. Unusually rapid movement of food through the digestive tract (shortened transit time) and diarrhea change the amounts and the relative composition of intestinal bacteria. Lactic acid bacteria supplements are available to help repopulate the intestine and help relieve symptoms of diarrhea. (See also ACIDOPHILUS.)

"When Bacterial Overgrowth Causes Malnutrition," *Emergency Medicine*, 26:1 (January 1994), pp. 45–46.

Gibson, Glenn R. and Roberfroid, Marcel B., "Dietary Modulation of the Human Colonic Microbiota: Introducing the Concept of Prebiotics," *Journal of Nutrition*, 125:6 (1995), pp. 1401–12.

bacterial toxins Complex substances produced by disease-causing bacteria. Toxins cause disease, especially food poisoning. Enterotoxins represent one class of bacterial toxins. These substances irritate the intestinal mucosa, causing diarrhea and intestinal muscle spasms leading to diarrhea. The two most common toxin-producing bacteria that contaminate food and cause FOOD POISONING by toxins are staphylococcus and clostridium. They produce protein enterotoxins and are a common cause of food poisoning in the United States and other countries. Other pathogenic bacteria, like SALMONELLA, cause illness by infecting the intestinal tract. Foods most likely to be involved in outbreaks of enterotoxin poisoning are contaminated, cooked foods such as HAM, POULTRY, BEEF, cream-filled pastry, FISH, SHELLFISH, potato salad, macaroni salad, and egg and milk products. Following contamination of a food, the staphylococcal bacteria require several hours of incubation at warm temperatures to form toxins. Sometimes large amounts of warm food placed in refrigeration cool so slowly that staphylococcal growth and toxin production occur. Brief reheating does not destroy enterotoxins.

Neurotoxins represent a second class of bacterial toxins. The most notorious neurotoxin causes BOTULISM, in a rare, though potentially deadly, form of food poisoning that occurs throughout the world. This disease is caused by the anaerobic, spore-forming bacillus *Clostridium botulinum*, which can produce a neurotoxin in inadequately canned or contaminated food. Botulinum toxins are heat-stable proteins that persist in cooked food. They are among the most poisonous natural toxins; only 2 micrograms can be lethal to an adult. Spores of clostridium botulinum are not killed at the temperature of boiling water, thus canning procedures must employ higher temperatures (230–250°F) for several minutes to assure destruction of this spore-forming bacteria.

Endotoxins are a third class of bacterial toxins. They represent a heterogenous group of products released from bacterial cell walls and protoplasm when bacteria die and disintegrate. They are normally excluded by the intestinal mucosal barrier and intestinal antibodies. However, with gut inflammation the intestinal lining becomes leaky and endotoxins may be absorbed to a limited extent. CYTOTOXINS are then capable of attacking cells of specific organs and causing disease. (See also FOOD TOXINS; LEAKY GUT.)

bagel A doughnut-shaped, dense roll made with high protein flour. The basic ingredients are typical of most BREADS: FLOUR, water, yeast and salt. Recent trends are to add sweeteners like sugar or honey. Most of the CALORIES come from CARBOHYDRATE, not FAT. Egg bagels contain additional fat and CHOLESTEROL derived from eggs. Bagels are traditionally eaten with cream cheese and lox. A typical plain bagel weighing 68 grams (2.4 oz) supplies 200 calories; carbohydrate, 38.2 g; protein, 7.5 g; and fat, 1.75 g. Larger bagels may weigh three times as much and supply 75 to 80 calories, and 1 to 2 grams of fat per ounce.

baker's yeast Strains of the yeast *Sacchromyces cervisia* used to leaven bread and other bakery items. The purpose of yeast is to metabolize carbohydrate and generate CARBON DIOXIDE, which when trapped as bubbles makes the dough rise. Yeast enzymes break down glucose released from the starch in dough. To maximize this leavening effect, strains of *Sacchromyces cervisia* have been selected for their ability to ferment sugar with maximum carbon dioxide formation and minimal ALCOHOL production. Thus baker's yeast differs from brewer's yeast, which maximizes alcohol production from sugar. Dried, easy blend baker's yeast is available in packets. It must be reconstituted in warm water before it is added to dough in order to activate yeast ENZYMES to generate carbon dioxide; the dehydrated yeast themselves cannot reproduce. Sugar fermentation is best carried out at 80° to 95°F, the temperature recommended to permit dough to rise.

baking powder A mixture of chemicals that generates CARBON DIOXIDE in dough, both in the mixing bowl and in the oven and without the intervention of yeast. Bubbles of carbon dioxide create pockets in the dough that make leavened bread and baked goods lighter. Baking powders typically contain three types of ingredients to maximize their effectiveness: sodium bicarbonate, an acidic chemical, and an anticaking agent like CORNSTARCH or calcium silicate to prevent caking in high humidity. In the presence of water, the acidic ingredient reacts with the basic salt, sodium bicarbonate, to generate carbon dioxide bubbles. Sodium bicarbonate is considered a safe food additive. Baking powder (and baking soda) contribute approximately 25% of the typical American's SODIUM consumption, and typical dietary guidelines recommend cutting back on sodium to minimize the risk of high blood pressure in susceptible people.

Three types of baking powders are available that are classed according to their acidic ingredients. Tartrate baking powders contain sodium or calcium tartrate. These acidic salts react quickly, and doughs containing them cannot be stored. Phosphate baking powders contain calcium acid phosphate, which can react in cold dough as well as releasing carbon dioxide during baking. Sodium pyrophosphate is sometimes added as an acidic ingredient. Studies suggest that pyrophosphate may harm fetal animals. Pregnant women may wish to avoid this particular food additive. Double-acting baking powders, designated (SAS), incorporate sodium ALUMINUM phosphate (or sulfate) and calcium acid phosphate. They generate carbon dioxide in cold dough, but they are most active when they contact the heated oven. A serving of cake prepared with these baking powders can contain 5 to 15 mg of aluminum. Aluminum was once thought to be a safe food additive, but its safety has been questioned because it has been shown to accumulate in the brains of senile patients. (See also ALZHEIMER'S DISEASE.)

baking soda A common leavening agent used in baked goods (bicarbonate of soda, sodium bicarbonate). Baking soda can be used in place of baking powder when an acidic ingredient is also added. Sour milk, molasses or CREAM OF TARTAR are sufficiently acidic to make dough and batter rise. The chemical reaction is the same as that occurring when baking powders are used, though baking soda produces more tender, lighter baked goods. Because bread and baked goods are so important in the American diet, baking powder and baking soda are major dietary sources of SODIUM: They contribute one-quarter of the average person's sodium intake. Excessive sodium intake increases the risk of high blood pressure in susceptible people. To test the effectiveness of any baking powder, mix a teaspoon of baking powder with a half teaspoon of hot water. A fully active powder will bubble vigorously. Baking soda is classified as a safe food additive. (See also BAKER'S YEAST.)

balanced diet A diet that supplies all essential nutrients in the appropriate amounts for optimal health throughout the life span. Food should provide VITAMINS, MINERALS, PROTEIN, CARBOHYDRATE, FAT, OILS and FIBER to meet individual needs. The calories consumed should match the amount used in order to stabilize body weight.

Variety characterizes a balanced diet, which emphasizes fresh, minimally processed or whole foods. Exchange lists, which can be found in some nutrition books, simplify making healthful food choices by supplying a variety of options; for example, among different protein sources. While not specifically a low-fat–low CHOLESTEROL diet, a balanced diet tends to have less saturated fat, refined carbohydrate and cholesterol. Diseases like CANCER, HYPERTENSION, OSTEOPOROSIS, diabetes and CARDIOVASCULAR DISEASE have reached epidemic proportions and are linked to unbalanced diets. A balanced diet definitely plays a role in preventing these and other chronic diseases.

Those who rely on PROCESSED FOOD, high in fat, sugar, salt and other FOOD ADDITIVES, run the risk of an unbalanced diet. Consumption of such foods increases the need for other foods in the diet that are very nutrient dense. However, the temptation is to eat more of the same processed foods, which may also be less nutritious because of the way they were grown, stored or processed. People who skip meals without replacing them with nutritious snacks, and who choose a weight loss diet, consuming less than 1,500 calories per day, are likely to have inadequate diets. Individuals with an increased risk of inadequate diets include low-income, pregnant or lactating women; low-income children and teenagers; elderly persons eating alone; and strict VEGETARI-

ANS, who may not consume enough needed nutrients. Pollution and job-related chemical hazards may increase nutrient needs beyond those supplied by the usual diet. Limiting food choices because of income or strict religious or philosophical preference requires planning to assure adequate consumption of all essential nutrients.

Replacing EMPTY CALORIES and sugary foods with more nutritious options represents a major challenge in achieving a balanced diet. Variety simplifies the task. Vegetables supply low-fat energy in the form of starch, vitamins, beta carotene, minerals and fiber. Dark-green leafy vegetables include CHARD, KALE and COLLARD, in addition to spinach. The cabbage family encompasses BROCCOLI, BRUSSELS SPROUTS, CAULIFLOWER and Chinese cabbage. Winter SQUASH, summer squash and YAMS represent yellow-colored vegetables. Whole grains are also important: WHEAT, CORN, MILLET, RICE, TRITICALE, RYE and BUCKWHEAT for starch and minerals, vitamins and fiber. LEGUMES supply fiber and protein: beans and peas, CHICKPEAS, lima beans and LENTILS. A balanced diet includes low-fat dairy products: low-fat CHEESE, low-fat or skim MILK, YOGURT, KEFIR and EGGS for protein and CALCIUM. Nuts and seeds provide plant oils: ALMONDS, sunflower and PUMPKIN seeds. Lean MEATS, POULTRY, FISH and SHELLFISH provide trace minerals, vitamins and AMINO ACIDS. A variety of fruits supply VITAMIN C, POTASSIUM and fiber. (See also DIETARY GUIDELINES FOR AMERICANS.)

balm (*Melissa officinalis;* lemon balm, garden balm, balm mint)   A lemon-scented herb native to Europe. Lemon balm is a perennial growing up to 2 feet in height with broad, dark-green leaves. Its pale, yellow flowers grow in clusters. Leaves and sprigs contribute a subtle lemon flavor to beverages (teas and lemonade), as well as to stuffings, sauces, fish, white meat dishes, soups and salad dressing. Balm also finds industrial use; the flowers are distilled to make perfumes and liqueurs.

bamboo shoot (*Arundinaria, Bambusa, Dendrocalamus*) The young, tender, sprouting stems of several types of bamboo that find use in Oriental cooking. This plant grows in tropical Asia. Edible shoots are white and conical in shape, averaging 25 inches in diameter and 4 inches in length. They are peeled of their tough outer sheaths and are sliced into strips before cooking. Boiling bamboo shoots removes a toxin (hydrocyanic acid). Canned bamboo shoots are precooked. Precooked bamboo shoots are used in soups, stir-fries and hors d'oeuvres and can accompany meat and fish. Salted, dried shoots are used as a seasoning. In Japan bamboo shoots are a spring vegetable. The shoots have a high water content. Canned bamboo shoots (1 cup, 131 g) provide 25 calories; protein, 2.3 g; carbohydrate, 4.2 g; fiber, 3.3 g; iron, 0.42 mg; with traces of vitamins, minerals and fat.

banana (*Musa paradisiaca*)   A seedless fruit of the banana tree, the most popular fruit in the United States. Their popularity is based on the fact that bananas have a pleasant taste and they are inexpensive, are easily chewed and are available year-round. The banana originated in India and is now cultivated in many tropical regions. The banana tree resembles a palm. Though there are many varieties of bananas, they fall into two major groups: fruit bananas are eaten raw and occasionally cooked; plantains are cooked as vegetables. Yellow bananas are the most common variety sold in the United States. These bananas are harvested green to avoid damaged, overripe fruit at the market. Green bananas will ripen at room temperature in a few days, and ripened fruit (solid yellow flecked with brown spots) can be refrigerated to prevent further ripening. Refrigeration darkens the skin but does not affect the flavor. Overripe bananas find use in breads, muffins and other baked goods. Bananas are a rich source of potassium. A single 8-inch banana (114 g) provides 105 calories; protein, 1.2 g; carbohydrate, 26.7 g; fiber, 3.3 g; iron, 0.35 mg; potassium, 451 mg; thiamin, 0.05 mg; riboflavin, 0.11 mg; niacin, 0.81 mg.

barbecued meat/charcoal broiled meat   Meat that is cooked over a gas, electric or charcoal grill. Cooking over charcoal is an ancient form of cooking, and most foods, including meat, fish and poultry, can be cooked on a grill. Foods acquire a distinctive flavor when grilled. Some meats are better flavored if they have been marinated beforehand. Vegetables like corn, potatoes, peppers and mushrooms can be wrapped in aluminum foil and cooked on a grill. Barbecued food can be served with any of a variety of traditional sauces. When brushed on during the last few minutes of cooking, sauces will prevent burning. To prevent food poisoning, defrost meat and poultry in the refrigerator. Discard leftover marinade. Never put cooked food back on a plate that held raw food. Likewise, wash all surfaces and utensils touched by raw foods. To reduce fat, trim meat free of visible fat and use leaner cuts. Grill poultry with the skin on to prevent drying, then remove skin before serving.

Barbecuing meat allows fat to drip on hot coals or hot metal, which forms cancer-causing agents (BENZOPYRENES). These vaporize, adhere to soot and deposit on the surface of the meat. To lessen the formation of potential CARCINOGENS from cooked food, avoid burning meat juices. Useful strategies include: covering the grill with foil prior to cooking; wrapping food with foil; cooking at a lower temperature; and broiling rather than grilling foods.

barbiturates   See ALCOHOL-DRUG INTERACTIONS.

barley (*Hordeum*)   A CEREAL GRAIN, related to WHEAT and other grasses. Archaeological evidence suggests that barley was the earliest cultivated grain. Several varieties of barley are cultivated; the inedible husk must be removed from all of them. Whole kernels are available as scotch barley. Pearl barley is polished; that is, it is drastically milled until it resembles small pearls to remove its outer husk. Pearl barley contains fewer nutrients; its COMPLEX CARBOHYDRATE content is high, its PROTEIN content moderate, and it is used primarily in soups, stews and broths. Because it contains little gluten, the sticky protein prevalent in wheat flour, barley is not a chief ingredient of bread. Its major commercial use is as a malting agent in beer, ale and whiskey manufacture.

Barley is a good source of beta glucan, a water-soluble form of fiber. Several studies suggest that barley can lower cholesterol levels as much as 15% in individuals who have very high cholesterol levels; the viscous fiber seems to retard fat and cholesterol absorption by the intestine. The fiber tends to bind bile salts, thus increasing cholesterol removal from the body, and fat soluble substances, tocotrienols, appear to suppress cholesterol synthesis by the liver. Pearl barley (raw) supplies 349 calories per half cup (100 g); protein, 8.2 g; carbohydrate, 79 g; fiber, 8.2 g; fat, 1 g; iron, 4.2 mg; potassium, 160 mg; zinc, 2.23 mg; thiamin, 0.14 mg; riboflavin, 0.05 mg; niacin, 4.0 mg.

barley malt   A natural sweetener derived from germinated barley. Barley malt tastes like blackstrap MOLASSES, which it can replace in a recipe. In the process of preparing barley malt, the grain is first sprouted. The sprouted barley supplies ENZYMES that then break down barley starch to the sugar, maltose. Although this sweetener contains a little THIAMIN (9% of the USRDA per tablespoon) and lesser amounts of other B COMPLEX, it represents a refined CARBOHYDRATE, classified as EMPTY CALORIES because it contains little else.

basal energy expenditure (BEE)   The increased energy requirements of patients recovering from disease or injury. In practice, BEE represents an estimate of the calories needed to sustain physiologic functions while a patient is at rest. BEE is measured without intervening emotional stress or physical exertion, at least an hour preceding the measurement, at a comfortable temperature several hours after a meal. The goal of recovering from illness, injury or surgery is to provide enough calories to meet energy needs and to maintain body weight and optimal metabolic function. In addition to BEE, a set of factors is used to predict the caloric needs required for healing various degrees of injury. An activity factor of 1.2 (for bedridden patients) or 1.3 (for ambulatory patients) is multiplied by injury factors: 1.2 for minor surgery; 1.35 for trauma; 1.6 for severe infection (sepsis); 2.1 for burns. Patients with burns have the longest period of increased energy needs.

basal metabolic rate (BMR)   The energy expended to maintain the body at rest. The BMR is measured in the morning for an awake, resting individual 12 to 18 hours after the last meal. Oxygen consumption (in liters of oxygen) for a defined interval is multiplied by 4.8 calories per liter of oxygen to yield the BMR, the heat produced during the timed interval. In practice it is easier to measure the resting metabolic rate (RMR), measured either sitting or lying down, in a comfortable environment several hours after a meal or significant physical activity. RMR avoids the overnight fast and is nearly equal to BMR. Normally this ranges from 1,200 to 1,800 CALORIES (5,000 to 7,600 kJ) per day. The BMR represents a considerable energy expenditure, accounting for 60% to 75% of the calories. This energy is used for normal functions of the body, such as glandular secretions and maintenance of cellular metabolism, as well as activation of the autonomic nervous system, which maintains heartbeat, breathing and other involuntary activity.

Many factors influence an individual's metabolic rate: diet history; degree of activity of the sympathetic nervous system; physical and emotional stress; body temperature; menstrual cycle; sleep; adaptation to altitude; occupation; race; and even the season of the year. Differences in metabolic rates due to differences in body size, sex or age largely disappear if the data are related to fat-free body mass. The decrease in basal metabolic rate observed with aging is pri-

marily due to decreased lean body mass. A genetic component also contributes to the differences in BMR among individuals. BMR is partially controlled by the THYROID GLAND; thus low thyroid activity may promote weight gain. BMR decreases with illness, FASTING and even stringent DIETING. This decrease is a temporary adaptation of the body to semi-starvation and accounts for the frequently observed decrease in the rate of weight loss a week into a dieting program. Recent studies indicate that after dieting, BMR rises to a new level that is appropriate for the new body weight.

Physical conditioning is another factor. Calories are burned more rapidly after exercising than not. The duration and intensity of aerobic exercise needed to secure this benefit is an important question still being studied. If the individual is sedentary, moderate exercise seems to cause a 10% increase in basal metabolism for several hours. A moderately active individual needs to do aerobic exercise such as swimming, aerobic dancing, and jogging a total of six hours per week to increase the metabolic rate for several days afterward. In addition, exercise increases muscle mass which burns more calories than fat does. Nicotine seems to boost metabolic rates in proportion to the level of physical activity. This may be a reason why smokers often tend to weigh less than non-smokers, and why smokers tend to gain weight when they stop smoking. (See also DIET-INDUCED THERMOGENESIS.)

Felber, J.P., Golay A., "Regulation of Nutrient Metabolism and Energy Expenditure," *Metabolism*, 44:2, supp. 2 (February 1995), pp. 4–9.

base   A substance that can accept hydrogen ions (protons) and thus neutralize acids. When added to water, bases raise the pH (the degree of a measure of acidity; a pH greater than 7.0 is considered to be basic). Typical mineral bases, such as sodium hydroxide (lye) and potassium hydroxide are caustic; they can cause severe burns and are classified as strong bases. Weak bases are much more common in foods and in the body. Ammonia and bicarbonate occur in the blood and body fluids and in other nitrogen-containing compounds. A very important weak base is BICARBONATE, which, in the blood and digestive juices, neutralizes acids, thereby increasing the pH. Bicarbonate plays an important role in buffering the blood. (See also BUFFER.)

basic food groups (Basic Four Food Groups)   A 35-year-old, simple guide for making food selections designed to assist consumers in planning a BALANCED DIET. This guideline emphasizes MEAT and dairy products to avoid undernutrition. It advises eating two servings of meat selections daily; two of MILK and dairy products; four of VEGETABLES and FRUITS; and four of GRAINS. There are several disadvantages. The Basic Four Food Group guidelines lack serving sizes and provide only the minimum numbers of servings. Overnutrition and nutritional imbalances are possible because they emphasize a diet high in animal FAT and lacking in FIBER. On the other hand, a diet with moderate quantities of low-fat dairy products, lean meat, poultry and fish can easily meet the needs for CALORIES, and minerals like IRON and CALCIUM. The basic food groups have been superseded by the FOOD GUIDE PYRAMID.

(See also DIETARY GUIDELINES FOR AMERICANS.)

Summary of the Basic Four Food Groups

Food Group	Main Nutrient Contributions
Meat and meat alternatives	Protein, iron, riboflavin, zinc, vitamin B_{12}, thiamin
Milk and milk products	Calcium, protein, riboflavin, zinc, vitamin B_{12}, thiamin
Fruits and vegetables	Vitamin A, vitamin C, thiamin, additional iron and riboflavin, fiber, folic acid
Grains (bread and cereal products)	Additional amounts of niacin, iron, thiamin, zinc in whole grains; fiber

basil (*Ocimum basilicum*)   A pungent herb; a member of the mint family. Its name is derived from the Greek *basilikos*, meaning royal, because once the king alone was allowed to harvest it. Each variety of basil differs in height, color of foliage, and taste. The leaves have a pungent lemon flavor. Of the six common varieties of basil, sweet basil and dwarf basil are most popular in the United States. Basil can be used fresh or dried as a seasoning in seafoods, salads, potatoes, soups and especially tomato-based dishes, and it is used extensively in Italian and Provencal cooking. In folk medicine basil has been used to remedy flatulence.

bass (*Micropterus*)   Refers to a number of different saltwater and freshwater species of spiny-rayed FISH. Bass is shaped like SALMON, but the flesh is very white. Both freshwater and saltwater varieties occur in North America. Freshwater game fish varieties include white or silver bass and yellow bass. Saltwater varieties, like sea bass and striped bass, are among the best known. Striped bass caught in polluted offshore waters can be contaminated with industrial pollutants. Fish farms are a major source of bass. The flesh has a delicate flavor and is served poached, braised or grilled. In order to keep the flesh intact during poaching, the scales are not removed.

basting   Spooning or brushing the cooking juices or melted butter over meat several times during cooking. This procedure keeps meat, particularly leaner cuts, moist during roasting or broiling. Basting brushes or a bulb-type baster simplify the operation. Roast turkey and meat cooked on a rotisserie are usually basted with fatty drippings or with butter to prevent them from drying out. If basting is performed with stocks or water, the resulting excess steam helps keep the meat moist. Prime cuts of meat contain so much fat that basting isn't necessary. Fat losses during cooking such meat may reach 40% of the weight.

bay (*Laurus nobilis*)   An evergreen shrub widely cultivated for its broad, aromatic leaves. The shrub is a species of laurel (bay laurel, true laurel). The edible bay should not be confused with the garden cherry laurel, *Prunus laurocerasus*, which is poisonous. Bay leaves are one of the most popular culinary herbs in North America. They can be obtained as dried leaves or in powdered form. Stews, soup stocks, marinades and ragouts incorporate this versatile seasoning. Because it is so pungent, small amounts are recommended. Bay leaf, together with parsley, thyme, cloves and celery are bound together as bouquet garni to flavor soups or stocks.

B complex (B vitamins)   A group of eight water-soluble VITAMINS, required in very small amounts to convert FAT, PROTEIN and CARBOHYDRATE to ENERGY. The B complex is not stored in the body, unlike fat-soluble vitamins, and adequate amounts must be supplied daily. The name originated from early nutritional research, when growth factors for organisms were designated as B_1, B_2, etc. As they were isolated and characterized chemically, each was found to serve as a parent of a specific enzyme helper (coenzyme): THIAMIN (vitamin B_1) forms thiamin pyrophosphate; NIACIN (vitamin B_3) forms NAD; RIBOFLAVIN (vitamin B_2) forms FAD; PANTOTHENIC ACID (vitamin B_5) forms COENZYME A; VITAMIN B_6 forms pyridoxal phosphate; VITAMIN B_{12} forms methylcobalamin; FOLIC ACID forms tetrahydrofolate; and biotin yields biocytin.

The amounts of vitamins required daily are quite low. Consider the REFERENCE DAILY INTAKE (RDI): folic acid, 400 mcg; niacin, 20 mg; riboflavin, 1.7 mg; thiamin, 1.4 mg; vitamin B_6, 2 mg; vitamin B_{12}, 6 mcg; biotin, 300 mcg; pantothenic acid, 10 mg. These qualities are so small that together they would weigh no more than a metal staple. Vitamins of the B complex work most effectively when all are present in the appropriate ratios. Common multi-vitamin supplements may not balance B complex vitamins when they provide small amounts of some B vitamins and large excesses of others.

On the average, men require more of the B complex than women because their larger bodies require more nutrients. The daily requirement of thiamin increases as more food is eaten, and drinking alcoholic beverages and eating SUGAR tend to deplete the liver's B vitamin supply. Populations with the greatest risk for B vitamin deficiency include people who are on weight loss programs and who skip meals; infants and children; the elderly; and pregnant teenage women. The daily intake of nutrients like folic acid is frequently inadequate with diets relying on highly processed convenience foods. Junk foods with an excess of calories or fat and with refined carbohydrates (white flour and sugar) displace whole, minimally processed foods that are more nutritious and contain fewer calories.

As many as 30% of people over the age of 65 may not consume an amount of vitamin B_6, vitamin B_{12} and folic acid adequate to prevent strokes and heart attacks, due to a build up of a potentially harmful amino acid byproduct called HOMOCYSTEINE. When homocysteine accumulates in the blood, there is an increased risk of damage to arteries. Only by consuming 400 micrograms of folic acid a day, twice the level specified by the RDA, do levels of homocysteine decline.

The richest sources of the B complex are organ meats like liver and kidney. Low-fat options for folic acid include cooked lentils, chickpeas, kidney beans and spinach; for thiamin, brewer's yeast, extra-lean meat, wheat germ, enriched breakfast cereals; for riboflavin, low-fat milk and other low-fat dairy products and enriched cereals; for niacin and vitamin B_{12}, fish, lean meat, poultry, and enriched cereals.

A diet that supplies adequate amounts of vitamins and minerals alone does not guarantee that a vitamin deficiency will not occur. There are several reasons for this. Foods must first be digested (broken down to amino acids, vitamins, sugars, fatty acids and so on) in order to release individual nutrients, and DIGESTION may be incomplete if the production of STOMACH ACID or of DIGESTIVE ENZYMES is low. Second, the products of digestion must be absorbed by the small intestine to be of any benefit. An unhealthy intestine will be able neither to complete digestion, nor to absorb individual nutrients effectively. (See also CARBOHYDRATE METABOLISM; CATABOLISM; MALABSORPTION; MALNUTRITION.)

"B Makes the Grade," *Consumer Reports on Health*, 7:6 (June 1995), pp. 61–63.

beach plum (*Prunus maritama*)

A member of the prune family. Beach plums grow wild in North America. When ripe the small fruit is dark purple with a tough skin. The flavor combines plum with cherry and grape flavors. Its sour flavor usually limits its use to jams and jellies.

bean curd

A highly nutritious source of plant PROTEIN, prepared from SOYBEANS. To prepare bean curd, soybeans are homogenized and the soy protein is coagulated by treatment with calcium sulfate or nigari, a mineral-rich liquid remaining after salt extraction of sea water. The precipitated protein is pressed into blocks for a low-fat, low-calorie alternative to meat. (See also TOFU.)

beans (*Phaseolus*)

Seeds of trailing vines, as well as bushy plants belonging to the legume family. Beans can be divided into two groups. One group yields edible pods, picked at an immature stage; another yields only edible seeds. In the former group are snap beans, yellow wax and green beans. Bush varieties grow as short plants and pods at the same time. Pole beans grow like vines. Each stem grows a single pod, and pods mature at different times. Green beans are usually blanched to maintain their fresh color. They supply BETA CAROTENE, FIBER and some minerals including IRON. Note that canned green beans contain a high level of SODIUM—340 mg per cup of drained beans as compared to 3 mg from raw beans. Green beans (one cup cooked, 125 g) provide 44 calories; protein, 2.4 mg; fat, 0.4 g; carbohydrate, 9.9 g; fiber, 3.1 g; calcium, 58 mg; iron, 1.6 mg; vitamin A, 583 retinol equivalents; thiamin, 0.09 mg; riboflavin, 0.12 mg; niacin, 0.77 mg; vitamin C, 12 mg.

In the second category of beans are various dried beans such as navy, pinto, lima, kidney (red) and fava or broad bean. Dried beans are excellent PROTEIN sources. One cup of cooked beans supplies between 12 and 25 g of protein (25% to 50% of the RECOMMENDED DIETARY ALLOWANCE (RDA). Shell beans are harvested halfway in their maturation to dried beans. They include SOYBEANS, BROAD (fava) BEANS and lima beans. Shell beans can be used interchangeably with dried beans in recipes. Bean protein, like most plant protein, is deficient in at least one essential amino acid. However, this "incomplete" protein is readily balanced by eating beans with whole grains, nuts or small amounts of fish, poultry, meat or dairy products. Dried beans contain STARCH, MINERALS (POTASSIUM, MAGNESIUM, iron and calcium) with little fat. Dried beans are also excellent sources of FIBER. For example,

a cup of cooked pinto beans supplies 18.9 g fiber. One cup of cooked lima beans (190 g) provides 260 calories; protein, 16.1 g; carbohydrate, 49 g; fiber, 9.7 g; calcium, 55 mg; iron, 5.9 mg; potassium, 116.3 mg; thiamin, 0.25 mg; riboflavin, 0.11 mg; niacin, 1.34 mg. Navy beans (one cup cooked, 190 g) contain 225 calories; protein 15 g; carbohydrate 40.1 g; fiber, 16.5 g; and calcium, 95 mg.

FLATULENCE after eating cooked, dried beans is a common experience. The culprits in gas-producing foods are a family of carbohydrate—raffinose, stachyose and verbascose that cannot be digested but are broken down by gut bacteria that release excessive gas. This problem is reduced by soaking beans in water for several hours, discarding the water after soaking. Beans are then boiled in water, which is again discarded, rather than incorporated into soup or chili. Over-the-counter preparations of an enzyme (alpha galactosidase) that can degrade these sugars are now available. (See COMPLETE PROTEIN; FIBER; FOOD COMPLEMENTING.)

London, Sheryl, and London, Mel. *The Versatile Grain and the Elegant Bean*. New York: Simon and Schuster, 1992.

beef

The flesh of steers, cows and heifers representing the ruminant family, *Bovidae*. The Aberdeen, Angus, Brahma, Hereford, Santa Gertrudis and Shorthorn represent typical breeds grown in North America for MEAT. Though beef consumption has declined significantly during the last two decades, beef is still America's most popular meat. The indirect costs of this preference are high, because the production of one pound of beef requires an estimated five pounds of GRAIN, and the energy equivalent of a gallon of gasoline.

Beef is an excellent source of PROTEIN, VITAMINS and MINERALS (except calcium). On the other hand, beef is rather high in fat, and the fat is saturated. The high consumption of animal fat correlates with increased blood cholesterol and increased risk of heart disease and cancer. Traditionally, cattle were bred for a high degree of "marbled" meat, heavily laden with fat, and the animals were fattened in feed lots before slaughter. Due to the recent consumer demand for leaner meat, there is a trend toward producing leaner animals. For example, a 3 oz (85 g) serving of round roast, which is about the size of a deck of cards, contains: calories, 205; protein, 23 g; fat, 12 g; cholesterol, 62 mg; calcium, 5 mg; iron, 1.6 mg; zinc, 4.7 mg; thiamin, 0.07 mg; riboflavin, 0.14 mg; niacin, 3 mg. Choice grades of several cuts of beef (cooked) provide the following calories per 3 oz serving: chuck roast (18% fat) = 257; rib roast (36% fat) = 400; sirloin steak (27% fat) = 240; canned corned beef (10 g fat) = 185; trimmed round roast (8 g fat) = 175.

Beef as HAMBURGER is the most commonly eaten meat in the United States and is a major contributor of saturated fat to the standard American diet. A 3 oz serving of hamburger contains 18 g fat (21% fat). "Lean ground beef" is a designation that does not need to meet USDA standards. Therefore, the fat content can range from 20% to 30%. The average fat in "lean ground beef" is 21%. In contrast, meat labeled USDA "lean meat" contains no more than 17% fat by weight, while "extra lean ground beef" contains 10% fat by weight. Supermarket brands of low-fat beef are designated as "light select" or "select" grades of beef and range from 5% to 15% fat.

Beef often contains chemical residues, such as growth promoters, ANTIBIOTICS like sulfa drugs, animal drugs and pesticides. The health effects of low-level exposure to such compounds are unknown. Some of these residues are potential cancer-causing agents. In 1989 the European Economic Community banned beef raised with growth hormones. Hormone-free beef is now commercially available in many areas of the United States. (See also FOOD LABELING; GRADED FOODS; MEAT CONTAMINANTS.)

Robbins, John. *Diet for a New America*. Walpole, Mass.: Stillpoint Publishing, 1987.

beef tallow   A hard fat, high in saturated fatty acids and cholesterol, which is rendered from trimmed meat (usually beef). Rendering is the process of melting fat out of fatty tissue, then filtering and purifying the melted fat. Tallow is more saturated than pork fat (lard) and chicken fat.

Tallow is often used in fast-food restaurants to cook french fries because consumers seem to prefer the flavor of potatoes fried in animal fat. The practical advantages of beef tallow are that it is relatively inexpensive and it does not break down at the high temperatures needed for frying. However, the cholesterol becomes oxidized with prolonged heating at high temperatures, and oxidized cholesterol is known to be a factor in the buildup of plaque in arteries. Beef tallow finds other commercial uses, including the manufacture of candles and soap.

bee pollen   The fertilizing element from flowering plants that is collected by bees and available as a food supplement. The composition of nutrients in bee pollen resembles that of legumes with varying amounts of B COMPLEX, such as thiamin, riboflavin, niacin, folic acid and pantothenic acid, PROTEIN and MINERALS. By weight it contains 50% CARBOHYDRATE and 25% protein. Bee pollen contains FLAVONOIDS, a type of plant pigment that helps normalize inflammation.

Bee pollen is widely marketed in health food stores as an aid in weight management and as an "energizer." There are no clinical studies that indicate bee pollen energizes the body, regulates weight, tones the skin or protects against heart disease. The official position of the American Dietetic Association is that such claimed ENERGY-boosting supplements ("ergoneic") are ineffective. Those who are sensitive to pollen may have an allergic reaction to bee pollen.

beer   An alcoholic carbonated beverage that is a product of FERMENTATION of grains such as WHEAT, MILLET and BARLEY. U.S. breweries ferment barley, CORN or RYE together with hops, with cultured yeast strains to provide the alcoholic content, carbonation and characteristic flavor of this beverage. Lager beer, the most popular American beer, is aged to mellow its flavor. The ALCOHOL (ethanol) content is typically 3.2%.

Beer is the oldest known alcoholic beverage and has the highest consumption of any alcoholic beverage worldwide. Hops were cultivated in the 1200s by monasteries in Germany for use in brewing. Brewing beer follows well-defined steps. In order for the starch in cereal grains to ferment, the grains are first processed. In malting, grain is soaked long enough to initiate germination, then is kiln-dried. The color of beer is related to the extent to which malt is heated. The malt is next ground and they mixed in hot water. Enzymatic degradation produces fermentable sugars from the starch. The insoluble material is separated and the resulting fermentable extract is called a wort. Flowers of hops are added to the headed wort, then yeast is added after cooling. Most lager beer production far exceeds that of ale. Lager fermentation usually lasts seven days, to give a beer flavored by hops and malt. Ale fermentation is typically carried out for three days at a higher temperature. Directly fermenting roasted grains yields more strongly flavored (stout) ale.

One serving of regular beer (12 oz) provides 116 calories (primarily alcohol), protein, 0.9 g; calcium, 18 mg; iron, 0.11 mg; niacin, 1.6 mg; and low levels of other B complex vitamins, indicative of its low nutrient density.

"Non-alcoholic" beverages are not strictly alcohol-free because they may contain 0.5% alcohol. With less alcohol, non-alcoholic beverages contain fewer calories than their alcoholic counterparts. However, beer with 2.5% alcohol can still be called "low alcohol" beer because it contains less alcohol than the usual 3.2% alcohol. (See also ALCOHOLISM; BREWER'S YEAST; WINE.)

beet (*Beta vulgaris*, garden beet)   A red root vegetable related to CHARD. Beets may be cultivated for their tops in addition to their roots. Common varieties include Crosby's Egyptian, Ruby Queen and Detroit Dark Red. Red beetroot is a food coloring agent. Beets in general have the highest sugar content of all other vegetables. White-rooted sugar beets are a major source of domestic sugar (SUCROSE). Cooked, fresh red beets are a source of a red pigment, betalaine a type of FLAVONOID, which is a class of plant products that have beneficial effects on the immune system, connective tissue and cellular metabolism. One half cup (cooked, 85 g) provides 26 calories; protein, 0.9 g; carbohydrate, 5.7 g; fiber, 1.96 g; iron, 0.53 g; potassium, 266 mg; niacin, 0.23 mg; and low levels of VITAMIN C and other B COMPLEX vitamins. Beet greens are an excellent source of fiber, beta carotene, calcium and iron. Cooked beet greens (one cup, 144 g) provides 40 calories; protein, 3.7 g; carbohydrate, 7.9 g; fiber, 3.0 g; calcium, 165 mg; iron, 2.74 mg; potassium, 1,308 mg; zinc, 0.72 mg; vitamin A, 734 retinol equivalents; vitamin C, 36 mg; thiamin, 0.17 mg; riboflavin, 0.42 mg; niacin, 0.72 mg.

behavior   See FOOD AND THE NERVOUS SYSTEM.

behavior modification   Considered a key to the successful treatment of EATING DISORDERS, OBESITY and ADDICTIONS, this form of therapeutic intervention relies on the premise that eating behavior is learned and that undesirable eating practices can be unlearned. Strategies to change behavior permanently include specifying a written commitment to achieving a goal, rewards for accomplishments, exercises to assist building self-esteem, support groups, changes in the availability of certain foods, changes in the location in which meals are eaten, changes in the social environment, and increased physical activity. A major concern with many weight management programs is that fat can be lost without adequate commitment and training that are necessary to assure eating patterns are changed permanently. (See also DIETING.)

Kern, P.A., Trozzolino, L., Wolfe, G., Purdy, L., "Combined Use of Behavior Modification and Very Low Calorie Diet in Weight Loss and Weight Maintenance," *American Journal of Medical Science*, 307:5 (1994), pp. 325–28.

benomyl A post-harvest FUNGICIDE that reduces fruit spoilage by killing MOLDS and fungi. BANANAS, APRICOTS, PEACHES, CHERRIES, PEARS, PLUMS and PINEAPPLES are among the commonly treated fruits. Benomyl has been linked to cancer and birth defects in experimental animals.

benzopyrene (benzo(a)pyrene) A multi-ringed organic compound related to benzene. Benzopyrene is classified as a polycyclic aromatic hydrocarbon, a member of a family of compounds that are potential mutagens (mutation-producing agents) and CARCINOGENS (cancer-causing agents). The liver converts ingested benzopyrene to highly reactive intermediates (epoxides) that can attack the DNA in cells. Traces of benzopyrenes occur in soil as the result of microbial activity. Plants can synthesize this hydrocarbon and may contain up to 10 mcg per kg of dry weight. However, far greater exposure comes from the incomplete burning (pyrolysis) of oil, fat and organic material from cooking, cigarettes, exhaust from industrial combustion and automobiles, and home heating. BARBECUED MEAT contains benzopyrenes due to the FAT dripping on charcoal or heating elements. MEAT cooked in frying pans, griddles or over open flames generates benzopyrenes. Benzopyrenes contaminate soot, which is deposited on meats on overlying grills. (See also CANCER.)

benzoyl peroxide A long-used FLOUR bleach. This chemical whitens flour without necessarily aging it. Used at a level of 50 ppm (parts per million) with a mixture of aging agents, benzoyl peroxide bleaches most flours within 24 hours. Along with destroying pigments, the peroxide destroys the vitamins in flour. The trade-off in producing white flour that makes excellent dough is decreased nutritional value. The breakdown product of benzoyl peroxide is benzoic acid, which remains in flour. This additive is classified as a safe FOOD ADDITIVE.

beriberi A condition, caused by chronic THIAMIN (vitamin B$_1$) deficiency, that affects peripheral nerves, the brain and the cardiovascular system. Early symptoms of thiamin deficiency include FATIGUE, irritability, poor memory, anorexia and sleep disturbances; with severe deficiencies, paralysis of limbs, cardiovascular abnormalities and edema appear. Beriberi rarely occurs in North America because wheat products and flour are enriched with thiamin. It is more common in developing nations among populations subsisting on polished rice from which much of the vitamins and minerals have been removed. (See also CARBOHYDRATE METABOLISM; ENRICHMENT; MALNUTRITION.)

beta blockers Drugs, used to control high blood pressure in salt-sensitive individuals, that may prevent fatal HEART ATTACKS. Beta blockers limit high blood pressure by preventing the kidneys from releasing angiotensin, a hormone that increases blood pressure. The drugs have other uses as well: to control migraine headaches and to reduce angina.

There are several precautions to be observed when using beta blockers. After years of use, they may promote heart repair, but they also may damage the kidney. Beta blockers increase the risk of severe allergy reactions in patients taking allergy shots. Possible side effects include depression (in patients with a history of depression or mood disorders), FATIGUE, fuzzy thinking, impotence, mood swings, increased blood CHOLESTEROL and diabetes-like symptoms. Use of alcoholic beverages while taking this medication can be fatal because the combination can cause a drastic drop in blood pressure. (See also ALCOHOL-DRUG INTERACTION; ALLERGY; IMMEDIATE; DIABETES MELLITUS; HYPERTENSION.)

beta carotene (provitamin A) A yellow-orange pigment that is converted to vitamin A in the body. The yellow-orange coloring in fruit and vegetables is mainly due to the presence of beta carotene. Commercially, beta carotene is used as a safe FOOD COLORING. Beta carotene is the most plentiful of the orange-yellow plant pigments (carotenoids) in foods, and it has the highest vitamin A activity. Because of differences in uptake, storage and chemical processing, only about one-sixth of the beta carotene in a plant food ends up as vitamin A (retinol) in the body. For this reason the vitamin A content in plant foods is usually given as "retinol equivalents," that is, the amount of vitamin A that could be derived from the carotene content. One RE (retinol equivalent) is defined as 1 mcg of (trans) retinol (vitamin A), 6 mcg of (trans) beta carotene, or 12 mcg of other carotenoids that can be converted to vitamin A. The other way of expressing the activity of carotenoids is in terms of international units, or IU. One IU of vitamin A is equivalent to 0.3 mcg and one IU of beta carotene is equivalent to 0.6 mcg of beta carotene. Thus 1 mg of beta carotene represents 1,667 IU. Beta carotene does not carry the risk of vitamin A poisoning because the body converts it to vitamin A only as needed. Some manufacturers of multiple vitamin supplements substitute beta carotene for vitamin A in their formulations to reduce the danger of vitamin A toxicity.

Beta carotene has a number of other functions that make it the most extensively investigated carotenoid. It is a very important ANTIOXIDANT as it can help prevent damage to tissues by FREE RADICALS—extremely reactive, damaging forms of oxygen and other chemicals. Beta carotene helps boost the IMMUNE SYSTEM, and it affects lipid metabolism in important ways: It lowers LOW-DENSITY LIPOPROTEIN (LDL), the undesirable form of cholesterol, and raises HIGH-DENSITY LIPOPROTEIN (HDL), the desirable form. The U.S. FDA has approved the use of beta carotene to treat a particular form of light sensitivity in patients who have a metabolic defect and overproduce pigments called porphyrins (erythropoietic porphyrias).

In exploring the role of carotenes in preventive health, attention has focused on the possibility of using beta carotene and vitamin A to reduce the risk of HEART ATTACKS in men with coronary heart disease and CANCER. Beta carotene reverses precancerous mouth lesions and population studies suggested that it may lower the risk of cancer of the lung, bladder, larynx, esophagus, stomach, prostate, cervix and colon. Several large-scale, long-term studies are under way or have recently been completed in the United States, Europe, China and Africa to test this idea.

Three large-scale studies on the effect of supplementation with synthetic (all trans) beta carotene on the risk of cardiovascular disease and cancer have been completed. The Alpha Tocopherol, Beta Carotene Cancer Prevention Study Group found that heavy cigarette smokers (high-risk subjects) receiving beta carotene had a slightly increased risk of lung cancer mortality than those not receiving supplements, although the group receiving beta carotene and vitamin E did not experience increased cancer. Both excessive smoking and alcohol consumption can lead to oxidative stress, which can transform beta carotene into potentially damaging materials. Protecting beta carotene by consuming other antioxidants seems prudent. It is interesting to note that among people without supplementation there was a lower cancer risk with increased dietary consumption of beta carotene, in keeping with the proposal that long-term consumption of carotenoid rich foods can protect against lung cancer.

In 1996, the Carotene and Retinol Efficacy Trial found an increased death rate among subjects who were taking beta-carotene. Also in 1996, the Physician's Health Study of over 22,000 male doctors (low risk subjects) reported no benefit in reducing the risk of cancer or cardiovascular disease with consumption of beta carotene, nor was there increased risk. The overall impression from the many previous studies is that beta carotene is not toxic and that it needs to be part of a balanced antioxidant picture, including carotenoids, in order to protect the body against oxidation and chronic disease. Diets high in fruits and vegetables supply a rich mixture of PHYTOCHEMICALS in addition to beta carotene that can be beneficial to long term health. Natural, mixed carotenoids as found in whole, minimally processed foods appear to be better antioxidants than synthetic beta carotene.

The optimal intake of beta carotene and natural carotenoids to afford maximum protection is not known. According to guidelines to food choices published by the National Cancer Institute and the U.S. FDA, the beta carotene intake should be the equivalent of about 6 mg daily. Actual consumption is about 1.5 mg per day. Thus the average American eats only 25% of the amount estimated to lower cancer risks. This means most Americans should increase their daily intake of foods containing the most beta carotene. One sweet potato contains 5 to 10 mg of beta carotene, representing 2,500 retinol equivalents. About 15 milligrams daily may be recommended if the diet is compromised by PROCESSED FOOD, or in cases of infection or diabetes.

Many good sources of beta carotene and carotenoids are eaten rarely in the typical U.S. diet though they are readily available. Good sources of beta carotene include SQUASH, CANTALOUPE, sweet potatoes, YAMS, CARROTS, yellow-colored fruit like NECTARINES, and dark-green, leafy vegetables like KALE, CHARD, greens (BEETS, COLLARD), spinach and BROCCOLI. Although tomatoes, lettuce and sweet corn are relatively poor sources of beta carotene, they contribute significantly to the total intake because Americans eat so much of them. (See also DIETARY GUIDELINES FOR AMERICANS; HYPERVITAMINOSIS.)

Gaziano, J.M. and Hennekens, C.H., "The Role of Beta Carotene in the Prevention of Cardiovascular Disease," *Proceedings of the New York Academy of Sciences*, 691 (1993), pp. 148–55.

beta hydroxybutyric acid   A simple acid produced by liver metabolism of fatty acids. Beta hydroxybutyric acid belongs to the family of KETONE BODIES, which are derived from fatty acid degradation and accumulate in the blood during conditions that promote extensive breakdown of body fat, including STARVATION, crash dieting, uncontrolled diabetes and ALCOHOLISM. Ketone body accumulation in the blood promotes KETOSIS (acid accumulation in body fluids.) (See also ACIDOSIS; ELECTROLYTES; FAT.)

betaine hydrochloride   A common supplemental form of hydrochloric acid used to increase stomach acidity. Betaine hydrochloride contains 23% hydrochloric acid, by weight. As a supplement to be taken with meals, betaine hydrochloride bolsters STOMACH ACID to help improve digestion in patients with HYPOCHLORHYDRIA and ACHLORHYDRIA (inadequate stomach acid production). Hydrochloric acid is a very strong acid. A thick mucous layer usually protects the stomach from typical amounts of GASTRIC JUICE. However, excessive use of betaine hydrochloride can irritate the stomach wall. Breaking capsules in the mouth releases acid, which burns the throat and dissolves tooth enamel.

Betaine is a nitrogen-containing compound related to CHOLINE. Its name comes from the fact that it occurs in *Beta vulgaris*, the common beet. Betaine helps to replenish the amino acid METHIONINE in the synthesis of compounds like the hormone epinephrine (adrenaline).

beta lipoprotein   See LOW-DENSITY LIPOPROTEIN.

BHA (butylated hydroxyanisole)   A very common synthetic ANTIOXIDANT used in the United States since 1947 to retard RANCIDITY in vegetable oils and foods containing them. BHA destroys FREE RADICALS (highly reactive chemical species), before they can break down the fat. Therefore this antioxidant is extensively employed to extend the shelf life of many processed foods containing fat or oil, such as baked goods, CHIPS, BREAKFAST CEREALS, pork SAUSAGES, as well as active dry YEAST and some CHEWING GUMS. The average American consumes several milligrams of BHA daily from these sources.

BHA is relatively non-toxic. Most animal studies indicate it is safe, although a 1982 study suggested it may cause CANCER in experimental animals at very high dosages. A review committee concluded that the cancer risk is slight and recommended that BHA not be banned, pending further investigation. Huge amounts of BHA (0.25 to 0.5% of diet) cause abnormal developmental behavior in the offspring of treated animals. Rarely does it cause allergic reactions. (See also BHT; FOOD ADDITIVES.)

BHT (butylated hydroxytoluene)   A synthetic ANTIOXIDANT in use in the United States since 1954. Like BHA, BHT helps prevent RANCIDITY in FATS, VEGETABLE OILS and PROCESSED FOODS that contain them. Both BHA and BHT block the oxidation of POLYUNSATURATED FATTY ACIDS by reacting with FREE RADICALS. These highly reactive forms of oxygen attack the double bonds of unsaturated fatty acids found in oils. They create off-flavor odors and break down products that are potentially damaging to cells. When included in the packaging material itself, BHT (and BHA) can migrate into the contents such as breakfast cereal, powdered milk and mixes, in addition to baked goods and chips. The U.S. FDA allows

BHT and BHA to be added to raw and cooked meat toppings for pizzas and meatballs.

A mixture of synthetic antioxidants is often more effective than single preservatives. Therefore many products contain BHA, BHT and PROPYL GALLATE, a third, less safe antioxidant. BHT is less expensive than BHA but is unstable when heated during PASTEURIZATION and baking.

The average American consumes 5 to 10 mg of BHT daily. BHT accumulates in human tissues, though the long-term significance of this is unknown. The safety of BHT has been questioned, and some individuals are allergic to it. It is known that BHT induces certain liver detoxifying enzymes (mixed function oxidases). This is viewed as a mixed blessing because an increased level of these enzymes can destroy some toxic materials, but they also can transform others into carcinogens (cancer-causing agents). The relationship of BHT to cancer is murky. Several reports suggest that BHT prevents cancer in experimental animals. Other studies suggest it has no effect; still others conclude BHT can cause cancer. Rats fed 0.1 to 0.25% BHT diets (about 10 to 20 times the typical American diet) developed behavioral changes. The U.S. FDA proposed removing BHT from the GENERALLY RECOGNIZED AS SAFE (GRAS) list of FOOD ADDITIVES; however, it has not been classified as a regulated food additive. In view of the concern about safety, some companies omit BHT from processed foods. (See also CYTOCHROME P450.)

bicarbonate   A common substance in the blood used to help regulate acid-base balance. Bicarbonate forms in the body when carbon dioxide dissolves in water or blood to form the weak acid CARBONIC ACID (H_2CO_3). Carbonic acid spontaneously yields bicarbonate. Together bicarbonate and carbonic acid form an effective physiologic buffer system to maintain the blood at a very narrow range, pH 7.3 to 7.4. Thus bicarbonate can neutralize modest amounts of acid that might occur through ingestion or metabolism.

Bicarbonate also occurs in BAKING SODA as sodium bicarbonate. In the presence of acidic ingredients like cream of tartar, bicarbonate forms carbonic acid, which spontaneously decomposes into water and carbon dioxide. It is this action that produces the gas bubbles that cause dough to rise.

bifidobacteria   A type of non spore-forming anaerobic (oxygen-sensitive) bacteria that ferments sugars to acids. Bifidobacteria ferment glucose, galactose and fructose to produce lactic and acetic acids. Bifidobacteria are often used in food preparation requiring the production of mild acids, in countries like Japan; in the United States lactobaccilli have been more widely used.

Bifidobacteria are normal, beneficial residents of the human colon. These bacteria colonize the intestine: *Bifidobacterium infantis* is the natural inhabitant of human infants. The bifidobacter strains acidify feces and produce antibacterial factors that limit the growth of undesirable bacteria and contribute to weight gain. Bifidobacteria get their start in the intestine, most readily through breastfeeding. Bifidobacteria are the predominant organisms in the large intestine of breastfed infants; they can account for up to 99% of the microflora.

In adults another strain of bifidobacteria (*Bifidobacterium bifidum*) populates primarily the lower regions of the intestine.

In healthy individuals the relative proportion of these bacteria remains rather constant. However, reduced gastric acidity, oral antibiotic therapy and other conditions can disrupt the gut microflora. Furthermore, the levels of bifidobacteria can decline with age. Bifidobacteria are available as supplements. The major beneficial functions of bifidobacteria are:

- prevention of colonization of the intestine by potential disease-producing microorganisms with which they compete for nutrients and attachment sites;
- production of short-chain fatty acids, which nurture the colon, from fiber fermentation;
- production of vitamins like biotin.

(See also ACIDOPHILUS.)

bifidus factor   A heat-stable factor in breastmilk that promotes the growth of the bacterium *Bifidobacter infantis* in the intestinal tract of infants. None of a variety of non-human milks favor the growth of these strains. Successful implantation of this acid-producing bacterium helps to establish normal intestinal flora and limit the growth of less desirable microorganisms. Bifidobacter play an important role in balancing intestinal flora. (See also ACIDOPHILUS.)

bile (gall)   The juice secreted by the liver and temporarily stored in the GALLBLADDER to aid fat DIGESTION. The hormone CHOLECYSTOKININ, released during eating, triggers the contraction of the gallbladder, which expels stored bile into the small intestine. There bile emulsifies FAT, permitting its digestion by a specific enzyme, LIPASE, secreted by the pancreas. The absorption of fat-soluble VITAMINS also requires bile emulsification.

Bile contains bile salts, natural detergents that are the principal emulsifying agents of fat. The liver synthesizes bile salts from CHOLESTEROL. Bile also contains the phospholipid LECITHIN to help dissolve fat and a small amount of free cholesterol, which is emulsified by bile salts and lecithin. If the ratio of water to lecithin to bile salt is altered, cholesterol can become insoluble in the gallbladder and form GALLSTONES in susceptible individuals. Bile also contains bilirubin, or BILE PIGMENT. Bilirubin is a waste product of hemoglobin metabolism from red blood cells and plays no significant role in digestion.

Once fat has been digested, bile salts are mainly reabsorbed by the intestine and recycled in the liver. A small amount is excreted in the feces. It is believed that some forms of fiber can lower blood cholesterol levels indirectly by binding bile salts so they cannot be reabsorbed. To compensate for this loss, the liver withdraws cholesterol from the blood to manufacture more bile salts, thus lowering blood cholesterol levels.

Bile salts may be decomposed by gut bacteria to potentially harmful products. A high FIBER diet helps to maintain a normal transit time to move waste out of the body. This action decreases both bile salt decomposition and exposure of the COLON to toxic materials. Such observations may explain why dietary fiber lowers the risk of colon CANCER. (See also ENTEROHEPATIC CIRCULATION.)

bile acids   The primary FAT emulsifying agents of BILE. Bile acids and their derivatives, the bile salts, are powerful detergents. They are released from the gallbladder in order to dissolve fat prior to its digestion by the INTESTINE. They emulsify fat-soluble VITAMINS and promote their uptake as well. The liver synthesizes bile acids from cholesterol. In this process, the liver first oxidizes cholesterol to primary bile acids like cholic acid. The sterol ring structure that typifies cholesterol remains intact. Subsequent steps couple cholic acid to the amino acids TAURINE and GLYCINE to form the more soluble bile salts, taurocholate and glycocholate. These so-called conjugated products are even more powerful detergents than bile acids. Once in the intestine, bacterial metabolism can further modify bile salts to secondary bile acids, such as deoxycholic acid. Bile acids are partially reabsorbed by the intestine and are returned to the liver via the portal vein to be recycled. A small fraction, normally about 5%, escapes in the stool. This fraction represents the primary pathway by which cholesterol can be metabolized to leave the body. (See also ENTEROHEPATIC CIRCULATION; FAT METABOLISM.)

bile pigment (bilirubin)   A yellow-brown pigment that is the end-product of HEMOGLOBIN breakdown. Bilirubin serves no functional role in digestion, although in the blood it acts as an antioxidant. BILE pigment is derived from HEME, the red pigment of hemoglobin. Bilirubin is produced by the spleen, which breaks down heme. In the process, the heme ring is broken to form a chain, bilirubin. Iron is then released to be recycled. Bilirubin is next transported in the blood to the liver, where it is absorbed and converted to a water-soluble form called conjugated bilirubin, which can be secreted. This pigment, together with bile salts and lecithin, forms bile. Colon bacteria further modify bilirubin to stercobilin, which colors the stool brown. JAUNDICE is a condition characterized by excessive bilirubin accumulation. Jaundice itself is not a disease, but is an indication of abnormal metabolism or processing limited by the liver.

bilirubin   See BILE PIGMENT.

bingeing   See COMPULSIVE EATING.

bingeing and purging   See BULIMIA NERVOSA.

bioavailability   The degree to which NUTRIENTS are effectively absorbed and assimilated by the body. To ensure adequate nutrition, three events must occur: Enough food must be consumed to provide enough essential nutrients. The foods must be adequately digested, and the released nutrients must be absorbed efficiently. If food is not efficiently digested or if nutrients are not absorbed, an individual can eat a well-balanced meal and yet be undernourished.

Many factors limit bioavailability:

1. Antinutrients, chemicals occurring in some foods, bind nutrients and prevent their use. For example, acidic derivatives (oxalates in vegetables and phytates in grains) can limit the uptake of trace minerals such as IRON and ZINC; RUTABAGAS contain materials that bind iodine.
2. Nutrient uptake can be blocked by competition with pollutants in food and water. As an example, LEAD blocks the uptake of CALCIUM. On the other hand, a high calcium intake does limit lead absorption.

3. Excessive amounts of nutrients can block the uptake of others. Thus excessive zinc blocks the uptake of COPPER and vice versa.
4. Inadequate DIGESTION may prevent the release of nutrients from food. Deficient STOMACH ACID (HYPOCHLORHYDRIA) reduces PROTEIN digestion. Inadequate BILE production limits FAT DIGESTION and uptake of fatty acids and fat-soluble vitamins.
5. A nutrient may not be in a suitably complexed form, for example, inadequate production of INTRINSIC FACTOR, a protein made by the stomach, limits VITAMIN B_{12} absorption in the intestine.
6. Inadequate intake of one nutrient can limit the bioavailability of another. Thus, too little VITAMIN D in the diet prevents the absorption of adequate calcium because vitamin D enhances the calcium uptake mechanism of the intestine.
7. An unhealthy intestinal lining limits nutrient absorption. The intestinal lining can be damaged by parasites (giardiasis). Allergy can cause intestinal edema and thus reduce trace mineral uptake. An extreme example is CELIAC DISEASE, a severe reaction to the cereal grain protein, GLUTEN. This disease causes severe damage to the intestine leading to MALNUTRITION, which is often associated with celiac disease. Food allergies can cause frequent spasming of the intestine, which can shorten the transit time of food through the intestine, thereby shortening the time available for nutrient uptake. (See also ANTIVITAMIN; GOITROGENS; SUBCLINICAL NUTRIENT DEFICIENCY.)

Dreosti, I.E., "Recommended Dietary Intakes of Iron, Zinc and Other Inorganic Nutrients and Their Chemical Form and Bioavailability," *Nutrition*, 9:6 (1993), pp. 542–45.

biochemical individuality   The molecular differences that exist among individuals of a population. Each person's need for nutrients like VITAMINS and trace MINERALS to achieve optimal health varies from the norm of the population. Consequently, some people need lesser amounts of essential nutrients than the average intake for optimal health, while others, especially those affected by the standard American DIET of highly processed foods, or who smoke or who are pregnant need larger amounts.

Tissue compositions differ in levels of ENZYMES, the metabolic machinery that operates cells, due to inherited differences, different medical histories and toxic exposures, diet and age. Molecular genetics has uncovered a far greater degree of genetic polymorphism in people than previously known. There may be many variants of a given gene, thus variants of the protein it codes for. Most variant proteins support normal functioning. In certain cases, however, the variant form of an enzyme may operate normally only as long as there is an abundant supply of an essential vitamin helper (COENZYME). When the concentration of the vitamin falls below a critical threshold, function could be impaired. Thus, perhaps 10% of the U.S. population may not be able to process HOMOCYSTEINE, a byproduct of the metabolism of METHIONINE, unless a sufficiently high level of folic acid is maintained in the diet. In other words nutrition can affect genetic expression (the phenotype). In extreme cases individuals may possess defective enzymes that cause genetic diseases such as phenylketonuria (PKU), an inherited inability to break down the amino acid PHENYLALANINE.

Differences in amounts of protective enzymes like antioxidant enzymes and detoxification enzymes of the liver can explain why some people are sensitive to environmental pollutants, while others can tolerate high exposures, and why individuals tolerate medications and anesthetics differently. A therapeutic dose effective for one person may be ineffective for the next. Biochemical individuality explains why only certain people experience side effects when exposed to a given food.

Individuals vary in their sensitivity to dietary salt, CHOLESTEROL, SUGAR, FAT or ALCOHOL. Perhaps one out of five Americans is sensitive to SODIUM and will tend to develop high blood pressure with a high salt diet, and approximately one in five will respond to a high sugar diet with elevated blood fat. An estimated one-third of Americans are sensitive to dietary cholesterol; their elevated serum cholesterol level puts them at high risk for developing clogged arteries. Biochemical individuality may explain, in part, why only a fraction of those who drink alcohol become addicted.

It is impossible to predict on an individual basis who will be sensitive to sodium, cholesterol, sugar or alcohol. In some people with high blood cholesterol, clinical laboratory testing may provide clues, such as elevated blood fat or LDL (low-density lipoprotein), the undesirable form of serum cholesterol. Family history often provides clues regarding susceptibility to illnesses like cancer, high blood pressure, heart disease and diabetes that are impacted by diet. With this information, prudent dietary and life-style choices can be made to lower the odds of chronic disease later in life. (See also ALCOHOLISM; ATHEROSCLEROSIS; CANCER; GENE; HYPERTENSION.)

Kadlubar, F.F., "Biochemical Individuality and Its Implications for Drug and Carcinogen Metabolism: Recent Insights from Acetyltransferase and Cytochrome P4501A2 Phenotyping and Genotyping in Humans," *Drug Metabolism Review*, 26:1–2 (1994), pp. 37–46.

bioimpedence analysis meter (BIA meter)   An electrical device sometimes used to check the amount of body fat. The BIA meter has been used in fitness centers and doctor's offices to adjust diets or to direct clinical treatment. The device attempts to measure body fat by measuring the flow of electricity between two electrodes attached at the ankle and the wrist when a very light current is applied. By gauging the resistance to the electrical current, the BIA meter can be used to estimate the water in tissues and thus fat content. There has not been an attempt to standardize measurements. Data are affected by body shape, moisture on the skin, the type of food or liquids consumed, muscle mass and adjacent electrical appliances. In 1994, a panel assembled by the U.S. National Institutes of Health concluded that the BIA meter can give distorted values that have little bearing on measuring relatively small changes in fat.

biological value (BV)   A measure of how efficiently the body uses dietary PROTEIN. The higher the biological value, the better the quality of food protein, that is, the more closely it supplies the optimal amounts of AMINO ACIDS for needed growth and maintenance. The intake of nitrogen for food protein is compared with loss of nitrogen under carefully controlled experimental conditions.

BV represents the percentage of food nitrogen retained by the body. It is defined as the amount of nitrogen from food protein retained by the body divided by the amount of nitrogen from food protein that was absorbed after digestion, expressed as a percentage.

Optimally, the BV could be 100%; all the nitrogen that is absorbed is used in amino acids to build proteins. In practice a protein with a BV greater than 70 (together with adequate calorie intake to meet energy needs) supports growth and represents a "complete" dietary protein. Most animal protein except gelatin has a high BV. A value less than 60 is considered low and represents "incomplete" protein. Many plant and grain proteins have low biological values because they are deficient in at least one essential amino acid. Typical CORN (maize) protein has a BV of 40% because it is low in the essential amino acid LYSINE, classified as a basic amino acid. High lysine strains of corn have been developed that have a higher biological value. LEGUMES are low in sulfur amino acids (CYSTEINE and METHIONINE). Other plant sources (including AMARANTH, QUINOA and SOYBEAN) provide protein that approaches the BV of meat.

The BV of plant protein can be improved by combining protein from different sources. When eating a variety of whole foods, VEGETABLES, GRAINS and grain products, BEANS and other legumes daily, the body averages its daily protein intake. Thus combining a food low in an essential amino acid with foods high in that amino acid raises the average for the day, and the net biological value is more than adequate. Knowledgeable vegetarians, or those on varied, high COMPLEX CARBOHYDRATE diets, can meet their protein needs with little or no meat. (See also DIETS, HIGH COMPLEX CARBOHYDRATE; DIETARY GUIDELINES FOR AMERICANS; FOOD COMPLEMENTING; NITROGEN BALANCE.)

biosynthesis   The formation of molecules by cells generally from smaller, simpler raw materials. Chemical reactions in cells require protein catalysts, known as ENZYMES, and biosynthetic reactions are no exception. Those enzymes employed in biosynthesis require energy and are said to be "anabolic." Frequently, larger biomolecules are assembled from smaller building blocks. Thus biosynthetic reactions produce PROTEINS (polypeptides) from AMINO ACIDS; GLYCOGEN and STARCH (POLYSACCHARIDES) from GLUCOSE, DNA and RNA (polynucleotides) from simple nucleotides; FATTY ACIDS and CHOLESTEROL from acetic acid; FAT from fatty acids.

Biosynthesis requires an input of two forms of chemical energy: ATP, the "energy currency" of cells, and a reducing agent, reduced nicotinamide adenine dinucleotide phosphate (NADPH). ATP and NADPH are produced by the oxidation of fuels, especially CARBOHYDRATES and fat. Therefore energy production is coupled to biosynthesis (energy consumption). Biosynthetic pathways are localized within cells. Some, like fat synthesis and protein synthesis, occur exclusively in the cytoplasm. Others such as DNA and RNA synthesis are restricted to the nucleus. (See also ANABOLISM; CARBOHYDRATE METABOLISM; NICOTINAMIDE ADENINE DINUCLEOTIDE (NAD, NADH)/NICOTINAMIDE ADENINE DINUCLEOTIDE PHOSPHATE (NADP, NADPH).

biotechnology   See GENETIC ENGINEERING.

biotin   A member of the B COMPLEX and formerly designated as vitamin H, this water-soluble VITAMIN assists in energy production in the body. It is essential for synthesizing saturated fatty acids from CARBOHYDRATE and for synthesizing BLOOD SUGAR from non-carbohydrate precursors like lactic acid and pyruvic acid during STARVATION and FASTING. Biotin functions as a protein-bound COENZYME, assisting primarily in reactions in which enzymes transfer carbon dioxide to compounds to create carboxylic acids (carboxylation reactions). The oxidation of the short-chain fatty acid, propionic acid, requires biotin, as does the breakdown of the essential amino acid leucine. The safe and adequate daily intake for adults, except for pregnant women, is estimated to be 100 to 200 mcg.

Intestinal bacteria supply biotin. Furthermore, biotin is very widespread in food, including egg yolk, liver, dark-green leafy vegetables and whole grains, so deficiencies are extremely rare. Deficiency symptoms include dermatitis, depression, pain and weakness. Biotin supplements are very safe: There is no known toxicity even with high doses. Biotin does not cure baldness, nor does it cure dermatitis, two purported therapeutic uses of this vitamin. AVIDIN is a protein in raw egg white that functions as an antimicrobial agent to protect the yolk. Avidin binds biotin tightly, and it has been used to induce biotin deficiency in experimental animals. Because large amounts of raw egg white are very rarely consumed avidin consumption is not an issue. (See also ACIDOPHILUS; FAT METABOLISM; GLUCONEOGENESIS.)

birth defects   Abnormalities that are apparent at birth. They may manifest themselves as physiological, structural or mental defects. The human embryo and fetus are sensitive to a wide variety of agents, ranging from chemicals, bacterial and viral infections and radiation to the nutritional state of the mother and hence the fetus.

The type of birth defect and the degree of severity, depend upon the type of external factor, the dose, as well as upon the developmental stage at which the factor was taken up. The first three months of pregnancy (embryonic development) are particularly critical. Brain development and the formation of organs, the skeleton and limbs occur in the embryo. Damage at this stage of human development may lead to severe structural birth defects. Agents that cause abnormal structural development in the embryo are known as TERATOGENS. They include maternal medications such as ESTROGENS, progestogens, certain anticancer drugs, some antibiotics, retinoic acid, VITAMIN D, and VITAMIN A (greater than 10,000 IU per day).

The terminal stages of pregnancy are also important. Fetal development (the last six months of pregnancy) involves integrating the ENDOCRINE SYSTEM and the elaboration of the nervous system. Certain medications may cause problems with the function of organ systems or with later development. These drugs are classified as "fetotoxic"; they include neosporin, several cardiovascular drugs, certain sedatives and tranquilizers, excessive VITAMIN K and the antibiotic tetracycline.

Infections can cause birth defects. If the mother contracts rubella (German measles) during pregnancy, the infant runs a greater risk of cataracts and severe abnormalities. TOXO-PLASMOSIS, an infection due to a common parasite, when con-

tracted during pregnancy can be transmitted to the fetus. This can cause severe problems after birth: epilepsy, blindness and mental retardation.

Maternal diet and nutrient status are critical for normal pregnancy and post-natal development. It is well established that nutritional deficiencies can lead to birth defects, mental retardation and slowed development. If it is balanced throughout her life, the woman's diet before pregnancy can also enhance prenatal development. Maternal protein MAL-NUTRITION can lead to smaller brains in infants, premature birth and difficulties after birth. ZINC is a key nutrient in maternal nutrition. Zinc deprivation can cause birth defects, delayed male sexual development and possibly slow learning. Spina bifida and NEURAL TUBE DEFECTS (birth defects of the spinal chord) are linked to FOLIC ACID deficiencies. A number of food-related agents affect embryonic and fetal development. Alcohol consumption during pregnancy can lead to mental retardation (FETAL ALCOHOL SYNDROME). CAFFEINE use by the mother during pregnancy can lead to abnormalities.

Many pollutants are implicated in birth defects and mental retardation. LEAD can affect mental development and learning. MERCURY can affect the nervous system of children, leading to mental retardation, seizures and learning disabilities. The banana pesticide BENOMYL, FUMIGANTS (thiabenazole) and HERBICIDES (Dinoseb and dioxin) can cause fetal abnormalities in experimental animals. Women consuming PCB in FISH have a greater risk of having low birth weight babies and infants with developmental disorders. Pregnant women are advised to avoid fish caught in polluted waters. Trace amounts of industrial pollutants, DTT, PBB, as well as PCB, are commonly found in breast milk. Their effects on infant health are unknown. Chemical pollutants occur in freshwater BASS, TROUT, white fish, walleye pike, CATFISH and fish from the Great Lakes and the Hudson River. Ocean fish caught from polluted waters, especially HALIBUT, MACKEREL, marlin, red snapper, sheepshead, TUNA, swordfish, BLUEFISH and striped bass are often contaminated by pollutants. (See also ALCOHOL; BREASTFEEDING; HEAVY METALS.)

Cordero, Jose F., "Finding the Causes of Birth Defects," *The New England Journal of Medicine*, 331:1 (1994), pp. 48–49.

biscuit   A flat, sweetened, dry baked food, usually containing a high percentage of fat. The term originated from the French and means "twice cooked." Heating fresh baked bread again in the oven dries it out. The hardened biscuit was a stable of military commissaries (sea biscuit, army biscuit) during the 19th century.

Biscuits contain varying portions of wheatflour, vegetable shortening, lard or butter, sugar and flavorings. Ship biscuits are simply prepared from flour, salt, shortening and water. Shortbreads are prepared from flour, butter or margarine, and sugar. Hot biscuits contain, in addition, milk and baking soda to create a tender dough. Biscuit flavorings vary with the menu, ranging from cinnamon and sugar to chives, parsley, cheese, fruit or nuts.

bitters   A family of aromatic beverages or tonics that have a bitter flavor. Bitters may or may not be alcoholic. Italian bitters are usually wine-based. Bitters can be served as aperitifs, and peach and orange bitters are often used as flavoring in alcoholic mixed drinks (cocktails). Bitters can also refer to a dry ale tasting strongly of hops. Several plants used in herbal medicine are bitter "tonics," including GOLDENSEAL, DANDELION, CHAMOMILE and gentian root. The physiologic actions include stimulation of glandular secretion to increase digestion, inhibition of inflammation and antibacterial effects.

blackberry (genus *Rubus*)   The conical fruit of a thorny shrub originating in Europe. A bramble of the rose family, the blackberry grows in Asia and Europe; in North America it grows from Alaska to Mexico and from Newfoundland to Florida. In the 1800s interest in blackberry cultivation lead to the development of many varieties from wild stocks for commercial growers and gardens. Like the RASPBERRY, this fruit is composed of small seed-containing fruits called drupelets. Blackberries ripen from August through October, and the ripened fruit is purple-black. Many hybrids are now cultivated, including boysenberries, loganberries and ollalieberries. Blackberries are used in jellies, tarts, pies, ice cream, syrups and jam. They are an excellent source of FIBER and contain VITAMIN C. One cup (144 g, uncooked berries) provides 74 calories; carbohydrate, 18.4 g; fiber, 9.7 g; potassium, 282 mg; traces of protein and fat; iron, 0.8 mg; trace of B vitamins and vitamin C, 30 mg.

blackcurrant oil   A seed oil used as a dietary supplemental source of essential fatty acids. Blackcurrant oil is unusual because it provides both families of ESSENTIAL FATTY ACIDS, omega-6 and omega-3. It also contains a high level of GAMMA LINOLENIC ACID, a fatty acid that is converted to hormone-like substances, PROSTAGLANDINS, believed to counterbalance pain, elevated blood pressure, blood clotting and inflammation. Gamma linolenic acid could help reduce blood clots and thus could potentially protect against STROKES and HEART ATTACKS. The conversion of gamma linolenic acid to prostaglandins may be inadequate when the diet contains excessive HYDROGENATED VEGETABLE OILS, excessive alcohol, or if the individual is diabetic or elderly.

blackstrap molasses   A semi-purified, thick, dark-brown syrup made from concentrated sugar juice. The preparation of molasses involves several steps. Sugar cane is cut close to the ground, where it is richest in sugar. The stalks are shredded, then pressed to extract the juice. The juice is boiled down to concentrate it to the point of crystallizing sucrose (table sugar). The sugar crystals are removed; the remaining liquid, or mother liquor, is blackstrap molasses—an important source of minerals. Light molasses is more purified and lacks the mineral content of blackstrap molasses. It contains per 2 tbsp. (40 g) 85 calories; carbohydrate, 22 g; calcium, 274 mg; iron, 10.1 mg; manganese, 103 mg; and potassium 1,171 mg. (See also NATURAL SWEETENERS.)

bladder infections (Urinary Tract Infections, UTI) Infections of the urethra or bladder, which increase the risk of a serious kidney infection. Cystitis refers to inflammation of the bladder. Ninety percent of patients with bladder infections are women; 20% of women have such infections at least

once a year. Bladder infections are not uncommon in children; 2% of girls have excessive bacteria in their urine. The prevalence increases with age.

The problem generally occurs when fecal bacteria or vaginal bacteria are introduced into the urethra. If the bladder is not voided completely, especially if there is infrequent urination or during the last stage of pregnancy, the risk of infection increases immensely. Unsweetened cranberry juice may lessen symptoms, but will not cure bladder infections; it contains hippuric acid, which retards bacterial growth and a carbohydrate that prevents coliform bacteria from adhering to the bladder and urethra lining, a step necessary before they can grow and cause infection. Garlic has been shown to have antimicrobial activity, including activity against bacteria associated with urinary tract infections. The care of a physician is strongly recommended in the event of bladder infections because of the risk of kidney infections. (See also CANDIDA ALBICANS.)

blanching   The process of exposing fruits and vegetables to boiling water or steam for a short time. Blanching both preserves color and inactivates ENZYMES that alter the texture and flavor of food. A typical procedure entails heating a vegetable up to three minutes in boiling water. Blanching CORN for two minutes before freezing helps preserve its flavor. Blanching TOMATOES and PEACHES simplifies peeling them. Blanched salad vegetables are softer than raw vegetables.

bleaching agents (flour)   Chemical oxidizing agents used to whiten FLOUR. Milled wheat flour is initially yellowish and does not form an elastic dough. Oxidation of flour protein, GLUTEN and pigments both whitens and matures flour so that it produces an elastic dough that is good for baking.

Consumer preference for white flour and white BREAD has lead the baking industry to use an unusual list of food additives. Before World War II, agene (nitrogen trichloride) was used extensively to bleach flour. In wartime England kennels increasingly used bread scraps to make up for the diminished supply of meat; dogs were observed to go into convulsions that mimicked epileptic fits. In severe cases the animals became crazed. In 1946 Sir Edward Mellanby reported the correlation between neurological symptoms and bleached flour. Later research demonstrated that the sulfur amino acid METHIONINE was converted to a potent inhibitor of a brain enzyme by agene, and the modified methionine could itself cause seizures. As a result of these findings, agene was banned in 1946. After exhaustive testing, chlorine dioxide was found to be a safe bleaching and maturing agent. Presently it is used mainly in the processing of fruit and vegetables. Instead of chlorine dioxide the baking industry now uses powdered bleaching agents that are simpler and less expensive to use. Benzoylperoxide can bleach flour in 24 hours, for example. Such bleaching agents leave innocuous residues in flour.

blood   The cell-filled liquid that circulates through the heart, arteries and veins. A 70 kg adult has a blood volume of 5 liters. Blood is regarded as a tissue in which red and white cells are suspended in a liquid (plasma) in the ratio of 45 parts cells to 55 parts plasma. This vital fluid performs many tasks. Blood supplies all tissues with nutrients and oxygen, and it transports waste such as UREA to the kidneys, and CARBON DIOXIDE to the lungs, for disposal. Blood is the medium for integration and coordination of tissues of the body through hormonal regulation. It maintains the chemical equilibrium of the body in terms of ELECTROLYTES (ionic substances) and polyelectrolytes (serum proteins), which in turn regulates water distribution in blood versus tissues. Blood pH is buffered to maintain a very narrow range at 7.35 to 7.45. Circulating antibodies, gamma globulin, represent blood aspects of the immune system and thus are the first line of defense against foreign substances. Blood also contains special cells, platelets, and protein clotting factors to form clots and thus limit blood loss. Fats, cholesterol and fat-soluble vitamins are transported in the blood by specialized structures (LIPOPROTEINS). Nutrients like vitamin A, iron and copper are carried by their own transport proteins. In terms of mechanical function, the bloodstream assures an even temperature for all regions of the body.

Most cells in blood are RED BLOOD CELLS (erythrocytes), which are specifically designed to transport oxygen. WHITE BLOOD CELLS (leukocytes) represent a much smaller fraction; as part of the immune system they protect against infection. Lymphocytes, which represent 20% to 50% of white cells, are derived from either bone marrow or from the thymus gland. They mount a cellular defense against foreign cells and materials. Plasma, the fluid remaining once cells are removed, contains fibrinogen. This inactive protein can be activated to form fibrin clots to plug holes in blood vessels. The fluid remaining after blood has clotted is called serum which lacks cells and clotting factors, but contains GLUCOSE and minerals like POTASSIUM, SODIUM and CHLORIDE, the most common electrolytes. These ions help maintain the appropriate ionic strength, pH and FLUID BALANCE of the body. Serum contains ALBUMIN and other proteins that help maintain ion concentrations in the blood, and it contains transport proteins, such as very low density (VLDL) lipoproteins for carrying fat and low-density lipoproteins (LDL) and high-density lipoproteins (HDL) to transport cholesterol.

Several types of nutrients support the circulatory system. For example, VITAMIN K and CALCIUM support the blood clotting mechanism. ZINC, IRON, MANGANESE, MAGNESIUM, VITAMIN B_6, FOLIC ACID, VITAMIN B_{12} and other nutrients support erythrocyte and leukocyte production. Vitamin C maintains strength and elasticity of capillaries. (See also BLOOD CLOTTING; ENDOCRINE SYSTEM; HEMOGLOBIN; IMMUNE SYSTEM.)

blood-brain barrier   A structural barrier that limits the passage of a variety of substances, including certain drugs and nutrients, from blood vessels into the brain and the central nervous system. This barrier consists of cells lining capillaries (endothelial cells). The attachments between these cells are called "tight junctions." However, the nature of the physical barriers and biochemical mechanisms for transporting materials across the barrier are complex and are not completely understood. Very small molecules like water and oxygen simply diffuse through cells and capillaries. GLUCOSE, the major fuel of the brain, is an example of a substance that can penetrate the blood-brain barrier, passing freely across the barrier, though other sugars do not. During star-

vation or crash dieting ketone bodies, small acidic compounds that accumulate in the blood during excessive fat degradation (a condition known as KETOSIS), can cross through capillary linings, pass into the brain and be burned for energy. In contrast, long-chain fatty acids that make up fat cannot penetrate the blood-brain barrier, and consequently fat cannot supply the brain with energy. Some nutrients rely on transport systems embedded in cell membranes to actively transport substances into the brain. Thus AMINO ACIDS enter by specific, energy-dependent processes (active transport) TYROSINE, PHENYLALANINE, LEUCINE, ISOLEUCENE, VALINE and TRYPTOPHAN compete for the same transport sites. Different sites are specific for other types of amino acids. (See also FOOD; NEUROTRANSMITTER.)

blood cells   See LEUKOCYTES; RED BLOOD CELLS.

blood clotting   The formation of a semi-solid mass from blood constituents. Exposure of blood to air, to foreign substances or to substances released from injured tissues (thromboplastin) stimulates blood clotting. Blood clotting is a complex process requiring the sequential activation of a series of clotting factors, which are protein modifying (proteolytic) enzymes. It culminates in the activation of thrombin, the terminal enzyme that catalyzes the conversion of fibrinogen, a soluble blood protein, to insoluble FIBRIN. Fibrin forms fibers that create a sticky mass that enmeshes blood platelets, a very small type of white blood cell, and RED BLOOD CELLS. This mass of fibers and cells forms a plug that covers the injured region of a capillary. The platelets fragment and release serotonin, a compound that causes the capillary to contract and the blood clot to retract. The net result is that the hole is patched and blood flow is reduced at the site of injury.

Nutrition status affects blood clotting. The maturation of prothrombin, the parent molecule of thrombin, and of other blood clotting factors (proenzymes) further up the clotting sequence of reactions, requires VITAMIN K and CALCIUM. A calcium deficiency effectively slows the activation of clotting enzymes because a calcium-prothrombin complex must first form in order to be activated to thrombin. Vitamin K deficiency slows clotting because prothrombin cannot be modified to bind calcium. STARVATION and protein MALNUTRITION reduce clotting because the LIVER synthesizes lesser amounts of the protein clotting factors and fibrinogen.

blood lipids   See CHOLESTEROL; TRIGLYCERIDES.

blood pressure   The pressure maintained in arteries and veins by the heart. Blood pressure usually refers to an indirect measurement of pressure of large arteries at the height of the pulse. Blood pressure reflects the resistance of blood flow in the capillary bed and arterioles as well as the elasticity of arteries themselves. The heart exerts pressure throughout the circulatory system. Ventricles of the heart contract (the systolic phase of the heartbeat), creating systolic pressure in the cycle of heart pumping. Ventricular relaxation between heartbeats creates the lowest pressure between heartbeats, the diastolic pressure. Like a barometer for measuring air pressure, blood pressure is measured in units equivalent to the height of a column of mercury. A pressure of 120/80 represents a systolic pressure equivalent to 120 mm of mercury and a diastolic pressure of 80 mm of mercury. A systolic pressure persistently greater than 140 and a diastolic pressure persistently greater than 100 indicate stages of HYPERTENSION (high blood pressure), a potentially serious condition.

The following factors correlate with increased blood pressure: overweight; age; emotional STRESS; physical activity; and male gender. Quiet sleep and female gender correlate with decreased blood pressure. Dietary factors and heredity are risk factors for susceptible individuals. Approximately 20% of adults will be adversely affected by overconsumption of SODIUM. Unfortunately, these salt-sensitive individuals cannot be readily identified. Eating a large meal can lower blood pressure quickly in older people when the stomach fills with food, and experiments show that such people may feel faint or have an angina attack unless they lie down. (See also HEART DISEASE.)

blood sugar   The level of glucose in the blood. RED BLOOD CELLS and most of the nervous system, including the brain, rely on this fuel to meet most of their energy requirements. The body strives to maintain blood sugar at a constant level. This reflects hormonal regulation and a delicate balance between diverse processes: CARBOHYDRATE DIGESTION and assimilation; tissue uptake of glucose; and release of glucose by the LIVER. During the fasting state, blood sugar levels remain relatively constant for an individual; the normal range of fasting blood sugar is 60 to 100 mg per 100 ml.

What Happens After a Meal?

Typically, blood sugar levels rise an hour or so after a meal containing carbohydrate, as the glucose produced by digestion of starch and complex sugars is absorbed by the intestine. Elevated blood sugar after a carbohydrate meal signals the endocrine PANCREAS to release INSULIN. This hormone lowers blood sugar by stimulating most tissues to take up glucose and metabolize it. The absorbed glucose is either stored as GLYCOGEN in muscle and liver, or it is converted to FAT by the ADIPOSE TISSUE and the liver. As a result blood sugar levels return to base line values several hours after eating.

What Happens Between Meals (Fasting)?

Glucose is constantly being consumed by the brain and other tissues. In response to a drop in blood sugar or to stress, the ADRENAL GLANDS release CORTISOL and EPINEPHRINE and the pancreas releases GLUCAGON. These hormones signal the release of glucose from glycogen stores in the liver, and the synthesis of glucose from amino acids by the liver, raising blood sugar levels to base line values.

HYPOGLYCEMIA refers to a sustained, abnormally low blood glucose level. If blood sugar drops too low, the brain does not function normally. This condition creates mood changes, irritability, fainting and fatigue. Reactive hypoglycemia refers to a drop in blood sugar levels that can occur several hours after eating. This is usually due to the abnormal functioning of insulin (dysinsulism). Severe hypoglycemia due to profound metabolic imbalances can lead to coma.

HYPERGLYCEMIA (elevated blood sugar) is at the other extreme and is characterized by sustained, elevated blood glucose as observed in DIABETES MELLITUS. Chronic high blood glucose, frequent in uncontrolled diabetes, has many unfortu-

nate ramifications. It can lead to the destruction of peripheral nerves and eye damage; lowered resistance to infections; toxemia during pregnancy; and heart and kidney disease. The excretion of excess sugar in the urine causes DEHYDRATION.

Life-style choices can help stabilize blood sugar levels and thus minimize wide swings in the changes brought about by the over- or underproduction of hormones. The body responds more efficiently to insulin with reduced intake of REFINED CARBOHYDRATES, COFFEE and ALCOHOL. Specific nutrients may help the body regulate blood sugar. Dietary CHROMIUM can help insulin work more effectively; STRESS, coffee and sugar consumption deplete the body of chromium. High levels of biotin seem to assist the liver with carbohydrate and fat metabolism. NIACINAMIDE, NIACIN, VITAMIN C, VITAMIN B_6, MANGANESE, MAGNESIUM, ZINC and SELENIUM have been shown to improve glucose tolerance in some instances.

Eating frequent, light meals that are high in protein often helps to avoid swings in blood sugar levels, and balanced meals with whole foods high in STARCH and FIBER are effective time-released sources of glucose. Stress reduction with meditation, yoga or biofeedback, regular exercise, and maintaining optimal body weight, also helps minimize blood sugar imbalances. (See also DIETING; GLUCONEOGENESIS; GLYCOGENOLYSIS.)

Gold, Paul E., "Role of Glucose in Regulating the Brain and Cognition," *American Journal of Clinical Nutrition,* 61:supplement (1995), pp. 987S–995S.

blueberry (*Vaccinium*)   Shrubs producing an edible, bluish berry. The blueberry is related to the heath family of plants that includes American laurel, rhododendron and broom. Varieties of blueberries include whortleberries and bilberries. They are an excellent source of fiber and anthocyanosides, blue-black pigments related to FLAVONOIDS. These pigments can help stabilize collagen structure. Blueberries also contain a carbohydrate that tends to prevent coliform bacteria from adhering to the walls of the bladder and urethra. (Attachment is the first step in infection.)

European bilberries are used in botanical medicine. Their flavonoids have many important effects on the body. They help decrease blood platelet aggregation; clumping of these small cell fragments of the blood is an essential step in blood clot formation, and excessive platelet aggregation increases the risk of strokes.

Bilberry flavonoids may benefit varicose veins by strengthening capillaries and vein structure. They also can strengthen the blood-brain barrier and limit uptake of harmful substances. They have been shown to help relieve day and night blindness and retinal degeneration. In folk medicine, bilberry leaf tea has been used to help normalize high blood sugar in diabetes.

Blueberries are eaten raw or cooked in pies, tarts and muffins as well as in ice cream, compotes and CHUTNEY. They are convenient to freeze. Frozen blueberries keep at least a year. One cup of blueberries (145 g) provides 82 calories; carbohydrate, 20.5 g; fiber, 4.9 g; vitamin C, 20 mg; and small amounts of protein, fat, minerals and vitamins.

bluefish (*Pomatomus saltatrix*)   A silver and blue fish from the Atlantic Ocean neighboring the coasts of North and South America. This fish runs in schools that migrate north in spring along the eastern seaboard of North America and return southward in autumn. It is both an important game fish and a commercial food fish. The annual catch ranges from 3,000 to 4,000 tons in U.S. waters. Bluefish typically weigh 3 to 5 pounds and have a delicate flavor. Like most fish, it is an excellent protein source. The baked fish (100 g) provides 159 calories.

blue food colors   Colors approved by the U.S. FDA for use in candy and soft drinks. Blue ARTIFICIAL FOOD COLORS can be mixed with yellows (FD&C No. 5 and No. 6) to create shades of green. The safety of these dyes has been questioned. FD&C Blue No. 1 may cause chromosomal damage. FD&C Blue No. 2 may cause brain tumors in experimental animals. (See also DELANEY CLAUSE; FOOD ADDITIVES.)

body fat   See FAT.

body fluids   The water-based components of the body. Approximately 60% of the human body is water. This water occurs within cells, the intracellular (cytoplasmic) compartment, and outside cells, the extracellular compartment. Typically, 20% of body weight represents intracellular water, and in normal, healthy adults it accounts for about 55% of total body water; trained athletes have a higher percentage. Extracellular water represents the sum of the lymph, blood plasma (the fluid of blood), the interstitial fluid (the water between cells and tissues) and the water bound to the skeleton and connective tissue. Plasma accounts for about 4% of body weight.

To function normally, cells maintain an appropriate osmotic pressure (the pressure generated by two solutions of different compositions separated by a partially porous membrane like the cell wall). Cells of the body generally maintain an osmotic pressure equal to that of blood. Cells are in danger of swelling and rupturing if excessive water enters them, and they will shrink and eventually collapse if excessive water moves out of cells. Cells regulate osmotic pressure by maintaining potassium ions inside and pumping sodium out. Water follows these ions, as well as the movement of chloride. Thus movement of these simple ELECTROLYTES plays a major role in water balance.

Circulating body fluids, the blood and the lymph, are buffered against extreme variation in pH (a relative measure of the degree of acidity and alkalinity of a solution) by proteins, inorganic ions, bicarbonate and phosphate, which bind an excess of acid (hydrogen ions) and neutralize bases. They help buffer the blood at a value of 7.3 to 7.4. A lower pH leads to acidosis (excessively low pH). A pH greater than 7.4 leads to alkalosis (excessively alkaline pH). Either imbalance can be dangerous.

body mass index (BMI)   A standard for body weight based upon the measurements of height and weight. This is one of the most useful relationships: It can be used to assess health risks associated with overweight and it can be used as a therapeutic guide. There is a high degree of correlation between BMI and body fat determined from density measurements. BMI is based upon surveys of lean adults between the ages of 20 and 29. To calculate this index of fatness, first divide the weight by the height in inches squared,

then multiply the result by 705. The normal BMI ranges between 20 and 25. A BMI under 20 is considered underweight. A value 30 or greater falls into the category of OBESITY. Nonetheless, there is no clear-cut, absolute standard for deciding if an individual is overweight or underweight. (See also ADIPOSE TISSUE; FAT; HEIGHT-WEIGHT TABLES; LEAN BODY MASS; OBESITY.)

bok choy (*Brassica chinensis*; Chinese mustard cabbage, pak-choi)   A type of Chinese cabbage resembling celery, with dark-green leaves. The leaves are smooth and elongated and are generally 8 to 18 inches long. Bok choy does not form a heart, unlike petsai, another commonly used Chinese cabbage. Bok choy has a mild flavor. It can be eaten raw in salads and coleslaw, like celery, or it can be cooked in stir-fries and as a condiment for pork, fish and shellfish. Bok choy is a good source of beta carotene, fiber and vitamin C. One cup (170 g) provides 20 calories; protein, 2.6 g; carbohydrate, 3 g; fiber, 3.4 g; calcium, 158 mg; potassium, 630 mg; beta carotene, 437 retinol equivalents; and vitamin C, 44 mg.

bologna   A processed all-meat product. This large, seasoned sausage contains minced turkey, pork, beef, veal or a combination of these meats. The meat is packed into a casing and is usually smoked. One slice contains 289 mg sodium. This high sodium content is typical of sausage. It is worth noting that about one-third of Americans have hypertension (high blood pressure), and many of those who restrict their sodium intake will experience lowered blood pressure. Furthermore, high dietary sodium increases the risk of hypertension in some susceptible people who may eventually develop this condition.

Most bolognas can be considered high fat foods. Two slices (2 ounces) of luncheon meat in a sandwich is the average serving, as determined by the USDA. A rule of thumb is that 2 ounces of meat should supply no more than 2 grams of fat. Saturated fat accounts for most of the calories in bologna. The high levels of fat, especially saturated fat, in the typical American diet is linked to an increased risk of heart disease. DIETARY GUIDELINES FOR AMERICANS recommends a diet with less saturated fat. The chemical sodium NITRATE is often added as a preservative to processed meats, including bologna, to prevent the growth of bacteria that can cause food poisoning. Nitrite can react in the stomach with nitrogen-containing compounds called amines to yield cancer-causing compounds called nitrosoamines. One slice of bologna (one ounce, [28 g]) contains 89 calories; protein, 3.3 g; carbohydrate, 0.55 g; fat, 8 g; cholesterol, 16 mg; calcium, 3 mg; iron, 0.4 mg; and small amounts of the B complex: vitamins.

bolus   The mixture of food and saliva produced by chewing (mastication). To be digested efficiently, food must first be pulverized by teeth and mixed with saliva to ease swallowing. This disperses and lubricates food particles and eases their passage into the stomach and initiates starch digestion by the enzyme, salivary amylase. The act of swallowing moves the masticated food past the epiglottis and down into the esophagus, which transports it into the stomach. The downward movement of food is carried out by PERISTALSIS, waves of contraction of smooth muscles encircling the esophagus. In the stomach, the bolus becomes chyme, partially digested food mixed with GASTRIC JUICE. (See also DIGESTION; DIGESTIVE ENZYMES.)

bone A structure of hard (osseous) tissue consisting of blood vessels, nerves, osteocytes (cells capable of bone synthesis), and a matrix of inorganic salts, protein and mucopolysaccharides (acidic and sulfated carbohydrate chains).

Bones provide support and define the shape of the body. There are two structural arrangements in bone: external, compact bone is dense and hard; internal or calcaneus bone is porous and is found in most flat bones and at the ends of long bones of the arms and legs. Red bone marrow fills the cavities and the ends of some long bones and most flat bones. In adults red marrow is the site of synthesis of red blood cells and certain white blood cells (lymphocytes of the immune system and blood platelets required for clotting). The periosteum is the membrane covering bone surface that supplies the bone with nerves and blood vessels. Osteocytes absorb CALCIUM, MAGNESIUM and other nutrients from blood, which is supplied by an exterior blood vessel and capillary system. These cells crystallize the ions as an insoluble matrix of hydrated calcium phosphate (hydroxyapatite) and calcium carbonate. In fact, bone accounts for 99% of the calcium in the body. While mature bones have a fixed size and shape and are composed of crystalline materials, their chemical composition is constantly changing. Short-term changes occur when calcium is deposited in the boney matrix and is again released into the blood. Longer-term changes occur in both the chemical and the structural makeup during the aging process.

Several nutrients besides minerals play important roles in bone metabolism. VITAMIN D stimulates cells of the intestinal mucosa to take up calcium. A chronic deficiency of this vitamin leads to RICKETS (in children) and OSTEOMALACIA (in adults). VITAMIN C plays a role in collagen synthesis, required for bone deposition. A chronic deficiency leads to impaired calcification. VITAMIN K is implicated in bone formation also. Maturation of RED BLOOD CELLS and WHITE BLOOD CELLS, both critically important, requires vitamins (FOLIC ACID, VITAMIN B_{12}, VITAMIN B_6, VITAMIN A) and minerals (IRON, ZINC, BORON, MOLYBDENUM, among others). (See also OSTEOPOROSIS.)

bone disease See OSTEOMALACIA; OSTEOPOROSIS.

bone marrow in meat See MEAT.

bone meal Powdered bone obtained from livestock, long used as a supplemental source of CALCIUM and MAGNESIUM. Bone meal is no longer recommended. Analysis of many commercial products has revealed extensive LEAD contamination. It is probable that the livestock that supplied the bones were contaminated by widespread lead pollution. The fetus, infants and children are especially sensitive to lead, which can retard growth and development. A dose of three teaspoons can result in a lead intake close to the acceptable maximum daily intake for infants and children between six months and two years. Pregnant women and nursing women and children should not use bone meal; safer calcium supplements are available. (See also HEAVY METALS.)

bonito (*thunnus*) Various medium-sized tuna, related to mackerel. A migratory species, bonito inhabits both Pacific and Atlantic oceans and is harvested on a large scale and sold canned or fresh. Tuna is the most popular seafood in the United States and is considered an oily high-fat fish, rich in vitamins A and D. It is a relatively good source of Omega-3 essential fatty acids, which help reduce the risk of blood clotting. A 3 oz serving of tuna, packed in oil and drained, provides 140 to 200 calories; when packed in water it provides 90 to 110 calories. Both provide protein, 21 g; fat, 1 g; cholesterol, 40 to 60 mg, and calcium, 10 mg. Typically, salt added in processing contributes 300 to 500 mg of sodium per serving. The DIETARY GUIDELINES FOR AMERICANS recommends that salt and sodium be used only in moderation because of a risk of hypertension (high blood pressure) in susceptible individuals. A substantial number of people with hypertension can lower blood pressure by restricting sodium intake. Nutrient content is the same as ALBACORE tuna.

borage (*Borago officianalis*) A perennial, whose beautiful flowers have been used in cooking and in herbal preparations since Roman times. In folk medicine, borage is used to induce perspiration. The leaves are used to flavor salads and pasta. They can also be used as cooked greens and mixed with spinach. The flowers are used in salads as a garnish or in making a fragrant tea. Borage oil is one of the three major supplemental sources of GAMMA LINOLENIC ACID, the important polyunsaturated fatty acid that serves as a precursor of PROSTAGLANDINS (PG_1). The prostaglandins are hormone-like compounds that help regulate diverse physiologic processes. Due to life-style and dietary habits, production of this family of prostaglandins may be deficient in many Americans. The PG_1 prostaglandin family is a factor in widening blood vessels, reducing the tendency of blood to form clots, lowering cholesterol production, and regulating the immune system. Borage oil contains up to 26% gamma linolenic acid, more than is found in evening primrose oil or black currant oil. It also contains 40% linoleic acid, the omega-6 essential fatty acid from which gamma linolenic acid is derived.

boron An essential mineral nutrient found in trace amounts in most tissues. Although its precise role is unclear, boron may function in bone formation in both women and men and may also help prevent CALCIUM and MAGNESIUM losses in postmenopausal women. Boron seems to aid in the formation of steroid hormones (estrogen) and vitamin D, and it improves COPPER metabolism. A magnesium deficiency accentuates the effects of boron. As yet there is no Recommended Dietary Allowance (RDA) for boron because a requirement has not yet been quantified. An estimated safe and adequate daily intake is 1 to 3 mg for adults. Sources of boron include legumes, leafy vegetables and fruit; APPLES, GRAPES and PEARS are good sources. A varied diet would be expected to supply adequate amounts of this mineral. Excessive use of boron supplements can cause a dangerous overdose of boron.

Newnham, R.E., "Essentiality of Boron for Healthy Bones and Joints," *Environmental Health Perspectives*, 102:supplement (November 1994), pp. 83–85.

borsch (borscht) A traditional eastern European beet soup. Its characteristic red color is based on beets, a major ingredient. Recipes may specify adding white kidney beans, mushrooms and various amounts of other vegetables such as shredded cabbage, carrots, parsley and onions to beef or other stock and vinegar. Borsch may be served with diced stewmeat, sausage and sour cream. It may be served hot or cold. Beer, rather than wine, is appropriate with this dish.

bottled water Commercially bottled drinking WATER that may or may not be carbonated. Presently one out of every six households relies on bottled water. This growth in bottled water consumption comes from the growing awareness of the widespread pollution of municipal water sources by pesticides, fertilizers and industrial chemicals. Most bottled water comes from wells or springs. Bottled "drinking water" may be filtered water or distilled water with some minerals added. Bottled water is disinfected by ozone, not by chlorine treatment. Bottled water is classified as a food product by the U.S. FDA, but producers are not required to list the source.

Although bottled water may taste better than tap water, it may be no more healthful. The EPA sets water quality standards for most of the drinking water sources. However, there is no guarantee that a bottled water will be safer or more wholesome, because bottled water is less regulated than is tap water. The issue of bottled water safety was publicized when analyses revealed a popular, imported brand was contaminated with the organic solvent benzene, a carcinogen. Spot checks have turned up traces of other organic solvents, NITRITES and toxic HEAVY METALS in samples of bottled water, and the SODIUM content can be high. Consumers can request the latest chemical analysis of their preferred brand of water from the bottler.

The most common types of bottled water are:

- Club soda, which refers to tap water that is filtered, carbonated with carbon dioxide, and treated with minerals to give it flavor;
- Distilled water, which is purified by condensing steam. It contains no minerals but may contain volatile organic contaminants. Unless calcium and magnesium are added back, distilled water has a flat taste;
- Mineral water, which refers to any water containing minerals, although there is no federal standard to regulate them. California has a standard for the amount of dissolved minerals in its "mineral water";
- Natural sparkling water, which is initially naturally carbonated, then is reinjected with carbon dioxide to increase carbonation; and
- Seltzer, which is carbonated water. Often seltzer is tap water that has been filtered to remove organic materials, and then treated with carbon dioxide to provide carbonation.

Ward, Elizabeth, "Safe Drinking Water: Is Bottled Really Better," *Environmental Nutrition*, 17:10 (October 1994), p. 2.

bottle feeding See INFANT FORMULA.

botulism (botulinus poisoning) A rare though deadly form of food poisoning due to ingestion of a toxin produced by the anaerobic soil bacterium *Clostridium botulinum*. Several strains of *Clostridium botulinum* produce one of the most deadly natural toxins. It is estimated that a few

micrograms of the toxin could kill an adult. Botulinum toxins are neurotoxins, nerve poisons, which explains symptoms such as nausea, vomiting, sudden weakness and difficulty in breathing, speaking and swallowing; blurred vision; and headache. Paralysis and death can occur in two to 10 days. Early detection is a critical factor to assure timely treatment with botulinum antitoxin.

Infant botulism was first recognized in the United States in 1976, and it is now the most common form of botulism. In susceptible infants, the botulinum bacterium can propagate before the development of normal intestinal flora that would inhibit it. HONEY has been implicated as the probable source of botulism spores in some instances.

Botulism is becoming more common with the use of microwave cooking, which may not sterilize food completely. Botulism is usually associated with canned food, especially improperly home-canned non-acidic vegetables, such as string beans, sweetcorn, beets, asparagus, spinach and chard. Toxin production is favored when contaminated food is stored at neutral or slightly alkaline pH at room temperature for 12 to 24 hours away from air, and then not reheated before serving. Improperly stored restaurant foods (potato salad, pot pies, stews, turkey loaf, preserved meat, fish and milk), have been reported as causes of outbreaks of botulism. Low-acid foods that are not canned, such as salami and other processed meats, depend upon a combination of treatments to inhibit germination of *C. botulinum* spores and bacterial growth: mild heat treatment, the addition of sodium nitrite and other additives; and refrigeration.

To prevent botulism: When in doubt about the safety of a food, it should be discarded. Commercially canned goods that are swollen and home-canned products that have bubbles, discolorations or are cloudy should also be discarded. These are signs of improper canning. Cooked foods should be refrigerated, especially foods that are in a tight wrapping (such as a baked potato in foil or food coated with fat or batter, like sauteed onions). Food should be reheated thoroughly; 10 minutes of high heat destroys botulinum toxin. (See also AFLATOXIN; SALMONELLA.)

Lund, Barbara M., "Foodborne Diseases Due to Bacillus and Clostridium Species," *Lancet*, 336 (October 20, 1990), pp. 982–86.

bouillabaisse A traditional fish stew from southern France. Freshly caught Mediterranean fish are cooked with tomatoes and herbs and served on a bed of vegetables. Originally, bouillabaisse was cooked by fishermen using the least suitable fish for market, such as rockfish and easily obtained shellfish like mussels and small crabs. According to legend, this fisherman's stew was divinely inspired and brought to humans by angels. A variety of whitefish and shellfish can be substituted for the traditional ones, including salmon, whiting, bass, lobster, crab, prawns and eel. The seafood is marinated in olive oil, tomatoes, onions, garlic, parsley, thyme, bay leaf, shredded orange peel, and salt and pepper before boiling.

bouillon The clear broth obtained from boiling vegetables, meat or poultry. Bouillon forms the base for a variety of dishes, soups and sauces. Commercially prepared bouillons contain high levels of sodium. Though they possess appetizing flavors, they are not nutrient-dense foods: Beef bouillon concentrate (one package) provides 15 calories; protein 1 g; carbohydrate, 1 g; fat, 1 g; and sodium, 1,019 mg; and only very small amounts of other minerals and vitamins.

bovine growth hormone (bGH; bovine somatotropin)

A genetically engineered hormone designed to increase MILK output from dairy cows. The U.S. FDA approved general use of bGH on cows; its assessment is that MEAT or milk from bGH-treated cows is nutritionally identical to milk from untreated animals. Controversy surrounding the application of this synthetic drug focuses on several issues. Though all milk contains growth hormone, the synthetic drug differs from the natural bovine growth hormone in structure, by 49 amino acids added from human growth hormone. (Bovine and human insulin-like growth factors are very similar and are not destroyed by pasteurization.) Differences in allergenicity (ability to cause an allergic reaction) can be expected, even though bGH itself seems to be biologically inactive in humans. The hormone increases the level of an insulin-like growth factor (IGF-1) in cow's milk, higher than that found in breastmilk, and its effects, if any, on children's upper GASTROINTESTINAL TRACT are unknown. Possible adverse effects in cows include mastitis (infected udders). This would require treatment with antibiotics that could get into the milk. The FDA has issued assurances that milk is tested for antibiotic contamination. (See also BREASTFEEDING; GENETIC ENGINEERING.)

National Institutes of Health Technology Assessment Conference Statements, "Bovine Somatotropin and the Safety of Cows' Milk," *Nutrition Reviews*, 49:8 (1991), pp. 227–32.

brain chemicals   See ENDORPHINS; NEUROTRANSMITTER.

bran, oat

The outer, protective coating of the oat kernel. Oat bran is a good source of SILICON, a trace mineral needed for healthy joints and for normal bone growth. Oat bran supplies a water-soluble form of FIBER called beta glucan. Like cellulose, oat fiber is a POLYSACCHARIDE composed of glucose units. Because of the manner in which the glucose units are joined, the carbohydrate chain is not digestible, and because of its "kinks," it is water-soluble and viscous. This differs chemically from water-insoluble fiber, like wheat bran, which is the kind of fiber usually found in bran breakfast cereals. Oat bran causes less bloating or diarrhea than is typical with an overdose of wheat bran.

Gel-like fiber often exerts physiologic effects. Soluble fiber reduces the rate of glucose absorption and insulin response after a meal, thus increasing glucose tolerance. Oat bran may help decrease blood FAT and blood CHOLESTEROL, especially the undesirable LOW-DENSITY LIPOPROTEIN (LDL) form, even in diabetics. Elevated LDL is associated with an increasing risk of heart disease. Regular consumption of oat bran and oat meal can lead to a modest reduction in blood cholesterol levels. Even a study purporting to show that oat bran lowers cholesterol by lowering fat intake suggested that a high oat fiber selectively lowered LDL, not HDL (the desirable form of cholesterol). The specific link between oat bran and lowered blood cholesterol has not been resolved. More generally, a diet high in fiber from vegetables, fruits, whole grains and legumes, together with healthy life-style habits, forms a foundation for heart disease prevention.

The ability of oat bran to lower blood cholesterol launched a health food fad that dramatically increased sales of oat and bran cereals. Though the data continues to suggest that including oats in the diet is beneficial, oat bran is only one of a large number of sources of water-soluble fiber. Barley, for example, contains fat-soluble substances called tocotrienols that suppress cholesterol synthesis by the liver. Furthermore, most foods contain both soluble and insoluble forms of fiber. Even oat bran contains 60% insoluble fiber. What seems clear is that eating more COMPLEX CARBOHYDRATES such as whole grains and cereal products, beans, vegetables and fruit, together with daily EXERCISE, can significantly lower blood cholesterol in most adults. (See also OATS.)

bran, wheat (roughage)

The outer coat of kernels of wheat. Though wheat bran contains vitamins, and minerals like CALCIUM and phosphate, most attention has focused on its FIBER content. Wheat bran represents a rich source of water-insoluble fiber that is mainly cellulose. Bleached flour is deficient in bran because bran is lost during milling and is not added back during ENRICHMENT. Wheat bran is typically included in bran breakfast cereals. Bran flakes (wheat cereals) contain approximately 40% bran.

Insoluble fiber is implicated in maintaining the health of the gastrointestinal tract in several ways. Bran adds bulk and relieves constipation because it absorbs water, making the stool soft. It reduces the transit time (the time taken for the passage of material from the mouth through the gastrointestinal tract). Dietary fiber also normalizes rapid transit time caused by diarrhea due to IRRITABLE BOWEL SYNDROME. Colon cancer is primarily a disease of developing countries. In searching for an explanation, investigations have shown that, in animals, diets high in fat and low in insoluble fiber are linked to colon cancer. Population studies indicate that countries whose populations are characterized by diets rich in grains and vegetables have lower cancer rates than does the United States. The standard American diet supplies only 30% to 50% of the soluble and insoluble fiber estimated to reduce the risk of diseases of the colon, including colon cancer. Nonetheless, the connection between colon cancer and fiber is not clear-cut. In some studies bran offered protection from colon cancer; in others, it had no effect. Researchers propose that fiber can bind bile salts and toxic materials and speed up their passage, with wastes, through the intestine. The toxins would then have less time to damage the colon. Another explanation is that about 50% of cellulose is degraded by colon bacteria, producing SHORT-CHAIN FATTY ACIDS, which have anticancer properties.

Individuals who choose to supplement with bran should add it to their diet slowly to allow the body to adjust. Suddenly increasing fiber intake can cause bloating, cramping and diarrhea. Individuals with serious diseases of the digestive tract, such as ulcerative COLITIS, should not supplement with fiber without consulting a specialist. A fiber intake exceeding 35 to 40 g daily may bind essential mineral nutrients like calcium and limit their absorption. One-half cup (18 g) of wheat bran provides 38 calories; protein, 2.9 g; carbohydrate, 11.1 g; fiber, 7.9 g; fat, 0.83 g; calcium, 21 mg; iron, 2.0 mg; zinc, 2.3 mg; thiamin, 0.14 mg; riboflavin, 0.06 mg; niacin, 4.9 mg. (See also BRAN, OAT.)

branched chain amino acids   A family of three essential dietary amino acids used as protein building blocks. LEUCINE, ISOLEUCINE and VALINE are classified as branched chain amino acids because they possess a branched structure. All three are essential amino acids because the body is unable to synthesize these structures. Branched chain amino acids are largely absorbed from the bloodstream and broken down by skeletal muscle in response to insulin. In the first step of their metabolism, amino (nitrogen) groups are removed by transamination, a process dependent upon vitamin B_6, leaving the carbon skeletons as keto acids. The keto acids are then oxidized in the mitochondria for energy production. The multienzyme complex that oxidizes the carbon skeletons of all three amino acids is more active with high protein diets. It has been proposed that the branched chain amino acids may enhance skeletal muscle adaptation to exercise training. Blood levels of branched chain amino acids are low in chronic renal failure and in encephalopathy, and supplemental amino acids have been used for critically ill patients.

Brazil nut (*Bertholletia excelsa*)   The large edible seed of an evergreen tree that grows wild in the Amazonian rain forest of South America. The tree is considered a renewable resource of the rain forest. The hard-walled fruit is 4 to 6 inches in diameter with several inch-long seeds arranged around a center, like the sections of an orange. The shell of the nut is triangular, and the very oily, creamy seed within has a rich flavor. Brazil nuts are available roasted in oil or dry roasted. One ounce (28 g, 7 nuts) provides 186 calories; fat, 18.8 g; protein, 4.1 g; carbohydrate, 3.6 g; fiber, 2.52 g; and small amounts of iron, zinc, thiamin and niacin.

bread   A baked food consisting of flour, water or other liquid as the main ingredients. The many varieties available indicate the ethnic diversity of bread: bagels, baguettes, crumpets, matzo, pumpernickel, sourdough, tortillas and whole wheat are a few of the varieties sold in the United States. Unleavened breads like matzo and tortillas were the first breads. The invention of leavened bread is attributed to the ancient Egyptians. As a staple of the standard American diet, leavened bread is prepared with yeast or baking soda to make the dough rise before baking.

Bread is one of the best sources of complex CARBOHYDRATE. The carbohydrate in bread is starch, its main ingredient. Complex carbohydrate digests slowly to the simple sugar glucose. The slow rise in blood sugar requires a modest output of the hormone insulin to regulate blood sugar levels. The current recommendations specify obtaining 50 to 60% of daily CALORIES from complex carbohydrates. Contrary to popular opinion, breads are not "fattening" unless you exceed your daily limit of calories from all sources needed to equal those burned for energy. Bread is much less fattening than high-fat foods like processed meats, cheese and fried foods. However, spreading BUTTER, MARGARINE or mayonnaise on a slice of bread doubles its calories. "Reduced calorie bread" contains half the usual calories, 20 calories a slice; bread may be made with powdered CELLULOSE as a non-caloric filler to lower calories.

Usually a bread is named after the grain from which the flour or meal is derived. An estimated 75% of Americans eat white bread and the remainder eat whole WHEAT and RYE. Wheat flour is ideal for leavened bread because wheat contains gluten, a protein that becomes sticky when mixed with water. Dough made from wheat flour is elastic enough to rise, as bubbles of carbon dioxide become trapped, thus creating light textured bread. In contrast, breads made with only low gluten flour will tend to be heavy (dense). The liquid used to prepare the dough affects the bread flavor and quality. Water produces bread with a stiff crust; milk produces a more tender crust and increases the nutritive value of bread. Added sugar helps brown the crust and helps yeast ferment, while fat may be added by bakers to make softer and lighter breads. Bread is a major contributor of carbohydrate, SODIUM, NIACIN, THIAMIN and IRON to the American diet, because so much of this enriched food is eaten. The sodium in bread comes from baking soda, the major ingredient of baking powder.

White bread is prepared from bleached flour, which is highly refined (purified). Milling and bleaching removes or partially removes over 22 important materials like FIBER, VITAMINS and MINERALS. To make up for a portion of this depletion, bakeries add back only four: thiamin, niacin, riboflavin and iron partially replace lost nutrients (ENRICHMENT). Other nutrients such as vitamin B_6 zinc, manganese and FOLIC ACID are not added. Because flour is so widely used, producers add iron to increase the daily intake of this mineral, and because white bread contains only half a gram of fiber a slice, bakeries sometimes increase the fiber content by adding dates, raisins or purified, powdered cellulose. Crystalline cellulose may not function in the body in the same way as the natural cellulose that occurs in the bran of whole wheat bread.

Whole-grain breads provide 2 to 3 grams of fiber per slice. Bread labeled "whole wheat" must contain 100% whole wheat as the first listed ingredient. Bread simply labeled as "wheat" or "cracked wheat" often contains white flour as the major ingredient; the brown color of such bread may be due to caramel coloring. Bread labeled "multigrain" may simply mean that the bread contains mainly refined wheat flour with small amounts of oatmeal, rye or whole wheat. The label should indicate whether caramel coloring has been added to give the bread a more wholesome appearance. One slice of whole wheat bread typically provides 70 calories; protein, 3 g; carbohydrates 12.7 g; fiber, 3.17 g; fat, 1.2 g; iron, 0.96 mg; sodium, 180 mg; thiamin, 0.1 mg; riboflavin, 0.06 mg; and niacin, 1.07 mg. One slice of white, enriched bread typically provides 65 calories; protein, 2.1 g; carbohydrate, 12.2 g; fiber, 0.68 g; fat, 1 g; iron, 0.71 mg; sodium, 129 mg; thiamin, 0.12 mg; riboflavin, 0.08 mg; and niacin, 0.94 mg.

breadfruit (*Artocarpus communis; A. altilis*)   The starchy fruit of a tree belonging to the mulberry family, which originated in southern Asia and Polynesia. Historically, breadfruit was a dietary staple among Asians and Pacific Islanders, and in Tahiti and other islands of the South Pacific breadfruit has a legendary importance. From its early origins in Southeast Asia it spread to Hawaii, and Europeans transported it to the Caribbean in the late 18th century. It is now grown from India to Jamaica. The closely related jackfruit is more widespread because it is hardier.

The egg-shaped fruit has a thick, pebbled skin and can weigh up to 5 pounds. The starchy flesh has a bread-like texture; its nutrient content is similar to that of wheat bread and it is eaten as a vegetable. The white to yellowish pulp sweetens as it ripens. When green, breadfruit tastes like potato. As it ripens breadfruit resembles the sweet potato and is used similarly. Canned or frozen breadfruit is available in markets catering to ethnic cuisines. Breadfruit with seeds can be eaten raw, or the seeds can be roasted like chestnuts. All seedless varieties must be cooked to be palatable. Breadfruit can be cooked like potatoes in recipes. It is boiled or roasted and can be added to stews and cooked as fritters. The ripened fruit can be baked as a pudding. Uncooked breadfruit (100 g) provides 114 calories; protein, 1.1 g; carbohydrate, 27.1 g; fiber, 1.5 g; fat, 0.23 g; thiamin, 0.34 mg; riboflavin, 0.17 mg; niacin, 2.1 mg; vitamin C, 26 mg.

breakfast   The first meal of the day, or morning meal, usually ends the 6- to 10-hour fast due to sleep. During slumber, blood sugar levels are maintained by the liver through the breakdown of glycogen (the storage polymer of glucose) and the synthesis of glucose from amino acids. Breakfast provides energy and replenishes glucose stores.

Meal skipping is an emerging pattern; roughly a quarter of the U.S. population claims to never eat breakfast. Breakfast skipping is most prevalent among 19- to 34-year-olds, while consistent breakfast eaters seem to be older. For those who eat breakfast, often it is a high calorie meal. Consider a typical American breakfast that provides more than 600 calories, with 40% of the calories from fat and more than 500 mg of cholesterol: two fried eggs (200 calories, 8 g fat), two slices of buttered white bread (220 calories, 9 g fat); coffee with 1 tablespoon cream with sugar (46 calories, 3 g fat); two slices of bacon (86 calories, 8 g fat)—rounded out with a glass of orange juice (90 calories). Such a breakfast can be converted to a low-fat meal with simple changes: two poached eggs (164 calories, 5.8 g fat); one cup of decaffeinated coffee with low-fat milk (12 calories); a large orange (58 calories); and two rice cakes (70 calories) or a slice of whole wheat toast without butter (70 calories)—total 304 calories, with 20% calories from fat. The cholesterol remains at 476 mg; this could be cut in half by eating a single egg.

The typical continental breakfast is a low-cholesterol meal: a cup of tea (no calories) or a cup of coffee with cream, 46 calories, 3 g fat; two buttered English muffins with honey or preserves, 373 calories, 7.6 g fat. Cholesterol from cream and butter amounts to 72 mg.

breakfast cereal   A food prepared from grains, WHEAT, CORN, RICE and OATS that is served hot or cold at breakfast. Cold breakfast cereals are one of the most common breakfasts. The basic ingredients of cold, ready-to-eat breakfast cereals remain unchanged from the 19th century, when they were invented. Only the processing of grain and the packaging has changed. Brands may add other grains, such as barley, quinoa or amaranth. Most flour used in breakfast cereals is still bleached. Grain is processed by being pressed into feeders, shredded and formed into biscuits, extruded into a shape that appeals to the consumer, or "pulped."

The label on breakfast cereals supplies nutritional information based on a serving size, usually 1 ounce or only a quarter cup. When estimating the actual amounts consumed by individuals, it is important to multiply the SODIUM, fat and sugar content by the number of servings actually eaten. Pouring half a cup of whole milk on a bowl of cereal adds 4 grams of fat and 75 extra calories. Skim milk adds 45 calories and no fat. Each adds 4 grams of protein.

Various additives are also used during processing. Sweeteners (including table sugar or corn syrup), salt, flavorings, preservatives, vitamins or minerals are added when enriched. Nuts and raisins are other nutritious additions to breakfast cereals. There is no nutritional need to add sugar (sucrose) to cereals, and several varieties do not contain added sugar: puffed rice, puffed wheat and shredded wheat. Ironically, these same cereals are the lowest in FIBER. At the other extreme are cereals designed to appeal to children's attraction to sweets. Fruit Loops, Marshmallow Crispies and Honey Smacks (Kellogg); Boo Berries, Count Chocula, Franken Berry (General Mills); and Fruity Pebbles, Super Golden Crisp (Post) provide about 13 grams (2.5 teaspoons) of sugar per ounce of cereal. Many other cereals contain more than 300 mg of sodium per ounce (more than potato chips). Often cereals with the most sugar contain the least salt.

The fiber in ready-to-eat breakfast cereals is mainly wheat bran, which is essentially insoluble fiber. The body needs both the insoluble and soluble forms of fiber provided by a balanced diet. At the top of the list of high-fiber cereals are All Bran (Kellogg) with extra fiber and Fiber One (General Mills), which provide 12 to 13 g of fiber per ounce. Other bran cereals provide 5 to 6 g of fiber per ounce. Some bran-enriched cereals also contain sugar, however. The amounts of fiber in other typical cereals made with refined flour and without bran are: cold oat cereals, 0.9 g per cup; crisp rice, 0.12 g; corn flakes, 0.4 g.

With the growing consumer awareness of the importance of whole grains, GRANOLAS have become popular. These typically contain vegetable oil to make them tastier. Thus a cup of commercially prepared granola can easily provide 600 calories or more. Such granolas often contain saturated fats and coconut and palm oils, though they can still be described as "100 percent natural cereal" on the label.

Hot breakfast cereals prepared from whole grains include oatmeal, creamed wheat, creamed rice, corn grits and whole wheat cereals. Unless fortified, the levels of calcium, vitamin A, thiamin, riboflavin and niacin in these cereals are generally less than in fortified, ready-to-eat cereals. On the other hand, hot cereals contain much less sodium, unless it is added during preparation. Only the quick cereals, which are simply added to hot water, contain substantial amounts of salt (240 to 260 mg sodium per packet). The fiber content varies depending upon the grain. Oatmeal or rolled oats provide 9.2 g of fiber per cup in a mixture of soluble and insoluble types of fiber. At the other end of the scale is creamed wheat, which provides much less fiber, 0.37 to 0.64 g per cup. (See also BRAN, WHEAT; FOOD LABELING.)

Liebman, Bonnie and Hurley, Jayne, "How to Pick a Cereal," *Nutrition Action Healthletter*, 22:5 (June 1995), pp. 11–13.

breast cysts (fibrocystic breast disease, chronic cystic mastitis)   Nodular breast cysts, usually affecting both breasts, are associated with premenstrual breast swelling and tenderness. Fibrocystic breast disease is the most common disorder of the breast. This condition accounts for more than half of breast surgery in the United States. An estimated 20 to 40% of women under age 50 have breast lumps. Fibrotic cysts are not malignant, but the only way to positively identify a lump is with a biopsy. The cause of this condition is unknown, although apparently an increased ratio of estrogen to progesterone favors fibrocystic disease. The occurrence of cystic breast disease often correlates with premenstrual syndrome (PMS), family history, exposure to estrogens from drugs and birth control pills, early menstruation, late menopause, cigarette smoking, glandular imbalances and a diet high in SATURATED FAT and calories.

Changing the diet may help prevent breast cysts. A COMPLEX CARBOHYDRATE diet, with reduced consumption of white FLOUR and SUGAR, and reduced FAT, especially SATURATED FAT and animal products, may be advised. Eliminating caffeine-containing beverages and foods (COFFEE, TEA, COLA SOFT DRINKS, CHOCOLATE and COCOA) has been reported to reduce breast tenderness. Caffeine and related theophylline and theobromine ALKALOIDS that stimulate production of fibrous tissue and cyst fluid. Vitamin E may relieve PMS symptoms, perhaps by helping to normalize blood levels of hormones. Iodine has been used to treat breast cysts. Thyroid hormone treatment may be helpful. High fiber normalizes bowel function, which may play a role in estrogen metabolism by increasing estrogen excretion. Vitamin B complex deficiency may also be linked to PMS and fibrocystic breast disease.

Vobecky J., Simard A., Vobecky J.S., Ghadirian P., Lamothe-Guay, M., Falardeau, M., "Nutritional Profiles of Women with Fibrocystic Breast Disease," *International Journal of Epidemiology*, 22:6 (1993), pp. 989–99.

Ghent, W.R. et al., "Choose Molecular Iodine to Treat Fibrocystic Breast Disease," *Modern Medicine*, 62 (April 1994), pp. 54–55.

breastfeeding (nursing)   Feeding an infant with breast milk. In general, health experts recommend breastfeeding for four to six months after an infant's birth, when breast milk can supply all the baby's requirements. The American Academy of Pediatrics recommends breastfeeding at least during the first one to two weeks after birth because the milk that is produced during this time, COLOSTROM, contains the mother's antibodies, which protect the baby while the immune system develops. Consequently, breastfed babies have a lower rate of diarrhea and respiratory infections. Colostrum also contains a unique blend of PROTEIN, FAT and CARBOHYDRATE for the newborn infant. Furthermore, initial breastfeeding may enhance the return of the mother's uterus and body to the non-pregnant state. Breastfeeding offers many advantages. Bonding between mother and child is enhanced by nursing, and studies indicate that this promotes the child's healthy development. Breastfeeding can help the infant's digestive system mature faster and take up nutrients more efficiently. Breast milk helps feed the infant's digestive tract with friendly bacteria to minimize intestinal infections. Breastfeeding and postponing the introduction of solid foods may decrease the risk of food allergies.

Breastfeeding affords advantages beyond infancy, including a decreased risk of childhood cancer, Crohn's disease, ear infections and respiratory infections. ALCOHOL, nicotine, CAFFEINE, marijuana and certain medications pass into breast milk and may affect a baby's development. Therefore medications not approved by a physician should be avoided if possible. Drinking more than a quart of cow's milk a day can introduce cow protein into the mother's own milk, causing an allergy. In some babies colic is caused by cow's milk proteins that pass through the mother's milk.

Milk production is a major metabolic burden. The nursing mother needs considerably more calories to produce milk composed of energy-rich nutrients, protein, fat and carbohydrate than non-lactating women. Together these nutrients represent an energy content of 670 to 770 calories per liter of human milk. Assuming a maternal efficiency conversion factor of 80% and a daily milk production of 750 ml (0.75 l), approximately 600 extra calories per day would be required by the lactating woman. The mother's physiology changes during breastfeeding so she can use her fat stores gained during pregnancy to help provide the extra calories needed for lactation. Consequently an average of 500 calories per day is recommended during lactation for women whose gestational weight gain was normal. This metabolic shift may explain the typical problem of weight gain after pregnancy.

Certain nutrient needs increase from their pregnancy levels. The nursing mother needs more protein (65 vs. 60 mg daily); more vitamin A (1,300 vs. 800 mcg); vitamin E (12 mg vs. 10 mg); more vitamin C (95 mg vs. 70 mg); and other vitamins and minerals. From the B COMPLEX, the nursing mother needs thiamin, 1.6 mg; riboflavin, 0.8 mg; niacin, 20 mg; vitamin B_6, 21 mg; folacin, 280 mg; and vitamin B_{12}, 2.6 mcg). Also needed are vitamin C (95 mg) and the MINERALS calcium, 1,200 mg; phosphorous, 1,200 mg; magnesium, 355 mg; zinc, 19 mg; iodine, 200 mcg; and selenium, 75 mcg; and vitamin D, 10 mcg; and vitamin K, 65 mg. The diet should include MEAT, FISH and POULTRY, dried beans and peas for protein, fat and minerals; fruits and vegetables for fiber and vitamins A and C; complex carbohydrates like pasta, brown rice and whole wheat bread for energy and trace minerals. Requirements for calcium may be too great to be met without supplements.

In spite of the clear-cut benefits of breastfeeding and the recommendation of health experts, breastfeeding declined in the 1980s in the United States. Among African-American women the rate fell from 33% to 23% during that time. Rather than a reflection of a larger percentage of women in the workforce, public health officials propose that other factors are involved: Hospitals do not provide enough support for breastfeeding, and free formula is provided to low-income mothers under the Women, Infants and Children Program. However, extra food coupons are also issued to women who are breastfeeding, and consultants are available to breastfeeding clients. The choice to breastfeed involves different behavior and possibly changes in attitudes that can simplify the process. Resources are available for the expectant mother, including the La Leche League International, and she can enlist the support of her family and medical staff. Many health-care professionals do not know the basics of breastfeeding management. Limited evidence seems to indicate that breastfeeding is declining in low-income countries worldwide. For example, weaning seems to occur earlier in Latin America. In some countries, Jordan and Kenya among them, the levels of breastfeeding may be low enough to impact child health and mortality.

Regarding introduction of cow's milk, experts recommend that infants receive either breast milk or INFANT FORMULA for the first 12 months. When the baby is 12 months or older, whole milk may be used to substitute formula or breast milk, though optimally cow's milk could be withheld until the infant is two years old. The high casein content of cow's milk can increase gastrointestinal bleeding and lead to ANEMIA if introduced too soon.

Angier, Natalie, "Mother's Milk Found to be Potent Cocktail of Hormones," *New York Times*, May 24, 1994.

Rasmussen, K.M., "The Influence of Maternal Nutrition in Lactation," *Annual Review of Nutrition*, 12 (1992), pp. 103–17.

breast milk   Breast milk is optimally balanced to nurture the infant during the first months. It is rich in sugar lactose and has substantial fat (3.8%) for efficient energy production. Human MILK contains both essential fatty acids (linoleic and linolenic), easily digested protein, and a high level of free amino acids and other non-protein nitrogen (25% of the total nitrogen). Special products like CARNITINE and TAURINE, believed to be important in infant metabolism, are present. The cholesterol content is relatively high, reflecting its importance in early development. Breast milk is relatively low in sodium and minerals, in accord with the limited capacity of the infant's immature kidneys to handle dissolved substances. The iron content, though low, is highly absorbable. Zinc, too, is better absorbed from breast milk. The calcium-to-phosphorus ratio is ideal for calcium absorption. The vitamin content (including vitamin C) to support infant growth is ample. Vitamin D content is low, though adequate for a normal-term infant.

The importance of omega-3 fatty acids in infant nutrition is suggested by the high level of the polyunsaturated fatty acid, DOCASOHEXAENOIC ACID (DHA), required in brain growth and development of the retina. DHA cannot be formed by preterm infants because their livers are not mature enough to synthesize it from essential fatty acids. Breast milk contains a complex mixture of hormones and growth factors, whose role in infant development is poorly understood. Thus milk contains unusually high levels of gonadotropin-releasing hormone, which could affect development of the newborn's sex organs. It also contains the hormone melatonin, possibly regulating the infant's internal clock; oxytocin, which could promote bonding between infant and mother; and thyroid hormones, which could stimulate the infant's immune system. Breast milk provides endorphins, which act as painkillers and growth factors—nerve growth factor, epidermal growth factor and insulin-like growth factor—that regulate development of the brain and digestive organs.

Pollutants in Breast Milk

Breast milk often contains traces of environmental pollutants, including pesticides and herbicides; industrial chemicals such as halogenated hydrocarbons (PBBs, PCBs, dioxin, cleaning solvents); and toxic heavy metals (cadmium, lead, mercury). These pollutants are insidious: They are odorless and colorless, they are not biodegradable, and they accumulate in animals and fish and in the people who eat them. Many pollutants slowly leave the body when there is no further exposure, while the body may accumulate halogenated hydrocarbons and toxic heavy metals (mercury and cadmium) throughout life.

The fetus and infant are very sensitive to halogenated hydrocarbons and toxic heavy metals. Significant exposure to these industrial chemicals increases the risk of cancer, abnormalities and learning disabilities in children. The effects of chronic exposure to trace levels of these materials and whether there are any additive effects due to exposure to mixtures of pollutants, are not known. The UN's World Health Organization, the EPA and the LaLeche League argue that the advantages of breastfeeding outweigh any potential disadvantages. Concerned mothers can have their milk tested at their local health department.

Pregnant and nursing women may be advised to minimize exposure to toxic pollutants by avoiding certain ocean fish (shark, ocean perch, halibut, striped bass, bluefish and swordfish) that are most likely to be contaminated. Among freshwater fish, catfish, brook and lake trout, freshwater perch and bass, walleye pike and whitefish caught in polluted waters are likely to be contaminated. Washing vegetables thoroughly and consuming homegrown produce or certified organic produce reduce exposure to pesticides. (See also ACIDOPHILUS; BIFIDUS FACTOR; INFANT FORMULA.)

brewer's yeast (*Saccharomyces cerivisiae*)   A single-celled organism, related to molds and fungi, that ferments sugars to ethanol (ALCOHOL) under anaerobic conditions (oxygen excluded). Brewer's yeast is a by-product of BEER and ale production. It is used as a nutritional yeast when grown in the presence of VITAMIN B$_{12}$ and other nutrients. This yeast is an excellent source of PROTEIN, B COMPLEX, IRON and other nutrients, including organically complexed chromium in the form of GLUCOSE TOLERANCE FACTOR. Unlike BAKER'S YEAST, which is not a rich source of vitamins and minerals, nutritional yeast does not contain living cells. Yeast products are not recommended for those with yeast infections. One tablespoon of dry brewer's yeast provides 25 calories; protein, 3.1 g; carbohydrate, 3.1 g; calcium 6 to 60 mg; iron, 1.4 mg; zinc, 0.63 mg; thiamin, 1.25 mg; riboflavin, 0.34 mg; and niacin, 3.16 mg.

brine   A concentrated solution of table salt (sodium chloride) used to preserve vegetables, FISH and MEAT. A pickling brine can be prepared by dissolving 50 g table salt in 500 ml (1 pint) of water. Vegetables such as cauliflower and cucumber soaked overnight are usually stored in pickling spices and vinegar. (See also SODIUM.)

broad bean (*Vicia faba*; fava bean, horse bean)   A large, flat bean resembling a lima bean. This legume is cultivated as a staple food, as well as fodder, worldwide. Its origins can be traced to Africa, where broad beans were cultivated by ancient Egyptians perhaps 4,000 years ago. Ancient Greeks recommended broad beans for improved athletic performance. Broad beans are a part of traditional Mediterranean cuisine and are a very popular food in the Middle East.

Broad beans occur in flat pods that can be very large, up to 18 inches long. Fresh, shelled beans should be thoroughly cooked, and the outer layer or skin is often removed. Varieties of broad beans may be green, brown or white after cooking. Young pods are cooked like green beans. Dried beans are usually soaked overnight and then cooked, with or without the skin. Broad beans are to be avoided by individuals who have an inherited sensitivity called FAVISM. This hemolytic syndrome (breaking down red blood cells) occurs in people of the Mediterranean regions (Sardinia, southern Italy, Greece, Turkey, Cyprus and Egypt), in Iran and in China. In severe cases ingestion of fresh broad beans can cause hemolytic anemia, an anemia caused by the rupture of fragile red blood cells. The toxic factors are apparently small, non-protein compounds, vicine and convicine. The dried flat beans are rich in protein, fiber, B vitamins and trace minerals. Uncooked broad beans contain (100 g): 76 calories; protein, 3.2 g; carbohydrate, 14.7 g; fiber, 1.7 g; fat, 0.5 g; calcium, 26 mg; vitamin A, 13.5 retinol equivalents; thiamin, 0.34 mg; riboflavin, 0.17 mg; niacin, 2.1 mg.

broccoli (*Brassica aleracea*)   A dark-green vegetable with small, tight heads (curds) mounted on stem-like buds. A member of the cabbage (Brassica) family of CRUCIFEROUS VEGETABLES, closely related to CAULIFLOWER and BRUSSELS SPROUTS. Broccoli is one of the most popular vegetables of this group. Both stems and heads are edible. Broccoli originated in Italy, where the name is derived from the Italian word *broccolo*, meaning a cabbage sprout, and was first cultivated in the 17th or 18th century.

Broccoli and other cruciferous vegetables produce nitrogen-containing materials called indoles and ISOTHIO-CYANATES that may reduce the risk of some forms of CANCER. Indoles seem to stimulate liver enzymes that modify the female hormone estrogen, making it less active and possibly reducing the risk of breast cancer. Broccoli and other cruciferous vegetables also contain isothiocyanates and sulfur compounds that stimulate the liver to produce detoxifying enzymes that help block the action of cancer-causing agents. Of particular interest is SULFORAPHANE, which specifically increases the level of so-called phase 2 detoxication enzymes, which attach highly water soluble chemicals such as glutathione, taurine, glycine and sugar derivatives to altered toxins so they can be more readily excreted. Broccoli is also an excellent source of FIBER, vitamin A precursor (beta carotene) and vitamin C, and it contains ample amounts of folic acid, niacin, iron and calcium. The most common kind in the United States is called Italian green broccoli. One cup chopped and cooked (156 g) provides 46 calories; protein, 4.6 g; carbohydrate, 8.7 g; fiber, 6.4 g; calcium, 178 mg; iron, 1.8 mg; vitamin A, 220 retinol equivalents; thiamin, 0.13 mg; riboflavin, 0.32 mg; niacin, 1.18 mg; and vitamin C, 98 mg.

bromelain   A protein-digesting enzyme from pineapple. This enzyme occurs in the stems and fruit. Commercial sources come from Taiwan, Japan and Hawaii. Because fresh pineapple contains this enzyme, neither fresh pineapple nor pineapple juice can be used in gelatin-containing desserts and salads; the gelatin would be broken down.

Bromelain is used as a MEAT TENDERIZER and as a digestive aid when taken with meals. Bromelain is an effective substitute for pancreatic enzymes when their production is inadequate. It may be more effective when combined with pancreatin, a preparation of digestive enzymes from hog pancreas, and bile. Bromelain can inhibit blood platelet aggregation and improve angina pain and several, inflam-

matory conditions. Orally administered bromelain seems to reduce swelling, bruising, pain and healing time due to injuries. Bromelain inhibits platelet aggregation and increases fibromolytic activity ("clot busting" effect), consequently it has been used to treat thrombophlebitis, a potentially dangerous condition due to blood clotting. In addition, it has been used also to treat respiratory congestion and rheumatoid ARTHRITIS. Bromelain could possibly increase the risk of bleeding in patients taking blood thinning drugs and aspirin. (See also DIGESTION; DIGESTIVE ENZYMES.)

brominated vegetable oil (BVO)   A FOOD ADDITIVE used by soft drink manufacturers to disperse flavoring oils in fruit-flavored beverages and to render them cloudy to create an illusion of thickness. Vegetable oils, including COTTONSEED OIL, CORN OIL and OLIVE OIL, can be chemically modified by bromine.

Long assumed to be safe, BVO was used extensively in North America until a Canadian report demonstrated that BVO has caused organ damage in experimental animals. BVO residues accumulate in human tissues, but the long-term effects are unknown. BVO is no longer classified as a GENERALLY RECOGNIZED AS SAFE food additive by the U.S. FDA, which had granted interim approval in 1970.

bronchi   The two main branches of the trachea that form the major air passageways of the lung. Each bronchus joins to bronchial tubes, smaller branches further into the lung. Each bronchial tube in turn branches into bronchioles, even smaller subdivisions of the air passageway, where gas exchanges occur. Oxygen required by the body is absorbed, while the waste product of oxidation, carbon dioxide, diffuses from red blood cells into expired air.

Foreign objects such as seeds, nuts or bran can lodge in the bronchi and cause diseases such as bronchitis or lung abscesses. ANAPHYLAXIS, shock due to a severe allergy attack affecting the entire body, can lead to labored breathing with spasming and contraction of smooth muscle surrounding the bronchioles. See also ALLERGY.

brown rice   Unpolished rice, after the husk has been removed. Brown rice retains bran and GERM, which provide most of the nutrients, as well as FIBER. Much of the fiber is cellulose and is found chiefly in the outer bran layer. Starch occurs in the internal portion (endosperm) of the GRAIN, which has much less fiber. The higher cellulose content is the major reason brown rice needs to be cooked about twice as long as white rice. Brown rice retains lectins, a class of protein that bind to cell surfaces. This protein may be the cause of the occasional allergic reactions to brown rice. Brown rice has a delicate nut-like flavor. The cooking time is approximately 45 minutes. One cup cooked (195 g) provides 233 calories; carbohydrate, 49.7 g; protein, 4.9 g; fiber, 3.9 g; calcium, 23 mg; iron, 1.17 mg; niacin, 2.73 mg; thiamin, 0.18 mg; riboflavin, 0.04 mg.

brown sugar   Table sugar colored with a little molasses or caramelized sugar. Classified as a refined CARBOHYDRATE, brown sugar supplies EMPTY CALORIES, like other purified sweeteners. Brown sugar is nutritionally equivalent to table sugar. The nutrient content of one tablespoon is 52 calories;

carbohydrate, 15.6 g; calcium, 12 mg; potassium, 48 mg; and only traces of other minerals.

brussels sprouts (*Brassica oleracea*)   A vegetable of the cabbage family (CRUCIFEROUS VEGETABLES), characterized by a stem with rows of small heads resembling miniature cabbages. Brussels sprouts are one of the seven vegetables developed from the wild cabbage native to northwestern Europe. The cruciferous vegetables in general possess cancer-inhibiting properties, as shown by experiments with animals and by population studies. This seems to be due to their content of materials that block cancer-causing agents: FIBER, VITAMIN C and BETA CAROTENE. In addition indoles, nitrogen-containing compounds occurring in cruciferous vegetables, seem to block the action of estrogen and reduce the risk of breast cancer, while ISOTHIOCYANATES, sulfur-containing compounds, stimulate liver enzymes that block the action of carcinogens. One cup (cooked, 156 g) contains 60 calories; protein, 6 g; carbohydrate, 13.5 g; fiber, 5.62 g; fat, 0.8 g; iron, 1.88 mg; beta carotene, 112 retinol equivalents; niacin, 0.95 mg; thiamin, 0.17 mg; riboflavin, 0.12 mg; vitamin C, 97 mg.

buckwheat   A seed with a nut-like flavor used like a cereal grain. Buckwheat is not a true grain, nor is it related to wheat, which belongs to the grass family. Buckwheat is native to Siberia and Manchuria and was grown extensively in China for thousands of years. Three common varieties are Silverhead, Tartary and Japanese. Regions of the former Soviet Union are a major producers; other important producers include Poland, France, Canada and the United States, where production has steadily declined in the last decade. Buckwheat can be a suitable wheat substitute for those sensitive to wheat protein (gluten). However, for patients with CELIAC DISEASE (severe gluten sensitivity) buckwheat may be excluded from the diet, in addition to the cereal grains. Buckwheat has a high level of fiber and protein, though not of the quality of AMARANTH or QUINOA. Buckwheat flour has a distinctive flavor that can add variety to grain dishes. In the United States, buckwheat flour is often used in griddle cakes (pancakes). Buckwheat groats (kernels from which the hull has been removed) are roasted and served like rice in a traditional dish called kasha in the Soviet Union and Poland. Food value of 1 cup (175 g) has: calories, 586; protein, 20.5 g; carbohydrate, 128 g; fiber, 15.6 g; fat, 4.2 g; calcium, 200 mg; iron, 6.7 mg; zinc, 4.4 mg; thiamin, 1.1 mg; niacin, 7.7 mg; riboflavin, 0.26 mg.

buffer   A substance that resists changes in the pH of a solution. A buffer system protects a solution against large fluctuations in hydrogen ion concentration by compensating for increased acidity (additional hydrogen ions that would normally lower the pH), as well as for increased alkalinity (due to bases that would raise the pH).

The constancy of the pH of body fluids is critically important for the normal functioning of enzymes. Small changes in hydrogen ion concentration (pH) can change the overall electrical charge on enzymes, alter their shape and thus usually inhibit their catalytic function. Other processes, such as the transmission of nerve impulses and ion transport across membranes into cells, are also exquisitely sensitive to changes in pH.

The major buffers in the blood are serum proteins, HEMO-GLOBIN, BICARBONATE and phosphate. They maintain the pH of blood and body fluids near neutrality (pH 7.4) and thus help regulate acid-base balance. The bicarbonate buffer system is constantly resupplied by the body from carbon dioxide produced by metabolism. Nonetheless, these buffers have limitations, and they can be overwhelmed by the excessive production of acid (ACIDOSIS) that accompanies starvation and uncontrolled diabetes or by excessively alkaline blood (ALKALOSIS) that accompanies hyperventilation (panting), for example. Persistent acidosis, alkalosis and imbalanced electrolytes can pose long-term health hazards and require medical attention.

bulgar   See WHEAT.

bulimia nervosa   An EATING DISORDER characterized by repeated binge eating often followed by purging. The number of cases of bulimia in the United States has increased dramatically since 1970. About 5 million Americans, and perhaps as many as 5% of adolescent women, binge and purge to some extent. Bulimics typically engage in repeated episodes of binge eating followed by self-induced vomiting, fasting, the use of LAXATIVES or DIURETICS and/or EXERCISE to lose weight. The use of laxatives or diuretics to lose weight is potentially life-threatening because these methods cause losses of ELECTROLYTES (sodium, POTASSIUM, CHLORIDE) and water that may severely affect brain and heart functions. A bingeing individual can consume the equivalent of three normal meals in an hour. The symptoms of bulimia include: bingeing and purging for months or years; a fear of not being able to stop eating; eroded tooth enamel and cavities from vomited STOMACH ACID; DEHYDRATION; antisocial behavior (such as eating alone); an obsession with food-related activities (like supermarket shopping or cooking); erratic eating; suppression of emotional vulnerability; chronic heartburn (from esophageal reflux); abdominal distension and gas; indigestion; undernutrition; and lower levels of body FAT.

There are about four times as many bulimics as there are anorexics. As in ANOREXIA NERVOSA, typical bulimic patients are young women obsessed with the fear of obesity. They fear being unloved, being judged in terms of their appearance and degree of success. Food, eating and weight control become obsessions, dwarfing other areas of their personal lives. Bulimics often have low self-esteem.

Evidence suggests a biochemical component in some instances of this disorder. Bulimics often do not reach satiation after eating, and some bulimic women seem to make less of CHOLECYSTOKININ, a hormone that promotes a sense of satiation. Eating may also increase the level of DOPAMINE, a neurotransmitter in a region of the brain (nucleus accumbens) that triggers pleasure and satiation. High levels of the hormone vasopressin (ANTIDIURETIC HORMONE) are found in women with bulimia. This hormone is normally released in response to stress.

Bulimia can be controlled. Physical assessment and a return to a balanced diet are important in increasing a person's sense of well-being. As with any compulsive behavior, a person with an eating disorder needs supportive therapy from professional counselors in dealing with social, psychological, familial, nutritional and physiologic factors. A nutritional program might entail these components: well-planned meals that are nutritionally balanced. Meals should provide adequate calories and avoid excess. Fat and fiber are included and needed for satiety after a meal. Nutritional deficiencies may be remedied by supplementation as needed. In this regard, subclinical ZINC deficiencies have been associated with eating disorders. The program specifies ongoing nutritional counseling to help the patient control behaviors that could trigger binge-purge behaviors. The American Anorexia/Bulimia Association and the National Association of Anorexia Nervosa and Associated Disorders provide resources. (See also COMPULSIVE EATING.)

Whitaker, Leighton C. and Davis, William N, eds. *The Bulimic College Student.* Binghamton, N.Y.: Haworth Press, 1991.

bulking agents   See FIBER.

butter
A saturated animal FAT (butterfat) obtained from MILK and cream. Butter is the fat from pasteurized cream and milk that has been solidified by churning. Butter contains 81% fat (butterfat), 16 to 18% water, and other ingredients like casein, lactose and salt. The salt content varies with the brand. The yellow color of butter is due to BETA CAROTENE, which comes from the plants eaten by the cow. In winter, fodder is more likely to be grain, which lacks beta carotene, and butter is white; the yellow coloring agents, such as beta carotene and ANNATTO seed extract, are added to maintain a yellow color year-round. Butter is graded by the USDA according to its flavor, butterfat content, purity and keeping quality, among other characteristics. U.S. Grade AA is a score of 93 and represents 80% or more butterfat.

As an animal fat, butter is classified as saturated fat. Average annual consumption is about 4 pounds for Americans, about a third as much as margarine. Butter is used in sauteing, frying and baking. Like all oils, butter should be refrigerated to prevent rancidity (oxidation and decomposition). Sweet butter or unsalted butter are available for those on a salt-restricted diet. Whipped butter contains air as a filler, yielding only two-thirds of the CALORIES of regular butter. Spreadable butter was developed by the dairy industry as an alternative to margarine. Like regular butter, this product is made from cream and milk and with beta carotene for coloring. However, it contains additional finely dispersed water. Because it has more water, spreadable butter has less fat, fewer calories and less cholesterol than butter or regular margarine. Typically the content of one tablespoon (14 g) of regular butter is 101 calories; protein, 0.12 g; carbohydrate, 0.08 g; fat, 11.5 g; cholesterol, 31 mg; vitamin A, 825 retinol equivalents; sodium, 933 mg.

butter, clarified (ghee)
A butter from which milk solids have been removed. Clarified butter is prepared by melting butter briefly to coagulate milk solids. Clarified butter is a basic ingredient of Indian cooking, and the term *ghee* or *ghi* is Hindustani for clear butter. It is stable for extended periods at room temperature and in hot climates without refrigeration. Ghee has been claimed to be more nutritious than butter, but clinical studies to back this claim are lacking. Clarified butter finds general use when cooking at higher temperatures because it is less likely to burn or scorch than

whole butter. On the other hand, clarified butter lacks much of the buttery flavor of casein, the protein component. One tablespoon contains 100 calories, like regular butter. Like butter, the fat is classified as saturated.

butterfat
The FAT of cow's MILK and cream, which is classified as a saturated fat because it contains 65% saturated FATTY ACIDS. It finds several uses in the food industry. Anhydrous butterfat, from which most of the water has been removed, is used commercially to reconstitute liquid dairy products and to prepare SHORTENING for special cooking purposes.

Fractional crystallization of butterfat can produce both a higher melting fraction and a lower melting fraction. The higher melting fraction is used to prepare ice cream and chocolate, while the lower melting fraction is combined with whole butter to increase its spreadability.

Butter-Flavored Granules
Several products (sprinkles or granules) are available that supply a butter flavor to foods with even fewer calories than diet margarine. These products can be used with moist foods such as vegetables and cooked cereals, rather than dry foods. They cannot be used in sauteing because the granules break down when heated, and they contain very little oil. Typical ingredients include salt, partially hydrogenated vegetable oil, and butter flavor with annatto and turmeric as coloring agents. One half-teaspoon provides 4 calories.

buttermilk
Originally, the sour liquid remaining after cream had been separated after churning. Modern preparation of buttermilk usually employs pasteurized skim milk to which lactic acid-producing bacteria are added to develop the characteristic flavor through fermentation. Lactic acid formed by fermentation precipitates milk protein, so buttermilk has a thicker consistency than regular milk. Cream or butter is added in commercial products. Buttermilk is often used in recipes in place of sour milk for biscuits, rolls, waffles and the like as well as in frozen desserts. One cup (245 g) provides 99 calories; protein, 8.1 g; carbohydrate, 11.7 g; and butterfat, 2.16 g.

butylated hydroxyanisole   See BHA.

butylated hydroxytoluene   See BHT.

butyric acid (butyrate)
An acid produced by the bacterial degradation of FIBER in the colon. Gut bacteria ferment undigested carbohydrate to a family of small saturated fatty acids, acetic acid and propionic acid in addition to butyric acid. A small amount of butyric acid is present in the diet. Butyric acid occurs in milk, and BUTTER contains 3.3% butyric acid. Butyric acid and other short chain fatty acids are taken up by the intestine to be used for energy. It is estimated that breakdown of short-chain fatty acids produced by colonic bacteria can satisfy 5 to 10% of the body's total energy requirements. Butyric acid is specifically an important energy source for the cells lining the COLON, where it seems to assist their normal development and maintenance. Butyric acid seems to reduce chronic inflammatory conditions of the colon, and high fecal levels correlate with decreased risk of colon cancer.

cabbage (*Brassica oleracea capitala*)   A widely cultivated CRUCIFEROUS VEGETABLE with a compact head and overlapping leaves, related to BROCCOLI and BRUSSELS SPROUTS. There are hundreds of varieties of cabbage that differ in shape, color and leaf texture. Some varieties have loose heads; others, firm. Colors range from white and green to purple. In the United States the most popular varieties are green, red, Savoy, bok choy and Napa. Cabbage was originally domesticated 2,500 years ago in western Europe, where wild cabbage still grows. It was first used as a medicinal herb. Sauerkraut, or pickled cabbage, has been in use at least since 200 B.C. in China, when it formed a staple of the diet for laborers building the Great Wall.

Cabbage and related vegetables contain compounds with potential anti-CANCER effects in experimental animals, such as ascorbic acid (VITAMIN C), an ANTIOXIDANT. A family of nitrogen-containing compounds called indoles may act as antioxidants; they also seem to speed the rate at which estrogen, a female hormone, is inactivated. (Estrogen can stimulate the growth of breast cancer.) On the other hand, cabbage also contains certain sulfur compounds called thiourea and thiocyanates, which may impede the assimilation of IODINE and THYROID hormone formation when consumed in excessive amounts. Raw cabbage juice has been used to heal ulcers.

Raw cabbage is used in coleslaw or cabbage salad. When prepared with mayonnaise, it can become high-fat fare. Cabbage can be cooked in many ways—baked, sauteed, stewed and steamed—and the leaves can be stuffed with meat or grains and tomatoes. To preserve its vitamin and mineral content, cabbage should never be overcooked. To avoid the disagreeable odor sometimes associated with cooked cabbage, cabbage should be young and fresh and cooked rapidly. Aluminum cookware should be avoided as it promotes the release of pungent compounds; older cabbage and stored cabbage acquire stronger flavors. Raw cabbage (shredded, 1 cup, 70 g) provides 16 calories; protein, 0.8 g; carbohydrate, 3.9 g; fiber, 1.6 g; iron, 0.4 mg; thiamin, 0.04 mg; riboflavin, 0.02 mg; niacin, 0.21 mg; and vitamin C, 33 mg. (See also FOOD TOXINS; GOITROGENS.)

cacao (*Theobroma cacao*)   An evergreen tree cultivated in tropical America that produces cacao beans, the source of COCOA and CHOCOLATE. Each pod contains 25 to 40 beans, which vary in shape and color, depending on the variety. Cocoa production begins when the harvested beans are stored in mounds to permit bacterial fermentation. This destroys the fruity pulp and germ and develops the characteristic color, aroma and flavor of the cacao bean. The beans are then washed, dried and roasted. The raw material for cocoa products and chocolate is cocoa paste, prepared by grinding the fermented beans.

cachexia   Severe wasting. A state of ill health characterized by the progressive loss of body fat and lean body mass (skeletal muscle). Profound weakness, anorexia (loss of appetite) and frequent anemia accompany this wasting syndrome. Its causes are unknown. A fever-induced, increased rate of metabolism may account for some of the weakness. Internal bleeding from intestinal defects may account for anemia, and reduced food intake is associated with anorexia and a change in the sense of taste. (See also CATABOLIC STATE; CATABOLISM.)

cactus   See PRICKLY PEAR.

cadmium   A toxic, HEAVY METAL pollutant. Cigarette smoke provides low levels of exposure. Drinking WATER can be contaminated when water leaches cadmium from galvanized or black polyethylene water pipes. Cadmium contaminates the food supply, a reflection of widespread low-level distribution from PESTICIDES, industrial waste and tires, in addition to smoke from incinerator plants and coal-fired plants. Oysters contain unusually high levels of cadmium; three to four parts per million have been recorded. It is a natural contaminant of phosphate fertilizers and is easily taken up by plants. Livestock grazing on these plants become contaminated with cadmium, and humans eating BEEF accumulate cadmium because it is not readily excreted in urine or feces. This is a concern because trace amounts of cadmium cause HYPERTENSION, heart abnormalities and toxic effects on reproductive organs in experimental animals. Severe symptoms (bronchitis, emphysema) develop in people exposed to cadmium at levels only 10 times more than the average daily exposure. Cadmium exposure may also increase bone loss in postmenopausal women, thus increasing the risk of OSTEOPOROSIS. The mechanism of cadmium toxicity is not understood, though it can block the use of the trace mineral nutrient, ZINC. (See also LEAD; MERCURY.)

caffeine   A bitter ALKALOID (methylxanthine) occurring in more than 60 plants, including tea leaves, COFFEE beans, cocoa beans and kola nuts. Up to 90% of the adults in North America consume caffeine regularly, provided mostly by coffee. Caffeine is the most widely consumed compound in the world that affects the nervous system.

Caffeine is water-soluble and is rapidly absorbed by the body. Caffeine consumption during pregnancy increases the risk of complicated deliveries and miscarriages. Caffeine also enters the placenta and can affect placental function. Caffeine even enters breast milk. Caffeine stimulates the ADRENAL GLANDS to produce EPINEPHRINE (adrenaline), which normally gears up the body for action in response to a threatening situation (FIGHT OR FLIGHT RESPONSE) by increasing the heart rate, stimulating the nervous system, increasing STOMACH ACID production, raising BLOOD SUGAR and increasing fat breakdown.

A cup of brewed coffee contains 80 to 115 mg of caffeine, while a cup of DECAFFEINATED COFFEE contains 2 to 3 mg. A cup of brewed tea contains 40 to 60 mg of caffeine. Per ounce, CHOCOLATE contains about 20 mg caffeine. In addition, cola beverages and some medications and over-the-counter drugs contain caffeine. Soft drinks can provide 30 to 72 mg caffeine per 12 oz serving.

Caffeine is classified as a GENERALLY RECOGNIZED AS SAFE food additive by the U.S. FDA, and moderate consumption of caffeine-containing foods does not seem to be harmful for the average adult. Most healthy individuals can tolerate 200 to 300 mg a day of caffeine as a mild stimulant. Side effects of excessive caffeine (800 mg or more) include anxiety, sleeplessness, agitation, shortness of breath, irregular heartbeat, nausea, HEARTBURN and headaches. Caffeine usage is linked to most, though not all, attributes of addiction (chemical dependency), including craving and withdrawal symptoms during abstinence. Withdrawal symptoms include irritability, vomiting and headaches. To break a caffeine dependency reduce consumption gradually over four or five weeks.

Caffeine consumption may be linked to symptoms resembling PREMENSTRUAL SYNDROME. Caffeine can intensify symptoms of HYPOGLYCEMIA. It may interact with medications (ANTIDEPRESSANTS, tranquilizers and antipsychotic drugs); aggravate arrhythmia (irregular heartbeat); and increase calcium loss in women treated with ESTROGEN to prevent bone loss after menopause. Pregnant women should minimize caffeine consumption. Women who consume the amount of caffeine in one and a half to three cups of coffee daily may increase their risk of miscarriage. Excessive caffeine consumption has caused birth defects in experimental animals. On the other hand, a normal daily intake of caffeine in coffee does not seem to increase the risk of fibrocystic disease, pancreatic CANCER or HYPERTENSION, as earlier believed. Cardiac risk begins to increase at five or more cups of coffee per day. (See also ENDOCRINE SYSTEM; STRESS.)

Chou, T. "Wake Up and Smell the Coffee. Caffeine, Coffee and the Medical Consequences," *Western Journal of Medicine*, 157:5 (1992), pp. 544–553.

calciferol vitamin D_2 (ergocalciferol, activated ergosterol)   A synthetic form of VITAMIN D derived from a cyclic lipid from a yeast and mold, ERGOSTEROL, used to fortify MILK. Exposure to ultraviolet light converts ergosterol to calciferol. One cup of milk routinely contains 100 IUs of vitamin D as calciferol, which contributes most of the vitamin D ingested by children. Infant formulas are fortified with the same amount. Fortified prepared breakfast cereals generally contain 40 IU of vitamin D per cup. (See also CALCIUM; ENRICHMENT.)

calcitriol   See VITAMIN D.

calcium   An essential mineral nutrient and the most abundant mineral in the body. Calcium represents approximately 2% of the total body weight; about 98% of this occurs in the bones and teeth. The small amount of calcium in body fluids and cells plays an important role in nerve transmission, muscle contraction, heart rhythm, hormone production, wound healing, immunity, blood coagulation maintaining normal blood pressure, and STOMACH ACID production. Calcium promotes blood clotting through the activation of the fibrous protein FIBRIN, the building block of clots. It lowers blood pressure in patients with spontaneous HYPERTENSION (not caused by kidney disease) because it relaxes blood vessels, and it may also diminish the symptoms of PMS (PREMENSTRUAL SYNDROME).

High intake of saturated fat tends to raise LDL-cholesterol (the less desirable form) and to increase the risk of colorectal CANCER. On the other hand, calcium binds saturated fats, preventing their uptake by the intestine; consequently, calcium-rich diets may reduce LDL-cholesterol. A high calcium intake also seems to reduce the risk of colon cancer.

If blood levels of calcium decrease in response to low calcium consumption, the body pulls calcium out of bones to use elsewhere. Thus bones are dynamic tissues, constantly releasing calcium and reabsorbing it to maintain their strength. The level of calcium in the blood is carefully regulated by hormones. Parathyroid hormone from the parathyroid gland stimulates bone-degrading cells to break down bone tissue to release calcium and phosphate into the bloodstream (a process called bone resorption). Parathyroid hormone also stimulates calcium absorption from the intestines by activating vitamin D, and stimulates calcium reabsorption from the kidney filtrate back into blood. This effect is counterbalanced by calcitonin, released from the thyroid gland when blood calcium levels are high. Calcitonin triggers bone-building cells (osteoblasts) to take up calcium from blood to lay down new bone.

During growth spurts more calcium is absorbed than lost. Therefore, adequate calcium intake in childhood and adolescence is critical for bone building. In addition, ZINC, manganese, fluoride, copper, boron, MAGNESIUM, calcium and vitamin D, together with EXERCISE, minimize bone loss after the age of 35. Calcium absorption requires the hormone calcitriol, formed from vitamin D.

An estimated 100 million Americans risk calcium deficiency. They include women, especially those who either avoid MILK or are postmenopausal or are pregnant. The average adult male obtains 75% of the calcium RDA; the average female, 50%. An estimated 87% of adolescent women and 84% of women between the ages of 35 and 50 are calcium deficient. Older people absorb less calcium and the calcium RDA should probably be increased for elderly persons.

Symptoms of prolonged calcium deficiency include insomnia, heart palpitations and muscle spasms, as well as arm and leg numbness. Chronic low calcium intake can lead to easily fractured bones due to bone thinning (OSTEOPOROSIS), and possibly hypertension. Severe deficiency symptoms are rare: convulsions, dementia, osteomalacia, rickets (bent bones and stunted growth in children) and periodontal disease.

In addition to age and heredity, many life-style and dietary factors increase the risk of developing calcium-related problems: age; heredity; chronic emotional STRESS; lack of exercise; dieting; excessive CAFFEINE, SODIUM, phosphorus (as found in processed foods and soft drinks) or dietary FIBER; high-fat foods; possibly high protein diets; low vitamin D intake; long-term use of corticosteroids; and cigarette smoking. Conditions like INFLAMMATORY BOWEL SYNDROME, low stomach acidity, LACTASE deficiency, kidney failure and diabetes increase the need for calcium, while mineral oil (laxative), lithium and some DIURETICS (water pills) block calcium uptake.

Dietary Sources of Calcium

The adult RECOMMENDED DIETARY ALLOWANCE (RDA) is 800 mg per day; for pregnant or nursing women the RDA is 1,200 mg daily. Some experts report that these levels are too low; the National Institutes of Health recommends 1,500 mg daily after menopause. Milk products like yogurt and CHEESE represent rich calcium sources. They need not be high in fat. Low-fat dairy products like skim or low-fat milk and low-fat

YOGURT contain about 300 mg calcium per cup. SARDINES and canned SALMON with cooked bones are high in calcium; plant sources include green leafy vegetables, COLLARD greens, CHARD, beet tops, BOK CHOY, spinach and BROCCOLI, as well as various seeds and SOYBEANS. The calcium in spinach is less easily absorbed. Two very good plant sources are TOFU, prepared with calcium to curdle soybean protein, and corn tortillas, prepared with lime. The following are examples of low-fat, high-calcium foods:

1% fat cottage cheese (half cup)	70 mg calcium
non-fat yogurt (half cup)	225
skim milk (1 cup)	300
cooked greens (1 cup)	100
cooked collard greens (1 cup)	280
cooked soybeans (1 cup)	450
tofu (1 ounce)	130
corn tortilla (1 ounce)	300
sardines (3 ounces)	370

Calcium Fortification

Calcium is added to foods and beverages. The food industry has responded to consumer fears of OSTEOPOROSIS (age-related thinning of bones) by adding calcium to a variety of foods and diet drinks, including some brands of orange juice, BREAKFAST cereals, whole milk, yogurt, cheese, sliced cheese, cottage cheese, white flour, bread and cocoa. Fortified or enriched foods can supply 25 to 100% of the calcium RDA per serving. Individuals prone to kidney stones might have problems with excessive calcium, and excessive calcium from any source can cause milk-alkali syndrome, which damages the kidneys. A very high calcium intake can block the uptake of MANGANESE, another essential mineral. (See also ENRICHMENT.)

Calcium Supplements

Forms of dietary CALCIUM containing higher amounts than usually found in foods. The advantages of obtaining calcium from food are twofold. First, calcium is better absorbed, and second, it is almost impossible to overdose on calcium from food. However, the typical U.S. diet provides only 450 to 550 mg of calcium daily, and individuals who avoid dairy products may encounter difficulty in obtaining adequate calcium from foods alone. Certain groups are more likely to develop calcium deficiencies: dieters, smokers, women past menopause or who have had hysterectomies, and those who drink several cups of coffee or several alcoholic beverages daily. For those who have a marginal calcium intake, calcium supplementation with vitamin D is a responsible alternative.

Most types of calcium supplements are effective, and calcium carbonate is inexpensive. Orange juice can aid calcium uptake from calcium carbonate. It is generally believed that chelated calcium (calcium citrate, lactate, gluconate, orotate)

may be more easily absorbed than calcium carbonate when stomach acid production is low, although this view has been challenged. Calcium tablets need to disintegrate in water for calcium absorption to occur.

There are several precautions to be aware of in using calcium supplements. Excessive calcium supplementation (3,000 to 8,000 mg per day) increases the risk of ZINC and MAGNESIUM deficiencies. Calcium supplements taken with meals may block the uptake of other minerals like COPPER, IRON and zinc. Overdosing with calcium supplements also increases the risk of kidney stones in susceptible people. Excessive calcium supplements can lead to vomiting, high blood pressure, DEPRESSION, excessive urination, muscle wasting and CONSTIPATION. (See also ANTACIDS; BONE; CORTISOL; GASTROINTESTINAL DISORDERS; HYPERTENSION; LACTOSE INTOLERANCE.)

NIH Consensus Development Panel On Optimal Calcium Intake, "Optimal Calcium Intake," *Journal of the American Medical Association*, 272:24 (December 1994), pp. 1942–48.

calcium blockers   Drugs prescribed to help prevent HEART ATTACKS. CALCIUM blockers lower blood pressure by preventing calcium from entering smooth muscles around veins and capillaries, thus keeping them from contracting in response to high SODIUM. Calcium blockers also inhibit chemical signals from the brain that normally speed up the heart when the patient becomes excited.

calcium propionate   The CALCIUM salt of PROPIONIC ACID, a short-chain fatty acid. This common, innocuous FOOD ADDITIVE is used in bread and rolls to prevent the growth of molds and bacteria. The level of propionate in baked goods (0.1 to 0.2%) is sufficiently high to alter the growth of microorganisms like bacteria and mold, but it does not kill them. Sodium propionate is also used in pies and cakes to prevent the interference of calcium with BAKING SODA or powder.

Propionate is a harmless additive occurring naturally in foods. For example, Swiss cheese contains 1% propionate, which serves as a natural preservative. Metabolic processes produce propionate from AMINO ACIDS and certain FATTY ACIDS. Furthermore, propionate is easily oxidized for energy. This process requires VITAMIN B$_{12}$. (See also BREAD; FOOD PRESERVATION; FOOD SPOILAGE.)

California Certified Organic Farmers (CCOF)   An agency that certifies organic produce and organic farms according to established standards in California. In particular, the CCOF label indicates the product has met limits of PESTICIDE residues lower than those set by the EPA. In general, unless organic produce is agency-certified, there is no guarantee it has been grown without the use of pesticides, HERBICIDES or chemical fertilizers. (See also ORGANIC FOODS.)

caloric value   The maximum amount of calories available from food. Caloric value refers to the number of calories released by completely oxidizing a gram of fuel nutrient, as FAT, CARBOHYDRATE or PROTEIN. Metabolic processes oxidize fat and carbohydrate completely to CARBON DIOXIDE and water, the same combustion products as found in the laboratory. The caloric yield is the same whether fuel is burned in

the body or in the test tube. The oxidation of GLUCOSE yields 3.7 calories per gram. STARCH yields 4.1 calories/gram; and SUCROSE, 4.0 calories/gram. Therefore an average yield of 4 calories per gram of carbohydrate is used by nutritionists. The oxidation of a monounsaturated fat like OLIVE OIL yields 9.4 calories per gram; of a more saturated animal fat like BUTTERFAT, 9.2 calories per gram. For simplicity an average value of 9 calories per gram of fat is used to approximate the caloric yield. AMINO ACIDS from protein contain nitrogen, which is not oxidized by the body but is excreted as UREA. Consequently the caloric yield of protein oxidized in the body is 4.1 calories per gram. This value is rounded off to 4 when used by nutritionists to calculate the caloric yield of food proteins. The key point is that fat contains more than twice as many calories as protein or carbohydrate.

calorie   A standardized unit of heat. The caloric yield of nutrients and the body's energy requirements are expressed as large calories, "kilocalories" in the medical literature, or simply "calories" in common usage. One kilocalorie is the amount of heat required to raise the temperature of 1 kg of water by 1°C. Another unit of energy used in some scientific articles is the kilojoule. One large calorie equals 4.124 kilojoules (KJ).

Calories are a measure of the energy released when the body burns any fuel including FAT, PROTEIN, CARBOHYDRATES and ALCOHOL. Calories from the oxidation of fuel nutrients maintain normal body functions such as the heart and circulation, as well as the (hormonal) endocrine system, nervous system and digestive system. Energy from food supports reproduction, growth, physical work, the uptake of nutrients, and the repair of wear and tear in cells and tissues. The actual number of calories used depends upon many factors, including body mass and the level of physical activity. A portion of the calories are released from food as heat to maintain body temperature. Women need fewer calories than men. Typically, women's needs range from 1,600 to 2,000 calories daily; men generally need 1,800 to 2,400 calories daily.

Caloric Balance

The relationship between caloric input and caloric expenditures is critical. Excessive calories, regardless of their source, may promote fat buildup because surplus calories are stored by the body rather than being destroyed. Contrary to popular belief, carbohydrates and STARCH are not high calorie NUTRIENTS; carbohydrates yield only 4 calories per gram. The distinction belongs to fat as a more concentrated source of calories (9 calories per gram). Calories derived from fat are linked to OBESITY because the conversion of dietary carbohydrate to body fat requires much more energy than the conversion of dietary fat to body fat. Consequently, it is harder to gain weight by eating large amounts of complex carbohydrates than by eating fat.

Common Sources of Excessive Calories

Popular high-calorie foods are cheeseburgers, soft drinks, processed meat and high-fat meats (SAUSAGE, BOLOGNA, etc.), FRENCH FRIES, doughnuts, cookies, cake, ice cream, fried food, cheeses, high-fat CRACKERS, CHIPS and alcoholic beverages. PROCESSED FOODS and CONVENIENCE FOODS often also contain added saturated fat (which increases the risk of atherosclerosis) and sucrose (SUGAR), which provides no nutrients other than carbohydrates. To put this in perspective, consider that you would need to walk one and a half hours to consume the calories provided by a single piece of pastry. Typical high-calorie items (HIGH-FAT FOODS) are easily replaced with low-calorie alternatives:

- one candy bar (500) vs. one cup of unbuttered popcorn (54)
- four pieces fried chicken (1,700) vs. one serving of broiled, skinless chicken (142)
- one slice of cheesecake (257) vs. one cup of strawberries (50)
- six ounces of potato chips (920) vs. one large salad, with a teaspoon of dressing (100)
- bread with two squares of butter (170) vs. one slice of bread (80)

Estimating Daily Caloric Needs

The following computation approximates daily caloric needs. Actual needs may differ depending upon age, gender, level of physical activity, personal METABOLISM, state of health, and stress level.

1. Divide body weight in pounds by 2.2 (to convert pounds to kilograms).
2. Choose appropriate energy factors: 1.0 for males, 0.9 for females or 0.8 for those over 50 years old.
3. To calculate the calories needed to maintain body weight: Multiply weight in kilograms by the appropriate energy factor times 24 hours. For example, a 123-lb. woman weighs 55.9 kg. She needs 55.9 kg × 0.9 × 24 hr. = 1,207 calories per day just for maintenance.
4. To estimate the daily calories required for physical activity: Choose the best estimate of activity level. Very light (e.g., desk job) = 0.6; Light (e.g., teacher) = 0.8; Moderate (e.g., a nurse) = 1.1; Strenuous (e.g., roofer) = 2.4. Multiply the hours per day spent on this major work activity by weight in kg. For example, for a woman with 7 hours of moderate work activity level: 55.9 kg × 7 hr. × 1.1 = 430 calories.
5. To calculate total calories, add Step 3 to Step 4. In our example, 1,207 calories plus 430 calories equals 1,637 calories, the estimate for a typical day.

Calorie Reduction Strategies

A knowledge of the calorie content of food is fundamentally important because a balanced diet must first provide adequate energy. Critical stages of life require more energy than usual. Pregnancy, lactation, growth during childhood and adolescence, and caloric restriction require medical supervision. Counting calories has long been a preoccupation of dieters. However, the most effective ways to lose weight require a change in behavior: Eating less high-fat food and exercising regularly. Specific dietary recommendations can be made to reduce calorie intake:

Dairy products Replace cream CHEESE or sour cream with low-fat YOGURT. Replace Camembert, Cheddar, Cheshire, feta, Limburger and provolone cheeses and cheese spreads, with lower fat cheeses like mozzarella or low-fat

COTTAGE CHEESE. Use skim MILK instead of whole milk or cream in recipes. Consume less ice cream, which can be 50 to 60% fat.

Meat and poultry Bake MEAT and POULTRY on a rack to drain fat. Remove fatty skin from poultry before eating. Select lean cuts of meat instead of prime or choice. Trim off all visible fat.

Processed foods Eat less processed foods. Often convenience foods provide high levels of saturated fat as butter, lard, shortening, hydrogenated vegetable oils, coconut and/or palm oils. Processed meats such as sausage, luncheon meats and hot dogs usually contain large amounts of SATURATED FAT. Substitute VEGETABLES and FRUIT for high-salt, high-sugar and/or high-fat snacks. Eat less fried foods, which contain 25 to 50% saturated fat. Drink less alcohol and sweetened soft drinks, which supply only calories. (See also DIETING.)

McDowell M. et al., "Energy and Macronutrient Intakes of Persons Ages 2 Months and Over in the United States: Third National Health and Nutrition Examination Survey, Phase 1, 1988–1991," *Advance Data No. 255* (October 24, 1994), p. 1.

campylobacteriosis A type of FOOD POISONING caused by the bacterium *Campylobacter pylori*; a leading cause of food poisoning in the United States. The bacterium occurs in livestock and can contaminate milk, raw MEAT and poultry. In 1987 the National Academy of Sciences concluded that half of the cases of campylobacter infections were attributable to contaminated chicken.

Campylobacteriosis has become an important cause of DIARRHEA from food during the last 15 years. Diarrhea is potentially a serious condition because it can prevent nutrient uptake and cause dehydration, leading to electrolyte imbalance. Other symptoms are fever, stomach cramps, and sometimes bloody stools. Symptoms appear two to five days after eating contaminated food and can last a week. To avoid contamination during meal preparation, the utensils and cutting board used to prepare raw meat should not come in contact with VEGETABLES or cooked meat. Consumption of untreated water or unpasteurized milk is not advised because of the increased risk of bacterial contamination from these sources. (See also GASTRITIS; HELICOBACTER PYLORI.)

cancer (malignancy) A broad category of diseases characterized by an uncontrolled, therefore virulent growth of cells. Cancer is classified according to the tissue of origin. The most common are carcinomas, which originate in epithelial tissues (tissues lining the body cavities and forming the outer surfaces of the body). Sarcomas develop from connective tissues, muscles, skeleton, circulatory and urogenital systems. Myelomas originate from bone marrow; lymphomas from the lymph system; and leukemia from blood-forming cells. Many cancers typically invade adjacent tissues. Such metastasizing tumors spread throughout the body via the circulatory and lymphatic systems.

Cancer is the second leading cause of death among Americans. An estimated one out of every three or four adults will die of malignancy or its complications. The chances of living longer once cancer is detected are better than ever, and the incidence of some forms of cancer has been dropping. However, the overall incidence of all cancer has been increased at an annual rate of 0.5% to 1% in the United States until 1990–95, when a slight decline in overall cancer mortality (31% over the five-year period) was observed, in spite of the extensive resources directed to cancer detection, treatment and prevention. A growing segment of the medical community believes cancer rates will not decline unless more effort is placed on cancer prevention. That cancer can be prevented to a large degree is borne out by recent analyses. Nutrition and life-style choices may account for as much as 90% of cancer in America. For example, cigarette smoking accounts for an estimated 25% to 40% of cancer cases, while flawed diets may cause roughly a third of cancer cases. Exposure to chemical pollutants (5 to 10%), infections (1 to 10%) and radiation are also significant causes. As an example of genetic influence on cancer vulnerability, people who lack a copy of a gene that codes for a carcinogen-detoxifying enzyme called glutathione transferase, and therefore lack this protective enzyme, have a four fold greater risk of a disease, myelodysplastic syndrome, that leads to leukemia.

Cancer Induction

CARCINOGENS are agents shown to cause cancer. The precise mechanisms of converting normal cells into cancer cells remain uncertain despite extensive research. According to one theory, the process requires several steps beginning with the chemical modifications of DNA, the genetic blueprint of cells. Most adults already have been exposed to cancer-causing agents, and their tissues already contain modified genes, which can remain dormant for years. Cancer may not show up unless the precancerous state is stimulated by other agents called promoters. These may be viruses, chemicals or agents in foods; excessive dietary fat is thought to be a cancer promoter. Consequently, carcinogens often manifest their effect many years after exposure. An additional requirement is that cell division be stimulated for cancer to occur. The body possesses powerful defenses. Efficient mechanisms repair DNA damages; however, they can be compromised by a poor diet, disease and age. The immune system wards off foreign cells, including cancer cells. Natural killer T cells and anti-cancer factors (tumor necrosis factor) are produced to destroy altered cells, but this surveillance declines with age.

Cancer and Diet

Perhaps as many as one third of all cancers are related to diet, and as many as 95% of colon cancer cases are diet related. Cancers of the prostate, breast, colon and lining of the uterus (endometrium) are most common in affluent nations, while cancers of the liver, cervix, esophagus and stomach are related to poverty. Although research and population studies suggest a correlation between specific nutrients and different types of cancer, most recommendations remain best guesses. Deficiencies of the following nutrients are linked to increased risk of cancer: amino acids (CYSTEINE, METHIONINE, TRYPTOPHAN, ARGININE), B complex vitamins (riboflavin, folic acid, vitamin B_6), fat soluble vitamins (vitamin A, vitamin E), minerals (calcium, zinc, copper, iron, selenium), other nutrients (choline, beta carotene) and other substances in foods that act as antioxidants or modify levels of liver detoxication enzymes (flavonoids, isothiocyanates, organosulfur compounds, phytoestrogens and others).

Meat and fat are closely correlated in the Western diet, making the separation of these two variables difficult. Most animal studies show that meat per se does not affect carcinogenesis. Human population studies do not link meat consumption with colon cancer, though meat intake may increase the risk of pancreatic cancer.

Fat and energy intake may be correlated with cancer. Geographic correlations suggest that a high-fat diet is a risk factor for cancers of developed countries. To decrease cancer risk, some experts believe that fat should be cut back to 20% or less of daily calories. In 1990 the National Cancer Institute evaluated existing data and concluded that both fat and surplus calories pose independent breast cancer risks. Diets high in fat enhance chemically-induced tumors in experimental animals. On the other hand, calorie restriction inhibits tumor growth even when the calorie-restricted animals ingest more fat than controls. One of the reasons animal studies have not strongly supported the risk of fatty diets and colon cancer may be that human high-fat diets usually include cooked foods. Cooking seems to increase the cancer risk of meat cooked in beef fat. Fiber-deficient diets have been correlated with colon cancer. Though not clear-cut, the data do suggest that a high-fiber, low–fat diet represents the best nutritional approach to reduce the risk of colon cancer. More generally, numerous studies indicate that high consumption of vegetables and fruits can lower cancer risk.

Vitamin deficiencies are implicated in some forms of cancer and several vitamins may lower cancer risk. Animal studies indicate that NIACIN deficiency is linked to cancer. Niacin helps repair damaged DNA, known to occur in the action of several carcinogens. Studies indicate that megadoses of FOLIC ACID (25 times the RECOMMENDED DIETARY ALLOWANCE) and VITAMIN B_{12} (160 times the RDA) can reduce precancerous lung tissue in some smokers. Folic acid has been used to treat cervical dysplasia (precancerous cervical tissue) in women taking oral contraceptives. Calcium deficiency is related to the risk of colon cancer. VITAMIN A and BETA CAROTENE therapy prevent the formation of precancerous areas in the mouth resulting from chewing tobacco.

Cancer prevention emphasizes proper nutrition, and increasing interest has focused on antioxidant nutrients in lowering the risk of free radical damage and cancer. Free radicals are highly reactive molecules that lack an electron and attack cell components like DNA and proteins. Selenium, vitamin C, beta carotene and vitamin E are all logical candidates as protecting agents because they squelch free radicals. Fruits and vegetables provide a wide assortment of other substances that can reduce oxidative damage. These include FLAVONOIDS, such as TANNINS and ANTHOCYANINS (blue, red, purple pigments of berries), terpenes, coumarins, CAROTENOIDS (such as beta carotene and lycopene), PHYTOESTROGENS (such as soy isoflavones), ISOTHIOCYANATES (found in cabbage family vegetables), organosulfur compounds (diallyl sulfide, others from oils, garlic) and diketones (curcuminoids from TURMERIC). Plant foods supply other materials that seem to bolster the body's ability to dispose of toxins and potential carcinogens or to repair damage they cause. Indeed, PHYTOCHEMICALS promise to play an increasingly important role in cancer prevention.

Other cancer prevention guidelines emphasize stopping all use of tobacco because smoking is linked to many forms of cancer; minimal use of ESTROGEN, because estrogen increases the risk of breast cancer; moderate consumption of ALCOHOL, because alcohol increases the risk of breast, mouth and esophageal cancer; practicing safe sex to minimize transmission of viruses that injure the immune system; reducing stress to bolster the immune system; avoiding sunburn to minimize the risk of skin cancer; and minimizing exposure to carcinogens in cigarette smoke, toxic materials such as dust, solvents, industrial chemicals, PESTICIDES and certain FOOD ADDITIVES like nitrates and artificial food colors.

The American Cancer Society notes that certain warning signs of cancer warrant medical attention: any unusual bleeding; a thickening lump, especially in the breast; a sore that does not heal; a persistent cough; hoarseness; a dramatic change in bowel movements or urination; indigestion; difficulty in swallowing; an unexplained weight loss; and a change in color or shape of a wart or mole. (See also CANCER-PREVENTION DIET; DELANEY CLAUSE.)

cancer-prevention diet The American Cancer Society recommends that Americans:

- Reduce total fat consumption. Diets high in animal fat, MILK and PROTEIN appear to be linked to colon, prostate, ovarian and possibly breast cancer, though the latter has been questioned recently. Studies indicate reduced intake of fatty foods may lower the risk of these cancers.
- Consume high-FIBER foods. FRUITS, vegetables and whole grains are useful substitutes for fatty foods and lower daily fat intake.
- Consume foods rich in CAROTENOIDS (such as BETA CAROTENE) and VITAMIN C daily. These foods include green leafy and orange vegetables, which contain nutrients that may protect against some forms of cancer.
- Consume more from the cabbage family, including BROCCOLI, BRUSSELS SPROUTS, KOHLRABI and CAULIFLOWER. They contain ingredients that may protect against cancers of the gastrointestinal and respiratory tracts.
- Reduce alcohol intake. Heavy drinkers who smoke have a high risk for cancers of the mouth, larynx and esophagus.
- Reduce consumption of cured food, including smoked, salt-cured and NITRITE-cured foods. Smoked fish, smoked ham and some smoked sausage absorb cancer-causing tars similar to those in tobacco smoke. Consumption of pickled or salt-cured foods seems to increase cancers of the stomach and the esophagus in susceptible individuals.
- Control weight. A 12-year study of over a million Americans indicates that cancer risks are higher among overweight women and men, especially those over the age of 40.

Cancer-Preventing Agents in Food

Certain nutrients are being studied for their effectiveness in preventing cancer: vitamin A, VITAMIN C, VITAMIN E, beta carotene, SELENIUM and fiber. Vitamin C, vitamin E, CAROTENOIDS (orange-red or yellow plant pigments like beta carotene) and selenium are ANTIOXIDANTS. They help pre-vent chemical damage by FREE RADICALS, mainly highly reactive forms of oxygen, such as superoxide, which occur from cellular metabolism as well as from exposure to environmental pollutants and to oxygen. Free radicals are treacherous because they damage DNA, the genetic blueprint of a cell. Alterations of genes seem to convert some cells to cancerous types; thus, free radicals can function as carcinogens. Antioxidants are widely distributed in fruits and vegetables. Foods rich in carotenoids like beta carotene are orange-colored vegetables like squash and dark-green leafy vegetables such as CHARD and broccoli. Fresh fruits provide vitamin C; vegetable oil, wheat GERM and nuts supply vitamin E; whole grains, selenium; and fruit, vegetables, grains and LEGUMES provide fiber.

A wide variety of other plant products seem to inhibit cancer formation, and their identification remains a very active area of research. These materials work in different ways. Flavonoids (complex multi-ring pigments found in many fruits and vegetables) serve as antioxidants, enhance the body's mechanisms for neutralizing toxic substances, and help regulate enzymes involved in malignancy. Ellagic acid, a flavonoid found in fruits, especially grapes, and in vegetables, seems to directly protect genes from chemical attack. Indoles (benzene-like compounds containing nitrogen) and flavones (flavonoids related to vitamin E) may serve as antioxidants. Certain phenolic compounds (oxygen-containing AROMATIC COMPOUNDS) also help neutralize carcinogens like NITROSOAMINES. Agents in the cabbage family may boost the liver's capacity to destroy CARCINOGENS. As an example sulfur compounds in broccoli and cauliflower called dithiolthiones stimulate the transfer of GLUTATHIONE, the cell's major sulfur-containing detoxifier, to make cancer-causing agents more easily excreted in urine and feces. Other agents include saponins, garlic products and fiber. Saponins and triterpenoids (unabsorbable carbohydrate derivatives) inhibit breast cancer in experimental animals. Soybeans contain ISOFLAVONES, plant substances that may decrease estrogen production in premenopausal women and thus apparently reduce the risk of breast cancer.

How much vegetables, fruits, legumes and whole grains to eat is not known. With the typical American diet, more is often better. Only an estimated 9% to 20% of Americans eat the recommended minimum five servings of fruits and vegetables daily. (See also AGING; BARBECUED MEAT; DELANEY CLAUSE.)

Dragsted, L.O., Strube, M., Larsen, J.C., "Cancer-protective Factors in Fruits and Vegetables: Biochemical and Biological Background," *Pharmacology and Toxicology*, 72:1 (1993), pp. 116–35.

Sporn, Michael B., "The War on Cancer," *Lancet* 347 (May 18, 1996), pp. 1377–81.

Valstar, E., "Nutrition and Cancer: A Review of the Preventive and Therapeutic Abilities of Single Nutrients," *Journal of Nutritional Medicine*, 4 (1994), pp. 179–98.

Candida albicans A disease-producing yeast belonging to the same family as molds and FUNGI. Candida flourishes in warm, moist environments that supply a nutrient source: Thus it can grow on moist tissues lining the body (mucous membranes). Traces of Candida and other yeasts may live in the intestine, but they are usually held in check by friendly gut bacteria and the immune system. Candida is an opportunistic organism that can spread when the immune system weakens and when secreted antibodies decline; when broad-spectrum antibiotics kill gut bacteria; and when the diet supplies excessive refined carbohydrate and sugar. *C. albicans* infection of the mouth (thrush) and esophagus occurs in infants and young children, and is also a sign of HIV (Human Immunodeficiency Virus)-induced conditions. Candida presents up to seven different forms for the body to suppress. This may partially explain its ability to exploit weaknesses in the body's defenses. Laboratory tests can discriminate *Candida albicans* from other pathogens. Candida resists typical antibiotics; therefore, treatment utilizes antifungal drugs like niastatin and botanical antifungal agents, such as berberine (goldenseal *Hydrastis*) and garlic extracts. (See also ACIDOPHILUS; CANDIDIASIS; FLORA, INTESTINAL.)

Challacombe, S.J., "Immunologic Aspects of Oral Candidiasis," *Oral Surgery, Oral Medicine and Oral Pathology*, 78:2 (1994), pp. 202–10.
Odds, F.C., "Candida Species and Virulence," *American Society of Microbiology News*, 60 (6) 1994, pp. 313–18.

candidiasis   A Candida (yeast) infection of the skin and mucous membranes of the body. Though CANDIDA ALBICANS is a common culprit, several Candida species produce disease. Typically candidiasis occurs in the colon, vagina, mouth (thrush), throat, lungs or nails. However, a serious systemic (body-wide) infection may occur when Candida invades the bloodstream. The symptoms of candidiasis syndrome attributable to intestinal infection can be extremely variable, ranging from headaches, confusion and loss of energy, to chronic fatigue, cramps, bloating, rectal itching and gas. It can be associated with lowered immunity. Because these symptoms fit many clinical conditions, it is imperative that diagnosis be confirmed by specific clinical lab tests based on specimen culture and analyses of anticandida antibodies in the bloodstream.

Several factors promote candidiasis: use of oral contraceptives and steroid hormones (which can suppress the immune system); long-term use of antibiotics (which kill bacteria that normally hold Candida in check); nutritional deficiencies, which weakens the immune system; chronic STRESS or viral (HIV) infection (which lowers immunity); low stomach acidity (which prevents sterilization of food and promotes maldigestion); high carbohydrate diet and diabetes (which increase sugar and support yeast growth).

In treating candidiasis, it is important to reduce the predisposing factors by:

- employing digestive aids;
- avoiding sugar and other refined carbohydrates;
- eliminating exposure to known allergens, which can weaken the immune system;
- bolstering the immune system with nutritional supplements;
- correcting low stomach acid production;
- repopulating the intestine with beneficial bacteria (lactobacillus species and bifidobacteria) to reestablish normal microflora.

Treatments specify any of a variety of antifungal agents. (See also ACIDOPHILUS; FLORA, INTESTINAL; HYPOCHLORHYDRIA.)

candy (confection)   A processed, sugar-based food, first produced in Venice in the 15th century. The United States produces the most candy worldwide, reflecting its regional popularity. The average American consumption in 1990 was about 20 pounds per person, representing over 2,000 different varieties of candy. The major ingredient is SUCROSE (table sugar), though candy may also contain MILK and milk products, GUMS, GELATIN, FAT and oils, STARCH, flavorings, fruit and nuts. In the United States CHOCOLATE is the major ingredient for the most popular brands of candy, the majority of which contain PEANUTS and peanut butter. Their high content of REFINED CARBOHYDRATES and SATURATED FAT indicates these are high-calorie, low-nutrient-density foods. Their "empty" calories are a concern for those who are attempting to improve their diet and eat more nutritious foods. Sugar-free candies are available to help satisfy a sweet tooth. They contain sugar derivatives such as SORBITOL and artificial sweeteners like ASPARTAME. Sugar-less candies are not calorie-free, however, because sorbitol and aspartame can be taken up and used for energy. (See also FLAVORS; NATURAL SWEETENERS; NUTRIENT DENSITY.)

canola oil   A monounsaturated vegetable oil derived from a relatively new variety of RAPESEED. The composition of canola oil resembles that of OLIVE OIL. It contains 32% polyunsaturated FATTY ACIDS, 62% monounsaturated fatty acids and only 6% saturated fatty acids. Monounsaturates are considered more healthful than saturated fats (animal fat, or COCONUT OIL and PALM OIL) because a diet high in monounsaturates and low in cholesterol tends to lower LOW-DENSITY LIPOPROTEIN (LDL), the less desirable form of blood cholesterol, while maintaining HIGH-DENSITY LIPOPROTEIN (HDL), the desirable form. Studies show that olive oil does not cause tumors in experimental animals, but long-term cancer studies have not been carried out with canola oil.

cantaloupe (*Cucumis melo cantalupensis*)   A variety of muskmelon with orange pulp and a fragrant taste. Most melons originated in the ancient Middle East, then spread to the Egyptian and Roman empires. The American cantaloupe's rind has a net-like appearance. Cantaloupe is the most common melon in the United States; Arizona, California and Texas are major domestic sources. Cantaloupe is an excellent source of BETA CAROTENE, to which it owes its orange color, as well as ASCORBIC ACID. One cup of cubed melon provides calories, 60; protein, 1.4 g; carbohydrate, 13 g; potassium, 495 mg; vitamin A, 510 retinol equivalents; fat, 0.4 g; ascorbic acid, 65 mg. Cantaloupe contains only low levels of other minerals and B vitamins.

canthaxanthine   A natural red food color belonging to the CAROTENOID family of plant pigment, which is related to BETA CAROTENE. Used in foods such as candy, sauces and margarines, canthaxanthine has no vitamin A activity, unlike beta carotene. Since it is fat-soluble, canthaxanthine can accumulate in fat tissue and the skin, although food is a source for only small amounts of this food colorant. However, it is marketed as a tanning aid, and canthaxanthine pills can supply more than 20 times the amount normally consumed in the diet. Accumulation can lead to blurred night vision, allergic skin reactions, hepatitis (inflamed liver) and, in extreme cases, ANEMIA.

capillary   A microscopic blood vessel. A network of capillaries connects the arterial and venous systems. Capillaries average 0.008 mm in diameter, slightly larger than the diameter of a RED BLOOD CELL. They connect with the smallest branches of the arteries (arterioles), and provide oxygenated blood and nutrients to cells within tissues. Capillary walls are sufficiently thin to permit rapid migration of oxygen and other nutrients from blood into surrounding tissues, and to permit waste products like CARBON DIOXIDE and LACTIC ACID to diffuse out of cells into the bloodstream. The total surface area provided by all capillaries for this transport function is huge: 6,300 square meters for an adult. (See also HYPERTENSION; PROSTAGLANDIN.)

caprylic acid   An acid classified as a medium-chain FATTY ACID, found in butter, goat and cow's MILK and in COCONUT OIL. Caprylic acid is classified as a saturated fatty acid because all carbon atoms are filled up with hydrogen atoms. Unlike the long-chain fatty acids typically found in fats and oils, medium-chain fatty acids are rapidly absorbed by the small intestine without the intervention of a special carrier (CHYLOMICRON) required to transport fats in the bloodstream. Medium-chain fatty acids can be readily used for energy by the liver and skeletal muscle. Oral caprylic acid products can combat intestinal yeast infections. Caprylic acid seems to block yeast cell-wall production. (See also CANDIDIASIS.)

capsaicin   The spicy, pungent compound of CHILI PEPPERS, and the most fiery of the pepper alkaloids. Capsaicin probably evolved to protect the pepper from being eaten by predators. In humans, this substance can help digestion by stimulating salivation, STOMACH ACID production and, perhaps, PERISTALSIS. Capsaicin has other potential benefits: It may also kill bacteria, reduce the risk of blood clots and serve as an ANTIOXIDANT. It seems to boost the production of intestinal IgA antibodies produced to exclude foreign materials from the intestine.

Capsaicin acts as a "counter-irritant," that is, it is a mildly irritating substance that blocks pain sensations. It seems to do this by interfering with sensory nerves that relay pain messages from the skin to the brain. In particular, capsaicin can deplete a chemical messenger called Substance P, which relays pain messages to the brain. Thus capsaicin "short-circuits" pain signals. This effect can be anti-inflammatory as well, and capsaicin-containing creams have been developed to reduce the pain of shingles and chronic foot and leg pain. There are several precautions when using these creams: Capsaicin irritates membranes of the eye and nose, though it does not injure the stomach, and capsaicin supplements may interfere with the functioning of anticoagulants. (See also IMMUNE SYSTEM; NEUROTRANSMITTER.)

Altman Roy D., et al., "Capsaicin Cream 0.025% as Monotherapy for Osteoarthritis: a Double Blind Study," *Seminars in Arthritis and Rheumatism*, 23:6, supp. 3 (1994), pp. 25–33.

capsicum pepper   See CHILI PEPPER.

captan   A useful, though potentially dangerous FUNGICIDE that retards the growth of molds, yeasts and fungi. Captan shows up frequently in grapes and is used generally for FRUIT (apples, peaches, strawberries) and VEGETABLES (beans, peas, carrots, corn, garlic, cabbage, lettuce, broccoli). Traces of captan have been detected in FAT and cooking oils. In use since the 1950s, the legal limit for captan was set before the discovery that it can cause kidney and intestinal CANCER in lab animals. Captan was named by the U.S. National Academy of Science as one of the most toxic PESTICIDES. The EPA has proposed banning captan because it is a suspected CARCINOGEN.

caramelized sugar   A brown food coloring prepared by heating table sugar (SUCROSE) without water. As sugar turns brown its sweetness is gradually replaced by a burnt flavor and aroma. Water is then added to create a brown syrup. Caramel provides a brown color to foods like pumpernickel bread, some partially whole wheat breads, and boeuf bourguignon. Vegetables like onion and carrots are glazed or lightly caramelized by being heated with sugar and water. The term caramel also refers to a type of brown, square-shaped CANDY with a chewy consistency. (See also ARTIFICIAL FOOD COLORS; FOOD ADDITIVES.)

caraway (*Carum carvi*)   A small, seed-like fruit used as an aromatic seasoning. This herb is related to CARROTS and PARSLEY. Dried caraway seeds are used to season rye bread, as well as pastry, soups, vegetables, meats and certain cheeses. It adds zest to potato salad and coleslaw. Caraway seed oil provides the distinctive flavor of kümmel, a liqueur. Fresh caraway leaves flavor soup, salad, cheeses, vegetables and meat.

carbohydrate   A large class of organic compounds that includes sugars, starches and fiber. Carbohydrates contain two hydrogen atoms and one oxygen atom (H_2O) for each carbon atom, and the name "carbohydrate" relates to the apparent "hydrated carbons" in their chemical formulas. Carbohydrates represent such a variety of substances that they are grouped into several categories.

Nutritionally important carbohydrates are categorized as simple and complex, according to their size. SIMPLE CARBOHYDRATES are referred to as sugars. Simple carbohydrates in the form of NATURAL SWEETENERS are among the most common FOOD ADDITIVES. Examples are SUCROSE, DEXTROSE, FRUCTOSE and CORN SYRUP, as well as any word on a food label that ends in "-ose." COMPLEX CARBOHYDRATES occur in plants as starch and fiber.

Nutritionists classify carbohydrates in foods according to their degree of processing. Refined carbohydrates, like sugar and white flour, are highly purified materials, containing little, if any, of the nutrients found in the whole food from which the carbohydrate was prepared; therefore, they supply mainly calories. Carbohydrates are also classified according to size: monosaccharides, dissacharides, oligosaccharides and POLYSACCHARIDES. The simplest are monosaccharides, which include simple sugars. The family of HEXOSES are monosaccharides containing six carbon atoms; glucose and fructose are examples. PENTOSES are simple sugars with five carbon atoms; ribose, the raw material for RNA, is the most common example.

The predominant carbohydrate of the body is glucose. Glucose in the blood is called BLOOD SUGAR and is a major fuel source for most cells of the body. The brain relies on glucose to meet its energy needs. Unless the diet supplies adequate carbohydrates, the body's metabolism switches to a STARVATION mode, in which body fat is burned to meet most energy needs. To fuel the brain during starvation, glucose is synthesized from AMINO ACIDS obtained by the breakdown of muscles.

Disaccharides contain two linked simple sugars. The most familiar is sucrose (table sugar). This disaccharide contains glucose and fructose. Fragments of complex carbohydrates are called oligosaccharides. As an example, food additives like maltodextrin are derived from starch and typically contain 3 to 10 glucose units. Because they are much smaller than starch molecules they are water-soluble.

The largest carbohydrates are polysaccharides, which are polymers (long chains) and contain many simple sugars linked together. STARCH and GLYCOGEN ("animal starch") are polysaccharides important in nutrition and metabolism. Unlike sugars, complex carbohydrates do not taste sweet, and they are often insoluble in water. Starch is composed of long chains of a thousand or more glucose units. The form of starch with many side chains or branches is AMYLOPECTIN; the unbranced form is called AMYLOSE. Starch functions as the plant storehouse of glucose. For example, when energy is needed during seed germination, the developing seed uses glucose from starch to grow into an embryonic plant. Starch is packed in granules that must be cooked to be edible. Digestion of starch yields glucose. Although glycogen is not an important food source of carbohydrate, it is the storage carbohydrate of tissues like muscle and the liver, and is broken down when fuel is needed.

Carbohydrates are classified as "macro nutrients" because they account for such a large part of the diet throughout the world. In the United States carbohydrates typically supply approximately 46% of the daily energy requirement. In Africa carbohydrates constitute almost 80% of dietary calories. The prevalence of carbohydrate in the diet is due to its ready accessibility from plant sources, its low cost and its ease of storage. Major sources of starch include cereal GRAINS, such as WHEAT, RICE, RYE, MILLET, sorghum and CORN. These grains contain 70% starch. Tubers, such as POTATOES and CASSAVAS, and root vegetables, such as parsnips, also supply starch. BEANS and seeds of legumes, rich sources of protein, also contain 40% of their weight as starch. Worldwide, wheat is the predominant crop source of dietary carbohydrate, followed by rice, corn and potatoes, and then by barley and cassava.

Fiber refers to indigestible complex carbohydrates found in plant cell walls and structures. The major classes of fiber possess different sugars as building blocks. CELLULOSE, one of the most common fibers, contains only glucose. HEMICELLULOSES, PECTINS, GUMS and LIGNIN are other important types. Humans do not produce digestive enzymes that can break down fiber, though colon bacteria can feast on them. The soluble forms of fiber, such as pectins and gums, and insoluble forms like cellulose assure a healthy intestinal tract and reduce the risk of diverticulosis, hemorrhoids, constipation, colon cancer and other intestinal disorders.

In the United States there is a long tradition of avoiding starchy food for weight control, out of a mistaken belief that carbohydrates are calorie-rich, but the opposite is actually true. Bread and pasta can help a dieter because carbohydrates contain only 4 calories per gram, less than half the calories in fat based on weight. In addition, carbohydrate calories are less efficiently stored as fat, compared to dietary fat. But, in general, excessive consumption of calories from any nutrient—whether PROTEIN, fat or carbohydrate—leads to fat accumulation. Every year Americans eat over 100 pounds of simple carbohydrates per person. This high sugar consumption contributes to excessive weight, promotes dental caries and leads to poor nutrition. Current dietary guidelines recommend increasing the amount of complex carbohydrate while decreasing sugar consumption by eating whole, starchy foods like LEGUMES, grains and fresh VEGETABLES to supply nutrients like MINERALS and FIBER, as well as plant substances that reduce the risk of cancer (isoflavones, ellagic acid, isothiocyanates, among others). (See also CARBOHYDRATE LOADING; CARBOHYDRATE METABOLISM.)

Asp, Nils-Georg, "Classification and Methodology of Food Carbohydrates as Related to Nutritional Effects," *American Journal of Clinical Nutrition*, 61:4 supp. (April 1995), pp. 930S–37S.

carbohydrate, available   The portion of dietary carbohydrate that can be digested to GLUCOSE and its storage form, GLYCOGEN. This fraction includes monosaccharides (such as glucose, FRUCTOSE, GALACTOSE, MANNOSE); disaccharides, which contain two sugars (LACTOSE, maltose, SUCROSE); starch fragments (DEXTRINS); and POLYSACCHARIDES (starches and glycogen, which contain hundreds of glucose units). Fiber is excluded from available carbohydrate because it cannot be digested. (See also DIETARY GUIDELINES FOR AMERICANS.)

carbohydrate digestion   The conversion of starch and dietary carbohydrates to simple sugars that can be absorbed and used by the body. Many carbohydrates in food are too large to be absorbed by the intestine, which normally absorbs only simple sugars. Starch digestion yields the simple sugar, glucose, through a complex series of events: Starch digestion begins in the mouth with an enzyme in saliva called AMYLASE as food is chewed. In the intestine amylase secreted by the pancreas digests starch to maltose, a sugar containing two linked glucose units. Intestinal enzymes, MALTASE and dextrinase, carry out the final step, the breakdown of small starch fragments to glucose. Sugars composed of simple sugars are also digested to their simple building blocks. Sucrose (table sugar) yields glucose and fructose by the action of the intestinal enzyme SUCRASE, and lactose (milk sugar) yields glucose and galactose by action of LACTASE, also an intestinal enzyme. (See also CARBOHYDRATE METABOLISM.)

carbohydrate loading (glycogen loading)   A procedure used by athletes who consume CARBOHYDRATES to force their muscles to increase the amount of stored carbohydrate, GLYCOGEN. Muscle glycogen represents emergency fuel because it is readily broken down to blood glucose and increasing glycogen content in muscles delays exhaustion and increases endurance. Modified regimen, six days before competition: days 1–3, normal diet with 50% carbohydrate. Day 1, 90-minute aerobic workout; days 2–3, 40-minute workout. Days 4–6, high carbohydrate diet with 70% carbohydrate. Days 4 and 5, 20-minute workout. Day 6, rest.

Carbohydrate loading will not increase endurance when exercising less than 1.5 hours. However, eating high carbohydrate meals the night before an athletic event and the day of the event can assist individuals participating in short events lasting up to 1.5 hours.

Carbohydrate loading is not recommended for athletes over 40, for adolescent athletes, or for people with kidney problems, heart disease or diabetes, nor is it recommended for anyone more than twice a year. After repeated episodes of loading, the glycogen in the heart increases. The additional water content of cells can adversely affect heart performance by altering the ability of those cells to perform work. (See also CARBOHYDRATE METABOLISM.)

Rauch, L.M., Rodger, I., Wilson, G.R., Belonje, J.D., Dennis, S.C., Noakes, T.D., Hawley, J.A., "The Effects of Carbohydrate Loading on Muscle Glycogen Content and Cycling Performance," *International Journal of Sport Nutrition*, 5:1 (1995), pp. 25–36.

carbohydrate metabolism   Cellular reactions that convert carbohydrates to the simple sugar GLUCOSE, and subsequently break down glucose to produce energy or raw materials for cell synthesis. Lactose (milk sugar) contains galactose, and sucrose (table sugar) contains fructose (fruit sugar); both must be converted to glucose prior to their being used by cells.

Glucose after Digestion

Following digestion, simple sugars absorbed by the small intestine are carried via the bloodstream to the liver, which converts fructose and galactose into glucose. After a carbohydrate meal, blood glucose rises rapidly. In response to elevated blood sugar levels, beta cells of the pancreas release the hormone INSULIN, which promotes glucose uptake by most tissues like muscle and fat cells. The brain and the liver do not require insulin to use glucose.

Glycogen Metabolism

In muscle and in the liver, surplus glucose can be linked up to form long, branched molecules called GLYCOGEN, the major energy reserve in these two tissues. Two hormones, EPINEPHRINE (adrenal glands) and GLUCAGON (pancreas), stimulate glycogen breakdown when energy is needed. The liver's role is to maintain adequate BLOOD SUGAR levels; when the diet does not supply enough carbohydrate the liver releases glucose from liver glycogen by a process called GLYCOGENOLYSIS. The liver also produces glucose from non-carbohydrate materials like AMINO ACIDS and LACTIC ACID through a branch of carbohydrate metabolism called GLUCONEOGENESIS.

Glucose as a Source of Energy

Once in the cell, glucose can be used in many ways. It can be burned for energy; it can be converted to glycogen (muscle and liver) for storage; it can produce an agent to supply hydrogen atoms used for biosynthesis, NADPH (reduced nicotinamide adenine dinucleotide phosphate), an enzyme helper based on the B vitamin niacin. The carbon atoms of glucose can be used to synthesize lipids. All cells of the body can oxidize glucose to produce ATP, the energetic currency of the cell.

A collection of enzymes work together to carry out the first part of this process, called GLYCOLYSIS, to yield PYRUVIC ACID, a three-carbon acid. Pyruvic acid is shortened to acetic acid and the carbon atom is removed as CARBON DIOXIDE. An activated form of acetic acid called acetyl COENZYME A is used to synthesize FATTY ACIDS and CHOLESTEROL. Alternatively, acetic acid can be oxidized completely to carbon dioxide by mitochondria, the cells' powerhouses. The oxidation of pyruvate and of acetyl CoA requires the B vitamins NIACIN, RIBOFLAVIN, THIAMIN and PANTOTHENIC ACID, which form key enzyme helpers (COENZYMES). The complete oxidation of each glucose molecule yields 38 ATP molecules. This is an excellent conservation of energy: it represents an overall efficiency of about 40%.

Glucose can also be oxidized by another route, a series of reactions called the Pentose Phosphate Pathway, to produce the NADPH needed in the formation of lipids like cholesterol and in other compounds, and to produce ribose, a simple sugar needed for DNA and RNA synthesis. (See also CARBOHYDRATE DIGESTION; FAT METABOLISM.)

Flatt, Jeane-Pierre, "Use and Storage of Carbohydrate and Fat," *American Journal of Clinical Nutrition*, 61: supp. (1995), pp. 952S–59S.

carbohydrate sweeteners   A variety of carbohydrates used in food production and home cooking as sweeteners. They include simple sugars (monosaccharides) such as FRUCTOSE and GLUCOSE, and the more complex disaccharides, like SUCROSE (table sugar).

Table sugar is highly purified from sugar cane or from beet roots. Other processed sugars are chemically prepared; corn sugar (glucose, "dextrose") yields high-fructose corn syrup. Syrup and molasses are partially purified mixtures. Even honey is considered a refined carbohydrate because it is processed by bees from nectar. Naturally-occurring sweeteners are found in fruits, fruit juices and some vegetables, like beets and carrots.

Carbohydrate sweeteners account for about 25% of the total calories of the typical American diet. Regardless of their source, carbohydrate sweeteners are converted to glucose before they can be burned as fuels. Because they are purified substances, not whole foods, they supply only CALORIES.

Two-thirds of the sugar consumption in America represents sugar added by food and beverage manufacturers and processors. Sucrose and fructose (FRUCTOSE CORN SYRUP) are the two most prevalent sweeteners and are among the most common FOOD ADDITIVES. Sucrose is added to foods ranging from catsup to gelatin desserts. Current U.S. guidelines recommend decreasing sugar consumption while increasing consumption of complex carbohydrates (starches and fiber). (See also ARTIFICIAL SWEETENERS; CONVENIENCE FOOD; EMPTY CALORIES.)

carbonated beverages   See CARBON DIOXIDE.

carbon dioxide (CO_2)   A colorless gas produced by the complete oxidation of organic compounds through the release of energy. Carbon dioxide is the endproduct when CARBOHYDRATE, PROTEIN and FATS are completely burned by the body to produce energy (respiration). This gas readily diffuses out of the cells where it is produced, dissolves in blood and is transported to the lungs. There, carbon dioxide migrates out into air, contained in the lungs, while oxygen diffuses into the blood to replace that used in respiration. The distance between blood and air at the lung tissue lining is exceedingly small, only 0.0001 cm—too small to slow gas exchange. Shallow breathing and lung diseases lead to excessive carbon dioxide buildup, which can create acidic conditions (ACIDOSIS).

Carbon dioxide in the blood is more than a waste product. It combines with water to form CARBONIC ACID, which breaks down to BICARBONATE, a major pH BUFFER to neutralize acids. The kidney also forms bicarbonate to help maintain the acid-base balance.

Industrial Uses of Carbon Dioxide

Carbonated beverages contain carbon dioxide maintained under pressure. Carbon dioxide is responsible for the bubbles in beer, mineral water and soft drinks and contributes to their slightly sour (acidic) taste. Carbon dioxide is used as a refrigerant (dry ice), a foaming agent, and as a growth promoter of plants in greenhouses. (See also CARBOHYDRATE METABOLISM; FAT METABOLISM; HEMOGLOBIN.)

carbonic acid   A weak ACID formed when CARBON DIOXIDE reacts with water in which it is dissolved. In beverages like champagne, beer, carbonated soft drinks and sparkling water, dissolved carbonic acid provides the fizz and the tart flavor.

Carbonic acid readily forms in the body when carbon dioxide, released as fuel, is burned, dissolves in the bloodstream. Carbonic acid breaks down to bicarbonate, and the mixture of bicarbonate and carbonic acid is maintained by RED BLOOD CELLS and the kidneys. Bicarbonate and carbonic acid buffer the blood at pH 7.35–7.45 by resisting changes in the hydrogen ion concentration. For example, bicarbonate neutralizes excess acids, while alkaline substances (bases) introduced into the bloodstream are neutralized by carbonic acid. (See also ACIDOSIS; ALKALOSIS.)

carboxylic acids   A large family of acidic compounds found in foods and produced by metabolic reactions. Carboxylic ACIDS are capable of releasing hydrogen ions and neutralizing bases. Carboxylic acids are classified as weak acids because they release only a small fraction of their hydrogen ions.

When these acids are neutralized, they produce "conjugate bases," salt forms of the parent acids. Carboxylic acids in cells, including LACTIC ACID, CITRIC ACID, and FATTY ACIDS like PALMITIC ACID and OLEIC ACID, have been neutralized and exist in cells only as their conjugate bases. They are called, respectively, lactate, citrate, palmitate and oleate.

The AMINO ACIDS can behave as acids, as the name suggests. Two amino acids possess extra carboxyl (acidic) groups and are classified as acidic amino acids: ASPARTIC ACID and GLUTAMIC ACID.

Many acidic compounds occur in foods as salts or conjugate bases. Common FOOD ADDITIVES include preservatives, SODIUM BENZOATE, potassium sorbate and CALCIUM PROPIONATE; acidifiers, SODIUM, hydrogen phosphate, potassium

tartrate, sodium citrate, FUMARIC ACID. (See also CARBOHYDRATE METABOLISM; FOOD ADDITIVES.)

carboxypeptidase   A pancreatic enzyme that digests food PROTEINS in the intestine. Carboxypeptidase breaks down proteins by clipping the links between AMINO ACIDS in proteins and is classified as a proteolytic enzyme. Carboxypeptidase, like many other enzymes, requires ZINC as the cofactor.

Proteolytic digestive enzymes, including carboxypeptidase, are synthesized by the pancreas in an inactive form to protect the pancreatic cell from digesting itself. Only when it is released into the intestine does it become fully activated. (See also DIGESTION; PANCREAS; ZYMOGEN.)

carcinogen   An agent or substance that causes CANCER in experimental animals or humans. Carcinogens occur in the environment as certain PESTICIDES, cigarette smoke, ozone or mold toxins. Some industrial chemicals cause cancer, though most do not. Four percent of the 10,000 chemicals that have been tested have been shown to cause cancer in animals. Carcinogens may be various forms of ionizing radiation: X rays, ultraviolet light in sunlight, and emissions from radioactive materials like radon.

Carcinogens may be produced within the body by normal processes. The liver may convert a foreign compound into highly reactive oxides in an attempt to render it more water-soluble, and hence excretable by the kidney. The BENZOPYRENE in cigarette smoke is such an example. Alternatively, carcinogens may form spontaneously in the body. The food preservative NITRITE reacts with amines, nitrogen-rich compounds in the digestive tract, to form NITROSOAMINES, which are carcinogens.

Trace amounts of carcinogens may inadvertently contaminate meat, dairy products, fruits and vegetables. These include insecticides, like Heptachlor; FUNGICIDES, like O-phenylphenol; and HERBICIDES like Alachlor. Several chemicals used as feed additives for livestock and poultry are suspected carcinogens (such as gentian green). Whether or not exposure to multiple low-level residues poses a tolerable risk is still being debated.

Plants have evolved multiple chemical defenses to protect themselves against predators, and a variety of plant agents occur naturally in foods that, when isolated in pure form, have been shown to cause cancer in experimental animals. Americans eat an estimated 1.5 grams of natural pesticides daily. About half have been found to be carcinogenic in animals. It has been proposed that naturally occurring carcinogens pose a greater threat than synthetic chemicals and pollutants. On the other hand, there is little evidence that foods themselves cause cancer. To the contrary, plant foods are a rich storehouse of potential anticancer agents: VITAMIN C, CAROTENOIDS like BETA CAROTENE and VITAMIN E. Substances like phenethyl isothiocyanate and indoles found in the cabbage family, and certain FLAVONOIDS such as ellagic acid, in strawberries and other fruits and vegetables, are powerful protective agents. More remain to be identified. Parsley, sage, oregano and rosemary prevent toxin-producing mold from growing, and garlic, onions, cumin, cloves and caraway possess compounds that reduce the effects of cancer-causing agents.

Examples of common foods that contain putative cancer-causing materials include: celery, parsley and parsnips, which contain a chemical, 5-methoxypsoralen, that can be a carcinogen when applied to the skin of experimental animals. It is unknown whether this causes cancer when consumed. The common supermarket white mushroom (*Agaricus bisporus*) and the false morel, a wild mushroom, contain agartine. There is limited evidence that its breakdown products may cause cancer in experimental animals; however, agartine is destroyed by cooking. Peels of oranges and other citrus fruits contain d-limonene. Studies of limonene are mixed: Some show that it did not cause cancer in lab animals, others that it acted as an anticarcinogen, and still others that it can cause cancer. Beets, lettuce, radishes, spinach and other dark-green leafy vegetables contain nitrate, which can be slowly converted to nitrite in the body, which can form carcinogenic nitrosoamines. The vitamin C and fiber present in these vegetables seem to counter this risk. The situation is more complex: for example a substance, such as capsaicin of chili pepper, can pose a low-level cancer risk to the gut and at the same time it may be an anticarcinogen elsewhere.

There is as yet no reliable data base upon which to estimate the daily intake of natural carcinogens. Furthermore, natural carcinogens are often less powerful than synthetic carcinogens. More research is needed to evaluate the net effect of natural carcinogens and anti-carcinogens together with fat, fiber and others implicated in foods. Overall, the predominance of evidence indicates that giving up smoking and improving the diet are the best defenses against cancer. The U.S. surgeon general and other experts recommend eating more fruits, vegetables and legumes and less fat to reduce the risk of cancer. (See also ARTIFICIAL FOOD COLORS; FOOD TOXINS; MEAT CONTAMINANTS; PESTICIDES; RISK DUE TO CHEMICALS IN FOOD AND WATER.)

cardamom (*Elettaria cardamomum*)   An aromatic spice, native to tropical Asia. Cardamom is a member of the ginger family, and cardamom seeds are sun-dried and marketed whole. Cardamom is used as a seasoning in curry, stews, processed meats like FRANKFURTERS and sausages, pickling spices, and even pastries. Cardamom seeds contain several substances with cavity-fighting properties—contributing to a growing body of natural substances that potentially can fight disease.

cardiovascular disease (CVD)   Chronic diseases of the heart and blood vessels associated with aging. CVD accounts for over 50% of all deaths in the United States. The epidemic of CVD appeared in the 1920s and mortality due to CVD increased until the 1960s, when the rate declined rapidly. In recent years the decline has slowed, yet this disease still affects nearly 66 million Americans; 1 million die each year, and most American men have a degree of arterial disease (clogged arteries).

The following are classified as cardiovascular diseases: ARTERIOSCLEROSIS (a general thickening or hardening of arterial walls), ATHEROSCLEROSIS (lipid accumulation on arterial walls), CORONARY ARTERY DISEASE (atherosclerosis of the arteries that supply blood to the heart), heart attack (damage to the heart muscle due to blocked arteries), STROKE (damage to the brain due to reduced blood flow because of blocked or damaged

arteries), HYPERTENSION (elevated blood pressure), peripheral vascular disease (varicose veins, thrombophlebitis, atherosclerosis of extremities) and congestive heart failure. Several conditions cause arterial disease. Aneurysms are weakened segments of vessels that fill with blood, causing the vessel to balloon outward. Disorders of the muscle sheath may cause arteries to constrict or to dilate. In atherosclerosis, deposits (PLAQUE) on the inner arterial wall may cause blockage.

Major risk factors for CVD have been identified. Risk factors simply increase the odds of developing CVD: They do not guarantee an individual will develop it, nor does the absence of risk factors guarantee that a person won't have a heart attack. They include high blood pressure (hypertension), cigarette smoking (one of the most important risk factors), elevated serum cholesterol (or, more precisely, elevated LDL, LOW DENSITY LIPOPROTEIN cholesterol), elevated serum TRIGLYCERIDES (fat levels), being overweight, diabetes, stress, lack of aerobic exercise, a family history of cardiovascular disease, being of the male gender, and increasing age. Recently, elevated blood homocysteine, an amino acid breakdown product, was found to be an independent risk factor for coronary heart disease. INSULIN resistance, that is, a lack of sensitivity to the hormone insulin, is as great a risk factor for obstructive artery disease as hypertension or cigarette smoking. These risk factors are more than additive; the combined effect of two or more risk factors is greater than it would be calculated by adding risks together. For an individual with three risk factors, the chances of heart disease are six times greater than when only one risk factor is present. The Centers for Disease Control found in 1992 that only 18% of Americans over age 18 were completely free of major risk factors for CVD. Among the least healthy were men between the ages of 50 and 64 and women over 65. Only 9% were reported free of major risk factors.

Some risk factors can't be changed: heredity, which includes racial tendencies toward diabetes and hypertension and a family history of CVD, gender, and increased age. Many other risk factors are controllable. Diet and lifestyle play critical roles, and personal choices can profoundly alter the probability of CVD and many other chronic diseases associated with AGING. The following steps have been recommended:

1. Stop smoking. Smoking contributes to atherosclerosis, hypertension, cancer and elevated blood cholesterol.
2. Control high blood pressure. Blood pressure above 120 (the larger number) increases the risk of heart attack.
3. Control DIABETES MELLITUS. Chronic elevated blood sugar and insulin predispose an individual to cardiovascular disease, in addition to cataract, infection, kidney disease and nerve damage.
4. Exercise. Regular aerobic exercise is the cornerstone of prevention of CVD. A sedentary life-style increases the risk of obesity and high blood lipids. Walking 30 to 60 minutes a day affords significant benefits for cardiovascular health.
5. Lose weight to help prevent adult onset diabetes, to lower blood pressure, lower LDL cholesterol and raise HDL cholesterol.
6. Consume less fat, especially saturated (animal) fat to lower LDL cholesterol and blood triglycerides, and to

lose or maintain desired weight. The content of unsaturated fatty acid is also important. A low polyunsaturated fat to saturated fat (P/S) ratio lowers blood cholesterol levels. Omega 6 polyunsaturated fatty acids (as found in most vegetable oils, such as safflower and soybean oil) and omega 3 fatty acids (as found in fish, fish oils, flax seed oils) decrease the risk of plaque formation and of blood clots. Minimize trans-fatty acids as found in hydrogenated vegetable oils to lower LDL cholesterol.

7. Reduce alcohol consumption. Two drinks per day for men, one drink per day for women can raise HDL cholesterol. More than this increases the risk of hypertension, cancer and abuse.

8. Cut back on cholesterol-rich foods to lower LDL cholesterol and triglycerides, especially if there is a family history of CVD and elevated blood lipids.

9. Eat more potassium-rich foods and less sodium. Eating more vegetables and fruits and decreasing high-sodium convenience foods can lower or stabilize blood pressure.

10. Consume at least five servings of fruits and vegetables daily. Choosing plenty of fruits, legumes and vegetables provides FIBER and PHYTOCHEMICALS, including ANTIOXIDANTS that promote vascular health.

11. Consider taking vitamin supplements. Supplements that provide folic acid and vitamin B_{12} may help decrease high levels of homocysteine to reduce the risk of stroke and heart disease. Consuming at least 100 IU of vitamin E seems to decrease the risk of heart attack, though the National Cholesterol Education Program believes the evidence so far is not strong enough to make a general recommendation.

A constellation of symptoms called SYNDROME X frequently appears in older people prone to cardiovascular disease. Syndrome X includes hypertension, insulin resistance, diabetes or prediabetic conditions, elevated serum triglycerides, low HDL-cholesterol and obesity (central body fat). By controlling hypertension, making a lifelong commitment to being physically active, consuming a semi-vegetarian diet (lower in fat, high in fruits and vegetables), syndrome X can often be controlled. It is now thought that the latest lipid deposits in arteries are those that are most likely to rupture and cause heart attacks. By eating less cholesterol and saturated fat, consuming a low-fat vegetarian diet with minimal animal protein, managing stress effectively and exercising regularly, these deposits can shrink. It is never too late to change life-style patterns to lower the risk of CVD. (See also CHOLESTEROL.)

Lee, Kyu Taik, Oike, Yasaburo, and Kanazawa, T., eds., "The Third International Conference on Nutrition in Cardio-Cerebrovascular Diseases," *Annals of the New York Academy of Sciences*, 676 (1992).

carnitine (L-carnitine)   A nutrient required for fat oxidation and energy production. Carnitine helps transport FATTY ACIDS into mitochondria, the cellular structure specialized for fuel oxidation. Carnitine may be necessary for the oxidation of certain amino acids (VALINE, ISOLEUCINE and LEUCINE) for energy. The daily requirement for L-carnitine for health is unknown. The body synthesizes L-carnitine from two essential amino acids, LYSINE and METHIONINE. The rate may be inadequate for: kidney patients on hemodialysis; patients with liver failure; strict VEGETARIANS; premature and low birth-weight infants; pregnant or lactating women; children with genetic predisposition to carnitine deficiency or who experience infection or malnutrition. Breast milk contains a high level of L-carnitine to nurture the infant, and it may be an essential nutrient for the newborn.

Carnitine deficiency causes muscle weakness, severe confusion, angina, and high blood lipids, including CHOLESTEROL. Carnitine deficiency is also linked to cardiac enlargement and congestive heart failure. Fatty acid oxidation is a major source of energy for the heart muscle, and carnitine deficiency causes extreme metabolic impairment. The normal heart stores carnitine, but if it does not receive adequate oxygen, carnitine levels drop. Supplementation with carnitine raises heart carnitine levels, allowing the heart to use a limited oxygen supply more efficiently. Thus carnitine has been used effectively to treat atherosclerosis, angina and coronary heart disease. Carnitine may reduce blood fat and LOW-DENSITY LIPOPROTEIN (LDL, undesirable cholesterol) and increase HIGH-DENSITY LIPOPROTEIN (HDL, desirable cholesterol). Carnitine also decreases blood fat. It may help patients with angina and CARDIOVASCULAR DISEASE, and with some types of muscle disease. A derivative of carnitine called acetyl L-carnitine appears to be neuroprotective. Supplementing with acetyl L-carnitine may improve cognitive defects associated with forms of senility and age-related depression. Low carnitine levels may be linked to chronic fatigue symptoms.

Good sources of carnitine are red meats and dairy products like milk. Tempeh and avocados contain some carnitine; however, most vegetables, fruits and grains are poor sources. Most soy-based infant formulas are supplemented with carnitine. While the naturally occurring form of carnitine, (L-carnitine) appears to be safe, high doses of synthetic carnitine (D, L-carnitine), a mixture of isomers, for many weeks can cause progressive weakness and atrophy of certain muscles. Symptoms disappear when supplementation with the mixture ceases. (See also FAT METABOLISM.)

Salvioli, G. and Neri, M., "L-acetylcarnitine Treatment of Mental Decline in the Elderly," *Drugs and Experimental and Clinical Research*, 20:4 (1994), pp. 169–76.

carob (*Ceratonia siliqua*; St. John's bread)   A CHOCOLATE substitute obtained from pods of a Mediterranean evergreen of the pea family. Carob pods contain many seeds, surrounded by an edible, fleshy pulp. A powder is prepared from the pods of the carob tree. Carob offers several advantages over chocolate: It is free of CAFFEINE-like stimulants and it contains only 1% FAT (0.18 calories per gram). In contrast, COCOA powder contains 23% fat. On the other hand, carob powder contains more sugar and TANNINS, bitter plant products, than chocolate. Carob CANDY may contain much more sugar and SATURATED FAT than chocolate bars, and may not be a low-calorie food. Carob candy provides an alternative for those with a chocolate allergy. Because carob powder is so sweet, the oven temperature should be decreased to minimize burning when used in recipes. (See also ALLERGY, FOOD.)

carob bean gum   A food thickener prepared from the bean of the carob tree. The GUM prevents a granular texture when added to ice cream. It is also added to thicken salad dressings, pie fillings, barbecue sauces and doughs. Carob bean gum is classified as a safe additive. It is also a mild laxative. (See also CANDY; FOOD ADDITIVES; THICKENING AGENTS.)

carotene   See BETA CAROTENE.

carotenemia   Elevated levels of carotene in the blood. A condition characterized by yellowed palms of the hands and soles of the feet. Carotenemia does not lead to coloration of the membranes that line eyes, unlike jaundice. The accumulation of BETA CAROTENE is not associated with the toxicity characterized by excessive VITAMIN A. Consumption of excessive amounts of yellow vegetables, carrot juice, dark-green leafy vegetables and beta carotene supplements can cause carotenemia in susceptible individuals. Supplementation with high levels of beta carotene when there is alcohol-induced liver damage can lead to toxic symptoms. (See also HYPERVITAMINOSIS.)

carotenoids   Yellow, orange and red pigments found in yellow and orange fruits and vegetables. Carotenoids also occur in dark-green leafy vegetables, where their color is masked by the green of chlorophyll. There are more than 500 carotenoids, all synthesized by plants; of these, 50 to 60 commonly occur in foods. Carotenoids are conveniently divided into carotenes and xanthophylls (oxygenated carotenes). The most famous carotenoid is beta carotene. Though most abundant in nature, it does not stand alone; in dark green leafy vegetables, xanthophylls can make up 90% of the total carotenoids.

Lobster and salmon are pink because they have ingested carotenoid-containing plants; the pigments color their tissues. Egg yolk derives its yellow color from carotenoids eaten by the hen. Yellow oils like peanut and corn oil reflect their carotenoid content. Several carotenoids are manufactured for use as food colors: BETA CAROTENE (orange to yellow); CANTHAXANTHINE (red); and apocaroenal (yellow). All three are approved food additives and are among the safest food colors. They are used in margarines, candies and sauces.

About 38 carotenoids can be converted to vitamin A (pro-vitamin A activity). Only a few of these occur in sufficient amounts to be significant in the diet. The most important pro-vitamin is beta carotene, followed by alpha and gamma carotene. Because of inefficiencies of absorption and conversion, beta carotene is one-sixth as effective a source as vitamin A itself. Conversion of the other carotenes is less efficient. Pure beta carotene used in supplements is the synthetic, all trans form. Foods supply mixed carotenoids, including cis forms. The *cis* forms of beta carotene rather than synthetic all *trans* beta carotene appear to be better antioxidants, suggesting that natural mixtures from foods may be more effective. Mild cooking generally improves beta carotene utilization. The yellow food additive canthaxin is an oxidized form of carotenoid from mushrooms that has no pro-vitamin A activity.

Multiple studies over the last two decades suggest that diets rich in carotenoid-containing foods decrease the risk of cancer and of cardiovascular disease. The beneficial effect of carotenoids in the prevention of cancer is believed to occur through protection against oxidative stress and enhanced immune function. In general carotenoids act as versatile antioxidants to block cellular damage due to free radical attack. Free radicals are highly unstable molecules or molecular fragments with one electron. They avidly attack any cell component they meet, damaging proteins, membranes and even DNA. Lycopene, the red carotenoid of tomatoes, red bell peppers and pink grapefruit, has no vitamin A activity in the body, but it serves as an antioxidant. Lutein, lycopene, cryptoxanthin and alpha carotene complement the antioxidant activity of beta carotene. These prevalent carotenoids occur chiefly in 50 commonly eaten fruits and vegetables. Various population studies and clinical trials have not supported the proposal that beta carotene alone prevents cancer and cardiovascular disease. Rather the emerging picture portrays beta carotene as only one ingredient of multiple antioxidants found in plant foods that work together to protect the body. Increased carotenoid levels have been associated with decreased oxidation of LDL, the less desirable form of cholesterol in the blood. Oxidized LDL is believed to play a key role in the initial events leading to clogged arteries. The only way to be sure of obtaining the full range of carotenoid antioxidants is to eat a variety of fruits and vegetables regularly. (See also FOOD ADDITIVES; FOOD COLORING, NATURAL.)

Canfield, L.M.; Krinsky; N.I. Olson; J.A., eds., "Carotenoids in Human Health," *New York Academy of Sciences*, 691 (1993).

carrageenan   A texturizer prepared from a seaweed (Irish moss) and classified as a dietary FIBER. This fiber has no nutritive value and is not absorbed. Irish moss, which grows along the shores of Maine and the Maritime provinces of Canada, the British Isles, Scandinavia and France, is often added to chocolate MILK. Carrageenan forms a mild gel with milk protein that prevents COCOA from settling. Carrageenan is used in frozen desserts like ice cream, syrups, GELATINS, soups, jellies, YOGURT and milk puddings. Carrageenan is added to some canned infant formulas to keep FAT and PROTEIN dissolved and is used to stabilize the BUTTERFAT suspended in evaporated milk. Carrageenan stabilizes the foam in BEER and gives body to soft drinks. Carrageenan is also a replacement for gelatin in the diet of vegetarians.

Unlike other plant polysaccharides, excessive carrageenan may be detrimental to health. Animal studies have shown that it can cause liver enlargement, birth defects and ulcerated colon. The United Nations World Health Organization concluded that it does not cause cancer. Carrageenan-containing products should not be given to premature infants in whom it may disrupt development of the gastrointestinal tract. (See also FOOD ADDITIVES.)

carrot (*Daucus carota*)   A root vegetable belonging to the parsley family that has been cultivated for at least 2,000 years. The wild carrot is a native of Europe and Asia. Orange-colored varieties were developed in the 19th century and owe their color to carotenoid pigment. Other varieties of carrots may have yellow, white or purple roots that may be blunt or nearly round. Carrots contain more sugar than any other vegetable except beets.

Carrot juice is an excellent source of BETA CAROTENE, the plant parent of VITAMIN A. There is no problem with moderate consumption of carrot juice, but an excess of carrot juice can saturate the body with beta carotene and turn the skin yellow-brown, indicative of CAROTENEMIA. If the body becomes saturated with beta carotene, the individual should cut back to avoid possible problems with other plant materials in the carrot juice. If the whites of the eyes turn yellow it may indicate JAUNDICE, a more serious condition. Carrots are used as a salad vegetable, in making stews and soups and stocks. Carrots (one half cup, 55 g, grated) provide: 24 calories; protein, 0.6 g; carbohydrate, 5.6 g; fiber, 1.55 g; potassium, 178 mg; vitamin A, 1,547 retinol equivalents, niacin, 0.67 mg; and low levels of other B vitamins.

casaba (*Cucumis melo inodorus*)   A group of large, pale-yellow winter melons that originated in Turkey. Casaba is a smooth-skinned melon with a globular shape, resembling muskmelon. The ripe fruit has white or yellow flesh that is sweet and juicy and a characteristic cucumber-like flavor. Casabas are extensively cultivated in California, where they were first introduced late in the 19th century. One slice (245 g) yields 38 calories; protein, 1.7 g; carbohydrate, 9.1 g; fiber, 1.2 g; vitamin A, 40 retinol equivalents; potassium, 351 mg; vitamin C, 18 mg; thiamin, 0.06 mg; riboflavin, 0.04 mg; niacin, 0.8 mg.

casein (sodium caseinate)   The principal PROTEIN of cow's milk. When milk curdles, the curd is mainly casein. Casein is used to improve the texture of frozen desserts such as ice cream, ice milk, frozen custard and sherbet. In NON-DAIRY CREAMERS, casein serves both as a whitener and as an agent used to suspend fat (emulsifier). Casein is added to boost the protein content of PROCESSED FOODS and is considered a safe FOOD ADDITIVE. It is a nutritious, high-quality protein because it contains large amounts of all essential AMINO ACIDS. In nutrient studies, casein is used as a reference for protein quality. For example, in calculating the Protein Efficiency Ratio (PER), the ratio of weight gained by young animals to the amount of protein consumed, the dietary protein is assumed to be adequate when it is equivalent to casein. In this case 45 grams of such protein provide 100% of the REFERENCE DAILY INTAKE (RDI) for protein.

cashew (*Anacardium occidentale*)   A mildly flavored, kidney-shaped nut that is the fruit of a tropical evergreen, native to South America. The world's leading producers of cashews are Brazil, China, East Africa and India. Cashew apples, the pear-shaped fruit, are used in jams and jellies. A double shell surrounds the kernel of the cashew nut, and between the two shells is a toxic oil that can blister the skin. The shell, acrid oil and skin are removed before cashews are marketed. Because they contain 45% fat, a high level, cashews may become rancid and taste stale with prolonged storage at room temperature. The high fat content increases when the nuts are roasted in oil. Cashews yield a delicate table oil. Roasted as well as unroasted cashews are available and are used as snacks and in cooking. Ground cashews make a pleasing nut butter. Cashews (per ounce, [28 g], dry roasted and salted) contain: 163 calories; protein, 4.3 g; carbohydrate, 9.3 g; fiber, 1.7 g; fat, 13.2 g; iron, 1.7 mg; potassium, 160 mg; sodium, 181 mg; thiamin, 0.06 mg; riboflavin, 0.06 mg; niacin, 0.4 mg.

cassava (*Manioc utilissima; Manioc dulcis aipi*)   The tuber of a shrubby perennial of Central and South America that is widely cultivated in tropical regions. The two most widely grown varieties are the bitter manioc, *Manioc utilissima*, and the sweet *Manioc dulcis aipi*. Manioc roots end in large reddish-brown tubers 3 feet in length and 9 inches in diameter, with a white pulp, and constitute a STAPLE food. Tubers of the sweet manioc, which has a chestnut-like flavor, can be roasted and eaten plain. Cassava tubers contain compounds that break down to cyanide but are rendered harmless when cooked and yield a bland, high starch flour. Cassava is used like sweet potato in recipes. Traditionally, it is baked in thin cakes and combined with beans to make a balanced protein meal. Cassava can replace wheat FLOUR in the diet. TAPIOCA is prepared from cassava pulp that has been heated to form granules. Cassava root, raw (per 100 g), provides 124 calories; protein, 3.1 g; carbohydrate, 27 g; fiber, 2.5 g; fat, 0.39 g; calcium, 91 mg; iron, 3.6 mg; thiamin, 0.23 mg; riboflavin, 0.10 mg; niacin, 1.4 mg; and vitamin C, 48 mg.

catabolic state   A physiologic condition characterized by rapid weight loss, associated with losses of body fat and muscle mass. A catabolic state often occurs when food intake does not provide enough calories to meet the body's energy needs. Conditions favoring the breakdown of the body's own stores of PROTEIN, FAT and CARBOHYDRATE for energy production frequently occur during STARVATION, CRASH DIET-ING, FASTING; uncontrolled diabetes; ALCOHOLISM; and recovery from severe burns, surgery, illness, and radiation or chemotherapy for cancer treatment. The average weight loss after surgery is about 10% of body weight, and typical weight loss during a week in the hospital amounts to 5% of body weight. Chronic stress can also place the body in a catabolic state.

Nutritional support is important when the catabolic state is prolonged and the patient has diminished nutritional reserves and lowered immunity. Body protein breakdown can be slowed by administration of calorie-rich foods and adequate protein. Specific nutrients may benefit the seriously ill patient.

Supplements of ZINC, IRON, VITAMIN A, VITAMIN C, VITAMIN K and the B COMPLEX may be recommended to help speed wound healing, to rebuild red blood cells quickly, to assist in blood clotting, and to build up the immune system. Specific amino acids may be used therapeutically. GLUTAMINE is usually classified as a non-essential amino acid, but the postoperative administration of glutamine decreases the rate of muscle loss and supports rapidly growing tissues like the mucosal lining of the intestine. In the kidney glutamine serves as a donor of ammonia to help regulate acid-base balance, and it is produced in muscle to help dispose of ammonia, a by-product of amino acid degradation. ARGININE can also benefit seriously ill patients by enhancing wound healing and increasing the activity of T-cells, thus increasing the immune response; it may also increase growth hormone and insulin levels. Supplemental essential fatty acids may modify the immune response and thus limit inflammation by stimulating the formation of regulatory substances (thromboxane A_3, leukotrienes B_5) that restrict inflammation. However, even aggressive nutritional support may not prevent body protein loss during severe catabolic illness, where there are utilization of body fat and breakdown of skeletal muscle protein. (See also CATABOLISM; FATTY ACIDS; OMEGA-3 FATTY ACIDS.)

catabolism The processes of METABOLISM by which FAT, CARBOHYDRATE and PROTEIN fatty acids, glucose and surplus amino acids are oxidized to release energy measured as CALORIES. The body requires vast amounts of energy each day. For example, every day the kidneys filter the equivalent of 425 gallons of fluid and the heart beats over 4,000 times. Most usual energy needs are met by carbohydrate and fat in the diet. Oxidation of these fuels occurs by increments with a series of ENZYMES that trap energy released in fuel oxidation as ATP. This energy "currency" is used by cells for growth and maintenance. Most untrapped energy is released as heat. ATP production occurs in MITOCHONDRIA, small subcellular structures that function as the cell's powerhouses where fuel is burned for energy. The ultimate breakdown products of catabolism are CARBON DIOXIDE and WATER.

Catabolic enzymes work together to catalyze reactions (speed up chemical reactions without being destroyed in the process). A series of functionally linked enzymes is called a enzymatic pathway. The following represent typical catabolic pathways: GLYCOLYSIS oxidizes glucose to a simple acid, pyruvic acid, which yields acetic acid. KREB'S CYCLE oxidizes acetic acid to carbon dioxide. Muscle and liver GLUCOSE is stored as a polymer, GLYCOGEN. In GLYCOGENOLYSIS, glycogen is broken down when glucose is needed to supply energy. Fatty acid oxidation yields the most ATP; consequently, fat is the most efficient form of energy storage. When insufficient calories are consumed, muscle protein is also broken down for many tissues. Muscle protein breakdown yields amino acids whose carbon atoms are either shunted into blood glucose by the liver or are oxidized by many tissues. In this case the catabolic end products are carbon dioxide, water and UREA (nitrogenous waste).

The B complex supports catabolic processes. NIACIN, RIBOFLAVIN, THIAMIN, PANTOTHENIC ACID, FOLIC ACID, VITAMIN B_6 and VITAMIN B_{12} are key players in catabolic pathways. These vitamins form specific enzyme helpers (COENZYMES). They do not provide energy; instead they help catalyze energy production, much as the spark plugs of a car engine activate gasoline combustion without themselves being consumed. (See also CARBOHYDRATE METABOLISM; CATABOLIC STATE; FAT METABOLISM.)

catalase A highly active ENZYME that destroys HYDROGEN PEROXIDE. Catalase is considered an antioxidant. Hydrogen peroxide is a powerful oxidizing agent occurring naturally in cells as a by-product of metabolism that can damage cells. It is formed by specialized oxidative structures within cells called peroxisomes. Catalase is widely distributed among tissues and fluids such as SALIVA, and it is concentrated in the lens of the eye, where it serves a protective function. Commercially, catalase is applied in food processing to degrade excess hydrogen peroxide that is added as an oxidizing agent. (See also CATARACT.)

cataract An opacity of the lens of the eye and/or of its capsule that impairs vision. As the only transparent tissue of the body, the lens depends upon the regular arrangement of crystalline proteins for its clarity. Nonetheless, cataracts and macular degeneration are the leading causes of blindness in older people. AGE-RELATED MACULAR DEGENERATION refers to the age-related degeneration of a tiny area of the retina responsible for seeing fine detail such as print. Cataracts affect about 60% of Americans over the age of 75. The cause of mature onset cataract formation is unknown. According to a recent hypothesis, age-related deterioration of the lens is the result of oxidative damage due to sunlight's UV light. The lens is particularly vulnerable to cigarette smoke and other forms of air pollution that contribute to oxidative damage. Damaged lens proteins cannot be replaced and they tend to clump and scatter light, rather than staying transparent. In animal models, cataract can be caused by oxidative stress, and can be prevented or delayed by ANTIOXIDANTS. The level of the general cellular antioxidant GLUTATHIONE decreases in the lens in aging animals and humans. Cataracts are linked to increased risk of ATHEROSCLEROSIS, and they can be classified as a degenerative disease associated with aging. Cataracts can also be the result of DIABETES MELLITUS and congenital defects in infants.

Current cataract research emphasizes the role of nutrition in prevention. A wide variety of clinical studies have shown that a CAROTENOID-rich diet decreases the risk of cataracts. Data from the Physicians' Health Study suggested a 27% decrease in the relative risk among doctors taking multiple vitamin supplements. The Nurses' Health Study found that women with the highest intake of VITAMIN C, VITAMIN E and CAROTENOIDS had 40% fewer cataracts. Those who supplemented with vitamin C for 10 years or more decreased their cataract risk by 50%.

In terms of prevention, a diet rich in fruits and vegetables, with restricted sugar usage, seems prudent. Sugars such as excessive glucose and galactose derived from milk sugar (LACTOSE) diffuse into the lens and are converted to sugar alcohols, such as sorbitol, that do not leave the cells as readily. Accumulation can cause water imbalance in the cell, and eventual damage. Lactose can increase the risk of cataract for those with genetic defects in galactose metabolism. Folic acid, vitamin C, vitamin E, carotenoids, selenium and zinc may decrease the risk of oxidative damage, particularly with deficiency of these nutrients. FLAVONOIDS, complex substances that protect plants form oxidation, such as QUERCETIN, inhibit the enzyme that converts glucose to sorbitol.

Christen, William Gerard, Jr., "Antioxidants and Eye Disease," *American Journal of Medicine*, 97 (supp. 3A: September 26, 1994), pp. 3A–17S.

Varma, S.D., Devamanoharan, P. S., Morris S. M., "Prevention of Cataracts by Nutritional and Metabolic Antioxidants," *Critical Reviews in Food Science and Nutrition*, 35:1 & 2 (1995), pp. 111–29.

catecholamines An important family of AMINES (nitrogen-containing compounds) derived from TYROSINE, an AMINO ACID. Dopamine, EPINEPHRINE (adrenaline) and norepinephrine constitute this family of amines whose functions depend upon their tissue of origin. Dopamine functions as a NEUROTRANSMITTER and serves as a raw material of norepinephrine. Norepinephrine is a HORMONE, produced by the inner region of the adrenal gland (adrenal medulla), which acts as a vasoconstrictor (increases blood pressure by closing down blood vessels). Elsewhere norepinephrine functions as a neurotransmitter. Norepinephrine is a precursor of epinephrine, itself a key adrenal hormone released in response to stress and to stimulation of the sympathetic NERVOUS SYSTEM.

catfish (*Ictalus punctatus*; channel catfish)   A large group of mainly freshwater FISH without scales. The barbels or feelers of this bottom feeder resemble a cat's whiskers, hence its name. Of the 2,500 or so species of catfish, only a small number are used for food. Originally a mainstay of Southern cuisine, catfish now ranks fifth in consumption in the United States, behind TUNA, shrimp, COD and Alaskan pollock. Previously caught in rivers, fish farms now supply 75% of catfish consumed. The farm-raised fish grow on a diet of soy protein, grains, fish meal and potatoes. In the wild, the catfish may become contaminated with industrial pollutants as it feeds from the bottom of streams and rivers. This tasty fish is sold fresh and frozen throughout the United States. Because the skin is hard to remove, fillets are preferable. While traditionally fried, catfish can also be poached, baked or grilled. A 3 ounce (100 g) serving provides 103 calories; protein, 15.5 g; fat, 3.6 g; calcium, 34 mg; thiamin, 0.038 mg; riboflavin, 0.09 mg; and niacin, 1.84 mg. (See also SEAFOOD.)

cauliflower (*Brassica oleracea*)   A vegetable closely related to broccoli. Cauliflower, a true flower belonging to the CABBAGE family, was originally grown in Cyprus. The white head, called a curd, represents immature buds and stems that form slightly rounded, compact flower buds. The head of white cauliflower is surrounded by blue-green leaves that protect it from light so that it doesn't turn green. A hybrid, cauliflower-broccoli, looks like cauliflower, but its head is pale green. It cooks more quickly and has a less marked taste than white cauliflower. Cauliflower and broccoli are cruciferous vegetables, believed to contain anticancer substances, like phenethyl isothiocyanate, which activate enzyme systems in the liver that can potentially destroy dangerous substances. Population studies suggest that consumption of cauliflower and its relatives decreases the risk of some forms of CANCER.

The strong odor associated with cooking cauliflower can be minimized by cooking this vegetable for a short time. Cooking this vegetable in an aluminum or iron pan will turn it off-color. Cauliflower can be used in soups, purees, cold salad and vegetable fondue, and it can be sauteed, braised or fried after it has been blanched. Food value of a cup of cooked cauliflower (180 g) is 34 calories; protein, 2.9 g; carbohydrate, 6.8 g; fiber, 3.9 g; ascorbic acid, 56 mg; calcium, 31 mg; iron, 0.74 mg; thiamin, 0.07 mg; riboflavin, 0.1 mg; niacin, 0.56 mg. (See also CANCER PREVENTION DIET.)

caviar   Sturgeon and fish roe that have been salted and pressed. Sturgeon of the Caspian Sea yield 90% of the world's caviar, though this source is endangered by overfishing and pollution. Eggs can account for 10% of the female sturgeon's body weight. To prepare caviar, washed, sieved eggs are placed in brine, then drained and packed. Less expensive versions of caviar are made from roe of SALMON, whitefish, HERRING and COD, among others. Various types of caviar differ in taste, color and texture. Caviar generally contains high levels of sodium, 300 to 700 mg per tablespoon

(16 grams). A tablespoon of caviar also contains 94 mg of CHOLESTEROL (one-third the recommended daily dose) plus 40 calories, protein, 4 g; carbohydrate, 0.64 g; and fat, 2.9 grams.

cayenne (*Capsicum frutescens* and *c. anum.*; long pepper)   A perennial derived from red pepper and a member of the nightshade family. Peppers were domesticated 5,000 years ago in South America, and some two dozen varieties are now cultivated. The long, dried fruit is ground to produce a pungent, red seasoning. This very hot pepper is used in seasoning SAUSAGE, curry, soups and pizza. CAPSAICIN is the predominant ingredient that accounts for the hot taste. This plant compound is an ALKALOID, an aromatic compound chemically related to vanilla, and has a history of use as a pain reliever. Currently, cayenne is used as a salve to relieve chronic pain due to arthritis or shingles, apparently by upsetting the chemical balance inside sensory cells that relay pain messages to the brain.

celeriac (*Apium graveolens var. rapaceum*)   A dark variety of CELERY with a bulbous root that is also known as celery root or celery knob. Celeriac originated in Europe, where it is still a popular vegetable. Like true celery, it is related to parsley. The cooked root is eaten in salads, soups and stews; it can also be marinated or eaten raw. Like celery, it is a low-calorie food. One half-cup (100 g, raw) provides 44.5 calories; protein, 1.5 g; carbohydrate, 9.2 g; fiber, 1.3 g; fat, 0.3 g; calcium, 43 mg; potassium, 300 g; thiamin, 0.03 mg; riboflavin, 0.03 mg; niacin, 0.03 mg; vitamin C, 6.3 mg.

celery (*Apium graveolens var. dulce*; true celery)   A biennial stalk vegetable, grown in temperate regions; a member of the parsley family. Celery is native to Europe, northeastern Africa and western Asia. Celery was used by the ancient Chinese as a medicinal plant, and the Greeks and Romans used it as a flavoring. First cultivated in its modern form in France early in the 18th century, this popular vegetable is now grown in the United States in California, Florida and Michigan. The Pascal variety does not have the characteristic stringiness of other varieties. Celery leaves, stalk and root are edible and are used raw in salads. They are cooked as a vegetable in soups, and celery leaves and seeds are used as a seasoning. Part of celery's popularity rests in its classification as a low-calorie food because of its high water content. Diced celery (raw, one half-cup, 60 g) contains 10 calories; protein, 2.2 g; carbohydrate, 2.2 g; fiber, 1.2 g; calcium, 22 mg; potassium 326 mg; vitamin C, 4 mg; thiamin, 0.03 mg; riboflavin, 0.03 mg; and niacin, 0.3 mg.

celiac disease (nontropical sprue, gluten-induced enteropathy)   A severe ALLERGY to cereal GRAINS, especially WHEAT. It is estimated that in the United States one person in 2,000–3,000 has celiac disease. Persons with celiac disease react strongly to GLUTEN, a grain protein common to wheat, OATS, RYE and BARLEY. Repeated exposure to gluten injures the cells lining the intestine, which are required to completely digest and absorb carbohydrates and sugars like table sugar (sucrose) and milk sugar (lactose), as well as FAT and protein. Consequently, celiac disease drastically reduces the uptake of fat, glucose and AMINO ACIDS, as well as IRON,

ZINC, and water-soluble vitamins, including VITAMIN B$_{12}$, and fat-soluble vitamins like vitamin A. Symptoms of celiac disease include weight loss, diarrhea associated with fatty stools (STEATORRHEA), MALNUTRITION, LACTOSE INTOLERANCE, ANEMIA, skin disorders, OSTEOMALACIA, sore tongue, abnormal bleeding and bleeding gums. Children with celiac disease grow poorly. Symptoms generally appear within the first year of life, when grains are introduced into the infant's diet. The cause of celiac disease is unknown. Family history plays a role, and breastfed babies have a decreased risk.

Gluten is the major protein fraction of wheat, composed of GLIADENS and glutenins, two protein fractions. Only gliaden is associated with the disease. Closely related proteins in other cereal grains cause similar symptoms. The closer a grain is related to wheat, the greater is its ability to activate celiac disease. Thus, rice and corn are not closely related to wheat and seldom activate the disease. Completely predigested gliaden does not activate the disease in susceptible individuals because it can no longer be recognized by the immune system as foreign.

Treatment programs specify a gluten-free diet; that is, a diet devoid of all wheat, rye, barley and oat products. Ninety percent of patients respond within two months. The problem of avoiding gluten is compounded by the fact that wheat and wheat products are so prevalent in food products, appearing in baked goods, CRACKERS, gravy, soy sauce, many PROCESSED FOODS, salad dressing and extenders used in ice cream. Gluten-free flours are available: QUINOA, AMARANTH, RICE, CORN and POTATO. At the beginning of treatment vitamin and mineral supplements can remedy deficiencies and rebuild nutrient stores. It is important that there be no underlying zinc deficiency, which will cause the disease to be unresponsive to diet therapy. Vitamin B$_{12}$ and FOLIC ACID are not well absorbed by patients with celiac disease if administered orally; they may be administered by injection. (See also ALLERGY, FOOD; GASTROINTESTINAL DISORDERS.)

Trier, Jerry S., "Celiac Sprue," *New England Journal of Medicine*, 325:24 (1991), pp. 1709–17.

cellulite   A pseudomedical term for FAT stored under dimpled skin of the thighs, hips and buttocks. There is no inflammation, though the skin may be quite tender. Subcutaneous tissue that binds the skin to underlying tissue contains fat cells, and this basic thigh tissue structure differs between females and males. The layer beneath the epidermis is thinner in females, and their fat cells are arranged in chambers, which have a vertical orientation not seen in the male. As women age, this layer thins as fat cells migrate into it. Subsequently, the connective tissue structure breaks down, allowing alternating depressions and protrusions to form; the number of supporting elastic fibers also decreases. Dimpled skin is more likely to occur in individuals with loose skin. Dimpled thighs are common in obesity and after menopause, while slim women and female athletes have little or no cellulite. EXERCISE and maintaining normal body weight are the best prevention of cellulite, and gradual weight loss permits gradual change in skin and connective tissue. Massage may be helpful in increasing circulation. It is often claimed that cellulite can be broken up by physical methods. However, body fat cannot be shaken, sweated or rubbed off. It must be burned by the body's metabolism. This requires an exercise regimen and diet management. (See also ADIPOSE TISSUE.)

cellulose   An insoluble form of dietary FIBER and a building block of plant cell walls and the woody parts of plants. Cellulose is the major ingredient of BRAN, the outer coating of seeds of cereal GRAINS. Cellulose is a linear polysaccharide (very long carbohydrate chain) in which glucose units are bound to each other in such a way that digestive enzymes cannot break down the chains.

Cellulose binds water. Thus, when wheat bran is consumed the cellulose it contains softens stools, reduces pressure on the colon, and can improve symptoms of constipation and diarrhea. Bran slows down carbohydrate digestion, thus aiding BLOOD SUGAR regulation. Cellulose does not seem to lower blood cholesterol levels, and excessive amounts may bind minerals like CALCIUM and limit their absorption. Cellulose and other dietary fiber is broken down extensively by colon bacteria to produce short-chain fatty acids, the preferred fuel of the gut lining.

Processed cellulose (microcrystalline cellulose) is a common FOOD ADDITIVE. It gives liquids a creamy consistency and improves the spreading properties of foods such as syrups and peanut butter. (See also COMPLEX CARBOHYDRATE; STARCH.)

cellulose, carboxymethyl (CMC, cellulose gum)   A chemically modified CELLULOSE that is the most widely used form of cellulose added to foods. Cellulose from wood pulp and cotton is treated with acetic acid to form CMC, which is neither digested nor absorbed. CMC is added to ice cream in conjunction with GELATIN or CARRAGEENAN; to BEER; to pie filling and jellies and to cake frosting. It holds moisture in bread doughs and prevents the sugar in candy from crystallizing. In diet foods, CMC adds bulk and helps to create a feeling of satiety without added CALORIES. It adds body to artificially sweetened soft drinks. Other types of modified cellulose improve the clarity of pie fillings, thicken foods and partially substitute for eggs in cake batter. (See also GUMS.)

ceramics and pottery   See LEAD.

cereal grains   The edible seeds of cultivated members of the grass family (*Gramineae*). They include RICE, RYE, WHEAT, BARLEY, CORN and OATS of the *Festucoideae* subfamily. MILLET belongs to a separate subfamily, *Panicoidacea*; thus it is more distantly related to wheat. BUCKWHEAT, AMARANTH and QUINOA are unrelated to wheat, though they are considered cereals. Cereal grains contain 7 to 14% protein and 70 to 80% carbohydrate in the form of STARCH. The protein from these sources is generally deficient in essential AMINO ACIDS, typically LYSINE. Millet is deficient in TRYPTOPHAN. Consequently, the BIOLOGICAL VALUE, the nutritional score that rates protein quality, for cereal protein is low. However, when cereal grains are eaten together with other foods containing ample levels of amino acids, which are low in grains, the overall quality of the combined protein increases and satisfies daily protein requirements. In wheat FLOUR gluten becomes sticky when moistened and creates resilient dough that can be used with leavening agents. Other types of flour are less suitable for baking because they contain little gluten. Gluten-containing foods, particularly wheat, must be avoided by patients with CELIAC DISEASE.

Worldwide, rice, wheat and corn are major dietary staples. Cereal grains are also used as feed for livestock and poultry that produce meat, dairy and poultry products. Industry uses grains to produce GLUCOSE, ALCOHOL (ethanol) and oils. Americans currently consume half as much cereal grains as they did in 1900. Grains provide about 20% of the daily calories of a typical American diet, primarily as starch (COMPLEX CARBOHYDRATE). Current dietary guidelines suggest increasing complex carbohydrate consumption.

Cereal grain kernels possess a tough outer coat (BRAN), associated with FIBER and MINERALS, the nutrient-rich GERM (embryo of the seed), the innermost part of the kernel and the starchy ENDOSPERM. Milling and refining remove the bran and germ, thus removing much of the fiber, minerals and vitamins, and leaving the starch. To replenish partially lost nutrients, wheat flour and products like BREAKFAST cereals are enriched with NIACIN, THIAMIN and RIBOFLAVIN, and are fortified with IRON. (See also BREAD; DIETARY GUIDELINES FOR AMERICANS; FLOUR.)

cereals See BREAKFAST CEREAL.

cerebrovascular accident (occlusive stroke) The formation or lodging of a clot in an artery of the brain, obstructing the flow of blood to a region of the brain. When an artery feeding the brain becomes blocked, the oxygen supply becomes very limited and brain function is severely affected, resulting in the most common form of STROKE. DIET affects the incidence of stroke and HEART ATTACK. The consumption of FISH and FISH OILS reduces platelet aggregation, a key step in clot formation. Blood platelets are small cell fragments essential for blood clot formation. If they become less sticky, the probability of clot formation decreases. ASPIRIN reduces the occurrence of stroke because it decreases the clot formation. (See also CARDIOVASCULAR DISEASE; ESKIMO DIET.)

certified food colors See ARTIFICIAL FOOD COLORS.

certified organic vegetables Vegetables certified to have been grown without pesticides and chemical fertilizers. Each U.S. state can set its own limits for levels of PESTICIDES in ORGANIC produce. For example, California permits up to 10% of the U.S. Environmental Protection Agency (E.P.A.) tolerance levels. Several state departments of agriculture offer organic certification programs. However, there is currently no uniform standard for organic farms, nor is there agreement on the best way to certify inspection of farms or to test produce for pesticide residues. Certification agencies, formed by regional trade associations, define standards for organic growers and certify farms that meet the standards. There are about 40 certification agencies in the United States and Canada, including the CALIFORNIA CERTIFIED ORGANIC FARMERS (CCOF), Independent Organic Inspectors Association (IOIA) and the Farm Verified Organic (FVO).

Commercial testing labs may be used by markets and growers to test their fresh vegetables and fruit for pesticide residues.

Congress passed the Organic Foods Production Act in 1990; however, the proposed regulations implementing this act have not yet been drafted (November 1996) by the Office of the Counsel General and members of the National Organic Program. Final evaluation by the Office of Management and Budget must then evaluate the costs of implementation. Until this occurs, the accreditation process cannot begin and there are no oversight or certifying agencies. Eventually, all products labeled as "organic" will have to be certified to one national standard, except for products from farms with annual sales less than $5,000. Several of the major U.S. food distributors now produce or market organic processed foods. (See also FOOD TOXINS; MEAT CONTAMINANTS.)

ceviche A raw fish dish, especially in Peruvian and Mexican cuisine. Various fish are marinated in lemon juice and served with LIMES, ONIONS or CORN. The acid content produced is strong enough to chemically soften the soft flesh of fish. However, to be effective at softening the fish, adequate marinating time must be allowed. Like other raw fish dishes, such as sushi, ceviche carries with it a risk of infection by parasitic worms. (See also SEAFOOD.)

challenge testing A strategy used to identify chemical and FOOD SENSITIVITIES. Sensitivities to foods are often difficult to pinpoint. A generally accepted way of identifying an offending agent in a food is to first eliminate exposure to suspected agents in order to permit the body's chemistry to reequilibrate. This may require several days to several weeks. After this time, suspected agents can be introduced one by one, and any response is noted. If symptoms reappear, the inference is that a particular food or agent is the culprit. (See also ALLERGY; ROTATION DIET.)

chamomile (*Matricaria chamomilla*) A medicinal plant with a long history in folk medicine. Chamomile contains several physiologically active ingredients, among them chamazulene, an anti-inflammatory agent that has been used to treat ulcers. In animal studies, chamomile infusions act as a mild central nervous system depressant, perhaps explaining the effectiveness of chamomile tea as a soothing relaxant. In addition, chamomile has antibacterial effects and has been used to stimulate liver function. Chamomile tea is obtained from the flowers of the plant and has a pleasing fragrance. Individuals who are allergic to ragweed and its relatives, aster and chrysanthemum, may react to drinking chamomile tea with hay fever–like symptoms and hives. (See also HERBAL MEDICINE.)

champagne A sparkling WINE named for the region in France where it originated; used in celebrations throughout the world. For champagne, Pinot Noir and Chardonnay grapes are often used.

In the 1600s a Benedictine monk developed the technique for producing and bottling champagne to maintain its effervescence. Wines in general release small amounts of CARBON DIOXIDE during a secondary FERMENTATION carried out in vats. For champagne, after the initial fermentation, a little sugar (GLUCOSE) is added and the wine is bottled before the second fermentation begins. Carbonation requires about three months. Substantial pressure builds up in the bottle during this time; therefore, care should be taken in uncorking the bottle. (See also ETHANOL.)

charcoal See ACTIVATED CHARCOAL.

charcoal-broiled meat See BARBECUED MEAT/CHARCOAL BROILED MEAT.

chard (Swiss chard; *Beta vulgaris cicla*) A dark-green, leafy vegetable that is a variety of beet. Chard is a common garden vegetable because it is hardy, prolific and tolerates both heat and cold. The leaves and stalks are well-defined, in contrast to the root, which is small and inedible. This biennial provides leaf stalks that can be boiled or steamed like spinach. Varieties of chard have either white stalks or beet red stalks. Unlike most cooking greens, the stalks don't have to be discarded; they can be sliced and cooked like asparagus. Chard is an excellent source of beta carotene (pro-vitamin A) and other caratenoids and a good plant source of iron and calcium. A half-cup, boiled (70 g), provides calories, 15; protein, 1.5 g; carbohydrate, 2 g; calcium, 55 mg; iron, 1.3 mg; vitamin A activity, 390 retinol equivalents; and small amounts of other vitamins.

cheddar See CHEESE.

cheese A solid food prepared from coagulated milk PROTEIN. Cheese is a popular food; the average annual consumption in the United State in 1992 was 28 pounds per person, twice that in the late 1960s. As is typical of dairy products, cheese is a high-FAT, high-calcium food. The flavor and texture of cheeses depend upon the source of the milk, the types of microorganisms used to ripen the cheese, and the ripening conditions. In cheese manufacture the enzyme RENNET is used to clot milk. The precipitate (curd) is then separated from the liquid (whey), salted and pressed into a block. Specific strains of molds and bacteria are added to ferment (ripen) the cheese.

Unlike MEAT, which can be trimmed of fat, the fat in cheese is hidden. Ten pints of whole milk typically make a pound of cheese, which retains most of the original fat. This mainly SATURATED FAT accounts for 65 to 75% of the CALORIES of most cheeses. In other words, two slices of cheese contain as much fat as 3.5 pats of BUTTER. Also unlike meat, cheese is an excellent source of CALCIUM. A slice of cheddar provides 204 mg or 20% of the calcium in the REFERENCE DAILY INTAKE (RDI). A half-cup of ricotta made from part-skim milk provides 700 mg of calcium, 70% of the RDI. Cheese is also a high sodium food, typically containing 200 to 400 mg of SODIUM per slice. Certain processed cheeses contain even more.

Food Labels for Cheese

A food label that states "made from partially skim milk" does not indicate how much cream has been added to make the final product. Most hard and soft cheese made from whole milk is quite high in fat. As an example, three ounces of cheddar cheese (18 grams fat or two slices) provides more fat than the same size sirloin steak. Fat contributes 70% of the calories of Muenster, blue Parmesan, American, provolone, Swiss, Roquefort, Monterey Jack and Colby cheeses, all of which contain 7 to 9 calories per ounce. Havarti provides 11 g fat per ounce. For reference, one ounce is equivalent to a one-inch cube of cheese. Fat accounts for 90% of the calories in cream cheese.

Using low-fat or non-fat milk allows cheese makers to produce cheese with less fat than usual (4 to 6 g of fat per ounce). Fat contributes 60% of the calories of part-skim mozzarella, whole milk ricotta, feta and creamed cottage cheese. The fat content of a food labeled "reduced fat" or "less fat" must be reduced by at least 25% per serving compared to the reference food.

"Low fat" cheese products are slightly lower in fat than the usual cheeses. For example, two slices of part-skim mozarella cheese provide 7 g of fat (55% calories as fat), while regular mozarella contains 9 g per two slices. "Low fat" indicates that a food provides a maximum of 3 g of fat per serving if the serving size is over 30 g (1.07 oz). If the serving size is the typical one-ounce slice (28 g), then the low-fat food must contain no more than 3 g of fat per 50 g (1.78 oz) of that food.

"Light" or "lite" cheese is a nutritionally modified food containing 33% fewer calories or at most 50% of the fat of the reference food when 50% or more of its calories come from fat. Most light cheese is labeled "cheese product" and contains 7 to 9 g of fat per ounce. Light cheese may contain more sodium than natural cheese.

For low-fat options, consider cheeses with less than 3 g of fat per ounce or those that supply less than half their calories as fat. Cottage cheese with 1% fat contains 1 g of fat per half-cup. Other options in this group are dry curd cottage cheese, several kinds of processed cheeses, part-skim ricotta, and yogurt cheese. Some "reduced fat" and "part-skim" cheeses can also be low-fat options. (See also DIETARY GUIDELINES FOR AMERICANS; FOOD LABELING; LACTOSE INTOLERANCE.)

cheese imitations (cheese substitutes) Products with less butterfat than natural CHEESE, as defined by a standard formulation (the USDA's STANDARD OF IDENTITY). Cheese substitutes made from vegetable oil and milk protein alone do not contain CHOLESTEROL. However, they may have just as much fat as real cheese because of added vegetable oil. The following terms are used on the food label if the product does not conform to the Standard of Identity for cheese: "cheese product," "cheese food" and "imitation cheese." "Lite" or "light" means that the cheese substitute represents a 50% reduction of its fat CALORIES when 50% or more of its calories come from fat. "Low SODIUM" versions of imitation cheese may mean the product contains only reduced sodium with the same high-fat calories.

cheese powders (spray-dried cheese powders) An additive used to create a CHEESE flavor in baked goods, chips and other convenience foods, salad dressings and soups. The desired cheese is dispersed in skim MILK or in a whey slurry. The suspension is homogenized, emulsified and spray-dried. Food manufacturers can select the flavor intensity, saltiness, and blend of whey or other milk protein in cheese powders. (See also PROCESSED FOOD.)

cheilosis Cracks at the corners of the mouth, and reddened lips and mouth, due to a deficiency of the B COMPLEX vitamins, particularly RIBOFLAVIN. Acute riboflavin deficiency is also accompanied by a glazed, shiny tongue (GLOSSITIS) and DERMATITIS. This condition often accompanies PROTEIN deficiency as well. In industrialized nations cheilosis is more likely to occur in alcoholics and in patients with chronic infection, cancer and other serious illnesses. Cheilosis can also be caused by VITAMIN A overdose or by an allergic response to food. Short-term, mild deficiencies and subsequent cheilosis may occur during pregnancy and lactation and during adolescence, when there is an increased vitamin requirement. (See also ARIBOFLAVINOSIS.)

chelate (chelating agent)   Usually an organic compound capable of binding metal ions by forming a very stable ring or cage-like molecular structure. Though chelated ions remain in solution, the chemical and biological properties of chelated metal ions differ from unbound ions. For example, ETHYLENEDIAMINETETRAACETIC ACID (EDTA) is a highly efficient chelate added to PROCESSED FOOD to trap metal ion impurities—ALUMINUM, COPPER, IRON, MANGANESE and nickel. Trace amounts of metals are inevitable because of the metal plumbing, grinders and processors used in food preparation. Chelating agents scavenge these metal contaminants, preventing reactions that would detract from the appearance and nutritive quality of the food. Large excesses of EDTA would trap CALCIUM, iron, ZINC and other essential mineral nutrients and prevent their assimilation. Chelates are used therapeutically; desterrioxamine, a chelate specific for iron, removes excess iron in HEMOCHROMATOSIS and HEMOSIDEROSIS, diseases of excessive iron accumulation, while British anti-Lewisite, a chelator of LEAD, is used in cases of lead toxicity. Many products of cellular metabolism like CITRIC ACID are chelating agents.

Chelated Minerals

Mineral nutrients like calcium, copper, iron, MAGNESIUM, manganese and zinc can be converted to water-soluble forms by combining them with chelating agents. In supplements, minerals are often chelated with citric acid (as citrate), ASPARTIC ACID (aspartate) and other AMINO ACIDS, orotic acid (as orotate), gluconic acid (as gluconate) and picolinic acid (as picolinate). These chemicals form stable complexes with positively charged metal ions. Chelated minerals often are more easily absorbed in the intestine; thus they are more "bioavailable." HEME is one of the most important iron chelates in the body because it functions in HEMOGLOBIN to transport oxygen in the blood. The uptake of iron in heme found in meat is about 30% efficient, while the uptake of non-heme iron, as supplied by vegetables, may only be 1 to 5%. Because the organic chelates contribute a larger percentage of the weight of the mineral compound than carbonates, for example, more milligrams of the chelated forms are needed to provide the equivalent amounts of minerals in a tablet compared to those containing a simple non-chelated form like carbonate. Chelation may increase mineral absorption in some individuals when stomach acidity is low, as is often the case for elderly people. For individuals sensitive to iron supplements, chelated iron is less likely to cause an upset stomach. (See also BIOAVAILABILITY; HEAVY METALS; TRACE MINERALS.)

chemical imbalance   The shift of chemical processes in the body away from equilibrium states. Imbalanced body chemistry underlies many disease processes, and a return to health entails a return to normal functioning. Acid-base balance, water balance, electrolyte balance and GLUCOSE sugar are carefully regulated by homeostatic mechanisms involving the brain (nervous system) and the endocrine (hormonal) system. They assure that combined systems will first maintain a relatively constant internal environment. The following examples of possible imbalances highlight the importance of nutrition.

Water   The body's main constituent. The cytoplasm of cells, the fluid between cells and the circulation, are watery environments. The normal functioning of cellular processes and waste disposal requires an adequate water supply at all times.

Minerals   Sodium, potassium, chloride and bicarbonate are required to maintain the appropriate ionic strength within cells and the circulation. Processes ranging from nerve transmission and kidney resorption to heart muscle contraction require the right balance of minerals. Excesses or deficiencies cause toxic symptoms.

Acid-base (pH) balance   Because enzymes are exquisitely sensitive to their ionic environment and require a limited range of hydrogen ion concentration to catalyze reactions, excessive acids or bases will alter enzyme function and, in the extreme cases, denature (irreversibly damage) them.

Blood sugar imbalance   A wide variety of foods can imbalance the body's chemistry. For example, excessive consumption of REFINED CARBOHYDRATES may trigger postprandial HYPOGLYCEMIA (low BLOOD SUGAR after a meal), when the pancreas releases the hormone insulin into the blood rapidly to compensate for the surge in blood sugar. Overcompensation by insulin causes blood sugar to plummet below normal levels until other hormonal compensating mechanisms take over.

Amino acids   Blood levels of certain AMINO ACIDS are linked to mood, thus affecting behavior. The brain and nervous system convert several amino acids to NEUROTRANSMITTERS, chemicals for nerve transmission. Low neurotransmitter production is believed to affect brain function. For example, DEPRESSION has been linked to low levels of the neurotransmitters dopamine and norepinephrine, formed from the amino acid TYROSINE. SEROTONIN is linked to decreased sensitivity to pain and to sleep and relaxation. This neurotransmitter is synthesized from the amino acid TRYPTOPHAN. The levels of dopamine, norepinephrine and serotonin in the brain also depend on the levels of precursor amino acids in the blood-stream, and this in turn depends to an extent on the type of foods consumed.

Trace minerals   A wide range of mineral imbalances are possible. Excessive COPPER and inadequate ZINC consumption correlates with periodic violent behavior in some individuals. Excessive zinc intake can suppress immunity temporarily and can block copper absorption. Excessive CALCIUM consumption can block IRON uptake, leading to FATIGUE.

Vitamin deficiencies   Deficiencies of most vitamins will affect behavior. Thus VITAMIN B_{12} deficiency is linked to memory loss in susceptible individuals; a classical symptom of NIACIN deficiency is DEMENTIA; severe THIAMIN deficiency is linked to nervous disorders.

Food allergies In addition to rapid responses like asthma, hives and runny nose, food allergies can cause slow-developing symptoms. Inappropriate immune responses can cause a large variety of symptoms ranging from headache to joint pain. The subsequent inflammation of the intestine can lead to the "leaky gut" syndrome, in which normally excluding antigens (foreign materials) can penetrate the body, setting the stage for multiple food allergies and malabsorption of nutrients.

Food sensitivities This broad term refers to any negative physiologic response to food. A common example is LACTOSE INTOLERANCE, which does not involve the immune system. It can cause diarrhea, bloating and intestinal upset. However, avoiding milk because of lactose intolerance can lead to calcium malnutrition.

Pollutants As an example of HEAVY METALS toxicity, LEAD poisoning is associated with a shortened attention span, slowed learning and development in children, ANEMIA and chronic fatigue. Toxic heavy metals also interfere with the uptake and the function of many trace mineral nutrients. PESTICIDES, flame retardants (PBBs) and transformer insulation (PCBs) can adversely alter METABOLISM, and in extreme cases cause chronic illnesses such as cancer.

Drugs Many prescription drugs can create imbalances profoundly affecting mood and behavior. VITAMIN B6 deficiency can be caused by drugs used to treat tuberculosis; HYPERTENSION (hydralzaine); Parkinson's disease (L-dopa), in addition to oral contraceptives. Folacin deficiency may be caused by cancer chemotherapy (methotrexate), malaria, epilepsy, edema and inflammation. Vitamin B12 deficiency can be caused by drugs used to treat diabetes, tuberculosis and high blood CHOLESTEROL. Tardive dyskinesia is a frequent side effect of anti-psychotic drugs. ALCOHOL modulates many physiologic processes and excessive use leads to malnutrition. This mood-altering drug is classified as a depressant. Alcohol imbalances liver metabolism, and over time, alcohol abuse will irreversibly damage the liver, as well as the brain. (See also ALLERGY, FOOD; CARBOHYDRATE; FOOD; MALNUTRITION; METABOLISM.)

chemical score A measure of the quality of a food PROTEIN based upon its amino acid content. The chemical score relies on a comparison of a food protein with a reference protein, rich in all ESSENTIAL AMINO ACIDS, such as egg protein. Specifically, the chemical score is the percentage of the essential amino acid found in the lowest concentration in the food protein, divided by the percentage of that same amino acid that occurs in the reference food protein. For example, a chemical score of 65 indicates that the limiting (less abundant) essential amino acid in the food protein is only 65% of the amount found in egg protein. The UN's World Health Organization has published tables of chemical scores for food proteins used throughout the world. The utility of the chemical score is that it permits a simple assessment of whether a particular protein source needs to be complemented. The data are easily obtained and amino acid analyses are inexpensive and convenient in comparison with the animal studies required to measure the BIOLOGICAL VALUE and PROTEIN EFFICIENCY RATIOS, other measures of protein quality. Hence nutritionists frequently employ chemical scores to express the adequacy of protein in a food. However, the chemical score does not assess the degree of digestion and assimilation of a particular food protein source, and suffers from this important limitation. Amino acid analysts cannot detect toxins or other materials in food that could limit protein bioavailability.

chemical sensitivity (multiple chemical sensitivity [MCS]) A sensitivity to environmental chemicals. An estimated 15% of the U.S. population may have adverse symptoms when exposed to chemicals. Susceptible individuals can react to food and FOOD ADDITIVES, drugs and medications, tobacco smoke and other particulate pollutants, plastics, formaldehyde, perfume and scents, detergents, solvents, hydrocarbons (auto and natural gas), PESTICIDES, animal dandruff, pollen, molds, mildew, synthetic fabrics and polyurethane insulation. Behavioral changes can occur after exposure to those materials causing reactions. Learning disorders, excessive FATIGUE, muscle pain, headaches, irritability, mood swings, breathing problems, irregular heartbeat and even chronic anti-social behavior have been reported.

Chemical and psychogenic causes may be involved in some cases of MCS. Syndromes once believed to be psychosomatic are now accepted as being chemically induced. "Sick building syndrome," found in occupants of sealed buildings, is due to toxicity of volatile chemicals released from construction materials, cleansers, furniture and office equipment, and new carpets. At home the list of chemicals includes pesticides, smoke and mothballs. Industrial workers, residents exposed to toxic dumps or pesticide spraying, and those who are susceptible to random exposure to certain foods, consumer goods, chemicals in the air or drugs may be at risk.

A U.S. National Academy of Sciences panel concluded in 1987 that hypersensitivity to low levels of potentially toxic chemicals and materials is a serious medical problem in the United States. This was explored in a workshop convened in 1991 by the National Research Council. The consensus was that more research emphasizing carefully controlled studies of patients' responses in clinical settings is needed, including double-blind, placebo-controlled studies. In such an investigation, neither the physician nor the patient know who is receiving a test sample and who is receiving an innocuous sample.

Environmental medicine is a branch of medicine dealing with people and factors in the environment causing illness. Clinical ecologists are physicians who deal with MCS. After consultation with a qualified health care provider a personal strategy for hypersensitive individuals might entail avoiding contact with materials that provoke a response; avoiding highly processed food and allergenic foods (to improve digestion and absorption of nutrients); taking VITAMIN and mineral supplements to remedy deficiencies and to normalize the body's chemistry and immune system. An immunologic treatment (desensitization) by an allergist also may be required. (See also CHALLENGE TESTING; FOOD POISONING; FOOD SENSITIVITY; ROTATION DIET.)

Terr, Abba I., "Multiple Chemical Sensitivity," *Journal of Allergy and Clinical Immunology*, 94 (1994), pp. 362–366.

Rea, William J. *Chemical Sensitivity*, vols. 1 and 2. Boca Raton, Fla.: Lewis Publishers, 1992.

chemoprevention   Refers to the policy supporting the dietary supplementation of specific nutrients in cancer prevention. The American Association for Cancer Research has issued a policy statement supporting chemoprevention. Chemoprevention differs from chemotherapy, which employs drugs to destroy infectious agents (parasites, bacterial or virus) or cancer cells. Potential anticancer dietary supplements are being clinically tested worldwide. They include VITAMIN A and its progenitor BETA CAROTENE and other carotenoids; CALCIUM, VITAMIN B$_6$, VITAMIN B$_{12}$, VITAMIN C and VITAMIN E; plus FOLIC ACID, SELENIUM and wheat bran. One of the largest studies involved over 22,000 male physicians who consumed 50 mg beta carotene or placebo for ten years (the Physicians Health Study). Because neither the subject physicians nor the officials administering the study will know who is receiving beta carotene and who is receiving a placebo (neutral substance) until the data are analyzed by a third party, this is a double-blind clinical study (placebo controlled), acknowledged to be the most objective approach. Such studies are least affected by preconceived ideas and expectations. After four years researchers involved in the study concluded that taking an aspirin tablet could lower the risk of first-time heart attacks. After 10 years, investigators found no evidence that synthetic beta carotene alone prevented cardiovascular disease mortality or cancer. In general studies of beta carotene and carotenoid-rich foods suggest that beta carotene must be protected by other ANTIOXIDANTS like vitamin E to be maximally effective, and that rather than acting alone, the combination of beta carotene with other carotenoids and plant substances as supplied in a diet well stocked with fruits, vegetables and legumes can lower the risk of cancer and heart disease. In addition, plant-derived antioxidants appear to be more effective in preventing the early stages of cancer induction, rather than in blocking later stages of tumor growth. (See also CANCER PREVENTION DIET; CLINICAL TRIAL.)

Wattenberg, Lee, Lipkin, Martin, Boone, Charles W., and Kelloff, Gary J. eds. *Cancer Chemoprevention*. Boca Raton, Fla.: CRC Press, 1992.

cherry (*Prunus*)   A small, long-stemmed red fruit. More than 600 varieties are cultivated for edible fruit or as ornamental trees and shrubs worldwide. Cherry trees are native to many temperate regions of the world. Leading producers of edible cherries are Germany, Italy, France, Turkey, the United States (Washington, Oregon, Utah and Michigan). Most edible cherries are hybrids of European varieties. There are two main types, sweet and sour. Sweet cherries, the most common type grown, belong to the species *P. avium*. Sweet cherries are firmer, larger fruit. Common sweet cherries include Bing, Black Tartarian, Coe, Elton, Giant, Lambert, Royal Ann, Seneca, Schmidt, Windsor and Yellow Spanish. Colors range from deep-red (Bing) to yellow-red (Royal Ann). Most sour cherries (*P. cerasus*) are either canned or frozen commercially, for use in pies and pastries. Morellos (Morello, Olivet) have a red juice, while anarellos (Montmorency, Early Richard, Carnation and English) have a colorless juice. Duke cherries are hybrids of sweet and sour varieties (May Duke, Late Duke, Royal Duke).

Cherries contain red-blue pigments, anthocyanins. The flavonoids (plant pigments) function as ANTIOXIDANTS, to prevent oxidative damage and help reduce inflammation. In terms of their nutrient content, cherries contain fruit sugar (FRUCTOSE). Sour cherries provide more vitamin C and less sugar than sweet varieties. However, the addition of sugar in sweetened cherries increases their calories. Ten sweet cherries (68 g) provide 49 calories; protein, 0.8 g; carbohydrate, 11.3 g; fiber, 1.25 g; fat, 0.7 g; potassium, 152 mg; vitamin C, 5 mg; thiamin, 0.03 mg; riboflavin, 0.04 mg; niacin, 0.3 mg; and low levels of other vitamins and minerals.

chervil (*Anthriscus cerefolium*)   A delicate herb with small leaves. Chervil resembles parsley with lacy leaves. An annual with small white flowers, chervil is used to season stews, soups or salads. It has a delicate parsley flavor and can be used in the same way as parsley. Turnip root chervil, *Chaerophyllum bulbosum*, is used as a root vegetable.

chestnut (*Castanea dentata*)   A dark-brown nut with a shiny shell that pops out of a spiny burr when ripe. Chestnuts were used as food by ancient Greeks, Chinese and Japanese and are today considered one of the most important tree crops. Almost all commercial chestnuts in the United States are now supplied by Europe. The chestnut (*C. sativa*) native to southern Europe, northern Africa and western Asia is fungus-resistant. The American chestnut, belonging to the beech family, was essentially destroyed by a European blight that began in 1904. The trees now grown in the eastern United States are blight-resistant crossbreeds of Chinese and Japanese chestnuts. (The horse chestnut is unrelated and is inedible.) Fresh chestnuts, in brown shells, are called roasting chestnuts and may be roasted, boiled or dried. They provide more CARBOHYDRATE, less PROTEIN and less fat than many other nuts. Roasted chestnuts (3.5 oz, 3/4 cup) provide 245 calories; carbohydrate, 53 g; protein, 3 g; fat, 2 g; potassium, 592 mg; thiamin, 0.2 mg; riboflavin, 0.2 mg; niacin, 1.4 mg; vitamin C, 26 mg.

chewing gum   A flavored product for chewing, usually made with synthetic gums. Chewing gum bases provide no nutritive value, although added sweetness may contribute calories (4 to 6 calories per stick). Gum bases include natural gums (such as chicle and natural rubber); synthetic gums (including butyl rubber, paraffin, polyethylene); and synthetic softeners (glycerated gum resin). MANNITOL is used to "dust" chewing gum sticks. It prevents gum from absorbing moisture and becoming sticky and is poorly absorbed by the body.

Sugarless gum is not calorie-free unless the label specifies "non-caloric." Most sugarless gum contains as many calories as sugared gum. Instead of sugar, SORBITOL may be used as a sweetener. This sugar derivative yields as many calories as sugar. Sugarless gum may also contain glycerol, hydrogenated glucose syrup, ASPARTAME, ARTIFICIAL FOOD COLORS and BHA. Nicotine gum can lessen the craving for tobacco when abstaining from smoking. However, overcoming a nicotine addiction requires abstaining from all forms of nicotine, whether in cigarettes or gum.

Chewing gum can reduce the risk of tooth decay. Chewing any gum seems to lower the amount of acids produced in the mouth because chewing increases saliva flow, which neutralizes acids produced by bacteria living on carbohydrates in the mouth. Neutralization prevents the acids from dissolving tooth enamel. (See also CANDY; NATURAL SWEETENERS; TEETH.)

chicken The most popular poultry in the United States and a dietary staple worldwide. Domestic chicken consumption has steadily increased since 1940 to about 49 pounds per year due to major changes in breeding and production geared to mass marketing. Such strategies have made chicken more affordable and plentiful. The increased popularity of chicken since the 1960s also reflects the shift away from beef, as consumers have become more concerned with saturated fat and its correlation with high blood cholesterol and heart disease. A 3- to 4-ounce serving of cooked chicken provides half the adult protein requirement. Chicken is a good source of B vitamins and trace minerals, but has less iron then red meat.

The modern chicken is fatter than before (80% of calories from fat), but much of the fat is associated with the skin. Trimming off visible fat and discarding the skin will reduce the fat content by up to 50%. Brown meat (thighs, wings) contains more fat (10 grams per 3.5-oz serving) but is more moist than breast meat. Roasting chicken at low temperatures melts away much of the fat. Chicken without the skin can be low-fat fare: A roasted, skinless chicken breast gets 19% of its calories from fat, well below the recommended guidelines of 30% of calories from fat. By comparison, the leanest steak gets about 37% of its calories from fat. Avoid breading chicken before frying; the coating absorbs fat and increases the calories.

A yellow chicken has been fed more yellow corn than a pale chicken. Some suppliers add yellow materials like marigold petals, which give chicken flesh an appealing golden color, though it does not improve the nutrient content of the meat.

Chicken is graded by the USDA on a voluntary basis, as is beef. USDA grade A represents higher quality, while lesser grades are used in processed meat products. The grading system for chicken is based upon appearance—a lack of tears or blemishes rather than on fat content—unlike the grading system for beef, which relies on fat content.

Fast-food chains have capitalized on consumer interest in chicken by offering more options, such as "nuggets" or "chunks"; their tastiness lies in their high fat and sodium content. A typical 4.4-ounce nugget provides 290 calories, of which 50% comes from fat. Ground chicken skin and breading used for frying are often major fat contributors. The sodium level can be as high as 500 mg per serving. Producers of convenience foods have followed suit by offering chicken "patties" and "rondelets," which contain ground chicken skin. They are breaded and fried and their fat content ranges from 50% to over 60% of calories.

With mass chicken production has come the increased risk of bacterial contamination. An estimated 25 to 33% of chickens and turkeys contain salmonella, a disease-producing bacterium. Half the cases of food poisoning caused by the bacterium campylobacter in 1987 in the United States were attributable to chicken. Conveyor lines in slaughterhouses have speeded up, leaving federal inspectors with only seconds to observe each bird. "Free range" chickens have been allowed to run more freely on farms, in contrast to mass-produced chickens raised in cages. They are processed the same way, and both are subject to bacterial contamination by fecal matter on the production line.

Although thorough cooking kills bacteria, the burden is on the consumer to minimize the risk of food poisoning. Safety tips: Poultry should be refrigerated or frozen as soon after purchase as possible to avoid bacterial growth. Avoid contaminating other foods by preventing chicken juice from contacting them. Wash everything that comes into contact with uncooked poultry and its juices, including cutting board and knife. Wear rubber gloves if you have a cut on your hands. Remove the skin before cooking; it is likely to be fatty and dirty. Cook poultry thoroughly—180°F to 185°F in the thickest part of the meat—to assure sterilization. Nutrient content: dark meat, 1 cup roasted (140 g) provides 286 calories; protein, 38.3 g; fat, 13.6 g; cholesterol, 130 mg; calcium, 21 mg; iron, 1.86 mg; thiamin, 0.1 mg; riboflavin, 0.32 mg; niacin, 9.2 mg.

Hurley, E.C., "The Skinny on Cooking Chicken," *Journal of the American Dietetic Association*, 95:2 (1995), pp. 167.

chickpea (*Cicer arietinum*, garbanzo bean, Spanish bean, ceci pea) A tan-colored legume the size of small hazelnuts. Pods grow on a small, bushy plant and produce one or two edible peas; different varieties produce white, black or red peas. Chickpea is native to Asia and has been cultivated since ancient times. Chickpea is now extensively cultivated in California, Latin America and the Middle East. Chickpeas are a rich source of fiber and protein and are often used as a vegetable in soups. They are a major ingredient of Middle Eastern, Latin American and Indian cuisine; hummus and falafel are typical Middle Eastern dishes that include chickpeas. Soaking overnight before cooking softens chickpeas and shortens the cooking time. One cup cooked beans (163 g) yields 270 calories; protein, 15 g carbohydrate, 45; fiber, 8.63 g; fat, 4.0 g; calcium, 90 mg; iron, 4.9 mg; potassium, 749 mg; zinc, 1.72 mg; thiamin, 0.25 mg; riboflavin, 0.13 mg; niacin, 1.3 mg. They do not contain vitamin C.

chicory (*Cichorium intybus*) A curly-leafed member of the endive family. Chicory is native to Europe and was cultivated by the Greeks and Romans. It can grow up to 6 feet high and possesses feathery leaves with dark-green edges. Chicory is now widely cultivated for its nutritious greens. The foliage is blanched to decrease the bitter taste and is used in salads. Plants given growth stimulants produce a crown of leaves (witloof); the greens are used as pot herbs. Chicory is an excellent source of beta carotene. Several varieties yield edible tap roots, which are roasted, ground and used as coffee extenders and coffee substitutes. The nutrient content of 100 g raw is 28.8 calories; protein, 1.7 g; carbohydrate, 4.7 g; fiber, 0.8 g; fat, 0.3 g; calcium, 100 mg; iron, 0.9 mg; potassium, 420 mg; thiamin, 0.06 mg; riboflavin, 0.1 mg; niacin, 0.5 mg; vitamin C, 24 mg.

chief cells Specialized cells in the stomach lining (gastric mucosa) that produce a digestive enzyme called pepsin.

Pepsin initiates protein DIGESTION in the stomach. Pepsin is secreted as an inactive precursor called pepsinogen, which is converted to pepsin by stomach acid. Glands of the main body of the stomach contain both chief cells and PARIETAL CELLS, which secrete hydrochloric acid (stomach acid) and INTRINSIC FACTOR required for intestinal uptake of vitamin B_{12}. These secretions mix with mucus and are released as gastric juices. (See also DIGESTIVE ENZYMES.)

children's vitamins   Supplements designed to help meet the growth requirements of children whose dietary intake may be compromised. The Recommended Dietary Allowances (RDA) for children are usually, though not always, lower than for adults because of their smaller body size. However, children grow rapidly, and their requirements for nutrients remain proportionately higher. As examples, the RDA for vitamin A for a typical five-year-old (500 mcg of vitamin A) is half the adult's RDA (1,000 mcg). The RDA for niacin is 12 mg for children (four to six years), while the RDA for an adult is 19 mg.

An estimated 10,000 children in the United States under the age of six mistakenly swallow large amounts of VITAMINS each year. This statistic reflects the need to educate children that vitamin pills are not snacks. When they look and taste like candy, chewable vitamins are a temptation for small children. The most serious consequence of overdosing on children's vitamins is an IRON overdose, the symptoms of which are vomiting and diarrhea. (See also HYPERVITAMINOSIS.)

chili pepper (*Capsicum frutescens;* capsicum pepper)   A spicy, hot PEPPER related to red bell peppers and the tomato. Hot peppers are unrelated to seasoning pepper, which comes from ground peppercorns and derives from Asia. Chili peppers were domesticated 5,000 years ago in the Americas. Some two dozen varieties are available in the United States, including poblano; Anaheim (long-lobed, either green or red); cayenne (a very hot chili used as a spice); habanero (lantern-shaped and the hottest domestic pepper); jalapeño (a very hot pepper that is canned, pickled and used in a wide variety of processed foods). Chili pepper is a good source of VITAMIN C, VITAMIN A and POTASSIUM. The hot ingredient, a family of chemicals called CAPSAICIN, is very concentrated in the white tissue of the pepper, not the seeds. Apparently capsaicin evolved to shield pepper plants against animal predation.

Research suggests that consuming chili pepper can lower the risk of heart disease by decreasing the risk of blood clots. Chili pepper also increases APPETITE and the production of digestive juices and it may help relieve congestion in the GASTROINTESTINAL TRACT. Capsaicin may stimulate the production of endorphins, brain chemicals responsible for the so-called "eater's high." Chili doesn't injure the stomach of most people, nor does it cause ULCERS. It can cause skin redness (a rubefacient), and chemically purified capsaicin has been used topically to reduce painful conditions like shingles and arthritis. Chili oil (hot oil), prepared from red chili pepper and sesame oil, is used in Asian cooking, including Thai and Szechuan dishes. (See also DIGESTION.)

China Project, The   A six-year study of diet and health in the People's Republic of China that is one of the most comprehensive studies of its kind. More than 6,000 Chinese in 130 villages in rural areas of the eastern half of China took part in this survey, which generated more than 100,000 correlations among diet, life-style and disease. In China, each region has retained traditional dietary patterns and generally relies on locally grown foods.

The study highlighted significant differences between the U.S. population and the Chinese. The average Chinese blood CHOLESTEROL level is 127, much lower than an American's average of 212. The average Chinese eats three times as much fiber as Americans, consumes many more FRUITS, GRAINS and vegetables, and eats MEAT only once a week. In countries such as the United States, where meat is frequently eaten, rates of CARDIOVASCULAR DISEASE are higher. For the Chinese, FAT accounts for an average 15% of daily CALORIES, while in the United States about 37% of calories come from fat. Although the Chinese consume 20% more calories than Americans, OBESITY is not a major health problem in China, as it is in the United States. The results suggest that a diet with 80% or more vegetables, grains and fruits—and low in fat—may be optimal for health and longevity.

Patterns of Chinese mortality also differ from those in Western nations. The rate of colon CANCER is 50% that of Americans, while the rate of heart disease among Chinese men is one-seventh that of their U.S. counterparts. Breast cancer is five times higher in the United States than in China. However, the leading cancer in China is stomach cancer, now rare in the United States. The high rate of cigarette smoking among the Chinese corresponds to the increasing prevalence of lung cancer.

In addition to diet, clearly heredity, exposure to environmental pollutants, quality of medical care, and other factors influence health. The Chinese in general are more physically active: They seldom depend on cars for transportation, bicycles are common, and the Chinese perform more physical labor throughout their lives. (See also AGING; DIETARY GUIDELINES FOR AMERICANS.)

chips   A baked convenience food often prepared from corn or other grains or potatoes. These snack foods include corn chips, tortilla chips and the well-known potato chips; carrot chips and apple chips are more recent products. Chips are generally high-fat foods. The best way to judge the fat content of a particular chip is to examine the percent of total calories that are derived from fat. Governmental agency guidelines recommend no more than 30% of calories from fat. Fat accounts for 60% of the calories in regular potato chips and 52% in corn chips.

"Light" chips, including fruit chips, generally get about 40% of their calories from fat and oils. Often manufacturers add "natural grains" to increase the nutritional value of chips. However, the main ingredients are often the same as that in the regular chip, with only a slight increase in fiber content. Chips are also high-salt foods; regular potato chips contain 133 mg sodium per 1-oz serving; regular corn chips, 233 mg; and regular tortilla chips, 140 mg. Some varieties are available with reduced sodium. (See also DIETARY GUIDELINES FOR AMERICANS.)

chive (*Allium schoenoprasum*)   An HERB that bears thin, hollow green shoots and is a small, hardy relative of onions and garlic. Chives are easily grown in a flower pot for a ready supply of fresh seasoning. The chive's attractive clove-like flower makes it an ornamental plant, in addition to being an herb. The slender, tubular leaves, fresh or dried, provide a mild onion flavor to meat, stews, eggs, salads, soups and vegetable dishes.

chlordimeform A common contaminant of COTTONSEED OIL. Chlordimeform was classified as one of the 10 most dangerous PESTICIDES by the National Academy of Sciences. Since the cotton plant is not grown as a food, permitted treatment with pesticides is less restrictive than for crops. Partially hydrogenated cottonseed oil is a frequent FOOD ADDITIVE in baked goods like corn chips and smoked oysters. (See also FAT; PROCESSED FOOD.)

chloride A major mineral NUTRIENT that occurs in body fluids. Chloride is prominent negatively charged ion (anion) and a predominant ion (ELECTROLYTE) of blood, where it represents 70% of the anions. Its negative charge balances positive charged ions (cations), SODIUM and POTASSIUM ions, to maintain osmolarity (total concentration of ions). For example, in serum the number of cations and anions both equal 155 milliequivalents per liter (MEq/L). The exchange of chloride and BICARBONATE between RED BLOOD CELLS and plasma, the cell-free fluid, helps regulate the pH and CARBON DIOXIDE transport by the blood. Chloride also functions with sodium and potassium in nerves to transmit electric impulses. Chloride is converted to stomach acid (hydrochloric acid) to maintain the acidity of the stomach; when stomach acid is neutralized, chloride is reabsorbed by the intestine and recycled.

Most dietary chloride comes from table salt (sodium chloride), which occurs both as a FOOD ADDITIVE and as a natural ingredient in food. Chloride is non-toxic, and a safe and adequate daily intake ranges between 1,700 and 5,100 mg. Chloride deficiency is rare because it is so plentiful in food. However, a chloride deficiency can occur with excessive perspiration, vomiting or diarrhea. Chloride deficiency symptoms resemble those of ALKALOSIS (alkaline blood): apathy, irritability and DEHYDRATION. Chloride is an essential nutrient for infants. Chloride inadvertently omitted from baby formula in 1978 led to poor muscle control, delayed speech and slowed growth in affected infants. (See also ELECTROLYTES; INFANT FORMULA.)

chlorinated hydrocarbons A family of very stable organic compounds that have become widespread food contaminants. This class includes PESTICIDES (DDT, heptachlor, aldrin, dieldrin); a wood preservative (pentachlorophenol); contaminants of processed paper products (DIOXIN); transformer coolants (PCB or partially chlorinated biphenyls); and cleaning solvents (carbon tetrachloride). Many are linked to cancer and chronic disease.

Chlorinated hydrocarbons in general are stable compounds due to their composition of carbon, hydrogen and chlorine. Because they are fat-soluble and are not effectively broken down in tissues, chlorinated hydrocarbons concentrate in fatty tissue. Chlorinated hydrocarbons gradually spread up through the FOOD CHAIN. Humans, carnivorous fish and birds of prey, which occupy the top of the food chain, possess relatively high levels in their tissues. Though many chlorinated hydrocarbons have been banned or their use drastically limited by the EPA, they persist in the environment and are detected in fish caught in polluted waters, in MILK and in livestock.

Most Americans carry trace amounts of the modified forms of DDT and dioxin in their fatty tissues. Traces occur in breast milk because this is one way the body can remove fat-soluble materials. Women are encouraged to breastfeed, however, the benefits to babies are greater than the small risk of their ingesting these contaminants. BEEF TALLOW (fat) often contains traces of chlorinated and brominated hydrocarbons due to contaminated animal feed and pastures. Exposure to chlorinated hydrocarbons in the home and workplace should be minimized; the cumulative effects of low exposure and the long-range effect of mixture of residues on human health are unknown. (See also BREASTFEEDING.)

Scheele, J., Teufel, M. Niessen, K.H., "A Comparison of the Concentrations of Certain Chlorinated Hydrocarbons and Polychlorinated Biphenyls in Bone Marrow and Fat Tissue of Children and Their Concentrations in Breast Milk," *Journal of Pathology, Toxicology and Oncology*, 14:1 (1995), pp. 11–14.

chlorine dioxide A BLEACHING AGENT used to produce white FLOUR. This agent works by releasing oxygen, which attacks pigments in flour. Concomitantly, it modifies AMINO ACIDS of PROTEIN and destroys much of the VITAMIN E content of flour. The use of chlorine dioxide was instigated after World War II to replace a bleaching agent found to cause convulsions in animals. By the 1980s powder bleaching agents had largely replaced chlorine dioxide because they are less expensive and are easier to manage than this toxic gas. The low level (14 ppm) of chlorine dioxide used to treat flour causes no adverse effects in laboratory animals, and it is considered safe as a bleaching agent. Since 1975 chlorine dioxide has been used in processing vegetables and fruits. (See also FOOD ADDITIVES.)

chlorofluorocarbons (CFCs) Very stable industrial compounds, once extensively used as refrigerants and as a propellant for aerosol cans. Applications included foams and sprays ranging from hair spray to whipped cream and frosting. The EPA banned the use of CFCs as propellants in 1978 after it was discovered that they had begun to deplete the ozone layer protecting the Earth from the massive ultraviolet radiation in sunlight. Substitutes now being used for foods that require propellants include carbon dioxide.

chocolate The extract of the cocoa bean of the cacao tree, which grows within 20 degrees of the equator. To make chocolate the beans are roasted, the shells are removed, and the meat of the bean is ground and extracted to obtain cocoa flavor, which is quite bitter. This extract represents the main ingredient of baking chocolate. Chocolate was consumed by the Aztecs in Mexico and the Mayans of Central America.

Chocolate CANDY originated in 1847. The candy contains 50% sugar, roasted cocoa and cocoa FAT, which is a saturated fat. Usually the darker the chocolate, the more fat it contains. The total amount of fat in chocolate is higher than in BEEF. Milk chocolate was developed in 1876. It contains BUTTERFAT, sugar and vanilla, among other ingredients. The slight differences in very low concentrations of flavor compounds like aldehydes and other compounds give distinctive flavor to various types of chocolate candy.

Chocolate is generally the food most frequently craved in those countries where it is available. It is a complex food with over 400 different compounds. Chocolate also contains stimulants, 20 to 30 mg of CAFFEINE and theobromine per ounce of dark chocolate. These stimulants can appear in breast milk. In susceptible individuals chocolate may cause irregular heartbeat. Chocolate contains TYRAMINE and phenylethylamine, substances that increase alertness and a sense of well-being. Chocolate contains significant MAGNESIUM (82 mg per oz), which is frequently low in the typical U.S. diet. These factors, together with fat and sugar, may account for chocolate's widespread popularity. Chocolate consumption has been linked to BREAST CYSTS, food allergies and heartburn. Despite notions to the contrary, chocolate does not cause ACNE, though psoriasis can be a symptom of an allergy to chocolate.

Chocolate sometimes develops a white discoloration due to improper storage, which could represent cocoa fat that has risen to the surface when stored too long at room temperature or sugar that has been drawn to the surface by condensation. One ounce of plain milk chocolate (28 g) provides 45 calories; protein, 2 g; carbohydrate, 16 g; fiber, 0.3 g; fat, 9 g; calcium, 50 mg; thiamin, 0.02 mg; riboflavin, 0.1 mg; niacin, 0.1 mg. (See also ACID INDIGESTION; ALLERGY, FOOD.)

chocolate substitute   See CAROB.

cholecalciferol (vitamin D$_3$)   The most common form of VITAMIN D, occurring naturally in MEAT and dairy products. (See also CALCIUM.)

cholecystitis   Inflammation of the GALLBLADDER. Chronic infection can change the lining of the gallbladder, altering its ability to keep calcium and CHOLESTEROL in solution. Lowered bile acids or less water promotes cholesterol stone formation. Chronic cholecystitis is far more common than acute disease. It is usually associated with GALLSTONE formation and occurs most often in middle-aged and older obese women. The cause is poorly understood, but bacterial infection may be involved. Crohn's disease, cystic fibrosis and parasitic infection of the gallbladder increase the risk of gallbladder disease. Acute cholecystitis, though rare, is more likely to involve a medical emergency. In most cases it is caused by the impaction of a gallstone in the neck of the gallbladder or the duct.

cholecystokinin (pancreozymin)   A HORMONE produced by the upper segment of the small intestine. Cholecystokinin is released into the bloodstream as food moves into the intestine from the stomach. This hormone also stimulates the gallbladder to release BILE and the PANCREAS to release DIGESTIVE ENZYMES. Cholecystokinin also causes the feeling of SATIETY after a meal; it directs the hunger center of the brain, located in the region known as the HYPOTHALAMUS, to stop sending "hunger" signals. This process requires about 20 minutes. Bulimia (binge eating) is linked in some bulimic women to abnormally low levels of cholecystokinin after eating. Nonetheless, APPETITE and CRAVING are complex phenomena, unlikely to be controlled by a single chemical signal. (See also BULIMIA NERVOSA.)

cholesterol   A waxy LIPID derived from food and from liver synthesis. Cholesterol is the substance from which all steroid hormones are obtained. Both cholesterol and FAT are classified as lipids because they do not dissolve in water. However, cholesterol differs from fat because it does not contain fatty acids and cannot be oxidized in the body for ENERGY. Fat represents the body's major energy reserve. Though cholesterol has the reputation of an unwanted, even dangerous substance, all cells of the body require cholesterol because it is an essential constituent of all cell membranes. Cholesterol forms sex HORMONES and hormones of the adrenal cortex, which regulate water and ELECTROLYTE balance, as well as the METABOLISM of CARBOHYDRATE, fat and PROTEIN. In addition the skin converts cholesterol to VITAMIN D, while the liver converts cholesterol to BILE salts, to digest and absorb fat. Bile salts are the primary way in which cholesterol leaves the body.

Cholesterol is not an essential nutrient because the body makes most of the cholesterol it needs. Liver synthesis produces approximately 50% of the cholesterol manufactured in the body. Cholesterol is constructed from a much smaller material, ACETIC ACID, used as an activated form (acetyl COENZYME A). INSULIN increases glucose utilization by tissues and stimulates cholesterol synthesis in the liver after a high carbohydrate meal.

Cholesterol Transport

Because cholesterol does not mix with water, specific carriers are required to transport cholesterol in blood, which is mainly composed of water. The liver exports cholesterol to tissues by a carrier known as LDL (LOW-DENSITY LIPOPROTEIN), which accounts for 60 to 70% of the cholesterol in serum, the clear liquid remaining after blood has clotted. LDL is considered the undesirable form of cholesterol because elevated levels have been linked to clogged arteries. LDL originates from VLDL (VERY-LOW-DENSITY LIPOPROTEIN), a carrier of fat synthesized by the liver. Peripheral tissues such as muscle absorb LDL at specific sites on cell surfaces. HDL (HIGH-DENSITY LIPOPROTEIN), the so-called "good cholesterol," plays a unique role in cholesterol metabolism. HDL acquires cholesterol from peripheral tissues and thus acts as a scavenger. HDL can exchange cholesterol with other lipid carriers, and it also transports cholesterol to the liver for disposal.

Cholesterol and Diet

Cholesterol occurs in animal products such as liver, eggs, CHEESE, animal fat (BUTTER, lard) and in fatty meats like PORK and beef. Contrary to popular opinion, updated analysis indicates that SHELLFISH like shrimp do not contain unusually high amounts of cholesterol. Vegetable oil, peanut butter, GRAINS and VEGETABLES do not contain cholesterol because plants don't make it. In 1993 the U.S. FDA approved the following definitions of cholesterol content on food labels: "Cholesterol free" implies the product contains less than 2 mg of cholesterol per serving. SAFFLOWER oil is an example of a cholesterol-free product. "Low cholesterol" implies the product contains less than 20 mg per serving. Low-calorie

MAYONNAISE is such a product. "Reduced cholesterol" simply means that the product contains 75% less than that in the original version.

Since 1960 the average daily cholesterol intake in the United States has dropped significantly, from 493 mg to 259 mg for women and from 704 mg to 376 mg for men. The typical American diet provides 500 mg of cholesterol daily, in addition to the amount the liver produces. Nonetheless, consumption of saturated fat remains high. While increased dietary cholesterol tends to raise cholesterol levels, the type of dietary fat also has a strong influence on the blood cholesterol level. SATURATED FAT, including hard fats like SHORTENING, lard, butter and hard MARGARINE, tend to raise LDL levels dramatically. Fats with a high content of saturated FATTY ACIDS, especially PALMITIC ACID, seem to stimulate cholesterol production. On the other hand, unsaturated vegetable oils tend to lower LDL and blood cholesterol levels.

In 1995 a survey of 38 clinical studies of the effects of soy protein concluded that eating soy protein significantly reduces moderate to high levels of blood cholesterol. For people with the highest cholesterol levels, the reduction averaged 24% with the consumption of an average of 31 to 47 g daily. Rather than simply adding soy protein to the diet, the recommendation is to replace animal protein with soy protein to decrease fat consumption.

LDL-Cholesterol and Cardiovascular Disease

Elevated blood cholesterol is considered to be a widespread public health problem in the U.S., and an estimated 40 million Americans have high blood cholesterol because of a faulty diet. People with high blood cholesterol are susceptible to heart disease due to clogged arteries (ATHEROSCLEROSIS). Furthermore, susceptible middle-aged American men may be prone to heart disease and colorectal cancer if their blood cholesterol is above 250. Since 1960 blood cholesterol levels, which represents predominantly LDL cholesterol, have dropped nearly 8% in the United States, most of this occurring since 1976 when public education programs geared toward lower dietary fat and cholesterol were initiated.

Whether elevated blood cholesterol increases the risk of coronary heart disease in older adults is not certain. Some reports have found a correlation between high cholesterol levels and increased risk of heart disease in elderly women but not in elderly men. For men over the age of 70 there is a progressive decline in cholesterol levels, more so than in women. There is also an age-related drop in HDL, a beneficial form of cholesterol, and this is a better predictor of heart disease and death.

Although high LDL cholesterol may increase the risk of cardiovascular disease in middle-aged men in the United States and northern Europe, increased HDL levels in the blood lower the risk. Apparently, high LDL cholesterol can promote fatty deposits within arteries (PLAQUE), and over time plaque buildup can block arteries, causing coronary heart disease, HEART ATTACK and STROKE. The actual culprit in damaging arteries may be rancid (oxidized) cholesterol and lipids in LDL, not fresh cholesterol in whole foods. Cholesterol in tallow used in some fast-food cooking, powdered eggs and FRENCH FRIES is oxidized. Oxidized cholesterol is also found in pancake mixes, powdered custards and powdered whole milk. LDL is a primary target of FREE RADICAL attack. Free radicals are highly reactive forms of oxygen that damage molecules by stealing their electrons. Therefore ANTIOXIDANTS in food such as vitamin E may lower the risk by preventing the oxidation of LDL lipids. (Many other factors increase the risk of cardiovascular disease, including inheritance, smoking, OBESITY, HYPERTENSION and DIABETES.)

Current guidelines advise reducing saturated fat consumption so that fat accounts for less than 30% of daily CALORIES. This translates to cutting back on fats and oils by one-quarter to one-third for the typical American diet. In addition exercise may be recommended. The last line of defense is anticholesterol drug treatment, which needs to be carefully monitored. The long-term effects of these drugs are not known.

Cholesterol Measurements

Monitoring total serum cholesterol is frequently used to screen high risk people. It has generally been assumed that the higher the cholesterol, the greater the risk of dying from heart disease. However, other indices such as LDL/HDL ratios or ratios of proteins that characterize each of these carriers, such as apolipoprotien B/apolipoprotein A, correlate much better with risk. Serum cholesterol is measured as milligrams per deciliter (a deciliter is equivalent to 100 ml or 3.3 oz) of blood. Regarding "normal" levels, the upper limit for normal is 180 for individuals under the age of 30; a cholesterol value below 200 is considered desirable for individuals over 30. Cholesterol between 200 and 239 is considered a "borderline-high" risk. Above 240, there is a high risk of coronary heart disease. An estimated 50% of American adults have elevated blood cholesterol by this criterion. For people with coronary artery disease, the total cholesterol value should be less than 160.

A single measurement of blood cholesterol is not reliable for diagnosis because of biological and test variation. Repeated tests help assure accuracy. Though the permitted uncertainty in cholesterol tests is currently 5%, the American Heart Association reported appreciable variation among different testing laboratories. Factors affecting serum cholesterol levels include the time of day, the meal time, the month (January and February are highest) and whether the patient is sitting or lying down. Generally blood is drawn before breakfast, with the client seated. Finger-stick cholesterol values are higher than the usual test in which a blood sample is taken from a vein.

According to federal guidelines, a simple total cholesterol reading does not provide enought information for diagnosis and treatment; a complete serum lipid analysis provides a more accurate assessment. This involves measuring high-density lipoprotein (HDL), low-density lipoprotein (LDL) and blood fat (triglyceride) levels in serum, the cell-free fluid remaining after blood has clotted. An average of several tests may provide more accurate assessment than a single test. LDL should be below 130 for people with fewer than two risk factors and without coronary heart disease (CHD). If the LDL value is between 130 and 159 (borderline high), the situation needs to be watched, while LDL above 160 is considered a high risk for people without CHD and who have fewer than two risk factors. With coronary artery disease,

LDL levels should be below 100. HDL is an important indicator of the risk of heart disease, and HDL levels of 35 or less increase the risk of heart disease. Values of 60 or more confer protection.

A complete lipoprotein analysis, which measures HDL to obtain a ratio of total cholesterol to HDL, is prudent for those whose cholesterol is 240 or above, and for those with several risk factors for heart disease. A ratio above four increases the risk of heart disease. The most discriminating cholesterol tests to assess the risk of heart disease measure the ratio of serum Apoprotein A-1 to Apoprotein B. This ratio correlates highly in the degree of coronary artery blockage. Apo A-1 is a specific protein marker for HDL and Apo B a specific for LDL. High levels of another cholesterol carrier called lipoprotein(a), a close relative of the LDL-cholesterol, are a risk factor for children who may develop heart disease later in life.

Cholesterol Education Program
(National Cholesterol Education Program)

Sponsored by the National Heart, Lung and Blood Institute, this program is designed to alert Americans to the presumed link between blood cholesterol and coronary heart disease. The message is that people over 20 should have their total blood cholesterol and HDL levels measured at least every five years. A person with a high blood cholesterol (240 or more), with coronary artery disease, or with borderline high cholesterol and two or more risk factors for heart disease, should get a complete blood lipid profile (total cholesterol, HDL and triglycerides). Heart disease risk factors are considered to be age, a family history of heart attacks, current smoking, high blood pressure, diabetes and HDL below 35. Even when total cholesterol is normal, a complete lipid profile is recommended when the HDL level is below 35 for women over 55 and men over 45. The desirable level of triglycerides is less than 200.

Adults with high blood cholesterol should change their diet and life-style as their first line of defense. Cutting back on saturated fat and avoiding excess calories are priorities. In 1991 a panel of specialists from the National Heart, Lung and Blood Institute of NIH further recommended that children older than two and adolescents limit their fat intake to 30% of calories or less, and saturated fat to 10% (about one-third less than current consumption).

Cholesterol and Children's Diets

American children have significantly higher blood cholesterol levels than children in other industrial countries. About 30% of U.S. children have high blood cholesterol and 5% of children between the ages of 5 and 14 years have very high blood cholesterol levels. Experts generally agree that atherosclerosis begins in childhood with the appearance of "fatty streaks" (fat deposits) in arteries that are thought to lead to clogged arteries in adult life. Clogged arteries can lead to heart disease, and one-third of U.S. adults will have a heart attack by the age of 60. Family history increases the odds of clogged arteries. Therefore if a parent has heart disease by the age of 55 or has high blood cholesterol, it may be prudent to check children's cholesterol levels. However, the U.S. Preventive Services Task Force does not support cholesterol screening for children.

In 1991 the National Cholesterol Education Program recommended that children older than two (but not younger) adopt a low-fat, low-cholesterol diet, with a maximum of 30% of calories from fat (down from a typical 35%) and only 10% of the calories coming from saturated fat (down from 14%). Many cardiologists, the American Heart Association, and the National Heart, Lung and Blood Institute recommend limiting a child's fat intake to less than 30% of calories from fat after the age of two, while providing a balanced diet with enough calories to support rapid growth. Only one-third of their dietary fat would come from saturated fat sources (palm kernel and coconut oils, fat fried foods, cheese, fatty meat like hamburger and ice cream). On the other hand, the American Academy of Pediatrics does not endorse the reduction of dietary fat and cholesterol for children because it does not consider the evidence strong enough to recommend this change for the whole population, particularly children.

A specialist should be consulted before any child is placed on a diet. Dietary changes should be moderate because severe, fat-restricted diets create the risk of slowed growth in children who do not have enough fat, cholesterol, vitamins and minerals to develop normally. Nutrition educators emphasize that parents can assist children in developing healthful, lifelong habits by providing nutritious meals and low-fat snacks and by supporting a healthful life-style.

Cholesterol-lowering Strategies

"Heart healthy" or cholesterol-lowering diets are designed to reduce LDL-cholesterol. The underlying assumption is that eating foods excessively high in cholesterol can increase blood cholesterol, leading to an increased risk for cardiovascular disease. Only about one-third of Americans are sensitive to cholesterol in their diets. These "responders" experience an increase in blood cholesterol levels when they eat large amounts of cholesterol as found in eggs, butterfat or meat. Another 25% respond to elevated saturated fat in their diets by increasing the level of blood cholesterol. There is no simple way to screen individuals unable to cope with high dietary cholesterol or fat.

The American Heart Association and the National Research Council of the National Academy of Sciences recommend strategies to lower the risk of cancer, heart disease and other chronic diseases. These recommendations were devised for adults, not children. A minority opinion holds that the "prudent diet" should be confined to those with a high probability of developing heart disease. The studies showing a benefit to lowering cholesterol levels have been conducted with middle-aged males, and recommendations for others are less clear. However, experts agree that the more risk factors an individual has, the greater the importance of lowering blood cholesterol using DIET and EXERCISE as the first line of defense.

Dietary Recommendations to Lower Plasma
Cholesterol Levels Include the Following

Step 1 recommended by the American Heart Association:

- Stay trim by maintaining appropriate body weight (obtained from HEIGHT-WEIGHT TABLES or the BODY MASS INDEX). Obesity is a risk factor for cardiovascular disease.

- Eat 30% or less of daily calories as fat. Excessive dietary fat is linked to elevated blood cholesterol, obesity and cancer.
- Saturated fat should account for no more than 10% of total calories. This means reducing consumption of butter, fatty meats, fried foods, oily or fatty PROCESSED FOODS, whole MILK and whole milk products like ice cream and cheese. A high intake of saturated fat increased blood cholesterol levels in susceptible individuals.
- Polyunsaturated fat should account for less than 10% of total calories. Emphasize monounsaturated fats like olive oil rather than saturated fat. Unsaturated fatty acids, especially monounsaturates, lower blood cholesterol levels without lowering the beneficial HDL (high-density lipoprotein). Fish and fat oils lower blood cholesterol.
- Do not consume more than 300 mg of cholesterol daily. Excessive dietary cholesterol can raise blood cholesterol levels in certain individuals.
- Limit ALCOHOL intake to no more than two drinks per day, if you drink at all. Very limited alcohol consumption seems to have a beneficial effect on cholesterol levels and reduces the risk of atherosclerosis a little. Because of the danger to the embryo and fetus, pregnant women are advised not to drink alcohol.
- Limit SODIUM intake to 3,000 mg daily (equivalent to 5 g of table salt, or 1 teaspoon of salt a day). Susceptible people will respond to a high dietary load of sodium with increased blood pressure. Hypertension is a risk factor for cardiovascular disease.
- Include at least five servings of vegetables (especially dark-green leafy plus yellow kinds) plus FRUITS daily.
- Eat at least six combined servings of grains, cereals and LENTILS to increase intake of COMPLEX CARBOHYDRATES like STARCH to at least 55% of daily calories. Such a diet lowers blood cholesterol for most people. Complex carbohydrates and fiber help displace fat from the diet. Soluble fiber present in legumes, lentils, oats, fruit and vegetables seem particularly effective at lowering LDL and raising HDL. Increased consumption of fiber-rich foods also helps. These include oatbran, rice bran, barley, lentils, beans and dried peas.

Step 2 is a more stringent program with the following modifications:

1. Dietary fat should account for less than 30% of total daily calories.
2. Less than 7% of total calories should come from saturated fat.
3. Cholesterol consumption should be less than 200 mg per day.

If a patient is already on a Step 1 diet, and the response is inadequate, the patient may be advised to incorporate Step 2 recommendations.

An estimated 75% of individuals with elevated cholesterol may decrease blood cholesterol levels by 10 to 15% by diet alone. Changes in cholesterol levels in response to dietary changes most often occur within three to four weeks. The decrease in cholesterol may continue for several months.

Reducing fat intake is more important than cutting back on cholesterol. To reduce animal fat consumption, eat less animal fat (red meat, dairy products like eggs, pastries, butter and lard, ice cream, whole milk and cheese); choose poultry and fish over meat; trim excess fat from meat; broil or bake rather than fry. Avoid fried foods generally. Simply avoiding eggs does not significantly lower blood cholesterol. Individuals may not need to avoid eggs if: the blood cholesterol is normal; they don't have risk factors for heart disease; and they have already reduced fat intake. Low fat, low cholesterol diets help reduce blood cholesterol more effectively when regular exercise is incorporated as part of their health regimens. Moderate exercise—jogging or brisk walking 45 minutes three times a week—is adequate. (See also DIETARY GUIDELINES FOR AMERICANS.)

"Cholesterol in Food: Tempest in an Eggcup?" *Consumer Reports on Health*, 7:4 (April 1995), pp. 42–43.

"Lowering Blood Cholesterol to Prevent Heart Disease," National Institutes of Health Consensus Development Conference Statement, 5:7.

Ulbricht, T.L.V. and Southgate, D.A.T., "Coronary Heart Disease: Seven Dietary Factors," *Lancet*, 338 (October 19, 1991), pp. 985–92.

cholesterol-lowering drugs Prescription drugs used to lower CHOLESTEROL levels in the blood. Very high blood cholesterol levels, together with a family history of HEART ATTACKS, greatly increase the risk of heart disease. In only 1 to 5% of persons with high blood cholesterol is the basic cause FAMILIAL HYPERCHOLESTEROLEMIA, a genetically determined high blood cholesterol. To lower blood cholesterol in these cases, medication may be prescribed, together with weight loss, EXERCISE and low-fat diet plans. The effectiveness of cholesterol-lowering drugs has been demonstrated only in middle-aged men with high blood cholesterol, and their effectiveness in elderly people and young men and women with mild to moderately elevated blood cholesterol has not been studied in clinics. Most people with high cholesterol levels will be able to control their problem with change in DIET after consultation with an expert, but drugs are not a panacea. All drugs have side effects, and they are expensive. The following medications will generally not be prescribed unless diet modification, exercise and weight loss are ineffective:

Bile-binding resins Cholestyramine (Questran or colestipol [Colestid] together with NIACIN may be the first choice for lowering elevated blood cholesterol due to family history. Cholestyramine binds BILE salts, forcing the liver to convert more cholesterol to bile salts. The high daily dose often causes constipation.

Niacin Niacin alone can reduce blood cholesterol. The high doses of this vitamin that are required may cause abnormal liver function, and consequently high niacin supplementation should be used only with medical supervision. Uncomfortable flushing caused by niacin can often be avoided by taking an aspirin tablet half an hour before the niacin dose. Most people with diet-resistant high cholesterol seem to tolerate niacin. However, niacin is not recommended for anyone with asthma, GOUT, COLITIS, GASTRIC ULCERS or abnormal heart rhythm. The use of colestipol (Colestid) with niacin is a standard treatment for very high blood cholesterol. This treatment can lower cholesterol levels 15 to 30%

and it has a long safety record. However, it can increase blood fat levels.

Enzyme inhibitors Lovastatin (Mevacor) inhibits cholesterol synthesis in the liver though its long-term safety is not known. It has possible harmful effects on the liver and eyes. Gemfibrozil (Lopid) reduced the occurrence of heart disease in middle-aged Finnish men. This drug seems to inhibit fat synthesis in the liver while raising HIGH-DENSITY LIPOPROTEIN (HDL) levels ("beneficial" cholesterol). On the other hand, it seems to increase the risk of GALLSTONES, liver toxicity and altered blood chemistry.

choline (trimethylaminoethanol) A nitrogen-containing substance that functions as a building block of an important lipid, LECITHIN, and an important brain chemical, ACETYL-CHOLINE. Lecithin is a phospholipid and a primary component of all cell membranes. As a membrane constituent, lecithin helps insulate nerves. As a NEUROTRANSMITTER, acetylcholine is one of the chemicals that carries impulses for cholinergic nerves. Choline is synthesized by most tissues from the essential AMINO ACID, METHIONINE.

Choline occurs in foods as a component of lecithin. Good sources of lecithin are egg yolk (1.5%); SOYBEANS (0.35%); beef liver (0.6%), as well as CAULIFLOWER, BEANS, LEGUMES, GRAINS and WHEAT germ. The typical Western diet supplies adults with 500 to 900 mg daily. A deficiency disease has not been demonstrated in humans, and it is not clear whether a dietary source of choline is required for optimal health.

Choline and lecithin supplements may improve short term memory in normal and in senile people. Specifically regions of brains of Alzheimer's patients are deficient in acetylcholine and choline and lecithin supplements may improve short-term memory in some patients with ALZHEIMER'S DISEASE in the beginning stages of the disorder. However, these supplements do not reverse or arrest Alzheimer's disease. Diet doesn't boost the level of choline in the brain very much.

Choline may help the liver mobilize fat deposits (fatty liver) that accompany a decline in normal liver function. Fatty liver occurs during STARVATION and ALCOHOLISM. Choline has been used to treat tardive dyskinesia, a twitching of facial muscles that can develop as a side effect of treatment with antipsycotic drugs. High doses of choline can cause dizziness, vomiting and a strong fishy odor.

Canty, D.J. and Zeisel, S.H., "Lecithin and Choline in Human Health and Disease," *Nutrition Reviews*, 52:10 (1994), pp. 327–39.

chromium A trace mineral nutrient, needed only in minute amounts to help increase the body's sensitivity to the hormone insulin for efficient utilization of surplus GLUCOSE. Chromium represents one of the most recently identified nutrients, and its role in metabolism was discovered in 1969. Chromium is converted in yeast and in tissues to GLUCOSE TOLERANCE FACTOR, in which chromium is complexed with nutrients like amino acids and niacin. In this form chromium can assist insulin. As a supplement, chromium may be effective in alleviating elevated blood sugar (hyperglycemia) in some elderly patients, and in some diabetics, as well as in healthy, non-diabetic people. It may protect against a form of non-insulin-dependent diabetes. However, clinical studies of this aspect have yielded mixed results. Chromium may protect against CARDIOVASCULAR DISEASE by helping to regulate FAT and CHOLESTEROL synthesis in the liver and by raising HDL ("desirable" cholesterol) and by lowering LDL ("undesirable") in the blood. Chromium also seems to help reduce high blood pressure (HYPERTENSION) in some cases.

Only the less oxidized form of chromium (Cr^{3+}) is biologically active and can be used by cells. The more oxidized form (Cr^{+6}) is a toxic industrial waste product, which is not formed in the body. The human body contains only very low levels of chromium (an estimated 6 mg or less). Chromium in food is poorly assimilated and only 1 to 5% of dietary chromium is absorbed. It is estimated that 90% of Americans consume less than 40 mcg of chromium daily, and many people may be chromium deficient, especially elderly persons, pregnant or lactating women, athletes, and healthy people who rely on PROCESSED FOOD. Chromium loss increases with injury, STRESS, AGING and strenuous EXERCISE. Consuming excessive SUGAR increases chromium losses from the body and lost chromium is slow to be replaced. Consequently chromium levels decline with age.

Chromium deficient animals exhibit weight loss, lowered male fertility, elevated blood sugar, ATHEROSCLEROSIS and nerve degeneration. Deficiency symptoms in humans include intolerance of ALCOHOL and a decreased ability to use insulin to help metabolize blood sugar, a pre-diabetic condition. Chromium supplementation, either as chromium chloride or as chromium picolinate, did not increase strength or improve body composition (in terms of increased muscle mass or decreased body fat) in male volunteers participating in an eight week weight-training program. Possibly the beneficial effects of chromium can occur when people are deficient in chromium. Chromium supplementation can lower iron transport and distribution in the body, possibly placing the individual at risk for iron deficiency.

The chromium intake for optimum health isn't known. A safe and adequate dose is thought to be 50 to 200 mcg daily. BREWER'S YEAST is the best food source. Other sources are liver, oysters, whole potatoes, egg yolks, prunes, mushrooms, WINE, BEER, MEAT and BEETS. Fruits are low in chromium; so are polished rice and bleached flour. Chromium levels in GRAINS and vegetables depend upon the amount of chromium in the soil in which they were grown; however, chromium in vegetables isn't well absorbed. Surprisingly, Calcium-fortified BREAKFAST CEREALS are often good sources of the mineral because added calcium contains chromium as a contaminant. Supplemental chromium is available as chromium chloride. When taken together with niacin, its effect on lowering blood lipids is significantly improved, and the combination is as effective as taking yeast glucose tolerance factor. Several organically complexed forms of chromium such as chromium picolinate may be more readily absorbed than chromium chloride as supplements. (See also GLYCEMIC INDEX.)

Mertz, Walter, "Chromium: History and Nutritional, Importance," *Biological Trace Element Research*, 32 (Jan.-March 1992), pp. 3–8.

chronic Lasting months or years. In medicine, a condition or illness of long duration, in contrast with acute conditions. The DEGENERATIVE DISEASES of AGING are typical chronic diseases. Thus, ARTHRITIS, OSTEOPOROSIS, PERIODON-

TAL DISEASE, CARDIOVASCULAR DISEASE are slow to develop, and they may go on for years before becoming debilitating.

chronic fatigue (chronic fatigue syndrome, CFS, myalgic encephalomyelitis, chronic fatigue immune dysfunction syndrome, CFIDS)

A complex syndrome with persistent flu-like symptoms with fever, lymph node swelling, joint and muscle pain, often with mood swings and other psychological symptoms. Though controversial, a clinical diagnosis of CFIDS may be confirmed by the following CDC criteria: fatigue causing a 50% reduction in activity for at least six months, exclusion of other illnesses that can cause chronic fatigue; presence of 8 of 11 symptoms that include mild fever; recurrent sore throat; painful lymph node; muscle weakness; muscle pain; prolonged fatigue after exercise; recurrent headaches; joint pain; neurological symptoms (sensitivity to bright light, forgetfulness, confusion, irritability and depression); sleep disturbances; and sudden onset of the above symptoms. Signs of CFIDS include low-grade fever, swollen lymph nodes and inflamed pharynx.

Though probably not a recent illness, CFIDS is a major public health concern in the United States and several other Western countries. The cause or causes of CFIDS remain unknown. Attention has focused on the possibility of a viral infection. Possible candidates include Epstein-Barr virus (EBV) which cause mononucleosis, herpes virus HHV-6 and enteroviruses (polio, Coxsackie and Echo) since these have been shown to be active in some patients. Evidence for the presence of an RNA-containing virus (HTLV), and the fact that the antiviral drug seems to benefit at least some patients, argues for the involvement of a virus as an infectious agent in CFIDS. Another hypothesis suggests that an immune disorder is the underlying cause of symptoms. A variety of immune system abnormalities have been observed in patients with CFIDS, including depressed natural killer cell and white cell activity. FIBROMYALGIA, a chronic musculoskeletal pain, is a closely related syndrome.

Fatigue is often the result of pre-existing conditions, including DIABETES MELLITUS, ANEMIA, CANCER, chronic pain, RHEUMATOIC ARTHRITIS, prescription drug use (such as tranquilizers, antihistamines, birth control pills), DEPRESSION, liver conditions, toxic exposure and HYPOTHYROIDISM. STRESS may also be involved in CFIDS and often patients are deficient in the adrenal steroid hormones, CORTISOL and DHEA. Many patients with CFIDS have food allergies, which can worsen fatigue symptoms. There is also a well-established connection between chronic fatigue and HYPOGLYCEMIA. LEAKY GUT SYNDROME, in which persistent intestinal inflammation leads to the uptake of potentially harmful substances, is sometimes implicated in CFIDS.

Stress reduction, moderate exercise and enhancement of the immune system are likely to be one of the most vital steps in achieving resistance and reducing susceptibility to viral infection. Nutritional support of the immune system includes trace minerals, particularly zinc, selenium, chromium and manganese; and vitamins, especially B_6, B_{12}, pantothenic acid and folic acid. Beta carotene is a potent antioxidant and is an effective booster of the immune system. Vitamin C helps increase the immune response. Magnesium deficiency has been suggested as a possible factor in CFIDS. Injections of this mineral, as well as mineral and vitamins may be beneficial. A diet that eliminates allergic foods and simple and refined carbohydrates can help balance the body's defenses. Alternatively chelated minerals (such as potassium, magnesium aspartate) may help alleviate fatigue. Siberian ginseng has a reputation for enhancing stamina. COENZYME Q and ANTIOXIDANTS can help support efficient energy production. Branched chain amino acids (VALINE, LEUCINE and ISOLEUCINE) are preferred fuels of muscles and have been prescribed. Certain supplements including, N-acetyl CYSTEINE and GLUTATHIONE, support liver disposal of toxic substances. Glutamine and folic acid can help normalize gut function. Antiinflammatory drugs and antidepressants may help. Therapeutic doses of steroids, hormones such as DHEA and cortisol may be beneficial when these hormones are low. Whole, minimally processed food including garlic and onions and fresh fruit may also assist in normalizing the immune system.

Bell, D.S., "Chronic Fatigue Syndrome Update," *Postgraduate Medicine*, 96:6 (1994), pp. 73–81.

Demitrack, Mark A., "Chronic Fatigue Syndrome; a Disease of the Hypothalamic-pituitary-adrenal Axis?" *Annals of Medicine*, 26:1 (1994), pp. 1–5.

chutney

A sweet-sour condiment prepared from a wide variety of fruit and vegetables. Chutney is cooked in vinegar and sugar and has the consistency of jam. Chutneys originated in Britain as an attempt to reproduce Indian recipes for a relish made of vegetables, sweet fruits and hot pepper. PLUMS, APPLES, raisins and unripened tomatoes are other examples that can be used. More exotic fruit like mango and tamarind can also be used. Chutneys can be seasoned with GINGER, GARLIC or CHILI PEPPER.

chylomicron

A lipid-protein particle that transports dietary FAT and fat-soluble vitamins to the liver, muscles and fat tissue via the lymph and the bloodstream. Chylomicrons keep water-insoluble lipids suspended in body fluids, which are mainly water. In this sense they can be considered emulsifying agents. Normally chylomicrons disappear from the blood within a few hours after a meal, as the fat they carry is consumed.

Chylomicrons demonstrate a complex metabolic history. After cells lining the small intestine (intestinal mucosa) absorb fatty acids from fat digestion, they convert them back to fat before packaging them as chylomicrons, to be released into the lymph. The lymph carries chylomicrons into the bloodstream. When chylomicrons reach the capillaries they encounter an enzyme that breaks down the fat molecules in chylomicrons to free fatty acids. Released fatty acids are quickly taken up by cells for energy or fat storage. The deflated chylomicron remnants carry vitamins and cholesterol to the liver for storage or processing. (See also HIGH-DENSITY LIPOPROTEIN; LOW-DENSITY LIPOPROTEIN; VERY-LOW-DENSITY LIPOPROTEIN.)

chyme

The homogeneous, semi-liquid mixture of masticated food and digestive juices found in the stomach. GASTRIC JUICE provides hydrochloric acid and PEPSIN to initiate protein digestion of chyme. PERISTALSIS, the rhythmic contraction of the stomach, and the periodic opening of the valve between the stomach and intestine (pyloric sphincter) move chyme from the stomach into the small intestine for complete DIGESTION and absorption of nutrients. (See also DIGESTION; STOMACH ACID.)

chymotrypsin   A potent digestive ENZYME secreted by the PANCREAS for protein digestion. Like other proteolytic (protein-degrading) enzymes, chymotrypsin is synthesized and secreted as an inactive form (ZYMOGEN) to prevent the pancreas from digesting itself. Pancreatic zymogens are activated only when they reach the intestine where their powerful digestive action breaks down food. An intestinal enzyme called enteropeptidase triggers this activation. Proteins are chains of amino acids linked together by peptide bonds, and chymotrypsin breaks bonds next to the amino acids PHENYLALANINE, TYROSINE and METHIONINE within protein chains. Other proteolytic enzymes clip protein chains at other amino acid links, so that food proteins are reduced to single amino acids. Therefore, chymotrypsin complements the activity of other major proteolytic enzymes. (See also DIGESTIVE ENZYMES.)

cider (apple cider)   The juice from pulped, pressed APPLES. Sweet cider refers to unfermented juice, while fermented or hard cider contains ALCOHOL and is carbonated; in Europe the term cider refers to fermented apple juice. In the United States and Canada homemade cider is unprocessed, with a sweet flavor. It will eventually ferment and turn into a vinegar. Basic cider preparation has changed little over the years: Whole apples are grated in a mill and the juice is extracted with a press. Preservatives are often added to commercially prepared cider, which is then pasteurized before being bottled. Frozen apple concentrate, first introduced in the 1960s, is a common household substitute for cider. Mulled cider has been heated with cloves and cinnamon sticks. Applejack refers to cider brandy, prepared by distilling hard cider. Cider VINEGAR is a mild, yellow vinegar, prepared from hard cider, containing between 5 and 6% ACETIC ACID; it is comparable to wine vinegar.

ciguatera poisoning   A fish-borne illness due to eating fish contaminated with a toxic substance ciguatoxin that is produced by a marine microorganism (algae). This toxin is carried through the food chain from the algae to certain fish that eat the algae. The toxin is not destroyed by cooking. It is most common in tropical seafood: Ciguatera poisoning has been most frequently associated with amber jack, grouper, goatfish, barracuda and snapper caught in Hawaii, Puerto Rico, the Virgin Islands, Florida and Guam. Symptoms appear within six hours after eating contaminated fish. They include headache and dizziness, blurred vision, joint and muscle pain, a metallic aftertaste and sensations of alternating hot and cold. Very rarely does it cause death. (See also FOOD POISONING; SEAFOOD; SEAFOOD INSPECTION.)

circulatory system   The system consisting of the cardiovascular system—veins, arteries, CAPILLARIES, the heart and the lymphatic system—devoted to transporting fluids though the body. The cardiovascular system is a true closed system because blood returns to its starting point, the heart. Pulmonary circulation refers to circulation of blood from the heart to the lungs and back to the heart in order to oxygenate the blood and to remove carbon dioxide loaded into the blood by tissue metabolism. Systemic circulation refers to blood circulating through the rest of the body. Arteries carry blood away from the heart to other tissues and veins carry blood back to the heart. Capillaries carrying oxygenated blood from the smallest arteries (arterioles) distribute blood to cells; blood then flows into the smallest veins (venules). Blood pumped out of the heart follows this sequence: from arteries, to arterioles, to capillaries, to venules, then to veins and back to the heart.

The cardiovascular system contains about 5 liters of blood in the average adult. It provides nutrients and OXYGEN to every tissue. Waste products are removed from tissue; generally they are processed by the LIVER and excreted by the KIDNEYS. Hormones are released into the bloodstream where they are transported to their target tissues, to regulate physiologic processes and maintain the internal environment of the body. The IMMUNE SYSTEM relies on circulation to effectively defend the body from invaders via ANTIBODIES and defensive cells. The circulation system assures an even temperature regulation for the entire body. With circulating hormones and nutrients, blood provides an avenue for communication between the endocrine system and the brain. In addition, the bloodstream contains a system to plug leaks in blood vessels (clotting factors).

The heart beats an average of 70 times per minute; this is equivalent to pumping about 4 liters of blood per minute. At this rate, the heart pumps 260 liters or 85 gallons an hour. Considering that the heart beats an average of 36 million times a year, it is capable of an astonishing amount of work in a lifetime.

The circulatory system is subject to disease, such as hardening of the arteries and CORONARY ARTERY DISEASES. The coronary arteries, two small branches of the aorta that deliver oxygenated blood to the body, supply the heart with nutrients. Two diseases of the coronary arteries are prevalent. Angina pectoris causes severe pain in the upper left portion of the chest when insufficient quantities of oxygen are carried by the coronary arteries. Nitroglycerine dilates these arteries and provides temporary relief. Myocardial infarction (heart attack) occurs when the heart does not receive enough oxygen, for example when a blood clot or cholesterol deposits (PLAQUE) clog arteries. Blockage of coronary arteries by plaque is a leading cause of heart disease.

The lymphatic system collects fluid that has leaked into tissues and body cavities. It serves a unique transport function by returning water, serum proteins and electrolytes, and by transporting dietary fat to the bloodstream. Unlike the cardiovascular system, the lymphatic system is not a closed circuit: Skeletal muscles contract and relax to propel lymph through the lymphatic ducts. This fluid enters lymphatic capillaries and moves into larger lymphatic ducts and finally returns to the blood in veins in the neck region. The lymphatic system also plays a key role in the body's defenses. Lymph nodes house bacteria and virus-destroying cells as part of the body's immune defense. (See also ATHEROSCLEROSIS; CARDIOVASCULAR DISEASE; RED BLOOD CELLS.)

cirrhosis (liver)   A serious LIVER condition involving extensive scarring and reduced liver functions. Scarring extends throughout the liver, altering tissue structure. This degeneration seems irreversible.

ALCOHOLISM is the leading cause of liver cirrhosis. Other causes include MALNUTRITION, chronic HEPATITIS, rare metabolic disorders leading to the deposition of IRON or COPPER, exposure to toxic chemicals and certain drugs, and a blocked bile duct. Destruction of liver tissue results in nausea, FATIGUE, low energy, susceptibility to bleeding, frequent infections and OSTEOMALACIA (soft bone disease). Liver failure can lead to death. Treatment entails abstinence from the damaging agent and nutritional strategies including vitamin supplements to bolster the liver (lipotropic agents). The prescription drug cholchicine has recently been used. Milk thistle (silymarin) is an herbal preparation reported to have a beneficial effect on liver metabolism.

A healthy liver is critically important to overall health. It produces most of the blood proteins like clotting factors (FIBRIN and prothrombin) and serum ALBUMIN as well as FAT, CHOLESTEROL and their LIPOPROTEIN carriers; BILE for DIGESTION; UREA to dispose of the toxic nitrogenous waste AMMONIA; KETONE BODIES to fuel the body during starvation; and carrier proteins for iron, copper, steroid hormones and others. The liver processes steroid hormones, drugs and toxic chemicals for excretion, and it maintains BLOOD SUGAR levels between meals so that the nervous system is adequately nourished. (See also CARBOHYDRATE METABOLISM; DETOXIFICATION.)

Britton, R.S. and Bacon, B.R., "Role of Free Radicals in Liver Diseases and Hepatic Fibrosis," *Hepato-Gastroenterology*, 41 (1994), pp. 343–48.

citric acid (citrate)   A common organic acid occurring in high concentration in citrus fruits and berries. For example, lemon juice contains up to 8% citric acid. Commercially, citric acid is produced by the mold *Aspergillus niger* during the FERMENTATION of MOLASSES from sugar beets. Citric acid is a key to energy production in plants and animals. Citric acid is the starting point of the KREB'S CYCLE, the final energy-producing pathway of CARBOHYDRATE, FAT and PROTEIN metabolism. Once citric acid is formed, a series of enzymic reactions converts it to CARBON DIOXIDE and OXALOACETIC ACID, a smaller acid that initiates the Kreb's Cycle.

Citric acid efficiently binds or traps metal ions. This process is called chelation and citric acid acts as a chelating agent. When ZINC and CALCIUM are chelated as citrates, these minerals are more efficiently absorbed by the intestine. Citric acid is used therapeutically to chelate heavy metals in the body and to prevent recurrent kidney stones.

Citric acid is one of the most common FOOD ADDITIVES. It adjusts acidity and contributes a tart flavor to fruit juice drinks and carbonated beverages. It also serves as an ANTIOXIDANT. It is often used with synthetic antioxidants which trap FREE RADICALS, highly reactive and damaging forms of oxygen. Citric acid traps metal ion contaminants that could promote SPOILAGE, RANCIDITY or discoloration of many processed foods. It helps preserve fresh FISH, instant potatoes and CHIPS. Citric acid is added to ice cream, sherbet, jellies, jams, canned fruit and vegetables, and CHEESE. Citric acid is used in wine making to react with traces of iron, which could precipitate TANNINS and make the wine cloudy. Citric acid, citrate salts and citrate esters are considered safe food additives. (See also CARBOHYDRATE METABOLISM; CHELATE; FAT METABOLISM.)

citric acid cycle   See KREB'S CYCLE.

citrus fruit   Fruits of the genus Citrus, including LEMONS, LIMES, ORANGES, tangelos, tangerines, GRAPEFRUIT, pummelo, ugli and KUMQUATS. They all share a flavorful rind that is sometimes used in flavorings and teas. Citrus fruits contain many juicy wedges and their tart flavor is due in part to the high amount of citric acid. Citrus fruits originated in southern Asia and are now cultivated throughout the world, especially in California and Florida of the United States and in Mediterranean regions (Spain, Italy, Israel). Citrus fruits are used extensively by the fruit juice industry. They are consumed as fresh fruit or as preserves or in baked goods. Oranges, lemons and limes are the most popular. The rind of lemon and grapefruit provides a commercial source of FLAVONOIDS, plant substances that enhance the effects of vitamin C. Citrus fruits are good sources of VITAMIN C and POTASSIUM. As an example, a medium-sized orange contains 80 mg of vitamin C; half a grapefruit, 47 mg; a tangerine, 26 mg. Several citrus fruits are more unusual. The Jamaican ugli is a hybrid of grapefruit and Mandarin oranges and is a popular citrus in Canada. It is more tender and juicy than other citrus fruits and has a sweet, unique flavor. Citron is used mainly for its very thick rind, which is often candied. Kumquats are the smallest of commercial citrus. They are the size of grapes with a bright orange rind. Blood oranges are closely related to Valencia oranges and other common oranges, except their pulp is scarlet red. Popular in Mediterranean countries, blood oranges are flavorful and have a sweet rind. The pummelo is quite large and resembles a grapefruit. It has a soft texture.

clam   A mollusk with two equal shells; a member of the invertebrate class, *Bivalvia*. More than 12,000 species are known, many of which are edible. The hard-shell clam or quahog is an edible clam found in North America. The northern quahog (*Mercenaria mercenaria*) is found from the Gulf of the St. Lawrence to the Gulf of Mexico and is the most important food clam in those waters. The southern quahog (*M. campechiensis*) is found from Chesapeake Bay to the West Indies. One of the larger edible clams on the West Coast is the geoduck (*Panopea generosa*), which grows along beaches lying between low tide and high tide from Alaska to Baja California. It can weigh up to 11 pounds and grows up to 20 cm in length. The soft-shell clam (*Mya arenaria*, steamer clam), found in oceans throughout the world, is used in soups and chowders. Other edible varieties include the donax or coquina clam (*Donax*). The northern species (*Donax fossot*) is found from Long Island to Cape May, New Jersey. The southern coquina (*Donax variabilis*) occurs in sandy beaches from Virginia to the Gulf of Mexico, while the razor clam is found on both the Atlantic and Pacific beaches of the United States. The Atlantic razor clam is *Ensis directus*.

In the United States the majority of seafood-related illnesses are brought on by eating raw, or partially cooked mollusks, including clams, which may be contaminated by harmful bacteria and viruses from seawater. Thorough cooking of mollusks is very important for anyone with liver, stomach or immune disorders. Red tides, caused by the overpopulation of microorganisms called dinoflagellates, can contaminate clams and their toxin can cause shellfish poisoning. Therefore, shellfish harvests may be banned at certain times of the year. Clams (mixed species, 100 g, raw) provide 74 calories; protein, 12.8 g; carbohydrate, 2.6 g; fat, 0.97 g; calcium, 46 mg; iron, 14.0 mg; sodium, 56 mg; riboflavin, 0.213 mg; niacin, 1.77 mg.

clarifying agents   A class of FOOD ADDITIVES added during processing to react with contaminants that would otherwise turn cloudy or coagulate. Examples of clarifying agents include enzymes and chelating agents, such as citric acid and EDTA, materials that remove minerals such as iron and copper from liquids. (See also PROCESSED FOOD.)

clay eating   See GEOPHAGIA.

clinical ecology   See ENVIRONMENTAL MEDICINE.

clinical trial   A carefully planned experiment, involving human subjects, to investigate the effects of a therapeutic agent or treatment. The experimental design typically incorporates a PLACEBO-controlled, double-blind procedure. In this case, neither physician nor subject nor patients know who has received a test material and who has received an innocuous substitute called a placebo until the study is completed. Those who receive the placebo are the control group and are used as a basis for comparison. Independent review boards must approve these studies, and participants are required to give their informed consent, based upon the risks and benefits of the treatment. Selection of subjects for either the control group or the test group is random.

Group studies, such as large clinical trials, have several important limitations. They generally ignore individual differences due to each person's unique genetic makeup (BIOCHEMICAL INDIVIDUALITY). Treatment protocols that are effective in group studies rarely apply to all individuals; some may actually be harmed by the treatment. In addition, treatments that are effective for a small subgroup will often be ignored and the treatment be judged ineffective in such clinical trials. Nutritional therapies usually require long periods of time, possibly years, in order to detect an effect. Chronic conditions such as degenerative diseases of AGING may have developed over decades. Therefore, studies must be performed over a sufficient period of time for an observable effect. On the other hand, when studies are carried out over many years, study groups may no longer be homogeneous and the therapeutic approach may become outdated (different dosage, different treatment substance may be more effective).

In addition, epidemiology notes a variety of possible pitfalls in clinical studies. It may be difficult to establish which factor is a cause and which is an effect after linkage has been demonstrated. For example, low serum cholesterol and cancer are linked, but it seems that cancer can lead to a drop in cholesterol, rather than low cholesterol being a cause of cancer. Often there are confounding factors, that is, many variables may be involved. Elaborate statistical procedures with their own limitations are used to sort out the contribution of each. The fact that a diet rich in fruits and vegetables is associated with a lowered risk of CANCER and CARDIOVASCULAR DISEASE may be due to increased consumption of fiber, trace minerals, antioxidant nutrients such as vitamin C, FLAVONOIDS,

CAROTENOIDS or any of a huge array of PHYTOCHEMICALS typical of these foods. People who eat more fruits and vegetables may also smoke less, exercise more and generally be more health conscious. Chance is another pitfall the research needs to be aware of. Typically, a result is called significant if the odds of it being due to chance are one in twenty. The odds of a finding being a fluke can be quite low, but not 100% eliminated. Bias can also influence the result. As an example, patient's preexisting health condition can be the major determining factor governing food choices.

Results obtained from this type of study are considered more reliable for groups of people than studies of single individuals or anecdotal information in which physician and patient know of the treatment and may have an expectation of its outcome. Knowing what treatment is being used and what results should be obtained to support an hypothesis can bias the evaluation by a physician or a patient. Clinical trials have been used to investigate the effectiveness of single drugs such as vaccines against polio, measles and rubella; food allergies; and the effects of cholesterol-lowering drugs. However, clinical studies are less appropriate for examining nutrients and ANTIOXIDANTS, which often function synergistically as members of complex interacting systems.

In contrast with the large-scale intervention study of a group of people, clinicians sometimes employ "N of 1" studies to examine the effectiveness of a nutritional treatment on single patients. The N of 1 study features the patient serving as his or her own control. According to one design, the patient randomly receives either an active substance or an inactive treatment. Optimally, neither the patient nor the physician knows the sequence of treatment until after the study is completed. Each treatment period needs to be long enough to establish an active response, and the intermediate period needs to be long enough to establish baseline values during the inactive period. N of 1 studies can be generalized to groups by repetition with many subjects. (See also RISK DUE TO CHEMICALS IN FOOD AND WATER.)

"Clinical Trials: Help Yourself by Helping Others," *Consumer Reports on Health*, 7:2 (February 1995), pp. 18–19.

Clostridium botulinum   See BOTULISM.

Clostridium perfringens   An anaerobic bacterium that is a potential source of FOOD POISONING. Strains of this bacterium produce toxins (enterotoxins) that can cause diarrhea, severe abdominal pain and flatulence 8 to 24 hours after eating. The symptoms usually end within a day, though older individuals can become seriously ill. *C. perfringens* occurs widely in raw and processed foods. *C. perfringens* can grow in food sealed in containers that are slowly cooled or kept warm for extended periods of time instead of being truly heated, such as gravies, stews and casseroles. Following what Grandmother would say, "Keep hot food, hot, and cold food, cold," warm cooked foods should be kept above 60° C (100° F) or cooled to below 10°C (50° F) within two to three hours after cooking. As an added precaution, chilled foods can be heated to a minimum of 75° C (170° F) immediately before serving to destroy toxin-producing bacteria. (See also FOOD TOXINS.)

clove (*Eugenia aromatica*)   An aromatic SPICE that is the dried flower bud of the clove tree. Clove is a member of the myrtle family and originated in the Molucca Islands. Cloves have been used since antiquity to season food. Cloves were used in ancient China for their medicinal properties and as a spice. They were introduced into Europe during the 4th century A.D. Whole or ground cloves find use in meat loaves, pork and ham, chili sauce, pickles, and in baked goods in combination with other sweet spices like gingerbread, spice-cake and pumpkin pie. In mulled wine, cloves are often combined with cinnamon. Cloves enhance the flavor of bean soups, baked beans and barbecue sauces. Clove oil has long been used to relieve pain of toothaches and tooth extractions. The oil contains 60 to 90% eugenol, an analgesic (pain killer). (See also HERBS.)

coagulated protein (precipitated protein)   Protein that has been cooked or otherwise treated to form curds or clumps. Soluble proteins in foods often clot when exposed to heat, extreme pH, enzyme action, organic solvents or extreme changes in concentration of the medium in which they are dissolved. Denatured or inactivated proteins are easier to digest because their amino acid chains are more accessible to attack by digestive enzymes. Cooked eggs and meat juices are visible examples of coagulation by heat. Whey is coagulated milk protein produced by acids of fermentation and by rennet during cheese manufacture. A protein like egg albumin in egg white is soluble before cooking because the protein molecule is folded tightly into a ball whose outer surface is negatively charged so that individual protein molecules repel each other. When the egg is cooked, heat breaks the tenuous links holding the globular structure together, exposing sticky regions that permit protein chains to bind randomly, forming a sticky mass. (See also COOKING; DENATURED PROTEIN.)

coal tar dyes   Synthetic dyes used to color fabrics, cosmetics and processed foods. Originally these dyes were synthesized from compounds isolated from coal tar, itself prepared by heating coal in the absence of oxygen. Modern manufacture prepares artificial dyes from compounds obtained from various sources including petroleum, rather than from coal tar. However, this descriptive name persists. (See also ARTIFICIAL FOOD COLORS; CANCER.)

cobalamin   The generic chemical name for VITAMIN B$_{12}$. Vitamin B$_{12}$, as it occurs in supplements and many foods, is called cyanocobalamin and contains a single cyanide ion bound to cobalt in cobalamin. The level of cyanide supplied by vitamin B$_{12}$ supplements is entirely safe because the dosage is minuscule. In the body, a water molecule displaces the cyanide of vitamin B$_{12}$ to form aquocobalamin, which is then converted to enzyme helpers (coenzymes). Methylcobalamin is an example of a coenzyme containing a bound single carbon atom. Cobalamin concentrate (USP grade) is used to treat vitamin B$_{12}$ deficiency. (See also ANEMIA; INTRINSIC FACTOR.)

cobalt   A TRACE MINERAL nutrient for bacteria. Its only established role in animals is as a component of VITAMIN B$_{12}$. Animals like ruminants that depend on bacteria for vitamin B$_{12}$ require inorganic cobalt as a nutrient. Only microorganisms are capable of incorporating cobalt into vitamin B$_{12}$.

The body cannot use unattached cobalt and cobalt supplements are therefore ineffective. Though cobalt has a low order of toxicity, overdosing with cobalt could lead to goiter and over-production of red blood cells in susceptible individuals.

Low concentrations of cobalt salts were once added to beer as an antifoaming agent. However, cobalt was incriminated in several epidemics of cardiac failure among beer drinkers. The typical American diet provides low levels of cobalt. Green leafy vegetables are the richest source, while dairy products and refined grain products are among the lowest. For example, spinach provides 0.4 to 0.6 mcg per gram, and white flour contain 0.003 mcg per gram. The oral intake of cobalt necessary to produce toxicity is many times greater than can be obtained by normal consumption of foods and beverages. (See also HEAVY METALS.)

cocoa   A powder prepared from cocoa beans that is the raw material for CHOCOLATE and chocolate-flavored beverages. The name cocoa is derived from the Aztec word, CACA HUATL, meaning the beautiful tree of paradise. The Aztecs attributed to cocoa the power to convey wisdom and to heal. Cocoa reached Europe in the 16th century; but it was not until the following century that cocoa became a popular beverage. To prepare cocoa, cocoa beans are dried, roasted, shelled and ground to yield cocoa paste, the starting material for cocoa and chocolate. Cocoa paste contains 45 to 60% FAT or cocoa butter; the fat (cocoa butter) is partially removed to produce cocoa. The remaining cocoa cake is ground to obtain cocoa powder, which contains 8 to 20% fat. Treatment of cocoa with an alkaline solution yields "Dutch process" cocoa with a dark color and rich flavor. Instant cocoa contains SUGAR, flavorings and an EMULSIFIER to suspend cocoa butter, in addition to cocoa powder. A cup of instant cocoa drink prepared with water contains 133 calories; protein, 4.8 g; carbohydrate, 30.2 g; fiber, 0.19 g; fat, 1.43 g; calcium, 118 mg; potassium, 300 mg; thiamin, 0.04 mg; riboflavin, 0.22 mg; niacin, 0.24 mg. Chocolate contains more sugar and more cocoa butter.

coconut (*Cocus nucifera*)   The fruit of a palm tree with an outer husk and a tough brown shell that encases a layer of white meat. The coconut probably originated in Polynesia, and it is now grown in tropical and sub-tropical regions worldwide. Marco Polo described the coconut, which had long been used as a food in Southeast Asia. Coconuts mature in a year. The hollow center of the coconut contains a sweet liquid called coconut milk. Coconut is a high-fat food, and COCONUT OIL is one of the most highly SATURATED FATS. Western recipes usually call for dried, shredded coconut meat when used in cakes, cookies and candy. In many regions of the world fresh coconut is used in condiments to season raw vegetables, and as an ingredient in stews. Coconut milk gives characteristic flavor to curries, sauces and rice. The coconut is an important ingredient in African, Indian, Indonesian and South American cooking. The nutrient content of 1 cup (80 g, shredded) of fresh coconut meat is 283 calories; protein, 2.7 g; fat, 34 g; carbohydrate, 12.2 g; fiber, 11.2 g; fat, 26.8 g; calcium, 12 mg; potassium, 285 mg; thiamin, 0.05 mg; riboflavin, 0.02 mg; niacin, 0.43 mg.

coconut oil A TROPICAL OIL obtained from coconut meat and used extensively as an additive in PROCESSED FOODS. Dried coconut pulp, called copra, is refined to produce this oil. Coconut oil is especially common in commercially prepared cookies, CHIPS and baked goods, as well as in NON-DAIRY CREAMER. A food label listing only "100 percent VEGETABLE OIL" will likely be high in coconut, palm or palm kernel oils—all classified as SATURATED FAT. Coconut oil is 92% saturated, one of the most saturated of dietary fats and oils. By comparison, BUTTERFAT is 65% saturated. (See also FOOD ADDITIVES.)

cod (*Gradus morrhua*; codfish) A large saltwater food fish from the North Atlantic. The adult cod averages 3 to 4 feet in length and weighs up to 10 pounds. Cod is classified as a very lean fish with a relatively low-fat oil content. Roe (fish eggs), which can account for half a female's weight, are a source of caviar. Cod is among the top five fish eaten in the United States. Haddock and pollack also belong to the cod family. Cod is a versatile fish and can be broiled, baked or used in chowder. A 3.5 oz (100 g) portion, poached, represents 94 calories; protein, 20.9 g; fat, 1.1 g; cholesterol, 60 mg; calcium, 29 mg; iron, 0.5 mg; zinc, 0.75 mg; and niacin, 3 mg. (See also SEAFOOD INSPECTION.)

cod liver oil An important FISH OIL and dietary supplement of VITAMIN A and VITAMIN D. Cod liver oil also contains polyunsaturated FATTY ACIDS, EICOSAPENTAENOIC ACID, docosahexaenoic acid and other omega-3 acids, that may help protect against CARDIOVASCULAR DISEASE and some CHOLESTEROL. A tablespoon of cod liver oil provides vitamin A, 12,000 IU; vitamin D, 1,200 IU; vitamin E, 3 mg; and cholesterol, 85 mg. Excessive consumption of cod liver oil can lead to vitamin A and vitamin D toxicity; these fat-soluble VITAMINS are stored and it is difficult for the body to rid itself of excessive amounts. The Recommended Dietary Allowance for vitamin A is 800–1000 mcg (2,667–3,333 IU). Doses 10 to 100 times greater than this over a period of months lead to nausea, cracked skin, headache and abdominal pain. Symptoms disappear when supplementation is stopped. (See also HYPERVITAMINOSIS.)

coenzyme An organic compound required by an ENZYME in order for it to function as a catalyst. Coenzymes are low molecular weight, often heat-stable substances, while enzymes are hundreds of times larger and are usually heat-sensitive. As enzyme activators, coenzymes combine with the inactive PROTEIN (APOENZYME) to form the active enzyme (HOLOENZYME). Vitamins of the B COMPLEX form coenzymes that are essential in metabolizing fat and carbohydrates for energy production. Each coenzyme serves a unique role in the body so that a surplus of one vitamin cannot correct for a deficiency of another. NICOTINAMIDE ADENINE DINUCLEOTIDE (NAD from NIACIN) transfers electrons in oxidations and reductions. FLAVIN ADENINE DINUCLEOTIDE (FAD, from RIBOFLAVIN) also transfers electrons. THIAMIN pyrophosphate (from thiamin) helps catalyze oxidations that create carbon dioxide from carbohydrate breakdown. COENZYME A (from PANTOTHENIC ACID) is used to carry fatty acids in metabolic pathways. BIOTIN attaches carbon dioxide to key intermediates while tetrahydrofolate (from FOLIC ACID) transfers single carbon fragments especially important in DNA

synthesis. Pyridoxal phosphate (VITAMIN B_6) transfers amino groups ($-NH_2$) in the first step of amino acid degradation, while coenzymes of VITAMIN B_{12} transfer carbon atoms and alter carbon chains of several compounds.

coenzyme A An enzyme helper based on the B vitamin pantothenic acid that prepares FATTY ACIDS and ACETIC ACID to participate in biosynthetic and degradative reactions of cells. For example, when fatty acids are oxidized as fuel, they are first attached to coenzyme A. The enzymatic breakdown of AMINO ACIDS, FAT and CARBOHYDRATE ultimately produces acetic acid, bound to coenzyme A (acetyl coenzyme A). In turn acetyl CoA is used to create new fatty acids, fat, CHOLESTEROL and other important lipids. Alternatively, acetyl CoA is shunted to the KREB'S CYCLE, the central oxidizing process used by tissues to produce energy. (See also CARBOHYDRATE METABOLISM; FAT METABOLISM.)

coenzyme Q (ubiquinone, coenzyme Q_{10}) A lipid oxidation-reduction agent found in MITOCHONDRIA, the powerhouses of the cell. Coenzyme Q helps mitochondria oxidize fuels like fat and carbohydrate to produce cellular energy (ATP) in a process known as OXIDATIVE PHOSPHORYLATION.

Because most cellular processes require energy, coenzyme Q is essential for health. Coenzyme Q can be viewed as a collector of hydrogen atoms removed during cellular oxidations. Coenzyme Q is liberally distributed in membranes of the cell and possibly serves as a membrane ANTIOXIDANT. A protective role for vitamin E in mitochondrial membranes appears likely. The body can synthesize coenzyme Q and therefore it does not have vitamin status. However, deficiencies can occur in patients with heart disease such as angina and congestive heart failure, as well as in older people with high blood pressure. There is as yet no simple clinical test to measure coenzyme Q deficiency.

Coenzyme Q has been prescribed for treatment for cardiovascular conditions, and it is a promising treatment for angina. Coenzyme Q supplements can aid cardiac patients, especially those with congestive heart failure who are deficient in coenzyme Q, and their use lowers high blood pressure. Coenzyme Q also bolsters the IMMUNE SYSTEM and helps protect against the effects of radiation and chemotherapy in cancer treatment. Very large amounts of coenzyme Q (several hundred mg per day) have been used in Europe for patients with soft tissue cancer such as breast cancer. No side effects have been reported for moderate doses. However, the issue of long-term safety of this supplement has not been explored. (See also CARBOHYDRATE METABOLISM.)

Folkers, K., Hanioka, T., Xia, L.J., McRee, J.T., Jr., Langsjoen, P., "Coenzyme Q_{10} Increases T4/T8 Ratios of Lymphocytes in Ordinary Subjects and Relevance to Patients Having the AIDS-related Complex," *Biochemical and Biophysical Research Communications*, 176:2 (1991), pp. 786–91.

cofactor A heat-stable enzyme activator. Most trace metal nutrients, including COPPER, IRON, ZINC, MANGANESE, SELENIUM, MOLYBDENUM and MAGNESIUM, function as enzyme cofactors. Many enzymes carrying out oxidation-reduction reactions require iron. An example is catalase, which degrades HYDROGEN PEROXIDE to water and oxygen. The mitochondrial enzyme complex that ultimately uses oxygen to burn fuels, CYTOCHROME oxidase, requires copper, while SUPEROXIDE DISMUTASE, an antioxidant enzyme that destroys a toxic form of oxygen, requires manganese, zinc and copper. Manganese is also required to operate the KREB'S CYCLE, the central enzyme system for oxidizing fat and carbohydrate for energy. The enzyme that destroys SULFITE preservatives (sulfite oxidase) and the enzyme that produces the nitrogenous waste URIC ACID (xanthine oxidase), require molybdenum as the cofactor. Magnesium and zinc are cofactors for hundreds of enzymes, including those for the synthesis of RNA and DNA required in cell division. (See also ANABOLISM; CATABOLISM.)

coffee   A popular, mildly stimulating beverage prepared from coffee beans. Coffee ranks as the second most popular beverage in the United States after soft drinks. As many as 96% of U.S. adults drink coffee, and the average annual consumption is nearly 30 gallons per person.

Coffee beans are imported from Central and South America. They are cured either by air-drying or FERMENTATION. The dried, hulled beans are then roasted and ground. The beverage is prepared by extracting ground coffee with hot water (brewing). Brewed coffee is a complex mixture of over 300 chemicals; CAFFEINE is perhaps the most notorious. A cup of coffee contains approximately 100 mg of this stimulant. Caffeine increases EPINEPHRINE (adrenaline) release, which stimulates the central nervous system, increases states of alertness and increases heartbeat.

Drinking coffee carries with it several risks. Coffee beans are grown abroad where fertilizer and PESTICIDES are not required to meet U.S. regulations; consequently there is an increased risk of contamination. Caffeine can be habit forming. Even a single cup of coffee a day contains enough caffeine to create the risk of withdrawal if it is suddenly eliminated in susceptible individuals. Coffee can cause heartburn by relaxing the muscle between the stomach and esophagus, allowing stomach acid to rise into the esophagus. Though coffee does not cause ulcers, it causes increased stomach acid production, which can exacerbate ulcers. On the other hand, drinking coffee does not seem to lead to HYPERTENSION, pancreatic CANCER or bladder cancer. The caffeine in coffee can block calcium and IRON absorption; coffee drinkers who avoid milk and dairy products need more calcium to minimize the risk of OSTEOPOROSIS.

Other associations are more controversial. Healthy men drinking three to six cups of coffee daily may experience a significant drop in blood pressure when they abstain from coffee. The Tromso Heart Study found that cholesterol levels were 14% higher among heavy coffee drinkers in Scandinavia drinking boiled coffee. Some studies have found the cholesterol of U.S. coffee drinkers, drinking more than nine cups daily, to be slightly higher than those drinking one cup; still other studies have found no consistent correlation between coffee and cholesterol. Caffeine itself does not seem to raise cholesterol levels. The American College of Obstetricians and Gynecologists recommends limiting coffee consumption because excess caffeine in coffee, tea or colas can increase the risk of miscarriage in pregnant women, even prior to conception.

The link between coffee and CARDIOVASCULAR HEART DISEASE (CHD) is even more uncertain. Some studies have found an increased risk of coronary heart disease among American men who drink five cups or more per day as compared to those who do not drink coffee. On the other hand, women who drink four cups per day may increase their risk of PREMENSTRUAL SYNDROME and non-malignant BREAST CYSTS (fibrocystic breast disease). However, the Framingham Study, a U.S. investigation spanning two decades and involving over 6,000 adults, did not find an association between coffee and coronary heart disease in smokers or non-smokers.

It is best to use a common sense approach to coffee: Drink it in moderation—which, according to the U.S. FDA, is one to two cups a day. People with high blood cholesterol levels, coronary diseases, heart arrhythmias and hypertension, and pregnant women may want to cut back on high coffee consumption and consumption of other beverages containing caffeine. Those who drink boiled coffee may want to switch to drip-filtered coffee. (See also ADDICTION.)

cola soft drinks   Beverages based on cola extract. The cola tree produces a fruit with many seeds (cola nuts). These seeds yield a brown extract that contains CAFFEINE and is a mild stimulant. Typical ingredients of cola SOFT DRINKS include: cola extract, caramel as additional coloring, carbonated water, additional caffeine, high-FRUCTOSE CORN SYRUP or ASPARTAME as sweeteners, and PRESERVATIVES. (See also EATING PATTERNS.)

cold-pressed vegetable oil   Vegetable oils that have been extracted from seeds under mild conditions. Consumers often assume that cold-pressed oils contain more essential nutrients like VITAMIN E and polyunsaturated FATTY ACIDS than more typical hot-pressed oils. This may not be true.

To prepare oils, seeds are first crushed and then pressed to expel oil. With the exception of olive oil, all vegetable oils are heated to varying degrees to increase their efficiency of extraction. Cold-pressed oils may be heated between 120° F and 150° F. Subsequently these oils are often purified, bleached and deodorized. These processes can involve further heating, possibly as high as 450° F, and such products possess compositions similar to hot-pressed oil. Seed oils containing high levels of the essential polyunsaturated fatty acids (such as evening primrose oil, borage oil and flax seed oil) need to be prepared under mild conditions that exclude air, heat and light in order to minimize rancidity. Vitamin E and beta carotene are often added to help stabilize these oils. (See also ESSENTIAL FATTY ACIDS; VEGETABLE OIL.)

colitis (ulcerative colitis)   A condition characterized by chronic inflammation and/or ulcers of the colon and rectum. Colitis is one of the two forms of INFLAMMATORY BOWEL DISEASE, affecting 1 to 2 million Americans. Colitis is more common in whites than in other groups and occurs more frequently between the ages of 15 and 35. The occurrence of colitis is increasing in Western societies while it is rare in populations consuming less refined, less PROCESSED FOODS. Symptoms include rectal bleeding, severe DIARRHEA, painful cramping, FLATULENCE, stomach ache and weight loss. The immune system is often imbalanced and colitis is considered an autoimmune disorder. The causes of colitis are unknown, though stress and viral or bacterial infections are implicated. FOOD SENSITIVITY may also be involved because many patients improve with intravenous nutrition and elemental diets (containing only pure nutrients), and symptoms can reappear when foods are reintroduced. Patients may be allergic to household dust and molds and they may be low in the steroid hormone DHEA.

For most people, colitis lasts for years and requires persistent medical attention. Patients are often malnourished due to a lack of appetite and inadequate nutrient uptake because of damage to the intestinal lining. Zinc, calcium, magnesium, iron as well as B vitamin intake may be low. Persistent diarrhea can upset the ELECTROLYTE balance. Inflammation and scarring can narrow the intestinal lumen, raising the possibility of obstruction. Colitis and similar diseases can increase the risk of colon and rectal cancer.

Recommendations for colitis include eliminating common food ALLERGENS, like WHEAT, CORN, citrus fruit, yeast or dairy products including EGGS, as well as eliminating refined sugar and alcohol while emphasizing vegetables and other FIBER-rich foods. Traditional medical treatment includes steroid hormones to reduce inflammation. The chronic use of steroids carries additional risks, however. Sections of the bowel may be removed surgically but the disease may flare up even after surgery. Butyrate (BUTYRIC ACID) enemas have proven effective in treating colitis. Butyrate is a short chain fatty acid naturally produced in the colon by bacterial fermentation of FIBER and undigested carbohydrate. Colonic cells use butyrate as a major fuel and it promotes normal structure and function of the intestinal lining. The National Foundation for Ileitis and Colitis can provide more information. (See also MALNUTRITION.)

Stenson, W.F. et al., "Dietary Supplementation with Fish Oil in Ulcerative Colitis," *Annals of Internal Medicine*, 116:8 (1992), pp. 609–14.

collagen   A fibrous, structural protein of connective tissue, skin, cartilage and BONE matrix, and the most prevalent PROTEIN of the body. The stability of collagen fibers requires the amino acids HYDROXYPROLINE and hydroxylysine. Hydroxyprotein synthesis from the amino acid proline requires VITAMIN C. Similarly LYSINE is converted to hydroxylysine. With prolonged vitamin C deficiency, neither hydroxyproline nor hydroxylysine may be formed in sufficient amounts for optimal collagen fiber formation. One consequence is weakened capillary walls, slow wound healing, bleeding gums and loose, painful joints—the symptoms of SCURVY.

Connective tissue and collagen content influence the toughness of meat. The more connective tissue, the tougher the meat. Slow moist-heat cooking, like braising and stewing, tenderizes flesh by breaking down connective tissue and converting collagen to GELATIN. Food processors prepare gelatin by boiling collagen in cartilage. High temperature has the opposite effect on muscle fibers and toughens meat. Two or three hours of moist heat at 180° F strikes a balance between softening connective tissue and minimizing muscle hardening.

MEAT TENDERIZERS soften tough meat by breaking down collagen with enzymes. Most powdered meat tenderizers use the plant enzyme PAPAIN as the tenderizing agent. This papaya product breaks down proteins of muscle, fibers and connective tissue to small fragments. Tenderizers generally work on the surface of the meat. As proteins, they are inactivated along with meat during cooking. (See also AMINO ACIDS; BIOLOGICAL VALUE.)

collard (*Brassica olercea*)   A dark-green leafy vegetable of the cabbage family. Like KALE, collard forms tall, broad leaves on long stalks but no head. Of the cabbage family, kale and collard have been cultivated the longest. In the southern United States collard greens are boiled with bacon or salt pork. Collard greens are relatively good sources of fiber, beta carotene, iron and calcium. A cup of collard, cooked (145 g), provides 20 calories; protein, 1.6 g; carbohydrate, 3.8 g; fiber, 4.1 g; calcium, 113 mg; iron, 0.59 mg; zinc, 0.93 mg; vitamin A, 322 retinol equivalents; folic acid, 55 mg; ascorbic acid, 14 mg; thiamin, 0.03 mg; riboflavin, 0.06 mg; and niacin, 0.34 mg.

colon (large intestine)   The lower part of the digestive tract, beginning with the end of the small intestine, the ileocecal valve, and ending at the rectum. The length is approximately 1.3 meters or 6 feet. Its divisions are the cecum, a pouch at the beginning of the colon, and the ascending, transverse, descending and sigmoid colon, which lies close to the anus. These sections form an inverted "U" surrounding the small intestine. The sigmoid is a common site of polyp formation and of colon cancer. Examination of this region is called a sigmoidoscopy. However, examination of the entire colon (colonoscopy), can reveal polyps and lesions that would be missed by a sigmoidoscopy. Colonic conditions affect millions of Americans; they include: bulges (DIVERTICULOSIS), inflamed pockets (DIVERTICULITIS), CONSTIPATION, ulcerated colon (COLITIS) and hemorrhoids. All are influenced by diet.

The ileocecal valve regulates the flow of food remnants from the small intestine into the colon. The colon is filled by the gastrocolic nerve reflex, by which food entering or leaving the stomach causes a discharge of contents of the ILEUM into the colon. The colon also fills four to five hours after a meal. Feces solidify in the colon during the next 24 hours. No digestion occurs during passage through the colon. The colon absorbs CALCIUM and electrolytes like sodium and potassium, as well as water and microbial products (see below).

The colon secretes mucus, which provides lubrication to ease the movement of fecal material and to serve as a physical barrier between the epithelial cells lining the colon and fecal matter. Pouch-like segments of the colon, haustra, slow the movement of fecal material through the colon. Nonetheless, peristaltic movement gradually pushes feces through the colon where fecal material is squeezed and mixed to permit more efficient absorption. When malfunctions do not allow adequate reabsorption of water, the feces appear watery, a condition known as DIARRHEA. If excessive amounts of water are removed from the feces, constipation results. The distal end of the colon is the rectum, and the valve keeping the fecal matter within the colon is the anal sphincter. Bowel movements are triggered by involuntary responses; however, muscles of the anal sphincter can be unconsciously contracted to delay bowel movement.

The colon houses a vast amount of bacteria and other microorganisms. Typically, the amount in an adult is about 4 to 6 pounds, and the total number of bacteria exceed the cells that exist in the body. This intestinal microflora forms a symbiotic relationship with the host. While deriving nutrients from undigested food supplied by the host, the beneficial bacteria supply the host with vitamin K, B complex vitamins, BIOTIN and SHORT-CHAIN FATTY ACIDS from the fermentation of fiber and undigested carbohydrate. These can supply several hundred calories daily. The beneficial bacteria limit the growth of potentially pathogenic bacteria and yeasts as well. (See also ACIDOPHILUS; CROHN'S DISEASE; IRRITABLE BOWEL SYNDROME.)

color additives   See ARTIFICIAL FOOD COLORS.

colostrum (pre-milk)   A thick, milk-like secretion produced by mammary glands, especially during the first two or three days after birth and before true lactation. This high-calorie fluid contains PROTEIN and FAT to nurture the infant. In comparison to mature milk it contains more protein and less milk sugar and fat. Its yellow color reflects a high content of beta carotene. Colostrum provides maternal ANTIBODY (IgA) and lymphocytes (white blood cells) to assist in protecting the infant's GASTROINTESTINAL TRACT. Some of the antibodies leak into the infant's bloodstream and provide additional protection. Colostrum provides BIFIDUS FACTOR, which helps beneficial bacteria populate the infant's intestine. Colostrum is sterile so the baby cannot contract bacterial infections, though the mother may have one. Colostrum changes to transitional milk between the third and sixth day after birth. By the tenth day, the major changes in milk composition are complete. (See also ACIDOPHILUS; BIFIDOBACTERIA; BREASTFEEDING.)

combining   See FOOD COMBINING.

comfrey (*Symphytum officinale*)   An herbal ingredient of teas, used in folk medicine as an astringent to close wounds or sores and a tonic for asthma, coughs and disorders of the gastrointestinal tract. This is an example in which a "natural" product is not necessarily safe. The comfrey leaves and roots contain substances, including allantoin, consolidine and pyralizidine alkaloids, that can injure the liver. Though symptoms may not show up until several months after use, liver damage can occur in a week. Infants are more susceptible to side effects. Comfrey leaves can cause cancer in experimental animals. (See also HERBS.)

complete protein   A food PROTEIN that contains all AMINO ACIDS in amounts adequate for normal growth and maintenance. Such proteins possess a high BIOLOGICAL VALUE (BV). Thus all protein building blocks are supplied simultaneously for optimal protein synthesis. If the diet does not supply adequate amounts of the dietary essential amino acids (that is, amino acids the body cannot make), then protein synthesis will be limited. Animal protein (dairy products, meat, poultry, fish, seafood) are excellent sources of complete proteins. In contrast, most plant proteins are deficient in one or more essential amino acids. Consuming a variety of protein from different plant sources helps the vegetarian meet the daily requirements for all essential amino acids. Certain plant proteins approach the quality of meat:

They include AMARANTH, QUINOA and SOYBEAN. (See also FOOD COMBINING.)

complex carbohydrate   Long-chained CARBOHYDRATES (POLYSACCHARIDES) that occur in plant-derived foods like fruits, vegetables and legumes. Nutritionists recognize two major classes of complex carbohydrate: STARCH and FIBER. Starch is the plant storage form of glucose, and it may be unrefined, as found in unprocessed foods such as brown rice, whole wheat flour, fresh vegetables, tubers and root vegetables. Whole foods provide VITAMINS, MINERALS and fiber that are removed more or less completely by refining, milling and other food processing. Refined starch appears in bleached FLOUR, white RICE and PASTA and lacks other nutrients.

Eating starch, particularly in minimally processed foods, offers many advantages. Starch digestion yields GLUCOSE, an excellent energy source. The digestion of starch in unprocessed foods generally yields blood glucose more slowly than from simple SUGARS. This diminishes the burden of the pancreas to produce INSULIN; thus whole foods are conducive to better GLUCOSE TOLERANCE. Glucose from carbohydrate digestion is converted to body FAT more slowly and with a greater expenditure of energy than are dietary fats and oils. Therefore, surplus starch calories are not as fattening as fat calories. Starch does not promote CHOLESTEROL build-up, unlike saturated fat. When following dietary recommendations for achieving a more healthful diet, the increased consumption of complex carbohydrates simplifies reducing fat intake.

The second type of complex carbohydrate is fiber, a diverse family of polysaccharides made up of various sugar constituents that serves as the outer protective layers of plant cells. Digestive enzymes do not attack fiber as they do starch. Though fiber is not digested, intestinal bacteria may break it down more or less completely, according to the type of food ingested. For example, short-chain fatty acids released by microbial metabolism can supply between 5 and 25% of daily energy requirements. Fiber can be divided into two general classes. Water-soluble fiber like PECTIN and GUMS form gels. Insoluble fiber, like CELLULOSE, HEMICELLULOSE and LIGNINS, provide bulk. They absorb water and soften stools. Research indicates that both soluble and insoluble fibers are essential for a healthy digestive tract. Abundant dietary fiber helps with weight management; reduces the risk of constipation, diarrhea, hemorrhoids, diverticulosis or pouching of the colon; reduces the risk of colon cancer and cardiovascular disease; and assists in the regulation of blood sugar and diabetic control.

Canadian and U.S. guidelines agree that increased consumption of foods containing more complex carbohydrates, and decreased consumption of concentrated sweets and fat, would be beneficial in most cases. Typically, Americans derive 25% of their calories from sugar. U.S. guidelines advise decreasing this to 10% while increasing complex carbohydrates to meet 50% of total energy intake. These additions would represent major additions to the DIET in terms of vegetables, grains, fruits and legumes. Americans generally need to increase their fiber intake. (See also BRAN, OAT; BRAN, WHEAT; BUTYRIC ACID; CEREAL GRAINS; DIETARY GUIDELINES FOR AMERICANS; GLYCEMIC INDEX; GLYCOGEN.)

Chinachoti, P., "Carbohydrates: Functionality in Foods," *American Journal of Clinical Nutrition*, 4S (1995), pp. 922S–929S.

compulsive eating (bingeing)   Episodes of excessive eating. Compulsive binge eating, BULIMIA and ANOREXIA NERVOSA are considered to be the three major eating disorders in America. Though most normal-weight individuals periodically overeat, compulsive behavior indicates an underlying problem.

Often compulsive eating is triggered by unresolved emotional issues. Like ADDICTION, abstaining from food may cause symptoms of distress. The failure to acknowledge personal feelings and to resolve personal pain may underlie compulsive eating. Identifying the feelings that are being shunned and working through alternative ways of dealing with emotions represent powerful first steps in recovery. Available programs provide a framework for change and a strong support system. One example is the 12-step program of Overeaters Anonymous, patterned after Alcoholics Anonymous. Individualized programs assist the client in feeling safer and more in control of eating behavior. Programs usually involve psychological counseling, providing emotional support, BEHAVIOR MODIFICATION, education about addictions, nutrition counseling, a BALANCED DIET and regular EXERCISE.

Behavior modification involves learning to eat only when hungry and to stop eating when hunger is satisfied. Counseling can help with attitudes toward food and self-nourishment. Affirming that the client has the choice of eating or not, without judgment, and that the client is in control at every bite, are valuable steps forward. During a binge, identifying underlying feelings may clarify whether food is being substituted for a deeper need, such as love and acceptance. Counseling also emphasizes a return to eating normally after bingeing and self-forgiveness in order to break patterns of guilt and self-defeat. A diet diary can reveal eating patterns and the accompanying feelings. Eating more whole, fresh foods and eating less highly processed CONVENIENCE FOODS moves the individual to a more balanced diet. As an added benefit, avoiding sugar and sweets may stabilize BLOOD SUGAR levels and moderate mood swings that can trigger a bout of bingeing.

condensed milk   A mixture of whole MILK and sugar (SUCROSE), concentrated by evaporation. Approximately 60% of the water is removed by heating. It is enriched with VITAMIN D (400 IU per pint). Sugar accounts for 40 to 45% of condensed milk. Because the high sugar content slows bacterial growth, condensed milk will keep somewhat longer than whole milk. Condensed milk is used in custards and pumpkin pies.

condiment   An extra flavoring for meat and vegetable dishes. Condiments are used to heighten natural flavors and to stimulate the appetite. They include relish, pickled fruit and vegetables. Unlike seasonings, which are added to foods during preparation, condiments are chosen to complement the main serving. They may be fresh, as onions, fresh herbs, cress or parsley, or they may be prepared, as sweet and sour sauces, purees, MUSTARDS, CHUTNEYS, catsup and capers. Condiment can also refer to natural coloring like beetroot and caramel, as well as extracts such as aniseed, almonds, some flowers and even cheeses.

conditioning   See FITNESS.

constipation   Infrequent or incomplete bowel movements with firm stools. One out of every ten Americans is constipated and 20% of those individuals over the age of 65 are chronically constipated. Chronic constipation is the cumulative result of a faulty DIET and inadequate fluid intake. Straining during bowel movements weakens muscles of the colon; they lose their tone (DIVERTICULOSIS) and, over time, pouches or bulges may develop in the walls of the colon. Many medications cause constipation. These include codeine; a CALCIUM BLOCKER (verapamil); ANTIDEPRESSANTS (Elavil and Toframil), especially in elderly persons; ANTACIDS containing aluminum or calcium; and some CHOLESTEROL-LOWERING DRUGS (Questran and Colestid). Some FOOD SENSITIVITIES, for example, to milk and dairy products, may cause constipation in sensitive people.

Constipation may be alleviated by drinking enough water and consuming more fiber-rich food like WHEAT bran, vegetables, prunes, FIGS, PEARS and BEETS. GUAR GUM and PSYLLIUM powder are other types of fiber that have been used as BULKING AGENTS to soften stools. Individuals need to consult their physicians before supplementing with fiber. Some people do not respond to dietary fiber because they have a slow rate of movement of waste through the intestine. Magnesium salts are traditional LAXATIVES and may help these persons. However, the long-term use of any laxative can lead to dependence upon it. Soap sud enemas are not recommended because they irritate the rectum and colon. (See also DIGESTION; GASTROINTESTINAL DISORDERS; GASTROINTESTINAL TRACT.)

convenience food   Foods that have been precooked or processed to minimize meal preparation at home. Convenience foods include cold BREAKFAST CEREALS, powdered soft drinks, prepared foods to be heated at home, canned foods and frozen foods (FROZEN ENTREES like pizza and tacos and TV dinners). Consumers may choose among gourmet microwave dinners; foods in pouches that need only to be mixed with water, warmed and served; snack foods; and a plethora of fast-food restaurants.

The number of different foods carried by a typical supermarket ranges between 15,000 and 40,000 and the variety continues to grow. Presently about 1,000 new food products are introduced each month. The abundance of convenience food does not necessarily mean that it is easier to make healthful choices among these products. Convenience foods are often highly processed and so are not as nutrient-dense as whole, minimally processed foods. The increased consumption of convenience foods has raised concerns because of the increased consumption of food additives like FAT and oils, salt and SUGAR. For example, frozen pizza, chips and snack foods often contain fat and oil, sugar, salt and other additives not present in whole foods and recipes prepared at home.

The basis for increased consumption of convenience foods lies in the changing attitude toward meals and meal preparation. Marketing surveys reveal that shoppers desire convenience in preparing tasty meals and snacks. Increasingly, more people are eating meals away from home, and busy work schedules dictate shorter meal preparation times. These desires have spawned a huge variety of foods that require a minimum of preparation and/or eating time. The degree to which consumer demand for convenience food has been shaped by ADVERTISING is debatable. Certainly children who watch TV commercials have a different attitude toward meals than their grandparents did. Home environments continue to change. Increased numbers of households in which both parents work, and of single-parent families, reflect important trends affecting family meal choices and meal preparation. (See also BALANCED DIET; EATING PATTERNS; FOOD ADDITIVES; PROCESSED FOOD.)

cooking Heating food to increase its nutritional quality and/or flavor. Accessibility to nutritive foods has played a dominant factor in human evolution. The use of fire for cooking preceded the domestication of plants and animals by perhaps 40,000 years. The importance of cooking cannot be over-emphasized because cooking causes profound changes in a food. The chemical changes soften, coagulate, break down or dissolve PROTEIN, ENZYMES and meat fiber. CELLULOSE and PECTIN fibers in plant materials are softened, thus increasing the digestibility of starch and other nutrients trapped within cell walls. All plant foods now used as staples require cooking for human consumption. These include grains, tubers, legumes and plants such as BREADFRUIT. FLOUR becomes edible when cooked because starch granules are made accessible to digestive enzymes. Cooking is no less important for MEAT. COLLAGEN is the main protein constituent of connective tissue. In a hot, moist environment collagen is gradually transformed to GELATIN as the connective tissue gradually dissolves. This makes the meat both more tender and more easily digested. Extensive cooking can also toughen meat as muscle fibers harden.

Cooking sterilizes foods; disease-producing viruses, parasites, yeast and bacteria are generally destroyed with adequate cooking times. Cooking often destroys "anti-nutrients," proteins that can block nutrient uptake (goitrogens) or inhibit enzymes (soybean trypsin inhibitor, an inhibitor of kidney beans). Cooking also can destroy toxic substances that are common in raw foods. Uncooked BROAD BEANS (fava beans) can induce hemolytic ANEMIA in susceptible individuals. OXALIC ACID crystals in RHUBARB, BEETS and SPINACH are broken down during cooking. Carbohydrate derivatives that release cyanide occur in the CABBAGE family, raw lima beans and CASSAVA. These are destroyed or reduced by cooking, especially by boiling.

Basic cooking techniques include frying (cooking in hot oil, which dramatically raises the fat content); poaching (simmering in hot water, a gentle technique for eggs and fish); pressure cooking (cooking with steam at high pressure); sauteing (a rapid pan-frying method); baking (a dry heat method); boiling (boiling water method, best for potatoes, beets and cabbage, rather than for green leafy vegetables); braising (slow moist-heat method for fish and poultry); broiling (oven-heated from the top, or grilled from the bottom, to provide a crisp outer layer on the cooked item while maintaining juices); steaming (an ideal way of cooking vegetables because foods are not immersed in water and nutrient loss is minimized); and microwaving (a rapid method that relies on generating microwaves to heat foods with little or no water, thus minimizing nutrient loss).

Cooking develops flavors that can be enhanced by HERBS and SPICES or marinating (treating the food before cooking with ingredients that permeate the food). Cooking also enhances the appearance of food, making it more palatable and appetizing. Glazing of vegetables is an example. Two or three hours of slow moist heat at 180° F is recommended to balance the softening of connective tissue, minimizing the hardening of muscle fibers and destroying bacterial contamination. (See also FOOD POISONING; MICROWAVE COOKING.)

copper An essential TRACE MINERAL. The body of an adult contains 100 to 150 mg copper. Though copper is present in all tissues, including RED BLOOD CELLS, the LIVER is the main site of copper storage. Most of serum copper is bound to ceruloplasmin, the copper transport PROTEIN synthesized by the liver. Ceruloplasmin also aids in IRON transportation and storage. Like most trace minerals, copper functions as an enzyme COFACTOR by activating certain key enzymes required to strengthen the structural protein COLLAGEN, which in turn strengthens cartilage, tendons, BONES, and blood vessels. Copper also serves as a cofactor of a protein in the blood that helps maintain lung tissue and prevent emphysema; and it is essential for insulating (mylination) nerve cells. As a cofactor for the enzyme superoxide dismutase, copper helps prevent oxidative damage by a highly reactive form of oxygen and thus is classified as an ANTIOXIDANT. Copper functions as a cofactor for CYTOCHROME oxidase of MITOCHONDRIA, the enzyme complex that ultimately transfers electrons from the oxidation of fat, carbohydrate and protein to oxygen for energy production. Copper also serves as a cofactor in the synthesis of norepinephrine, an important NEUROTRANSMITTER and adrenal hormone.

The estimated safe and adequate daily intake of copper for normal adults is 2 to 3 mg. About 30% of dietary copper is assimilated. Good sources of copper include liver, kidneys, SHELLFISH, nuts, seeds, FRUIT and dried LEGUMES. Cow's MILK is low in copper. The standard American diet is copper-deficient and between 66 and 75% of the U.S. population do not consume enough copper. Dieters, elderly persons and chronic alcoholics are especially vulnerable. The following factors increase the need for copper: excessive dietary FIBER, high zinc supplements (50 mg or more daily), CADMIUM, excessive VITAMIN C and excessive sugar (fructose) intake (at least in rats).

Low copper consumption increases the risk of high blood CHOLESTEROL and coronary heart disease, lowered immunity, GOUT, diabetes, high blood pressure, ANEMIA, nervous disorders, decreased pigmentation of skin, fragile bones and erratic heartbeat. Low dietary copper is linked with an increased risk of HEART ATTACK. Evidence also links copper deficiency with increased oxidative damage to cell membranes. Levels of norepinephrine in the brain are decreased with copper deficiency but may be restored by supplemental copper. There are certain precautions to keep in mind for copper supplements. Consumption of 10 to 15 mg of copper daily can cause side effects. Patients with a rare copper accumulation disease (Wilson's disease) should not use copper supplements. An excessive copper overload has been linked to various psychiatric syndromes. A green stain in the sink from a faucet drip, or in a tea kettle, suggests excessive copper in drinking water, leached from copper plumbing. (See also FERRITIN; ZINC.)

Prohaska, Joseph R. and Failla, Mark L., "Copper and Immunity," in *Human Nutrition—A Comprehensive Treatise*, vol. 8 of *Nutrition and Immunology*, Klurfeld, David M., ed. New York: Plenum Press, 1993.

corn (*Zea mays*; maize)   A high-carbohydrate CEREAL GRAIN. Corn originated in Central America 5,000 to 6,000 years ago and its cultivation spread throughout the Americas. After its discovery by Europeans, corn spread throughout the world. Americans eat about 25 pounds of corn per person annually. Although it is often considered a vegetable, corn is actually a grass. Field corn refers to non-sweet varieties with a high STARCH content. Dried kernels are used as livestock feed, and are processed to yield CORN-STARCH, high-fructose corn syrup, whiskey, and non-food products ranging from paper to plastics. Popcorn is a type of field corn with thick kernels. When heated, steam is generated within dried kernels, which causes them to pop.

Corn is closely related to millet and cane sugar. Sweet corn is the most popular variety of corn and has a high sugar content. Super-sweet varieties with even higher sugar content have now been bred. The sugar, GLUCOSE, begins to be converted to starch as soon as it is harvested. However, cold storage retards this process. In addition to sweet corn, hundreds of varieties of corn have been developed that may be yellow, white or multicolored. Those with yellow color contain a small amount of beta carotene. Corn is considered a significant source of this important antioxidant because so much of it is consumed. Corn contains ample amounts of protein; however, corn PROTEIN is low in the essential AMINO ACID, LYSINE. This contributes to the low protein quality of this grain. New high-lysine strains have been bred to remedy this deficiency.

PELLAGRA, the NIACIN deficiency disease, occurs among low-income people on inadequate, corn-based diets that provide very little niacin or the essential amino acid TRYPTOPHAN. Inclusion of high quality animal protein, an excellent source of tryptophan, or of niacin supplements, abolishes the disease. Under normal conditions, the body converts some tryptophan to niacin. Niacin is not easily released from corn protein unless premixed with alkaline substances. For example, in Mexico, corn flour is traditionally treated with slaked lime (calcium hydroxide, an alkali) in the preparation of tortillas. This procedure releases protein-bound niacin, and pellagra does not occur. One half-cup, as kernels (cooked, 82 g), provides: calories, 67; protein, 2.5 g; carbohydrate, 16.8 g; fiber, 3.9 g; fat, less than 0.1 mg; vitamin A, 20 retinol equivalents; thiamin, 0.11 mg; riboflavin, 0.04 mg; niacin, 0.96 mg. (See also BIOLOGICAL VALUE; CORNMEAL; CORN OIL; CORN SYRUP.)

corn chips   See CHIPS.

cornmeal   Ground corn kernels. Corn kernels consist of bran or hull, hominy or ENDOSPERM, and GERM, which contains oil. Traditionally, dried whole kernels were ground to prepare cornmeal. This cold-processed cornmeal contains more oil and BETA CAROTENE than in the "new process." In this latter procedure both the hull and germ of the kernel are removed before milling. New-process cornmeal keeps better because it contains less fat. Corn flour represents more finely ground corn. Both yellow corn and blue corn are available as meal and flour; neither contains GLUTEN, the sticky protein occurring in wheat, oats and, to a lesser extent, in rye. Corn does contain protein that may cause food allergies in susceptible people. Cornmeal: whole-ground, 1 cup (122 g), provides 435 calories; protein, 11 g; carbohydrate, 90 g; fiber, 9 g; fat, 5 g; potassium, 346 mg; vitamin A, 62 retinol equivalents; thiamin, 0.46 mg; riboflavin, 2.4 mg; and niacin, 2.4 mg. (See also CEREAL GRAINS.)

corn oil   A polyunsaturated vegetable oil. Corn oil is often used in deep-fat frying and in the preparation of margarine. To prepare corn oil, the germ is first separated from the starchy endosperm by steaming, milling and sifting and is then heated and pressed to yield oil. Corn oil is rich in unsaturated fatty acids, that is, fatty acids whose carbon atoms are deficient in hydrogen atoms. It contains 59% polyunsaturated FATTY ACIDS and 24% monounsaturated fatty acids. Corn oil has a high level of LINOLEIC ACID, an ESSENTIAL FATTY ACID, but lacks ALPHA LINOLENIC ACID, the other essential fatty acid. This issue becomes relevant in powdered infant formulas that are corn oil–based and lack DHA (DOCASAHEXAENOIC ACID), an omega-3 fatty acid derived from alpha linoleic acid and believed to be essential for normal brain and nervous system development. (See also INFANT FORMULA.)

cornstarch   A form of starch purified from corn kernels and used as a food additive. Cornstarch thickens gravies, sauces and puddings. Cornstarch is a more effective thickener for acidic fruits than wheat FLOUR. However, overcooking breaks down this thickening agent. New varieties of corn yield waxy cornstarches that are used to stabilize frozen sauces and fillings. Non-food uses of cornstarch include incorporation in laundry starch.

Starches in general are long chains of glucose, and cornstarch is no exception. Starch breakdown yields glucose syrup, a NATURAL SWEETENER. Glucose syrup in turn is enzymatically converted to high-FRUCTOSE CORN SYRUP, a popular sweetener that is sweeter than table sugar. (See also CARBOHYDRATE; THICKENING AGENTS.)

corn syrup   A sweetener prepared by digesting cornstarch with acid to yield the simple sugar building block, glucose. Corn syrup is an inexpensive sweetener, used extensively in PROCESSED FOODS like PEANUT butter, ketchup, NON-DAIRY CREAMER, imitation fruit drinks and mixes. Corn syrup has replaced maple syrup as the main ingredient in most commercial syrups. Together with its derivative, high-fructose corn syrup, it is rapidly replacing sucrose (table sugar) as the major carbohydrate sweetener in processed foods and beverages. As with other refined sugar sweeteners, corn syrup represents EMPTY CALORIES. It lacks important nutrients found in unrefined foods. The dramatic increase in the consumption of sweeteners in the United States during the 1980s was mainly due to the increased use of corn sweetener additives. (See also CALORIE; FOOD ADDITIVES; NATURAL SWEETENERS.)

coronary artery disease (CAD)   A pathologic condition caused by the narrowing of coronary arteries, the major arteries feeding heart muscle, to the point where they cannot adequately supply the heart with blood. HEART ATTACK is the leading cause of death in the United States accounting for 20% of death in people over 65. A frequent cause is ATHERO-SCLEROSIS, where fatty deposits and cellular build-up containing CHOLESTEROL (PLAQUE) create arterial thickening and partial blockage of blood flow. Such constrictions can close off the artery completely or they can trigger the formation of blood clots that can lodge in such constrictions. Blockage of coronary arteries in either case causes heart attacks in which a lack of oxygen damages heart muscle.

Coronary Heart Disease (CHD)

This disease is the result of damage to the heart muscle (myocardium) due to an inadequate blood supply. A heart attack refers to the sudden blockage of an artery supplying blood to the heart. Diseased arteries can be blocked by blood clots (thrombosis) or by accumulated cholesterol (plaque build-up) or by a combination of both processes.

Risk Factors for CAD and CHD

As with any chronic disease, the incidence of CHD is the product of dietary, environmental and inherited risk factors. Risk factors simply increase the odds of developing CAD; they do not guarantee a person will have a heart attack. Likewise, the absence of known risk factors is no guarantee a person will not have a heart attack. The cumulative effect of risk factors is greater than if individual risks were simply added together. Thus a person with three risk factors has a sixfold increase in his or her risk of heart attack.

Major risk factors for CAD have been identified. They include life-style factors such as smoking; lack of physical exercise; chronic emotional stress, and certain personality traits that relate to coping with stress; overeating, weight gain and high fat diet.

Medical history can dramatically increase the risk of heart disease: high blood pressure (HYPERTENSION), DIABETES MELLITUS, GOUT, OBESITY, high LDL-cholesterol (the less desirable form of blood cholesterol) and low HDL-cholesterol (the more desirable form of cholesterol). Premature menopause without hormone replacement therapy is another risk factor related to medical history. Elevated levels of HOMOCYSTEINE, a breakdown product of the amino acid METHIONINE, has been shown to be an independent risk factor for heart attacks and strokes.

Other risk factors relate to inheritance and cannot be altered:

- Gender. Males are more likely than females to develop heart attacks before the age of 55. After 75 or 80, the rate of developing CAD is the same for both men and women.
- Racial background. Certain groups face greater odds for heart attacks, including African Americans, who are more at risk for developing hypertension, and Pima Indians, who are more likely to develop diabetes.
- Aging. The occurrence of CAD increases dramatically after the age of 65.
- Family history of premature or coronary heart disease. A heart attack or sudden death in father, brother or son before the age of 55 or a heart attack or sudden death in a mother, sister or daughter before the age of 65.

Effect of Diet on CAD and CHD

A high fat DIET, especially one with large amounts of animal or saturated fat, is linked to diseases of arteries and heart. Certain saturated FATTY ACIDS seem to promote plaque buildup, including lauric acid (with 12 carbons), myristic acid (with 14 carbons) and PALMITIC ACID (with 16 carbons). Palmitic acid is the most common saturated fatty acid in animal fat and it is the most atherogenic (promoting plaque accumulation). In addition, the lauric, myristic and palmitic acids seem to promote blood clot formation. Diets high in the longer fatty acid, STEARIC ACID (with 18 carbons, a common saturated fatty acid in animal fat), do not raise serum cholesterol. Nonetheless, foods are mixtures of nutrients, and fats consist of both stearic acid and palmitic acid. A second point to consider: fats and oils contribute more than twice as many calories as carbohydrate and protein, therefore, the total number of fat calories consumed per day is a determining factor for risk of obesity, coronary heart disease and cancer. Meat consumption alone, especially red meat consumption, shows no apparent correlation with CHD among individuals in 26 European countries.

Other dietary factors that may protect against CAD and CHD include unsaturated oils. Most vegetable oils contain polyunsaturated fatty acids related to LINOLEIC ACID, an ESSENTIAL FATTY ACID, and classified as omega-6 fatty acids. These oils are called "polyunsaturates" because their fatty acid structures possess several double bonds and are deficient in hydrogen atoms. (Saturated fats are filled up with the maximum number of hydrogen atoms.) In a reduced fat diet, in which less than 30% of calories come from fat, polyunsaturates reduce serum cholesterol levels when the polyunsaturates account for more than 10% of calories. However, they also lower HDL cholesterol, the beneficial form of cholesterol, an undesirable effect. Polyunsaturates reduce platelet aggregation, i.e., blood clotting, thus reducing the risk of dangerous blood clots. Monounsaturates contain monounsaturated fatty acids with a single double bond and are much less susceptible to oxidation (lipid peroxidation) than are polyunsaturates. Olive oil and related monounsaturated oils may lower LDL without lowering HDL when total fat consumption is high. TRANS FATTY ACIDS in hydrogenated vegetable oils such as stick margarine and vegetable shortening may increase the risk of cardiovascular disease, even though consumption of trans fatty acids is estimated to be approximately 15 g/day.

Cold water ocean fish in the diet are important because they provide omega-3 polyunsaturated fatty acids, DHA (DOCOSAHEXAENOIC ACID) and eicosahexaenoic acid, which are related to a lowered risk of heart disease. These omega-3 fatty acids seem to lower blood fat and LDL-cholesterol levels when blood cholesterol is high, while increasing HDL levels. They also lower mildly elevated blood pressure and reduce the risk of blood clot formation.

People with high blood levels of HOMOCYSTEINE, an amino acid byproduct, often do not consume enough B vitamins, especially FOLIC ACID, VITAMIN B_{12}, and VITAMIN B_6. Eating enough foods rich in folic acid—including beans, green, leafy vegetables and liver, to obtain 400 mcg of folic acid daily—may reduce the risk of heart disease and, incidently, this may lower the risk of BIRTH DEFECTS.

Fiber consumption is another factor. Reports of the effects of dietary fiber on CAD and CHD are conflicting. Oats and oat bran can lower serum cholesterol in men with raised cholesterol levels. In middle-age American men, the risk of fatal and non-fatal heart attack were found to be 41% less common among those who consumed at least 28 g of fiber per day, as compared to those eating the level typically found in the standard diet (12 to 13 g per day). These effects may pertain to women as well. The benefits of fiber lie beyond increasing satiety and reducing fat intake. Diets rich in fiber from fruits and vegetables provide antioxidants and other important nutrients. Wheat bran cereals, which supply mainly insoluble fiber, reduces the risk of heart disease. Other sources of mixed fiber include legumes like kidney beans, peas, apples, grapefruit, broccoli and leafy vegetables.

ANTIOXIDANTS protect against heart disease by squelching *free radicals*, which are highly reactive forms of oxygen and other chemicals that lack a single electron. Free radicals attack cells indiscriminately and can damage genetic material, DNA, and even proteins. Dietary antioxidants include: vitamin C, vitamin E, BETA CAROTENE and related orange-red plant pigments (CAROTENOIDS), trace minerals like COPPER, SELENIUM and MANGANESE, and FLAVONOIDS (complex plant substances), together with certain compounds made by the body like GLUTATHIONE, bilirubin and uric acid. Vitamin E and selenium may also be important in regulating platelet aggregation and clot formation as well as serving as important antioxidants. Current attention focuses on the possibility that free radicals oxidize LDL cholesterol (LOW DENSITY LIPOPROTEIN), which in turn induces plaque deposits and clogged arteries. Thus inadequate antioxidants can promote the development of CHD by increasing LDL oxidation. Several recent studies indicate the protective role of vitamin E. Patients enrolled in the Cambridge Heart Antioxidant Study who had severe heart disease and who received either 400 or 800 IU of vitamin E daily for 17 months experienced significantly lower risk of developing heart attacks than controls who received a PLACEBO (blank pill). Vitamin E appears to slow down the accumulation of plaque in arteries with vitamin E supplementation. With increased consumption of essential fatty acids, more vitamin E is needed to protect them from oxidation.

The "French Paradox" refers to the observation that some European populations such as the French who consume plenty of animal fat (saturated fat) and large amounts of red wine have a lower prevalence of cardiovascular disease than seen for the U.S. Moderate alcohol consumption (one or two drinks per day) can raise the levels of HDL-cholesterol, the most beneficial form, regardless of the source of alcohol, thus the paradox may be more apparent than real. Drinking to reduce cardiovascular risk is not recommended, because the risks of addiction and alcohol abuse are so great.

Recommendations to Modify Controllable Risk Factors for CAD

A comprehensive program that entails very low fat diets, providing ample fruits, vegetables, grains and restricted amounts of animal protein and used in conjunction with exercise, stress reduction and group support have caused a decrease in plaque accumulation (atherosclerotic lesions) in some coronary patients.

An optimal life-style can retard the progression of CHD and possibly prevent heart disease.

- Stop smoking. This is perhaps the single most important preventive action a person can take.
- Prevent hypertension, or control existing hypertension. With each drop in one point in the diastolic blood pressure reading (the larger of the two blood pressure measurements), the risk of CAD declines by 2 or 3%.
- Make a lifelong commitment to stay physically fit. Sedentary people can decrease their risk of CAD by an estimated 35 to 55%. Even walking or other low intensity exercise, when done regularly for years, can lower lifetime risk.
- Maintain a healthy body weight. Being overweight doubles or triples the risk of CAD for adults at any age. Fat accumulation around the waist is more risky than fat around the thighs.
- Prevent diabetes, or control existing diabetes. Non-insulin dependent diabetes increases the odds of CAD in men by a factor of 2 or 3, and in women, by 3 to 7.
- Eat plenty of fruits and vegetables, while getting plenty of antioxidants, including vitamin E, vitamin C and beta carotene and carotenoids, from ample servings of vegetables and fruits. Population studies in Europe suggest that a high intake of antioxidants from foods reduces the risk of CAD. Consuming enough B vitamins, especially folic acid, vitamin B_{12} and vitamin B_6 is also prudent.
- Manage stress effectively. Suppressed anger, hostility and a sense of lack of control at work can increase the risk of heart attack. Emotional support is an important factor.

For Those with High Blood Cholesterol

Perhaps as many as one third of Americans are extremely sensitive to dietary cholesterol; their blood levels rise significantly when they eat cholesterol-rich foods. These individuals should limit their dietary cholesterol to no more than 300 mg per day. Particularly those with a family history of early heart disease or high cholesterol levels need to be watchful. The following step program outlines an approach to modifying the diet.

Step 1: Dietary fat should account for less than 30% of total daily calories. Less than 10% of total calories should come from saturated fat and daily consumption of cholesterol should not exceed 300 mg per day. If a patient is already on a Step 1 diet, and the response is inadequate, the patient may be advised to incorporate Step 2 recommendations.

Step 2: While dietary fat should account for less than 30% of calories, less than 7% of total calories should come from saturated fat, and cholesterol consumption should be less than 200 mg per day. (See also AGING, CARDIOVASCULAR DISEASE, DEGENERATIVE DISEASES, DIETARY GUIDELINES FOR AMERICANS.)

Gaziano, J. Michael, "Antioxidant Vitamins and Coronary Artery Disease Risk," *American Journal of Medicine*, supp. 3A: (1994), pp. 18S–21S.

Schaefer, E.J. et al., "Lipoproteins, Nutrition, Aging and Atherosclerosis," *American Journal of Clinical Nutrition*, 61:supplement (1995), pp. 726–40S.

Ulbricht, T.L.V., Southgate, D.A.T., "Coronary heart disease: seven dietary factors," *Lancet* 338 (October 19, 1991), pp. 985–92.

cortisol (cortisone, hydrocortisone)   A steroid hormone produced by the inner portion of the ADRENAL GLANDS (adrenal cortex) in response to stress. Unlike EPINEPHRINE, which is released by the outer region of the adrenal gland (adrenal medulla) as a rapid response to stress, cortisol alters METABOLISM over a period of hours and days, rather than minutes. Cortisol stimulates the body's catabolic processes, such as increasing protein degradation and fat breakdown. It stimulates the LIVER to build GLUCOSE from AMINO ACIDS (GLUCONEOGENESIS), which appears as BLOOD SUGAR. Cortisol also reduces inflammation. Cortisol levels in the blood normally follow a circadian rhythm, reaching a maximum concentration in the morning before breakfast and reaching a nadir in the evening.

Chronic stress, which may cause excessive cortisol production, can suppress the immune system. This in turn may increase the risk of chronic infections and promote FOOD SENSITIVITIES. Higher than normal cortisol production could also increase blood cholesterol and cause blood sugar fluctuations. With prolonged stress the precursor steroid, pregnanolone, can be diverted to cortisol synthesis, rather than to sex hormones and DHEA. Subsequently DHEA levels in blood can drop, leading to increased insensitivity to insulin and decreased ability to maintain normal blood sugar levels.

In late stages of stress adaptation to chronic, severe stress, the fatigued adrenal glands no longer respond adequately to stimuli or follow the normal circadian rhythm. With lowered cortisol output the body becomes even more prone to inflammation, excessive fatigue and HYPOGLYCEMIA.

Aerobic exercise and stress reduction strategies such as meditation are keys to normalizing adrenal function. Nutritional support for adrenal glands includes vitamin C, pantothenic acid, niacinamide, coenzyme Q, as well as the minerals magnesium, manganese, zinc and potassium. For low cortisol output, thiamin, CARNITINE and OCTOCOSANOL in addition to the above may be beneficial. In general, essential fatty acids from flaxseed, borage or black currant seed oils may help reduce inflammation and antioxidants such as FLAVONOIDS may be effective. Sulfur amino acids, methionine and taurine may help the liver detoxify accumulated waste products. It is also important to avoid sugar, caffeine and nonsteroidal antiinflammatory drugs. The diet should favor whole grains and fresh vegetables. (See also CATABOLISM.)

cottage cheese   A high-PROTEIN, low-fat CHEESE prepared from curdled milk (curds). The curdling process leaches CALCIUM from the curds into the liquid, called whey, which is removed. Consequently cottage cheese retains only 25 to 50% of milk calcium. Cottage cheese is prepared with varying amounts of FAT. It is highest in creamed small curd cheese (4.2% fat), while low-fat cottage cheese contains 1 or 2% fat, and dry curd cottage cheese has 0.5% fat. Cottage cheese is usually salted, but unsalted versions are available. One cup (210 g) of small curd, 1% cottage cheese, provides: calories, 164; protein, 28 g; carbohydrate, 5.6 g; fat, 2.3 g; calcium, 138 mg; sodium, 850 mg; vitamin A, 101 retinol equivalents; cholesterol, 31 mg; thiamin, 0.04 mg; riboflavin, 0.34

mg; niacin, 0.27 mg. For comparison, one cup of creamed cottage cheese (210 g) provides: calories, 215; protein, 26.2 g; carbohydrate, 5.6 g; fat, 8.93 g; calcium, 126 mg; cholesterol, 31 mg; sodium, 1,850 mg; vitamin A, 101 retinol equivalents; thiamin, 0.04 mg; riboflavin, 0.34 mg; niacin, 0.23 mg.

cottonseed oil   A polyunsaturated oil derived from cotton. Cotton is not classified as a food, therefore pesticide use in its cultivation is not as restricted as for vegetables, and cottonseed oil may be contaminated. This oil contains 52% polyunsaturated FATTY ACIDS, 18% monounsaturated fatty acids and 26% saturated fatty acids. The ratio of unsaturated to saturated fatty acids is 2.7:1. The higher degree of saturation makes cottonseed oil less prone to oxidation and rancidity than soybean, corn or safflower oils. It is thus a useful additive in salad dressings and in processed foods such as CHIPS, where shelf life stability is important. Like all oils and fat, cottonseed oil provides 9 calories/gram. (See also CHLORDIMEFORM; FOOD ADDITIVES; PROCESSED FOOD.)

cow's milk   See MILK.

crab   A broad-backed crustacean related to lobster and shrimp, with five pairs of legs. One pair is enlarged for foraging. The head and thorax are fused and are covered by a hard armor-like plate called a carapace. True crabs can be divided into two categories: swimming crabs (the blue crab) and walking crabs (rock crab). They represent 4,500 species although only a few types are common. Edible crabs that are important seafoods commercially are found in Europe (*Cancer pagurus*); along eastern coasts of the United States, (*Callinectes sapidus*, blue crab or soft-shell crab; and the Florida stone crab); and along the Pacific Coast of the United States (*Cancer magister*, Dungeness crab). The largest crab is the Alaskan king crab.

Crab meat is delicate and is available fresh, cooked, canned or frozen. It is used for crab salad, stuffed crab, aspics and souffles. Because this seafood is so expensive, imitation crab is sometimes substituted. This fish-based product (SURIMI) has been processed to have the same consistency as crab meat and flavored by small amounts of crab products. Alaskan king crab (100 g, edible portion) provides 84 calories; protein, 18.3 g; fat, 0.6 g; iron, 0.59 mg; calcium, 46 g; potassium 204 mg; sodium, 836 mg; thiamin, 0.043 mg; riboflavin, 0.043 mg; niacin, 1.10 mg.

cracked wheat   See WHEAT.

cracker   A thin, flat biscuit usually made of wheat flour. Chips and crackers are popular processed snack foods. Unless the food label specifically states "whole wheat" as the first and only wheat ingredient, the cracker contains between 50 and 90% bleached flour. Words like "stone ground" do not guarantee whole wheat. Crackers often contain substantial FAT or vegetable oil such as the highly saturated tropical oils (coconut or palm kernel oils). The fat content in crackers can vary by a factor of 10. For example: wheat wafers contain 1.1 to 2 g of fat per ounce; cheese-flavored, fat-rich crackers, 8.0 g; and corn chips and potato chips, up to 10.0 g. The typical fat content of cheese-flavored crackers is 40 to 55%. If the cracker leaves a grease spot on a paper napkin, it has a high fat content. A sense of fat content can be obtained from the list of ingredients on the food label. The lowest in calories are crisp breads and matzo-type crackers.

Rye crisp or rye flat bread may provide 2 to 4 g of fiber per half-ounce serving, equivalent to one or two peaches, with 40 to 70 calories. By comparison, a whole wheat cracker can provide only half a gram of fiber for the same serving size. Note that "unsalted" crackers still contain some sodium. "Low sodium" or "low salt" means that the food cannot contain more than 140 mg of sodium per serving, while "sodium free" can appear on food labels that contain less than 5 mg of sodium per serving.

cranberry (*Vaccinium*) A tart, bright red berry produced by a shrub that is a member of the heath family. Both American and European varieties are cultivated in the United States. Cranberries are used in relish, canned sauce, pies and preserves. Because cranberries are so sour, sugar is usually added to these products. One cup (95 g) of fresh cranberries provides 46 calories; protein, 0.37 g; carbohydrate, 12 g; fiber, 1.14 g; potassium, 67 mg; thiamin, 0.029 mg; riboflavin, 0.019 mg; niacin, 0.095 mg; and vitamin C, 44 mg.

Cranberry Juice

Cranberry juice has been recommended for BLADDER INFECTIONS because it contains a carbohydrate that inhibits the growth of disease-producing bacteria. This material prevents the bacteria from binding to the lining of the urinary tract, a preliminary step in infection. Because it limits bacterial growth, cranberry juice is considered "bacteriostatic" rather than "bactericidal," which refers to agents that kill bacteria. Used by itself, cranberry juice doesn't prevent or cure urinary tract infections. Often the infection flares up when the juice is no longer used. Cranberry juice is a DIURETIC and promotes urine production. Cranberry juice is so sour that juice producers add large amounts of sweeteners, and consequently it is high in CALORIES (145 calories per 8-oz serving). VITAMIN C is added; one serving provides 90 mg. One cup of cranberry juice cocktail provides 145 calories; carbohydrate, 36.6 g; fiber, 0.76 g; fat, 0.1 g; potassium, 45 mg; thiamin, 0.02 mg; riboflavin, 0.02 mg; niacin, 0.09 mg; and vitamin C, 90 mg.

Avorn, Jerry et al., "Reduction of Bacteriuria and Pyuria after Ingestion of Cranberry Juice," *Journal of the American Medical Association*, 271:10 (March 9, 1994), pp. 751–54.

crash dieting See DIETING.

craving A strong desire for a food. A food craving is a stronger need for food than HUNGER and is specific for a particular food. Though craving food may suggest a dependency, usually the desire to eat a specific food declines once it has been eaten. Women generally experience more food craving than men; however, by middle age this difference disappears. There probably is no single mechanism underlying food craving. Social factors are involved since taste and appearance of food are learned and profoundly influence food choices. It is also possible that craving sweets represents a desire for gratification. Food craving by women may be hormonally driven. Studies have shown that cravings for sweets and fatty foods are associated with PREMENSTRUAL SYNDROME, DEPRESSION and seasonal mood changes.

A biochemical imbalance may promote food craving. This model focuses on the NEUROTRANSMITTER, SEROTONIN, a chemical that helps in the transmission of nerve impulses. Brain serotonin is lowest before menstruation. Brain centers requiring serotonin regulate APPETITE, as well as thirst, mood and sleep. Certain individuals may produce abnormally low serotonin due to their unique genetic makeup or due to dietary imbalance. Thus craving sweets could be a form of self-medication. According to one hypothesis, carbohydrate consumption stimulates the brain to increase synthesis of the serotonin from its raw material, the amino acid TRYPTOPHAN, and that low serotonin levels can trigger the urge to eat sweets. However, brain serotonin levels may not influence carbohydrate food choices on an ongoing basis.

Alternative explanations have been offered for food craving. Thus craving may be based upon brain peptides, ENDORPHINS, that decrease pain perception. Endorphin production increases during ovulation and drops during menstruation. Endorphin formation and release are stimulated when fat and carbohydrate are eaten together. The craving for chocolate associated with premenstrual syndrome may be explained by chocolate's high content of phenylethylamine, a compound that can promote relaxation and affect mood. Food craving is a possible sign of a FOOD SENSITIVITY, in which the body may gradually tolerate an allergy-producing food to the extent that omitting that food from the diet could create a craving (withdrawal) similar to a physical dependency. A disturbance in the body's HOMEOSTASIS could create biochemical imbalances in the brain and in the endocrine system. Thus changes in hormone levels, nutritional deficiencies, disease states and addictions can be predisposing factors to these imbalances. For example, it is known that low blood-sugar levels can trigger cravings for carbohydrates and sweets. There could also be a link with the consumption of junk food: CONVENIENCE FOOD is high in sugar and fat, which slows down digestion, slowing signals to the brain to shut off hunger signals, which could in turn induce people to eat more junk food than they would normally. Food craving increases the risk of cigarette smoking and alcohol and drug abuse. (See also ADDICTION; BULIMIA NERVOSA.)

creamer See NON-DAIRY CREAMER.

cream of tartar (potassium tartrate) A widely used food additive that serves many roles. As an ingredient in BAKING POWDER, tartrate provides an acidic environment that converts the BICARBONATE in baking powder to CARBON DIOXIDE, which creates bubbles in dough of leavened baked goods. Cream of tartar serves as an anticaking agent to keep powdered materials from clumping. Sodium tartrate and sodium potassium tartrate are added to stabilize emulsified foods and to control pH in such foods as cheese, jam and jelly. Cream of tartar also provides tartness to beverages, CANDY, ice cream, baked goods and gelatin desserts. Tartaric acid is a natural ingredient of fruits such as GRAPES and is a by-product of wine production. (See also BUFFER; FOOD ADDITIVES.)

cress   A green leafy vegetable of the mustard family. The most popular is watercress (*Nasturtium officinale*), a hardy perennial native to Europe and now widespread in the fresh running water of many regions. Watercress's pungent leaves are used as seasoning, garnish and as a salad green. Garden cress or pepper cress (*Lepidium sativum*), native to western Asia, is cultivated and is used as a garnish like parsley. As a member of the cruciferous vegetables, cress supplies nutrients and plant substances with anticancer properties. Cress (100 g, raw) provides: calories, 32; protein, 2.6 g; carbohydrate, 5.5 g; fiber, 1.10 g; fat, 0.70 g; calcium, 81 mg; potassium, 606 mg; thiamin, 0.08 mg; riboflavin, 0.26 mg; niacin, 1.0 mg; vitamin C, 69 mg.

Crohn's disease (ileitis)   A chronic inflammatory condition in which the intestinal tract is ulcerated. It is characterized by deep sores in the lower part of the SMALL INTESTINE, the COLON and other regions of the digestive tract. The inflammatory condition often involves all layers of the bowel wall, and granular growths often occur. Crohn's disease is one of two forms of INFLAMMATORY BOWEL DISEASE, which collectively affect 1 to 2 million Americans. Crohn's disease is most prevalent in developed, Western societies. This disease most often affects people between the ages of 12 and 40, and the incidence is highest among teenagers.

Symptoms include low-grade fever, cramps, gradual weight loss, anorexia, flatulence, weakness, MALNUTRITION, persistent bouts of DIARRHEA, possibly ARTHRITIS, skin inflammation, abdominal tenderness, vaginal and urinary inflammation and rectal bleeding. Crohn's disease causes malabsorption, and nutrient deficiencies can delay development in children. Diarrhea accompanying Crohn's disease upsets ELECTROLYTE balance and also limits nutrient availability, while abdominal pain may limit food intake.

Whether infectious agents are involved is still debated. Viruses like Epstein-Barr rotavirus and cytomegalovirus are mentioned as candidates. Among bacteria, chlamydia is another candidate. Family history is a risk factor. Possibly this is an AUTOIMMUNE DISEASE, in which antibodies attack the mucosal lining of the lower intestinal tract. Processes regulating immune activation of the intestine seem to be imbalanced in Crohn's disease, creating an exaggerated inflammatory response. Crohn's disease may also be associated with increased intestinal permeability, thus increasing the penetration of foreign materials into the body leading to increased inflammation and tissue injury.

To uncover possible causes of Crohn's disease, patients' diets have been analyzed. Crohn's disease patients typically consume more refined SUGAR and eat less raw fruit, vegetables and FIBER than healthy individuals. Deficiencies of minerals (CALCIUM, MAGNESIUM, IRON, ZINC, SELENIUM), of water soluble vitamins (VITAMIN B$_{12}$, VITAMIN C, FOLIC ACID) and of fat-soluble vitamins (vitamin A, vitamin D, vitamin K) may cause some of the symptoms of this disease. It is important to rule out FOOD SENSITIVITIES; which may be a contributing factor. Food allergies contribute to increased gut permeability. A variety of nutrients support healing of the small intestine. They include the amino acid GLUTAMINE, zinc and folic acid. Improving DIGESTION can help absorption, decrease the burden of food antigens and help decrease intestinal inflammation. Other dietary modifications include avoiding seeds, nuts, greasy food, CAFFEINE and sugar. If lactose intolerance has developed, the patient may be advised to avoid milk and milk products. Eliminating allergenic foods has been an effective approach in treating inflammatory bowel disease.

Crohn's disease is a serious condition and treatment requires a broad-based approach. Emotional support is needed by patients with Crohn's disease, especially if the person is young. Hydrolyzed protein formulas and ELEMENTAL DIETS, which combine simple nutrients rather than protein or starches, are more easily absorbed and have been used during acute phases of the disease. Oral intake of food may be withheld temporarily while IV feeding is used in order to normalize the bowel. As the client progresses, an oral diet that is nutrient-rich and well-balanced may gradually be tolerated.

There is presently no drug available to cure Crohn's disease. Medical treatments have included surgery and steroid treatment. Surgery does not necessarily impede the progress of the disease, and it can contribute to weight loss and malabsorption. Steroids reduce inflammation, but their side effects include increased risk of bone loss, high blood pressure, BLOOD SUGAR fluctuations and suppressed immunity—all limiting their effectiveness. (See also CATABOLIC STATE; COLITIS; GASTROINTESTINAL DISORDERS; LEAKY GUT SYNDROME.)

Wantke, F., Gotz, M., Jarisch, R., "Dietary Treatment of Crohn's Disease," *Lancet*, 343 (Jan. 8, 1994), p. 113.
Wu, Scott et al., "Intense Nutritional Support in Inflammatory Bowel Disease," Digestive Diseases and Sciences, 40:4 (April 1995), pp. 843–52..

cruciferous vegetables   A large family of vegetables that help protect against some forms of CANCER. Members include BOK CHOY, BROCCOLI, BRUSSELS SPROUTS, CABBAGE, CAULIFLOWER, Chinese cabbage, COLLARD, greens, horseradish, KALE, KOHLRABI, mustard greens, RADISH, RUTABAGA, turnip greens and watercress.

Population studies show that consumption of cruciferous vegetables lowers cancer risk. Cruciferous vegetables are very good sources of VITAMIN C, FOLIC ACID and BETA CAROTENE, in addition to FIBER—all of which inhibit certain cancers. Furthermore, vegetables of this group also contain protective substances called dithiothiones, indoles and isothiocyanates. These seem to help activate the liver to destroy cancer-causing agents. Cruciferous vegetables contain ANTIOXIDANTS that can inhibit oxidative damage to DNA. It is probable other substances with anticancer activity remain to be characterized as members of this versatile group of vegetables.

To avoid the possible off-taste and odor of cruciferous vegetables when cooked, they should be cooked for as short a time as possible. Note that acids in lemon juice and VINEGAR turn the rich green color of cabbage-family vegetables to an unappetizing olive drab. (See also CANCER PREVENTION DIET.)

crude fiber   See FIBER.

cucumber (*Cucumis sativus*)   A long, cylindrical, crisp green vegetable produced by a vine related to squash. Cucumbers have a shiny skin with a watery, crisp flesh. The cucumber once grew wild in the foothills of the Himalayas and was domesticated at least 3,000 years ago in India. Used in ancient times by Egyptians, Hebrews, Greeks and Romans, it has had a long history in the West. Presently there are several varieties differing in texture, size and shape. The larger, "slicing" varieties are eaten fresh, while smaller, lighter varieties are pickled. The very large cucumbers that grow on string vines are adapted to growing on frames or trellises. In mild climates cucumbers are grown as a field crop. The European cucumber tends to be smooth-skinned, long (1 to 2 ft.) and seedless. In Europe and Canada cucumbers are grown in greenhouses. If the skin has a sheen, it has probably been waxed. All waxed cucumbers should be peeled. Though it has a low nutrient content, cucumber's characteristic flavor makes a useful addition to salads. Freshly picked cucumbers are best. The skin can be bitter and is often peeled before eating in salads. Sometimes raw cucumbers are salted and drained to remove bitterness. Cucumbers are cool and crisp because their water content is high (96%). Cooked cucumbers can be sauteed, cooked au gratin or they can be stuffed. Gazpacho (cold tomato soup) incorporates grated cucumber. Cucumber is one of the vegetables that can cause flatulence.

Several varieties of cucumbers like the Kirby (dill pickles) and gherkins are pickled in salt. Pickling incorporates pickling salt, white vinegar and pickling spices. Grape and cherry leaves help maintain the firmness of pickled cucumber. A cup of fresh sliced cucumber (104 g) provides 14 calories; protein, 0.56 g; carbohydrate, 3.0 g; fiber, 0.62 g; vitamin A, 46 retinol equivalents; thiamin, 0.032 mg; riboflavin, 0.02 mg; niacin, 0.32 mg.

cumin (*Cuminum cyminum*)   A seasoning that is the principal ingredient of curry powder, a blend of powdered Indian spices. Cumin is a member of the parsley family and cumin seeds resemble caraway seeds. The aromatic seed has a characteristic strong, slightly bitter taste. Traditionally cumin has been used to flavor cheese, sauerkraut, unleavened bread, marinades, chili and tomato sauce.

cyanocobalamin   See VITAMIN B₁₂.

cyanogen (cyanogenic glycosides)   A family of sugar derivatives found in many plants that can break down to cyanide in the intestines. Cyanogens occur in varying amounts in lima beans, sweet potatoes, YAMS, peas and fruit (seeds of apricots, cherries, plums). Usually, the levels are so low as to pose no hazard, and these foods contribute significantly in creating a balanced diet low in fat and high in complex carbohydrate. Furthermore the content varies with the strain, and most cultivated strains contain little cyanogen; for example, American strains of lima beans contain little cyanide. CASSAVA, which does contain cyanide, is traditionally prepared in a manner that destroys cyanogens. Small, non-fatal doses of cyanide lead to headaches, a sensation of tightness in the throat, palpitations and weakness. (See also COOKING; FOOD TOXINS.)

cyclamate (sodium, calcium cyclamate)   An ARTIFICIAL SWEETENER used until 1970 as a food and beverage additive. Cyclamate is 30 times sweeter than table sugar (SUCROSE) but does not contribute calories. Cyclamate also lacks the aftertaste commonly experienced with SACCHARIN.

Cyclamate was banned because evidence linked it to bladder CANCER in rats and mice. Its safety was reexamined in 1985 and the National Academy of Sciences/National Research Council concluded that cyclamate by itself does not cause cancer, but it could still be a tumor promoter, that is, it could enhance the effect of cancer-causing agents. The evidence that it causes genetic damage and testicular atrophy continues to be examined. (See also DELANEY CLAUSE; FOOD ADDITIVES.)

cysteine (cys, L-cysteine)   A sulfur-containing AMINO ACID that serves both as a building block of proteins and as an ANTIOXIDANT to prevent oxidative damage within cells. Most individuals manufacture ample amounts of cysteine from METHIONINE, an essential sulfur-containing amino acid; thus cysteine is not generally essential when the diet provides ample, high-quality protein. However, cysteine may become a conditionally essential amino acid for the newborn infant when its synthesis by the immature liver is limited. Cysteine is the only amino acid with a free sulfur group, and in proteins sulfur groups from neighboring cysteines link up to stabilize the protein structure to enhance biological activity; for example, cysteine links stabilize the hormone INSULIN, the digestive enzyme CHYMOTRYPSIN and the protective protein keratin, found in hair, nails and skin.

Cysteine is a raw material for the important cellular antioxidant, GLUTATHIONE, made in large amounts by most cells. Glutathione represents a key in the defense against FREE RADICALS, highly reactive molecules that are suspected culprits in the initiation of CANCER. Both cysteine and glutathionine lessen tissue damage due to radiation therapy, perhaps through their antioxidant activity. Glutathione also helps boost immunity.

Cysteine seems to reduce chemical toxicity: In experimental animals cysteine reduces toxicity to certain anti-cancer drugs, ACETAMINOPHEN (a common analgesic drug), certain PESTICIDES, industrial compounds (acrylonitrile) and even ALCOHOL (ethanol). A derivative, N-acetyl cysteine, can decrease abnormal thick mucus (mucolytic activity) and has been used to raise glutathione levels in the liver. It may be a therapeutic agent for cardiovascular disorders and AIDS. There is evidence that cysteine stimulates B cells, a part of the IMMUNE SYSTEM that is responsible for antibody production. Cysteine should be used only with medical supervision. Excessive cysteine may interfere with insulin, a critical hormone for regulating blood sugar in diabetics. More generally, very little is known about safe doses and long-term effects of cysteine supplements. There is a possibility of causing kidney stones when cysteine is oxidized; VITAMIN C may counteract this effect. (See also HOMOCYSTEINE.)

cystine   The oxidation product that forms spontaneously from the sulfur-containing AMINO ACID, CYSTEINE. Cystine itself is not a protein building block and is not considered one of the 20 basic alpha amino acids. Cystine is quite insoluble and can precipitate (crystallize) in the urine, forming stones in the kidneys and the bladder.

cystitis   An inflammation of the bladder and one of the most common ailments of the urinary tract. (See also URINARY TRACT.)

cytochrome P450   A family of iron-containing enzymes, primarily responsible for the ability of the LIVER to modify potentially dangerous chemicals and to neutralize normal products of metabolism. Unlike cytochromes found in MITOCHONDRIA, cytochrome P450 occurs as part of the membranous system (ENDOPLASMIC RETICULUM) of liver cells, as well as intestinal and kidney cells, which help detoxify chemicals.

Repeated exposure to pollutants and drugs stimulates the liver to form high levels of cytochrome P450. While the increased activity allows the liver to dispose of a greater toxin load, it also increases the likelihood that the liver will produce highly reactive by-products and FREE RADICALS that are potential MUTAGENS and CARCINOGENS. Thus pollutants can increase the oxidative damage associated with AGING, CANCER and DEGENERATIVE DISEASES such as ATHEROSCLEROSIS.

The levels of cytochrome P450 enzymes in the liver vary greatly among individuals. Low levels or high levels of certain cytochrome P450s can reflect the inherited ability of the body to synthesize certain of these enzymes. A person with high levels of these detoxifying enzymes may process toxins quickly, creating free radicals and potentially damaging compounds in the process and creating a drain on antioxidant defenses. Alternatively, those who produce very low levels may be very sensitive to environmental toxins due to their limited ability to clear them from the body. "Rapid detoxifiers" may need a higher dosage of drug or anesthetic; slow detoxifiers may need less. Diagnostic tests are being developed to distinguish these situations. Riboflavin, niacin, vitamin B_6, phospholipids like lecithin, as well as FLAVONIDS support the function of the cyctochrome P450 detoxication. (See also ANTIOXIDANT; CHOLESTEROL; FOOD TOXINS.)

cytochromes   A family of iron-containing PROTEINS that function in important oxidation reactions of cellular chemistry (METABOLISM). Cytochromes possess a helper compound, HEME, a red oxidation-reduction pigment containing IRON. Cytochromes play a key role in cellular RESPIRATION, in which FAT and CARBOHYDRATE are burned (oxidized). Cytochromes belong to a group of electron carriers, the ELECTRON TRANSPORT CHAIN, that function in mitochondria, the energy-producing particles of cells. Electrons pass sequentially from one cytochrome to another, like a bucket brigade, and simultaneously energy released from burning metabolic fuels is harnessed as ATP, the energy currency of cells. Other cytochromes are key constituents of the liver's battery of drug-destroying enzymes. These enzymes attack drugs, pesticides, pollutants and other foreign chemicals to inactivate them and to make them water-soluble so they can be excreted. (See also CYTOCHROME P450; DETOXIFICATION.)

cytolithiasis   The formation of stones (calculi) in the urinary bladder and kidneys. The occurrence of kidney stones is steadily increasing worldwide, paralleling the occurrence of CARDIOVASCULAR DISEASE, diabetes and HYPERTENSION. Over 5% of males and 10% of females experience a kidney stone during their lifetime. Kidney stones account for one out of every 1,000 hospital admissions in the United States. There are usually no apparent symptoms of cytolithiasis until a stone blocks the urinary tract, when the pain can become excruciating as the stone passes down the urinary tract. In the first half of the 20th century, stone formation occurred almost exclusively in the bladder. Presently in the United States, stones form more often in the upper urinary tract or kidney.

Conditions for the formation of kidney and bladder stones include increased rate of excretion of CALCIUM, OXALIC ACID and URIC ACID in the urine. With DEHYDRATION, the concentration of excreted calcium oxalate can increase to the point where calcium oxalate crystallizes. To prevent all types of stones, dilution of urine is critical; this is best accomplished by drinking 2 liters of fluids daily. The formation of calcium-containing stones, the most prevalent kind, is associated with consumption of low-FIBER, highly REFINED CARBOHYDRATE, high-FAT, high-SODIUM, and high-CALCIUM foods. A high VITAMIN D intake, excessive MILK consumption and ALUMINUM salts, in addition to kidney disorders and glandular conditions like hyperthyroidism, may also play a role. Many patients with GOUT have a higher risk of kidney stones due to their excessive build-up of uric acid. A high oxalic acid intake from black tea, COCOA, SPINACH, beet greens and RHUBARB promotes stone formation. Poor fat absorption, possibly excessive VITAMIN C and VITAMIN B_6 deficiency, increase the risk of stone formation, and ANTACIDS containing calcium carbonate, when overconsumed, can lead to kidney stones in susceptible people.

Prevention of Gallstones

Vegetarians have a lowered risk of developing kidney and bladder stones, suggesting that diet plays a role in the etiology. To the extent this is true, then most kidney stones may be preventable. Eating more FRUITS and VEGETABLES, controlling weight and minimizing SUGAR intake helps avoid high urinary calcium. Adequate MAGNESIUM in the diet limits the crystallization of calcium oxalate as kidney stones. Vitamin K is required to form a urinary glycoprotein that inhibits calcium oxalate crystallization in the bladder, while vitamin B_6 reduces the production of oxalates. Furthermore many patients with recurring stones show abnormal B_6-dependent enzyme levels. CITRIC ACID binds calcium and retards stone formation, consequently citrate supplementation may prevent recurrent kidney stones. (See also GALLSTONES.)

cytoplasm   The gel-like liquid that fills all cells, excluding organelles like the nucleus and MITOCHONDRIA. The cytoplasm is surrounded by the cell's outer boundary, the plasma membrane, and consists primarily of WATER, in which ions (especially POTASSIUM and CHLORIDE) and ENZYMES are dissolved. The cytoplasm houses all of the protein synthesizing machinery including messenger RNA, AMINO ACIDS and ribosomes, as well as enzymes of carbohydrate metabolism (GLYCOLYSIS) and fatty acid synthesis. An elaborate array of subcellular protein fibers, such as actin, myosin, microfilaments and microtubules, assist in cell movement and help direct the flow of materials to the cell membrane. HORMONES affect cellular function via cytoplasmic messenger molecules. Embedded in the cytoplasm is a system of smooth membranes, called the ENDOPLASMIC RETICULUM, which, in the liver, completes FATTY ACID synthesis, synthesizes steroid hormones and destroys drugs and pollutants. (See also FAT METABOLISM; FATTY ACIDS.)

cytosine A nitrogen-containing compound that is a building block of DNA and RNA. Cytosine is one of the four nitrogen-containing compounds used by DNA to define the genetic code. Cytosine is synthesized by all cells with nuclei from the amino acids aspartic acid and GLUTAMINE, together with BICARBONATE, and therefore is not an essential nutrient.

Cytosine is degraded to CARBON DIOXIDE, ammonia and smaller fragments, all of which are water-soluble and do not contribute to the URIC ACID load in the bloodstream. Therefore cytosine breakdown does not promote GOUT. (See also PURINE.)

cytotoxins (cytotoxic agents) A diverse family of chemicals capable of destroying cells and tissues. Cytotoxins can be antibodies or they can be toxic agents from bacteria, mold or mushrooms that attack a particular organ. Examples include AFLATOXIN, a liver carcinogen from grain mold; botulinum toxin, a bacterial neurotoxin responsible for BOTULISM, a deadly form of food poisoning; and toxins in shellfish that accumulate during "red tides," a brownish-red coloration of tidal water due to the growth of huge numbers of microscopic organisms. Other cytotoxic agents include by-products of lipid oxidation, for example in rancid FATS and oils, as well as oxidized CHOLESTEROL formed when animal fat is heated at high temperature. Foods fried in lard contain oxidized cholesterol, as do powdered whole MILK and powdered egg products. Oxidized cholesterol may damage cells lining arteries (ATHEROSCLEROSIS).

Cytotoxic agents also include a family of drugs developed to kill cancerous cells. The strategy of chemotherapy lies in selecting cancerous, diseased cells as targets, while sparing other normal, rapidly dividing cells such as cells of the immune system. As an example, methotrexate and aminopterin, drugs that resemble the B vitamin FOLIC ACID, are used to inhibit cell division in leukemia cells. (See also ANTIOXIDANTS; CANCER; VEGETABLE OIL.)

Daily Reference Values (DRVs)   A set of new dietary reference values established for nutrients for which no standards have previously existed for food labels. Into this category fall fat, saturated fat, cholesterol, total carbohydrate, protein, fiber and potassium. The DRVs for nutrients that produce energy, including fat, protein, carbohydrate and fiber, are based on a 2,000 calorie a day diet, unless listed otherwise for a 2,500 calorie diet.

DRVs are calculated according to the following guidelines:

fat: 65 g, based on 30% of calories and saturated fat 20 g, based on 10% of calories
total carbohydrate: 300 g, based on 60% of calories
fiber: 25 g
protein: 50 g, based on 10% of calories. (This DRV for protein is for adults, except for pregnant women and nursing mothers, and children over the age of 4 years: The DRV for infants under 1 year is 14 g; for children between 1 and 4 years, 16 g; pregnant women, 60 g; and nursing mothers, 65 g.)

The DRVs for cholesterol, sodium and potassium do not change with the calorie level because they do not yield energy:

cholesterol: 300 mg
sodium: 2,400 mg
potassium: 3,500 mg

Kurtzweil, Paula, "Daily Values Encourage Healthy Diet." In Food and Drug Administration, *Focus on Food Labeling*, Washington, D.C.: Department of Health and Human Services, 1993 pp. 40–45.

Daily Values (DVs)   A set of new reference values designed to help consumers use food labels and assist them in planning a healthful diet. They appear on food labels and are comprised of two sets of nutrient reference values, the Daily Reference Values (DRVs) and the REFERENCE DAILY INTAKES (RDIs), as the basis for declaring the nutrient content on a food label. Food labels now provide the amount of key nutrients as percentages of the DVs for each nutrient provided by one serving. DVs also provide a basis for thresholds in such descriptions as "high fiber" or "low fat." Thus the term "high fiber" designates the fiber content in a serving of food providing 20% or more of the Daily Value for fiber, that is, 5 g or more. (See also REFERENCE DAILY INTAKE.)

dairy-free frozen desserts   Ice cream substitutes that contain no milk, cream, lactose (milk sugar) or cholesterol. TOFU and soy-milk frozen DESSERTS, frozen natural fruit confections, and even frozen rice desserts are now marketed. Usually these desserts lack CALCIUM, ARTIFICIAL FLAVORS and artificial colors, artificial stabilizers, preservatives or the SATURATED FAT found in ice cream. On the other hand, frozen desserts generally contain large amounts of SUGAR or other sweeteners (FRUCTOSE CORN SYRUP, FRUCTOSE or HONEY). Rice-based frozen desserts may contain maple syrup and fermented rice sweetener in addition to rice.

Some brands of frozen desserts also contain VEGETABLE OIL. Tofu-based frozen desserts are usually high-calorie, high-fat foods. The calories in dairy-free desserts range from 128 to 247 per half-cup serving, and the fat or oil content of soy-derived desserts ranges from 6 to 14 g per serving, which is equivalent to ice cream. The amount of tofu varies from brand to brand and can be less than 10% of the ingredients.

Fruit-based frozen desserts are prepared from whipped fruit juices and fruit purees. Some brands contain only 9% fruit and fruit juices and may contain GUMS and PECTIN. Sugar or fat are not usually added, so fruit-based desserts are lower in fat and total calories than the tofu frozen desserts or ice cream. They generally provide 63 to 80 calories per 4-oz serving. Sorbet and fruit ices are almost fat-free, but they contain more sugar, including corn syrup.

Sometimes people who are sensitive to cow's milk react to foods labeled as "non-dairy" or "pareve" (containing neither milk nor milk products). Traces of milk protein have been found in samples of frozen soy and rice desserts. This is an important consideration because an estimated 0.1 to 7.5% of children have adverse reactions to cow's milk. (See also BALANCED DIET; PROCESSED FOOD; SOYBEAN.)

dandelion (*Taraxacum official*)   A green leafy plant that is a member of the sunflower family. Though gardeners have long confronted the dandelion, dandelion greens are a nutritious food. Like other vegetable greens they are a rich source of IRON and CALCIUM. The beta carotene content of dandelion greens exceeds that of carrots. Dandelion greens also provide INULIN and PECTIN (soluble fiber). Herbalists throughout the world use dandelion to improve liver function and bile flow and for liver conditions such as hepatitis and jaundice. Dandelion also seems to act as a diuretic (increases water loss).

Cultivated dandelion greens are more tender than wild greens. Wild dandelions may have been sprayed with a weed killer or fungicide, and plants growing next to roads with a high volume of traffic may have been contaminated by exhaust pollution. A cup of chopped, cooked dandelion greens contains 35 calories; protein, 2.1 g; carbohydrate, 6.7 g; fiber, 1.4 g; calcium, 147 mg; iron, 1.89 mg; vitamin A, 1,229 retinol equivalents; and vitamin C, 19 mg.

date (*Phoenix dactylifera*)   The fruit of the date palm tree. Dates are actually a single-seeded berry. They have been cultivated in North Africa and regions of the Middle East since 2,000 B.C. or earlier. The Middle East still supplies most of the world's date crop, although Arizona and California supply U.S. domestic needs. Unripened dates are green. When ripened, they are yellow or red with a thick, syrupy flesh. Dates are harvested, ripened and dried before shipping. Dates are good sources of dietary fiber and iron though, unlike most fruits, dates do not contain significant amounts of VITAMIN C. The most common variety of date produced in the United States is the Deglet Noor, which is semisoft. Semisoft dates can be stored up to eight months if refrigerated. Dry dates contain little moisture and are often pasteurized to inhibit mold growth. Dates are a very sweet fruit, they can contain up to 70% SUGAR. Ten pitted dates provide 228 calories; protein, 1.6 g; carbohydrate, 61 g; fiber, 7.23 g; potassium, 540 mg; iron, 1 mg; niacin, 1.83 mg; thiamin, 0.07 mg; riboflavin, 0.08 mg. Most of the CARBOHYDRATE is in the form of sugar.

DDT   (dichloro-diphenyl-trichloroethane, chlorophenothane) One of the first powerful, synthetic PESTICIDES to be used worldwide. DDT has been used against a wide range of insects, especially Japanese beetle and European cornborer, as well as louse, mosquito, bed bug, fly, flea and cockroach. DDT is classified as a CHLORINATED HYDROCARBON, a type of compound that is neither easily degraded in the environment, nor readily broken down in the body. The first pesticides were designed to persist in the environment in order to control pests longer. This decision has had profound ramifications. First, the widespread use of DDT rapidly led to DDT-resistant insects. Second, DDT and other chlorinated hydrocarbons accumulate in the FOOD CHAIN because they are not readily biodegradable. Birds, including the American eagle, and fish suffer well-documented toxic effects from DDT, and in 1972 the United States banned DDT except for public health use (to control insects that can spread disease) and for crop protection where no alternative pesticide was available. In spite of the ban on DDT, high levels were reported in fish caught off California coastal waters nine years after its manufacturing was terminated. Individuals eating polluted fish have more DDT in their blood.

DDT causes cancer in mice, but the effects that chronic exposure to small doses has had on human health are unknown. Breast cancer rates in the United States have risen steadily, and an increased environmental exposure to pollutants has been implicated. A Kaiser Foundation Research Study of 57,000 women did not find a link between DDT exposure and increased risk of breast cancer. In the United States a mother's milk can contain DDT at a level that is one and a half times more concentrated than in the woman's blood. For an average infant this represents a daily intake of about 50 mcg of DDT—on a weight basis, equivalent to about 10 times the average adult intake. The long-term effects on childhood development of this exposure are unknown. (See also GREEN REVOLUTION.)

decaffeinated coffee   Coffee from which most caffeine has been extracted. The process of decaffeination causes a small loss in flavor and aroma. Decaffeinated coffee is not caffeine-free; it contains low levels of caffeine, 1 to 5 mg per cup, compared to 100 to 150 mg for a cup of regular. This level may be enough to trigger cravings in those attempting to overcome caffeine addiction. Some producers extract caffeine from roasted ground coffee with organic solvents, either methylene chloride or ethyl acetate. Following solvent extraction, the decaffeinated beans are steamed to remove residual solvent. The excess moisture is removed and the decaffeinated beans are roasted. Ethyl acetate seems to be a safe solvent for caffeine extraction, though concern was raised about the use of methylene chloride because it is a weak carcinogen. The U.S. FDA has ruled that the trace amounts of these solvents present in some decaffeinated coffee pose no health threat.

To avoid organic solvents altogether, caffeine can be extracted with water, followed by charcoal filtration. In this process, beans are first steamed, then soaked in water for long periods to remove 97% of the caffeine. They are then dried and roasted to develop aroma and flavor. Tea can also be decaffeinated. Typically, solvent extraction either with ethylacetate or with carbon dioxide at high temperature and pressure can remove most of the caffeine from tea. Decaffeination affects the flavor of tea more than coffee.

decalcification   The removal of CALCIUM from BONES. A deficiency of calcium or inadequate VITAMIN D required for calcium uptake, and an imbalance of certain hormones (parathyroid hormone and calcitonin), can cause mineral loss from bone (dissolution). Calcium usage in the body and bone loss depend upon complex interactions. If calcium levels in the blood begin to decrease, the parathyroid glands secrete parathyroid hormone, parathormone, which increases calcium levels by activating osteoclasts (cells that break down bone) while decreasing calcium excretion by the kidney and increasing calcium uptake by the intestine. Parathormone stimulates the kidneys to convert vitamin D to the hormone, CHOLECALCIFEROL.

It is believed that a deficiency of the female sex hormone ESTROGEN, after menopause causes osteoclasts to be more sensitive to parathormone, resulting in increased bone breakdown and elevated blood calcium levels. Elevated blood calcium in turn would decrease parathormone output, decrease vitamin D activation and thus further increase excretion of calcium. Estrogen replacement therapy is ultimately aimed at maintaining bone mass in postmenopausal women.

Calcium losses are influenced by the diet. High protein intake, high phosphate intake (from soft drinks) and excessive sugar consumption increase calcium loss in the urine. Calcium is also lost when excessive dietary FIBER is ingested. MAGNESIUM, VITAMIN B_6, FOLIC ACID, VITAMIN B_{12}, BORON and STRONTIUM have been shown to stabilize bone calcium and bone density. Boron seems to increase estrogen levels in postmenopausal women; it may also help activate vitamin D. (See also HORMONE; OSTEOMALACIA; OSTEOPOROSIS.)

decoction The extraction of water-soluble materials and flavors from meat and vegetables by boiling in water for varying times. BOUILLONS are prepared in this way. In botanical medicine, essences may be extracted from plant material by boiling in water. Decoction differs from an infusion, in which boiling water is poured on a plant material; extraction continues without further boiling. A common example of infusion is TEA steeped in hot water. Because the act of boiling is more vigorous and occurs at a higher temperature, decoction extracts more material than infusion.

deficiency, subclinical The state of being marginally nourished. In contrast with overt malnutrition, which causes identifiable diseases, mild or moderate nutrient deficiencies need not reveal obvious signs of illness. Nonetheless, subclinical deficiencies lead to lowered immunity and decreased resistance to viral, bacterial and fungal infections; difficult pregnancies, low birth-weight infants and delayed growth and development; learning problems; short-term memory loss and a host of vague symptoms ranging from fatigue to depression.

A marginal nutrient deficiency can lead to inadequate reserve to meet emergencies. For example, a woman who diets, especially a teenage woman whose body is growing, may not have enough iron reserves to support a pregnancy adequately. Subclinical malnutrition can have long-term consequences. Subclinical deficiencies can set the stage for DEGENERATIVE DISEASES that include CANCER, HEART DISEASE, high blood pressure, diabetes, OSTEOPOROSIS, ARTHRITIS, PERIODONTAL DISEASE, AUTOIMMUNE DISEASES and SENILITY.

For optimal health the body needs more than minimum amounts of vitamins and minerals to prevent full-blown disease. However, the nutrient requirements for optimal health are unknown for most nutrients. The RECOMMENDED DIETARY ALLOWANCES (RDAs) are standards designed to maintain health for a healthy population and do not define the optimal amount for each of the nutrients for individuals. As a general guideline, an intake of a given nutrient that is consistently two-thirds of the RDA or less increases the risk of malnutrition. When several nutrients fall substantially below the RDA there is a much greater risk of malnutrition and its consequences.

Problem Nutrients

Surveys in the United States and Canada indicate the most common nutrient deficiencies are: CALCIUM, IRON, MAGNESIUM, ZINC, VITAMIN A, VITAMIN C, VITAMIN B_6 and FOLIC ACID, among certain groups. In developing countries protein-calorie malnutrition is the major nutritional disorder, followed by vitamin A deficiency. In developed countries the most obvious cause of subclinical nutrient deficiency is an inadequate diet. Reliance on highly processed foods can lead to inadequate intake of key nutrients beyond those used as food enrichment or fortification.

Causes of Subclinical Deficiencies

Historically, poverty, illiteracy and malnutrition are intertwined. Infants and children in low-income families, pregnant teenagers, elderly persons and institutionalized clients are most likely to be inadequately nourished in the United States. Nutritional deficiencies can occur even with an adequate diet. Inadequate stomach acid and DIGESTIVE ENZYMES limit nutrient assimilation. A diseased or inflamed intestine will not be able to complete DIGESTION, nor will it absorb individual nutrients effectively, especially if transit through the gastrointestinal tract is too rapid for efficient absorption, as during diarrhea.

Strategies to Correct Marginal Nutrition

Even if the amount of each nutrient needed for optimal health were known for the average person, the amounts needed by individuals would still differ, due to the unique biochemical makeup of each individual. Variations in nutrient needs reflect different genetic compositions, overall health, diet histories, life-styles, ages, and exercise patterns. Therefore individualized nutrition counseling is a most effective strategy to overcome nutritional deficiencies. Nutrition counseling relies on evaluating how well the body is stocked with nutrients and on dietary planning to correct nutritional imbalances. Optimally, the physician and nutritionist work as a team in evaluating results of diagnostic tests, comprehensive physical examinations and medical history, as well as assessment of nutrient intake, to work out an individualized program that meets the client's needs, including patient education. (See also BIOCHEMICAL INDIVIDUALITY; DIETING; MALABSORPTION.)

Goldschmidt, Millicent C. et al., "Reduced Bacteriocidal Activity in Neutrophils from Scorbutic Animals and the Effect of Ascorbic Acid on These Target Bacteria in Vivo and in Vitro," *American Journal of Clinical Nutrition*, 54:6 supp. (December 1991), pp. 1214S–20S.

deficiency disease A disease state caused by inadequate nutrient uptake and assimilation. Modern nutrition has its origins in the repeated demonstration that severe diseases can be the result of severe, chronic nutrient shortages and are treatable with the appropriate vitamins and minerals. In this respect the importance of VITAMINS to human nutrition was well established before 1940. Most outright nutrient deficiency diseases have vanished in the United States, though worldwide they are all too prevalent. It is worth noting that nutritional deficiencies can occur with maldigestion and MALABSORPTION even if the diet supplies adequate amounts of vitamins and minerals. Foods must be digested and nutrients must be absorbed to be effective.

Conditions related to severe vitamin deficiencies:

- NIACIN deficiency causes PELLAGRA.
- THIAMIN deficiency causes BERIBERI.
- VITAMIN B$_{12}$ deficiency leads to PERNICIOUS ANEMIA.
- VITAMIN A deficiency promotes NIGHT BLINDNESS.
- VITAMIN D deficiency causes RICKETS and bone disease.
- VITAMIN B$_6$, VITAMIN E, vitamin A and FOLIC ACID deficiencies can cause ANEMIAS.
- VITAMIN C deficiency causes SCURVY.

Conditions related to mineral deficiencies:

- CALCIUM deficiency leads to bone disease and bone malformation (OSTEOPOROSIS, OSTEOMALACIA, RICKETS).
- Zinc deficiency causes BIRTH DEFECTS.
- IRON and COPPER deficiencies cause deficiency anemia.
- IODINE deficiency causes GOITER.
- ESSENTIAL FATTY ACID deficiencies cause skin conditions and can contribute to heart disease.

Conditions Related to Protein-Energy Malnutrition

An inadequate intake of protein and energy is the most important nutritional problem in developing nations. Protein and energy deficiencies cause STARVATION syndromes, KWASHIORKOR and MARASMUS, as extremes. Children bear the brunt: The World Health Organization has suggested that a minimum of 500 million children suffer from nutritional deficiencies. The effects of starvation and semistarvation on children are profound: anemia, infections due to depressed immunity, chronic DIARRHEA, stunted growth, and failure to thrive. Growth retardation may be irreversible. (See also BALANCED DIET; DIETARY GUIDELINES FOR AMERICANS.)

degenerative diseases Diseases commonly associated with aging in Western, developed countries. They include CARDIOVASCULAR DISEASE (ATHEROSCLEROSIS or clogged arteries; ARTERIOSCLEROSIS or hardening of the arteries, coronary heart disease, STROKE, HEART ATTACK); OSTEOPOROSIS (brittle bones); SENILITY (dementia, ALZHEIMER'S DISEASE); adult diabetes; PERIODONTAL DISEASE; AUTOIMMUNE DISEASES (rheumatoid ARTHRITIS, sprue, insulin-dependent diabetes); and CANCER. Several of these diseases are now epidemics of industrialized nations. Cardiovascular disease, cancer, diabetes and others are linked to OBESITY, itself a potential harmful condition characteristic of affluent societies.

Although a history of inherited tendencies plays a role, degenerative diseases are not necessarily inevitable because life-style choices profoundly affect susceptibility to chronic diseases. Often many can be prevented, or at least reduced in their intensity, with a life-long commitment to EXERCISE, wise food choices, to emotional well-being and to avoiding exposure to harmful substances. Therefore you have a major impact on your health through healthful choices.

Many degenerative diseases respond to nutritionally sound practices. Moderate calorie intake and WEIGHT MANAGEMENT help prevent obesity, diabetes and hypertension, while adequate CALCIUM, trace minerals and VITAMIN D intake and exercise help prevent later bone loss. Moderate SODIUM consumption lowers the risk of hypertension and related heart and kidney diseases, and adequate fiber intake helps maintain the health of the digestive tract and lowers the risk of colon cancer. ANTIOXIDANTS as found in fruits and vegetables like VITAMIN C, VITAMIN E, BETA CAROTENE and CAROTENOIDS decrease the risk of some forms of cancer, cataracts, mental aging and heart disease. Moderation is a key: Moderate sugar consumption lowers the risk of dental caries; moderate alcohol consumption helps prevent liver disease; and moderate fat consumption lowers the risk of obesity, heart disease and some forms of cancer. (See also AGING.)

Ames, Bruce N., Shigenaga, M. K., Hagen, T.M., "Oxiadants, Antioxidants and the Degenerative Diseases of Aging," *Proceedings of the National Academy of Sciences* (U.S.), 90 (September 1993), pp. 7915–22.

deglutition The process of swallowing, especially foods. Deglutible refers to a substance that can be swallowed. In the first stage of swallowing, chewing pulverizes food and mixes it thoroughly with SALIVA. The tongue forces the BOLUS (wad) of food back into the mouth and into the upper part of the throat. In the involuntary or automatic stage of swallowing, the bolus moves into the ESOPHAGUS, the tube leading to the stomach. The bolus triggers nerve signals to the deglutition center in the brain stem. In turn, the brain signals the palate to close the nasal passage. Breathing is interrupted for about two seconds and the palate again reopens. PERISTALSIS, rhythmic contractions, conducts the bolus through the esophagus to the stomach.

Gulping food can lead to swallowing an excessive amount of air, which in turn can cause an excessive air build-up in the stomach, which is one cause of heartburn. Chewing food thoroughly not only eases swallowing but also aids digestion because pulverized food is more easily broken down. Furthermore, up to 20 minutes may elapse before the stomach senses that food has entered the stomach itself and relays that signal to the brain. The brain responds by triggering the release of hormones that stimulate the release of stomach acid and digestive enzymes. (See also DIGESTIVE TRACT.)

dehydrated food Refers to a wide range of dried foods. The removal of most of the water content of foods is an ancient form of preservation. Modern dehydration methods employ freeze-drying technology to remove the water rapidly and to preserve nutrients and food quality. Microbial breakdown and many chemical reactions are minimized in dehydrated foods. However, light-induced reactions and lipid oxidation can still occur. Therefore dehydrated foods are generally sealed both from air and from light, as well as from moisture.

Freeze-drying works best with foods that can be frozen quickly and can be spread in thin layers. For example, soups, vegetables and stews are quick-frozen at very low temperature, then subjected to a vacuum (reduced pressure). Under reduced pressure ice evaporates (sublimes), leaving behind the powdery residue minus the weight of water.

On the other hand, sliced fresh fruit, like pears, plums, apples, apricots and other watery fruit, can be dried in an evaporator that blows warmed air over the food. Dates, figs, currants and raisins are traditionally sun-dried. Modern production of dried vine fruit employs blown hot air over the fruit on racks.

Dehydrated milk, powdered eggs and cheeses are commercially dehydrated. They are first blown through a nozzle to create a mist of fine droplets, which is sprayed into a heated chamber for drying. Studies indicate such processes create oxidized forms of CHOLESTEROL, which promotes PLAQUE build-up in arteries in experimental animals. (See also ATHEROSCLEROSIS.)

dehydration   A condition resulting from excessive WATER loss. The importance of adequate water for health cannot be overemphasized. The body is a watery environment containing 60% water, and blood is 90% water. The internal environment of the cell, the cytoplasm, is primarily water. Water also functions in digestion and absorption. Water helps maintain the ELECTROLYTE balance, the balance of dissolved ions in body fluids. Water is the medium for acid-base balance, so that the appropriate pH can be maintained. Water helps dispose of wastes. The kidney requires water to filter wastes out of the blood, and the liver requires water to remove toxic materials and waste products. Water evaporation helps regulate body temperature.

During dehydration, the kidneys do not filter out wastes efficiently, and toxic products such as ammonia can accumulate in the blood. Extreme dehydration can lead to coma, and even death.

COFFEE, TEA, BEER and COLA SOFT DRINKS can increase water loss through increased urination. People with busy life-styles often do not drink enough water. THIRST may not be a good indicator of how much water is needed because the sensation of thirst lags behind real need. Consumption of eight to ten glasses daily of water and other beverages will replace water lost through urine, sweat and wastes. Food supplies the equivalent of about four glasses of water daily.

Many situations can lead to dehydration. Dehydration can affect athletes (especially during prolonged exertion in hot weather); individuals working in a hot environment; elderly people who gradually lose their sense of thirst; and institutionalized patients. Other situations causing dehydration are prolonged vomiting or DIARRHEA; use of DIURETICS (water pills) that cause excessive urination; and excessive sweating. (See also ANTIDIURETIC HORMONE; EXERCISE.)

Coyle, Edward F. and Mountain, Scott J., "Benefits of Fluid Replacement with Carbohydrate during Exercise," *Medicine and Science in Sports Exercise*, 24 (September 1992, supp.), pp. S324–S330.

dehydrocholesterol (7-dehydrocholecalciferol)   A substance formed by the skin that can be converted to VITAMIN D. As the name implies, dehydrocholesterol is closely related to its parent compound, CHOLESTEROL. The skin and other tissues convert cholesterol to dehydrocholesterol. Exposure to ultraviolet light in sunlight converts this cholesterol derivative into vitamin D. In northern latitudes (Scandinavia, Canada, northern United States) winter skin exposure to sunlight may be inadequate for vitamin D formation. Institutionalized patients who are not exposed to sunlight and who do not drink vitamin D-fortified milk are also prone to the effects of vitamin D deficiency because of inadequate formation of vitamin D from dehydrocholesterol. (See also CALCIUM; MALNUTRITION.)

Delaney Clause   An amendment to the federal drug and cosmetic act banning the addition of cancer-causing additives to processed food, cosmetics and drugs. This legislation reflected the belief that there is no safe limit of exposure to a CANCER-causing material (CARCINOGEN). Controversy has surrounded the Delaney Clause since it came into being in 1958. In the 1980s reinterpretation of the existing law directed the U.S. FDA to permit the low level use of known carcinogens. The Food Quality Protection Act of 1996 supersedes the Delaney Clause and it amends the Federal Insecticide, Fungicide and Rotenticide Act by establishing a single health-based standard for PESTICIDE residues in all foods. The new safety standard is defined as "a reasonable certainty that no harm will result from aggregate exposure to the pesticide chemical residues." This act will allow the use of additives that present a negligible risk. The EPA will have authority to require chemical manufacturers to disclose information about their pesticides. Prior existing pesticides will be reviewed in light of the new standard and all existing tolerances for pesticides will be reviewed within 10 years. Provisions to ensure the safety of children are included. When the evidence for safety is questionable, then the allowable levels will be lowered to permit up to 10-fold more protection for children. The act also requires distribution of health information about pesticides in foods by food stores nationwide.

Clearly only a fraction of chemicals cause cancer. Identifying the risks of cancer due to new additives and chemicals, as well as to food additives introduced prior to the legislation in the 1960s, are major goals of medical research. A fundamental issue lies in the estimated number of cancer-related deaths that are tolerable when balanced against the benefits of using a given additive. An additional complication is a result of modern technology. Chemical analytical techniques are now ultra-sensitive so that carcinogens at extremely small concentrations, a few molecules in a billion or less, are routinely measured. The consequences of exposure to such minute amounts of carcinogens, pollutants and possible additive effects, are areas of active research. (See also EPIDEMIOLOGY; CHEMICALS.)

Weisburger, J.H., "Does the Delaney Clause of the U.S. Food and Drug Laws Prevent Human Cancers?" *Fundamental and Applied Toxicology*, 22:4 (1994), pp. 483–93.

dementia (senile psychosis)   A permanent mental deterioration that characterizes decreased mental functioning. Psychiatrists specify five indicators of senile psychosis: impairment of judgment, memory, orientation, intellectual functioning and changeable emotional response. General mental deterioration often occurs after the age of 70 with a gradual onset. Dementia occurs more often in women than in men. Typically dementia brings short-term memory lapses, loss of interest in life, fitful sleep, mood swings and confusion. It can progress to tantrums, paranoia, severe depression and refusal to eat. The patient may become incontinent and unable to feed herself.

There is no single cause of senility. Decreased blood supply to the brain is often a culprit. With hardening of arteries (cerebral ARTERIOSCLEROSIS) the brain becomes deprived of oxygen and nutrients. This condition may happen quickly. Senility is also linked to HYPERTENSION (high blood pressure). In addition, nutrient deficiencies, including severe deficiencies of VITAMIN B$_{12}$ and NIACIN, can produce symptoms resembling mental aging.

Certain illnesses can create apparent senility: heavy metal poisoning (like lead poisoning); alcoholism; high fever due to infections; disorders of the liver and kidney; hormonal imbalances. Many common medications can produce apathy, weakness, depression and mental confusion; this is an increasing problem among the elderly, who often take multiple medications. (See also AGING; AIDS; ALZHEIMER'S DISEASE; PELLAGRA; SENILITY.)

denatured protein   A PROTEIN that has lost its biological function or activity. Typically, ENZYMES become inactive and no longer serve as catalysts. Proteins are fragile molecules; their biological function depends upon the maintenance of a single shape or conformation, which can be altered by a wide variety of agents, including heat; extreme acid or alkaline conditions; foaming; oxidation; and removal of ions from solution. Organic solvents and detergents are also denaturing agents. BLANCHING vegetables denatures enzymes that cause changes in texture, color and flavor of food. Cooking protein-rich foods like meat, eggs and legumes denatures the protein, making it more accessible to DIGESTIVE ENZYMES and speeding DIGESTION. Stomach acid (hydrochloric acid) also serves as a protein denaturant, significantly increasing digestion. (See also COAGULATED PROTEIN.)

dental caries   See TEETH.

dental fluoridosis   A light brown mottling of tooth enamel due to excessive FLUORIDE consumption during tooth maturation and before the tooth has erupted from the gum. The mottling of teeth is not considered a health risk, though cosmetically it may be important. Continued exposure to high levels of fluoride may be related to a risk of bone fractures later in life. (See also FLUORIDATED WATER.)

dental plaque   Transparent deposits of bacteria and debris adhering to tooth surfaces. Dental plaque precedes tooth decay and PERIODONTAL DISEASE, which are bacterial infections of teeth.

Diet clearly has an important role in the formation of plaque, and sugar remains the leading dietary cause of tooth decay because it is a particularly effective food for the bacteria. Bacteria responsible for dental plaque, such as *Streptococcus mutans*, ferment sugars in food to organic acids, which dissolve the minerals in teeth. Tooth enamel cannot repair itself. Bacteria can then infect pockets in enamel, leading to cavities. In addition, several strains of bacteria can infect gums. Plaque build-up and periodontal disease may be prevented by proper flossing, brushing and periodic cleaning by a dental hygienist and by limiting consumption of sugar-rich foods like candy and sweets. Brushing immediately after eating such foods limits plaque formation. (See also CANDY; CARBOHYDRATE.)

deoxycholic acid   See BILE ACIDS.

deoxyribonucleic acid   See DNA.

deoxyribose   A simple sugar building block of DNA, the genetic material of cells. The DNA molecule consists of very long chains with a "backbone" of deoxyribose. Deoxyribose is not an essential nutrient because the body makes ample amounts from ribose, a common sugarcontaining five carbon atoms. (See also CARBOHYDRATE META-BOLISM; GLUCOSE.)

depression   A feeling of overwhelming sadness. Beyond experiencing sadness after a loss, clinical depression is prolonged and disproportionate. Possible manifestations include an inability to feel pleasure, loss of appetite, weight loss or weight gain, excessive guilt, diminished ability to concentrate, sense of hopelessness, lethargy, insomnia, suicidal thoughts and persistent headaches. Chronic and severe depression can lead to psychosis and suicide. Depression is a serious health problem; an estimated 4% of Americans are severely depressed. Depression may indirectly increase the risk of clogged arteries by increasing the risk of cigarette smoking, which raises levels of a clotting protein (fibrinogen).

Causes

Depression is a complex, not fully understood phenomenon and there is no single cause. Depression is associated with premenstrual syndrome, chronic viral infections and seasonal affective disorder, a seasonal tendency to depression. Food allergy and environmental sensitivies as causes of psychological symptoms remains controversial. However, in some cases food allergies or chronic exposure to toxic chemicals, solvents and toxic metals causes mental disturbances. Nutritional deficiencies, hormonal imbalances and reactions to medications contribute to depression.

Many nutrient deficiencies can cause depression. A deficiency of the essential amino acid TRYPTOPHAN, and several mineral deficiencies, including calcium, iron, magnesium and potassium, lead to depression. Certain vitamins are specifically associated with behavioral changes: These include VITAMIN C, BIOTIN, VITAMIN B$_{12}$, FOLIC ACID, NIACIN, RIBOFLAVIN, PANTOTHENIC ACID, VITAMIN B$_6$ and THIAMIN. Folic acid and vitamin B$_{12}$ status are low in some patients suffering from depression; 30% of psychiatric patients in the United States may be deficient in folic acid. In the brain, folic acid and vitamin B$_{12}$, together with the essential amino acid methionine, seem to raise levels of the neurotransmitter SEROTONIN, which acts as an antidepressant.

Circumstantial evidence links thiamin deficiency and depression. Thiamin deficiency alters brain chemistry, and thus, upon admission psychiatric patients are frequently found to be thiamin deficient. Depression is one of the symptoms of chronic niacin deficiency (PELLAGRA).

Hormone Imbalances

Imbalances of the PITUITARY, HYPOTHALAMUS, THYROID and/or ADRENAL GLANDS have been implicated in depression. Depression is an early symptom of hypothyroidism (low thyroid output), and adrenal gland malfunction can lead to excessive cortisol production, which can produce depression, nervousness and insomnia. The brain is very dependent upon blood sugar (glucose) for energy, and severely emotionally disturbed patients are prone to HYPOGLYCEMIA (low blood sugar). A gradual onset of hypoglycemia can lead to depression, blunted mental functioning and emotional instability.

Medications

Depression can be induced by corticosteroids, beta blockers and blood pressure medications that disrupt the normal balance of neurotransmitters, the chemicals that convey nerve impulses. Oral contraceptives can induce deficiencies of vitamin B_6, presumably resulting in lowered serotonin production in the brain, which can affect mood.

Approaches to the Treatment of Depression

Normalizing swings in blood sugar levels is often helpful in treating depression. Small, frequent meals that are high in protein and complex carbohydrates, while eliminating sweets and refined carbohydrates are useful strategies. To correct a faulty diet, minimize junk food and convenience foods with low amounts of nutrients. Nutritional supplements can help ameliorate depression associated with nutrient deficiencies.

Much research has focused on neurotransmitter imbalances associated with depression, especially serotonin. Supplementing nutrients that are raw materials for neurotransmitters, particularly the amino acids tryptophan, PHENYLALAMINE and L-TYROSINE, together with vitamin B_6, has been used therapeutically with inconsistent results. Most likely to benefit are those with manic depression. These nutrients may enhance the effects of antidepressants in some cases. The use of gram amounts of amino acids requires the supervision of a physician skilled in nutrition. In 1990 the U.S. FDA withdrew tryptophan as an isolated nutritional supplement. St. John's Wort (*Hypericum perforatum*) has been used historically to elevate mood in cases of mental disturbance.

Aerobic exercise can improve mood, and increased physical activity is strongly associated with decreased malaise, depression and anxiety. In addition to dance, movement therapy and improved sleep patterns, light therapy (for seasonal affective disorder) and psychotherapy are among the non-nutritional approaches that have been recommended. (See also ALLERGY, FOOD; CHRONIC FATIGUE.)

Maurizi, C.P., "Why Not Treat Melancholia with Melatonin and Tryptophan and Treat Seasonal Affective Disorders with Bright Light?" *Medical Hypotheses*, 27, (1988), pp. 271–76.

Potter, W.Z., Rudorfer, M.V., Manji, H., "The Pharmacologic Treatment of Depression," *New England Journal of Medicine*, 325:9 (1991), pp. 633–42.

dermatitis A range of skin conditions involving inflammation, with redness and swelling, itching and other abnormalities. Contact dermatitis is caused by exposing the skin to an irritating substance. Poison ivy and poison oak are classic examples of agents causing contact dermatitis. Regular exposure to mild irritants can cause the skin to become red, dry, scaly, cracked or flaking. Cosmetics (hair care products, colognes, antiperspirants), antibiotics, and kitchen chemicals like detergents and cleansers can be causes of contact dermatitis in susceptible people.

ATOPIC DERMATITIS is associated with more severe symptoms, such as ECZEMA, with skin eruptions, blisters and crusts. This condition runs in families. About 3% of infants have atopic dermatitis, which often clears up by 18 months of age. Food allergy is often implicated as a possible cause. In adults, itchiness, redness and swelling may worsen with STRESS and FATIGUE. An allergy to wool, excessive exposure to oils and soaps, and a deficiency of any vitamin of the B COMPLEX can cause atopic dermatitis. (See also ALLERGY, FOOD.)

dessert The last meal course. In the United States dessert is likely to be a high-sugar, high-fat food: pastry-like cookies; cakes and pies; ice cream or other frozen dessert; custards or puddings; and gelatin desserts. In Britain, meals often end with nuts, fruit and a dessert wine like port. In France, meals traditionally end with fruit, cheese and a wine. In northern Europe elaborate cakes and tarts are famous desserts. In Spain and Latin-America, flan, a custard, is traditional. Dessert may also include milk-based sweets with fruits. In India, sweet puddings and cakes flavored with honey, nuts and rose water are dessert items. In many other cuisines, fresh fruit, tea and coffee end the meal, without a sweet course. (See also DAIRY-FREE FROZEN DESSERTS.)

detoxification The chemical modification of foreign substances and waste products in order to help the body dispose of potentially harmful substances. Detoxification refers to treatment protocols designed to help the body rid itself of waste and toxic materials. The LIVER is a key actor in detoxication. Its battery of protective enzymes can oxidize and inactivate toxic compounds to increase their water-solubility so they can be excreted more readily. Liver enzymes perform (Phase 1 reactions) oxidations (adding oxygen); hydrolysis (breaking bonds); demethylation (removing carbon atoms); and conjugation (Phase 2 reactions) reactions (attaching highly water-soluble materials [like amino acids and sugar derivatives] to a wide range of compounds). Common examples of substances detoxified by the liver include ALCOHOL, oxidized to a derivative of acetic acid, AMMONIA, the toxic by-product of amino acid degradation, converted to non-toxic UREA, steroid hormones and pollutants.

CYTOCHROME P450 refers to a major class of oxidizing enzymes of the liver, requiring IRON and RIBOFLAVIN. Cytochrome P450 enzymes can add oxygen atoms to otherwise very resistant compounds, including a variety of drugs and cyclic hydrocarbons. A genetic defect in this cytochrome system, in an estimated 20 million Americans, reduces their ability to break down drugs. Individuals with this defect are more likely to develop side effects when administered common prescription drugs such as pain killers at typical dosages.

Detoxification Procedures

A variety of treatments have been designed to help rid the body of toxins and environmental pollutants. The recommended approach entails a lifelong commitment to a healthful diet and regular physical exercise. With a substantial loss of body fat through supervised fasting or weight loss programs, there will be less fat available to accumulate fat-soluble contaminants like pesticides. In addition drinking plenty of WATER helps the kidneys work efficiently to cleanse the blood and to excrete waste products. At least two quarts of water should be drunk daily. The diet should emphasize whole, minimally processed foods with fruits and vegetables and should supply adequate antioxidants including VITAMIN C, plus COPPER, MANGANESE, SELENIUM and ZINC, needed by the body's detoxication enzymes to function optimally. Additional antioxidants, including vitamin E, may be prudent. Cabbage family vegetables (CRUCIFEROUS VEGETABLES) boost detoxifying enzyme levels. "Lipotropic" factors like CHOLINE, a nitrogen-containing compound used as a raw material for the phospholipid lecithin and for brain chemicals, and the essential sulfur-containing amino acid, METHIONINE, may help liver metabolism especially with fat-soluble materials. Milk thistle (*Silybum marianum*) and other botanical preparations have also been used to support liver metabolism.

Of course, limiting exposure to toxic agents is critically important. Gel-forming fibers like psyllium husk, guar gum, pectin and oat bran can help bind ingested toxins and prevent their absorption. These can be combined with toxin-binding materials such as bentonite clay. The PESTICIDE burden can be reduced by eating organic produce and peeling waxed fruits and vegetables. Exposure to toxic chemicals, including drugs, should be minimized. Since many organic solvents are easily absorbed through the skin, direct contact with paint and solvents should be avoided. (See also ORGANIC FOODS.)

Parke, Dennis V., "Nutritional Requirements for Detoxication of Environmental Chemicals," *Food Additives and Contaminants*, 8:3 (1991), pp. 381–96.

detoxification in recovery programs Supervised programs designed to assist in the recovery from a drug or an alcohol ADDICTION. Detoxification in this context involves abstaining from the addictive substance to allow the body to recover, while supplying support and counseling during critical phases. Withdrawal symptoms often initially accompany abstinence: CONSTIPATION, FATIGUE, irritability, headache, joint ache and perspiration. Severe withdrawal symptoms may accompany abstinence from ALCOHOL, tranquilizers or sleeping pills and may require medical supervision. After a detoxification program has been completed exposure to even small amounts of the offending material may set off a strong reaction. In addition to abstinence, nutrition counseling is recommended. Eating nutritious meals with less fat, COFFEE, alcohol, white bread, pastry and SUGAR forms a key part of the recovery process.

Programs may recommend certain vitamins, amino acids and ANTIOXIDANTS to diminish withdrawal symptoms and to boost the body's ability to dispose of toxic materials. (See also ALCOHOLISM; BEHAVIOR MODIFICATION.)

dextrin (maltodextrin) A sweetener containing a mixture of STARCH degradation products. Dextrin is obtained commercially by treating starch with enzymes, alkali or acid. The source of starch is usually corn, but potato and other starches are also used. Because starch is composed of glucose as building blocks, dextrin yields glucose during digestion.

Dextrin prevents sugar in candy from crystallizing and also serves as a thickening agent. Dextrin is used to encapsulate flavors used in powdered mixes. Dextrin holds water in foods and is used in baked goods, as well as gravies and sauces. It is incorporated into electrolyte-replacement sports drinks, where it serves as a readily used energy source.

dextrose (glucose, grape sugar, corn sugar) A simple sugar used commercially as a sweetener. In foods glucose occurs in fruits and HONEY. Dextrose contributes to the brown color of bread crusts and baked goods. Dextrose is less sweet than sucrose and is often used as a food additive when over-sweetness is a problem. Dextrose is 75% as sweet as sucrose, and is used as an additive in soft drinks to increase the flavor and thus make the beverage more appealing to the consumer. Dextrose is a refined carbohydrate and consequently adds only calories, and no other nutrients like vitamins and minerals, to food.

Glucose, whether ingested as a dextrose sweetener in processed food, or produced by starch digestion in the intestine, enters the blood very quickly and rapidly raises BLOOD SUGAR. Elevated blood sugar stimulates the pancreas to release INSULIN; in turn, this hormone causes tissues to absorb glucose, so that it can be burned for energy or converted to fat. (See also CARBOHYDRATE METABOLISM; GLYCEMIC INDEX.)

DHEA (dehydroxyepiandrosterone) A hormone made by the adrenal glands, testes and ovaries. Like other steroid hormones, DHEA is fabricated from cholesterol and is released into the bloodstream where it is the most abundant of this hormone class. However, unlike the other steroid hormones, production of DHEA peaks between the ages of 25 and 30, then declines with increasing age. DHEA possesses complex, multiple roles in health and disease; however, its physiologic role is still not clear. Research suggests that low blood levels of DHEA are linked to CARDIOVASCULAR DISEASE in men. Animal studies provide an insight as to how this can occur: DHEA treatment decreases fat synthesis and the formation of LDL (LOW-DENSITY LIPOPROTEIN, the less desirable form of cholesterol). In addition, DHEA may reduce the risk of OSTEOPOROSIS and several forms of cancer. DHEA also can prevent the development of diabetes in mice with a predisposition to this disease. On the other hand, high DHEA levels in postmenopausal women can lead to increased abdominal fat, resistance to the blood-sugar lowering action of INSULIN and increased risk of cardiovascular disease.

DHEA supports a healthy immune response. Low DHEA blood levels increase the risk of infection. DHEA may be effective against autoimmune diseases like RHEUMATOID ARTHRITIS and lupus, in which the immune system attacks the body. DHEA apparently increases the levels of a growth factor (Insulin-like Growth Factor) that boosts cell metabolism and helps regulate immunity. In men DHEA administration may activate T-cells called natural killer cells that combat viruses. Current research suggests that this powerful hormone plays a role in the aging process, and administering DHEA to older men and women can increase the sense of physical and mental well-being. However, this hormone does not prevent aging. (See also ADRENAL GLANDS; ENDOCRINE SYSTEM; IMMUNE SYSTEM.)

Ebeling, Peretti, and Koivisto, "Physiological importance of dehydroepiandrosterone," *Lancet*, 343 (1994), pp. 1479–8.

diabetes, gestational (maternal hyperglycemia)

Persistently elevated BLOOD SUGAR that may occur during pregnancy. Gestational diabetes occurs in about 2% of pregnancies. In most cases the mother's carbohydrate regulation generally returns to normal after birth. The American College of Obstetrics and Gynecology recommends that all pregnant women be screened for diabetes. Gestational diabetes seems to be caused when the hormones of pregnancy prevent INSULIN from acting normally. Like non-insulin dependent DIABETES MELLITUS, gestational diabetes results from reduced insulin sensitivity in muscle and other tissues. It increases the risk of difficult pregnancies, stillbirths, high birth weights and birth defects. Women at risk include those with a family history of the disease or with HYPERTENSION; with previous difficult pregnancies; who are older than 30 to 35; or who are obese. (See also CARBOHYDRATE METABOLISM; GLUCOSE TOLERANCE; GLYCEMIC INDEX.)

diabetes insipidus

A rare disease characterized by excessive urine production without glucose excretion. The resulting copious water loss creates an intense thirst (POLYDIPSIA). This condition is caused by the inadequate secretion of ANTIDIURETIC HORMONE from the PITUITARY GLAND, unlike DIABETES MELLITUS, which is caused by an imbalance in carbohydrate utilization. Diabetes insipidus can be associated with pituitary cancer, inflammation of the pituitary or hypothalamus, meningitis and even tuberculosis. Likewise, antidiuretic hormone production may be diminished after surgical or radiation damage to the pituitary gland, severe head injuries or unknown (idiopathic) causes. (See also DEHYDRATION; ELECTROLYTES).

diabetes mellitus

A common disease characterized by excessive BLOOD-SUGAR levels after a meal and by excessive production of urine containing an abnormal amount of GLUCOSE. When the body does not effectively absorb GLUCOSE from blood, blood sugar remains elevated for an abnormally long time. (In diabetes insipidus, altered kidney function leads to excessive urine production.) Diabetes is one of the most prevalent degenerative diseases in the United States, where it strikes one out of every 20 people. It is increasing at the rate of 5% per year in epidemic proportions and is the third major killer in the United States. Significantly, half of those with diabetes are undiagnosed because the disease does not cause painful symptoms. Early symptoms include fatigue, numbness or cramping of legs, feet or hands, and slowed wound healing. There are many complications of this disease: DEHYDRATION, with increased thirst, ELECTROLYTE imbalance, muscle weakness, increased infections of the urinary tract, early ATHEROSCLEROSIS and HYPERTENSION, poor blood supply to arms and legs potentially leading to gangrene, eye problems and blindness, kidney disease, and shortened life span. A GLUCOSE TOLERANCE TEST would reveal abnormally high blood sugar levels if they remain elevated three to six hours after ingesting glucose. When blood sugar levels increase to about 180 mg/dl, the kidney passes glucose into the urine; extra water is drawn into the urine, resulting in frequent urination and excessive thirst.

In diabetes two sorts of events may occur: Either microscopic cells of the pancreas (beta cells) produce too little INSULIN, the hormone needed by tissues to take up glucose, or the released insulin may be ineffective when tissues depending on it for the uptake of glucose become resistant to its normal action. During untreated, severe diabetes mellitus, the inability to use blood sugar creates a state resembling STARVATION. The body responds by degrading stored fat for energy, which can lead to excessive KETONE BODIES, acids from fat metabolism that produce acidic conditions (ACIDOSIS), mineral imbalance and frequent urination.

Insulin-dependent Diabetes Mellitus (IDDM)

IDDM is also known as Type I diabetes or juvenile onset diabetes. Patients with IDDM require insulin injections to lower blood sugar because the PANCREAS is damaged and cannot produce insulin. IDDM often begins suddenly and primarily children are affected, though it may affect adults. IDDM appears to be an AUTOIMMUNE DISEASE in which malfunction of the immune system destroys insulin-producing cells. One of the earliest indications is the production of an antibody capable of attacking the insulin-producing cells. Viral infections such as (measles, mumps, flu, hepatitis), chemicals or other agents may trigger the immune system to backfire. There are no known means of preventing IDDM and there is no cure.

Non-insulin-dependent Diabetes Mellitus (NIDDM) (Type II, Adult Onset Diabetes)

NIDDM is also designated as adult onset diabetes or Type II diabetes. In general, NIDDM patients do not depend on insulin injections; thus NIDDM is a less severe form of the disease. NIDDM occurs five times more frequently than insulin-dependent diabetes. It slowly progresses from beginnings in the teen years with prolonged elevation of blood glucose and often is detected only in its later stages, when it affects primarily adults over the age of 40. The problem often lies in the body's inability to use insulin efficiently. As an example, the number of insulin attachment sites on tissues diminishes with OBESITY, a condition to which NIDDM is frequently related. Inheritance can play a role; having relatives with diabetes increases the risk of developing NIDDM, possibly related to an inherited defect in sugar metabolism. Without treatment, patients gradually become increasingly resistant to insulin action, and they may reach a point at which they can no longer compensate for elevated blood sugar.

Treatment

The treatment of diabetes focuses on stabilizing blood sugar at normal levels (60–160 mg/dl of blood), improving nutritional status, implementing a weight management strategy and preventing secondary conditions: eye disorders, cardiovascular disease, kidney disease, nerve degeneration, reduced circulation and infections. In IDDM insulin must be administered and blood sugar and insulin must be balanced throughout the day especially with carbohydrate meals. Excessive insulin administration can lead to severe HYPOGLYCEMIA.

General dietary guidelines include eating regular meals and snacks; minimizing consumption of sugar and sugary foods and sweets; minimizing high-fat foods and emphasizing whole or fresh or minimally processed foods. These steps can minimize a rapid increase in blood sugar, permit more effective regulation by insulin, and permit better utilization of fat.

Syndrome X is a constellation of signs and symptoms often related to NIDDM: obesity, (especially "apple" or android obesity), elevated blood sugar, elevated insulin (HYPERINSULINEMIA), elevated blood pressure, high LDL-cholesterol and low HDL-cholesterol. High carbohydrate diet contributes to the appearance of Syndrome X, which carries the risk of CARDIOVASCULAR DISEASE.

Recent discoveries shed light on mechanisms of weight control and diabetes. Defects in a gene (beta$_3$ adrenergic acceptor) that codes for the binding site for norepinephrine a brain chemical (NEUROTRANSMITTER), increase the risk of middle-age obesity and NIDDM. According to one model, fat tissue secretes LEPTIN, a protein that travels to the hypothalamus (brain). There it could decrease production of neuropeptides that trigger appetite, and also activate sympathetic nerves that release norepinephrine. Normally this neurotransmitter directs fat cells to boost their metabolic rate to burn more fatty acids, but if their coupling site for norepinephrine is inefficient, fat calories may not be burned so easily. The question remains, does diabetes cause obesity or does obesity cause diabetes?

Several recommendations have been made to minimize the effects of non-insulin-dependent diabetes: If overweight, weight loss and weight control is the primary means of prevention as well as treatment. If these prove ineffective, oral hypoglycemic (blood-lowering drugs) may be prescribed. Often patients who lose weight also reduce their need for medication. Regular aerobic EXERCISE and fitness programs help the body burn glucose. Elevating the heart rate for at least 30 minutes three times weekly is recommended to burn glucose and increase the efficiency of insulin action.

While moderate amounts of SUCROSE (table sugar) in a simple meal may be tolerated by diabetics, over time sucrose consumption can have undesirable effects on metabolism. SUGAR increases blood fat (TRIGLYCERIDES) and CHOLESTEROL levels in some people, and diabetics are prone to HEART DISEASE, which is linked to high lipid levels. Sugar-rich foods often contain extra fat and oils. The current recommendation is to minimize sucrose consumption and to monitor individual response. Fructose has a lower glycemic response than sucrose; however, large amounts can raise LDL-cholesterol and there is no clear-cut advantage to using fructose.

Regarding fat consumption, a reasonable approach is to limit fat intake to no more than 25–30% of daily calories, with no more than a third coming from animal fat and hydrogenated vegetable oils. Increasing complex carbohydrate and increasing fiber from fruit and vegetables to 50% or more of daily calories, with reduced intake of refined carbohydrate, seems prudent. Weight loss diets need to be tailored carefully for the individual.

During the last decade, the major emphasis has been on high complex carbohydrate–low-fat diets with increased FIBER for diabetics. For example, the American Diabetic Association recommends a high COMPLEX CARBOHYDRATE diet, provided that blood LIPIDS are also monitored during medical supervision. Such diets can increase the risk of heart disease in some people. Apparently the high insulin levels required to process a high carbohydrate diet can increase blood triglycerides in some people. Consult a specialist before increasing dietary fiber because it may lower medication or insulin requirements, and a high fiber diet (above 30 g/day) may not be tolerated well.

Specific nutrients have been shown to help improve the body's ability to dispose of blood sugar, especially when deficiencies are present: vitamins including NIACIN, NIACINAMIDE, VITAMIN B$_6$, BIOTIN, VITAMIN C; and minerals such as CHROMIUM, VANADIUM, COPPER, MANGANESE, MAGNESIUM and SELENIUM. Chromium supports the action of insulin and biotin supports glucose and fatty acid metabolism by the liver. Magnesium and vitamin B$_6$, zinc and niacin have been found to improve the nutritional status of diabetics. Antioxidants, including vitamin E, vitamin C and selenium, may help in preventing cataracts. Essential fatty acids containing GAMMA LINOLENIC ACID as supplied by borage, primrose or black currant seed oils may be correct imbalances in essential fatty acids.

Sorbitol accumulation within cells is believed to be a major contributing factor in diabetic-related damage. This glucose derivative, once formed within cells, tends to disturb water balance and disrupt cell function. Sorbitol formation can be inhibited by vitamin C. In addition, vitamin C and other antioxidants slow the rate at which excess blood sugar attaches to proteins, a detrimental process that accelerates with elevated blood sugar levels. FLAVONOIDS work with vitamin C to enhance capillary strength and connective tissue integrity, which may be compromised in diabetics. Vitamin B$_{12}$ can help prevent both neuropathy and retinopathy associated with diabetes. In older diabetic patients, digestive function may be compromised and digestive aids may be appropriate.

Helmrich, Susan P. et al., "Physical Activity and Reduced Occurrence of Non-insulin-dependent Diabetes Mellitus," *New England Journal of Medicine*, 325:3 (1991), pp. 147–52.

Olefsky, J.M. and Nolan, J.J., "Insulin Resistance and Non-insulin-dependent Diabetes Mellitus: Cellular and Molecular Mechanisms," *American Journal of Clinical Nutrition*, 61:supp. (1995), pp. 980S–986S.

diarrhea A condition characterized by frequent, loose bowel movements. Diarrhea may be chronic, lasting for weeks or months, or it may occur abruptly and last a short time (acute diarrhea). Acute diarrhea, is usually due to an intestinal viral disease or parasitic infection (dysentery), excessive fruit consumption or a FOOD SENSITIVITY. Too much roughage or bulk in foods like fruit, bran, prunes, apples and pears; psyllium products marketed as natural laxatives; chemical poisons; and certain medications like erythromycin and tetracycline may cause diarrhea.

Diarrhea involves several different mechanisms:

- Osmotic diarrhea refers to excessive fluid retention in the intestines due to the increased concentration of water-soluble materials in the intestine. This can be caused by laxatives containing magnesium (milk of magnesia, epsom salts), carbohydrate malabsorption such as LACTOSE INTOLERANCE; excessive non-metabolized sweeteners like SORBITOL; excessive VITAMIN C; and excessive consumption of legumes, like beans.
- Secretory diarrhea results from excessive secretion of ions into the intestine, which draws water into the stool. Laxative abuse, fat malabsorption syndromes, infection by bacteria that produce toxins (poisons) often trigger bouts of diarrhea.
- Inflammatory disease, such as COLITIS, CROHN'S DISEASE, bacterial infection, parasitic infection.

Re-establishment of normal intestinal bacteria may be important in treating diarrhea. Friendly bacteria like lactobacillus and BIFIDOBACTERIA limit the growth of disease-causing bacteria and have antifungal and antiviral activity. It is important to drink plenty of fluids during bouts of diarrhea to prevent DEHYDRATION. If diarrhea persists more than several days, or if it is accompanied by fever or weakness, a physician should be consulted for a detailed diagnosis and treatment plan. (See also ANTIBIOTICS; GIARDIASIS.)

Fernandez, C.F., Shahani, K.M. and Amer, M.A., "Control of Diarrhea by Lactobacilli," *Journal of Applied Nutrition*, 40:1 (1988), pp. 32–43.

diastolic blood pressure

The least fluid pressure in arteries when the heart relaxes after its contraction (between heart beats). The range for normal is 60 to 90 mm of mercury. Elevated diastolic pressure can result from constriction of arterioles (the smallest vessels carrying oxygenated blood to the capillaries) of the circulatory system, as during a response to stress.

Elevated diastolic pressure is a prime indicator of HYPERTENSION, (high blood pressure), one of the leading risk factors for CARDIOVASCULAR DISEASE. In adults systolic pressure of 160 mm/Hg (the pressure during heart contraction) and a diastolic pressure of 95 mm/Hg (expressed as the ratio, 160/95) is considered indicative of hypertension. (See also BLOOD PRESSURE; CAFFEINE; SODIUM.)

dicoumarin (dicumarol)

An oral anticoagulant used to treat abnormal clotting in blood vessels. Dicoumarin is classified as an ANTIVITAMIN; it interferes with the complex process of BLOOD CLOTTING by preventing VITAMIN K from activating clotting factors in the blood, thus retarding the activation of FIBRIN, the blood protein that forms the foundation of a blood clot.

Do not take dicoumarin if there is any bleeding disorder, ulcerative colitis, CROHN'S DISEASE, or an ulcer in the stomach or intestine. Alcohol consumption can either raise or lower dicoumarin's anticoagulant properties. Foods that contain high levels of vitamin K, especially liver, and green leafy vegetables like spinach can decrease the anticoagulant effect of this drug.

diet The portions and types of foods and beverages consumed on a regular basis. A BALANCED DIET provides all nutrients at levels needed for growth and maintenance of health. A diet can also be a prescribed meal plan, specifying food consumption for a particular health condition or disease state. Four examples are bland diets, clear liquid diets, ELEMENTAL DIETS and LOW-FAT DIETS.

Bland diets Bland diets are traditional nutritional approaches to the treatment of peptic ulcers. They are built around milk, soft-fiber foods, milk toast, poached eggs, creamed cereals, strained cream soups, white crackers, rennet milk pudding, custard and gelatin desserts, bananas, cooked vegetables as tolerated, fruit juice, cooked or canned fruit, potatoes, pasta, butter or margarine. They omits foods that may cause distress: strongly flavored seasonings, olives, pickles, caffeinated beverages and COFFEE, fried pastries and rice, salad dressings, bran cereals, nuts, raw vegetables, most fresh fruits and gas-forming foods (brussels sprouts, cabbage, cauliflower, cucumber and the like).

Clear liquid diets Clear liquid diets contain foods that remain clear and liquid at room temperature. They are used to provide fluids and electrolytes and to prevent dehydration. This diet would contain BOUILLON, broth, carbonated beverages, coffee, filtered or strained fruit juices, gelatin desserts and commercially prepared clear-liquid formulas.

Elemental diets Elemental diets are chemically defined formulas. They contain nutrients in their simplest forms; for example, AMINO ACIDS may be included in the form of protein hydrolyzates rather than as proteins. Elemental diets are appropriate in those who cannot digest food adequately and therefore require simple nutrients.

Low-fat diets When a group of American men with blocked arteries followed a diet providing no more than 10% of total calories as fat, coupled with exercise, support groups, meditation and counseling, their blocked arteries were cleared. They were able to keep off an average of 22 pounds from four to eight years afterward. It is not clear whether such a low-fat diet is generally appropriate for adults. Children and young adults into their early twenties continue to grow and have greater nutritional needs unlikely to be met with very low intake of fat. By eating mostly fruits, vegetables and grains, and avoiding high calorie food, people will often tend to lose weight. However, approximately 10% of Americans respond to a high carbohydrate diet by increasing blood fat (triglyceride) levels, which can increase the risk of adult onset diabetes and possibly increase the risk of heart disease. (See also DIETING; ROTATION DIET.)

Downer, Nelda and Gregory, Janet, "Nationalizing Nutrition Education," *School, Foodservice & Nutrition*, June/July 1994, pp. 88–93.
Woteki, Catherine E. and Thomas, Paul R. eds. *Eat for Life*. Washington D.C.: National Academy Press, 1992.

diet, high complex carbohydrate

A high-fiber diet that typically emphasizes whole, fresh and minimally processed foods to provide 60% or more calories as CARBO-HYDRATE, mainly as COMPLEX CARBOHYDRATE, 10 to 15% as PROTEIN and 30% or less as FAT. A high complex carbohydrate diet resembles a typical Oriental meal. The fat comes from whole GRAINS, VEGETABLE OILS, lean MEAT and FISH, low-fat dairy products, and nuts and seeds; the protein comes from grains, lean meat, plus low-fat dairy products. Starchy foods like BEANS and lentils add protein and FIBER. Lentils also increase BLOOD SUGAR slowly, thus potentially increasing GLUCOSE TOLERANCE (the body's ability to dispose of blood sugar rapidly and effectively).

A high-fiber, high complex carbohydrate diet often helps improve the body's ability to manage blood sugar. Such a diet is associated with lower fasting blood sugar levels and lower insulin requirements. Dietary fiber slows the rate of DIGESTION by slowing the rate of food passing through the intestines, and water-soluble fiber seems to reduce the rate of glucose absorption.

High-fiber diets supplemented with fiber up to 50 g daily, have been used to lower blood lipids and to lower blood cholesterol. On the other hand high-fiber diets can raise blood lipids and/or blood sugar among diabetics, cause excessive insulin production and lower the desirable kind of blood CHOLESTEROL, HIGH-DENSITY LIPOPROTEIN (HDL). Therefore, a high complex carbohydrate diet may not be advisable for some non-insulin-dependent diabetics and patients with high blood pressure. People who eat a high complex carbohydrate diet should monitor their blood fat and blood cholesterol. Other individuals may not tolerate a high-fiber diet because it can cause gas, cramping and diarrhea. Obese diabetics should lose weight and exercise in addition to changing their diet. The combined strategy pays greater long-term dividends. (See also DIABETES MELLITUS; GLYCEMIC INDEX.)

Hirsch, J., "Role and Benefits of Carbohydrate in the Diet: Key Issues for Future Dietary Guidelines," *American Journal of Clinical Nutrition*, 61:4, supp. (1995), pp. 996S–1000S.

diet, low carbohydrate   A diet providing inadequate CARBOHYDRATE with normal to high fat and protein consumption. Many "eat all you want" diets specify high-fat and protein, with little carbohydrate (less than 100 g a day). Without enough carbohydrate in the diet, METABOLISM switches to a STARVATION mode, regardless how much fat or protein is eaten. There is no evidence that this form of DIETING leads to permanent weight loss, and weight that is lost tends to be muscle rather than fat. Weight lost quickly represents water loss, accompanied by lost ELECTROLYTES.

The brain and nervous system require GLUCOSE (BLOOD SUGAR) for energy. When the diet does not provide enough carbohydrate, muscle protein breaks down to supply AMINO ACIDS. The liver converts them to glucose, which is released to raise blood sugar. Massive fat breakdown promotes the accumulation of KETONE BODIES in the blood, and disposal of these acids can cause DEHYDRATION and electrolyte imbalances. Side effects of low carbohydrate diets include nausea, low blood pressure and fatigue. Fat may deposit in the liver because the normal fat-burning machinery is overwhelmed by extensive fat degradation. Children, pregnant women, and patients with a history of GOUT should not diet to lose weight without medical supervision. (See also DIETING: CRASH PROGRAMS; FAT METABOLISM; GLUCONEOGENESIS; KETOSIS.)

diet, very low calorie (VLC diet, liquid protein diet)   Packaged, generally powdered formulations, with low CARBOHYDRATE and CALORIES. VLC DIETS supply PROTEIN and carbohydrate to provide 300 to 600 calories a day, but without adequate protein and carbohydrate in the diet, the body will lose 2 oz of muscle protein a day. VLC diet products available today represent improvements over earlier versions because they supply high-quality protein together with the required amounts of vitamins and minerals. These modifications help prevent the dangerous losses of heart muscle that sometimes accompany complete FASTING. Liquid or powdered formulations should meet the RECOMMENDED DIETARY ALLOWANCES (RDAs) for protein (AMINO ACIDS), VITAMINS, ELECTROLYTES and TRACE MINERALS. Including a modest amount of carbohydrate in the formulation minimizes muscle breakdown and loss of lean body mass.

Many commercial weight management programs use VLC diets to get a client's weight loss program off to a fast start. However, their use is a severe strategy, to be followed for a short time only. VLC diets require supervision by qualified personnel, experienced in monitoring weight management. Optimally, supervision is coupled with behavior modification and nutrition education programs. VLC liquid protein diets are designed for obese adults who are at least 30% above their optimal body weight and for whom OBESITY creates a medical risk.

The drastic reduction in calories characteristic of very low calorie diets can damage heart muscle and can lead to HEART ATTACKS in susceptible individuals. Clinicians cannot predict who is most at risk. Furthermore, these diets induce DEHYDRATION and electrolyte imbalance. Side effects can be nausea, dry skin and intolerance to cold. Drastic, short-term weight loss programs require routine monitoring by qualified professionals.

If the liquid protein formulation is to be used as a total weight loss diet, the label must warn that its use without medical supervision can lead to severe illness or death. If it is to be used to supplement a diet with more than 400 calories, the label must warn that the product cannot be used in weight loss diets supplying less than 400 calories a day.

VLC diets are not advised for infants, children, pregnant or nursing women, nor for patients with insulin-dependent diabetes or severe mental problems. (See also DIABETES MELLITUS; DIETING; DIETING: CRASH PROGRAMS.)

Prasad, Neni, "Very Low Calorie Diets," *Postgraduate Medicine*, 88:3 (1990), pp. 179–88.

dietary fiber   See FIBER.

Dietary Guidelines for Americans   Governmental recommendations to prevent disease and overnutrition, first published by the U.S. Department of Agriculture and the U.S. Department of Health and Human Services in 1980 and updated in 1995 (fourth edition). The following seven recommendations for all healthy Americans two years of age or older, together with examples of the rationale offered in those recommendations, are quoted as follows:

1. Enjoy eating a variety of foods.
Get the many nutrients your body needs by choosing among the varied foods you enjoy from these groups:

grain products, vegetables, fruits, milk and milk products, protein-rich plant foods (beans, nuts) and protein-rich animal foods (lean meat, poultry, fish, and eggs). Remember to choose lean and lowfat foods and beverages most often.

The Food Guide Pyramid illustrates [see p. 189] the importance of balance among food groups in a daily eating pattern. Most of the daily servings of food should be selected from the food groups that are the largest in the picture and closest to the base of the Pyramid.

- Choose most of your foods from the grain products group (6–11 servings), the vegetable group (3–5 servings), and the fruit group (2–4 servings).
- Eat moderate amounts of foods from the milk group (2–3 servings) and the meat and beans group (2–3 servings).
- Choose sparingly foods that provide few nutrients and are high in fat and sugars.
- Choose different foods within each food group.

2. Balance the food you eat with physical activity—maintain or improve your weight.

Try to maintain your body weight by balancing what you eat with physical activity. If you are sedentary, try to become more active. If you are already active, try to continue the same level of activity as you age. More physical activity is better than less, and any is better than none. If your weight is not in the healthy range, try to reduce health risks through better eating and exercise habits. Take steps to keep your weight within the healthy range (neither too high nor too low). Many Americans gain weight in adulthood, increasing their risk for high blood pressure, heart disease, stroke, diabetes, certain types of cancer, arthritis, breathing problems and other illness. Therefore, most adults should not gain weight. In order to stay at the same body weight, people must balance the amount of calories in the foods and drinks they consume with the amount of calories the body uses. Less sedentary activity and more vigorous activity may help you reduce body fat and disease risk. Try to do 30 minutes or more of moderate physical activity on most—preferably all—days of the week. Weights above the healthy weight range are less healthy for most people.

Location of body fat: Research suggests that the location of body fat also is an important factor in health risks for adults. Excess fat in the abdomen (stomach area) is a greater health risk than excess fat in the hips and thighs. Extra fat in the abdomen is linked to high blood pressure, diabetes, early heart disease, and certain types of cancer.

(Note: The 1995 guidelines recommend for the first time that adults should maintain a single healthy weight, and conclude that weight should not be gained with aging. The guidelines include weight ranges for specific heights, taking into account individual variation in bone, muscle and fat. The guidelines recommend a slow rate of weight reduction: one-half to one pound per week. This is far less than what is touted by many weight loss programs.)

3. Choose a diet with plenty of grain products, vegetables and fruits.

Grain products, vegetables, and fruits are key parts of a varied diet. They are emphasized in this guideline because they provide vitamins, minerals, complex carbohydrates (starch and dietary fiber), and other substances that are important for good health. They are also generally low in fat, depending on how they are prepared and what is added to them at the table. Most of the calories in your diet should come from grain products, vegetables and fruits. The antioxidant nutrients found in plant foods (e.g., vitamin C, carotenoids, vitamin E, and certain minerals) are presently of great interest to scientists and the public because of their potentially beneficial role in reducing the risk for cancer and certain other chronic diseases. Scientists are also trying to determine if other substances in plant foods protect against cancer. Eat more grain products (breads, cereals, pasta, and rice), vegetables, and fruits. Eat dry beans, lentils, and peas more often. Increase your fiber intake by eating more of a variety of whole grains, whole-grain products, dry beans, fiber-rich vegetables and fruits such as carrots, corn, peas, pears, and berries.

4. Choose a diet lean in fat, saturated fat, and cholesterol.

To reduce your intake of fat, saturated fat, and cholesterol, follow these recommendations, as illustrated in the Food Guide Pyramid, which apply to diets consumed over several days and not to single meals or foods.

- Use fats and oils sparingly.
- Use the Nutrition Facts Label to help you choose foods lower in fat, saturated fat, and cholesterol.
- Eat plenty of grain products, vegetables, and fruits.
- Choose low-fat milk products, lean meats, fish, poultry, beans, and peas to get essential nutrients without substantially increasing calorie and saturated fat intakes.

Specific recommendations for a diet low in fats and cholesterol:

- Use fats and oils sparingly in cooking and at the table.
- Use small amounts of salad dressings and spreads such as butter, margarine, and mayonnaise. Consider using low-fat or fat-free dressings for salads.
- Choose vegetable oils and soft margarine most often because they are lower in saturated fat than solid shortenings and animal fats, even though their caloric content is the same.
- Check the Nutrition Facts Label to see how much fat and saturated fat are in a serving, choose foods lower in fat and saturated fat.
- Choose low-fat sauces with pasta, rice, and potatoes.
- Use as little fat as possible to cook vegetables and grain products.
- Season with herbs, spices, lemon juice, and fat-free or lowfat salad dressings.

- Choose two to three servings of lean fish, poultry, meats, or other protein-rich foods, such as beans, daily. Use meats labeled "lean" or "extra lean." Trim fat from meat; take skin off poultry.
- Limit intake of high-fat processed meats such as sausages, salami, and other cold cuts.
- Limit the intake of organ meats (three ounces of cooked chicken liver have about 540 mg of cholesterol); use egg yolks in moderation (one egg yolk has about 215 mg of cholesterol). Egg whites contain no cholesterol and can be used freely.
- Choose skim or low-fat milk, fat-free or lowfat yogurt, and lowfat cheese.
- Have two to three low-fat servings daily. Add extra calcium to your diet without added fat by choosing fat-free yogurt and lowfat milk more often.

Partially hydrogenated vegetable oils, such as those used in many margarine and shortenings, contain a particular form of unsaturated fat known as trans-fatty acids that may raise blood cholesterol levels, although not as much as saturated fat.

5. Choose a diet moderate in sugars.

Scientific evidence indicates that diets high in sugars do not cause hyperactivity or diabetes. Avoiding sugars alone will not correct overweight. To lose weight reduce the total amount of calories from the food you eat and increase your level of physical activity. For very active people with high calorie needs, sugars can be an additional source of energy. However, because maintaining a nutritious diet and a healthy weight is very important, sugars should be used in moderation by most healthy people and sparingly by people with low calorie needs. This guideline cautions about eating sugars in large amounts and about frequent snacks of foods and beverages containing sugars that supply unnecessary calories and few nutrients. Use sugars in moderation—sparingly if your calorie needs are low. Avoid excessive snacking, brush with a fluoride toothpaste, and floss your teeth regularly.

6. Choose a diet moderate in salt and sodium.

Sodium has an important role in the body. However, most Americans consume more sodium than is needed. The Nutrition Facts Label lists a Daily Value of 2,400 mg per day for sodium (2,400 mg sodium per day is contained in 6 grams of sodium chloride [salt]). In household measures, one level teaspoon of salt provides about 2,300 mg of sodium. Most people consume more than this amount. There is no way at present to tell who might develop high blood pressure from eating too much sodium. However, consuming less salt or sodium is not harmful and can be recommended for the healthy normal adult.

To consume less salt and sodium

- Read the Nutrition Facts Label to determine the amount of sodium in the foods you purchase. The sodium content of processed foods—such as cereals, breads, soups, and salad dressings—often varies widely.

- Choose foods lower in sodium and ask your grocer or supermarket to offer more low-sodium foods. Request less salt in your meals when eating out or traveling.
- If you salt foods in cooking or at the table, add small amounts. Learn to use spices and herbs, rather than salt, to enhance the flavor of food.
- When planning meals, consider that fresh and most plain frozen vegetables are low in sodium.
- When selecting canned foods, select those prepared with reduced or no sodium.
- Remember that fresh fish, poultry, and meat are lower in sodium than most canned and processed ones.
- Choose foods lower in sodium content. Many frozen dinners, packaged mixes, canned soups, and salad dressings contain a considerable amount of sodium. Remember that condiments such as soy and many other sauces, pickles and olives are high in sodium. Ketchup and mustard, when eaten in large amounts, can also contribute significant amounts of sodium to the diet. Choose lower sodium varieties.
- Choose fresh fruits and vegetables as a lower sodium alternative to salted snack foods.

7. If you drink alcoholic beverages do so in moderation.

What is moderation? Moderation is defined as no more than one drink per day for women and no more than two drinks per day for men.
Count as a drink—

- 12 ounces of regular beer (150 calories)
- 5 ounces of wine (100 calories)
- 1.5 ounces of 80-proof distilled spirits (100 calories)

Who should not drink?
Some people should not drink alcoholic beverages at all. These include:

- Children and adolescents.
- Individuals of any age who cannot restrict their drinking to moderate levels. This is a special concern for recovering alcoholics and people whose family members have alcohol problems.
- Women who are trying to conceive or who are pregnant. Major birth defects, including fetal alcohol syndrome, have been attributed to heavy drinking by the mother while pregnant. While there is no conclusive evidence that an occasional drink is harmful to the fetus or to the pregnant woman, a safe level of alcohol intake during pregnancy has not been established.
- Individuals who plan to drive or take part in activities that require attention or skill. Most people retain some alcohol in the blood up to 2–3 hours after a single drink.
- Individuals using prescription and over-the-counter medications. Alcohol may alter the effectiveness or toxicity of medicines. Also, some medications may increase blood alcohol levels or

increase the adverse effect of alcohol on the brain. When you drink alcoholic beverages, do so in moderation, with meals, and when consumption does not put you or others at risk.

(See also DENTAL CARIES; DIETING; EXERCISE; FOOD; HEIGHT-WEIGHT TABLES; HYPERTENSION; TEETH.)

dietetic foods   Convenience foods processed especially for certain kinds of diets. Low-CHOLESTEROL, low-SODIUM and low-CALORIE dietetic foods are typical. For a diabetic, several dietetic products may be helpful, including artificially sweetened soft drinks, ARTIFICIAL SWEETENERS, and sieved fruit packed in water, not syrup.

The following terms now have specific meanings:

"Low fat" means that the food contains no more than 3 g of fat per serving; or the food contains no more than 3 g of fat per 50 g of food (if the serving size is less than 30 g or 2 tablespoons).

"Low sodium" means that the food provides no more than 140 mg sodium per serving. If the serving size is 30 g or less, or no more than 2 tablespoons, the food will provide at most 140 mg of sodium per 50 g of food.

"Low cholesterol" means that the food provides less than 2 mg of cholesterol (and no more than 2 g of fat) per serving. If the serving size is 30 g or less, or no more than 2 tablespoons, the food provides at most 2 mg of cholesterol per 50 g of food.

In contrast with the above established definitions, specifying foods as "dietetic" has no precise meaning because there are no standards to which food manufacturers must adhere for this designation. Dietetic foods may have reduced, though still appreciable, calories. The consumer often has difficulty in determining how well the product fits a given diet plan because determining the contents from food labels can be difficult. (See also DIABETES MELLITUS; FOOD LABELING; FOOD PROCESSING.)

diet foods   Processed foods marketed for individuals requiring low CALORIE, reduced calorie or calorie-restricted diets according to FDA guidelines. These products often reduce calories by incorporating ARTIFICIAL SWEETENERS that provide little or no calories. (See also DIETETIC FOODS; DIETING.)

diethylstilbestrol (DES)   A hormone analog of ESTROGEN, which is a female sex hormone. As a prescription drug, DES is used to treat symptoms of menopause (replacement therapy for estrogen deficiency) and menstrual cycle irregularities. It should not be used during pregnancy. DES has been shown to increase the possibility of toxicity when combined with tricyclic antidepressants. VITAMIN C can increase the estrogen effect of DES. Because DES can cause CANCER, it is not permitted in food. DES is a banned growth promoter of livestock. Occasionally DES residues have been detected in meat due to illegal use in livestock. The human health hazards of exposure to traces of DES in meat are unknown. (See BEEF; MEAT CONTAMINANTS.)

diet-induced obesity   See YO-YO DIETING.

diet-induced thermogenesis (specific dynamic effect) Heat produced in the body as a result of digesting food and absorbing nutrients. Heat is normally produced as the body uses energy for any of its activities. In other words, thermogenesis is proportional to the total CALORIES used daily. The portion used for DIGESTION and assimilation accounts for 5 to 10% of total calories. Glandular secretions, synthesis and release of DIGESTIVE ENZYMES, uptake of nutrients by the intestine, and transport of fat and lipids in the blood account in part for this energy expenditure. The energy required to operate body functions while at rest (BASAL METABOLIC RATE) accounts for another 60 to 70%. The remainder represents energy needed for physical activity. (See also ENERGY; EXERCISE.)

Visser M. et al., "Resting Metabolic Rate and Diet-induced Thermogenesis in Young and Elderly Subjects: Relationship with Body Composition, Fat Distribution and Physical Activity Level," *American Journal of Clinical Nutrition*, 61:4 (1995), pp. 772–78.

dieting   Restricting food intake in order to control weight. Dieting is a major preoccupation in the United States where the term "dieting" implies changing one's physical appearance to fit society's image of beauty. This raises issues of high expectation, self-esteem, sacrifice, guilt, and denial of underlying emotional problems. At any given time an estimated one out of every six Americans is dieting to lose weight. A 1994 Family Circle Nutrition Report found that 40% of women and 25% of men were dieting to lose weight on any given day. Some studies show that as many as four out of five preadolescent girls believe being thin is attractive and are eating to lose weight and that girls as young as 10 years old are dieting. This attitude may explain in part the modern epidemic of BULIMIA NERVOSA and ANOREXIA NERVOSA in young women.

Women's metabolism generally seems to run slower than men's by an average of 50 calories daily. This means they burn fewer calories. In addition, women's bodies have higher levels of enzymes for storing FAT, and lower levels of enzymes for burning fat, than men do. Hypothetically, these differences in metabolism favor child-bearing and fetal development.

Various methods are available to estimate an "appropriate" body weight based upon health standards, rather than an "ideal" body weight, which does not exist. Generally it is healthier to be within 10 pounds of appropriate body weight than overweight. Recent evaluations support the premise that thinner individuals (down to 10 pounds below the average weight of their group in height and build) may live longer, provided they are healthy and do not smoke.

Individuals with health problems, pregnant and lactating women, and children should not undertake self-prescribed popular weight-loss diets. The choice of dieting other than dieting for medical reasons depends upon diet history, distribution of body fat, activity level, health status, personal reasons for losing weight and degree of motivation. Heredity is another consideration; an estimated 25% of differences in body fat are due to genetic predisposition and family history.

How successful are diet programs once a desired body weight has been achieved? Estimates of dieters' success rates, for those who lose weight and maintain the new weight for at least a year, vary anywhere from 2 to 25%.

General studies provide clues as to why diets frequently fail:

1. Often the dieter's eating habits did not change while undergoing the dieting program. Without changing eating patterns the weight lost in a dieting program returns as soon as the dieter resumes usual eating patterns.

2. Many obese people underreport the amount of food they consume. Careful analysis of caloric intake and fat deposition reveals that they may eat more that normal-weight people.

3. STARVATION or semi-starvation is not a successful weight loss strategy. Drastically reducing food intake promotes a loss of 5 pounds a week, but it represents mainly water loss, not fat loss, and the body regains the water immediately when the diet ends. Losing more than two pounds a week, unsupervised, is not recommended because consuming fewer than 1,000 calories per day throws the body's physiology into a defensive mode for starvation. The BASAL METABOLIC RATE slows down to use fewer calories more efficiently. The body tends to keep the same amount of fat or to gain more weight later. Furthermore, starvation diets are too low in essential nutrients like vitamins and minerals, and chronic dieting can lead to serious health problems and malnutrition.

4. Often dietary goals are unrealistic and set up the person for failure. People who keep weight off tend to do it for their own satisfaction, rather than for an external expectation or pressure.

5. In YO-YO DIETING (a cycle of on-again, off-again dieting) the body can adapt to periods of low calorie intake by increasing its energy efficiency, although the effect on metabolism is not firmly established. Some people find it easier to gain weight and harder to lose it, even without overeating. Negative psychological effects of yo-yo dieting include negative body image, problems with interpersonal relationships and depression.

6. Some obese people cannot make permanent reductions in weight, even with severely restricted diets, without emotional repercussions. Some researchers have proposed that certain obese people have an altered metabolism. OBESITY may be locked into the number of an individual's fat cells, because children tend to follow the body build and fat cell distribution of their parents. Formerly obese individuals tend to store dietary fat as body fat rather than burning it. Recent research has demonstrated the presence of a hormone, LEPTIN, produced by fat cells that affects the appetite center in the brain to increase satiety and to curtail eating. In humans obesity seems to be linked more frequently to the decreased sensitivity of the brain to leptin than to the inability to produce leptin. Nonetheless it is unlikely that a single substance will treat obesity. Genes that are involved in weight control act together with diet and exercise, and probably no drug will substitute for either.

7. The lack of physical exercise is perhaps the most important factor in regaining lost fat. Exercise temporarily increases the body's metabolic rate even at rest, and it helps maintain lean body weight when dieting. It also seems to increase the sensitivity of the appetite control center, which tends to be blunted by a sedentary lifestyle.

8. Overweight people tend to prefer the taste of fattier food, and people who gain weight often eat high-fat foods like chips, fatty meats, fried foods, CHEESE and ice cream. Calories from fat are converted to body fat with a cost of 3% of calories. By comparison, 25% of calories from STARCH (GRAINS, LEGUMES, VEGETABLES, FRUIT) are burned in their conversion to fat.

What are typical recommendations for dieting to lose weight?

1. Avoid yo-yo dieting or diet cycling, crash dieting, and reliance on diet beverages and ARTIFICIAL SWEETENERS. They are ineffective weight loss strategies. Artificial sweeteners do not help with weight control and they may actually promote weight gain, perhaps by creating a craving for sweets, or by creating a false sense of security in eating calorie-laden food.

2. Choose a well-balanced, low-calorie diet providing about 1,200 calories per day for women and about 1,600 calories per day for men for prudent weight loss. The diet should allow for a mixture of whole, fresh foods. A diet plan should be developed and followed after weight loss in order to subsequently maintain the current weight.

3. Eat whole foods, instead of convenience foods, in order to stock up on COMPLEX CARBOHYDRATES, while cutting back on fat. Eating fruit instead of fruit juice and whole grains instead of white flour products provides more fiber. Chewing FIBER-rich foods puts a damper on hunger. Fiber also helps fill the stomach, which leads to a feeling of satiation.

4. Eat less fat, which provides more than twice as many calories as carbohydrates. Eat enough PROTEIN (40 to 50 g per day) to help lose fat, not muscle. An example would be eating 4 oz of MEAT, FISH or POULTRY and two glasses of skim MILK a day. Sweet and salty foods typical of many convenience and snack foods can stimulate HUNGER without satisfying it, and they may not satisfy hunger until excessive amounts have been eaten.

5. Cut back on refined sugars, which can increase hunger and promote weight gain. They boost the body's INSULIN level and this may be a hunger signal for the brain. Whole food snacks like unbuttered popcorn, apples and bananas will not stimulate hunger. The fat in fatty foods such as doughnuts, ice cream and pie is easier to convert to body fat than is complex carbohydrate.

6. Use supplements when needed. Many popular diet plans do not provide the RECOMMENDED DIETARY ALLOWANCE (RDAs) of VITAMINS and MINERALS, and supplements may be needed when the diet plan provides only 1,000 to 1,200 calories per day.

7. Make breakfast the main meal of the day rather than supper. Eating heavy meals at breakfast, followed by a medium lunch and a light supper, while consuming the usual amount of calories for the day, may assist some overweight people to lose 5 to 10 pounds per month without restricting their calories. Eating only when hungry, and eating smaller meals, can be important dietary modifications.

8. Obtain psychological support. A support group and a qualified counselor can help define and support individual goals. BEHAVIOR MODIFICATION can help change deep-set patterns. Exposure to cues that trigger eating can be controlled. Hostile and anxious people have higher than usual blood cholesterol and greater risk of heart disease, perhaps related to their tendency to burn fat more slowly and make more cholesterol.

9. Exercise regularly. Thirty minutes of aerobic EXERCISE will burn 300 calories. With regular exercise body fat can eventually be replaced with lean muscle, which burns calories at a higher rate. Because exercise increases the calories spent, calories are consumed rather than being stored as fat. Regular exercise helps maintain body weight at the end of the diet program because it counterbalances the body's adaptation to decreased food intake with lowered basal metabolic rate.

Dieting While Dining Away from Home

Eating out poses a challenge for anyone on a reduced calorie diet. The following suggestions may help in maintaining a diet plan when eating out or eating while traveling.

- EXERCISE before eating out to help burn calories and take the edge off HUNGER.
- Eat a light snack if dinner will be served later than usual. This will help avoid nibbling high-calorie snacks such as CHEESE, dips and cold cuts.
- Screen restaurants ahead of time to find those that offer low-calorie options.
- Trim off fat and skin from POULTRY to reduce fat intake.
- Drink less ALCOHOL and fewer soft drinks, which provide surplus calories. Choose mineral water or select non-alcoholic BEER or WINE. Drink more water to quench thirst.
- Share the order or order two appetizers or a soup and salad rather than ordering a full-course meal.
- Eat whole foods such as vegetables and legumes to obtain COMPLEX CARBOHYDRATE instead of fatty foods, which represent surplus calories.
- Order baked, steamed or poached foods, rather than fried or braised foods, which are cooked with fat or vegetable oil and supply surplus calories.
- Minimize BUTTER, sour cream or salad dressings that are essentially fat. Skip rich, high-fat desserts for the same reasons.

(See also BODY MASS INDEX; DIETING: CRASH PROGRAMS; FAT METABOLISM; HEIGHT-WEIGHT TABLES.)

Papazian, Ruth, "Never Say Diet," *FDA Consumer*, 28:8 (1991), pp. 9–12.

Perri, M.G., Nezu, A.M., Viegener, B.J. "Improving the Long-term Management of Obesity," New York: John Wiley & Sons, 1992.

dieting: crash programs   Drastically reducing CALORIES to lose weight rapidly, often by using APPETITE SUPPRESSANTS (AMPHETAMINES and DIURETICS) and by purging. Not only is there no evidence that crash DIETING leads to permanent weight loss, crash dieting is medically unsafe. Excessive weight loss, up to five pounds a week, represents mainly water loss, not FAT loss, and the water returns when the diet ends. STARVATION diets do not provide adequate levels of essential nutrients like CARBOHYDRATE, PROTEIN, VITAMINS and MINERALS. Without enough carbohydrate and protein, muscle protein can be lost at the rate of 2 oz per day.

The body adjusts to starvation conditions by burning stored fat for ENERGY. In this process, it can overproduce KETONE BODIES, a readily transported form of fat calories. Excess ketone bodies acidify the blood (ACIDOSIS) and cause dehydration and ELECTROLYTE imbalance. Crash dieting can lead to YO-YO DIETING, a cycle of on-again, off-again dieting. The body may responds by storing fat, not losing it. Crash dieting for several days can also lead to critical losses of fluids and electrolytes.

Rather than crash dieting, consider eating 1,500 calories a day to lose a maximum 1 to 2 pounds a week (adult male), and 2,000 calories a day to maintain weight. For adult females, consider 1,100 calories a day to lose 1 to 2 pounds a week, and eating 1,500 calories a day for stable weight.

(See also BALANCED DIET; CONVENIENCE FOOD; KETOSIS; OBESITY.)

dietitian (Registered Dietitian, R.D.)   A health professional who provides dietary advice and plans and manages food preparation, and has successfully completed a course of study leading to professional certification. A dietetics educational program is in tune with conventional medical practice and typically emphasizes nutrition; food science; food preparation; assessment and dietary management for common clinical situations, such as pregnancy; diabetes and weight control; as well as management training. Much of the dietitian's training occurs in clinic/institutional environments. Program variations may also emphasize mental health or other specialty areas. College preparation to become a registered dietitian involves a four-year B.S. program, which qualifies graduates to take the certification examination administered by the American Dietetics Association. About half of the states require licensing. Applicants for licensing exams must be well prepared, with a degree in dietetics, food service management, nutrition or the equivalent from an accredited institution. Alternatively, a master of science degree program that meets eligibility requirements for the certification exam, can qualify an individual for state-approved certification.

diet margarine   See MARGARINE.

diet pills   A variety of drugs used to suppress HUNGER. AMPHETAMINES (Benzedrine, Dexedrine) are stimulants that have been prescribed for short-term weight loss (10 pounds or less). Newer drugs, such as mazindol, phentermine and diethylpropion, are safer than amphetamines. They mimic the effects of EPINEPHRINE (adrenaline) and block hunger signals in the brain so the patient will eat less food. Nonetheless, these drugs alone are not effective for large-scale weight loss because they do not lead to permanent changes, alter eating patterns or deal with food-related emotional issues and exercising—essential ingredients of successful weight loss programs. Because the use of these drugs does not lead to a permanent change in behavior the lost weight often returns when medication ceases.

Amphetamine-type drugs gradually lose their effectiveness so that higher doses are required to get the original effect. Side effects of amphetamines include nervousness, irritability, insomnia, a false sense of well-being, dry mouth and dizziness. Less common are blurred vision, vomiting, irregular heartbeat, HYPERTENSION and impotence. An important consideration is that they are habit-forming. Furthermore, amphetamines are dangerous in combination with monoamine oxidase inhibitors or with other APPETITE SUPPRESSANTS because the combination can severely increase blood pressure. They should not be used by patients with kidney disease, glaucoma, heart problems or a history of drug abuse or bouts of DEPRESSION.

Other diet pills incorporate DIURETICS, BULKING AGENTS or thyroid hormone preparations. Diuretics are drugs that increase water excretion by the kidneys; therefore, they are used to control edema, water accumulation in the body, and they do not affect fat loss. Bulking agents add volume to food without calories. They contribute to a sense of feeling full (satiety); so theoretically less food is eaten. Thyroid hormones speed up metabolism; however, the fuel that is burned seems to be muscle protein rather than fat. Their use for weight control is controversial. Other discoveries have paved the way to newer weight-loss drugs. Fenfluramine and phentermine have long been available. They increase the level of brain chemicals to diminish appetite and craving in seriously overweight patients, thus helping them avoid overeating. The drug close to dexfenfluramine (Redux) is representative of a new generation of drugs to control weight. Approved by the U.S. FDA in 1995, the drug is controversial. It works by increasing brain levels of the neurotransmitter serotonin, as does the popular antidepressant Prozac. There is a concern that Redux could cause problems in mood regulation. Fenfluramines can casue side effects, including drowsiness, constipation, memory loss and confusion. Rarely, they can cause a fatal lung disorder (primary pulmonary hypertension). No drug yet devised is completely safe and effective for treating OBESITY and for weight loss. (See also BEHAVIOR MODIFICATION; DIETING; MAO INHIBITORS; WEIGHT MANAGEMENT.)

diet record (diet diary)   A complete inventory of the kinds and amounts of all foods, beverages and supplements consumed for one or more days in order to assess adequacy of nutrient intake. A DIET record can be used to obtain an individualized estimate of daily calories. Typically, a record is kept for three days, one of which includes a weekend, or for a week. The amounts of food are recorded in terms of the number of ounces, slices, cups or tablespoons. For example, a piece of meat the size of a deck of cards is about 2 ounces. A NUTRITIONIST uses food composition tables compiled by the USDA to calculate the average daily consumption of essential nutrients, including vitamins, minerals, protein, carbohydrate and fat. Sodium, CHOLESTEROL, SUGAR and dietary FIBER can be calculated. Age, risk factors for disease, medical history, overall health and life-style, and dietary goals are other important parameters in evaluating the adequacy of a diet. (See also DIETING.)

digestibility (coefficient of apparent digestibility)   A measure of nutrient uptake, based upon the difference between the amount ingested and the amount recovered in feces in healthy individuals. The index of digestibility, the "coefficient of digestibility," represents the percentage of a nutrient assumed to be absorbed. Typical values for PROTEIN, CARBOHYDRATE and fat in the standard American diet are 92%, 97% and 95% respectively, indicating efficient digestion of major, energy-producing nutrients under normal conditions. These are approximations because intestinal microflora ferment undigested nutrients.

digestion   The breakdown of food to simple nutrients in the gastrointestinal tract. Food is a complex mixture of many nutrients, and during digestion it undergoes both physical and chemical changes to make these nutrients available to the body. In terms of physical changes, food is pulverized and mixed with SALIVA as a lubricant. STOMACH ACID produces further changes by denaturing (curdling) protein molecules. FAT, oils and lipid-soluble materials are emulsified by detergent-like BILE salts. These physical changes make substances in foods more accessible to the action of digestive enzymes. Each of the major sources of energy—CARBOHYDRATE, FAT and PROTEIN—undergoes HYDROLYSIS to release smaller molecules during digestion: PROTEINS yield AMINO ACIDS; fat and oils yield FATTY ACIDS and GLYCEROL; and STARCHES yield the single sugar GLUCOSE. Even table sugar (SUCROSE) must be broken down to its building blocks, glucose and FRUCTOSE. As food is digested, it is mixed, squeezed and pushed down the GASTROINTESTINAL TRACT by the action of the muscle of the intestine alternately contracting and relaxing in a wave motion.

Many enzymes are required to digest food. The mouth initiates digestion. Saliva contains the enzyme AMYLASE, to begin starch digestion. The second site of digestion is the stomach. The stomach produces hydrochloric acid (stomach acid) to sterilize food as it is kneaded to a thick liquid. Protein digestion begins in the stomach with the enzyme PEPSIN, released by tiny gastric glands in the stomach wall and activated by stomach acid. The stomach also manufactures INTRINSIC FACTOR, a protein that binds VITAMIN B_{12} to facilitate absorption of this vitamin.

The SMALL INTESTINE completes digestion and absorbs most nutrients. In this process the pancreas plays a key role. Pancreatic juice enters at the beginning of the small intestine (DUODENUM), providing a battery of enzymes to break down fats, oils, starch and protein, as well as minor food constituents like PHOSPHOLIPIDS, the building blocks of cell membranes. Secreted BICARBONATE neutralizes stomach acid. The intestine produces an activator of the protein-digesting enzymes. Bile released from the gallbladder emulsifies fat, prior to fat digestion by pancreatic LIPASES. In the last phase of digestion the intestine produces a battery of enzymes that completely digest PEPTIDES (protein fragments), starch fragments (maltose, DEXTRINS), fat fragments (diglycerides), LACTOSE (milk sugar) and table sugar (sucrose). FIBER is not digested in the small intestine because the body does not manufacture enzymes capable of hydrolyzing this type of COMPLEX CARBOHYDRATE.

A family of hormones work together to regulate digestion. These hormones are produced in many different tissues and affect the gastrointestinal tract in different ways. The following are representative: GASTRINS from the lower region of the stomach stimulate the secretion of pepsin and hydrochloric acid (stomach acid) from gastric glands. Gastrins also stimulate the secretion of bile from the GALLBLADDER and of digestive enzymes from the pancreas. CHOLECYSTOKININ from the DUO-DENUM, the initial section of the small intestine, also stimulates bile release from the gallbladder and enzyme secretions by the pancreas. SECRETIN from the duodenum stimulates BICARBON-ATE secretion from the pancreas to neutralize stomach acid and pepsin release in the stomach. Gastric inhibitory protein from the small intestine blocks stomach acid secretion, while stimulating INSULIN production by the pancreas. Motilin from the intestine stimulates gastric and intestinal peristalsis (the rhythmic contraction and relaxation of muscles around the gastrointestinal tract), while enteroglucagon from the intestine blocks intestinal peristalsis. Vasoactive intestinal peptide from the intestine promotes digestive enzyme secretion by the pancreas and intestine, while inhibiting stomach motility.

Individual amino acids, simple sugars and fatty acids, together with vitamins and minerals freed by digestion, are efficiently absorbed by the villi, the fuzzy, rough surface of the small intestine. Most of these nutrients pass on directly to the bloodstream. Fatty acids are an exception. They must be reassembled into fat molecules (TRIGLYCERIDES); together with fat-soluble materials like cholesterol and fat soluble vitamins, they are packaged as CHYLOMICRONS (fat transport particles), then released into the lymph, which carries them to the bloodstream.

The COLON (large intestine) completes the digestive process. It absorbs WATER and minerals like CALCIUM and MAGNESIUM, and forms feces. It is the home of beneficial bacteria that supply VITAMIN K and BIOTIN and other nutrients while limiting the growth of undesirable microorganisms. Much of the fiber in ingested food is degraded by the gut microflora. They produce short-chain fatty acids, which nurture the colon.

Diarrhea, and intestinal disorders like CELIAC DISEASE and CROHN'S DISEASE, reduce intestinal absorption of nutrients. Intestinal inflammation due to FOOD SENSITIVITIES, medications and infections can make the intestine porous, permitting foreign materials and toxic materials to penetrate the body.

The surfaces of the MOUTH, ESOPHAGUS, STOMACH and INTESTINES possess important barriers to unwanted materials and pathogenic microorganisms. Cells lining these passageways secrete MUCUS, a slippery viscous material that tends to trap foreign particles. Mucus production especially in the intestine declines with STRESS. In addition to the physical barrier, the immune system is important. For example, cells beneath the intestinal lining secrete an ANTIBODY (secretory IgA) that can neutralize the huge load of foreign materials to which the intestine is subjected daily. Stress and inflammation can limit antibody production, thus setting the stage for infections and multiple food sensitivities. (See also DIGESTIVE ENZYMES; LEAKY GUT; PANCREAS; PERISTALSIS.)

Ciprandi, G. and Canonica, G.W., "Incidence of Digestive Diseases in Patients with Adverse Reactions to Foods," *Annals of Allergy*, 61 (November 1988), pp. 334–36.

digestive disorders   See GASTROINTESTINAL DISORDERS.

digestive enzymes   A collection of enzymes secreted by tissues that degrade foods and release nutrients. Four regions produce digestive enzymes: the mouth, the stomach, the PANCREAS and the intestine.

AMYLASE (ptyalin) is a salivary enzyme that hydrolyzes STARCH to sugars.

GASTRIC JUICE from the stomach wall contains PEPSIN together with hydrochloric acid (STOMACH ACID). Pepsin initiates PROTEIN digestion and releases protein fragments. In the stomach, inactive pepsins (pepsinogens) released in gastric juice are rapidly activated by stomach acid.

The pancreas secretes many digestive enzymes into the intestine: Amylase completes starch DIGESTION initiated in the mouth. TRYPSIN, CHYMOTRYPSIN and CARBOXYPEPTIDASES A and B represent a battery of proteolytic enzymes that digest proteins to amino acids. LIPASE hydrolyzes fats and oils to fatty acids. Phospholipase degrades PHOSPHOLIPIDS to free fatty acids. Deoxyribonuclease and ribonuclease break down DNA and RNA respectively. An intestinal enzyme called enteropeptidase activates trypsin, which in turn activates other proteolytic enzymes. Therefore, the health of the small intestine is important in protein digestion.

The small intestine provides important enzymes that complete digestion, peptidases that degrade protein fragments called PEPTIDES to free amino acids and to very small peptides containing just two or three amino acids. All of these products of protein digestion are absorbed readily. Likewise sugars assembled from smaller sugars (disaccharides) must be hydrolyzed to their constituents in order to be absorbed. LACTASE digests milk sugar (LACTOSE); MALTASE digests maltose; SUCRASE digests table sugar (SUCROSE); and small fragments (DEXTRINS) are digested to glucose by destrinase. Inadequate pancreatic enzyme levels lead to malabsorption of nutrients and eventually to malnutrition. Inadequate levels of digestive enzymes lead to maldigestion and malabsorption of nutrients. Cystic fibrosis and chronic inflammation of the pancreas (pancreatitis) can decrease pancreatic output of digestive enzymes. Low stomach acid production plays a role in disease processes: Normally an acidic mixture of food paste leaves the stomach and stimulates pancreatic secretion, while an alkaline mixture does not, leading to maldigestion and malnutrition. Parasitic infections, bacterial infection, celiac disease, inflammatory bowel disease and intestinal resection can diminish the absorptive surface of the small intestine, decrease sucrase and lactase production, and produce lactose or other carbohydrate intolerances. None of the digestive enzymes in humans possess the appropriate specificity to hydrolyze fiber like CELLULOSE or PECTIN, so they are fermented by colonic bacteria to varying degrees. (See also DIGESTIVE TRACT.)

digestive tract (digestive system, alimentary tract) The continuous cavity extending from the mouth to the rectum, together with accessory digestive organs devoted to food ingestion, DIGESTION, nutrient ABSORPTION and waste elimination. These represent a huge task: During a lifetime, approximately 20 tons of food pass through the body.

The digestive tract consists of the mouth, esophagus, stomach, SMALL INTESTINE and colon. Digestion begins in the mouth. Chewing (MASTICATION) breaks food into particles and mixes it with SALIVA. Saliva contains AMYLASE to begin STARCH digestion. It also provides MUCIN, which acts as a lubricant for swallowing. The ESOPHAGUS is the long tube that connects the mouth to the stomach. A muscular valve separates the esophagus from the stomach's acidic contents. Acid indigestion occurs when the valve stays open for a period of time, allowing stomach acid to back up into the esophagus.

The stomach is located on the left side of the body, below the diaphragm. It produces the enzyme PEPSIN to initiate protein digestion and hydrochloric acid (STOMACH ACID) to sterilize masticated food and to catalyze pepsin activation. The stomach also produces GASTRIN, a hormone that increases acid production, and INTRINSIC FACTOR, essential for VITAMIN B$_{12}$ absorption in the small intestine. PERISTALSIS, wave-like contractions of muscles around the stomach and INTESTINE, moves chyme (a mixture of food paste and digestive fluids) through the stomach and intestine.

The intestine, a tube about 20 feet long, extends from the stomach to the rectum. The small intestine represents the upper three-fourths of the intestinal tract and begins at the pyloric valve, which regulates partially digested food leaving the stomach. The larger intestine or colon represents the last 5 feet of the intestine. The small intestine contains microscopic glands that produce enzymes to complete carbohydrate and protein digestion. Its enzymes also break down sugars like milk sugar, LACTOSE (with LACTASE) and table sugar (with SUCRASE) to simple sugars. It also digests small protein fragments (with aminopeptidases) to amino acids.

The small intestine consists of three regions. The first section, within a foot of the stomach, is called the DUODENUM, where BILE and pancreatic secretions flow into the intestine. Bile drains from the GALLBLADDER, after synthesis by the LIVER. The pancreatic enzymes are activated at this point. The JEJUNUM or middle region of the small intestine follows the duodenum. It is about 8 feet in length and ends with the ILEUM, which is about 12 feet long. The ileum joins the large intestine at a musclebound valve called the ileocecal valve.

Most nutrient absorption occurs in the small intestine. The highly folded surface is lined with a fuzzy coating, projections called VILLI, that creates a velvet-like appearance of the intestinal wall. The number of villi, 10 to 40 per square millimeter, dramatically increases the surface area to maximize absorption. Furthermore, each absorptive cell possesses many microscopic, hair-like projections called MICROVILLI that further increase the surface area. Nutrients taken up by intestinal cells pass into capillaries and lymphatic vessels. Any undigested or unabsorbed material enters the colon.

The colon represents the last 5 feet of the intestine. It is shaped like a hoop around the mass of the small intestine. The upward leg of the hoop represents the "ascending colon"; top of the hoop represents the "transverse colon"; the downward leg represents the "descending colon." The sigmoid colon is the last short section before the rectum. No digestive enzymes are produced by the colon. It absorbs mainly water minerals like calcium and magnesium and short-chain fatty acids from the bacterial fermentation of undigested carbohydrate plus fiber, and it condenses undigestible wastes as feces. The colon houses several pounds of bacteria; most serve useful functions. In particular they ferment fiber to produce short-chain fatty acids required by colon cells as fuel for normal growth. Other useful functions: Colonic bacteria produce vitamins and limit growth of disease-producing microorganisms. (See also CANCER; COLITIS; DIGESTIVE ENZYMES; MALABSORPTION.)

diglycerides A common type of FOOD ADDITIVE related to FAT and used to suspend fatty materials. Diglycerides pre-vent bread from going stale by blocking starch alterations; they also make bread soft. Diglycerides improve the stability of MARGARINE, and they improve the consistency of cake dough to make cakes fluffy. This additive also prevents the oil in peanut butter from separating. Diglycerides are common food additives and Americans eat more than a half-pound of glyceride additives per person per year. Glyceride additives account for about 1% of the normal fat intake.

Diglycerides are composed of two FATTY ACIDS linked to glycerol, while fat and oils are TRIGLYCERIDES, containing three fatty acids bound to glycerol. Diglycerides are readily digested and are considered safe food additives. A variety of additives related to glycerides have been created by food technology. Ethoxylated monoglycerides and diglycerides are used as dough conditioners to improve the texture of baked foods. Sodium sulfacetate monoglycerides are used as an antispattering agent and as an emulsifier in margarine. Acetylated monoglyceride and diglycerides are waxy materials used in jelly beans and chocolate coatings. Glycerides are also coupled to LACTIC ACID, CITRIC ACID and SUCCINIC ACID to form other emulsifiers.

dill (*Anethum graveolens*; false anise) An aromatic herb. Dill was cultivated by ancient Mediterranean civilizations; the Romans regarded dill as a symbol of vitality. Dill leaves and seeds can season sour cream, fish dishes ranging from salmon to crayfish, as well as bean, cucumber, potato and cabbage dishes. Bread and cheese may also be flavored with dill. In vinegar, dill is used in pickling.

dimethylpolysiloxane (methylsilicone, methylpolysilicone) An organic derivative of silicon. These silicon compounds are insoluble in water and chemically very stable. They find limited use in food manufacture compared to their widespread use in industry and in medicine. Dime-thylpolysilicone prevents foaming during steps in the manufacture of refined sugar, GELATIN, chewing gum and wine. Methyl-silicone is added at 1 to 10 parts per million to VEGETABLE OILS to prevent foaming when these oils are used in cooking. Silicones are inert in the body and are classified as safe FOOD ADDITIVES, although dimethylpolysiloxane contains trace amounts of formaldehyde as a preservative. (See also EMULSIFIERS.)

dioctyl sodium sulfosuccinate (DSS) A FOOD ADDITIVE whose detergent-like properties improve the suspension of powders in water. Many powdered materials like starch, cocoa and fatty acid derivatives tend to float on top of water. By coating these materials with DSS and similar detergent-like molecules, they more easily dissolve. DSS is used with thickening agents, powdered soft drink mixes and cocoa milk beverages (to dissolve cocoa butter). DSS is also used as a detergent to clean fruit and vegetables, and in sugar manufacture. In 1984 the U.S. FDA recommended additional health studies on this additive.

dioxin A widespread toxic pollutant. Dioxin refers to a family of chlorine-containing organic compounds that are industrial by-products; the most toxic member is TCDD. Dioxin now contaminates all populations in Western societies. Dioxin is a contaminant of commercial herbicides and the wood preservative pentachlorophenol, and it is created in wood stoves, in municipal incinerators and wood pulp waste from pulp mills.

Trace amounts of dioxin have been found in people not directly exposed to dioxin. The average American carries five parts per trillion TCDD in fat tissue; and it is present in the breast milk of nursing mothers. Despite this finding, experts of the U.S. EPA, the World Health Organization and the La Leche League advise that the advantages of BREAST-FEEDING outweigh potential disadvantages.

Dioxin occurs in meat, eggs, poultry and FISH. Fish likely to be contaminated include Great Lakes fish, walleye pike and bass caught from polluted waters. It is found in root crops like carrots, potatoes and onions grown in soil contaminated by spreading pulp mill sludge. Traces of dioxin contaminate paper and paper products like coffee filters, tampons, food packaging, milk cartons, teabags and disposable diapers. Dioxin appears to migrate into microwaved meat from paper trays. Often the amounts of dioxin are extremely small, 5 to 13 parts per trillion. This is equivalent to adding one drop to the water carried by the tank cars of a 10-mile train. However, exposure to one part per billion is considered a potential hazard.

Dioxin's toxicity varies with the animal species. When digested by some species of animals, like rats and guinea pigs, TCDD is toxic to the fetus; it causes cleft palate and kidney abnormalities, damages the immune system in newborns, and disrupts the hormone system causing feminization of male offspring. In some animal studies, dioxin causes CANCER in liver, thyroid, skin and respiratory tract.

Human toxicity of dioxin is controversial. Although the U.S. EPA considers dioxin the most potent known animal carcinogen, until recently there was little evidence for specific toxic effects in humans other than serious ACNE. In 1991 German and U.S. studies indicated that at fairly high exposures, as experienced by chemical workers, dioxin is a human carcinogen. The possibility of long-term, subtle effects remains. A 1994 EPA review suggests that dioxin can lower immunity in humans.

To reduce exposure to dioxin: Drink filterless coffee. This reduces exposure due to bleached paper products. Consume organic produce or homegrown produce that has minimal contact with PESTICIDES. Peel or thoroughly wash fruit and vegetables in soapy water. Avoid freshwater fish caught from polluted waters. Eat less fatty portions of meat, and dairy products with high BUTTERFAT. Dioxin is a fat-soluble contaminant and accumulates in fat. (See also BIRTH DEFECTS; RISK DUE TO CHEMICALS IN FOOD AND WATER.)

dips High-fat spreads used as appetizers and snack foods. Commercial snack dips typically contain high levels of sodium and saturated fat (cream cheese, sour cream, hydrogenated vegetable oil, palm and coconut oils). This is important because OBESITY remains a major health problem in the United States, and fat is more easily stored as body fat than as carbohydrate. Saturated fat is considered a risk for ATHEROSCLEROSIS in susceptible people. Excessive dietary sodium can increase the risk of HYPERTENSION in sodium-sensitive people. Home-prepared dips based on low-fat yogurt or low-fat cottage cheese can cut the fat content by 90%. (See also DIETARY GUIDELINES FOR AMERICANS; PROCESSED FOOD.)

direct calorimetry A laboratory procedure to measure the number of CALORIES in a food. Food is burned completely in the presence of pure oxygen in a "bomb calorimeter," a sealed chamber immersed in water. Heat released is absorbed by the water. The increase in temperature is measured and converted to calories. A large calorie (kilocalorie) is defined as the amount of heat required to raise the temperature of 1 liter of water at 15° C by 1 degree. The amount of heat released when food is oxidized completely to carbon dioxide and water is the same whether the process occurs in the body or in the laboratory. The amount of heat released—the calories burned—can also be measured directly by immersing a subject in water in an insulated chamber. (See also ENERGY.)

disodium guanylate (GMP, guanosine monophosphate) A FLAVOR ENHANCER used commercially since 1940. GMP contains GUANINE, a nitrogen-containing bicyclic organic compound (base). GMP is found in high concentrations in several species of fish and mushrooms. GMP has little taste of its own; rather it accentuates natural food flavors. In particular, this FOOD ADDITIVE increases meat flavor without adding more expensive natural flavoring.

GMP appears in instant soups, chicken salad spreads, canned vegetables and processed meat. GMP is degraded to the waste product URIC ACID and excreted. Individuals with GOUT (uric acid accumulation in joints) and with certain rare genetic diseases (related to PURINE metabolism) should not eat these foods. Otherwise it is considered a safe food additive. (See also MONOSODIUM GLUTAMATE.)

disodium inosinate (IMP) A FLAVOR ENHANCER used commercially since 1960. Flavor enhancers accentuate food flavors without contributing their own taste. IMP occurs in a wide variety of fish and animals where it contributes to the meat flavor of these foods. IMP is often used with DISODIUM GUANYLATE and MONOSODIUM GLUTAMATE (MSG), which act synergistically to produce a meaty flavor. By adding flavor enhancers, food manufacturers can use smaller amounts of expensive meat extracts in powdered soup mixes, ham and chicken salad spreads, sauces, and canned vegetables, which may contain IMP and disodium guanylate at levels ranging from 0.003 to 0.05%. Individuals with GOUT (uric acid accumulation in joints) and those who must avoid PURINES for genetic conditions should avoid this additive because the body converts it to uric acid. (See also FOOD ADDITIVES.)

distilled liquors Alcoholic spirits or liquors produced by distillation of products of FERMENTATION. Distillation concentrates ALCOHOL and characteristic essences of the material fermented. Thus distillation of fermented sugar cane and juice, syrup or molasses yields rum; fermented grain mashes yield whiskey and rye whiskey comes from wheatmash. Rum and whiskey rely on fermentation of mashes by special strains of distiller's yeast (*Saccharomyces cerevisia ellipsoideus*), which produce high alcohol concentrations. Aging distilled liquors in charred oak barrels further modifies the composition. It is important to realize that the alcohol content of one shot (1.5 fluid oz) of 80 proof gin, vodka or rye whiskey contributes about 100 calories—and no other nutrients (EMPTY CALORIES). (See also DIETARY GUIDELINES FOR AMERICANS.)

distilled water   See WATER.

diuresis   The excretion of large amounts of urine. Normally the pituitary gland (neurohypophysis) produces the hormone ADH (ANTIDIURETIC HORMONE), which causes the kidney to remove water from urine and return it to the bloodstream, thus conserving body water. A deficiency of ADH causes DIABETES INSIPIDUS, characterized by excessive, dilute urine. This condition should not be confused with DIABETES MELLITUS, which is a disorder of insulin production and utilization and yields excessive urine with a high level of sugar (glucose) due to high blood sugar. The large quantities of unreabsorbed glucose hold water in kidney tubules, thus causing increased urine output.

Ingestion of certain drugs (DIURETICS), ALCOHOL, CAFFEINE and large volumes of liquids increases urine output. In contrast, pain, stress, exercise and anxiety increase ADH production and decrease urination as do morphine, nicotine and common medications (clofibrate, carbamazepine and chlorpropamide). (See also ELECTROLYTES.)

diuretics (water pills)   Agents that increase urine production. Diuretics are prescribed to treat EDEMA (water retention) and HYPERTENSION (high blood pressure). These powerful drugs help the kidney lose sodium and water, so they increase the frequency of urination. Some of the safest and most effective are the thiazide diuretics. ALCOHOL and CAFFEINE also increase urine output, and thus are also classified as diuretics.

Thiazide diuretics should not be taken together with alcohol because the combined effect is a dangerous drop in blood pressure. This imbalance is potentially harmful to the heart. Thiazide-type diuretics can cause ELECTROLYTE imbalance, because they may increase the loss of POTASSIUM from the blood. Thiazides may also increase urinary excretion of MAGNESIUM, ZINC, RIBOFLAVIN and CALCIUM. Triamterene can increase loss of SODIUM and lower blood levels of VITAMIN B_{12} and FOLIC ACID. Furosemide can increase losses of calcium and sodium, and lower serum levels of potassium.

Recent studies link the use of diuretics to mild diabetes, increased blood CHOLESTEROL and an increased risk of HEART ATTACK; and they should not be used as weight loss aids. The rapid weight loss they promote is water loss, not fat loss. (See also BULIMIA NERVOSA; DIETING; CRASH PROGRAMS.)

diverticulitis (diverticular disease)   Inflammation of pouches or bulges (diverticula) in the COLON. Diverticulitis is a potentially serious condition when the contents of the colon are forced into pouches, leading to stagnation of fecal matter, infection and inflammation. This disease does not, however, seem to lead to cancer. Diverticulitis can be aggravated by FOOD SENSITIVITIES such as to MILK, WHEAT and CORN. Symptoms include: cramps, alternating DIARRHEA and CONSTIPATION, gas, bloating and indigestion.

Life-style changes may help prevent diverticulitis. Drinking plenty of WATER and eating enough FRUIT, vegetables and whole grain foods can prevent complications by keeping the intestine toned and by keeping material flowing through the intestine at a normal rate. The diet should minimize SUGAR and refined CARBOHYDRATES. Increased FIBER intake up to 30 g daily may be helpful; however, a patient with acute diverticulitis, ulcerative COLITIS or CROHN'S DISEASE should avoid fiber supplements because they may aggravate these conditions. Allergenic foods, foods causing gastrointestinal symptoms, and fruits with tiny seeds, such as STRAWBERRIES, RASPBERRIES and TOMATOES, can irritate the colon. LAXATIVES and enemas can irritate the colon. Regular physical exercise may help some patients. (See also ALLERGY, FOOD; DIVERTICULOSIS; GASTROINTESTINAL DISORDERS.)

Gabel, Lawrence, et al., "Dietary Prevention and Treatment of Disease," *American Family Physician*, 46:5 (Supp.) November 1992, pp. 41S–48S.

diverticulosis   A non-disease condition featuring diverticula (bulges) in colon without symptoms. Hernias (bulges) in the muscle wall of the intestine are very common later in life, and about two or three in 10 Americans develop this condition by the age of 60. The bulges are caused by straining to propel stools during constipation. A small fraction of individuals with diverticulosis develop inflamed bulges and pouches leading to cramps, alternating DIARRHEA and CONSTIPATION, gas, bloating and indigestion. Measures to prevent constipation include increased FIBER (roughage) consumption and drinking plenty of water. This means eating more vegetables of all kinds, LEGUMES, FRUIT and whole GRAINS. Safe, mild laxatives can also help avoid constipation. (See also DIVERTICULITIS.)

DNA (deoxyribonucleic acid)   The chemical that contains the genetic information of the cell and thus controls heredity. Genes are informational units of DNA that determine the individual's structural and biochemical traits, which are passed from one generation to the next. DNA specifies the structure of all proteins in the body, as well as the mechanisms for duplication and repair of DNA. DNA synthesis require many nutrients, including ZINC, MAGNESIUM and B vitamins like FOLIC ACID and VITAMIN B_{12}.

The structure of the DNA molecule is unique; human DNA is a meter long, yet it is tightly compressed into the cell's nucleus. DNA exists as compact clusters called chromosomes. DNA is classified as a polynucleotide, consisting of a sequence of four different kinds of cyclic compounds, resembling beads in a chain. The building blocks are called THYMINE and CYTOSINE, ADENINE and GUANINE. Their sequence defines (codes for) the sequence of amino acids in a protein.

Pairs of DNA chains twist about each other to form a double helix, resembling a double-railed spiral staircase with the steps composed of purine and pyrimidine extending inward. The sequences of bases in each DNA strand of the double helix are complementary to each other: a base of one DNA strand specifically pairs with its complementary base of the neighboring strand. The rule for complementary base pairing is simple: Adenine always pairs with thymine; guanine, with cytosine. DNA replication produces exact copies for new cells by using the parent DNA to serve as a template for synthesizing identical DNA chains.

Chemical agents in the environment as well as ionizing radiation can attack DNA, causing mutations, structural alterations in genes. The mutated DNA is passed on to successive generations. Changes in DNA structure alter the coding for specific amino acids, yielding mutant proteins with abnormal structures. Protein variants are common. For example, there are over 500 variants of HEMOGLOBIN in which a single amino acid is replaced by another. Most of these mutations are "silent" because the altered amino acid sequence does not impair biological activity. On the other hand, mutant proteins may be more or less inactive and can cause genetic diseases. Sickle-cell anemia, favism (sensitivity to broad beans) and familial HYPERCHOLESTEROLEMIA (inherited tendency for high blood CHOLESTEROL) illustrate the possible consequences of specific mutations. On the average 10,000 DNA "hits" per cell are repaired daily. Consequently mutations are infrequent events. As the organism ages, the DNA repair mechanisms become less effective. DNA damage accumulates in the cell nucleus as well as in the mitochondria, which contain a tiny chromosome. Cumulative DNA damage is believed to underlie the decline in immune function and the increased frequency of cancer associated with aging. (See also CARCINOGEN; GENE; GENETIC ENGINEERING; MUTAGEN; PROTEIN.)

Hartmann, Andreas, et al., "Vitamin E Prevents Exercise-induced DNA Damage," *Mutation Research*, 346:4 (1995), pp. 195–202.

docosahexaenoic acid (DHA)   A large polyunsaturated FATTY ACID that is concentrated in cold-water oceanic FISH and their oils. DHA, together with its relative, EICOSAPENTAENOIC ACID (EPA), seems to lower the risk of coronary heart disease, possibly by reducing blood fat and CHOLESTEROL levels (when initial levels are high) by slowing the production of LDL (LOW-DENSITY LIPOPROTEIN), the less desirable form of cholesterol. Both acids reduce the synthesis of APOPROTEIN B, a key component of LDL.

DHA and EPA also reduce blood clot formation. EPA seems to block the formation of thromoxane A_2, a factor that causes blood platelets to stick together, by slowing its production, while DHA seems to alter cell membrane properties. DHA and EPA may also reduce inflammation associated with AUTOIMMUNE DISEASE. DHA is necessary for normal development of the eye (retina) and the brain. Premature babies fed DHA-deficient formula have poorer vision six months after birth than similar infants fed DHA-supplemented formula. FISH OIL supplements help improve visual activity of DHA-deficient infants. DHA is a constituent of human milk, suggesting its importance in development. DHA levels are decreased in pregnant women with TOXEMIA and in the elderly.

DHA belongs to the omega-3 family of fatty acids derived from the ESSENTIAL FATTY ACID, alpha linolenic acid. It is a complex fatty acid with six double bonds and 22 carbon atoms. DHA and EPA can be synthesized to some extent by the liver from alpha linonelic acid. However, the intake of this fatty acid may be low, and its conversion may be diminished by dietary factors such as an excess of the more common essential fatty acid, LINOLEIC ACID. Consequently, the consumption of fish oils and fish can be beneficial. (See also ESKIMO DIET.)

Nettleton, Joyce A., "Are n-3 Fatty Acids Essential Nutrients for Fetal and Infant Development?" *Journal of the American Dietetic Association*, 93:1 (1993), pp. 58–64.

dolomite   A CALCIUM and MAGNESIUM mineral supplement. This supplement is a combination of calcium and magnesium carbonates. Since dolomite is a mineral, its composition varies depending upon the source. Because analyses indicate that dolomite may contain traces of LEAD, it is not recommended for children and pregnant women. (See also OSTEOPOROSIS.)

dopamine   The parent compound of EPINEPHRINE (adrenalin), a key stress hormone and a brain chemical. In the ADRENAL GLANDS, dopamine is converted to the hormones, norepinephrine and epinephrine. In the brain, dopamine serves as a NEUROTRANSMITTER, a chemical that relays nerve impulses. PARKINSON'S DISEASE, an uncontrollable shaking of hands and arms, is caused by the degeneration of a part of the brain (substantia nigra) producing dopamine. Dopamine cannot penetrate the BLOOD-BRAIN BARRIER and therefore cannot serve as a therapeutic agent. However, its precursor, L-dopa, can get into the brain, and it has had some success in treatment of this disease.

double-acting baking powder   See BAKING POWDER.

double-blind experiments   Clinical experiments in which neither the investigator nor the subject or patient knows who is in the experimental group that will receive the test substrate and who is in the control group until after the experiment has been completed. This approach attempts to eliminate the effects of preconceived ideas about a group's performance that could affect the study's results.

Carefully designed experiments employ subjects who are matched in terms of age, sex, health, status or other appropriate factors that could alter the results. In a typical scenario, subjects are randomly assigned to a control group and an experimental group. In a "placebo-controlled" experiment, the experimental group is administered a substance whose effect is being examined, while the control group receives an inert substance. (See also CLINICAL TRIAL; EPIDEMIOLOGY; PLACEBO.)

drug/nutrient interaction   The ability of medications to interfere with the uptake or utilization of a nutrient. Interactions between foods and drugs are very common. Elderly persons are more susceptible to drug/nutrient interactions because they are more likely to be taking multiple medications; also, they do not break down and inactivate drugs as effectively as younger people because their detoxifying enzymes are less active.

Drugs can affect nutrients themselves or they can increase the requirement for a nutrient by blocking its uptake or interfering with its normal function. The following are examples of drugs affecting specific nutrients.

- Analgesics (pain relievers). ASPIRIN competes with FOLIC ACID for uptake by the intestine. Chronic aspirin users need more VITAMIN C. Excessive use promotes gastrointestinal bleeding and an increased IRON requirement.
- Antibiotics that are not absorbed (such as neomycin) can promote LACTOSE INTOLERANCE.
- The use of ANTACIDS based on aluminum hydroxide to decrease stomach acid can reduce CALCIUM, phosphate, VITAMIN A and VITAMIN D uptake.

- Anticonvulsive agents and sedatives like diphenylhydantoin, phenobarbital and glutethimide increase vitamin D and VITAMIN K metabolism. They can create folic acid and VITAMIN B$_{12}$ deficiencies as well.
- Resin-type CHOLESTEROL-LOWERING DRUGS (such as Questran) interfere with the absorption of fat-soluble VITAMINS.
- DIURETICS (to treat edema) such as chlorthiazide increase MAGNESIUM and POTASSIUM excretion.
- LAXATIVES. Mineral oil interferes with the uptake of fat-soluble vitamins like vitamins A, D and E. Bulking agents and psyllium gum can interfere with RIBOFLAVIN absorption.
- Medication for Parkinson's disease. Levodopa increases the need for vitamin B$_{12}$, vitamin C and VITAMIN B$_6$.
- Corticosteroids (cortisone, prednisone) have multiple effects. They increase urinary losses of ZINC, potassium and vitamin C. They increase the need for vitamin B$_6$ and vitamin D and they can create blood sugar dysregulation.
- Hypotensive agents like hydralazine deplete vitamin B$_6$ stores.
- Oral contraceptives (conjugated estrogens, ethinyl estradiol) reduce bone loss and calcium excretion but deplete folic acid and vitamin B$_6$.
- Lithium (to treat manic depression) reduces SODIUM (salt) uptake. Conversely, a high sodium intake interferes with lithium.

Foods Can Also Interfere with Medications

- Milk and dairy products can bind some antibiotics like chloramphenicol used to treat infections and prevent their uptake. Wait two hours after taking these drugs before eating dairy products.
- Avoid liver, large amounts of cabbage and dark-green leafy vegetables including spinach when taking anticoagulants, drugs used to thin blood and prevent blood clots. Their high vitamin K levels can promote blood clotting. Limit alcohol and caffeine consumption.
- ANTIDEPRESSANTS (monoamine oxidase inhibitors) to treat depression, high blood pressure. Avoid aged, sharp cheeses; chianti and red wine; pickled herring, yogurt, chicken liver, bananas, avocados, pastrami, pepperoni, salami, meat tenderizer and yeast. Cut back on chocolate, cola beverages and coffee. These products contain TYRAMINE, which can lead to severe high blood pressure in combination with the monoamine oxidase inhibitors.
- Thyroid medications (to increase thyroid function). Avoid brussels sprouts, soybeans turnips, and cabbage. An ingredient in these vegetables can counteract this medication.

(See also ALCOHOL; CYTOCHROME P450; DETOXICATION.)

Roe, Daphne A. *Drug-induced Nutritional Deficiencies.* 2nd ed. Westport, Conn. AVI Publishing Co., 1985.

dry milk   See MILK.

dry weight (dry matter)   The weight of a food after water has been removed. Water accounts for much of the weight of foods; the water content ranges from 40 to 90%. To standardize contents, ingredients or compositions are often expressed as a percentage of dry weight to provide a more accurate basis for comparison.

duodenal ulcer   An open sore or lesion in the wall of the duodenum, the first 12 inches of the small intestine. Duodenal ulcer is one of the two ulcerative disorders of the upper gastrointestinal tract. Duodenal ulcers occur four times more frequently in men than in women. The most common symptom is chronic pain below the stomach, usually occurring 45 to 60 minutes after meals and that can be relieved by ANTACIDS and by food. This condition may be aggravated by excessive exposure to stomach acid and pepsin, the digestive enzyme produced by the stomach. Patients with duodenal ulcers have twice the number of acid-secreting cells in their stomachs as individuals without ulcers. Other factors implicated in ulcer formation include food allergies, cigarette smoking, stress, aspirin and other non-steroidal analgesics, alcohol and coffee.

An infection by the bacterium *Helicobacter pylori* is associated with over 90% of cases of duodenal ulcer. Eradication of the bacterium in duodenal ulcers protects against relapses. Conventional treatment entails bismuth salts and antibiotics.

Patients with ulcers in the digestive tract need medical attention, and complications such as perforation and hemorrhage present medical emergencies. A diet rich in whole foods that are high in COMPLEX CARBOHYDRATES can promote tissue healing. VITAMIN A, VITAMIN E and ZINC may be beneficial. Liquorice has been reported to help with duodenal ulcers. (See also ALLERGY, FOOD; DIGESTION; GASTRIC ULCER; GASTROINTESTINAL DISORDERS.)

duodenum   The first 12 inches of the small intestine. This region spans the upper region of the small intestine between the pylorus (the lower stomach opening) and the JEJUNUM (the middle section of the small intestine). It begins with the pyloric sphincter (valve) that regulates the flow of chyme into the stomach. BILE and pancreatic secretions flow into the intestine at this location through the common duct. The duodenum secretes an alkaline mucus to protect the intestinal wall from stomach acid and digestive enzymes. Chyme, acidic food paste released by the stomach, contains fat, partially digested protein and hydrochloric acid and stimulates the small intestine to produce SECRETIN and CHOLECYSTOKININ, hormones that stimulate pancreatic secretions. In terms of disease states, the duodenum is often the s ite of ulcers. (See also DIGESTION; DIGESTIVE TRACT; DUODENAL ULCER; HELIOBACTER PYLORI.)

dysbiosis   See INTESTINAL FLORA.

dyspepsia   Indigestion or abdominal pain that occurs during a meal or shortly after eating. The symptoms include heartburn, nausea, belching, feeling stuffed and flatulence. Many factors cause dyspepsia. It may be the result of a gastrointestinal disease such as FOOD POISONING, or it may be caused by nerve response to a disturbance in the abdominal cavity. Alternatively, food sensitivities, overeating, eating too quickly, eating under stress, and gulping air when swallowing, are functional causes of dyspepsia. (See also ACID INDIGESTION; ANTACID; HIATUS HERNIA.)

dysphagia   A difficulty in swallowing. Symptoms include food sticking in the throat, and coughing during swallowing. Dysphagia is associated with depression and anxiety. Food lodging in the lungs can promote respiratory infections. Possible causes of dysphagia include abnormalities in the structure of the mouth, throat or esophagus as caused by a tumor; infection and inflammation (e.g., tonsillitis); paralysis obstruction in the pharynx or esophagus, for example, following a stroke; diseases that affect nerves stimulating peristalsis, the wave-like contraction of the DIGESTIVE TRACT that propels food downward; and physical injury to the throat. (See also DEGLUTITION.)

eating disorders A class of diseases based upon obsessive behavior related to eating: ANOREXIA NERVOSA, BULIMIA NERVOSA and compulsive overeating. Eating disorders affect people from all socioeconomic classes and ages range from 12 to 60. Although both men and women can develop eating disorders, predominantly women are affected.

Though factors vary among individuals, the cycle of eating disorders seems to be initiated by psychological injury, including physical and psychological abuse among family members, reduced self-esteem, oppression, social isolation and nutritional insults, including faulty diet, abuse of drugs, alcohol and medications, and food intolerance. The resulting behavioral changes and altered eating can lead to a cycle of altered diet, altered APPETITE and hunger mechanisms worsened by nutritional imbalances, leading to further eating changes and compulsive behavior.

Anorexia nervosa, self-induced starvation out of an intense fear of becoming obese, was first described 100 years ago. It now occurs in an estimated 1% of American women. Although there is a genetic predisposition, social factors play key roles in determining the occurrence of anorexia nervosa. Symptoms include a markedly distorted body image and self-restricted dieting, leading to extreme weakness, muscle wasting and loss of 25% of original body weight, and cessation of menstruation. Anorexia nervosa is potentially life-threatening.

Bulimia nervosa is characterized by recurring episodes of binge eating (rapid, excessive eating), followed by purging. Most bulimics are women. Bulimia was first described in the United States in 1980 and the incidence in America is increasing. It is characterized by frequent attempts to lose weight by severely restricted diets, followed by episodes of bingeing, followed by deliberate vomiting or abuse of diuretics or laxatives, to lose weight. Bulimics generally possess low self-esteem and fear an inability to stop eating. Frequent fluctuations in body weight are common.

The third category is compulsive overeating, which refers to episodes of excessive overeating or bingeing in secret. Compulsive overeating is accompanied by repeated attempts to lose weight and diet. The increased occurrence of compulsive overeating among American teenagers parallels their increased prevalence of OBESITY. Compulsive overeating can substitute for confronting life issues and dealing with emotions and their sources.

Hazards associated with eating disorders other than obesity include starvation, electrolyte and fluid imbalances, liver damage, kidney damage, stroke, cessation of menstruation, diabetes, internal bleeding and ultimately death.

Eating disorders are complex conditions that profoundly affect health, and therapy entails multiple approaches including psychological counseling, support groups, nutrition counseling and, in extreme cases, medical intervention. Strategies that focus on weight reduction or diet modification alone are of limited effectiveness in treating eating disorders because they fail to resolve underlying psychological issues. The most comprehensive treatment programs address emotional, social, physical and spiritual components. Extended aftercare services as well as active participation in self-help groups support recovery.

Farley, Dixie, "Eating Disorders Require Medical Attention," *FDA Consumer*, 26:2 (1992), pp. 27–29.

eating patterns   Trends in food consumption in the United States; patterns of eating behavior, reflecting food choices based on personal habits, taboos, customs and family traditions. Food costs and food availability profoundly influence day to day food choices. Many personal values affect food choices: political conviction, such as conviction about the environment, or religious preferences (for example Catholic, Muslim or Jewish); perceptions of social status; conditioning through advertising. Food purchases are often made according to health concerns, thus recent trends in eating fewer EGGS, less whole MILK and less red MEAT are based in part upon consumers' concerns about CHOLESTEROL and clogged arteries.

The typical American diet, indeed the common pattern in industrialized nations, is low in fresh FRUIT and VEGETABLES and relies upon meat and upon highly processed food that is high in FAT, sodium and sugar. Such a diet does not supply adequate FIBER, TRACE MINERALS, VITAMINS and substances in plant foods whose antiaging and anticancer properties are still being discovered. Sweets and alcohol displace nutrient-rich foods, and lifestyle choices such as cigarette smoking and lack of EXERCISE alter nutrient needs.

Meal time has changed from eating at home with family, to eating quick meals away from home. For many Americans half of every dollar spent on food goes to outside meals. Generally, the odds of eating a less nutritious meal increase the more meals are eaten away from home. Often the choices rely on convenience foods and snack foods that contain high levels of fat, sugar and sodium. Teenagers often obtain 20% of their food from such snacks, which has a long-term impact on their health.

The typical United States diet is imbalanced due to nutrient inadequecy and nutrient excess:

1. Nutrient inadequacy. The typical diet provides less than half the recommended FIBER and inadequate amounts of key minerals (CALCIUM, IRON, ZINC, MANGANESE, SELENIUM, COPPER and CHROMIUM) and VITAMINS (VITAMIN B$_6$, FOLIC ACID, VITAMIN C) for specific populations, including low-income children, pregnant teenage women and the elderly.
2. Nutrient excess. The typical diet supplies too many CALORIES and too much FAT. Sweeteners in soft drinks, snacks, candy, ice cream and pastry supply 25% of the calories. Each succeeding generation of Americans appears to get fatter, and 27% are obese (1994). The typical diet supplies more fat than recommended to lower the risk of cancer and of heart disease. Paradoxically women often have a problem in finding diets that will provide all the vitamins and minerals they need, while lowering their fat and calorie intake.

Comparisons of United States food consumption patterns between 1970 and 1991 reveal how eating patterns have changed over the last two decades.

Meat   After reaching a peak consumption of about 85 pounds per person in 1975, annual beef consumption dropped to about 63 pounds by 1991. Though Americans ate less red meat, it still represented over half of the meat-fish-poultry total. Pork consumption fluctuated between 1970 and 1985, then stabilzed at about 47 pounds per person annually.

Chicken   CHICKEN consumption climbed to 43.9 pounds per person per year in 1991, exceeding pork consumption, following a steady rise over the last 20 years. Much of this increase represents high-fat food such as fried chicken, chicken nuggets and similar fast food. Ironically chicken as a convenience food is often considered low-fat fare.

Turkey   Consumption was 14.2 pounds per person per year in 1970, it more than doubled in the following 20 years. The increased availability of ground TURKEY, turkey breast and other easily prepared cuts probably accounts for the rise.

Fish and shellfish   FISH and SHELLFISH consumption remained steady at about 15 pounds per person per year after 1985. Fish prices have risen sharply in recent years, perhaps explaining the modest increase in fish consumption over the years. The most popular fish in the United States is TUNA, which is usually canned.

Eggs   The consumption in 1991 was 231 eggs per person annually. Egg consumption has declined steadily since World War II.

Butter   BUTTER consumption declined from 5.4 to 4.2 pounds per person per year.

Milk   Low-fat milk (1% fat) intake increased 340% from 29.8 to 99.9 pounds per person per year. More low-fat milk is consumed than whole milk. Whole milk consumption has steadily dropped from 213.5 pounds to 84.8 pounds per person per year. Skim milk (non-fat milk) consumption doubled from 1970 to 23.8 pounds in 1991.

Cheese   Since 1970 the annual consumption of high-fat hard CHEESES has more than doubled to 25.2 pounds per person. In part this increase is due to the popularity of pizzas and cheeseburgers.

Ice cream   Since 1970 annual ICE CREAM consumption declined only slightly from 17.8 to about 16.4 pounds per person. Ice milk consumption also remained nearly constant at about 7.7 pounds per person annually.

Grains   The annual consumption of flour and cereals increased from 135.3 pounds to 184.7 pounds per person per year, equivalent to 8 oz daily. Wheat flour was by far the greatest contributor to the diet, at 136 pounds in 1991. The consumption of corn products was 21.9 pounds per person yearly, while rice consumption was 17 pounds in 1991. Despite these increases, Americans ate only half as much cereal, bread, pasta and GRAIN products as their forebears did in 1910.

Vegetables   Americans ate 145 pounds of fresh vegetables per person annually in 1991 and 20 percent more produce than 20 years earlier. Potato consumption increased from 121.5 to 130.5 pounds per person annually and made up nearly 40% of the fresh vegetables consumed. However, fast-food baked potatoes and french fries contributed to much of this increase. Canned vegetable consumption declined to about 80 pounds per year per person, while frozen vegetables accounted for 60 pounds per person in 1991.

Fruits   Fruits (90.6 pounds) increased. Bananas were the most popular fruit, with an annual consumption of 25.3 pounds per person in 1991, up from 17.4 in 1970, while oranges decreased from 16.2 to 8.3 pounds per person per year. Apples increased from 17.0 to 18.7 pounds per person annually.

Caloric sweeteners   The average consumption of table sugar (SUCROSE) was 64.9 pounds per person per year, down from 101.8 pounds in 1970. The increased consumption of CORN SYRUP and high FRUCTOSE CORN SYRUP, 73.9 pounds, exceeded the decline in sugar consumption. The net consumption of sweeteners of all kinds was 140.2 pounds a year per person in 1991, amounting to a daily intake of over a third of a pound of refined sugar.

Beverages   The number one beverage in the United States was soft drinks, with the average American consuming over 43.2 gallons annually in 1991. Coffee consumption declined steadily from 53.4 to 26.8 gallons. Milk is the second most popular beverage at 25.7 gallons per year. Milk consumption slightly exceeded coffee consumption in 1991.

Fats and oils   At 4.2 pounds of butter per person per year, Americans were eating 25% less butter in 1991 than in 1970. In general there has been a switch from animal fat to VEGETABLE OILS (salad oil and cooking oil). Annual consumption of oils rose steadily from 15.4 to 25.2 pounds per person. Consumption of shortening (hydrogenated vegetable oil) increased from 17 to 22 pounds per year per person, while lard consumption declined to about 1.7 pounds per person yearly. In contrast, Americans ate more than twice as much MARGARINE (10.6 pounds per person) as butter and 13 times as much shortening (22.1 pounds) as lard.

Results of Surveys

Surveys provide insight about what Americans are eating and how they make food choices. Recent polls to discover whether Americans are becoming more concerned about nutrition offer conflicting results. On the one hand, many Americans realize that diet is a factor in health risks, while on the other hand, some results suggest that Americans have become less concerned about limiting high cholesterol food and obtaining adequate nutrients like vitamins. While heads of households have become more interested in many foods high in fiber and lower in fat and CHOLESTEROL, many also say that their health habits have not significantly changed. As many as 65% of Americans may be eating at least one high-fat snack daily. Although fat intake has declined from 41% of calories in 1981 to 37% of calories in 1993, this is far from the recommended 30% or less. Only 10% to 20% of adults reported eating the five daily servings of fruits and vegetables recommended to lower the risk of disease (1991). Currently Americans eat an estimated 2.5 to 3.5 servings daily.

Recent data indicate that Americans are getting fatter, and are doing less about it. In 1993 fewer Americans followed key dietary guidelines than in the previous 10 years, including eating enough fiber and avoiding overconsumption of fat. A 1994 survey by the Centers for Disease Control showed that 27% of Americans were obese; one-third of men and one-quarter of women fell into this cate-gory. The number of overweight people who were dieting in 1994 was 53%, down from 56% reported in 1985.

That the average American now weighs more than 20 years ago is perhaps related to the fact that food consumption has increased 20 pounds per person. As it stands now, Americans annually consume 55 pounds of fat and oil and 50 pounds of cake and cookies each year. While cutting back on obviously fat foods like butter, eggs and red meat, the average person is eating more invisible fat (salad dressing, MAYONNAISE, pasta toppings, pasta salad, fried fast foods, and baked goods like CRACKERS, cookies and CHIPS). The consumption of SATURATED FAT in food declined 16% between the 1960s and 1990, the most recent data available. Sources include saturated vegetable oils added to foods: COCONUT OIL, palm kernel oils and HYDROGENATED VEGETABLE OIL. Saturated fat increases the risk of CARDIOVASCULAR DISEASE.

Eating healthier means changing one's life-style. A number of experts recommend gradual change and moderation, with ample information to enable people to make and support wise choices. A variety of food substitutions can be implemented in a stepwise fashion to achieve a gradual change to healthier alternatives. The following illustrates initial substitutions:

Food	Healthy Alternative	Healthier Alternative
whole milk	low-fat milk	non-fat milk
cottage cheese	low-fat cottage cheese	non-fat cottage cheese
sugar cereal	non-sugar cereal	whole-grain cereal, non-processed
fruit drink	orange juice	whole orange
soft drink with sugar, caffeine	diet soft drink	sparkling water or fruit juice
white bread	brown bread	100% whole-wheat bread
bologna	ham	turkey

(See also DIETARY GUIDELINES FOR AMERICANS; FAT, HIDDEN.)

Liebman, Bonnie, "The Changing American Diet," *Nutrition Action Healthletter*, 22:5 (1995), pp. 9–10.
Woteki, Catherine, "Consumption, Intake Patterns and Exposure," *Critical Reviews in Food Science and Nutrition*, 35:1,2 (1995), pp. 143–47.

echinacea (*Echinacea augutifolia; E. purpurea*)   A perennial herb that stimulates the body's immune system. Echinacea is native to North America, from Texas to the prairies of Canada. Native American tribes have long used this herb as an antiseptic and as an analgesic (pain reliever). The dried root is used most often. It contains echinacin, a polysaccharide (complex carbohydrate) that speeds wound healing and helps maintain connective tissue. Echinacea contains inulin, a polysaccharide composed of fructose that activates the "alternative" complement pathway, a system that increases defenses against viruses and bacteria, and speeds the migration of defensive white cells (such as neutrophils, monocytes and lymphocytes) to injured or infected regions.

Echinacea stimulates T-lymphocytes, which help direct immune defenses. It also stimulates the production of interferon (antiviral defense) and of lymphokines, chemicals of the immune system that stimulate natural killer cells and scavenger cells (macrophages). Echinacea is regarded as a safe herb.

eclampsia (toxemia of pregnancy)   A serious medical condition that can accompany pregnancy. "Preeclampsia" is the early stage characterized by high blood pressure, headache, protein in urine and swelling (EDEMA) of legs and feet. If untreated, the patient may develop true eclampsia.

Eclampsia develops in 0.5% of patients with preeclampsia. Convulsive seizures can occur between the 20th week of pregnancy and the first week after birth; eclampsia is usually fatal if untreated. In addition to the symptoms of preeclampsia, symptoms of eclampsia include severe headaches, dizziness, abnormal pain, nausea, convulsions and possibly coma. The kidney, liver, brain and placenta are affected. The causes of eclampsia are unknown. HYPERTENSION and kidney disease contribute to the problem. Treatment of eclampsia is medical. Salt restriction is not part of the treatment, and the use of DIURETICS may simply mask signs and symptoms.

Poor nourishment may predispose a woman to preeclampsia. Multicenter studies by the U.S. National Institutes of Health are underway to determine whether calcium supplements or low doses of aspirin can prevent preeclampsia.

Anyaegbungm, A., and Edwards, C., "Hypertension in Pregnancy," *Journal of the National Medical Association*, 86 (April 1994), pp. 289–93.

Walsh, Scott W., "The Role of Fatty Acid Peroxidation and Antioxidant Status in Normal Pregnancy and in Pregnancy Complicated by Preeclampsia," *World Review of Nutrition and Diet*, 76 (1994), pp. 114–18.

eczema (atopic dermatitis)   Persistent itchy and inflamed skin, often with scales, crusts, scabs or small blisters. Eczema may be dry or there may be a discharge; the condition is not infectious. Allergies may be involved; many eczema patients test positive for allergies and they may exhibit hay fever symptoms. Emotional upset and stress can aggravate itching. Contact with chemical irritants can trigger eczema. Inheritance is a risk factor for eczema and dietary factors are involved.

The Role of Diet

Often eczema symptoms improve with an ELIMINATION DIET in which suspected allergy-producing foods are avoided, suggesting a linkage to food allergy in some cases. In infants, cow's milk is the most common food allergy associated with eczema. ESSENTIAL FATTY ACIDS can help limit the inflammatory process. Omega-3 fatty acids are the essential fatty acids found in flaxseed oil and fish oils, while omega-6 fatty acids are found in EVENING PRIMROSE OIL and BORAGE oil. Vitamin C and FLAVONOIDS, plant substances that serve as ANTIOXIDANTS, appear to help control or limit inflammatory processes also. Vitamin A plays a key role in skin development and maintenance, and deficiencies should be corrected. Many eczema patients are ZINC deficient and zinc

supplementation may be helpful. This may be linked to the fact that low stomach acid is very common in patients with eczema, and low stomach acid contributes to mineral malabsorption, ultimately leading to eczema. Zinc is necessary to convert essential fatty acids to PROSTAGLANDINS, hormone-like substances that regulate inflammation, among other processes.

The diet of eczema sufferers should minimize convenience foods that supply high levels of fat, sugar and other additives, while emphasizing whole foods, particularly fresh fruit and vegetables. Increasing consumption of polyunsaturated FAT (like SAFFLOWER oil) and FISH OIL may help decrease inflammation and boost the immune system. (See also ACNE; ALLERGY, FOOD; BREASTFEEDING; LEUKOTRIENES.)

Ursell, Amanda, "Dietary Manipulation in Eczema," *Practitioner*, 238 (April 1994), pp. 284–88.

edema (dropsy)   The swelling of any part of the body due to fluid accumulation. Allergies can cause edema when the allergic response releases HISTAMINE and other inflammatory agents that make capillaries porous so that fluid from BLOOD can then leak into surrounding tissue, causing puffy eyes and a swollen face, for example. Edema is also one of the symptoms of pre-eclampsia in pregnancy. Generalized edema can result from serious medical conditions such as HYPOTHYROIDISM, kidney failure, liver disease and congestive heart failure.

Nutritionally related causes of edema include excessive SODIUM, certain nutrient deficiencies and food allergies. Excessive sodium can cause edema in about 20% of the American population who are sensitive to high salt intake. Edema is also associated with severe nutritional deficiency diseases such as BERIBERI (due to a deficiency of THIAMIN) and with protein MALNUTRITION. Edema is often treated with DIURETICS (water pills), which increase urine production to remove water and salt from the body. The use of diuretics is considered potentially dangerous during pregnancy. Reduced salt intake can be helpful and low-sodium diets may be prescribed. (See also ALDOSTERONE; ECLAMPSIA; HYPERTENSION; KWASHIORKOR; SODIUM.)

edible portion (e.p.)   The portion of food usually consumed. For example, husks, hulls, rinds, peels, seed, bones, gristle and the like are usually excluded from weight measurements and nutrient compositions.

EDTA (ethylenediaminetetraacetic acid; disodium EDTA)   A FOOD ADDITIVE used as an ANTIOXIDANT and a preservative to trap unwanted metal ion contaminants. As an antioxidant, EDTA blocks the formation of highly reactive forms of oxygen that attack fats and oils. Attack of food molecules by oxygen requires metal ions as catalysts. When metal ion contaminants are trapped by EDTA, they do not form free radicals. EDTA is often combined with butylated hydroxytoluene (BHT) and PROPYL GALLATE, which work together as antioxidants in processed foods.

EDTA is added to salad dressings, MARGARINE, MAYONNAISE, potatoes, peas and vegetables. EDTA traps metal ions in canned SHELLFISH that would promote off-color and altered taste. In BEER it prevents excessive foaming and turbidity. Soft drink producers use EDTA to stabilize ARTIFICIAL

FOOD COLORS. Excessive EDTA would trap essential nutrients in the body, such as trace mineral nutrients and CALCIUM, and therefore typical usage is 0.01% in foods and beverages. The body absorbs only about 5% of an oral dose, and absorbed EDTA is excreted in the urine. EDTA is considered a safe additive. In medicine, EDTA is used to treat metal (LEAD) poisoning and as an alternative treatment in cardiovascular disease. (See also CHELATE.)

EFA   See ESSENTIAL FATTY ACIDS.

egg   As food, typically the ovum of domestic fowl. Eggs are an inexpensive, nutrient-rich food that provides high-quality protein with all essential amino acids. Egg protein is often used as a reference protein in nutritional studies because it is readily digested and supplies a well balanced mixture of amino acids that are readily absorbed. A popular food, non-fertile chicken eggs are mass-produced, inexpensive, readily available and are easily prepared. Hen's eggs contain an inner fluid, the egg white, which contains half of the PROTEIN but no cholesterol. It contains several proteins that protect the yolk from bacteria. One example is AVIDIN, which tenaciously binds the B vitamin, BIOTIN. Bacteria requiring this vitamin cannot grow in the egg white.

The yolk provides many nutrients like minerals, vitamins, all of the CHOLESTEROL (213 mg) and 5 g of fat. The yellow color of the yolk is due to the plant pigment, xanthophyll (lutein). This material is distinct from BETA CAROTENE and it does not supply VITAMIN A. The egg yolk is also rich in LECITHIN, a phospholipid used to emulsify other lipids. As food, eggs have limitations: Their CALCIUM content is low and they lack VITAMIN C. In recipes, egg yolks can often be substituted by using double the amount of egg white. Most commercial EGG SUBSTITUTES use egg whites only.

Eating more than a few eggs a week can raise blood cholesterol in sensitive people. On the other hand, moderate consumption seems safe for most healthy people. Perhaps as many as one third of Americans are extremely sensitive to dietary cholesterol; their blood levels rise significantly when they eat cholesterol-rich foods. These individuals should limit their dietary cholesterol to no more than 300 mg per day. Particularly those with a family history of early heart disease or high cholesterol levels need to be watchful. More important than monitoring cholesterol in the diet, is limiting fat consumption, especially consumption of SATURATED FAT. With a low-fat diet, egg cholesterol seems to have little impact on blood cholesterol levels.

Organic chicken eggs, farm fresh eggs and mass-produced eggs contain the same amount of cholesterol, although mineral and vitamin content can vary according to the chicken feed. Efforts are being made to increase the content of ESSENTIAL FATTY ACIDS of eggs by varying the hens' diets. Eggs can be contaminated by trace amounts of PESTICIDES from feed, so purchasing organic eggs might be desirable. Eggs should be cooked well (poaching, hard-boiled or easy over). Because raw or undercooked eggs can transmit food poisoning (SALMONELLA), discard cracked eggs and cook eggs thoroughly. Keep eggs refrigerated to prevent bacterial contamination and age-related changes. One chicken egg (58 g) contains 79 calories; protein, 6.1 g; fat, 5.6 g; cholesterol, 213 mg; calcium, 28 mg; iron, 1.04 mg; zinc, 0.61 mg;

vitamin A, 78 retinol equivalents; thiamin, 0.04 mg; riboflavin, 0.15 mg; niacin, 0.03 mg. (See also BIOLOGICAL VALUE; ORGANIC FOODS.)

egg allergies   A very common type of food allergy, usually due to a sensitivity to egg whites. Egg allergies may be fast-reacting, with symptoms such as hives, asthma, watery eyes, edema and nausea shortly after the egg is consumed. Alternatively, a delayed sensitivity, with symptoms such as headaches, DIARRHEA or CONSTIPATION, can develop hours after the food is consumed. Because eggs are so common in processed foods, read food labels of baked goods carefully before purchase to avoid egg-containing products. (See also ALLERGY, FOOD; BIOLOGICAL VALUE; FOOD SENSITIVITY.)

eggplant (*Solanum melongena*; aubergine)   A large, pear-shaped vegetable closely related to the POTATO. The eggplant is a member of the NIGHTSHADE FAMILY that includes tomatoes and peppers. It probably originated in India and has been cultivated since antiquity. Eggplant is often dark purple with a glossy skin, but white, yellow and striped varieties are also cultivated. It is a good source of fiber and is an ingredient in many Middle Eastern dishes. Ratatouille, a dish based on eggplant, is part of southern French cuisine. Unripened eggplant may contain the toxic alkaloid SOLANINE, which also occurs in green potatoes. Solanine can cause neurological symptoms and damage red blood cells. One cup of cooked eggplant (160 g) contains 45 calories; protein, 1.3 g; carbohydrate, 10.6 g; fiber, 6 g; calcium, 10 mg; iron, 0.56 mg; potassium, 397 mg; vitamin A, 10 retinol equivalents; thiamin, 0.12 mg; riboflavin, 0.03 mg; niacin, 0.96 mg; vitamin C, 2 mg.

egg substitutes   Cholesterol-free alternatives to eggs. By eliminating the yolk, food manufacturers have developed several cholesterol-free products. Egg substitutes usually contain egg white (egg albumin); a partially HYDROGENATED VEGETABLE OIL like CORN OIL; together with ARTIFICIAL FOOD COLORS, GUMS, EMULSIFIERS and several VITAMINS and MINERALS found in a typical egg. Soy protein-based egg substitutes are also marketed.

eicosapentaenoic acid (EPA)   A large, complex POLYUNSATURATED FATTY ACID found in fish and fish oils. EPA belongs to the omega-3 family of polyunsaturates, derived from the ESSENTIAL FATTY ACID, ALPHA LINOLENIC ACID. EPA, with 20 carbons and five double bonds, is the parent compound for PROSTAGLANDINS (PGE_3 series) and thromboxane A_3, hormone-like substances that help counterbalance inflammatory processes triggered by other prostaglandins (PGE_2 series) and other thromboxane A_2. The latter come from ARACHIDONIC ACID, an omega-6 polyunsaturate prevalent in meat. Therefore EPA and fish oil tend to balance some of the effects of a high meat diet. Recent research has focused on the relationship between EPA and heart disease.

Population studies indicate that death due to heart disease is lower among those who consume an average of 30 g of fish daily, as compared with those who eat meat daily. Other studies have yielded mixed results. While the results are suggestive it is not yet clear which of the constituents of fish oils are more important. EPA could reduce the risk of coronary heart disease by several mechanisms: EPA can inhibit clot formation indirectly. It blocks the formation of thromboxane A_2, a potent factor that causes platelets to clump. Clumping of these cellular fragments in the blood helps form blood clots within vessels. EPA is also converted to PGI_3, a prostaglandin that directly blocks platelet aggregation. EPA and related lipids seem to lower blood fat levels. They may lower serum cholesterol, if initial levels are elevated and diets are high in saturated fat, by depressing the formation of LDL (LOW-DENSITY LIPOPROTEIN), the undesirable form of cholesterol. EPA and its relatives may also block the early stages of atherosclerosis. The improvement of glucose utilization in diabetics who use fish oil supplement remains controversial.

Using fish oil as a supplemental source of EPA carries potential hazards. Depending upon the source, it may contain industrial pollutants. Fish liver oil may contain high levels of VITAMIN A and vitamin D, which can be toxic in high doses, as well as pesticides and other contaminants. Guidelines regarding the optimal intake of EPA or of fish oil have not yet been established. (See also ESKIMO DIET; OMEGA-3 FATTY ACIDS.)

elastin   A fibrous PROTEIN found in the lung, in large blood vessels and in other elastic connective tissue such as ligaments. Elastin differs from other fibrous proteins like COLLAGEN in that it is capable of undergoing a two-way stretch, like a trampoline net. Synthesis of elastin requires copper, and an inherited inability to absorb copper (Menke's syndrome) causes defective arteries.

electrolyte replacement   See SPORT DRINKS.

electrolytes   Electrically charged atoms or molecules occurring in the blood and other body fluids and in solutions in general. Electrolytes control the distribution of water among the blood, cells and tissues, and the spaces between them; thus electrolytes help regulate blood volume and composition. The electrical charge of electrolytes enables them to function in the transmission of nerve impulses and in muscle contraction, including heart muscle. Electrolytes also help regulate ACID-base balance to maintain the pH of body fluids close to neutrality.

Electrolytes consist of positively charged ions (cations) and negatively charged ions (anions). The predominant cations are POTASSIUM, SODIUM and MAGNESIUM, while the major anion is CHLORIDE. These electrolytes are not evenly distributed: Sodium and chloride are concentrated outside cells, while potassium and magnesium are concentrated in the cytoplasm (within cells).

Sodium, potassium and chloride are nutrients. Low levels are excreted daily, and they must be regularly replaced through foods and beverages. The kidneys reabsorb these electrolytes and play an important role in regulating electrolyte balance. Electrolytes are secreted by the GASTROINTESTINAL TRACT in digestive juices and bile. For example, chloride is secreted by stomach glands as hydrochloric acid and pancreatic secretion, and the small intestine releases sodium and bicarbonate. However, much of sodium and chloride is reabsorbed and recycled.

The body malfunctions when electrolytes are lost—through vomiting, diarrhea, excessive urination caused by certain medications (diuretics) or uncontrolled diabetes, or through excessive perspiration. Too little sodium causes fatigue, muscle weakness or even convulsions. Potent diuretics most frequently cause potassium losses because they rid the body of excess water. Diabetes, severe burns and dietary deficiencies can also cause low potassium. Symptoms of potassium loss include a weak pulse, general weakness and low blood pressure. Magnesium deficiency can be the result of diarrhea, chronic alcoholism, inflamed pancreas (pancreatitis), kidney disease and inadequate diet. Chloride loss can occur with diarrhea and intestinal disease. Because chloride helps prevent excessive bicarbonate, which is alkaline, low chloride can cause the body to become excessively alkaline.

Mild losses of sodium and chloride are easily replaced by common beverages and processed foods. Potassium and magnesium are obtained from whole grains, green leafy vegetables, and fruits and juices. The loss of electrolytes and water can lead to life-threatening situations more rapidly than for losses of any other nutrient. With prolonged electrolyte imbalance the brain, heart and lungs do not function normally, and medical attention is required to replace fluids and electrolytes intravenously. (See also BULIMIA NERVOSA; DEHYDRATION; KETONE BODIES.)

electron transport chain (terminal respiratory chain)   A collection of ENZYMES responsible for the final stages of oxidation of FATTY ACIDS, CARBOHYDRATES, AMINO ACIDS and other fuels in the presence of oxygen. The electron transport chain is part of the machinery of the MITOCHONDRIA, the cell's powerhouses. The oxidation-reduction enzymes are called CYTOCHROMES. Electrons pass sequentially from one cytochrome to the next like a bucket brigade. Nutrients like iron and coenzyme Q are required for this process. In the last step, the enzyme cytochrome oxidase transfers electrons to molecular oxygen to yield water. Cyanide poisons cytochrome oxidase, accounting for the toxicity of this substance.

An essential feature of electron transfer between cytochromes is the simultaneous synthesis of ATP, which is the cell's energy currency. Chemical energy trapped in ATP meets almost all energy requirements of cells. (See also KREB'S CYCLE; OXIDATIVE PHOSPHORYLATION.)

elemental diet (defined-formula diet)   A defined DIET in which nutrients are present in their simplest, least combined forms. Free AMINO ACIDS and the simple sugar GLUCOSE are typical ingredients. Generally they contain no FIBER and very little FAT. Elemental diets require minimal digestive action in order to be absorbed and utilized by the body. Elemental diets are prescribed for INFLAMMATORY BOWEL DISEASE and other conditions in which the digestive and absorptive functions of the gastrointestinal tract are severely compromised: preparation for gastrointestinal surgery, treatment of burn victims, pancreatitis and severe diarrhea. (See also DIGESTION; GASTROINTESTINAL DISORDERS.)

elimination diet/challenge test   A simple way of detecting food allergies. During the initial (recovery) phase of an elimination diet all foods suspected of causing allergies are avoided for 5 to 14 days, to provide time for the IMMUNE SYS-TEM to recover from the irritant. During the recovery phase, the diet is limited to "safe" foods and might include foods generally considered to be non-allergenic, such as lamb, rice, pears and pure springwater or a chemically defined meal replacement that incorporates hydrolyzed protein such as rice protein. When symptoms have diminished or disappeared, individual foods are added back to the diet, one at a time, for example, every two days. During this challenge period, the patient is instructed to record the recurrence of allergy symptoms when a questionable food is added back to the diet. This is a practical way to identify the offending food. However, patients should not stay on an elimination diet for a long time because it is too restrictive, and patients on such a diet risk inadequate intake of vitamins and minerals. This method is also cumbersome when there are multiple food allergies and requires patience and persistence. For severe food allergy symptoms, medical supervision should be obtained before eating any suspected food. (See also ALLERGY, FOOD.)

Ferri, Clodoveo, et al., "IgA Nephropathy: Preliminary Results of a Low Antigen Content Diet Treatment," *Archives of Internal Medicine*, 152 (1992), pp. 429–38.

ELISA Enzyme-linked immuno-absorbant assays—sensitive analytical methods used in clinical diagnostic testing. These highly sensitive lab tests use manufactured ANTIBOD-IES (monoclonal antibodies), which bind with great specificity to a particular class of molecules, such as steroid HORMONES, tumor markers, viral antigens, parasitic antigens and even other types of antibody molecules. The antibody used in the test is tagged with marker enzymes to permit measuring the degree of its binding. ELISA assays provide a previously unattainable window for assessing nutrient conditions and fundamental physiologic mechanisms, like circadian rhythm of hormone secretion, food allergies and disease processes such as HIV (Human Immunodeficiency Virus)-related conditions. (See also ALLERGY, FOOD.)

emaciation An extensive loss of body fat and muscle mass. Potential causes of emaciation are STARVATION, undiagnosed ANOREXIA NERVOSA, CANCER, uncontrolled diabetes, parasites, HYPERTHYROIDISM, nutrient MALABSORPTION due to GASTROINTESTINAL DISORDERS, such as chronic diarrhea and obstruction of stomach or esophagus. (See also CROHN'S DISEASE; INFLAMMATORY BOWEL DISEASE.)

Emden—Meyerhoff pathway See GLYCOLYSIS.

emesis Vomiting of stomach contents, and possibly of intestinal contents in severe situations. Potential causes of emesis include conditions such as food poisoning; chemical poisoning; viral infections; drug side effects; and nervous conditions like brain injury, migraines, meningitis, seasickness; stimulation of the brain's vomiting center; gastric conditions such as cancer and peptic ulcers; and intestinal disorders like intestinal obstruction. Aggravating factors include excessive pain, sensitivity to certain foods, and toxic chemicals. Odors, shock, nervousness, anxiety, hysteria, morning sickness, coughing, and irritation of the pharynx can cause reflexive vomiting. Chronic vomiting can lead to ELECTROLYTE loss and tooth erosion due to gastric acid, DEHY-DRATION and MALNUTRITION. (See also BULIMIA NERVOSA; EATING DISORDERS.)

emetic Any agent causing vomiting. Chemicals such as ipecac syrup, mustard and zinc sulfate induce vomiting by local stimulation. Chemical emetics may be dangerous in pregnancy, GASTRIC ULCERS, CARDIOVASCULAR DISEASE or hernia. Drinking large amounts of warm water can also induce vomiting. (See also BULIMIA NERVOSA; STOMACH ACID.)

empty calories (junk foods) Calories derived from burning food that provide excessive FAT, sugar and/or white flour but contain far fewer key nutrients than found in minimally processed foods. In particular, trace minerals, vitamins, protein and fiber are likely to be deficient. Foods supplying empty calories are said to have low NUTRIENT DEN-SITY. Alcoholic beverages, soft drinks, natural sweeteners like syrup and sugar, many manufactured foods, pastry, DESSERTS, CHIPS and similar high-fat snacks lack the balance of nutrients found in whole foods and tend to crowd out more nutritious foods.

Most healthy people can tolerate an occasional splurge on junk food. However, problems arise when eating empty calorie foods becomes a habit. The greater the consumption of less nutritious foods, the more important it is for the remainder of the diet to supply important nutrients to make up for the deficiency. All too often nutrient deficiencies such as folic acid, iron, calcium, even fiber occur. High-fat foods provide excessive calories, which favors weight gain. OBESITY is a growing problem for both American adults and children. Excessive fat and inadequate ANTIOXIDANT nutrients like VIT-AMIN C, vitamin E and BETA CAROTENE are linked to CARDIO-VASCULAR DISEASE, AGING and CANCER. (See also CONVENIENCE FOOD; DEGENERATIVE DISEASES; EATING PATTERNS; FAST FOOD; REFINED CARBOHYDRATES.)

emulsified vitamins Fat-soluble VITAMINS like vitamins A, D and E that are processed as water-soluble emulsions. While not true solutions, emulsions consist of microscopic particles uniformly dispersed and stabilized so that oil and water do not separate. Like fat, these vitamins are normally insoluble in water. Emulsified fat-soluble vitamins are absorbed directly by intestinal cells. Emulsification facilitates their uptake, an important consideration for individuals with MALABSORPTION. (See also VITAMIN A; VITAMIN D; VITAMIN E; VITAMIN K.)

emulsifiers (stabilizers, surfactants) A class of FOOD ADDITIVES widely used in manufactured foods to suspend oily materials in water. These chemicals, related to detergents, can suspend oils and lipids (water-insoluble materials) such as dyes in water as tiny droplets that do not coalesce or separate upon standing.

The most common commercial emulsifiers are DIGLYC-ERIDES, MONOGLYCERIDES, LECITHIN, POLYSORBATES and sorbitan mono-stearate. Emulsifiers are used to keep bread from becoming stale; to stabilize fat in NON-DAIRY CREAMERS for COFFEE; to keep cakes fluffy; to suspend flavors and food coloring in processed foods; and to stabilize ice cream. Egg lecithin is used to emulsify vegetable oils and vinegar to create MAYONNAISE. (See also CONVENIENCE FOOD.)

endive (*Cichorium endivia*)   This biennial or annual herb is a member of the aster family. It was used by ancient Egyptians and Romans and may have originated in India. Endive was adapted as food in France in the 14th century and is cultivated as a salad plant. Endive is closely related to CHICORY, which it resembles. It is a slightly bitter salad green. The leaves are finely divided and curly (curly endive) and are clustered in a loose head. The leaves taste somewhat bitter. To decrease their bitterness, the leaves are covered several weeks before harvest. It is an excellent source of BETA CAROTENE. Nutrient content of 1 cup (50 g) is 28 calories; protein, 0.6 g; carbohydrate, 1.7 g; fiber, 0.46 g; calcium, 30 mg; 1.026 retinol equivalents; vitamin C, 3.2 mg; niacin, 0.49 mg; and small amounts of other nutrients.

endocrine system   The collection of ductless glands that secrete hormones, chemical regulators of the body that travel to their target tissues via the bloodstream. As members of the body's system of checks and balances, ENDOCRINE glands respond to signals from the brain and to changes in chemicals in the blood, including BLOOD SUGAR, calcium and hormones.

The endocrine system consists of the ADRENAL GLANDS, PITUITARY (hypophysis), endocrine PANCREAS, THYROID, PARATHYROID, testes and ovaries, the pineal gland and the thymus. The placenta also secretes hormones. Each endocrine gland produces a characteristic hormone, or set of hormones. Endocrine malfunctions create serious imbalances. Hyposecretion, in which inadequate levels of hormones are secreted, and hypersecretion, in which excessive amounts of hormones are secreted, cause many pathological conditions ranging from diabetes to excessive FATIGUE and CATABOLIC STATE.

The *hypothalamus* is the nerve tissue that links the brain with the pituitary gland. The hypothalamus indirectly controls many functions. It integrates and controls the autonomic nervous system, the grouping of nerves that regulates involuntary processes such as smooth muscle contractions (for example, the movement of food through the GASTROINTESTINAL TRACT and glandular secretions). In response to signals from the brain, and its own sensing mechanisms, the hypothalamus releases hormones that regulate the release of six hormones from the pituitary. The hypothalamus also forms two hormones, oxytocin and ANTIDIURETIC HORMONE (ADH), which travel to the posterior pituitary where they are released.

The functions of individual endocrine glands can be summarized as follows:

Pituitary   Though it is only the size of a pea, the pituitary is considered the "master" endocrine gland because it regulates the activity of so many different glands throughout the body. ADH regulates SODIUM and WATER balance while oxytocin stimulates uterine contraction and the ejection of milk from mammary glands. The anterior pituitary makes "trophic hormones," hormones that activate other glands of the endocrine system. Trophic hormones include melanocyte-stimulating hormone (MSH) to regulate pigmented cells (melanocytes); PROLACTIN for milk secretion in females and for TESTOSTERONE production in males; interstitial cell stimulating hormone (ICSH), for testosterone production (males); lutenizing hormone (LH), for ovulation and progesterone production (females); follicle stimulating hormone (FSH), for development of ova and estrogen production (females) and sperm production in testes (males); thyroid stimulating hormone (TSH) for release of hormones from the thyroid gland; GROWTH HORMONE for tissue repair and maintenance; and ADRENOCORTICOTROPIC HORMONE (ACTH) for cortisol release from the adrenal cortex. The hypothalamus regulates the release of growth hormone, thyroid stimulating hormone, ACTH, FSH and LH, and prolactin from the pituitary.

Adrenal glands   In response to ACTH, the adrenal glands produce the stress hormones EPINEPHRINE and NOREPINEPHRINE from the inner region of the adrenals (medulla) to increase blood sugar, raise blood pressure, increase pulse rate, and similar effects that adapt the body to stress. The outer region of the adrenals (cortex) produce steroids, like GLUCOCORTICOIDS, which raise blood sugar, increase the rate of breakdown of protein and fuels, and MINERALOCORTICOIDS, which conserve sodium and water.

Thyroid gland   Thyroid hormones regulate the rate of energy production of cells, the rates of tissue growth and development, and they regulate activity of the nervous system. Calcitonin lowers blood calcium levels.

Parathyroid glands   Parathyroid hormone raises calcium and phosphate ions and activates bone degradation.

Thymus   Thymic hormones, thymosins, activate the immune system by promoting the proliferation of T cells, a major type of white blood cell.

Islets of Langerhans   Clusters of endocrine cells scattered throughout the pancreas. The islets contain the alpha cells that produce GLUCAGON to increase blood glucose; and the beta cells that produce INSULIN to lower blood glucose.

Ovaries   ESTROGENS (from the follicles) are female sex hormones that control the growth and development of female reproductive organs and secondary female characteristics and protein synthesis. They also produce PROGESTERONE (from the corpus luteum), which helps prepare the endometrium for implantation of a fertilized egg, and promotes milk production.

Gonads   Produce testosterone in males. This hormone controls growth of male sex organs, body growth, secondary male characteristics and sperm development.

Pineal gland   Produces melatonin, which has an inhibitory effect on ovaries. The pineal gland helps regulate circadian rhythms and may inhibit reproductive activities.

Placenta   Serves as a temporary endocrine gland until birth. During pregnancy the placenta secretes chorionic gonadotropin, a hormone capable of stimulating the growth and function of the gonads, as well as estrogen and progesterone. (See also HOMEOSTASIS.)

endogenous carbohydrate   Glucose that is synthesized in the body from non-carbohydrate compounds, excluding FATTY ACIDS, rather than obtained from the diet. The process, called GLUCONEOGENESIS, converts most AMINO

ACIDS to glucose; thus approximately 50% of dietary PROTEIN may be metabolized to glucose under normal (non-fasting) conditions. GLYCEROL from FAT breakdown yields glucose as does LACTIC ACID, PYRUVIC ACID, and such carboxylic acids of the KREB'S CYCLE as CITRIC ACID, SUCCINIC ACID and OXALOACETIC ACID. (See also CARBOHYDRATE METABOLISM; FASTING.)

endoplasmic reticulum   A membrane system found within the cytoplasm of many cell types. The endoplasmic reticulum functions in the synthesis, transport and storage of a wide variety of exported products, such as DIGESTIVE ENZYMES. The endoplasmic reticulum of the LIVER also houses enzymes for cholesterol synthesis, for completion of long chain FATTY ACIDS, and for powerful oxidizing enzymes (detoxifying enzymes) needed to modify toxic molecules and products of normal metabolism such as steroid hormones, to convert them to water-soluble materials that are more readily excreted. Long-term adaptation to repeated drug exposure produces a growth of "smooth" endoplasmic reticulum with increased levels of detoxifying enzymes in the liver. The portion of the endoplasmic reticulum devoted to protein synthesis machinery is called the "rough" endoplasmic reticulum. The cytoplasm of cells that manufacture huge amounts of protein, such as the PANCREAS and liver, is packed with rough endoplasmic reticulum to support their export of proteins. (See also CHOLESTEROL; CYTOCHROME P450; DETOXIFICATION.)

endorphins (opioid peptides)   Brain chemicals that block the awareness of pain, that is, they produce analgesia. Endorphins are chains of about 40 AMINO ACIDS, shorter in length than proteins. Endorphins are produced by the body in response to pain, stress and emotions, and they regulate the release of pituitary hormones, including growth hormone, ADRENOCORTICOTROPIC HORMONE (which triggers hormone release from the adrenal glands), and thyroid-stimulating hormone, among others. Endorphins also regulate cells of the immune system, lymphocytes (white blood cells), antibody producing cells and natural killer T cells.

Endorphins are 50 to 100 times more potent than morphine as pain killers (analgesics). Beta endorphins may suppress pain by blocking the release of substance P, a material in nerves that conducts pain-related nerve impulses to the central nervous system.

Endorphins bind to specific sites in the brain associated with pain perception and sedation. They may also assist in memory, learning, sexual drive, regulation of body temperature and decreased blood pressure. Increased endorphin levels may be related to an increased sense of well-being or euphoria, much like the effects of morphine and other opiates. According to one hypothesis, individuals with chronic pain may have less brain endorphins than usual.

EXERCISE may cause a natural "runner's high," a sense of euphoria and insensitivity to pain, when the brain is stimulated to form endorphins. Endorphins may regulate APPETITE; and possibly certain foods like sweets may trigger the brain to produce endorphins, causing an "eater's high." Bulimics often binge on food, especially CARBOHYDRATE and sweets, and their CRAVING may represent the need to feel better by eating food that triggers endorphin production in the

brain. Thus a craving may be a form of "self-medication." Similarly, people with chemical dependencies may be deficient in certain neuropeptides and thus crave substances that stimulate endorphin production or opiate drugs, which substitute for them, because of their increased need for endorphin stimulation.

Enkephalins

Brain compounds that block pain were first discovered in 1975. Enkephalins are smaller than endorphins and contain only a few amino acids. Enkephalins are concentrated in the hypothalamus, parts of the limbic system of the brain, and in the spinal cord. They too are more potent analgesics than morphine. It is believed they inhibit pain pathways of the nervous system like endorphins. (See also ADDICTION; BULIMIA NERVOSA; NEUROTRANSMITTER.)

endosperm   The starchy portion of kernels of CEREAL GRAINS that is concentrated in flour. During germination the endosperm would normally supply the growing plant embryo with energy. In the production of flour, the milling of grains removes FIBER and GERM from kernels to yield a STARCH fraction that can be decolorized and bleached to yield white flour. (See also BREAD; WHEAT.)

energy   The capacity to carry out work. In nutrition, energy is measured in large CALORIES (or kilocalories), defined as the amount of heat required to increase the temperature of 1 liter of water by 1° C—or in terms of kilojoules, a less common measure of energy used in medical literature.

There are two principal kinds of energy: potential energy (stored energy, such as chemical energy) and kinetic energy (motion). Energy takes many forms. Radiant energy is characterized by wave motion; heat and light are common examples. Chemical reactions involved in the breakdown of nutrients release some energy as heat, which cannot be used for cellular work. Electrical energy, based upon the flow of ions or electrons, is the form of energy essential for nerve impulses and for muscle cells.

The law of conservation of energy states that energy cannot be created or destroyed, only changed to other forms. This holds true for energy considerations of the body, where energy storage equals the difference between food consumed and energy output.

Energy is released when organic compounds are oxidized or broken down. On the other hand, the formation of bonds when biomolecules are assembled requires energy. Reactions involved in building processes (biosynthesis) require the input of energy supplied by the breakdown and oxidation of foods. Therefore the body requires fuel to produce energy to drive all of the processes of growth, maintenance and repair of the body.

The major fuels are FATS, CARBOHYDRATE and, to a lesser extent, PROTEIN. Their oxidation yields a large amount of energy released as heat or trapped as chemical energy in the form of ATP, the energy currency of the cell. The end products of the complete oxidation of fuels are water and carbon dioxide. The process is quite efficient: Up to 40% of the energy released during glucose oxidation is trapped as chemical energy in the form of ATP. The amount of ATP present at any moment is very small; it is not a storage form of energy. Instead the body stores energy primarily as fats (triglycerides) in adipose tissue.

The total number of calories in a food can be determined in the laboratory by a process called direct calorimetry. In this procedure, a food is completely oxidized in a sealed chamber immersed in an insulated water tank. The heat released or the oxygen consumed are measured to obtain total calories. However, the calories in a food determined by direct calorimetry exceed the caloric yield in the body because not all food constituents are oxidized by the body to carbon dioxide and water. Tables of caloric values of foods are corrected for this discrepancy. Food energy values can be calculated using general energy conversion factors (4 calories per gram of protein or carbohydrate; 9 calories per gram of fat) and adding up the calories contributed by carbohydrate, fat and protein. Most tables list physiologically available energy values based on specific energy conversions.

Energy Balance

Energy balance refers to the difference between calories consumed in food and the energy used for work and lost to the environment as heat and an increased state of disorder or randomness (increased entropy). The body requires a steady input of chemical energy to maintain all energy-requiring processes of the cell.

At "energy equilibrium," energy released from food consumed equals the work performed. There is no surplus, and body weight is stable. If the number of calories consumed exceeds energy needs, the excess energy is stored primarily as body fat and, therefore, weight increases.

Weight loss occurs when ingested food provides fewer calories than required to fuel the body, that is, when fuel expenditure exceeds intake. This fact is exploited by calorie-reduction diets, which are designed to assure that fuel intake is less than energy needs. The difference is made up by burning fat deposited in ADIPOSE TISSUE; muscle protein may also be broken down when calories are restricted. With gradual weight loss, the pounds lost represent the consumption of body fat.

The total number of calories in food consumed represents the energy intake. Energy expenditure consists of three categories. The resting energy expenditure (REE) is defined as the energy required to breathe, to pump blood, to keep the neurons of the brain active, in general to maintain all body functions and normal temperature while at rest, awake and at a typical room temperature. It represents the largest contribution to total energy requirements. REE accounts for approximately 60% of the energy output and reflects lean body mass. This accounts for the observed differences in REE between men and women, and between younger and older adults. In practice, the REE is easier to measure than the BASAL METABOLIC RATE (BMR), which is measured 12 hours after a meal, and soon after awakening in the morning. REE differs from BMR by only 10%, and for convenience REE is often used.

A second category of energy expenditure is a heat factor called the thermic effect of food (TEF), which represents the energy cost of digesting food and absorbing nutrients. This factor is small, approximately 5–10% of total energy expenditure.

Energy expended for physical activity represents the third category of energy output. This is the only component readily modified by life-style. Activity factors have been developed that correlate with different activity levels. The representative activity factor for resting (asleep) is 1.0; for very light work, 1.5; for light work, 2.5; for moderately heavy work, 5.0; and for heavy labor, basketball, football, soccer and the like, 7.0.

The RDA (RECOMMENDED DIETARY ALLOWANCE) for energy takes into account differences among people based on their sex, body size, age, pregnancy, lactation and activity level. For example, an average energy allowance for a healthy male between the ages of 25 and 50 and weighing 174 lbs is 2,900 calories per day. For females weighing 143 lbs, the average energy allowance is 1,900 calories per day. (See also DIETING; EXERCISE; FASTING; WEIGHT MANAGEMENT.)

Diamond, Jared, "The Athlete's Dilemma," *Discover*, August 1991, pp. 78–83.

enrichment The addition of nutrients to foods as established by federal standards. In 1980 the U.S. FDA established guidelines for the addition of nutrients to food: decrease a nutritional deficiency for a given population; restore nutrients lost in processing; and improve the nutritional quality of food substitutes and imitations. Though enrichment is not required, the FDA has established standards for those enriched foods that include VITAMIN A, VITAMIN D, iodine, THIAMIN, RIBOFLAVIN, NIACIN, IRON and calcium. The term "fortification" is often used synonymously with enrichment, although fortification originally meant the addition of specific nutrients to foods, in excess of those usually found in those foods. These additions are usually in moderate amounts.

England and Canada have enrichment programs similar to the United States. Nutrients are commonly added to salt, milk, margarine and cereal grain products including bleached flour and pasta, white rice, cornmeal and bread and buns. FDA standards of enrichment include iodine in salt at a level of 7.6 mg per 100 g; vitamin D is added to milk at a level of 400 IU per quart; and vitamin A is added to margarine at a level of 15,000 IU per pound (the average vitamin A content of butter throughout the year). Thus, a cup of bleached white flour can contain 45% of the RECOMMENDED DIETARY ALLOWANCE (RDA) of thiamin, 25% of the RDA of riboflavin, 25% of the RDA of iron and 30% of the RDA of niacin. Bread may also be enriched by the addition of enriched flour, pure nutrients or nutritional yeast with iron. Fortified beverages include vitamin A- and vitamin D-fortified milk; calcium- and vitamin B_{12}-fortified soy milk. Calcium is added to some orange juices and VITAMIN C is added to some synthetic beverages. (See also ERGOCALCIFEROL; FOOD ADDITIVES; FOOD FORTIFICATION.)

enteritis Inflammation of the intestine, particularly the layer of cells lining the intestine (mucosa) and also the underlying connective tissue. (See also INFLAMMATORY BOWEL DISEASE.)

enterohepatic circulation The absorption of nutrients and other materials by the INTESTINE, their transport to the LIVER and reutilization. A variety of substances released into the intestine can be reabsorbed by the intestine. Thus

BILE salts released from the GALLBLADDER are absorbed by the small intestine, where they pass into the capillaries and then are transported to the liver via the portal vein. Bile salts can be taken up by the liver and released again in bile. Less than 1% of bile salts escape this recycling process daily. This small loss nonetheless represents the major route by which CHOLESTEROL is altered and lost by the body. (See also FAT DIGESTION.)

enteropathy A general medical term refering to the broad class of intestinal disease. Typical examples are CROHN'S DISEASE, CELIAC DISEASE, INFLAMMATORY BOWEL DISEASE and infectious DIARRHEA. Enteropathies can affect the small intestine, the colon or both portions of the intestine.

enteropeptidase (enterokinase) An intestinal enzyme responsible for activating protein-degrading enzymes from the pancreas. The pancreas secretes enzymes that digest proteins as inactive precursors in order to prevent the pancreas from digesting itself. These inactive enzymes encounter enteropeptidase, which triggers the following cascade of events. Enteropeptidase activates trypsin, a powerful digestive enzyme. Trypsin in turn activates all other protein-digesting enzymes of the pancreas. Severe milk intolerance is linked to enteropeptidase deficiency, inadequate pancreatic enzymes and, ultimately, to maldigeston. (See also DIGESTIVE ENZYMES.)

enterotoxin Bacterial products released or produced in the intestine that can cause illness. Certain bacterial species produce chemicals that cause food poisoning, including enterotoxin-producing strains of ESCHERICHIA COLI that can contaminate undercooked or raw meat. Staphyloccocal FOOD POISONING is caused by ingestion of bacterial toxins in contaminated food, usually in custards, milk products and unrefrigerated meats, while *Shigella* species cause dysentery (very severe DIARRHEA) by releasing toxins at sites of infection. In contrast, the bacterium SALMONELLA causes food poisoning through rapid intestinal growth without the production of enterotoxins. (See also ACIDOPHILUS.)

environmental medicine (clinical ecology) A branch of medicine that focuses on the role of environmental factors in illness. Allergies or sensitivities to chemicals in food, water and air, at home and at work, are relevant topics. Exposure to substances that cause symptoms can be physical or chemical, and usually symptoms are chronic and cyclic. Environmental ecologists believe that environmentally induced illness is the most common cause of chronic symptoms. Multiple organ systems are often involved. Treatment involves avoidance, control of air and water quality and immunization therapy to control adverse responses and rotation diets.

Rosenstock, L., Rest, K.M., Benson, Jr., J.A., et al., "Occupational and Environmental Medicine," *New England Journal of Medicine*, 325:13 (1991), pp. 924–27.

enzymes A class of proteins that catalyze (speed up) the chemical reactions of cells. Enzymes are extremely important and dynamic proteins. The body carries out more than 100,000 different chemical reactions, and each of these requires a specific protein catalyst to speed up and control reactions. Because catalysts are not used up as they do their work, tiny amounts of enzymes can form a huge amount of products from substrates.

Enzymes play major roles in METABOLISM. They are required for DIGESTION, energy production, nerve function, muscle contraction and regulation of blood pH. They help form all cell structures such as RNA and DNA—and much, much more. Chemical compounds that react in enzyme-catalyzed reactions are called substrates. A classic model is helpful to visualize how enzymes work: A key (substrate) fits into a carefully constructed keyhole where chemical bonds are made or broken. The names of enzymes often use the suffix "-ase," for example, CATALASE, dehydrogenase, AMYLASE and oxidase.

Like all PROTEINS, enzymes are long chains of amino acids (POLYPEPTIDES) composed of the 20 AMINO ACID building blocks. Each type of enzyme possesses a unique amino acid sequence, which is encoded in genes. The amino acid sequence determines both the structure and the function of a given enzyme. Mutations in genes are due to chemical modifications of DNA that lead to the production of proteins with altered amino acid sequences. Mutant proteins may not function as well as the unaltered protein; in the most severe cases, mutations can lead to completely non-functional enzymes and genetic diseases. PHENYLKETONURIA, an inherited inability to break down the amino acid phenylalanine, is an example.

The thousands of different enzyme reactions fall into just six categories. "Hydrolases" break chemical linkages in molecules by adding water (hydrolysis). Amylase (STARCH digestion), LIPASE (FAT digestion) and proteolytic enzymes like trypsin (protein digestion) are examples. "Transferases" move a group of atoms from one compound to another, for example, transaminases transfer amino (-NH_2) groups to carboxylic acids in order to form new amino acids. "Lyases" break bonds between carbon and carbon atoms, between carbon and nitrogen atoms (and carbon and oxygen atoms) of compounds without adding water molecules or oxygen. "Isomerases" catalyze rearrangements of atoms within molecules. Several reactions in glucose breakdown require isomerizations. "Ligases" utilize the energy of ATP to create new carbon compounds. Energy-requiring steps play key roles in the synthesis of fat from FATTY ACIDS, of proteins from amino acids, of complex carbohydrates from simple sugars. And finally, "oxido-reductases" carry out oxidation-reduction reactions. These enzymes are called "dehydrogenases" or "oxidases," for example, lactate dehydrogenase, which produces LACTIC ACID in the muscle during strenuous exertion.

Metabolic Pathways

Enzymes often participate in functional sequences of reactions called metabolic pathways. In metabolic pathways the product of one enzyme becomes the substrate for the following enzyme, which modifies the intermediate product before passing it on to the next enzyme, much like a bucket brigade. A typical sequence can be illustrated as A→B→C→D, in which enzyme 1 catalyzes the reaction A→B; enzyme 2 catalyzes B→C; enzyme 3 catalyzes C→D and so on.

Regulation

Enzyme pathways are often carefully regulated. The first enzyme committed to the pathway often controls a bottle-neck step, limiting the flow of material through the pathway. Such rate-limiting enzymes can be activated to speed up the pathway or they can be inhibited, to slow it down. Thus entire metabolic pathways can be turned on or off by regulating such key enzymes.

The body regulates enzymes in other ways as well. The amount of enzymes in tissues can be increased, for example, during adaptation to a carbohydrate-rich diet; fasting; embryonic and fetal development; pregnancy; and when taking drugs or medications. These changes are slow because they alter protein-forming machinery. Certain hormones are often enzyme inducers: Insulin induces biosynthetic enzymes associated with glycogen and fat formation for energy stores, while cortisol can increase levels of enzymes for fat degradation. Other hormones, such as the stress hormone EPINEPHRINE, can activate or inhibit enzymes quickly. The flow of molecules within cells can activate or block metabolic pathways quickly. In a common scenario a build-up of the products of a pathway can inhibit the first step of the pathway (FEEDBACK INHIBITION) to slow the flow of materials. As examples, ATP can shut down GLYCOLYSIS (glucose breakdown) and NADH (reduced NICOTINAMIDE ADENINE DINUCLEOTIDE) can shut down the KREB'S CYCLE, the central pathway in energy production of the cell's powerhouses (mitochondria).

Coenzymes and Cofactors

Many enzymes require non-protein components to be active. TRACE MINERALS and the vitamins of the B COMPLEX assist in enzyme function. Trace mineral nutrients (like MAGNESIUM, MANGANESE, IRON, COPPER, ZINC, SELENIUM and MOLYBDENUM) function as enzyme COFACTORS. For example, zinc helps DNA polymerase, the enzyme that makes DNA. Iron helps CYTOCHROMES, responsible for mitochondria production of ATP, with the transfer of electrons to oxygen to form water.

The body modifies vitamins of the B complex to form COENZYMES (enzyme helpers). An enzyme combined with its coenzyme is called a holoenzyme, while an APOENZYME lacks its coenzyme and consequently is completely inactive. NIACIN yields NAD (nicotinamide adenine dinucleotide), and RIBOFLAVIN forms FAD (FLAVIN ADENINE DINUCLEOTIDE) for oxidation reduction reactions, for example, in oxidizing fuels for energy. THIAMIN forms thiamin pyrophosphate, used in oxidation of carbohydrate. PANTOTHENIC ACID forms COENZYME A, used to carry fatty acids and acetic acid through reaction sequences. BIOTIN forms biocytin for reactions in which carbon dioxide is attached to compounds to form new acids, while FOLIC ACID forms tetrahydrofolate, used in shuttling single carbon atom fragments between molecules. VITAMIN B6 forms pyridoxal phosphate for transferring nitrogen group, and VITAMIN B12 forms methylcobalamin used to regenerate the essential amino acid methionine, among others. As an example of the critical role that vitamins play in metabolism, consider that thiamin, riboflavin, pantothenic acid and niacin are essential to burn fuels to produce ATP in the Kreb's cycle, the central energy pathway of mitochondria. A deficiency of any one of these vitamins impairs this pathway, and hence the ability of cells to produce energy.

Enzyme Inactivation (Loss of Enzyme Activity)

Enzymes are fragile and can be poisoned or destroyed by chemicals. Toxic HEAVY METALS like LEAD and MERCURY are poisons because they bind to enzymes. Enzymes are also sensitive to pH. If blood is too acidic (ACIDOSIS) or too basic (ALKALOSIS), enzymes may be inactivated. Heat, as used in cooking food and blanching vegetables, destroys enzymes. Soap destroys enzymes by causing the protein molecules to unfold and unwind. Oxidation and other chemical reactions can also irreversibly alter enzyme structure with loss of function.

Variability in Enzymes Among Individuals

Each person has somewhat different enzyme levels in his or her tissues. These slight but important differences in the enzyme makeup are the result of differences in heredity, age, sex, exercise pattern, diet history, state of health, life-style, exposure to environmental pollutants, medications and drugs. The level of enzymes may increase as the body adapts to change. Thus drug-destroying enzymes of the liver will increase after prolonged drug exposure. (See also BIOCHEMICAL INDIVIDUALITY; CARBOHYDRATE METABOLISM; CARCINOGEN; FAT METABOLISM; TRACE MINERALS.)

EPA (Environmental Protection Agency) A federal agency established in 1971 to form and enforce laws to protect the environment and to control pollution. It is the largest independent regulatory agency of the federal government. The EPA administers clean water programs, clean air and solid waste disposal programs, and toxic waste clean-up; and PESTICIDE research and programs to establish pesticide standards. The EPA establishes tolerance levels for toxic materials, pesticides and even excessive noise. It also monitors radioactivity levels in the home and workplace. The EPA is responsible for setting limits based on lifetime exposure to toxic materials such as DIOXIN, LEAD, air pollutants and pesticides found in FOOD, air and WATER. It has outlawed a variety of pesticides and instigated reductions of sulfur dioxide and lead from automobile and industrial stack emissions. Two examples illustrate current efforts. Lead is a regulated toxic metal. It is generally recognized that lead poisoning is one of the most serious problems for children in the United States, primarily from eating lead-based paint and breathing automobile exhaust. The EPA banned lead in house paint and lead in gasoline is being phased out; consequently, nationwide lead levels have declined to 5 mcg per deciliter of blood. In 1986 the EPA proposed lowering the "threshold of concern" for lead because a level of 20 mcg per deciliter of blood, the existing threshold, can cause women to deliver low birthweight babies and result in IQ deficiencies in children. The Centers for Disease Control now advises governmental agencies to initiate lead awareness campaigns where children have lead blood levels of 10 mcg per deciliter or higher.

As a second example, the EPA presents an annual report on national water quality. In 1990 it concluded that about 75% of all surface water, as assessed by states, met water quality standards. That report noted that 87% of municipal sewage treatment plants and 97% of major industrial facilities met federal and state pollution control requirements. The EPA issued standards for 85 water contaminants, including industrial chemicals and pesticides like NITRATE,

CADMIUM, fluoride, endrin, lindane, 2,4-D, methoxychlor and radioactivity in 1992. (See also FDA; USDA.)

epidemiology   The study of factors in populations that determine the frequency of diseases and their distribution in populations. Epidemiology requires the collection of data for groups of people to establish RISK factors and associations. "Retrospective" studies examine medical records to learn about past events. As an example, comparison of the occurrence of cancer in high-risk areas with low-risk areas where people rarely get a given type of cancer suggests that 80–90% of human cancer is preventable. One problem with linking diet to disease is that such studies usually depend upon diet recall, that is, what people remember they ate, especially years ago when the initial events may have occurred. "Prospective" studies start with the selected group and follow a characteristic of that group for a period of time.

Several concepts are used in epidemiology. The "prevalence" of a disease or condition is like a "single snapshot" of a population; it answers the question: How many individuals are affected at a given moment. The "incidence" of a condition is a rate; it predicts the number of individuals who will be affected per unit of time, typically a month or a year.

Epidemiology demonstrated the link between cigarette smoking and increased risk of cancer, and the link between diets with ample fiber, fresh vegetables and fruits and decreased risk of cancer. In addition to cancer, epidemiology has uncovered other associations between environment (diet) and disease. For example, diets high in FISH and marine lipids are linked to a decreased risk of heart attack, in the United States, diets high in SATURATED FAT are linked to an increased risk of CARDIOVASCULAR DISEASE; alcohol consumption increases the risk of FETAL ALCOHOL SYNDROME. Nonetheless, correlations between two variables alone cannot prove cause and effect because they deal with probabilities. Epidemiology can help calculate the probability, or odds, but it cannot predict events for a given individual. (See also FRAMINGHAM STUDY; RISK DUE TO CHEMICALS IN FOOD AND WATER.)

epinephrine (adrenaline)   A HORMONE released by adrenal glands in response to STRESS. Epinephrine and a related hormone, norepinephrine, are synthesized from the amino acid TYROSINE by the inner portion of the adrenal gland (medulla). Epinephrine synthesis requires many nutrients in addition to tyrosine: COPPER, IRON, VITAMIN C, VITAMIN B_6, VITAMIN B_{12} and METHIONINE.

The "flight or fight" response to physical stress or to situations perceived as threatening involves stimulation of the sympathetic division of the autonomic nervous system, the branch of the nervous system that controls involuntary responses. When epinephrine is released into the bloodstream in response to nerve stimulation, it constricts CAPILLARIES and reduces circulation in hands and feet, causing cold hands and feet. Epinephrine slows DIGESTION, increases heart rate and relaxes bronchial smooth muscles to open air passageways and increase the oxygen supply to the lungs.

Epinephrine mobilizes the body's energy stores: It stimulates the release of FATTY ACIDS from ADIPOSE TISSUE into the bloodstream, and it stimulates the release of GLUCOSE from liver GLYCOGEN to increase BLOOD SUGAR so they can be burned for quick energy. Epinephrine also triggers muscle glycogen breakdown to release glucose as an immediate fuel for muscle.

epithelial tissue (epithelium)   The tissues lining the cavities and ducts of the body and all body surface. The epithelium forms the skin, the lining of the GASTROINTESTINAL TRACT and ducts of secretory tissues like the LIVER and PANCREAS, the urinary tract, the reproductive system, the respiratory tract and the blood vessels.

There are several fundamental types of epithelium. Simple squamous epithelium forms a single layer of flat cells, like a tiled floor, and lines the lungs, kidneys, heart, blood vessels, lymph vessels and CAPILLARIES. Epithelial cells of the digestive tract (stomach, intestines, pancreas, liver, gallbladder) secrete digestive juices, a process controlled by long, columnar cells. Often they secrete complex polysaccharide, which forms MUCUS or a protective barrier. Epithelial cells of the gastrointestinal tract have a relatively short half-life. They constantly slough off, their protein is degraded and their amino acids are recycled in digestion.

Multi-layered squamous epithelium functions as protection. A tough protective layer (keratinized tissue) form the outer layer of skin while softer, non-keratinized tissues with moist surfaces are found in the mouth, tongue, ESOPHAGUS and vagina. Glandular epithelium secretes products into ducts; these ducts include mammary glands, digestive glands like salivary glands, and the pancreas. Endocrine epithelium secretes hormones into blood. Examples are the pituitary gland, thyroid gland, ADRENAL GLANDS, ovaries and testes and thymus gland. (See also DIGESTIVE TRACT; ENDOCRINE SYSTEM.)

ergocalciferol (calciferol, vitamin D_2)   A common supplemental form of vitamin D. Ergocalciferol is readily manufactured from a plant lipid, ERGOSTEROL, by exposure to ultraviolet light. Ergocalciferol is the most common form of vitamin D used to fortify foods because it is readily available. Routine vitamin supplements containing more than 400 IU of vitamin D are not recommended because vitamin D can accumulate to toxic levels with excessive consumption; 1,800 IU of vitamin D (45 mcg) can cause symptoms in young children who are particularly susceptible. The levels of vitamin D in milk can vary widely and adults consuming several glasses of vitamin D-fortified milk daily may receive substantially higher levels of vitamin D. (See also HYPERVITAMINOSIS; RICKETS.)

ergogenic supplements   Supplements that purportedly increase the potential for physical work by improving energy production, or energy efficiency during EXERCISE. Ergogenic supplements are said to increase endurance and the capacity for exercise. However, in general supplementation of specific nutrients above dietary allowances for healthy athletes does not improve athletic performance. According to a position paper of the American Diabetics Association, nutritional supplements such as BEE POLLEN or vitamins neither provide energy nor boost athletic performance when there is no deficiency. So-called vitamin B_{15} or PANGAMIC ACID, mixtures of free AMINO ACIDS, ALCOHOL, bee pollen, GELATIN, HONEY, wheatgerm oils and inosine do not appear to consistently increase athletic performance.

Other substances have been periodically called "ergogenic." Tryptophan at large doses can increase growth hormone levels, but its effect in athletes has not been measured. In 1990 the U.S. FDA banned the sale of this amino acid supplement due to a toxic contamination. Aspartates, particularly potassium and magnesium aspartates, derived from the amino acid ASPARTIC ACID, have shown some positive effects in double-blind, PLACEBO-controlled trials in which neither the investigator nor the subject knew who received aspartate and who received an inactive substance (placebo). Large doses of single amino acids can cause imbalances in susceptible individuals because the excess consumption of one can affect uptake of another.

CAFFEINE is a stimulant and may facilitate the use of fat stores for energy during exercise. Its use is permitted by the International Olympic Committee in limited amounts. An estimated dose of 5 mg caffeine per kilogram of body weight could provide a stimulant effect, yet be legal by IOC rules. (See also ARGININE; CARNITINE; OCTACOSANOL.)

Thein, L.A., Thein, J.M., Landry, G.L., "Ergogenic Aids," *Physical Therapy*, 75:5 (1995), pp. 426–429.

ergosterol   A plant lipid found in yeasts and molds. This white, waxy substance is used commercially to synthesize vitamin D₂. Irradiated ergosterol or other forms of VITAMIN D are commercially added to MILK to ensure an adequate intake of this vitamin and to avoid vitamin D deficiency disease. (See also ERGOCALCIFEROL; FORTIFICATION; HYPERVITAMINOSIS.)

ergot   A toxic substance produced by a fungus, *Claviceps purpurea*, which can infect rye and other grains. Ergot poisoning may occur from eating bread made from flour contaminated with this fungus, now a rare occurrence in developed nations. Historically outbreaks of ergot poisoning were known as St. Anthony's Fire. Ingestion of ergot can cause tumors in experimental animals. (See also AFLATOXIN; FOOD POISONING; FOOD TOXINS; MOLD.)

erucic acid   A monounsaturated fatty acid found in seed oils such as RAPESEED and MUSTARD seed, with 22 carbons. Research conducted in Canada and elsewhere in the 1960s demonstrated that consumption of large amounts of rapeseed oil by experimental animals resulted in impaired growth and pathological changes in heart muscle. Human toxicity was not reported; apparently erucic acid can be broken down normally in humans. Nonetheless new varieties of rapeseed (*Canadian brassica*) were developed that contain little or no erucic acid. BORAGE oil contains a low level (1 to 3%) of erucic acid. (See also FATTY ACIDS; OLIVE OIL.)

eructation   Belching. The noisy release of gas from the stomach. Drinking carbonated beverages, gulping food with excessive swallowing of air, and fermentation processes in the stomach can cause belching. (See also ACID INDIGESTION.)

erythema   The redness of skin produced when CAPILLARIES close to the skin surface expand. Erythema is caused by inflammation, including allergies; reaction to food poisoning and to certain drugs; contact with toxic substances; and environmental factors such as heat, cold and sunburn, as well as emotional upsets. (See also ALLERGY, FOOD).

erythorbic acid (sodium erythorbate)   A FOOD ADDITIVE used to protect processed foods against oxidation. Although it is a close relative of VITAMIN C, it is poorly absorbed. As an ANTIOXIDANT, erythorbic acid prevents undesirable changes in the color, aroma and taste of processed foods.

Erythorbate and vitamin C are added to non-citrus fruits like apples, pears and bananas, as well as vegetables such as eggplant, potatoes and yams, to retard deterioration and browning reaction during processing.

Erythorbate is added to BEER after FERMENTATION to help prevent its darkening, turbidity and taste deterioration. In cured meats such as SAUSAGE, HAM and BACON, this antioxidant helps stabilize color and inhibit the formation of NITROSOAMINES, which are CARCINOGENS. (See also BHA; BHT; FREE RADICALS.)

erythrocytes   See RED BLOOD CELLS.

erythropoiesis   The formation of mature RED BLOOD CELLS (erythrocytes) from immature precursors ("stem" cells). Erythropoiesis is stimulated by the HORMONE, erythropoietin, which is created by the kidneys when they are subjected to low oxygen levels. The kidneys respond by releasing a factor that converts a blood protein to erythropoietin. This hormone targets the bone marrow where immature precursor cells (erythroblasts) are induced to synthesize massive amounts of HEMOGLOBIN, the oxygen transport protein of red blood cells. Erythroblasts become reticulocytes, immature red blood cells released into the bloodstream where they mature into erythrocytes, full-fledged red blood cells, in one to two days. (See also ANEMIA; CIRCULATORY SYSTEM.)

Escherichia coli   A rod-shaped bacterium that normally inhabits the colon (large intestine). *E. coli* is considered one of the friendly gut bacteria in fecal matter. By occupying an ecological niche, it can prevent potentially harmful organisms from growing. The presence of this bacterium in water and milk indicates fecal contamination. Normally non-pathogenic (non-disease producing), *E. coli* can cause URINARY TRACT infections when it infects that tissue. Certain strains of *E. coli* are pathogens (disease-producing microorganisms). A pathogenic strain causes at least 40% of traveler's DIARRHEA.

E. Coli 0157:H7

This strain of *E. coli* was discovered as a human pathogen in 1982. It damages the intestine and produces a toxic substance that can penetrate the body, damaging blood vessels and kidneys. It is the leading cause of bloody diarrhea in the United States. *E. coli* 0157:H7 also causes severe abdominal cramping. Infection by this strain of *E. coli* is the most common cause of hemolytic uremic syndrome, a serious disease that can cause kidney damage and death in children. The Centers for Disease Control considered this to be the most serious public health problem relating to foodborne illness (1994). Estimates range from 200,000 cases per year; more states are requiring that cases of *E. coli* 0157:H7 be reported by doctors, so the picture will become clearer. Children under five are the most susceptible; infection can be spread by fecal contamination at day-care centers or preschools.

Rare or uncooked meat, especially hamburger and ground beef, is a common source of E. coli 0157:H7 because fecal material often contaminates animal carcasses in meat packing plants. To be safe, meat must be cooked thoroughly until pinkness is gone and meat juices are clear. (See also ACIDOPHILUS; BIFIDOBACTERIA; FOOD POISONING.)

Foulke, Judith, "How to Outsmart Dangerous E. coli Strain," *FDA Consumer*, 28 (January–February 1994), pp. 7–11.

Eskimo diet A "heart healthy" diet that includes cold-water ocean FISH, in addition to FAT and CHOLESTEROL from marine animals. This diet is enriched in oils of coldwater fish; such oils contain high levels of omega-3 FATTY ACIDS. The rate of HEART ATTACK of Greenland Eskimos is only 10% that of United States adults. Omega-3 fatty acids lower blood CHOLESTEROL, reduce the tendency for blood to clot, and lower the risk of thrombosis. These factors in turn prevent cholesterol accumulation in arteries and therefore protect against heart disease. For Americans, eating fish regularly may help lower cholesterol only if fish is substituted for red MEAT, not added to a diet already high in SATURATED FAT. Although they have a lowered risk of heart disease, the health of Greenland Eskimos is threatened by mercury pollution in the fish and marine mammals they eat; by ARTHRITIS; and by a high rate of stroke (brain hemorrhage). (See also DOCOSAHEXAENOIC ACID; EICOSAPENTAENOIC ACID; ESSENTIAL FATTY ACIDS; FISH OIL.)

esophagus The tube connecting the mouth and the upper end of the STOMACH. In the process of swallowing, chewed food is transported down the esophagus by the involuntary wave-like contraction and relaxation of smooth muscle walls (PERISTALSIS). The valve between the stomach and esophagus may not close properly (due to a reaction to food, or gulping air with food). When this occurs, stomach acid can back up into the esophagus, a condition called esophageal reflux, which causes ACID INDIGESTION or heartburn. (See also ANTACID; DIGESTIVE TRACT.)

essential amino acids Eight of the 20 AMINO ACIDS that are protein building blocks and must be supplied by the diet through the digestion of food proteins. The essential amino acids are the following: TRYPTOPHAN, PHENYLALANINE, METHIONINE, LYSINE, THREONINE, VALINE, ISOLEUCINE and LEUCINE. Two other amino acids, HISTIDINE and ARGININE, are essential under special circumstances. Histidine supports growth in young children and arginine supports newborns and adults with damaged livers. When the diet does not provide adequate methionine, CYSTEINE becomes an essential amino acid because it is synthesized from methionine. These amino acids are therefore "conditionally essential" amino acids.

Because essential amino acids must be supplied in the diet on a daily basis, their levels in food are important to a balanced diet. The relative proportions of essential amino acids in a food protein determine whether it is "high" or "low" quality protein. Thus a high-quality protein is one that supplies adequate levels of all essential amino acids to meet the body's requirements. POULTRY, FISH and MEAT,

together with milk products and EGGS, are the most common sources of high-quality protein in industrialized nations. Although there is no perfect protein, chicken eggs provide a mixture of essential amino acids in close to optimal amounts for healthy people and are the international standard by which other protein sources are measured. Plant protein is often relatively low in lysine, tryptophan and methionine.

The following deficiencies are noted: corn (tryptophan and threonine); grain cereals (lysine); legumes (methionine); rice (tryptophan, threonine); soybean (methionine). Therefore the limiting amino acids need to be complemented by mixing with plant protein sources. Thus combining rice protein and bean protein can satisfy the body's need for essential amino acids. Surplus essential amino acids from digestion as fuel are burned for ENERGY or are converted to FAT. (See also BIOLOGICAL VALUE; NET PROTEIN UTILIZATION; PROTEIN COMPLEMENTATION.)

essential fatty acids (EFA, vitamin F) Two fatty acids that cannot be synthesized by the body and must be provided by the diet. The essential fatty acids LINOLEIC ACID and ALPHA LINOLENIC ACID are polyunsaturated FATTY ACIDS, that is, they possess two or more double bonds and lack several hydrogen atoms found in saturated fatty acids. They differ in their location of double bonds, that is, bonds between carbon atoms that are deficient in hydrogen atoms. This small chemical difference has a huge nutritional impact. Linoleic acid contains 18 carbon atoms and belongs to the omega-6 family of fatty acids, in which the first double bond occurs at the sixth carbon atom of the molecular chain. Linoleic acid serves as the parent of a large polyunsaturated fatty acid, called ARACHIDONIC ACID. Arachidonic acid in turn forms PROSTAGLANDINS (PGE_2) and thromboxanes (TXA_2), hormone-like lipids that tend to promote blood clotting, induce pain and inflammation and cause smooth muscle contraction. Another pathway converts arachidonic acid to LEUKOTRIENES, one of the most powerful inflammatory agents. Events triggering inflammation stimulate cells to synthesize prostaglandins (PGE_2) and thromboxanes (TXA_2). As a component of membrane lipids, linoleic acid helps maintain flexibility of cell membranes. Arachidonic acid is not a dietary essential unless a deficiency of linoleic acid exists.

The second essential fatty acid, alpha linolenic acid, is the major polyunsaturated fatty acid of plants. It contains 18 carbon atoms and three double bonds and belongs to the omega-3 family of fatty acids, in which the first double bond occurs at the third carbon of the fatty acid. Alpha linolenic acid is converted to a very long fatty acid, EICOSAPENTANEONIC ACID (EPA), which forms prostaglandins (PGE_3) and thromboxane (TXA_3) that counterbalance the effects of proinflammatory products derived from arachidonic acid by reducing the tendency to clot, reducing pain and inflammation. Dietary alpha linolenic acid will tend to inhibit arachidonic acid conversion to inflammatory agents, and thus further limit inflammation. Alpha linolenic acid occurs in high levels in BORAGE oil and flax seed oil, while EPA occurs in high levels in fish and shellfish.

If the diet lacks adequate amounts of either linoleic or alpha linolenic acid, deficiency symptoms will develop that include scaly skin, hair loss and slow wound healing. Omega-3 fatty acid deficiency leads to impaired brain and retinal development in experimental animals and possibly in premature births.

Polyunsaturated seed oils and fish oils supply the essential fatty acids in the typical U.S. diet. There is no RECOMMENDED DIETARY ALLOWANCE for linoleic acid or alpha linolenic acid. However, the amount of linoleic acid and related omega-6 fatty acids needed to prevent deficiency in adults is estimated to be 1 to 3% of calories, equivalent to approximately 6 g/day. Linoleic acid in typical American diets ranges from 5 to 10% of calories due to a high consumption of vegetable oils. It has been proposed that alpha linolenic acid represent 0.25 to 0.54% of daily calories for optimal health. Large amounts of polyunsaturated fatty acids may increase the requirement for antioxidants like VITAMIN E to prevent their chemical degradation. (See also DOCOSAHEXAENOIC ACID.)

essential nutrients   Substances in FOODS that are indispensable for growth and maintenance and must be supplied by the diet. About 40 essential NUTRIENTS have been identified. For healthy adults the essential nutrients include eight AMINO ACIDS, two ESSENTIAL FATTY ACIDS (LINOLEIC and ALPHA LINOLENIC ACIDS); VITAMINS (13 are so classified); MINERALS, including trace minerals and water. Foods must supply 15 minerals; none can be generated in the body. A certain minimal input of digestible CARBOHYDRATE is required to prevent excessive muscle protein and fat breakdown. Dietary FIBER maintains normal bowel function. The amounts of these materials required for optimal health have not been specified.

A number of nutrients are best classified as conditionally essential, because under certain circumstances, the diet may not supply adequate amounts to meet the body's needs for growth, maintenance or repair and healing. The amino acids asparagine, histidine, methionine and cysteine fall into this category. The need for nutrients such as TAURINE, a sulfur-containing compound derived from the sulfur amino acid cysteine, COENZYME Q_{10}, CHOLINE and CARNITINE, a compound needed to degrade fatty acids, can increase during heart disease and other conditions. There is a growing awareness that vegetables and fruits supply a wide range of substances that support health beyond those traditionally recognized nutrients. These include complex aromatic compounds called FLAVONOIDS that affect liver detoxication, limit inflammation, strengthen capillary walls and serve as antioxidants. Dark green leafy and orange vegetables and fruits supply orange-yellow pigments called CAROTENOIDS that act as antioxidants and enhance the immune system. It may well be the case that such plant products are essential components of a balanced diet over a lifetime to prevent or retard chronic disease. (See also RECOMMENDED DIETARY ALLOWANCES.)

esterase   An enzyme that breaks down esters. LIPASES are esterases that degrade fats and oils (TRIGLYCERIDES) to FATTY ACIDS and GLYCEROL during FAT DIGESTION and in LIPOLYSIS, the process of breaking down stored fat. Phospholipases digest PHOSPHOLIPIDS to fatty acids. An esterase plays a key role in the transmission of nerve impulses. Acetylcholine esterase breaks down the neurotransmitter ACETYLCHOLINE to its constituents, CHOLINE and ACETIC ACID. (See also DIGESTIVE ENZYMES.)

esters   A class of organic compounds that includes fragrances, fruity flavors, FATS, OILS and WAXES. Esters contain two types of building blocks—acids and alcohols. Esters that evaporate easily account for aromas and flavors of apples (methyl butanoate); oranges (octylacetate); pineapple (ethylbutanoate); and rum flavor (ethylformate). Artificial fruit flavors are primarily mixtures of low molecular weight esters.

Fats and OILS are triple esters containing the complex alcohol and long-chain FATTY ACIDS plus the triple alcohol, GLYCEROL, and are called TRIGLYCERIDES; they represent the most abundant LIPIDS. Digestion of fats and oils yields fatty acids that are readily absorbed.

Whether a triglyceride is a solid depends upon its fatty acid composition. Triglycerides containing unsaturated fatty acids, such as OLEIC ACID and LINOLEIC ACID, are liquid at room temperature and are called oils. Corn oil, soybean oil and wheatgerm oil contain approximately 80% unsaturated oil and therefore these substances are liquids. On the other hand, triglycerides rich in saturated fatty acids, such as PALMITIC ACID and STEARIC ACID, are semi-solid or solid at room temperature and are called fats. For example, beef fat (BEEF TALLOW) contains approximately 41.5% saturated fatty acids and is a waxy solid.

Naturally occuring waxes such as beeswax are esters containing a fatty acid combined with a large alcohol with a chain length from 16 to over 30 carbon atoms. Waxes are harder, more brittle and less greasy than fats, and they are used in cosmetics, ointments and time-release nutrient supplements, and are also used to coat produce in order to reduce moisture loss and to create a shiny appearance.

Other types of esters are important in cellular formation. Simple sugars like glucose must be esterified with phosphate before they can be used. Once phosphate is attached, sugars cannot leak out of the cell. Phosphate esters are also represented by a class of lipids called phospholipids, such as LECITHIN, which form cell membranes. Phosphate esters also link the building blocks of DNA and RNA. (See also CARBOHYDRATE METABOLISM; ESTERASE; FLAVORS; SUGAR.)

estrogen   A class of steroid HORMONES that function as female sex hormones. Estrogens are formed by the follicles of ovaries. They serve many functions: They increase protein synthesis in targeted tissues; they are responsible for secondary female characteristics (such as the development of breasts and the deposition of fat); and they stimulate regeneration of epithelial tissue of the uterus. Estrogen levels increase in the postmenstrual phase of the menstrual cycle. Together with progesterone, estrogen prepares the endometrium for ovulation. Women's overall eating patterns are affected by the menstrual cycle, thus a decline in food consumption corresponds to a rise in estrogen levels at the time of ovulation.

Estrogen retards bone loss, and after menopause, estrogen may be used therapeutically to reduce the risk of OSTEOPOROSIS. Minimal doses are required to reduce the risk of estrogen-induced cancer in older women. Estriol is an estrogen that does not appear to promote cancer. Most studies suggest that estrogen replacement therapy lowers the risk of CARDIOVASCULAR DISEASE. (See also CALCIUM; ENDOCRINE SYSTEM; TESTOSTERONE.)

Hileman, Bette, "Environmental Estrogens Linked to Reproductive Abnormalities, Cancer," *Chemistry and Engineering News*, (Jan. 31, 1994), pp. 19–23.

Seachrist, Lisa, "What Risk Hormones?" *Science News*, 148 (August 1995), p. 94–95.

ethanol (ethyl alcohol, grain alcohol)   An ALCOHOL traditionally produced in the fermentation of carbohydrates and starches. Ethanol is present in fermented beverages and distilled liquors. Absolute alcohol contains 99% ethanol and 1% water. Ethanol is rapidly absorbed by the stomach and small intestine, and it is destroyed at a constant rate by the liver. Oxidation yields 7 calories per gram.

Ethanol is oxidized by ethanol oxidizing systems (EOS), an enzyme system that may be more active among heavy drinkers. Nonetheless, excessive alcohol can block the liver's ability to synthesize GLUCOSE, leading to low blood sugar (HYPOGLYCEMIA). Persistent over-consumption of ethanol can deplete the liver of vitamins and can lead to fatty liver and eventually to CIRRHOSIS.

Ethanol has several commercial uses; it is employed to extract herbal essences and is used in several patent medicines. Denatured alcohol is alcohol that has been rendered unfit for human consumption by the addition of a toxic substance; it is used commercially as a solvent. (See also ALCOHOLISM.)

ethylenediaminetetraacetic acid   See EDTA.

ethyl formate   A food additive used in artificial flavors including artificial lemon and strawberry. Ethyl formate serves as a fungicide and as an agent to kill insect larvae in cereals and dried fruit.

etiology   The cause of a disease or health condition. (See also EPIDEMIOLOGY.)

evaporated milk   Concentrated milk, prepared from homogenized whole MILK through heating and evaporation. Each pint of evaporated milk is enriched with 400 IU of VITAMIN D. Upon dilution with water, evaporated milk provides the same food value and fat content as fresh milk. Evaporated skim milk is also available. Condensed milk is more concentrated than evaporated milk; in addition it is sweetened with sugar. (See also PASTEURIZATION.)

evening primrose oil   The oil prepared from seeds of the evening primrose, which is used as a supplemental source of essential fatty acids. It contains 72 to 75% LINOLEIC ACID, an ESSENTIAL FATTY ACID; 9% GAMMA LINOLENIC ACID; and 9% OLEIC ACID, the non-essential fatty acid. The first metabolic conversion of linoleic acid to PROSTAGLANDINS, hormone-like fatty acid derivatives, is the transformation to gamma linolenic acid. This conversion is partially blocked by excessive saturated FATTY ACIDS, TRANS-FATTY ACIDS in

processed vegetable oils, ALCOHOL and zinc deficiency, and the process slows during diabetes and AGING. Dietary gamma linolenic acid can bypass this blocked step; furthermore it is metabolized to a type of prostaglandin (PGE$_1$) that inhibits the formation of pro-inflammatory prostaglandins, thus helping to reduce allergy symptoms and atopic ECZEMA in some cases. Both linoleic acid and gamma linolenic acid seem to have other diverse effects, including boosting the immune system and reducing symptoms of premenstrual syndrome, lowering blood CHOLESTEROL, and slowing BLOOD CLOTTING. (See also ALLERGY, FOOD; ALPHA LINOLENIC ACID.)

exchange lists (U.S. exchange system)   Food lists devised to help consumers plan nutritious, balanced meals. Exchange lists emphasize variety, freshness, fat, calorie control, and whole foods rather than processed foods. In the U.S. Exchange System, six groups categorize foods according to a similar content of CALORIES, CARBOHYDRATE, FAT and PROTEIN: MILK; low-calorie VEGETABLES; FRUIT; grain products like BREAD and PASTA plus starchy vegetables like lima beans and corn; a MEAT group including CHEESE and PEANUT butter; and fat, including oils.

This system simplifies the balancing of calories because each serving of a given food group has the same number of calories and the same amount of carbohydrates, protein and fat, and interchanges within the group of foods are simplified. A further advantage is that fat content in foods is emphasized. For example, meats and cheeses are broken down into low-, medium- and high-fat content foods. Meat items are given in terms of one-ounce portions, while a more typical portion size is 3 oz or more. Exchange lists are available for diabetics, for those on weight loss programs, and for individuals on salt-restricted, cholesterol-restricted or fat-restricted diets. (See also BASIC FOOD GROUPS; DIABETES MELLITUS.)

Boyar, Andrea P. and Loubridge, Janet R., "The Fat Portion Exchange List; a Tool for Teaching and Evaluating Low Fat Diets," *Journal of the American Dietetic Association*, 85 (May 1985), pp. 589–94.

excretion   Processes by which the body eliminates waste products. Not only must the body take in nutrients, it must also rid itself of wastes. The body eliminates gaseous waste products (carbon dioxide, ACETONE) through the lungs and water-soluble wastes through the kidneys (urine); feces through the INTESTINE and perspiration through the skin. Typical waste products include CARBON DIOXIDE and UREA, from the oxidation of foodstuffs, and also BILIRUBIN (from HEMOGLOBIN degradation) and URIC ACID (from DNA and RNA breakdown). The kidneys excrete urea, uric acid, creatinine, end products of hormone metabolism, in addition to processed drugs and ingested chemicals, for example, metal ions like ALUMINUM. Urea is the major nitrogen-containing waste product from protein degradation, while creatinine is a waste product of muscle. A variety of materials are absorbed but cannot be utilized by the body so they too are excreted in the urea. Several plant carbohydrates, sugar derivatives like mannitol, as well as the artificial sweeteners CYCLAMATE and SUCRULOSE are examples. Plant LIGNIN, a form of fiber that is neither digested nor absorbed by the COLON, is excreted in the feces.

Substances produced in the body in excessive amounts can be excreted in urine. Urinary excretion of KETONE BODIES during acute STARVATION, and GLUCOSE excretion during uncontrolled DIABETES MELLITUS, reflect excessively high blood levels of these substances. Overconsumption of substances such as water-soluble vitamins, VITAMIN C and the B complex, beyond what the body can use or store, is also excreted. Alternatively, fat malabsorption or maldigestion can lead to the appearance of unusually large amounts of fat in feces. (See also ARTIFICIAL SWEETENER; CATABOLISM; DETOXICATION; FIBER.)

exercise   Physical activity to maintain FITNESS or to strengthen the body. Regular aerobic physical exercise strengthens the oxygen delivery system (heart and lungs), increases endurance and lowers the pulse rate, so the heart doesn't have to work as hard. Exercise assists in coping with emotional STRESS, and individuals who exercise are healthier and live longer than those who are sedentary. They maintain their body weight more easily. Active people tend to weigh less than sedentary people.

Moderate exercise, 30 minutes daily, promotes these beneficial effects: It increases HDL (the desirable form of cholesterol), insulin responsiveness to BLOOD SUGAR, bone strength and antibody production. It lowers blood pressure and the risk of blood clots, cancer, abdominal FAT and cardiovascular disease. Sedentary people who start exercising might reduce their risk of dying from HEART DISEASE. Vigorous exercise strengthens the heart and blood vessels. Strenuous exercise (endurance events), however, can temporarily suppress the immune system.

Regular exercise helps keep lost weight off after DIETING. There are several factors involved. Exercise increases muscle mass, and muscle burns calories more efficiently than fat tissue does. Examples of moderate exercises that burn 100 CALORIES include walking a mile, jogging a half-mile, swimming one-third of a mile, cycling a quarter of a mile.

Calories are also burned more rapidly after exercising than not, though the duration and intensity of exercise needed to secure this benefit is an important question still being studied. If the individual is sedentary, moderate exercise seems to cause a 10% increase in basal metabolism for several hours. A moderately active individual may need to do aerobic exercise such as swimming, aerobic dancing and jogging a total of six hours per week to increase the metabolic rate for several days afterward.

Exercise also seems to diminish the desire for fatty foods and increase the likelihood of eating CARBOHYDRATES, which contain fewer calories. Fat is a potential problem in the diet because the body more easily converts fat in food to body fat.

Carbohydrates are the best fuel during short, intense exercise such as sprinting, when muscles rely on GLUCOSE as fuel. During low to moderate intensity exercise, fat supplies about half the energy, while GLYCOGEN and blood SUGAR supply the rest. Fat is the major fuel during medium to intense exercise, when exercise lasts more than one to one and a half hours. Stored fat can supply as much as 70% of calorie needs for moderate exercise lasting four to six hours, especially when muscle glycogen stores are low. Afterward, PROTEIN supplies 5 to 15% of a person's energy needs.

APPETITE often stays the same with regular, moderate exercise (for example, 15 miles a week of jogging or walking). The appetite may increase to make up for the extra calories burned. Athletes burn more calories; while training for competition, the appetite of athletes increases because so many more calories are needed for strenuous physical activity.

Nutritional Needs During Exercise

Water   Adequate water is essential for the body to use food and for the kidneys to dispose of waste. Perspiration controls body temperature. Drinking one to three cups of water or non-caffeinated beverage before exercise is recommended. Dehydration and overheating can be problems with prolonged exercise, especially during warm weather. Replacement of water losses may be needed before thirst is sensed, and adult athletes should drink 500 to 600 ml (16 to 20 oz) of fluid during the two hours before exercise and up to 500 ml of fluid 10 to 15 minutes before an event.

Plain water or fruit juice is usually adequate; ELECTROLYTE replacement sports drinks are not necessary. During prolonged strenuous exercise, remedy weakness due to low blood sugar by drinking diluted carbohydrate beverages containing fruit sugar or glucose every 10 to 15 minutes, 150 to 250 ml (4 to 6 oz). Fruit juices should be diluted to prevent delayed gastric emptying. Glucose-electrolyte sports drinks should contain between 6 to 10% carbohydrate for optimal uptake. Some contain maltodextran, short starch fragments that leave the stomach faster than plain sugar.

After an event, replace each pound of lost weight with 500 ml (16 oz) of fluid. Caffeinated and alcoholic beverages should be avoided. Alcohol and CAFFEINE act as diuretics, and dehydrate the body. The International Olympic Committee has banned the use of large doses of caffeine in athletes.

Protein   The typical U.S. diet probably supplies up to twice as much protein as needed to maintain the body. However, it is important that the intake of calories be adequate. If calories are restricted, then protein needs will increase. For a sedentary adult, 0.8 g protein per kilogram of body weight per day is required to avoid deficiencies. Endurance athletes have increased protein requirements, estimated to be 1.5 g/kg/day. Athletes engaged in strength training may need as much as 2g/kg/day. This protein requirement would be met by balanced diets providing 12 to 15% of their calories as protein. Loading up on protein powders or meat may promote calcium losses in female athletes. A high-protein diet tends to be high in SATURATED FAT, potentially harmful for the heart. A better approach is a diet with a mixture of carbohydrate, fat and adequate protein.

Amino acids are a significant fuel source during endurance exercise, especially branched chain amino acids; and they have been used as supplements. However, single amino acids in large doses can cause amino acid imbalances, and the margins of safety are unknown. Large amounts of the amino acids ORNITHINE and ARGININE have been hypothesized to stimulate GROWTH HORMONE release and thus stimulate fat loss and protein build-up. However, reports on the anabolic effects of these amino acids remain inconclusive, and most available amino acid mixtures supply much lower doses of those amino acids than are found to be effective in some studies.

Carbohydrate During strenuous exercise (marathon running, for example) muscle glycogen becomes depleted; when this occurs, exhaustion sets in. For example, glycogen depletion can occur during exercise that requires near maximal bursts of effort (basketball, football and soccer). Alternatively, glycogen depletion can occur gradually with repeated heavy workouts, in which glycogen breakdown exceeds its role of replacement. "Staleness" and FATIGUE can be due to overtraining and to inadequate carbohydrate consumption.

Complex carbohydrate The typical American diet supplies only 46% percent carbohydrate, judged inadequate to meet increased energy needs of someone in training. Exercising for more than an hour per day increases the need for complex carbohydrates: whole GRAINS and CEREAL GRAINS, BREAD, VEGETABLES, LEGUMES and FRUIT. Extra carbohydrate should supply 55 to 60% of calories. This means covering approximately two-thirds of a plate with carbohydrate foods at each meal. No more than 15% of calories should come from sugar. To prepare for strenuous exercise lasting more than an hour and a half by building up glycogen stores, a high carbohydrate diet (60 to 70% of daily calories) may be required for three days prior to the event together with a reduction in training. Carbohydrates eaten soon after strenuous exercise can refuel muscles with glycogen stores. Simple carbohydrates in juices and fruit will work best for the first few hours after a workout, followed by high complex carbohydrate meals.

Fat Fat is a significant source of energy during moderate intensity exercise. Its utilization increases with duration. Although animal studies suggest that high-fat diets increase endurance, human studies have failed to reveal any advantage. There are many disadvantages to high-fat, low-carbohydrate diets. They tend to raise blood cholesterol levels, which is linked to the increased risk of CARDIOVASCULAR DISEASE. They are hard to follow. High-fat diets increase the risk of OBESITY, because fat calories are more readily stored as body fat than carbohydrate. The National Research Council (U.S.) recommends that fats and oils should account for less than 30% of the calories for adults and saturated fat (animal fat, tropical vegetable oils) be limited to one-third of the total. Avoid fatty foods before exercise because they require three to four hours for digestion.

Supplements A BALANCED DIET supplying extra calories is adequate for increased needs due to exercise, although supplements can remedy nutrient deficiencies. Athletes on low-calorie diets to reduce body fat run the risk of malnutrition because they may not consume adequate VITAMIN E, VITAMIN D or vitamins of the B COMPLEX like FOLIC ACID, CALCIUM and IRON. Marginal VITAMIN C deficiency can impair performance. Iron intake for many women is marginal and exercising can worsen an iron deficiency, leading to ANEMIA.

There is no special set of recommended dietary allowances for vitamins and minerals for athletes. Some studies indicate an increased need for certain nutrients. Requirements for B complex and zinc may increase with exercise, and female gymnasts may be low in VITAMIN B_6, folic acid, calcium, iron and zinc. Teenagers who are long-distance runners may be anemic because some blood is lost to the intestine through jarring. Eating mainly processed foods worsens the problem. POTASSIUM losses in perspiration are negligible, except under severe conditions, and are easily replaced by foods after a workout. Sodium replacement is also accomplished by the typical diet except for long, strenuous events and when the temperature is high or when additional electrolytes may be needed. However, salt pills can be dangerous because they can supply excessive SODIUM too rapidly. Sodium and electrolytes lost through sweating are easily made up with salt in food and by drinking diluted fruit juice. Recent studies indicate that vigorous physical exercise increases oxidative damage to the body due to the generation of free radicals and other reactive types of chemicals. The effects of moderate exercise are less clear. In any event depletion of antioxidant defenses increases the body's vulnerability to oxidation, therefore the consumption of sufficient antioxidants is important. Ample vitamin C, vitamin E, trace minerals such as zinc, copper, selenium and manganese, and sulfur-containing amino acids are keys to maintaining antioxidant defenses. Whether people who exercise at moderate intensity need extra antioxidants is controversial. Endurance training has been shown to deplete body vitamin E in subjects consuming a normal diet.

Clearly vitamin and mineral deficiencies will impair performance. Vitamin C, vitamin E and B vitamins will not increase energy production or utilization by the body unless there is a deficiency. Vitamins and mineral supplements cannot be used to patch up a faulty diet—one based on fatty, fried or convenience foods.

Meals before competition A light meal (300 to 800 calories) two to four hours before running may be recommended. The meal should be served in a comfortable setting; it should be easily digested and low in fat and protein. Eating during the hour before competition and consuming excessive sugar before exercise could stimulate insulin production, possibly leading to lower blood sugar (HYPOGLYCEMIA) during the event and hindering performance. Symptoms of hypoglycemia include feeling light-headed and shaky, blurred vision and fatigue. Avoid foods and beverages with simple sugar sweeteners such as soft drinks, candy and fruit juices, within an hour of exercising.

(See also CARBOHYDRATE METABOLISM; FAT METABOLISM; GLYCOGEN LOADING.)

Berning, Jacqueline R. and Steen, Suzanne Nelson. *Sports Nutrition for the '90s.* Gaithersberg, Md.: Aspen Publishers, 1991.

Clarkson, Pricilla M., "Antioxidants and Physical Performance," *Critical Reviews in Food Science and Nutrition*, 35:1,2 (1995), pp 131–141.

Katzel, Leslie I., et al., "Effects of Weight Loss vs Aerobic Exercise Training on Risk Factors for Coronary Disease in Healthy, Obese, Middle-aged and Older Men—A Randomized Controlled Trial," *Journal of the American Medical Association* 274:24 (December 27, 1995), pp. 1915–21.

extracellular fluid   Fluid that lies outside of the cells of the body. The human body is 60% WATER, by weight. Water is indispensable because it forms a major constituent of every tissue and every cell and is the medium for nearly all functions and chemical transformations. Water in the body distributes itself in two general compartments. Water within cells is considered INTRACELLULAR FLUID, which represents 60% of the body's water content. Extracellular fluid includes fluids between cells and tissues and in the circulatory systems. Less than 20% occurs in blood and lymph systems. (See also BODY FLUIDS; CYTOPLASM; DEHYDRATION.)

FAD   See FLAVIN ADENINE DINUCLEOTIDE.

fad diets   Drastic weight reduction programs. Fad diets are potentially dangerous because they employ one or more of the following flawed strategies:

Severely restricting calories   With less than 1,000 CALORIES a day the body adapts to semi-starvation by burning its fat and muscle, regardless of whether or not a little PROTEIN or CARBOHYDRATE is consumed. This adaptation raises the possibility of excessive water loss and excessive build-up of acidic products of fat metabolism (KETOSIS). Water loss disrupts fluid and ELECTROLYTE balance, which can harm the heart. The harmful aspects of severe caloric restriction are worsened by the use of laxatives, DIURETICS or induced vomiting, which can cause electrolyte imbalance and flush water out of the body. The resulting weight loss represents water loss, not fat loss.

Consuming no carbohydrates   Without dietary carbohydrate, the body switches into a CATABOLIC STATE in which stored fat is oxidized and KETONE BODIES (metabolic acids) accumulate, a situation called ketosis. As excessive ketone bodies are excreted in the urine, extensive water losses promote DEHYDRATION, while the loss of sodium causes electrolyte imbalance. The brain requires GLUCOSE for ENERGY, and when carbohydrate is not supplied by the diet, BLOOD SUGAR must be synthesized from AMINO ACIDS, derived from muscle protein breakdown.

Consuming only one kind of food for an extended period of time   Unless the diet supplies adequate amounts of protein and carbohydrate, body chemistry switches over to fat and muscle breakdown. No single food or supplement supplies all the required nutrients in the appropriate ratios needed to maintain health.

Using appetite suppressants   This class of compounds includes benzocaine, BULKING AGENTS and PHENYL-PROPANOLAMINE, a commonly used APPETITE SUPPRESSANT in diet pills. Benzocaine numbs the taste buds without bringing about a long-term change in eating behavior, while phenylpropanolamine causes only a temporary appetite reduction and may raise blood pressure. (See also AMPHETAMINES; DIET, LOW CARBOHYDRATE; DIET, VERY LOW CALORIE; DIETING: CRASH PROGRAMS; FASTING; GLUCONEOGENESIS.)

familial hypercholesterolemia   An inherited tendency to have elevated serum CHOLESTEROL levels. This trait greatly increases the risk of coronary heart disease. About 1 in 500 people carry a defective gene causing a two- to three-fold increase in serum cholesterol from birth. Individuals who possess the defective gene in both sets of chromosomes are much more severely affected. Their cholesterol may be five to six times normal, and they may have heart attacks by the age of 20 due to clogged arteries (ATHEROSCLEROSIS). Therefore, a family history of premature coronary heart disease greatly increases a person's risk.

One form of hypercholesterolemia is characterized by the inability of tissues to remove LOW-DENSITY LIPOPROTEIN cholesterol (LDL) from circulation. LDL transports cholesterol to the various tissues of the body where it must bind to specific docking sites on cell surfaces. As a result, LDL cannot be effectively taken up by cells. Recent investigations have revealed that this condition is often the result of mutations of the gene for the LDL receptor. Patients with familial hypercholesterolemia are likely to be placed on low-cholesterol diets and to be given medications in order to lower their cholesterol levels. (See also CHOLESTEROL-LOWERING DRUGS; HYPERLIPOPROTEINEMIA.)

FAO   See FOOD AND AGRICULTURAL ORGANIZATION.

fast food   Meals that are mass-produced and often sold by franchised restaurant chains. Typical offerings include fried CHICKEN, chicken nuggets, pizzas, fried FISH, roast BEEF, HOT DOGS, HAMBURGERS, FRENCH FRIES, nachos, tacos, chili, pasta salads and doughnuts. There are currently about 160,000 fast-food restaurants in the United States, where it is often possible to order a meal and eat it within 10 to 15 minutes.

Nearly one out of every four Americans eats fast food every day, and more than half of the money spent on meals away from home goes for fast food. The immense popularity of fast foods rests on convenience, dependable quality and moderate expense. Two-income households have less time for home chores, including cooking, and they have more money to spend. Busy schedules for each member of the family place a premium on time spent in planning, preparing and eating a meal. Fast food is also appealing to travelers and commuters. The fast-food industry has expanded overseas sales as well as branching out into hospitals, airports, colleges and airline in-flight meal service.

Fast-food chains have responded to nutrition awareness of consumers. Many now offer salad bars, low-fat roast beef, low-calorie salad dressing, corn on the cob and baked potatoes. Several chains reduced the CALORIES and FAT in their hamburgers. It is now often possible to obtain a "heart healthy" meal with less salt, less SATURATED FAT and more vegetables and fresh fruit than before. Several restaurant chains provide nutritional information about calories, fat and SODIUM content, as well as additives such as SULFITES, MONOSODIUM GLUTAMATE (MSG) and LACTOSE. Nutritional information has not yet found its way to labels on fast-food products, however.

With prudent selection from a fast-food menu, most healthy people can eat fast foods occasionally without compromising their health. The health costs of relying on fast foods, however, are high.

Overnutrition   Many fast-food items contain excessive fat (especially saturated fat), SUGAR, salt and calories. Fast food supplies 20% of the fat in American diets and much of it is saturated. A single meal can easily supply all the calories and sodium needed for an entire day.

Although fish, chicken and POTATOES alone are relatively low-calorie foods, they become high-fat, high-calorie foods when dipped in batter and fried. In addition, chicken skin, which is essentially fat, is added to chicken nuggets. If the fat used in cooking is BEEF TALLOW, fried foods—regardless of

their source—are also high in CHOLESTEROL and in saturated fat, believed to promote clogged arteries. Several fast-food chains have switched to soybean oil or to saturated vegetable oils to avoid the potential problems and negative image of animal fat. Pasta salads are usually high in fat because of added dressings, cheese or processed meat toppings. A typical 3/4-cup serving can provide fat equal to the amount in a fast-food cheeseburger (nearly four teaspoons). (See page 166.)

Undernutrition   Many menu options that are high in sugar and fat calories are often low in critical nutrients. These include FIBER, vitamins (like VITAMIN A, VITAMIN C, vitamin E and FOLIC ACID) and minerals (like chromium, manganese, magnesium, ZINC and IRON). There is a growing appreciation of the importance of the non-nutrient constituents in plant foods called phytochemicals, which seem to protect against chronic diseases associated with aging, such as cancer. Between 10 and 20% of the U.S. population consumes the minimum recommended five servings of fruits and vegetables daily.

Poor digestion   Eating a meal in 10 minutes may not provide enough time for adequate digestion. Adequate chewing is a signal to start the digestive juices flowing, and minimal chewing means less efficient breakdown and assimilation.

To cut down on fat while still enjoying fast foods:

1. Eat less fried food.
2. Peel off the batter coating of fried fish or chicken, which retains the fat.
3. Select the salad bar but cut back on salad dressing, pasta salad, bacon bits and potato salad. These contain extra fat. Add flavor with low-fat COTTAGE CHEESE, pepper, spices or KETCHUP.
4. Substitute a baked potato for french fries, which retain much of the fat and oil they were fried in.
5. Omit sour cream, CHEESE and BUTTER (all high in saturated fat) on salads and baked dishes.
6. Select roast beef instead of hamburger. A lean roast beef sandwich plus a salad without heavy dressing or a seafood salad provides a balanced meal.
7. Eat less butterfat. Croissants, sweet rolls, milk shakes and ice cream are all sources of saturated fat.

(See also ADVERTISING; ATHEROSCLEROSIS; BALANCED DIET; CONVENIENCE FOOD; EATING PATTERNS; MALNUTRITION; OBESITY.)

Jacobson, Michael F. and Fritschner, Sarah. *The Fast-food Guide*. New York: Workman Publishing Company, 1986.

fasting   Choosing not to eat. Fasting for a day with adequate water is generally safe for healthy adults. Children are more susceptible to problems associated with fasting because their energy reserves of GLYCOGEN and FAT are smaller; prolonged fasting causes major metabolic changes that can eventually be harmful.

On the first day of fasting, carbohydrate stored in the liver (glycogen) is broken down to supply blood GLUCOSE. During the first week, body fat begins to be broken down to meet the energy requirements of the body. Muscle protein breakdown yields AMINO ACIDS, which the liver converts to BLOOD SUGAR

Hidden Fat in Fast Foods

	weight (g)	calories	fat (g)	percent calories from fat
McDonald's Arch Deluxe™	247	570	31	49
McDonald's Big Mac	215	530	28	48
Wendy's Single (plain) Sandwich	133	360	16	40
Burger King Whopper	270	614	36	53
Arby's Regular Roast Beef	154	388	19	44
Hardee's Chicken Fillet Sandwich	215	480	18	34
Wendy's Spicy Chicken Sandwich (regular)	216	470	20	38
McDonald's Chicken McNuggets® (6 pieces)	106	290	17	53
KFC Original Recipe Breast	115	283	15	48
KFC Extra Tasty Crispy Thigh	119	406	30	66
Hardee's Big Roast Beef Sandwich	184	460	24	47
Wendy's Big Bacon Classic Sandwich	280	570	29	51
Arby's Fish Fillet Sandwich	220	529	27	46

Hidden Fat in Typical Fast Foods

	weight (g)	calories	fat (g)	percent calories from fat
beef taco	81	195	11	51
hot dog and bun	85	260	15.3	53
corndog	111	330	20	55
beef and bean burrito	175	390	17.5	40
cheese pizza (1/8 of 15-in diameter)	120	290	9	28
french fries cooked in vegetable oil (10)	50	158	8.3	47
vanilla milk shake (10 fl oz/1.25 cup)	283	314	8.4	24
ice cream, rich, vanilla 16% fat (1 cup)	148	349	23.7	62
doughnut, glazed, 3.5-in diameter	50	210	12	46
fried apple pie (apple turnover)	85	255	14	49
apple pie (1/6 of a pie)	158	408	17.5	39

Jacobson, M., *The Fast-Food Guide,* 2nd ed.,. New York: Workman Publishing, 1991.

(GLUCONEOGENESIS) to fuel the brain. With prolonged fasting, the body's metabolic rate slows in order to conserve energy and fuels are used more efficiently. With excessive fat breakdown, KETONE BODIES (water-soluble acids derived from fatty acids) can accumulate in the blood. They acidify the blood and cause excessive urination, which in turn causes DEHYDRATION and loss of ELECTROLYTES. Severe imbalance of ions in the blood can lead to heart failure.

Three commonly stated reasons for fasting include:

- Weight loss. Fasting is not a recommended weight loss strategy. Fasting causes considerable weight loss initially (up to 5 pounds per week), but this represents extensive water loss, not fat loss. Such lost weight will be regained rapidly upon return to the usual DIET. Studies show that during fasts muscle is lost, as well as fat, and lost muscle may be rapidly replaced by fat at the end of the fast.

- Detoxification (a procedure for the removal of toxins). As body fat is consumed, materials trapped or stored in fatty tissue may be released. Weakened cells in tissues are selectively destroyed by the immune system. The build-up of toxic materials released into the bloodstream can create an additional metabolic burden and oxidative stress for the liver, which is responsible for disposing of toxic materials.
- An altered state of consciousness. During fasting, individuals sometimes experience a greater clarity of mind, and fasting has traditionally accompanied forms of meditation.

Precautions regarding fasting:

1. No one should fast more than a day or so without medical supervision.
2. Pregnant or lactating women, children, adolescents whose bodies are growing, and diabetics should not fast.
3. It is important to drink plenty of liquids; the production of metabolic wastes continues at a high rate during fasting. A juice fast is safer than drinking water alone because the carbohydrate, vitamins and electrolytes of fruit juices help maintain body functions more adequately, and the carbohydrate they contain is needed to fuel the brain.
4. To end a fast, resume eating food with several small meals rather than with one large one. Fatty foods should be added back slowly because fat is harder to digest than carbohydrates and protein.
5. During fasting the production of ketone bodies in the urine can be monitored by using a "dip stick" available at drug stores. The presence of ketone bodies in urine indicates a state of KETOSIS, excessive fat breakdown.

(See also ACIDOSIS; DIET, VERY LOW CALORIE; DIETING: CRASH PROGRAMS.)

"Insights into Fasting," *Lancet*, 339 (January 18, 1992), pp. 152–53.

fasting blood sugar The blood glucose level that is maintained between meals. Normally BLOOD SUGAR is maintained at a concentration between 60 and 100 mg per deciliter. An elevated fasting blood sugar level can indicate a diabetic or pre-diabetic condition. Adequate blood sugar is maintained by the liver, which breaks down GLYCOGEN, a starch-like carbohydrate synthesized from glucose after a meal. Maintenance of blood sugar is controlled by hormones. GLUCAGON and GLUCOCORTICOIDS help raise blood sugar levels by directing the liver to synthesize glucose from AMINO ACIDS released from muscle and INSULIN stimulates glucose uptake after a meal. (See also GLUCONEOGENESIS; GLUCOSE TOLERANCE TEST.)

fat (triglyceride, triacylglycerol) An oily nutrient that is the most concentrated form of ENERGY, supplying 9 calories per gram, more than twice as much energy as in CARBOHYDRATE or protein. Fat is one of the most abundant nutrients in foods, and it is a major fuel for the body. Dietary fat supplies about 36% of total calories in the standard American diet. Current recommendations are to decrease fat consumption to supply less than 30% of daily calories. Fat serves two other functions: It carries flavors in foods and helps fat-rich foods create a feeling of satiety (feeling full) by slowing the rate of stomach emptying.

Fat is classified as a LIPID because it dissolves in organic solvents like hexane rather than in water. Although often considered a "fat," cholesterol is a very different compound, though they are both insoluble in water and thus are both lipids. Fat functions as an energy reserve; it is usually broken down to carbon dioxide to supply energy, while cholesterol is converted only to steroid hormones and BILE salts. From a dietary perspective, a low-cholesterol diet also lowers saturated fat intake because both fat and cholesterol occur in meat.

Fats and oils contain three FATTY ACIDS bonded to GLYCEROL (glycerin) like streamers hung from a flagpole. During digestion fat is broken down by the enzyme pancreatic lipase and is released into the intestine. Fat can also be broken down in the test tube by a process called saponification in which fats and oils react with alkali to produce soaps.

Fats are classified as saturated or unsaturated, according to their fatty acid compositions. Saturated fat is solid at room temperature; examples are LARD and HYDROGENATED VEGETABLE OIL (VEGETABLE SHORTENING). Saturated fat contains relatively high levels of saturated fatty acids (40% for lard, to 50% for BEEF TALLOW, to 62% for butterfat). If a fat contains less than one-third saturated fatty acids, it is considered unsaturated.

Oils contain more unsaturated fatty acids, or they contain smaller than usual saturated fatty acids (medium-chain fatty acids). Examples of the oils with higher amounts of unsaturates are vegetable oils (corn, safflower, soybean, sunflower, olive oils) and FISH OIL. Examples of saturated-fat oils are PALM OIL and palm kernel oil. Several unsaturated oils contain relatively high levels of unsaturated fatty acids (89% for sunflower oil, 91% for safflower oil, 86% for olive oil and 87% for corn oil).

Fat calories in food are not the same as carbohydrate calories because the body converts dietary fat to body fat much more efficiently than it converts carbohydrate to fat. That is, 23% of the calories in starches and sugars are consumed in converting them to fat, while only 3% of the calories in dietary fat are expended in converting it to stored fat.

Many authorities recommend fat intake of less than 30 calories daily. To estimate the amount of dietary fat represented by 25% of daily calories, as an example: Add together all the calories consumed for a day using food-calorie tables (available at supermarkets and health food stores). This will require that you estimate how much of each food you ate. Divide the total calories by 4 to obtain 25% of calories as fat. Then divide by 9 to obtain the number of grams of daily fat, because there are 9 calories in each gram of fat. As an example, for a woman eating 1,600 calories daily, the limit for fat would be 44 g (3 tablespoons). For a man eating 2,400 calories per day, the limit would be 67 g of fat. To help visualize this, five tablespoons of any vegetable oil or three-quarters of a stick of butter equals 70 g of fat. (See also DIETING; DIET RECORD; FAT, TISSUE; OBESITY.)

Mayfield, Eleanor, "A Consumer's Guide to Fats," *FDA Consumer*, (May 1994), pp. 15–19.

fat, hidden The invisible FAT in foods. Visible fat is readily identified and measured, in such foods as butter, margarine, lard and cooking oils. The National Research

Council of the U.S. National Academy of Sciences estimates that between 1970 and 1990 overall fat consumption by Americans did not change greatly. Despite documented cutbacks on obvious fat sources like fatty red meat, butter and whole milk, the average consumption of fat in prepared foods and other high-fat foods significantly increased.

Fats and oils are found in most cheeses and spreads; in salad dressing; corn, potato and wheat CHIPS; cookies, muffins, pastries and CRACKERS; fried FISH and fried CHICKEN; FRENCH FRIES; GRANOLA; and whipped cream substitute. Non-dairy coffee whitener often has more SATURATED FAT than butter because it contains coconut oil. HAMBURGER legally can contain up to 30% fat. CHEESE and dairy products are high-fat foods. Hidden fat can supply 60 to 75% of their calories; BEEF and PORK have much more fat than chicken or fish. However, when fish and chicken are breaded and deep-fat fried, their calorie content increases dramatically due to hidden fat. Processed meats such as HOT DOGS, SAUSAGE, BOLOGNA and luncheon meats are generally extremely fatty. (See chart p.166.)

Food labels can help sort out high-fat foods. The U.S. FDA has instituted wide-ranging changes in food labels, including listing the number of fat calories. To calculate the percentage of fat calories, divide calories from fat by the total calories per serving and multiply the product by 100. Governmental dietary guidelines recommend that fat calories not exceed 30% of the total calories.

Claims such as "98 percent fat-free" on a food label have been misleading, and such claims are not permitted under the revision of food labels. "Fat free" means the food contains less than 0.5 g fat per serving. "Low fat" means the food contains 3 g or less per serving, while "reduced fat" or "less fat" indicate the food contains at least 25% less fat per serving than the reference food. (See also CONVENIENCE FOOD; EMPTY CALORIES.)

fat, tissue Fat found in ADIPOSE TISSUE, which is the only tissue specialized to store fat, the major fuel of the body. Body fat also insulates the body against changes in cold and serves as a shock absorber for sensitive organs like the kidneys. Stored fat comes from two different sources. It can be made from carbohydrate or ethanol or even from an excess protein, carbohydrate meal, or it can come from excessive dietary fat.

Body fat accumulates during early childhood and adolescence, when the number of fat cells increases. At other times, fat is deposited in preexisting fat cells when caloric intake exceeds calories spent. For example, METABOLISM slows and people tend to EXERCISE less, while continuing to eat high-calorie food as they get older. This accounts for the weight gain often seen at middle age.

Body fat can be burned up when the diet does not provide adequate calories. In response to stress, ADRENAL GLANDS secrete EPINEPHRINE, which signals fat cells to break down their stored fat to fatty acids, which are released into the bloodstream, absorbed by muscle and oxidized for energy production. Women have greater levels of enzymes for storing fat and lesser amounts of enzymes to degrade fat than men do. This may help to partially explain why some women have greater difficulty in dieting and maintaining body weight than men do. Chronically hostile and anxious people may burn fat more slowly than less upset and more emotionally balanced people who do not suppress anger.

A person's optimal amount of body fat depends upon many factors, including inheritance, body build, sex and age. Women's average body fat is about 20 to 25% of their body weight, while men's weight is typically 15 to 20% fat. Women usually have more fat than men because fat is important in pregnancy and lactation. Athletes who train vigorously (like marathon runners) have less fat. Fat may be 7% of a male athlete's body weight and 10% of a female athlete's weight. The distribution of excessive body fat is linked to HEART DISEASE. Fat around the middle (abdominal obesity) is a greater risk for heart disease than fat accumulated around hips and thighs (the "pear" profile).

To lose body fat, eat nutritious meals while reducing calories and exercising regularly. DIETING without exercise results in slower fat loss since muscle burns more energy per pound than adipose tissue. Avoid YO-YO DIETING (repeated episodes of dieting alternated with eating regular meals) because this may condition the body to store surplus calories as fat. (See also CELLULITE; FAT DIGESTION; FAT METABOLISM; LIPOSUCTION; SET POINT; STRESS.)

fat and chronic disease There is a general consensus that excessive fat consumption is a contributing factor in OBESITY, CANCER and HEART DISEASE. The prevailing medical opinion is that Americans eat too many fatty foods. Excessive fat consumption has been singled out as the number one dietary problem in the United States; average fat consumption is 130 pounds a year per person, which includes animal fat, VEGETABLE OIL, SHORTENING, MARGARINE and partially HYDROGENATED VEGETABLE OILS. This consumption is about twice as much fat and oil as is considered healthy by some experts. The DIETARY GUIDELINES FOR AMERICANS (U.S.) recommend cutting back on fat by at least 25%, so that total fat accounts for no more than 30% of daily calories for adults.

Fat contributes to obesity in part because it is easier to gain weight from eating excess fat than it is from eating excess CARBOHYDRATE. The body's metabolism is not efficient in converting sugar to fat; about a quarter of the calories in sugar are lost in the conversion. On the other hand, only 3% of the calories in consumed fat is expended in converting dietary fat to body fat.

Cancer

A high-fat intake is one of the strongest risk factors for cancer, after cigarette smoking. For example, lung cancer risk increases with diets high in saturated fat. High-fat diets decrease the ability of the IMMUNE SYSTEM to destroy cancer cells, and eating less animal fat and vegetable oil lowers the risk of colon, prostate and, possibly, breast cancer.

Overconsumption of fat increases the risk of heart disease in American populations. A diet with too much animal fat tends to raise blood CHOLESTEROL. On the other hand, polyunsaturated vegetable oils help lower blood cholesterol levels, believed to decrease the risk of heart disease. FISH and FISH OIL also seem to protect against heart disease. A special ingredient of fish oil, OMEGA-3 FATTY ACIDS, balances the immune system and decreases inflammation. Fish and fish oils slow down blood clotting, lower serum fat and perhaps cholesterol levels, and may reduce the risk of heart attacks. People who are generally angry or anxious have higher cholesterol levels; they degrade fat more slowly than their peers who are not angry or anxious. Consequently, slow fat breakdown may be one of the risk factors in heart attacks.

A very-low-fat diet, with 10% of calories from fat, was incorporated into a program to reduce the risks in people with heart disease. The program included exercise, stress reduction, counseling and support groups. Men who changed their life-style managed to reverse clogged arteries and to keep off lost weight for four to eight years.

Recommendations to Reduce Fat Calories

- Eat less fat by eating fewer servings and smaller portions. Be realistic about your expectations rather than totally eliminating favorite fatty foods. Dairy products like BUTTER and sour cream and plant-derived fat, like COCONUT OIL, palm and PALM kernel oil, shortening, margarine and CHOCOLATE, are sources of saturated fat. Vegetable oils such as SAFFLOWER oil, CORN OIL, SOYBEAN oil and mayonnaise represent unsaturated fat. Substitute low-calorie margarine and low-calorie mayonnaise. Use spices, vinegar or lemon juice rather than oily salad dressing.
- Reduce consumption of fat in meat by trimming off visible fat or by using only lean MEAT ("select" or good quality beef). Eat fewer hot dogs, hamburgers and sausage. Drain fat after browning meat. Remove skin from chicken and turkey. Broil, bake, poach or steam food rather than eating fried foods.
- Chill soups and discard coagulated fat. Cook vegetables in water and herbs instead of sauteing them in butter. Eat tuna packed in water, not oil. Bake fish with lemon juice instead of butter.
- Avoid pastry and rich desserts like ice cream.
- Use skim milk, non-fat yogurt and low-fat cottage cheese rather than products derived from whole milk. Avoid adding sour cream and cheese toppings to baked potatoes.

(See also ATHEROSCLEROSIS; BODY MASS INDEX; DIETING; EATING PATTERNS.)

fat digestion The breakdown of fat to its building blocks: FATTY ACIDS and the polyalcohol GLYCEROL. Fat DIGESTION is primarily an intestinal process requiring LIPASES, fat-splitting enzymes secreted by the pancreas. The pancreatic protein colipase assists in this process.

After digestion, fat follows a complex route through the body. BILE released from the gall bladder provides bile salts needed to absorb fatty acids into the intestine, where they are reassembled into fat, then packaged as CHYLOMICRONS, a lipid-protein complex that transports dietary fat first through the lymphatic system, then through the blood stream.

Fat in chylomicrons is degraded by a special lipase in capillaries to fatty acids, which are absorbed by muscle to be oxidized for energy and by adipose tissue to be stored as fat.

In contrast to usual dietary fats and oils, a fat containing medium-chain fatty acids (MEDIUM-CHAIN TRIGLYCERIDES) is used therapeutically with compromised digestion and maldigestion syndromes, because it passes directly into the bloodstream without chylomicron formation and is delivered to the liver, where it can be used immediately. (See also DIGESTIVE ENZYMES; DIGESTIVE TRACT.)

fatfold test (skinfold test) A convenient method of estimating body FAT. This test relies on a measurement of the width of a fold of skin on the back of the upper arm or other part of the body. Skin fold measurements, together with measurements of waist and hip circumference, have been used to estimate bone growth and changes in muscle mass during weight loss or weight gain. A caliper that applies a fixed pressure is used to measure skin fold thickness. A fatfold of over an inch wide reflects OBESITY. The fat at the back of the arm or from the upper back is roughly proportional to total body fat. When fat is gained, or lost, the fatfold increases and decreases proportionately. The test requires an experienced assessor for reliable results.

The distribution of fat is important in considering the risk of CARDIOVASCULAR DISEASE because abdominal fat, not hip fat, is correlated with an increased risk. Abdominal fat seems to be more easily metabolized by the liver and converted to LDL (LOW-DENSITY LIPOPROTEIN), the undesirable form of CHOLESTEROL. (See also BODY MASS INDEX; HEIGHT/WEIGHT TABLES; LEAN BODY MASS.)

fatigue Feelings of persistent tiredness and lethargy, unrelieved by rest. This is a multifaceted condition and may be the result of MALNUTRITION, fluctuations in BLOOD SUGAR levels and allergic reactions. Glandular imbalances, depression, cancer, infections, autoimmune diseases, diabetes, heart disease, AIDS, parasites, chronic pain, drugs and liver disease can also cause fatigue. Deficiencies of most VITAMINS, MINERALS, CARBOHYDRATE and PROTEIN promote fatigue as do conditions that affect the delivery of oxygen to tissues. These include ANEMIA, emphysema and other respiratory problems. Fatigue is also a symptom of HYPOTHYROIDISM, which lowers basal metabolism and contributes to the sluggishness of many functions, including muscular activity. The overproduction of CORTISOL, a steroid hormone produced by the ADRENAL GLANDS, can be the result of adaption to chronic stress and can cause fatigue. Inadequate cortisol production contributes to low blood sugar (HYPOGLYCEMIA), which leads to fatigue. (See also: CHRONIC FATIGUE; STRESS.)

fat metabolism (post-digestion) Reactions in the body encompassing the synthesis of FATTY ACIDS and FAT, as well as fat degradation and fatty acid oxidation. Fat stored in the body (ADIPOSE TISSUE) is constantly synthesized and constantly broken down. When the number of calories consumed exceeds the energy needs of the body, the surplus fuel is converted to fat for energy storage. Consumption of an excess of ALCOHOL, CARBOHYDRATE, PROTEIN or fat can therefore lead to weight gain. Alternatively, when fewer calories are consumed than needed for extended periods, stored fat is gradually depleted as it is needed for energy production.

Fat (Triglyceride) Synthesis

Fat synthesis occurs after a high-carbohydrate meal. Fat is made mainly in the liver and fat cells (adipose tissue in response to the hormone INSULIN, but not in muscle. The liver and adipose tissue convert GLUCOSE, the simple sugar with six carbon atoms, into acetic acid, which contains only two carbon atoms and represents the raw material for fat synthesis.

In the next phase, eight molecules of activated acetic acid are chained together to create a long saturated fatty acid with 16 carbon atoms (C–C–C–C–C–C–C–C–C–C–C–C–C–C–C–C), known as PALMITIC ACID. The enzyme system that performs this complex conversion is called fatty acid synthetase. The B vitamins BIOTIN and NIACIN are required to synthesize fatty acids. In the final step of fat synthesis, three fatty acids are attached to GLYCEROL, a three-carbon fragment of glucose, to form a fat molecule known as a triglyceride.

Palmitic acid can be lengthened to produce STEARIC ACID, a common saturated fatty acid containing 18 carbon atoms. The body can also make simple monounsaturated fatty acids such as OLEIC ACID, which is deficient in two hydrogen atoms and possesses one double bond (C–C–C–C–C–C–C–C–C=C–C–C–C–C–C–C–C–CO_2H) from saturated fatty acids. To summarize, neither palmitic acid, nor stearic acid, nor oleic acid are dietary essentials. On the other hand, the body cannot create most fatty acids with multiple double bonds, such as the ESSENTIAL FATTY ACIDS; LINOLEIC ACID C–C–C–C–C–C=C–C–C=C–C–C–C–C–C–C–C–CO_2H and ALPHA LINOLENIC ACID C–C–C=C–C–C=C–C–C=C–C–C–C–C–C–C–C–CO_2H.

Fat synthesized by the liver is transported in the bloodstream as a water-soluble carrier particle called VDL (VERY-LOW-DENSITY LIPOPROTEIN), which delivers newly formed fat molecules to fat cells where it can be stored.

Fat Degradation

When too few calories are consumed to meet the body's energy needs, the body breaks down stored fat, its primary stored fuel. The hormone EPINEPHRINE (adrenaline) activates an enzyme in fat cells called LIPASE, which cleaves stored fat molecules to free fatty acids; these enter the bloodstream and are carried to tissues.

Tissues rapidly absorb circulating fatty acids, which last only a few minutes before being absorbed. Muscle cells oxidize this fuel to produce ATP to meet their energy needs. In contrast glucose is the major fuel for the brain, because fatty acids do not cross the BLOOD-BRAIN BARRIER.

To be oxidized, fatty acids are first transported into MITOCHONDRIA, the cell's energy producing factory, using a carrier molecule called CARNITINE. Carnitine may be an essential nutrient for elderly people and patients with heart disease. In mitochondria fatty acids are completely oxidized (burned) to carbon dioxide for energy by the KREB'S CYCLE, the central energy-producing mechanism of mitochondria. Fatty acid oxidation requires enzyme helpers from three B vitamins: PANTOTHENIC ACID, niacin and RIBOFLAVIN. Mitochondria trap energy as ATP. The amount of ATP from the oxidation of fatty acids is more than double the amount from glucose oxidation. This reflects for the fact that fat provides more than twice as many calories per gram as carbohydrate. (See also ELECTRON TRANSPORT CHAIN; METABOLISM; RESPIRATION, CELLULAR.)

Norum, K.R., "Dietary Fat and Blood Lipids," *Nutrition Reviews*, 50:4 (1992), pp. 30–37.

fat substitute   A FOOD ADDITIVE that partially replaces FATS and oils in processed foods. Fat substitutes are classified as protein-, carbohydrate- or lipid-based. Their presence tricks the mouth into sensing flaky, tender baked goods or creamy foods without the presence of fat and its associated calories. Carbohydrate- and protein-based fat substitutes break down at high temperature and cannot be cooked.

Among carbohydrate fat replacers are the following:

- DEXTRINS and maltodextrins. These STARCH fragments prepared from WHEAT, TAPIOCA, POTATO, CORN or OAT flour, are used in salad dressing, puddings, frozen desserts, dairy products, margarine, spreads, fillings.
- Modified food starch. Chemically treated starch is prepared from corn, potato, wheat, rice or tapioca and used in processed meat, salad dressing, frosting, frozen desserts.
- Microcrystalline CELLULOSE. This highly purified form of cellulose is prepared from wood pulp and ground into tiny particles. It is used in dairy products, sauces, frozen desserts.
- GUMS. Plant gums including xantham gum, guar gum, locust bean gum and carrageenan, are used in reduced calore and fat-free salad dressing and processed meats.
- Fruit fiber. Fiber from apples, figs and prunes is used in baked goods.

Fat substitutes can also be classified in terms of their digestibility. Digestible fat substitutes yield calories, while nondigested fat substitutes do not. An example of a digestible fat substitute is SIMPLESSE, approved in 1990 by the U.S. FDA as the first synthetic fat substitute for the U.S. market. This product is derived from EGG white and milk PROTEIN by a process of blending and heating. Simplesse is digested and used by the body as protein. Simplesse cannot be used in cooking because frying or baking causes it to lose its creamy consistency. It may appear more frequently in products like frozen desserts, MAYONNAISE, salad dressing and cheese spreads.

SUCROSE POLYESTER (Olestra) is an example of an indigestible fat substitute and does not yield calories. Its structure resembles fat, except that it has a molecule of sugar at its core instead of glycerol and has eight attached fatty acids instead of three. It has a new structure that cannot be digested and it has been the center of controversy. Sucrose polyester has been recently approved by the FDA as a new food additive. Long-term animal studies suggest that it might cause liver problems and could interfere with the absorption of fat-soluble vitamins; other studies indicate it is safe. It is being marketed with supplemental fat soluble vitamins, in potato chips and snack foods.

Oatrim is made from oat flour and contains soluble fiber. It was developed by the USDA in 1993 and is being used in cheeses and ground beef, cookies and muffins. Other products are being developed. Oatrim supplies 1 calorie per gram, in contrast with fat, which supplies 9 calories per gram. Like any other high-fiber food, it can cause gas and bloating.

Modification of the structure of the fat molecule has yielded another family of digestible fat replacers. These products employ short-chain fatty acids, like acetic acid and propionic acid, which provide fewer calories than the usual fatty acids found in fats. These modified triglycerides provide 5 calories per gram.

Whether fat substitutes will help people eat less fat is unknown. By analogy to ARTIFICIAL SWEETENERS, fat substitutes may contribute to a false sense of security, leading consumers to eat additional amounts of high-calorie foods. artificial sweeteners do not help people change their diets significantly. Even if Simplesse were incorporated into all foods for which FDA approval was sought, it would reduce fat intake by at most 14%, assuming no further change in the diet. Many low-fat foods contain sugar, while sugar-free foods may contain fat. The reason is that it is difficult to take both sugar and fat out of a food and have it taste good. In the final analysis, no fat substitute or other food additive can replace wise food choices and regular exercise for weight control.

fatty acids   A class of organic acids (CARBOXYLIC ACIDS) containing short, medium or long chains of carbon atoms. Fatty acids are the major constituent of fat and represent the major energy source of the body. When oxidized for fuel, fatty acids yield 9 calories per gram, more than twice as much energy as from sugar.

Short-Chain Fatty Acids

Short-chain fatty acids contain two, three and four carbon atoms; they are, respectively, ACETIC ACID, PROPIONIC ACID and BUTYRIC ACID. These acids are products of microbial digestion of fiber in the gut and are a significant energy source, especially for intestinal epithelial cells. The oxidation of protein, fat and carbohydrate for energy production yields acetic acid, attached to a carrier called COENZYME A, which plays a central role in energy production.

Medium-Chain Fatty Acids

Medium-chain fatty acids are saturated fatty acids containing five to 12 carbon atoms. An example is CAPRYLIC ACID, with eight carbons. Medium-chain fatty acids are commonly bound to GLYCEROL to form medium-chain triglycerides. Commercially, medium-chain triglycerides are prepared primarily from coconut and palm oils. They have long been used in parenteral (intravenous) formulations for patients who do not absorb fat efficiently. Medium-chain triglycerides are digested by pancreatic lipase to free acids in the intestine and are transported in the blood and rapidly absorbed by tissues for energy production. Medium-chain fatty acids do not require special transport mechanisms, unlike usual fats.

Long-Chain Fatty Acids

Long-chain fatty acids are common building blocks of fats and oils and therefore are the major fat components in a typical diet. Long-chain fatty acids may be either saturated or unsaturated. Saturated fatty acids are filled up with hydrogen atoms; PALMITIC ACID (16 carbon atoms) and STEARIC ACID (18 carbon atoms) are the most abundant saturated fatty acids in the body.

Unsaturated fatty acids lack pairs of hydrogen atoms and contain one or more double bonds, and this difference sets them apart from saturated fatty acids. Those with a single double bond (monounsaturates) are represented by palmitoleic acid (16 carbon atoms) and OLEIC ACID (18 carbon atoms), which is the most common. Polyunsaturates contain two or more double bonds. Because the typical unsaturated fatty acids possess a bent shape, they do not pack together

easily to form solids at room temperature and therefore tend to be liquids. Fats high in unsaturated fatty acids are oils. Saturated fatty acids lack built-in kinks and they tend to stack together in parallel, like cords of wood, and they solidify easily. Therefore, fat containing mainly saturated fatty acids is solid at room temperature.

Two types of polyunsaturated fatty acids must be supplied in the diet because the body cannot fabricate them: LINOLEIC ACID and ALPHA LINOLENIC ACID. Certain details like the position of the double bonds are important distinctions for these fatty acids because the body is very selective in how they are used.

Both linoeic acid and alpha linolenic acid possess 18 carbon atoms: The former possesses two double bonds, while the latter possesses three double bonds. Linoleic acid belongs to the omega-6 family of polyunsaturates, with double bonds beginning at the sixth carbon atom from the end of the fatty acid; while alpha linolenic acid belongs to the omega-3 class, with double bonds beginning at the third carbon atom from the end of the fatty acid. Omega-3 fatty acids and omega-6 fatty acids cannot be converted one to another. In general, the ESSENTIAL FATTY ACIDS can be converted to more complex fatty acids and hormone-like substances such as PROSTAGLANDINS, compounds that can stimulate or inhibit many physiologic processes, and LEUKOTRIENES, very powerful inflammatory agents.

Omega-6 Fatty Acids

The smallest member of the omega-6 "family" is linoleic acid, an essential fatty acid. Linoleic acid is converted to more complex omega-6 fatty acids, including GAMMA LINOLENIC ACID, which can give rise to the PGE$_1$ series of prostaglandins that help counterbalance inflammatory processes and return the body to normal. The conversion to gamma linolenic acid is hampered in cases of zinc deficiency, ALCOHOLISM or diabetes. Human milk contains a high level of gamma linolenic acid, suggesting an important role in growth and development.

Linoleic acid is also converted to the largest member of the omega-6 family, ARACHIDONIC ACID, which yields the PGE$_2$ series of prostaglandins, the 2 series of thromboxanes (TXA$_2$) and leukotrienes that increase physiological responses to stress. The PGE$_2$ prostaglandins increase inflammation, especially involving joints and skin; produce pain and fever; increase blood pressure; and induce blood clotting.

Deficiency symptoms of linoleic acid include DEPRESSION, irritability, rough skin, ECZEMA, ACNE, psoriasis, dandruff, hair loss, slow wound healing, ANEMIA, blurred vision and lowered immunity. Deficiencies have been linked to an increased risk of multiple sclerosis, HYPERTENSION, some forms of CANCER and HEART DISEASE.

Dietary omega-6 fatty acids have long been known to reduce serum CHOLESTEROL and thus may lower the risk of ATHEROSCLEROSIS. Chronic low intake correlates with an increased risk of heart attack among Americans. The general conclusion is that a modest increase in dietary omega-6 fatty acids can help protect against cardiovascular disease. Consequently dietary strategies to lower cholesterol have often specified lowering the intake of saturated fatty acids while increasing the intake of omega-6 unsaturated fatty acids. Although such diets can lower LDL (LOW-DENSITY LIPOPROTEIN), the undesirable form of cholesterol, they also lower HDL (HIGH-DENSITY LIPOPROTEIN), which protects against coronary heart disease.

In the United States linoleic intake ranges from 5 to 10% of calories. The U.S. National Research Council recommends a maximum 10% of calories as omega-6 fatty acids. Common sources of linoleic acid include vegetable oils like SOYBEAN oil, sunflower and SAFFLOWER oil (safflower oil is the richest source). A tablespoon of polyunsaturated vegetable oil daily meets the daily requirement. EVENING PRIMROSE OIL and BLACKCURRANT OIL are common supplemental sources of gamma linolenic acid.

All polyunsaturated fatty acids are susceptible to oxidation. Oxidized fatty acids contain lipid peroxides, which can generate free radicals, can damage cells and can cause cancer. Therefore, increased consumption of polyunsaturates increases the need for VITAMIN E as an ANTIOXIDANT.

Omega-3 Fatty Acids

The smallest member of the omega-3 fatty acids is alpha linolenic acid, an essential fatty acid that is the building block for all other longer chain omega-3 fatty acids. It occurs in certain plants, pumpkin seeds and walnuts. FLAXSEED OIL and FISH OIL are used as supplemental sources. This fatty acid also occurs in phytoplankton, which are consumed by coldwater ocean fish. They convert alpha linolenic acid to larger members of the omega-3 family, EICOSAPENTAENOIC ACID (EPA), 20 carbon atoms, 5 double bonds (20:5), and DOCOSAHEXAENOIC ACID (DHA), 22 carbon atoms, 6 double bonds (22:6), which are found in highest concentrations in fish and fish oil.

A growing body of evidence indicates that a diet enriched in omega-3 fatty acids conveys significant health benefits, though this area is controversial. They may decrease inflammation common to degenerative diseases like rheumatoid arthritis. At the molecular level the body converts omega-3 fatty acids to families of regulatory substances including prostaglandin (PGI$_3$), thromboxane (TXA$_3$) and leukotrienes, which counterbalance products of omega-6 fatty acids that promote platelet aggregation, blood clotting and inflammation. EPA is a source of prostacyclin PGI$_3$, a substance that decreases blood platelet clumping, an important step in blood clot formation (thromobogenesis). In addition, omega-3 fatty acids can block the formation of substances that trigger inflammation.

Fish and fish oils that are enriched in EPA and DHA seem to lower the risk of heart attack by lowering blood cholesterol, if the initial levels are high. They generally lower the level of blood fat and VLDL (VERY-LOW-DENSITY LIPOPROTEIN), which transports fat in the blood. The mechanism seems to involve blocking the synthesis of VLDL and LDL, the undesirable forms of serum cholesterol.

A deficiency of the omega-3 fatty acids is associated with retarded growth, retarded retinal development in infants, and abnormal brain development in experimental animals. Furthermore, anyone whose diet relies on highly processed foods might be deficient in omega-3 fatty acids. The omega-3 fatty acids in general, and alpha linolenic acid specifically, are deficient in the standard American diet. There is little or none in fast foods, including fried fish, fried chicken or hamburgers. Processing removes or destroys omega-3 fatty acids because they are susceptible to rancidity and shorten the shelf life of processed foods. Furthermore, the high levels of omega-6 fatty acids in conventional American diets, which emphasize meat, block the production of EPA from alpha linolenic acid.

Optimal levels of alpha linolenic acid in the diet are unknown, though recommended daily intakes range from 1 to 2.5% of daily calories. The recommendation of the American Heart Association is to eat several servings of fish weekly. The optimal ratio of omega-6 to omega-3 fatty acids is not known. In the traditional Japanese diet the ratio is 4:1; in the American diet, the ratio is more like 10:1 and may be too high. With increased consumption of polyunsaturated fatty acids there is an increased need for fat-soluble antioxidants like VITAMIN E.

Fish oil and flaxseed oil are very susceptible to rancidity and are often packaged with vitamin E as an antioxidant. To minimize their oxidation, refrigerate fish oil supplements as well as any unsaturated oils in capped containers. Never use flax oil or other highly unsaturated oil for cooking because they are too easily oxidized when heated.

Wainwright, Patricia E., "Alpha Linolenic Acid, Long Chain n-3 Fatty Acids and Neonatal Brain Development," *Nutrition*, 7:6 (1991), pp. 443–46.

Wallingford, J.C. and Yetley, E.A., "Development of Health Claims Regulations: the Case of Omega-3 Fatty Acids and Heart Disease," *Nutrition Reviews*, 49:11 (1991), pp. 323–29.

fatty liver A deposition of FAT in LIVER tissue. Normally lipids are transported out of the liver. With a massive breakdown of fat during STARVATION, DIABETES MELLITUS, crash DIETING and chronic ALCOHOLISM, the fat tissue releases free fatty acids into the bloodstream. They enter liver cells and are converted back to triglycerides (fat), leading to lipid deposits in the liver. Decreased fatty acid oxidation by the liver during alcoholism further adds to fat accumulation in the liver.

Chemical poisons (hepatoxins), like carbon tetrachloride, alcoholism and protein malnutrition slow the liver's ability to export fat and increase fat accumulation. Over time accumulated fatty deposits impair liver function. Eventually, if liver cells die and are replaced by scar tissue leading to irreversible damage, the result is liver scarring. (See also CIRRHOSIS; FAT METABOLISM.)

favism A condition that causes the rupture of red blood cells—a hemolytic syndrome. Favism occurs in genetically susceptible individuals when they ingest seeds or inhale pollen of *Vicia faba*, the BROAD BEAN (fava bean). The disease occurs in Mediterranean and Middle Eastern countries and in western China. Children are more susceptible to favism than adults. The acute stage associated with fever, abdominal pain, headache, ANEMIA and, in severe cases, coma, lasts 24 to 48 hours and symptoms usually diminish. Favism is linked to a deficiency of an enzyme that supports the antioxidant system required to maintain the structure in red blood cell membranes (glucose-6-phosphate dehydrogenase). Enzyme deficiencies make red blood cells more susceptible to damage by external agents. (See also FOOD SENSITIVITY.)

FDA (U.S. Food and Drug Administration)   A federal agency, founded in 1927, that is responsible for enforcing the Federal Food, Drug, and Cosmetic Act, together with its amendments, the Fair Packaging and Labeling Act, and sections of the Public Health Service Act. The FDA inspects, tests, approves and sets standards for most foods, including imported foods, drugs, cosmetic products like lipstick, perfume, shampoo, deodorant and toothpaste. Similarly, the FDA approves and monitors medical devices such as thermometers, sunlamps, artificial body parts and drug testing kits. The FDA approves and monitors prescription drugs, as well as labels for over-the-counter drugs. The FDA assures the efficiency and long-term effects of drugs such as heart medications, vaccines, over-the-counter medications, AIDS drugs, cancer drugs, breast implants and drugs that treat baldness and skin conditions. (MEAT, POULTRY and EGGS are regulated by the U.S. Department of Agriculture.)

The FDA is responsible for verifying the contents of drugs, foods and supplements. With regard to foods, the FDA regulates food handling to assure sanitary, safe foods, free of harmful chemical contaminants and spoilage. Low levels of additives and pesticide residues that may cause cancer are permitted, provided the risks are negligible, according to the Food Quality Protection Act of 1996, which supersedes the DELANEY CLAUSE of the amended Food, Drug and Cosmetic Act. The FDA monitors pesticide residues in foods, including illegal drug use in livestock and chemicals released from food packaging. If pesticide or chemical residues are too high, the FDA can order a crop destroyed. The FDA monitors more than 2,800 FOOD ADDITIVES currently approved for foods. It regulates new food additives and reviews additives already in use. The FDA also regulates interstate food shipment.

The FDA is concerned with new food products and nutritional claims. It also sets and maintains standards for safe and adequate food labeling. In 1990, Congress passed the Nutrition Labeling and Education Act, which gave the FDA the responsibility of creating a national FOOD LABELING standard. The FDA issued its proposals in 1991; they became law in 1993. (See also FOOD LABELLING.)

FD&C-approved food colors   Synthetic color additives approved for food and beverages. The abbreviation stands for Food, Drug and Cosmetics to designate intended use. Ninety percent of all dyes are synthetic and employ FD&C designations such as "FD&C No. 1," "FD&C No. 2" and so on. (See also ARTIFICIAL FOOD COLORS.)

fed state   Refers to changes in energy production and physiologic processes in response to a meal. The fed state favors the synthesis of protein, fat and glycogen, a chain of GLUCOSE molecules that serves as an energy storage mechanism. In contrast, fat degradation, fatty acid oxidation and glycogen breakdown are blocked after a meal.

A complex series of events unfolds at the end of a meal. After eating carbohydrate, digestion produces glucose, which is absorbed by the small intestine into the blood-stream. BLOOD SUGAR rises more or less rapidly, then gradually declines to the fasting level maintained between meals. The hormone INSULIN dominates the body's response to an increased blood sugar. This hormone is released by the pancreas in response to elevated blood sugar and promotes glucose uptake by most tissues, thus lowering blood sugar levels. Muscle converts surplus glucose to glycogen, the liver forms glycogen and fat, and adipose tissue forms fat. In addition, insulin stimulates muscle to take up circulating amino acids, particularly BRANCHED CHAIN AMINO ACIDS (LEUCINE, ISOLEUCINE and VALINE) for protein synthesis.

After eating a fatty meal, digested fat is absorbed by the intestine and packaged as CHYLOMICRONS, water-soluble fat carriers that distribute fat to tissues via the bloodstream. The short-term rise in serum fat level after a meal is termed "postprandial hyperlipidemia." Dietary fatty acids released from fat in chylomicrons are taken up by many tissues and burned for energy. Adipose tissue also absorbs and reincorporates fatty acids into fat for storage. (See also ANABOLISM; CATABOLIC STATE.)

feedback inhibition   A common control mechanism in the regulation of biochemical reactions of the body and/or a mechanism for maintaining processes within normal limits (HOMEOSTASIS). Feedback inhibition can refer to a way of regulating a system of enzymes that operate to create a final product (metabolic pathways) or it can refer to hormonal regulation. In a metabolic pathway, very often the first unique step is catalyzed by a "bottleneck" enzyme, which regulates the rate at which material flows through the pathway.

In feedback inhibition of a metabolic pathway, the build-up of the final product of that pathway shuts down the bottleneck or regulating enzyme. When the product is consumed, inhibition is released and more product can be synthesized by the pathway. This type of regulation is quite common. As an example, HEME, the iron pigment of hemoglobin in red blood cells, is an end product of a system of enzymes devoted to its synthesis. If levels of heme build up due to overproduction or a slowdown in consumption, heme inhibits the key enzyme regulating heme synthesis. As another example, an excess of ATP, the cell's energy currency, blocks GLYCOLYSIS, the pathway that degrades GLUCOSE to produce energy.

Feedback is a common occurrence in the regulation of endocrine glands that secrete certain hormones that stimulate other glands to release hormones. As an example, the anterior pituitary secretes thyroid-stimulating hormone (TSH), which in turn stimulates THYROXINE (thyroid hormone) production by the thyroid gland. When the blood level of thyroxine build up to an optimum level, the anterior pituitary senses this level and stops secreting TSH. Consequently the thyroid stops producing excess thyroxine and the blood level falls. (See also CATABOLISM; ENDOCRINE SYSTEM.)

Feingold diet   A diet based on the studies of Benjamin Feingold, M.D., a pediatric allergist who in 1973 proposed treating HYPERACTIVITY and learning disorders with diet modifications instead of medications. He evolved a diet that eliminates foods containing synthetic colors and flavors, as well as the antioxidant preservatives BHA and BHT. It also eliminates foods, beverages and medications containing salicylates, which are compounds related to ASPIRIN. Naturally occurring salicylates are found in ALMONDS, APPLES, APRICOTS, berries, CLOVES, COFFEE, NECTARINES, ORANGES, PEACHES, PLUMS, TANGERINES, TEAS, TOMATOES and oil of wintergreen.

The Feingold diet is a controversial plan. Parents who use it successfully for hyperactive children stoutly defend it, although a panel of experts of the U.S. National Institutes of Health concluded there aren't enough clinical studies to grant official approval. While the Feingold diet has been effective in some cases, it is very restrictive for children. Eating away from home while maintaining this diet is difficult; common foods like luncheon meats, sweets, and even non-food items like toothpaste, are artificially colored and flavored. As with any diet modification program, there must be a supportive home environment for a permanent dietary change to occur in children. (See also ARTIFICIAL FOOD COLORS; FOOD ADDITIVES.)

Goldstein, Sam and Goldstein, Michael. *Managing Attention Disorders in Children.* New York: Wiley, 1990.

fennel (*Foeniculum vulgare*) An aromatic vegetable belonging to the parsley family that is native to Mediterranean regions. Common fennel is a perennial with characteristic bright-green feathery leaves and stalks resembling celery. Its flavor is similar to anise, though less pronounced. Fennel leaves and bulbs are used for seasonings, soups, stews and salads, while fennel seed is a spice in cooking, candy and certain liqueurs. Fennel oil extracted from seeds is used in perfumes, soaps and several medications.

fermentation The microbial degradation of CARBOHYDRATE, particularly simple SUGARS. Characteristics of the fermentation depend upon the nature of the carbohydrate, the type of microorganism and conditions such as degree of acidity and the amount of available oxygen. Bacteria, molds and yeasts commonly carry out fermentations by degrading sugars without the direct participation of air or oxygen (anaerobically).

Alcoholic fermentation Under anaerobic conditions specific strains of yeast ferment sugar (GLUCOSE) to alcohol in the preparation of alcoholic beverages. In WINE making, yeast ferments the sugar in grape juices. Alcohol can be prepared by the fermentation of other fruit juice. ALE and BEER are the product of fermentation of sugar from starch in malted grains. In this case partly sprouted grains produce enzymes that release sugars from starch. In VINEGAR manufacture (acetic acid fermentation) the alcohol in wine and beer is further oxidized by microbial fermentation to ACETIC ACID.

Lactic acid fermentation Lactic acid-producing bacteria (lactobacillus strains) ferment LACTOSE in MILK to sour milk. In cheese production, the enzyme RENNET is used to clot milk, and the resulting curdled milk protein is fermented with bacteria or mold strains to ripen cheese. YOGURT is milk that has been boiled and then inoculated with lactic acid-producing bacteria.

The many other fermented foods include the dough in leavened baked goods containing yeast enzymes; SAUSAGE; fermented vegetables such as SAUERKRAUT, BORSCH and kimchi. Far Eastern fermented foods are prepared from SOYBEANS, RICE, LEGUMES and FISH. Other types of fermentations produce citric acid from glucose (citric acid fermentation) and oxalic acid from glucose (oxalic fermentation).

Colon bacteria ferment undigested carbohydrates in dried beans, lactose (due to LACTOSE INTOLERANCE) and FIBER. Excessive fermentation can cause FLATULENCE or DIARRHEA. Normally much of dietary fiber is fermented anaerobically to produce short-chain fatty acids: ACETIC ACID, PROPIONIC ACID and BUTYRIC ACID. These fatty acids are absorbed and are the preferred fuel of cells lining the colon. (See also ACIDOPHILUS.)

ferritin An iron storage PROTEIN in tissues that represents the major form of stored iron in the body. Ferritin accounts for 20% of the total iron in adults. Ferritin functions both in iron absorption and iron recycling. APOFERRITIN, the protein portion of ferritin, is formed by intestinal mucosa, LIVER, spleen and bone marrow. These tissues combine apoferritin with inorganic iron (ferric phosphate and ferric hydroxide) obtained from iron carried in the blood by the serum protein TRANSFERRIN. Iron released from ferritin can be transported to other tissues via the bloodstream.

During early stages of iron deficiency a decreased serum ferritin level is the first sign of decreased iron stores. On the other hand, many conditions elevate serum ferritin: inflammation, cancer, infections and liver disease. Iron overload disease, HEMOCHROMATOSIS, a potentially damaging condition, is associated with iron build-up in tissues. (See also ANEMIA.)

ferrous gluconate Iron salt of gluconic acid, an acidic derivative of glucose. Ferrous gluconate is used to darken OLIVES to a uniform black color. As a nutritional supplement, it is a readily absorbable form of ferrous IRON. (See also CHELATE; VITAMIN.)

fetal alcohol syndrome (FAS) A congenital condition in children whose mothers drank ALCOHOL during their pregnancy. One in 300 to 500 babies are born with FAS. It is characterized by mental retardation; facial deformities, particularly of the upper lip and eyelids; hyperactivity; low birth weight; and heart problems. Some children may be permanently brain damaged, and the average IQ of adults with fetal alcohol syndrome is 68. While the dosage of alcohol that can damage the fetus is unclear, even moderate alcohol consumption during pregnancy can affect the newborn, and the American College of Obstetricians and Gynecologists recommends abstaining from alcohol completely during pregnancy.

FAS can have long-term effects as well. Mental deficiencies and emotional problems make it difficult for adults with FAS to adapt to normal living, and there is an increased need for society to prevent the dysfunctional living, chronic mental illness and homelessness so frequently observed in older patients with this disorder. (See also BIRTH DEFECTS.)

Spohr, Hans-Ludwig et al., "Prenatal Alcohol Exposure and Long Term Developmental Consequences," *Lancet*, 341 (April 10, 1993), pp. 907–10.

fiber (roughage, bulk) Undigested plant residues that represent the outer coating or plant wall material of VEGETABLES, GRAINS, seeds and FRUITS. Fiber is considered essential to maintain a healthy digestive tract. A low-fiber diet has been associated with CONSTIPATION, colon CANCER, spastic colon, HIATUS HERNIA, varicose veins, hemorrhoids, HEART DISEASE, HYPERTENSION, GALLSTONES, diabetes, OBESITY, COLITIS and CROHN'S DISEASE. Fiber can help curb appetite because the stomach feels full. Fiber-rich foods require longer chewing, which stimulates digestive juices and helps digestion. Fiber displaces fat calories and slows fat digestion and absorption by binding bile salts and therefore it may help control OBESITY. Fiber helps fight heart disease. In a study of over 40,000 U.S. middle-aged men, researchers have found that heart attacks were 41% less common among men who consumed at least 28 g fiber daily compared with men who ate less than 13 g daily as typical of the usual U.S. diet. It is estimated that fiber-deprived men reduced their risk of heart attack by 20 to 44% for each 10g of additional fiber, without lowering their fat intake. The largest reduction was among men who ate wheat bran, which represents mainly insoluble fiber.

Regular fiber consumption may also help prevent colon cancer. Most of the evidence comes from population studies or case studies with fiber-rich foods. While the connection is not clear-cut, several factors may be implicated: Fiber may dilute and bind carcinogens and promoters; it may modify gut bacteria metabolism to a more beneficial pattern; and it may modify the metabolism of CARCINOGENS by gut microorganisms. The fermentation of fiber by gut microflora produces small fatty acids (short-chain fatty acids) that are used as energy sources and that promote normal growth of mucosal cells of the colon.

It is estimated that Americans consume only one-third to one-half the optimal amount of fiber daily. The National Cancer Institute recommends doubling or tripling fiber intake from 12 g to 20 to 35 g per day. At this level there is minimal interference with nutrient ABSORPTION, while assuring normal maintenance of intestinal function. However, there is as yet no formal RECOMMENDED DIETARY ALLOWANCE for fiber because the exact amount required for health has not been established.

"Dietary fiber" refers to the fiber content in plant foods that resists digestion by enzymes of the GASTROINTESTINAL TRACT, and dietary fiber is the usual designation for fiber content in foods. Lab methods for measuring dietary fiber are more gentle than those for crude fiber, which measure only material that resists strong acid treatment. Values for dietary fiber can be up to four times higher than for crude fiber contents. New food labels (May 1994) are required to list the amount of dietary fiber as a percentage of daily value, based upon the needs of a 2,000 calories per day diet. Listing the amount of soluble and insoluble fiber is voluntary.

Major Types of Fiber

Fiber consists of a mixture of very different non-starch complex carbohydrate and non-carbohydrate materials. The major classes of dietary fiber are cellulose, HEMICELLULOSES, PECTIN, mucilage, GUMS, algal materials and LIGNIN.

- Cellulose is a linear chain (polymer) of glucose units.
- Hemicelluloses are highly branched structures found in plant cell walls. They are a diverse group with varying sugar compositions, including the simple sugars MANNOSE, GLUCOSE, GALACTOSE, xylose, arabinose, and an acid derived from glucose called glucouronic acid. Some hemicelluloses are water-soluble.
- Pectins function as a glue that holds plant tissues together, and they contain an acidic sugar derived from galactose, galacturonic acid, in the primary chains, with side chains or branches containing less common sugars: arabinose, fucose and xylose.
- Gums are plant secretions and contain acidic sugars.
- Algal polysaccharides are products of edible seaweed.
- Lignin is a non-carbohydrate insoluble material and a principal structural material of wood.

Insoluble Fiber

It is convenient to break down fibers according to whether they are insoluble or water-soluble. Insoluble fiber includes CELLULOSE and lignin. This type of fiber swells in water, increases stool weight (bulk) and stool frequency, and helps prevent constipation, colonic inflammation (diverticulitis) and hemorrhoids, by softening stools and speeding up the movement of waste through the intestine. Cellulose is not digested, although colon bacteria break down 40 to 80% of cellulose. Lignin is not degraded and passes through the digestive tract unchanged. Lignin softens stools, increases regularity and may lower blood cholesterol.

Bran is the most common source of insoluble fiber, derived from the outer husk of kernels of WHEAT and other CEREAL GRAINS. It contains cellulose and other cell wall materials and slows the rise in blood sugar after a meal and may help prevent the occurrence of precancerous polyps in the colon. Bran can protect against heart disease in middle-aged men; oatmeal is also effective, though more may need to be consumed to get the same effect as wheat bran.

Soluble Fiber

This type of plant fiber swells in water and forms glue-like gels. Soluble fiber is made up of non-cellulose carbohydrates, including pectins, gums, algal polysaccharides and some types of hemicellulose. Soluble fiber has important physiologic effects. It becomes viscous, thus softening stools and slowing the rate of stomach emptying. Soluble fiber also slows starch digestion and glucose uptake, in turn lowering the amount of insulin needed to process blood glucose after a meal, and it may help diabetics. Eating oat BRAN (2 oz) regularly each day may effectively lower blood sugar levels. Despite the popularity of oat bran as a source of water-soluble fiber, it provides both water-soluble and insoluble fibers.

The water-soluble fibers are completely degraded by intestinal microorganisms to SHORT-CHAIN FATTY ACIDS, which are used as fuels to help maintain the intestinal lining.

Soluble fiber may bind potential carcinogens and toxins, and thus lower the risk of colon cancer. Soluble fiber also seems to lower blood CHOLESTEROL. Regular consumption of oat bran and legumes may lower blood cholesterol. Fiber binds bile salts in the intestine, which could reduce their resorption, thus forcing the LIVER to remove more cholesterol from the blood to make more bile. Pectin, guar gum and locust bean gum have been reported as effective in this regard. Because it believes that long-term health benefits are not yet proven, the U.S. FDA does not permit health claims linking fiber consumption with the prevention of either heart disease or certain types of cancer.

Good sources of fiber include dried BEANS, LENTILS, lima beans, pinto beans, SWEET POTATOES, BROCCOLI, BRUSSELS SPROUTS, SPINACH, ALMONDS, CORN, wheat, oat bran and fruit (blackberries, pears, apples). In general the less processed a food is, the more fiber it has. Therefore, eating whole, minimally processed foods assures a mixture of soluble fiber and insoluble fiber; both kinds are needed for health.

Sources of insoluble fiber include skins of vegetables and fruits, whole grains (not white flour), high-fiber cereals, dried beans, broccoli, bulghar wheat. Bran is a common and inexpensive source of insoluble fiber. Cold bran cereals have more insoluble fiber than hot cereals. Bran is lost in preparing white flour and it is not replenished by ENRICHMENT.

Good sources of soluble fiber are fruits, cooked dried beans, CHICKPEAS, BARLEY, LENTILS, navy beans, vegetables such as SQUASH and CARROTS, plus barley, oat and rice bran. GUAR GUM, GLUCOMANNAN and pectin are common soluble fiber supplements.

When increasing fiber consumption, the recommendation is to begin gradually because excessive fiber intake causes bloating, gas, cramps, nausea and DIARRHEA. A month may be required to adapt to a high-fiber diet. Initial steps can be eating whole fruit instead of juices; popcorn instead of potato chips; whole WHEAT instead of white BREAD; and a baked potato with its skin instead of mashed potatoes. Consult a physician when planning to take fiber supplements if you have a serious digestive disease, or if you plan a daily consumption over 35 g of fiber. By following the FOOD GUIDE PYRAMID, which specifies eating six to eleven serving of grain-based foods and two to four servings of fruits and three to five servings of vegetables daily, you automatically consume the recommended fiber intake.

Fiber Supplements

Supplements are a popular way of increasing dietary fiber intake, although the National Cancer Institute recommends increasing fiber intake through whole, fiber-rich foods. Fiber supplements often contain bran, guar gum, pectin or PSYLLIUM. Since they swell in water and help create a feeling of being full, fiber supplements have been used in weight reduction programs to control APPETITE. It is not clear that they help with permanent weight loss, however. Fiber from psyllium seeds is the primary ingredient of several popular brands of non-chemical LAXATIVES.

Patients with serious intestinal disorders such as DIVERTICULITIS, ulcerative colitis or Crohn's disease should avoid taking fiber supplements without medical supervision. Consult a physician before consuming more than 35 g of fiber supplements a day; high levels of fiber can block the uptake of IRON, CALCIUM, ZINC, COPPER and other minerals and cause calcium losses. Avoid fiber supplements that also contain APPETITE SUPPRESSANTS like phenylpropanolamine, which can cause side effects.

Dietary Fiber Content of Selected Foods

	dietary fiber	grams
cereals:		
wheat bran	(1 oz)	8.4
shredded wheat	(" ")	2.6
oat meal	(" ")	0.5
grains:		
wheat germ	(3 tbsp.)	3.9
barley	(1/2 cup)	3.0
corn	(" ")	2.9–3.9
whole wheat bread	(slice)	1.5–2
white enriched bread	(slice)	0.5
oat bran	(1/3 cup)	4.0
vegetables:		
brussels sprouts	(1/2 cup)	2.3
cauliflower	(")	1.1
chickpeas	(")	8.0
kidney beans	(")	8.0
lettuce	(")	0.3
potato	(")	2.5
sweet potato	(")	4.0
fruit:		
apple	(1)	2.8
orange	(1)	3.0
prune	(1)	1.0
raspberries	(1/2 cup)	4.6
strawberries	(1/2 cup)	1.7
banana	(1)	2.2
figs (dried)	(3)	4.6

Eastwood, Martin A., "The Physiological Effect of Dietary Fiber: An Update," *Annual Review of Nutrition*, 12 (1992), pp. 19–35.

fibrin　An insoluble, fibrous protein that forms a gel-like blood clot to seal openings in blood vessel walls. Fibrin is produced from its precursor in the blood, fibrinogen, by the enzyme THROMBIN, one of a series of coagulation factors that are protein-degrading enzymes. BLOOD CLOTTING is a vitamin-K-dependent process because the vitamin is required in the processing of thrombin. Therefore, a vitamin K deficiency can increase the tendency to bleed (hemorrhage).

Individuals with disorders that prevent fat absorption may experience uncontrolled bleeding because vitamin K uptake is inadequate to produce enough thrombin. Calcium is also required for thrombin activation. In the final step of the clotting pathway, thrombin produces fibrin, a fibrous protein that forms insoluble clumps at a site of injury. Cell fragments called blood platelets embed themselves in the fibrin clot to complete the blood clotting process. Once a clot is formed it plugs the ruptured area of the vessel, preventing hemorrhaging. Fibrin threads gradually retract because platelets pull on them. This helps close the hole in the vessel by pulling the edges of the wound closer together.

fibrocystic disease   See BREAST CYSTS.

fibromyalgia syndrome (fibrositis)   A condition characterized by widespread aching pain with tenderness in both sides of the body. The prevalence of fibromyalgia is about 4% for adults after the age of 60, and it occurs more frequently in females than in males. Common complaints include persistent pain in the neck, shoulders, low back and hips, morning stiffness, fatigue and fitful sleep patterns. There may also be numbness in hands and feet, headaches and intolerance to heat or cold. At a cellular level, energy production may be sub-par.

Patients with fibromyalgia syndrome may have food allergies and sensitivities to toxins and chemicals in the environment. One common denominator is LEAKY GUT, in which inflammation makes the intestine more permeable (leaky) to materials that should normally be excluded, such as incompletely digested food proteins and bacterial breakdown products. A leaky gut can result from the destruction of beneficial intestinal bacteria during prolonged use of antibiotics or non-steroidal anti-inflammatory agents. Patients with fibromyalgia may be helped by avoiding materials to which they are sensitive, for example, household chemicals (like cleansers) and food allergens. Supplementation with nutrients that support antioxidant defenses and energy production—including minerals (ZINC, SELENIUM, MAGNESIUM, MANGANESE), and enzyme helpers (COENZYME Q, VITAMIN C and the B complex vitamins)—may help. Patients may also benefit from an individualized plan that includes exercise, physical therapy and manipulation, and dietary options to meet all of their nutritional needs. (See also FATIGUE; STRESS.)

fibrous proteins   Highly elongated, water-insoluble PROTEIN that helps protect and support the body. Fibrous proteins form static, insoluble rigid rods (hair) or sheets (skin, connective tissue), which are stabilized by crosslinks between protein segments. In contrast, proteins such as ENZYMES and ANTIBODIES are dynamic: They attach to other molecules for biological function and generally they are globular in shape and water-soluble. Extended arrays of fibrous proteins form the structure of skin, tendon, bone and connective tissue, while KERATIN is the protein of hair and outer layers of the skin. COLLAGEN is the primary fibrous protein of connective tissue, and MYOSIN forms fibers that cause muscle contraction. Two other fibrous proteins are worth mentioning. FIBRIN forms blood clots, while ELASTIN forms ligaments and the valves of large blood vessels.

The insolubility and high degree of cross-linking of fibrous proteins in connective tissue limits their digestion in meat. COOKING softens myosin fibers in muscle and gelatinizes collagen, making meat more digestible.

fig (*Ficus carica*)   The pear-shaped fruit of the fig tree. The fig is native to southwestern Asia; approximately 700 varieties are now cultivated throughout the Mediterranean area. California is the source of most domestic figs. Red, purple, white and green figs are the basic types. Figs possess a tough skin and a soft pulp. Because the fresh fruit has a short life span, 90% of household figs are either dried or canned. Dried figs are a rich source of sugar, dietary fiber and minerals. The Calimyrna, Black Mission and Brown Turkey are the most popular dried figs. Figs are among the sweetest of all fruits. Food value for 10 dried figs (187 g) is 477 calories; protein, 5.7 g; carbohydrate, 122 g; fiber, 24 g; calcium, 269 mg; iron, 4.2 mg; magnesium, 11 mg; potassium, 1,331 mg; zinc, 0.94 mg. Figs contain moderate amounts of B vitamins; thiamin, 0.13 mg; riboflavin, 0.13 mg; niacin, 1.3 mg.

fight or flight response   The physiologic response to real or perceived stress. Stress may be physical (exposure to disease-producing organisms and to toxic agents, or injury) or psychological (fear or joy associated with a crisis). There are three phases of adaptation to stress; each is regulated by the adrenal glands.

The body initially responds to stress with an "alarm" that mobilizes the body for immediate physical activity—to confront or flee from a threatening situation. The brain perceives the threat and activates the ADRENAL GLANDS to secrete norepinephrine and EPINEPHRINE (adrenaline). These hormones, released by the adrenal medulla, stimulate energy production and promote a state of alertness, increase the heart rate to pump more blood to the brain and muscles, and increase blood pressure. Blood is channeled to muscles and brain and away from the skin and the organs, except the lungs and the heart. Epinephrine and norepinephrine increase the rate of breathing to supply more oxygen to the heart, skeletal muscles and the brain. The hormones promote BLOOD CLOTTING, increase BLOOD SUGAR rapidly and mobilize stored fat to increase free FATTY ACID levels in blood. The release of digestive juices drops and PERISTALSIS slows to severely restrict digestive processes, and perspiration increases.

In the second phase of adaptation to stress, the resistance reaction allows a more sustained adaptation to a stressor to enable the body to carry out strenuous work, cope with emotional upsets and ward off infection. In response to ACTH (adrenocorticotropin) from the pituitary gland, the adrenal cortex produces steroid hormones to adapt the body to long-term stress. Glucocorticoids like CORTISOL stimulate catabolic (degradative) processes and favor the breakdown of muscle protein to amino acids, which are converted by the liver to blood sugar. Glucocorticoids stimulate fat breakdown as well.

Continued high cortisol output contributes to fatigue. High cortisol also suppresses the immune system and antibody production, thus increasing the risk of infection, and alters bone metabolism. Normally cortisol output follows a circadian rhythm: Levels are highest in the morning, dropping to a plateau between noon and 4 to 5 P.M. and reaching a nadir at midnight. This pattern can be disrupted in chronic stress.

To manage stress, EXERCISE, relaxation techniques and nutritional support are preeminently important. Regular exercise leads to an increased ability to deal with stress and also reduces the risk of stress-related conditions such as heart disease and depression. Relaxation through prayer, yoga, meditation or biofeedback reverses the physiologic effects of the fight or flight response. Nutrients that are required to support adrenal function include vitamin C, the B complex VITAMINS, especially VITAMIN B₆ and PANTOTHENIC ACID, and zinc and magnesium. POTASSIUM losses reduce adrenal function, therefore potassium levels need to be maintained. (See also CATABOLISM; GENERAL ADAPTATION SYNDROME.)

firming agents   Food additives that maintain firmness and crispness of vegetables and fruits when canned or pickled. CALCIUM and ALUMINUM compounds are added to pickles and maraschino cherries, as well as to canned peas, tomatoes, potatoes, and apples. Examples of firming agents include aluminum sulfate, calcium lactate and calcium chloride. (See also FOOD ADDITIVES.)

fish   An aquatic cold-blooded vertebrate used as a food source since prehistoric times. Edible bony fish fall into two categories: saltwater fish and freshwater fish. Important saltwater fish include COD, FLOUNDER, HALIBUT, HADDOCK, HERRING, MACKEREL, SALMON, sole, swordfish, sea bass and TUNA; freshwater fish include BASS, CATFISH, pike, sturgeon, PERCH and TROUT. Fish contribute high-quality protein to the diet and supply MAGNESIUM, COPPER, ZINC, IODINE and B vitamins, together with modest amounts of IRON and CALCIUM. Fish can replace red meat in a healthy diet because it does not contain high levels of saturated fat. Coldwater ocean fish and their oils contain high levels of essential fatty acids, polyunsaturated FATTY ACIDS derived from the omega-3 family. These fatty acids are believed to lower serum fat and cholesterol levels, to lower the risk of blood clots and of CARDIOVASCULAR DISEASE. Fish and FISH OIL also seem to reduce inflammation associated with chronic disease. Oily fish and fish liver oils contain significant amounts of VITAMIN A and VITAMIN D.

A variety of studies have demonstrated the benefits of fish on health. The Multiple Risk Factor Intervention Trial involving 13,000 U.S. men showed that the risk of dying from heart attack was 40% less for those eating the most fish. Dutch studies have shown that men eating fish several times weekly were less likely to die of heart attack or stroke. An American study, the Physician's Health Study, did not observe a connection between fish and heart attacks.

Besides replacing saturated fat meals with unsaturated fat, the addition of fish to the diet may reduce platelet stickiness, making these cell fragments less likely to form clots; may lower high blood fats (triglycerides) that may indirectly promote cholesterol-clogged arteries; and may help stabilize heart muscle and prevent deadly, abnormal heart rhythms during heart attacks.

On the other hand, fish oil impairs blood clotting, possibly increasing the risk of stroke due to bleeding into the brain (hemorrhagic stroke).

The optimal amount of fish in the diet is unknown, although eating average servings (4 oz) of fish instead of red meat several times a week seems to offer protection against heart attacks. Health benefits seem to increase when total dietary fat, especially saturated fat, consumption decreases, and more polyunsaturated fats are consumed. Consider coldwater ocean fish, like salmon, cod, mackerel, halibut, canned sardines, smelt, herring, bluefish and albacore tuna. Shark, SHELLFISH, rainbow trout and striped bass are fair to good sources of omega-3. To preserve the essential oils in fish, poach, steam or bake fish at medium temperatures. Fast-food fish contain almost no omega-3 fatty acids.

Fresh frozen seafood has generally a better flavor and texture than canned or frozen fish because it is frozen within four hours after being caught. Fresh fish sold in supermarkets may be 10 days old by the time it is purchased by the consumer. Fresh fish has almost no odor; if fish smells after cooking, don't eat it. Fresh fish should be refrigerated and eaten soon after purchase. Store frozen fish no more than a month. Clean freshly caught game fish as soon as possible to eliminate major bacterial contamination.

Seafood Safety Issues

A small percentage of the fish and seafood consumed in the United States is currently inspected, and the adequacy of SEAFOOD INSPECTION programs has been questioned. Seafood safety is a prominent issue because fish spoil more rapidly than most other foods and may be contaminated by hard-to-degrade pollutants because they are at the top of the aquatic FOOD CHAIN. To meet increased consumer demand, fish and shellfish are being harvested closer to shore, where pollution levels are higher. Fish that scavenge food from sediment lake beds and the sea floor may be likely to contain industrial contaminants deposited in sediments. Great Lakes fish, freshwater fish grown in polluted water, and certain predatory species like swordfish, tuna and walleye pike and fatty fish, are more likely to contain fat-soluble pollutants like pesticides, PBBs, PCBs and mercury. These could harm a fetus and increase the risk of cancer (PCBs). Tuna can accumulate mercury and swordfish and lake whitefish tend to be high in mercury or PCBs. Sole and flounder may contain less pollutants, and fish harvested from relatively clean areas like the Northern Pacific may be even less contaminated. The general recommendation is to eat a variety of fish several times weekly.

Raw fish can contain worms (*Aniskis simplex* and *Pseudoterranova decipiens*). Adequate cooking or freezing destroys these parasites. However, partial cooking and short-term microwave cooking may not kill worms or their eggs. Sushi is a raw fish dish from Japan. Its growing popularity in the United States raises questions about the safety of eating raw fish. In the United States fish has traditionally been smoked or cooked before eating. If you eat sushi, rely on sushi bars of reputable restaurants. Salting, smoking or marinading may not kill all parasites. Symptoms of parasitic infections include vomiting, diarrhea and stomach cramps. Parasitic diseases are difficult to diagnose. Their diagnoses may usually relies on analyses of stool specimens or blood specimens. (See also BREASTFEEDING; OMEGA-3 FATTY ACIDS; PARASITES IN FOOD AND WATER).

Hurley, Jayne and Liebman, Bonnie, "Seafood: What a Catch," *Nutrition Action Healthletter*, 21:9 (November 1994), pp. 1, 6–8, 9.

fish oil Supplements containing lipids from coldwater fish. These fish accumulate large, highly unsaturated fatty acids—EICOSAPENTAENOIC ACID (EPA) and DOCOSAHEXAENOIC ACID (DHA)—belonging to the omega-3 family of essential fatty acids. In fact, fish and fish oils are the major concentrated source of these polyunsaturated fatty acids, which form a class of hormone-like substances (PROSTAGLANDINS and thromboxanes) of the omega-3 series that reduce pain and inflammation and counterbalance inflammatory processes in the body and help restore equilibrium in the body after stress and injury. (In contrast red meat supplies ARACHADONIC ACID, which generates pro-inflammatory prostaglandins and thromboxane.) Eating fish seems to lower the risk of cholesterol-clogged arteries, and fish oils may do the same. Population studies suggest that the more ocean fish consumed, the lower the risk of HEART DISEASE, even when consumption of CHOLESTEROL is high, as is the case for Greenland Eskimos. Eating oily fish several times per week provides about 0.5 g of omega-3 long-chain fatty acids. Modest amounts of fish oil can reduce levels of blood fats known as VLDL (VERY-LOW-DENSITY LIPOPROTEIN), which transports fat in the bloodstream in healthy people as well as type II diabetics. It may also reduce LDL (LOW-DENSITY LIPOPROTEIN, the less desirable form of serum cholesterol) in normal people (if the diet is high in saturated fat). The issue is by no means clear-cut because fish oils sometimes raise rather than lower LDL levels in people with high blood fat levels.

Fish oil is a complex mixture of lipids, and the relative importance of each constituent in lowering the risk of heart disease is not presently known. In some studies, beneficial effects reported for people with high fish intake could be due to other dietary modifications. Negative results with fish and fish oils are sometimes explained by the fact that olive oil, used as a control, itself may lower the risk of heart disease and is not a neutral substance.

Other possible effects of fish oils are wide ranging. Together with ASPIRIN and anticoagulants, fish oil capsules help preserve the effects of coronary artery widening. Fish oils have potent anticlotting effects: They inhibit the production of a blood protein called fibrinogen, which triggers clot formation when activated. High fibrinogen levels are a risk factor for heart diseases. Fish oils also reduce the stickiness of platelets, small cell fragments in the blood that promote blood clotting. Fish oils also seem to block the action of a substance called thromboxane TXA_2, which promotes blood clot formation. In addition, EPA generates the prostaglandin PGI_3, which inhibits clumping of blood platelets and reduces the risk of blood clots.

Fish and fish oils reduce inflammation and may lessen symptoms of AUTOIMMUNE DISEASES like rheumatoid ARTHRITIS, lupus erythematosus, and other diseases related to an abnormal response of the immune system, such as psoriasis and multiple sclerosis. Eating fish regularly reduces the risk of chronic bronchitis and emphysema among cigarette smokers. In terms of inflammation, fish oils and omega-3 fatty acids appear to block the production of LEUKOTRIENES and other potent inflammatory agents like prostaglandin PGE_2.

Fish oils may help prevent fatal changes in heart rhythm (ventricular fibrillation) following a heart attack. Very large doses many have a modest effect on high blood pressure. Fish oil-fortified formula seems to help visual development of premature infants. Standard infant formula does not include fish oil or the long-chain OMEGA-3 FATTY ACID, docosahexaenoic acid, which normally accounts for a third of the fatty acids in the retina and the gray matter of the brain. The system for fabricating this fatty acid is ineffective in infants, and DHA can be considered a "conditionally" essential nutrient for preterm babies.

Basic questions about fish oil supplements remain unanswered. It is not known how much fish oil to take, why it needs to be taken, who should take it, or how long it should be taken. For these reasons, the American Heart Association does not recommend fish oil for treatment of heart disease nor does the U.S. FDA permit health claims to be made regarding fish oil and disease.

There are several precautions to be taken in using fish oil supplements. Those with high blood fat (TRIGLYCERIDES) or high blood cholesterol levels should not self-medicate; consultation with an expert on heart disease is warranted. Diabetics need to be aware that larger doses of fish oil can increase blood sugar and therefore blood sugar should be carefully monitored when using these supplements. Asthmatics who cannot tolerate aspirin can experience more frequent asthma attacks after taking fish oil supplements. Some fish oils (including COD LIVER OIL) contain significant amounts of cholesterol. Fatty fish can be contaminated with industrial chemicals like MERCURY, PCB, PBB and PESTICIDES. Cod liver oil is a very concentrated form of VITAMIN A and VITAMIN D. It is easy to overdose with these vitamins because they are stored by the body. Large amounts of fish oils increase bleeding tendencies and they may decrease the ability of white cells to fight infections. Excessive fish oil increases the need for vitamin E. (See also BREASTFEEDING; DDI; ESKIMO DIET.)

Nordoy, A., et al., "Individual Effects of Dietary Saturated Fatty Acids and Fish Oil on Plasma Lipids and Lipoproteins in Normal Men," *American Journal of Clinical Nutrition*, 57 (1993), pp. 634–39.

fish poisoning (scromboid fish poisoning) A FOOD POISONING that occurs within an hour after eating species of spoiled fish that populate tropical oceans, including TUNA, MACKEREL, skipjack, BONITO, HERRING, mahi-mahi, SARDINES and anchovies. An important clue to contamination is that infected fish taste metallic and peppery. Symptoms of poisoning include flushing, sweating, nausea, vomiting, diarrhea, headache and dizziness. Antihistamines relieve the symptoms. Scromboid fish poisoning can be prevented by keeping fresh fish on ice or refrigerated until it is cooked. (See also FOOD TOXINS.)

fish protein concentrate (FPC) An inexpensive protein FOOD ADDITIVE. The flesh of less desirable commercial fish is minced, defatted and dehydrated to produce the powdered protein concentrate. It is added to bread, cookies and tortillas to increase their PROTEIN quality. When 5 to 10% FPC is added to wheat flour or corn flour that is low in several ESSENTIAL AMINO ACIDS, the protein quality matches that of milk, which is high quality. (See also NET PROTEIN UTILIZATION; TEXTURIZED VEGETABLE PROTEIN.)

fish toxin (*Ciguatera*)   A toxin produced by a species of algae that contaminates fish eating the algae. Fish from Hawaii, the Caribbean and Florida are increasingly contaminated by ciguatera. Red snapper (rock fish), grouper, jack and barracuda are the most often affected. Ciguatera is odorless, has no flavor and is not destroyed by cooking. Symptoms of toxicity include nausea, tingling, itching, burning pain and change in taste perception. In extreme cases, ciguatara poisoning is lethal. (See also FOOD POISONING; SEAFOOD INSPECTION.)

fitness (conditioning)   The physiologic adaptation to physical exertion. Fitness implies increased muscular endurance or the ability of muscles to sustain repeated contractions, which correlates with strength. Regular, sustained EXERCISE significantly increases the body's ability to use and store ENERGY efficiently. At maximal exertion skeletal muscles increase their overall metabolic rate by over tenfold. Conditioning increases the ability of muscles to oxidize FAT because muscle cells produce more of the fat-metabolizing machinery, MITOCHONDRIA, to meet the increased demand for energy due to increased work. As a result, muscles burn fat more rapidly even between periods of exercise, which assists in weight control. Conditioned muscles will burn fat longer before beginning to use muscle carbohydrate stores (glycogen), thus contributing to endurance.

Regular physical exertion increases the capacity of the lungs and heart to deliver oxygen. Well conditioned individuals typically have a lower heart rate than sedentary people, which means the heart does not need to work as hard during physical exertion. Regular aerobic exercise lowers LOW-DENSITY LIPOPROTEIN (LDL), the less desirable form of cholesterol, and increases HIGH-DENSITY LIPOPROTEIN (HDL), the desirable form, thus decreasing risks associated with CARDIOVASCULAR DISEASE. Exercise has also been found to help in recovery from heart attacks. Even moderate exercise stimulates the immune system. (See also FAT METABOLISM.)

flatulence   The production of gas in the stomach and INTESTINES. Excessive flatus gas in the digestive tract is responsible for bloating and gas pains after eating. Normally the intestine produces gases from colon bacteria, fermenting undigested SUGARS, CARBOHYDRATES and FIBER. Products of fermentation are carbon dioxide, methane, hydrogen, and volatile sulfur and nitrogen-containing compounds from protein degradation, which have an unpleasant odor (skatole, putrescine and others). Little research has been carried out on the causes of gas, or on its remedy. Individuals differ in their tolerance to foods, and tolerance can change daily. Possible causes of gas and bloating include:

Swallowed air   When chewing gum or gulping food, excessive air may be swallowed.

Lactose intolerance   Individuals with the inability to digest milk sugar should avoid MILK and milk products such as ice cream. When undigested, LACTOSE can be fermented by colonic bacteria. Alternatively, LACTASE, an enzyme that degrades lactose to simpler sugars GLUCOSE and GALACTOSE, can be used in digesting milk sugar. Preparations of lactase are commercially available as tablets or drops.

Flatulence-causing foods   Foods likely to cause gas include APPLES, BEANS, BAGELS, BRAN, BROCCOLI, BRUSSELS SPROUTS, CABBAGE, CAULIFLOWER, CITRUS FRUIT, ONIONS, RAISINS, GRAINS like WHEAT and OATS, CARROTS, prunes and APRICOTS. These foods contain fiber and other undigested carbohydrate that can be broken down by bacteria. Less of a problem are BREAD, pastries, radishes, EGGPLANT, BANANAS, CELERY, lettuce, POTATOES and CORN. It is best to modify the diet to avoid those foods that provoke a reaction. To remove the bulk of flatulence-producing sugars in beans (stachyose and raffinose), soak the beans four to eight hours in hot water, then discard water and cook in fresh water.

Carbonated beverages   These can worsen a gas problem because of released carbon dioxide in the beverages that one drinks.

Fatty foods   Fat slows down gas moving through the digestive tract and should be limited.

Stress   Prolonged STRESS can alter gastrointestinal function.

Whether medication helps reduce flatulence remains uncertain. The U.S. FDA judged simethicone safe and effective for relieving gas. On the other hand, a panel of experts later concluded that no safe ingredient of any presently marketed medication is effective for flatulence. (See also ACID INDIGESTION.)

flavin adenine dinucleotide (FAD)   A type of enzyme helper (COENZYME) formed from RIBOFLAVIN (vitamin B$_2$). FAD functions as an electron carrier in key oxidation-reduction reactions in energy production by mitochondria, the cellular powerhouse. Specifically, FAD assists enzymes in the Kreb's Cycle, the central energy-yielding pathway ultimately responsible for oxidizing fat, carbohydrate and protein breakdown to carbon dioxide; in the oxidation of fatty acids. In addition, FAD helps to detoxify potentially harmful molecules like cigarette smoke and pesticides.

Flavin Adenine Mononucleotide (FMN)

FMN is a type of coenzyme formed of riboflavin that serves a more limited oxidation-reduction role than FAD. FMN assists enzymes participating in the oxidation of certain AMINO ACIDS and in the ELECTRON TRANSPORT CHAIN, the bucket brigade sequence of enzymes that ultimately consumes oxygen and produces ATP in mitochondria when fat and carbohydrate are oxidized. (See also CARBOHYDRATE METABOLISM; CATABOLISM; GLYCOLYSIS.)

flavonoids (bioflavonoids)   A large family of widely distributed plant substances, formerly designated as vitamin F. However, flavonoids are not classified as essential nutrients, nor do they have a vitamin status. These compounds are often pigments and occur in high concentrations in all fruits, especially CITRUS FRUITS; purple berries and apples; as well as in VEGETABLES, including onions; tea; and whole grains. They are responsible for astringency of certain fruits and tea.

Flavonoids include flavones (such as QUERCETIN), ISOFLAVONES (from soybeans), FLAVANONES (such as naringen and HESPERIDIN and RUTIN from citrus), ANTHOCYANINS (blue, purple, red plant pigments) and flavononols (including catechins, ellagic acid and TANNINS). Typical examples of major flavonoids and common sources are listed in the accompanying table.

Research before World War II demonstrated that vitamin C taken with flavonoids (called "vitamin F" at that time) strengthens capillaries, and in the 1950s flavonoids were frequently prescribed for bleeding. Subsequently the U.S. FDA ruled that they were ineffective despite medical experience to the contrary. Flavonoids have been used as supportive treatment for menstrual bleeding, bruising, frostbite and cold sores.

Flavonoids can also strengthen the blood-brain barrier to increase protection of the nervous system against foreign substances and they help reduce damage due to inflammation, thereby reducing allergy symptoms and allowing tissues to normalize. They accomplish this in the following ways: Flavonoids strengthen and repair connective tissue by stimulating the synthesis of COLLAGEN, the fibrous protein of the connective tissue that holds cells together and by inhibiting collagen breakdown. Furthermore these plant materials slow the infiltration of neutrophils, immune cells that can cause damage, into an inflamed area. Flavonoids also stabilize defensive cells in tissues (mast cells), making them less likely to release substances such as histamine, protein-degrading enzymes and LEUKOTRIENES that initiate inflammation. Flavonoids can even block the production of proinflammatory PROSTAGLANDINS as well as leukotrienes and they act as ANTIOXIDANTS to prevent FREE RADICAL damage and lipid oxidation that triggers inflammation. Free radicals are highly reactive molecules that tear electrons away from neighboring molecules to make up for their own deficiency.

Populations studies indicate that consumption of flavonoids from tea, onions and apples by northern European men can decrease the risk of heart attack, and the consumption of black tea is associated with a lower risk of STROKE. Two properties may account for these effects. Flavonoids make small blood cells called platelets less sticky, thus they can reduce the risk of dangerous blood clots. Flavonoids also act as antioxidants, possibly preventing the oxidation of LDL-cholesterol, believed to be an initiating event in atherosclerosis. Other studies suggest that certain flavonoids block cancers (anticarcinogenic activity). They can activate or inhibit various DETOXICATION enzymes in the liver, thus they may prevent the activation of carcinogens.

The amounts of key flavonoids in foods and beverages have been determined and dietary intakes can be computed. How much of a given flavonoid needs to be consumed to achieve a protective effect is uncertain, though a diet that provides 25 to 50 mg of key flavonoids offers a degree of protection against heart disease. How flavonoids are processed in the intestine by gut bacteria, how they are absorbed and how they are assimilated remain largely unknown factors. Very likely combinations of flavonoids together with other factors in foods will be most beneficial. The long-term effects of purified flavonoids on health have not been fully investigated. It should be pointed out that certain flavonoids can actually increase oxidation (prooxidant effects) and that high levels could inhibit the thyroid gland. (See also PHYTOCHEMICALS).

Hertog, Michaël G.L., Feskens, Edith J.M., Hollman, Peter C.H., Katan, M.B., and Kromhouty, D., "Dietary Antioxidant Flavonoids and Risk of Coronary Heart Disease: The Zutphen Elderly Study," *Lancet*, 342 (October 23, 1993), pp. 1007–11.

Flavonoids That May Benefit Health

Flavonoid	Typical Sources	Possible Beneficial Effects
Anthocyanin	Blueberries, blackberries, raspberries, (grapes, eggplants, red cabbage, wine)	Antioxidants. May dilate blood vessels.
Ellagic acid	Strawberries, grapes, apples, cranberries, blackberries, walnuts	Antioxidant. May block damage of DNA from carcinogenics.
Catechin	Green tea, black tea	Antioxidant. May stimulate detoxication enzymes and protects liver. Strengthens capillaries. Blocks inflammation. May inhibit tumor formation.
Tannin	Green tea, black tea	Antioxidant. May stimulate detoxication enzymes and strengthen capillaries. Blocks inflammation. May inhibit tumor formation.
Kaempferol	Strawberries, leeks, kale, broccoli, radishes, endives, red beets.	Antioxidant. May stimulate detoxication enzymes and strengthen capillaries. Blocks inflammation. May inhibit tumor formation.
Quercetin	Green tea, onions, kale, red cabbage, green beans, tomatoes, lettuce, strawberries, sweet cherries, grapes.	Antioxidant. May stimulate detoxication enzymes and strengthen capillaries. Blocks inflammation. May inhibit tumor formation.

flavor enhancers   FOOD ADDITIVES used to increase the effect of certain flavors. Enhancers themselves contribute little flavor to a food. First used in fish and meat dishes, they now intensify desired flavors and mask unwanted ones in beverages, processed fruit and vegetables, and baked goods like breads and cakes. Flavor enhancers work to enhance each other; therefore, mixtures are usually used. MONOSODIUM GLUTAMATE (MSG), DISODIUM GUANYLATE and DISODIUM INOSINATE are common examples. (See also HYDROLYZED VEGETABLE PROTEIN.)

flavors (flavorings)   One of the largest groups of FOOD ADDITIVES. About two-thirds of all additives are flavors or FLAVOR ENHANCERS. Flavors stimulate the sense of taste and/or smell. Except for sweet, bitter, salty and sour taste sensations, flavors are the result of odor perception. In spite of their wide usage, only tiny amounts of flavorings are consumed yearly (about an ounce per person) in the United States. Therefore, the U.S. FDA has less stringent regulations for them than for other food additives. Despite the small quantity consumed individually each year, food manufacturers use flavors extensively in manufactured foods because they can either replace natural flavors lost in processing, or they can replace expensive natural flavors with less expensive ingredients.

Most natural flavorings are either extracted or derived from plant products. SPICES, HERBS, YEAST, FRUIT, leaves, buds and roots of certain plants are used to provide natural flavors. Examples of natural flavors are allspice, bitter ALMOND, ANISE, balm, BASIL, caraway, cardamom, cinnamon, celery seed, chervil, citron, CLOVES, coriander, CRESS, CUMIN, DILL, FENNEL, fenugreek, GINGER, LEMON, LICORICE, MARJORAM, mint, MUSTARD, NUTMEG, OREGANO, PAPRIKA, PARSLEY, ROSEMARY, SAGE, savory, tarragon, thyme, TURMERIC, VANILLA, wintergreen.

Artificial Flavors

Artificial flavors are manufactured; their chemical structure may be the same as those flavors that occur naturally. For example: Artificial vanilla contains vanillin, the same compound as from vanilla beans. Artificial flavors may be new flavors or they may be new compounds that create familiar flavors. They have several advantages: Synthetic flavors can withstand processing; they cost less than natural flavors; they are readily available; and they are consistent in quality. Flavors are often very complex mixtures of ingredients, whether naturally occurring or created from synthetics, and food technologists have gone to great lengths to assure that the blend of synthetic flavors will meet with consumer acceptance. A wide variety of synthetic flavors are used in processed foods. Artificial flavors (like artificial cherry, raspberry, strawberry, watermelon and vanilla) can cover up the absence of more expensive ingredients in manufactured foods like mixes and soft drinks.

There are hundreds of flavoring compounds. These examples illustrate their versatility:

- allyl butyrate: pineapple odor, apple taste;
- allyl cinnamate: berry flavors, grape and peach;
- bornyl acetate: minty flavor;
- cinnamaldehyde: cinnamon, cola blends;
- cyclohexyl propionate: banana, rum;
- 2-ethyl butyraldehyde: chocolate, cocoa;
- hexyl hexanoate: strawberry, vegetable flavors;
- 5-hydroxy-4-octanone: butter, cheese, nuts;
- lactic acid: dairy flavors;
- d-limonene: citrus flavor;
- menthol: mint flavor, toothpaste;
- myrcene: citrus imitation, fruit blends;
- nonanoic acid: coconut;
- nonyl isovalerate: fried fatty food aroma and flavor;
- phenethyl isovalerate: apple, pineapple, pear, peach mixtures;
- 4-phenyl-2-butanol: melon flavors;
- 2-thienyl mercaptan: coffee-roasted flavors;
- valeraldehyde: chocolate, coffee, nut flavors;
- vanillin: vanilla, chocolate;
- zingerone: spice, root beer, raspberry.

(See also FAST FOOD; PROCESSED FOOD.)

flaxseed oil   A rich source of ALPHA LINOLENIC ACID, one of two ESSENTIAL FATTY ACIDS. Flaxseed oil contains 57% alpha linolenic acid, 16% LINOLEIC ACID (the second essential fatty acid) and 18% oleic acid, a non-essential fatty acid. Essential fatty acids are polyunsaturated FATTY ACIDS, that is, they lack pairs of hydrogen atoms and are sensitive to oxidation. They cannot be manufactured by the body and therefore must be supplied by foods or supplements. Alpha linolenic acid belongs to the omega-3 family of fatty acids. This family is converted to certain PROSTAGLANDINS, hormone-like lipids that normalize key processes of the body. For example, the omega-3 fatty acids help balance the immune system, decrease inflammation, decrease blood pressure and decrease the tendency to form blood clots. The typical diet supplies twice as much omega-6 oils as needed while supplying little omega-3 fatty acids. Most of the plant oils Americans consume—CORN OIL, peanut oil, SAFFLOWER oil and sunflower oil, to name a few—are omega-6 oils. A deficiency of omega-3 fatty acids is associated with several health problems. Omega-3 oils may improve conditions associated with *heart disease*, diabetes, inflammatory conditions such as allergies, and rheumatoid ARTHRITIS.

There are several advantages to obtaining omega-3 fatty acids from plant sources. Flaxseed oil has none of the cholesterol, vitamin A or vitamin D that occur in fish liver oils and can accumulate in the body. Fish oil may be contaminated with pesticides and industrial chemicals, depending upon where the fish lived. However, there is no clear evidence to indicate how much flaxseed oil is optimal.

Flaxseed oil is very easily oxidized and should never be used as cooking oil. To avoid rancidity, this oil needs to be refrigerated and protected from light and oxygen. BETA CAROTENE and VITAMIN E are often added to flaxseed oil as ANTIOXIDANTS. Note that linseed oil for wood finishing is prepared from flaxseed by a different process and is not fit for human consumption.

flora, intestinal   Bacteria that normally inhabit the intestinal tract. More bacteria live in the human intestinal tract than there are cells in the body. By far most live in the large intestine (colon). Lactic acid-producing bacteria, LAC-

TOBACILLUS ACIDOPHILUS and *L. bifidus*, are important examples of "good" bacteria. Optimally the relationship between intestinal bacteria and the host is symbiotic: Beneficial bacteria produce VITAMIN K, BIOTIN and other nutrients, which are absorbed. They provide the intestinal lining with a substantial part of its energy. Intestinal microorganisms promote localized acidic, anaerobic environments that inhibit the growth of potential disease-producing (pathogenic) organisms. Lactic acid-producing bacteria *L. acidophilus* and *L. bifidus* are important in this regard. Beneficial gut bacteria can also produce antimicrobial substances that limit the growth of pathogenic organisms and stimulate the IMMUNE SYSTEM.

The composition of colonic bacteria varies with the composition of the diet, the transit time (the speed with which food passes through the GASTROINTESTINAL TRACT), and use of antibiotics. A low-fiber diet contributes less carbohydrate for bacterial fermentation. Products of fermentation include short-chain FATTY ACIDS that are primary fuels for cells lining the colon. A short transit time limits the ability of acid-producing bacteria to create an acidic environment to inhibit growth of potential pathogenic organisms. Broad-spectrum antibiotics destroy beneficial bacteria as well as pathogenic bacteria. This alteration of the intestinal environment can permit opportunistic organisms such as yeast to proliferate causing disease (See also ACIDOPHILUS; BIFIDOBACTERIA; CANDIDA ALBICANS.)

flounder   A large family of saltwater FISH that includes gray sole, lemon sole and winter flounder. Flounder are bottom feeding fish, that is, they feed off the ocean floor. Their flattened bodies, with eyes on top of the head, are adaptations to this mode of feeding. This important food fish is lean and delicate. A 3-oz (8.5 g) serving of baked flounder provides 80 calories and: protein, 17 g; fat, 1 g. It contains moderate amounts of iron, 1 mg; cholesterol, 75 mg; calcium, 34 mg; niacin, 2.9 mg; riboflavin, 0.1 mg; and small amounts of other vitamins. (See also SEAFOOD INSPECTION.)

flour   Finely ground powder generally prepared from cereal GRAIN, although flours are also prepared from legumes, vegetables and fish. Flour is the primary ingredient in baked goods. It provides starch (complex carbohydrates) and varying amounts of protein and other nutrients. In cooking, flour thickens soups and gravies, and batters (mixtures of flour, water and oil) are used in sauteeing and frying foods. Flour is prepared by milling (grinding with steel rollers and sieving) grains to separate the larger starchy layer (ENDOSPERM) of the kernel from its hard outer layer (BRAN) and the oil-rich germ. In whole-grain flours, bran and endosperm are added back at this point. Wheat flour is further purified by removing oil to prevent rancidity, bleaching to remove a yellow endosperm color, and then aging by chemical treatment to produce white flour for baking.

Twenty-two nutrients are more or less removed or destroyed at most of these preparation steps: trace minerals (ZINC, MANGANESE, MAGNESIUM); vitamins (VITAMIN B_6, FOLIC ACID, RIBOFLAVIN, THIAMIN, NIACIN); ESSENTIAL FATTY ACIDS; VITAMIN E; both soluble and insoluble FIBER, and even proteins to an extent. Most states require that white flour be enriched with thiamin, riboflavin and niacin, plus iron to partially compensate for the loss of nutrients. Minerals like zinc and manganese, vitamins like folic acid, vitamin B_6 and fiber, are not added back, however.

Wheat flour is favored throughout the world because it forms elastic doughs that contribute a light texture to baked goods with yeast or other leavening agents. Wheat flour contains GLUTENS, a family of proteins (GLIADEN and glutein) that gives dough its elasticity. Aging partially oxidizes the protein and creates a flour that yields an even more elastic dough for baking. "Hard" wheat contains more protein than "soft" wheat. Most flours are blends. All-purpose flour has a higher percentage of soft wheat, while bread flour has a higher protein content. Biscuit flours are produced from soft wheat, as are cake flours.

Whole wheat flour, milled from the entire wheat kernel, contains many of the nutrients of the whole grain. Consequently whole wheat BREAD is generally more nutritious than white bread. Because it contains oils, whole wheat flour can become stale unless it is refrigerated. It does not create a fine pastry flour; often a 50/50 mixture of whole wheat to white flour is appropriate for baking.

"All-purpose" flours are used for baking bread or pastries and in thickening. All-purpose flour is enriched and may be bleached or unbleached, and some such flours contain more protein than others. Flour with 11 g or more of protein per cup will yield more tender yeast breads. Bran and cracked wheat flour, as well as oat flour, are all-purpose flours that contain wheat flour plus another grain. Pastry flour is not as coarse as all-purpose flour nor as finely milled as cake flour; it is suitable for pastry doughs. Bread flour is milled from hard wheat and has more protein, making a stronger dough. Self-raising flours also contain chemical leavening agents and salt; they are suitable for quick breads, cakes and cookies. SEMOLINA, made from durum wheat, is a granular flour, suited for pizza dough because of its high protein content.

Other flours are available at health food stores and supermarkets, including arrowroot, RYE, BUCKWHEAT, SOY, CORNMEAL, OAT, TAPIOCA, POTATO and AMARANTH flours. Amaranth and buckwheat flour are alternatives for those with grain allergies; they belong to plant families unrelated to the grass family, of which wheat is a member. (See also BAKING POWDER; BAKING SODA; ENRICHMENT.)

flour substitute (imitation flour)   A FOOD ADDITIVE used as a flour filler to reduce calories and to increase the FIBER content of bread and baked goods. A flour substitute consists of CELLULOSE that has been highly purified from wood, corn husks and other plant materials. Though purified, finely ground cellulose can be classified as a form of insoluble fiber, it probably doesn't reduce the risk of CONSTIPATION, colon CANCER or high blood cholesterol as well as the cellulose in whole foods. LEGUMES, GRAINS, fruits and vegetables can also provide additional fiber for bread. (See also IMITATION FOOD.)

fluid balance   Regulation of WATER distribution in the body. Water is the most prevalent compound in the body, accounting for approximately 60% of body weight. Body water exists within cells (cellular water), in tissues (between cells), in body cavities and in the circulation (blood and lymph). The water content in each of these compartments is carefully regulated to assure normal function of all systems.

Water diffuses freely through cell membranes and capillary walls. Excessive water distends cells, altering their membrane properties; inadequate water interferes with metabolism, which relies on a watery environment for normal function.

Water distribution is regulated by serum PROTEINS, highly charged proteins that normally do not cross the membranes of cells and capillary walls, and by ELECTROLYTES, ions whose transport across membranes is carefully regulated. Water follows the distribution of these ions, and they work together to maintain appropriate osmotic pressure. The kidneys filter 180 liters of fluid daily while producing about 2 liters of urine a day. Therefore, a liter of fluid must be ingested to make up for this loss. Kidney malfunction can alter the fluid composition of the body, which is under hormonal control. For example, ALDOSTERONE from the adrenal glands regulates SODIUM levels in the blood by directing the kidneys to take up sodium from urine. Since water follows the movement of sodium, aldosterone regulates water retention by the kidneys as well. Excessive water loss, through DEHYDRATION, DIARRHEA, bleeding and vomiting, upsets water and electrolyte balance. (See also EXTRACELLULAR FLUID.)

fluoridated water   WATER treated with controlled amounts of sodium fluoride. About half of the municipal water supplies in the United States are fluoridated. In 1988 half of the children in the United States between the ages of 5 and 17 had no cavities. The reduction in cavities in people drinking fluoridated water has been consistently observed, although this effect is not as large as earlier believed. The increased use of fluoride dental treatment, of fluoride mouth washes and toothpaste, as well as consumption of fluoridated water, could explain the reduction in dental caries in recent years. The reduction could also be due to a complex array of factors including diet changes, oral hygiene and, perhaps, increased immunity.

Fluoridation remains a controversial issue. Those opposed to fluoridation often view it as a personal rights issue, in which exposure to a potentially toxic agent is a health risk about which they should have a choice. The American Academy of Pediatrics, the U.S. Public Health Service and the American Dental Association traditionally support fluoridation of water as an effective way of reducing tooth decay. They recommend fluoride supplements for children, if drinking water does not contain fluoride. They feel there are no harmful effects at the optimal level of 1 mg of fluoride per liter of water. A committee of the National Research Council concluded in 1994 that at the presently allowed level in drinking water, fluoride does not increase the odds of cancer, bone disease or kidney failure. On the other hand, high levels can adversely affect the nervous system, a possible link to learning problems. Some tooth pitting and discoloration are possible at somewhat higher levels. With a high intake, fluoride can alter BONE structure. Evidence indicates that patients with kidney disease have an increased RISK of bone abnormalities due to fluoridation. (See also CALCIUM; FLUOROSIS; TEETH.)

fluoride   An essential TRACE MINERAL required to build strong bones and teeth. Fluoride is the ionized form of the element fluorine. The estimated safe and adequate daily dietary intake of fluoride for adults is 1.5 to 4 mg. Most research regarding fluoride has focused on the relationship of fluoride to preventing tooth decay because fluoride hardens tooth enamel. Fluoride is absorbed by gums and incorporated into the structure of developing teeth as a fluoride-containing mineral, fluorapatite. This mineral strengthens the enamel and dentine, making them more resistant to bacterial decay. Fluoride is part of BONE structure and fluoride may protect against OSTEOPOROSIS. Traces of fluoride also occur in soft tissues but its role there is unclear.

Adult intake of fluoride in the United States from various sources may reach 0.5 to 1.0 mg daily. Seafood and tea are especially good sources of fluoride. Low levels are present in many foods and in drinking water. Two fluoride-containing compounds, stannous fluoride and sodium fluorophosphate, are common ingredients of toothpaste and mouth rinse. Most toothpastes contain one milligram of fluoride per gram of paste, and a fluoride overdose is possible. Do not swallow fluoridated toothpaste.

Side effects of chronic fluoride overdose include stomach ulcers, stress-induced bone fractures and swollen joints. Questionable evidence for fluoride being a carcinogen in rats was found by the Natural Toxicology Program in 1990. A 1991 review by the U.S. Public Health Service (PHS) concluded that there is no evidence that fluoride causes CANCER in humans. The incidence of bone cancer in males below the age of 20 has risen since 1973, but the panel concluded that this is not related to fluoridation. The PHS review recommended further study to determine the relationship between fluoride intake and bone fractures. The National Research Council also concluded that current levels of fluoride in drinking water do not increase the risk of kidney disease, birth defects or intestinal problems. (See also FLUORIDATED WATER; TEETH.)

Li, Y., "Fluoride: Safety Issues," *Journal of the Indiana Dental Association*, 72:3 (May–June 1993), pp. 22–26.

fluorosis   A disease resulting from excessive FLUORIDE consumption, which can lead to the mottling of tooth enamel during tooth development. The ingestion of fluoride at levels 100 times the optimal level may lead to fluoride toxicity, characterized by bone overgrowth, brittle bones and stiff joints. Excessive fluoride in drinking water can cause fluorosis. However, fluorosis does not occur in communities where fluoride is added to drinking water because the level is raised to only 1 mg/liter. (See also TEETH.)

folacin   See FOLIC ACID.

folic acid (folacin, folate)   A water-soluble vitamin and a member of the B COMPLEX family. Folic acid is essential for cell division (especially in RED BLOOD CELLS and the immune system), for growth and for reproduction. The Reference Daily Intake (RDI) for folic acid is 400 mcg for adults while the RDA (RECOMMENDED DIETARY ALLOWANCE) is 200 mcg for men and 180 mcg for women (who are not pregnant or lactating). Approximately half of women of childbearing age consume less than the RDA for this vitamin.

Folic acid deficiency is one of the most common vitamin deficiencies worldwide, and Americans are likely to eat too little folate containing foods. Specific groups more likely to be folate deficient include: alcoholics; women taking oral contraceptives or who are pregnant; people who rely on convenience foods; and elderly people. A variety of drugs interfere with folic acid uptake and utilization: oral contraceptives, GLUCOCORTICOIDS, barbiturates, ANTACIDS, ASPIRIN, dilantin for epilepsy, and some anticancer drugs.

Deficiency symptoms include fatigue, sore tongue, mental disturbances, megaloblastic anemia, digestive disturbances and growth problems. Mild folate deficiency that does not cause anemia has been linked to NEURAL TUBE DEFECTS (SPINA BIFIDA), TOXEMIA of pregnancy, some types of CANCER (lung, esophagus, breast, colon) and cervical dysplasia, a precancerous state. Researchers have found that the risk of heart attack and heart disease is greater with low folic acid consumption. The link seems to be HOMOCYSTEINE, a byproduct of the amino acid METHIONINE. High homocysteine levels in blood increases the risk of atherosclerosis, leading to heart attacks and strokes. Homocysteine accumulates with suboptimal folic acid intake and homocysteine possibly injures blood vessels. Most people's level of homocysteine drops with supplemental folic acid, at least 400 mcg daily. There is yet no clinical study demonstrating that lowering homocysteine levels protects against heart disease.

In the body folate forms an important enzyme helper (COENZYME) called tetrahydrofolate. This coenzyme transfers single-carbon fragments from amino acid breakdown to create building blocks (PURINES and THYMINE) of DNA and RNA. Inadequate supply of these building blocks reduces the rate of DNA synthesis, hence of cell replication. Tetrahydrofolate also plays an important role in recycling METHIONINE, an essential AMINO ACID, from homocysteine. Methionine is required to synthesize CHOLINE (employed in neurotransmitter synthesis to help carry signals between nerve cells) and EPINEPHRINE (a hormone synthesized by adrenal glands to help adapt the body to stress).

Sources of folic acid include dark green leafy vegetables, BEANS (legumes), BROCCOLI, SPINACH, citrus fruits, breakfast cereals, nuts, LIVER, SALMON and whole GRAINS. Cooking and food processing destroy this fragile vitamin. It has not yet been added back to processed foods.

Doses of folic acid in the range of 5 to 10 mg per day may reduce the risk of some kinds of cancer. A randomized, double-blind prevention trial performed in the United Kingdom (Medical Research Council Vitamin Study, 1991) concluded that folic acid supplementation starting before pregnancy can be recommended for women at high risk of having a pregnancy with neural tube defects. The U.S. government recommended that women of child-bearing age take 400 mcg of folate daily. The U.S. FDA proposed in 1993 that bread and grain products such as cornmeal, flour, rolls, rice and noodles be fortified with 0.14 mg folic acid per 100 g (3.5 oz) serving, or 40 to 70 mcg per slice of fortified bread. This level is below the amount needed by women.

Folate supplements are not considered to be toxic at the usual therapeutic doses. Huge doses (10 to 20 g per day) may induce convulsions in epileptics. Folate supplementation may mask a VITAMIN B$_{12}$ deficiency, common in older Americans, and this can lead to nerve damage. Consequently, folate and vitamin B$_{12}$ are administered together when used therapeutically (See also BIRTH DEFECTS; ECLAMPSIA.)

Morrison, H.J., Schaubel, D., Desmeules, M., and Wigler, D.T., "Serum Folate and Risk of Fatal Coronary Heart Disease," *Journal of the American Medical Association*, 275 (June 26, 1996), pp. 1893–96.

food Edible substances that provide nourishment for growth and maintenance of health. Foods are mixtures of NUTRIENTS—broadly classified as MINERALS, VITAMINS, CARBOHYDRATES, PROTEINS, FATS and OILS—and WATER. FIBER is essential for a healthy intestinal tract.

Foods are neither "good" nor "bad." To evaluate the appropriateness of a particular food for an individual, it is important to know its nutrient content; the quantity being consumed and the frequency of consumption; the overall DIET and the effects of life-style on the diet; the health and nutritional status as well as the age. Genetic susceptibility to CANCER, HEART DISEASE, HYPERTENSION and diabetes need to be taken into account. Specific foods can either reduce or increase the risk of disease. A given food may be undesirable for those with FOOD SENSITIVITIES, food allergies or inherited conditions such as PHENYLKETONURIA (an inherited inability to process acid phenylalanine.) Most healthy people can tolerate splurging occasionally on cookies, CHOCOLATE or ice cream. However, moderation and a variety of fresh, whole (minimally processed) foods are hallmarks of a BALANCED DIET.

The question of whether foods and specific nutrients can prevent or minimize the effects of degenerative diseases cannot be answered in detail; this area is being researched vigorously. Clearly a reliance on highly PROCESSED FOODS can lead to health problems because such a diet does not provide adequate nutrition. On the one hand, such a diet may supply inadequate vitamins and minerals, while on the other, some nutrients are provided in excess—typically, salt, SUGAR, SATURATED FAT and TROPICAL OILS, together with HYDROGENATED VEGETABLE OIL. These additives can pose problems in susceptible individuals. Consequently, a "junk food" diet with a surplus of calories and minimal trace nutrients is not recommended. (See also CHOLESTEROL; DEGENERATIVE DISEASE; DIETARY GUIDELINES FOR AMERICANS; SODIUM.)

food additives Substances intentionally added to food products. Food additives are used for a variety of reasons: to make food look more appealing to consumers; to maintain freshness; to make food safer or more nutritious; or to ease food manufacture or processing. Unintentional (incidental) food additives are inadvertently present in foods. They have no planned function in food, but become incorporated during processing, packaging or storing. There are nearly 3,000 intentional additives. Many are derived directly from foods, like LECITHIN, a lipid related to fat. Clearly certain additives are needed to prevent spoilage and to maintain freshness of foods that must be distributed to consumers far from the point of manufacture or origin. Paradoxically, scientists' ability to detect food additives in foods, whether intentional or incidental, exceeds their ability to interpret the results in terms of human health.

The Federal Food, Drug and Cosmetic Act (1938) is the basic food law; it gives the U.S. FDA the responsibility for the safety of foods. Three amendments strengthened this act in 1954. The Miller Pesticide Act provided for establishing safe tolerances for pesticides in raw agricultural products.

The Food Additives Amendment of 1958 required pre-marketing clearance by the FDA for food additives. It includes the DELANEY CLAUSE, which made it illegal to add cancer-causing chemicals to foods. The Color Additive Amendment (1960) regulated the certification of food colors. The FDA legally classified substances added to food into four categories: food additives, GRAS (GENERALLY RECOGNIZED AS SAFE) substances, prior sanctioned items, and food colors. Hundreds of food additives were classified as GRAS in 1958, based on common experience and apparent safety record. These include SUGAR, salt, SPICES, VITAMINS, MINERALS, milk and egg protein. The GRAS list is periodically updated as new safety data are available. Thus CYCLAMATE, SULFITES, several food colors and SACCHARIN were removed when their safety was found wanting. Prior sanctioned additives are those agreed upon before 1958. NITRITE used as a preservative for processed meat is an example. That a food is prior-sanctioned or that it is on the GRAS list does not assure safety; it must be evaluated in light of more current knowledge and more advanced technology.

Excluding salt, sweeteners and sugar, the average yearly U.S. consumption of food additives like flavors, preservatives and colors is 5 to 10 pounds per person. Food additives are used extensively by the food industry to help create a huge variety of processed foods. These manufactured foods tend to have a high level of fat and oil, salt, sugar, preservatives and artificial coloring, and lower levels of several important nutrients.

Common functions of food additives:

1. ANTICAKING AGENTS are added to powdered or crystalline products to prevent lumping, e.g., silicon dioxide, CORNSTARCH, calcium silicate.
2. Antimicrobial agents preserve foods by preventing growth of bacteria, molds and yeasts, e.g., CALCIUM PROPIONATE, sodium benzoate.
3. ANTIOXIDANTS retard deterioration or rancidity and discoloration due to oxidation, e.g., VITAMIN C (ascorbic acid), VITAMIN E, BHA, BHT, propyl gallate.
4. Curing and pickling agents provide characteristic flavors and increase shelf life, e.g., sodium NITRATE, sodium nitrite.
5. Emulsifiers establish a uniform dispersion, e.g., lecithin, carrageenan.
6. Enzymes can improve food processing, e.g., glucose oxidase, MEAT TENDERIZERS.
7. FLAVOR ENHANCERS increase original taste without imparting their own flavors, e.g., DISODIUM GUANYLATE, DISODIUM INOSINATE, HYDROLYZED VEGETABLE PROTEIN.
8. Flavorings impart a taste or aroma to food, e.g., SODIUM chloride, SUCROSE and many artificial flavoring agents.
9. Flour treatment agents are bleaching and maturing agents added to flour, e.g., BENZOYL PEROXIDE, AZODICARBONAMIDE.
10. Food colors or color adjuncts are used to enhance a color or impart a color to a food, e.g., canthoxanthin, caramel, FD&C colors (Blue No. 1, Red No. 3, Yellow No. 5 and others), grape skin extract. Certain chemicals can stabilize or fix a food color.
11. HUMECTANTS absorb water and help keep foods moist, e.g., invert sugar, DEXTROSE, glycerin (GLYCEROL).
12. LEAVENING AGENTS produce CARBON DIOXIDE in baked goods, e.g., sodium BICARBONATE, yeast.
13. ARTIFICIAL SWEETENERS have less than 2% of the caloric value of sucrose (table sugar) when used at the same level of sweetness. They include saccharin and ASPARTAME.
14. Nutrient additives like IRON, THIAMIN and RIBOFLAVIN enrich white flour and partially replace some of the nutrients lost in preparing bleached flour. Iodide (the chemical form of iodine) is used to fortify salt.
15. Nutritive sweeteners include sucrose, dextrose, CORN SYRUP and high FRUCTOSE CORN SYRUP.
16. Many pH control agents change or maintain the acidity or alkalinity of a food. These include ACIDS, BASES and BUFFERS like dihydrogen phosphate, ACETIC ACID, phosphoric acid and citric acid.
17. Processing aids include clarifying agents, clouding agents and crystallization inhibitors. Filter aids are used to clarify beer, for example.
18. Propellants are used to expel a product. Carbon dioxide and other gases have replaced chlorofluorocarbons in foams and aerosols.
19. Sequestrants combine with metal ions to form complexes. This action improves product stability, e.g., CITRIC ACID, ethylenediaminetetraacetic acid (EDTA).
20. Thickeners produce viscous solutions while stabilizers form stable suspensions (emulsions). They impart "body" to foods or beverages, e.g., CAROB BEAN GUM, AGAR and alginates, as found in salad dressing, whipped cream, cheese, pudding and frozen desserts.
21. Surface finishes increase palatability, preserve gloss and inhibit food discoloration, e.g., polishes, waxes and glazes.
22. Texturizers alter the appearance and "mouth feel" of food; e.g., PECTINS, GUM GHATTI and GUM ARABIC.

Safety

The most questionable additives are artificial food colors because they may cause cancer and/or allergic reactions and their use is strictly cosmetic. Consumer advocates claim they could be eliminated without altering the nutritional value of the food. Other food additives are potentially harmful; for example, sodium nitrite, a preservative, can be converted to a class of compounds (in the stomach and intestine) that cause cancer. Saccharin, an artificial sweetener, also causes cancer in lab animals. Its use has been continued through congressional action, though saccharin-containing food must bear a warning label.

Nutritive sweeteners like sugar (sucrose) and salt are by far the most common food additives. Sweeteners represent EMPTY CALORIES because they do not supply minerals, vitamins, protein or fiber. Americans eat 28 billion pounds of sweeteners each year; the yearly per capita consumption is 130 to 150 pounds. There is consensus that excessive sugar consumption contributes to tooth decay and to obesity, now considered a leading disease in the U.S. Salt (sodium) is often added to processed foods because they lack flavor. The yearly U.S. consumption of salt per person is 10 to 15 pounds. A high-sodium diet contributes to high blood pressure in some people, who have an increased risk of dying from heart disease. There is no easy way to identify those who are sensitive to sodium ahead of time.

To minimize exposure to food additives, decrease your consumption of foods containing artificial food colors, excessive amounts of fructose corn syrup, hydrogenated vegetable oil, modified cellulose, nitrites, propyl gallate, sulfites and other synthetic antioxidants, and saccharin, as determined from the food label. Eat a variety of fresh or minimally processed foods, and eat less convenience food to limit your exposure to any one additive. (See also CHELATE; DIETARY GUIDELINES FOR AMERICANS; EATING PATTERNS; FAST FOOD; HYPERTENSION; NITROSOAMINES; PROCESSED FOOD.)

Thayer, Ann M., "Food Additives," *Chemical and Engineering News*, 70 (June 15, 1992), pp. 26–44.

food advertising   See ADVERTISING.

Food and Agricultural Organization (FAO)   A branch of the United Nations that has long been concerned with worldwide nutrition and health. It presents a world forum for dealing with international problems concerning food, agriculture and fisheries, and helps developing nations with agriculture and food production. As examples of its nutrition-related activities, the FAO has published standards for nutrient intakes, similar to the RECOMMENDED DIETARY ALLOWANCES of the United States. The FAO sets world standards for key nutrients such as PROTEIN and has published tables based on egg protein as the standard for evaluating the compositions of ESSENTIAL AMINO ACIDS of food proteins. The FAO has also developed regulations and standards for PESTICIDES, an important function because pesticide use is increasing worldwide and is not monitored carefully on a global basis. (See also EPA; HUNGER; PROTEIN QUALITY).

food allergy   See ALLERGY, FOOD.

food banks   Organizations that provide donated free food. Since the 1970s many grassroots organizations have sprung up in the United States to help combat hunger in communities. Food can be donated by private citizens, large food distributors like supermarkets, and the U.S. Department of Agriculture. Surplus commodities like RICE, BUTTER, FLOUR, HONEY, CORNMEAL and MILK have been provided free by the USDA, as specified by the Temporary Emergency Food Program of 1983. A food bank may be administered by a larger agency, offering a variety of services ranging from clothing assistance to pre-employment training. Eligibility requirements vary depending upon the particular agency or organization. Typically, individuals and families needing assistance can obtain a sack of groceries several times a week.

food-borne arthritis   Chronic joint inflammation and degeneration resulting from food poisoning due to the bacterium SALMONELLA (salmonellosis), one of the fastest growing food-borne illnesses. Salmonellosis can cause ARTHRITIS as a long-term side effect, as well as other chronic illnesses. In both the United States and Canada cases of salmonellosis have steadily increased since the 1970s. Salmonella is estimated to cause between 790,000 and 3,690,000 cases annually in the United States (1992). *Salmonella typhimarium* is the most frequent pathogen and has been responsible for the largest food-borne outbreaks. (See also AUTOIMMUNE DISEASES; EGG; FOOD POISONING.)

food chain   The linkage of the feeding habits of animals to each other and to the plants they consume. As the ultimate consumer of foods, humans are at the top of the food chain. Livestock, which live on grain and grasses, are slaughtered for human consumption. Carnivorous food fish, like tuna, live on small fish that, in turn, live on plankton.

The food-chain concept has several important ramifications: The higher up the food chain, the less efficiently a species uses the energy in food. According to the "10% rule," animals at each rung on the ecological ladder use approximately 10% of the energy trapped by life forms in a lower rung. In other words, cattle use about 10% of the energy trapped in GRAIN, and humans utilize only 10% of the energy trapped in BEEF. Thus, 3,000 calories of energy (gas, oil, cultivating, planting, harvesting, fertilizer and PESTICIDES) are required to produce one pound of sweet corn, which contains the equivalent of 375 calories. A cow has to eat approximately 80 pounds of corn (representing 29,500 calories) to produce 5 oz of beef, which then contributes 375 calories in a meal. By eating foods lower down on the food chain, people can conserve energy and resources like water because less of each is needed to produce plant foods. In terms of energy conservation and global awareness, a greater reliance on plant food would decrease the demands on the world's resources of water and fuel (energy).

A second ramification of the food chain is that materials not effectively degraded by microorganisms in the environment tend to accumulate in plants and small organisms and therefore in the animals that eat them. In this way, pollutants can be passed up the food chain, to be concentrated in the species highest on the food chain, whether bird, carnivorous fish or mammal, which are therefore the most susceptible to the toxic effects of accumulated pollutants. Falcons and hawks have been most damaged by DDT in their food supply. Ocean fish like swordfish and tuna are often contaminated with MERCURY, while walleye pike, a freshwater species, is contaminated with many industrial wastes. Scavengers like crabs and catfish are more likely to be contaminated when they consume foods that are themselves laden with pollutants. Humans are especially vulnerable because of the consumption of many other species likely to possess high concentrations of fat-soluble waste chemicals that are poorly degraded and poorly excreted. As one consequence, nearly all Americans carry traces of CADMIUM, LEAD and mercury, as well as pesticides, DIOXIN, PBB, PCB and other chemicals in their tissues without having been directly exposed to these pollutants. (See also CHLORINATED HYDROCARBONS; HEAVY METALS.)

food coloring, natural   Food colors are derived from plants, insects and, historically, even minerals. Plant colorings approved by the U.S. FDA include ANNATTO, BETA CAROTENE, PAPRIKA, SAFFRON and TURMERIC. Their colors range from yellow to red. Caramel (burnt sugar) and roasted cottonseed flour create brown colors. Powdered algae, yellow corn oil and tagetes (Aztec marigold) are added to chicken feed to yellow chicken skin and augment the color of egg yolk. Fruit JUICES and vegetable juices can be used to color foods. As examples, grape extract can be used to create purple-red foods, dehydrated beets contribute a dark red, while carrot oil and a related plant pigment CAN-THAXANTHINE create orange-colored foods. Insect pigments appear rarely. Carmine comprises 10% of the extract of cochineal insects; about 2,000 pounds are used annually in the United States.

Certain inorganic compounds are approved by the U.S. FDA as coloring agents. Ferrous gluconate develops a black color in ripe OLIVES, and titanium oxide can be used up to 1% in foods as a whitener. Sodium NITRITE contributes pink color to processed meats like HOT DOGS and HAM and processed meat products, but it is considered a preservative.

Only about 5% of food coloring currently being used is derived from natural products. The rest represents artificial dyes, synthesized from petroleum products. Careful studies (lasting more than a year) have not been carried out on most of these plant-derived coloring agents. While there is no evidence so far that they are in any way harmful, the question of their long-term safety remains unanswered. (See also ARTIFICIAL FOOD COLORS; FOOD ADDITIVES.)

food combining   Eating certain foods in combinations based on the belief that PROTEIN-rich foods should not be eaten with fruits, vegetables or starchy foods. There is little evidence to support the contention that protein DIGESTION and CARBOHYDRATE digestion would interfere with each other. In the first place, most foods are mixtures of protein and carbohydrates, and normally the body is well suited to efficiently digesting both nutrients simultaneously. Both pancreatic AMYLASE and pancreatic proteolytic enzymes are secreted simultaneously. Carbohydrate consumed within four hours of protein can enhance protein breakdown and can provide raw materials for nonessential AMINO ACIDS that can help increase protein synthesis. In this respect, adequate supplies of dietary fuels, carbohydrates and FAT lower the dietary requirement for protein; consequently, amino acids from food protein are retained more effectively to be utilized in building new protein. For people with multiple food allergies or with maldigestion problems, there may be a benefit to following such guidelines.

food complementing   Eating a variety of VEGETABLES, GRAINS and LEGUMES in order to supply the body with the appropriate amounts of amino acids that it cannot make (essential amino acids). Individual plant foods are often deficient in one or more essential amino acid. When eating a variety of plant foods it is unnecessary to determine the amino acid composition or the grams of protein in each type of food, nor is it necessary to eat a mixture of protein sources with each meal. Simply eating generous portions of a variety of foods that represent each of the vegetables, legumes and grains families each day assures an adequate supply of essential amino acids. (See also BIOLOGICAL VALUE; COMPLETE PROTEIN; VEGETARIAN.)

food composition tables (Handbook 8, USDA publication) Tables prepared by the U.S. Department of Agriculture defining the nutrient compositions of many foods. These tables describe the caloric content, the content of PROTEIN, CARBOHYDRATE, FIBER, and FAT together with the content of VITAMINS, MINERALS and CHOLESTEROL. Typically, CALCIUM, IRON, MAGNESIUM, PHOSPHOROUS, POTASSIUM, SODIUM and ZINC are included. These tables usually omit certain trace nutrients such as IODINE, COPPER, SELENIUM and chromium.

Among water-soluble vitamins, THIAMIN, RIBOFLAVIN, NIACIN, VITAMIN B_6, FOLIC ACID, and VITAMIN C and one fat-soluble vitamin, vitamin A, are routinely listed. Other fat-soluble vitamins (VITAMIN D, VITAMIN K and VITAMIN E) and certain water-soluble vitamins (VITAMIN B_{12}, BIOTIN and PANTOTHENIC ACID) are omitted. The tables indicate the portion size, whether the food has been trimmed (edible portion) or whether the food is fresh or raw.

Many factors influence the reported nutrient values: mineral content in the soil in which the food was grown, method of processing, method of storage, genetic characteristics of the harvested plant, time of year the food was harvested, methods used for nutrient analysis, different moisture contents of the food, methods of cooking and the like. Therefore the nutrient data are close approximations, rather than exact values. The Government Accounting Office reported in 1994 that some of the information is flawed, due to inconsistent collection of data and lack of information on quality assurance procedures pertaining to data submitted to the USDA. Some values of nutrients in food are underreported while other nutrients may be overreported.

To obtain more information, request "U.S. Department of Agriculture, Nutritive Values of Foods," Home and Garden Bulletin No. 72. These tables are appended to most nutrition textbooks. Additional detailed information and more complete entries are found in USDA's Handbook 8 series. The nutrient content of fast foods is available from the Center for Science in the Public Interest. Request "The Fast Food Guide." This type of information is also available for brand-name items, including canned food, TV dinners, cookies and snack food. For ethnic foods, request "Composition of Foods Used by Ethnic Groups—Selected References to Sources of Data" from the Food and Diet Appraisal Group of the Consumer and Food Economics Institute, U.S. Department of Agriculture, Agricultural Research Service. (See also DIET RECORD.)

Food, Drug and Cosmetic Act (U.S.)   The basic food law that gives the Federal Drug Administration the responsibility for the safety of foods. The first Food and Drug Act (1906) was designed to prevent the use of toxic preservatives and dyes in foods and to regulate the safety of patent medicines. In 1927 the Food, Drug and Insecticide Administration was formed, which later became the Food and Drug Administration. In 1938 the Federal Food, Drug and Cosmetic Act broadened the scope of the 1906 act by including coverage of medical devices and cosmetics, and requirements for assuring the safety and efficacy of new drugs; by setting tolerances for unavoidable toxic materials in food; by setting standards of identification for certain foods; by authorizing food manufacturing and processing factory inspections and providing for court injunctions with regard to seizures and possession.

Three amendments strengthened this act. The Miller Pesticide Act (1954) provides for establishing safe tolerances for pesticides in raw agricultural products. The Food Additives Amendment (1958) requires premarketing clearance by the FDA for food additives; it includes the DELANEY CLAUSE, which made it illegal to add CANCER-causing chemicals to foods. The Color Additive Amendment (1960) regulates the certification of food colors. In 1958 the term "food additive" was legally defined to exclude PESTICIDES, food colors, new animal drugs and substances listed on the GRAS (GENERALLY RECOGNIZED AS SAFE) list. (See also CARCINOGEN; USDA.)

food fortification   The addition of nutrients to foods without the intention of adding back nutrients lost in preparation. The added nutrient may or may not have been present in the original food. If normally present in the food, the amount of the nutrient added could be well above the amount found naturally. Often the term fortification is used synonymously with enrichment, that is, addition of a nutrient to levels at or near the original food before processing. General criteria for a nutrient to be used in fortification are as follows:

The consumption of the nutrient in question should be low in the diets of a significant number of people. The food to be fortified should be frequently consumed. The nutrient should be readily absorbed and it should not become inactive during processing and storage. It should not interfere with the nutrient qualities of the food. There should be no toxicity of the nutrient associated when an excess of the food is eaten. And the nutrient should not contribute to a nutritional imbalance.

Many new products are being fortified, including fruit juices (with calcium and vitamin C and other antioxidants), peanut butter (with vitamins and minerals), non-fat yogurt (with vitamins, minerals and lactic acid–producing bacteria), and a wide range of herbal products and beverages. Processed foods and synthetic beverages may be fortified and, at the same time, still be deficient in other nutrients. Enriched white bread contains added IRON, niacin, riboflavin and thiamin, but lacks the VITAMIN B$_6$, MANGANESE and FIBER found in the original food, for example. Whole, minimally processed foods are more nutritious options.

To improve health and minimize the risk of nutrient deficiencies, salt is generally fortified with IODINE (sodium iodide) at a level of 76 mcg iodine per g and MILK is fortified with VITAMIN A (50 IU per cup) and VITAMIN D (80 IU per cup). CALCIUM is now added to several juices and beverages. Iron is added to FLOUR and GRAIN products; otherwise grains are poor sources of iron. Enriched white bread contains 0.7 mg iron per slice (25 g); enriched cornmeal, 1.1 mg per 25 g meal; enriched breakfast cereals, 4 to 11 mg per 25 g (1 cup). The U.S. FDA has proposed that folic acid be added to bread and grain products such as pasta, grits, breakfast cereals and rolls. The level proposed, 140 mcg per 3.5 oz serving, is much less than the REFERENCE DAILY INTAKE of 400 mcg, which is considered protective. Iron is now added to so many products there is a concern that excessive dietary iron over the years might promote iron accumulation disease (HEMOCHROMATOSIS) in susceptible people, especially men. (See also ENRICHMENT; SODIUM.)

food grading   A process used to classify foods according to standard criteria. Usually sensory qualities are used, including flavor, texture and appearance or color. A higher grade does not imply a higher nutritional content. As an example, maple syrup can be graded Fancy, Grade A or Grade B. Grade B is the darkest and most strongly flavored. Graded food meets standards set by the U.S. Department of Agriculture for MEAT and POULTRY products, while the National Marine Fisheries Service grades FISH and fish produce similarly. USDA grades are not based on nutritional content. MILK and milk products generally carry a "Grade A" label, based on FDA recommended sanitary standards for milk production and processing. This grade does not refer to nutrient content, though the FDA requires specific levels of VITAMIN A and VITAMIN D for certain milk products.

food guide pyramid   A food guide plan released in 1991 by the USDA. This new plan is designed to replace the "Basic Four Food Groups," in use since 1956. The pyramid attempts to demonstrate graphically the relative importance of food groups as layers on a pyramid. Minimal daily servings are given. At the bottom of the pyramid are GRAINS, including BREAD, CEREAL, RICE and PASTA (9 to 11 servings). The next layer up consists of VEGETABLES (3 to 5 servings) and FRUITS (2 to 4 servings). By depicting produce and grains as the dietary foundation, the federal government is moving away from viewing MEAT as the dietary foundation, as it was in the old four food groups. The larger areas also stress foods that have less fat. Recommended consumption of fruits and vegetables is therefore a minimum of 5 servings daily. In 1993 less than 10% to 20% of the U.S. population ate this much. The third layer up consists of dairy products: MILK, YOGURT and CHEESE (2 to 3 servings for men and 3 to 4 servings for women) and red meat, POULTRY and FISH. Included is another group of high-protein foods: dry BEANS, EGGS and NUTS (2 to 3 servings). The peak of the pyramid, covering the smallest area, indicates food items to be used sparingly: FAT, oils, sweets, ALCOHOL, BUTTER, MARGARINE, CANDY, cookies, cakes and SOFT DRINKS.

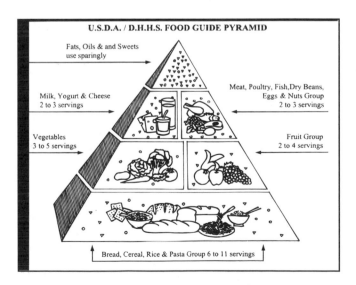

Food Guide Pyramid

The old Basic Four guide considered only PROTEIN, CALCIUM, THIAMIN, NIACIN, RIBOFLAVIN, VITAMIN A and VITAMIN C as "leader NUTRIENTS." The belief was that when people consumed enough of these nutrients, the consumption of more than 40 other nutrients would also be adequate. As early as 1974 it was shown that DIETS based upon the Basic Four were low in many key trace nutrients. The importance of fiber in the diet was not acknowledged in the Basic Four, nor was that guide designed to prevent overnutrition. A high-fat, low-fiber diet is linked to increased risk of HEART DISEASE and may be linked to the most common cancers unrelated to smoking: prostate, breast and colon.

There are several caveats attached to the food guide pyramid. The USDA's first edition poster depicted PEAS and LENTILS together with high-fat foods like meats. Though they provide protein, LEGUMES are low-fat foods that are rich in fiber and should not be classified as fats, nor should they be restricted because of fat content. Later posters will correct this error. The serving size is not clear; potato represents two servings, while a slice of bread counts as a single serving.

The food guide pyramid is based on the 1990 DIETARY GUIDELINES FOR AMERICANS, which recommends decreasing fat consumption to less than 30% of daily calories. Many nutritionists recommend that less than 25% of food calories should be derived from fats and oils. It may well be that no more than 20% of total calories should come from fat for maximum protection from chronic disease. Furthermore, non-animal sources of calcium can provide extra calcium, and they may be more beneficial than high-fat dairy products.

Achterberg C., McDonnell E., Bagby R., "How to put the Food Guide Pyramid into practice," *Journal of the American Dietetic Association*, 94:9 (Sept. 1994), pp. 1030–1035.

food handling and public health   Foods that are extensively handled and are not thoroughly reheated before serving represent possible health hazards. Most items in kitchens are not sterile, and manipulation of food will contribute to the risk of food contamination. For example, handlers of raw MEAT and animal products may be asymptomatic carriers of bacteria and viruses that can cause disease. Staphyloccal infections can be spread easily because they occur frequently in the nose and skin. Many disease-producing microorganisms are transmitted by fecal contamination; HEPATITIS A outbreaks in restaurants have been traced to poor personal hygiene of employees. Food handlers with gastric enteritis caused by salmonellosis can spread this disease because of the increased risk of fecal organism contamination with DIARRHEA. Careful attention to personal cleanliness, the use of disposable gloves, separate work areas and personnel to handle raw and cooked foods, rigorous cleaning schedules and disinfectant procedures can minimize microbial contamination. (See also FOOD POISONING.)

food interactions   See DRUG/NUTRIENT INTERACTION.

food intolerance   Physiologic reactions to foods that can be the result of toxins, metabolic diseases or enzyme deficiencies. There are two broad categories of food intolerances: those based upon a response of the IMMUNE SYSTEM and those independent of the immune system. In the former situation, food-derived molecules can trigger an allergic reaction and activate the immune system. Food allergens can be absorbed by the intestine if it is inflamed and if the protective mucosal barrier is inadequate. True food allergy attacks can be immediate (immediate onset food allergy) or delayed (delayed onset food allergy), with symptoms occurring hours after exposure to the provoking substance.

Food intolerances not regulated by the immune system include the following types of situations. Avoidance of the provoking substance(s) is important in recovery from this form of food intolerance.

Reactions to FOOD ADDITIVES, such as ARTIFICIAL FOOD COLORS (e.g., FD&C yellow No. 5), MONOSODIUM GLUTAMATE (MSG) and SULFITES.

Reactions based upon natural substances that behave as drugs. Some substances affect blood vessels (vasoactive amines) and mimic hormones. Examples are tryptamine and TYRAMINE (in aged cheese and cured meats); phenylethylamine (in CHOCOLATE); HISTAMINE and amines (in red WINE, oranges, plums, pineapples and tomatoes). Other active substances are methylxanthines such as CAFFEINE (in COFFEE, TEA, colas, chocolate and COCOA). These can cause headache, palpitations, anxiety or vomiting.

Reactions based on a metabolic imbalance or a metabolic defect (enzyme deficiency) or altered body chemistry. LACTOSE INTOLERANCE due to a deficiency of LACTASE, the enzyme responsible for digesting milk sugar, is the most common of this type. PHENYLKETONURIA is an example of an inherited metabolic disease based upon an intolerance of PHENYLALANINE due to a deficiency of an enzyme required to degrade this amino acid. Sugar sensitivity or HYPOGLYCEMIA are metabolically-based conditions that may reflect hormonal imbalances.

Reactions classified as FOOD POISONING. Bacterial toxins (BOTULISM) and mold toxins (AFLATOXIN) are possible causes. (See also: ALLERGY, FOOD; ALLERGY, IMMEDIATE; ELIMINATION DIET; ENTEROTOXIN.)

food irradiation   Sterilization of food using radiation. The intent of food irradiation is to extend the shelf life of a food and to kill potentially dangerous microorganisms and insects. Another advantage is that irradiation can also delay ripening and inhibit sprouting of POTATOES and WHEAT. Food irradiation in the United States is currently approved for SPICES, WHEAT, fresh FRUIT like strawberries, fresh vegetables including POTATOES, PORK, fresh poultry and frozen, uncooked poultry, medical supplies and some drugs. Irradiation of chickens is permitted in order to kill salmonella bacteria, which can cause food poisoning. Irradiated foods are required to be labeled as such; the warning symbol is a floral emblem. Prepared foods do not need to be labeled, though they may have been irradiated. Presently, no law requires labeling fast foods.

Proponents argue that irradiation could replace postharvest PESTICIDES on fruit and vegetables and reduce the threat of salmonella food poisoning in CHICKEN. However, irradiation is turning out to be more expensive and sometimes less effective than predicted. The only foods being irradiated worldwide are GRAINS (eastern Europe) and potatoes (Japan). Irradiated food does not become radioactive, though it may be exposed to radioactive elements. The irradiation process breaks up molecules in pests as well as in the food itself, and VITAMIN C and VITAMIN E plus THIAMIN are thus destroyed. The high doses of radiation required to kill pests create new substances (called radiolytic products) from the production of molecular fragments (free radicals). The radiolytic products are potential CARCINOGENS, and critics of irradiation argue that not enough testing has been done to establish long-term safety of irradiated food.

The presently permitted irradiation dose does not completely sterilize grains and nuts, thus leaving them susceptible to potentially dangerous molds when stored for extended periods. Opponents of food irradiation contend that the salmonella problems should be corrected through more sanitary processing in slaughterhouses and meat-packing facilities. On the other hand, food irradiation is endorsed by the World Health Organization and the U.S. National Academy of Sciences, which believe the production of harmful chemicals is negligible. (See also FOOD PROCESSING.)

Webb, T., Lang, T., Tucker, K. *Food Irradiation*. Rochester, Vt.: Thorsons Publishers, 1987.

food labeling   Consumer information required by the U.S. FDA and the Food Safety and Inspection Services for about 90% of processed foods. Nutrition labeling and nutrient lists are required of most foods regulated by the FDA, excluding restaurant foods and foods served for immediate consumption on airplanes, in hospitals and by food service vendors; deli and bakery goods prepared on-site; foods sold in bulk and not for resale; foods produced by small businesses; medical foods, such as those designed for specific patient needs; plain coffee and tea; and products for export. Foods in small packages (less than 12 sq. in., such as a candy bar 1-in. thick, 2 in. wide and 6 in. long) need not have nutrition information unless a nutritional claim is made. Labeling for meat and poultry products is regulated by the U.S. Department of Agriculture (USDA).

Nutrition Facts	Amount/serving	% DV*	Amount/serving	% DV*
Serv. Size ⅓ cup (56gf)	Total Fat 1g	2%	Total Carb. 0g	0%
Servings about 3	Sat Fat 0g	0%	Fiber 0g	Ê0%
Calories 80	Cholest. 10mg	3%	Sugars 0g	
Fat Cal. 10	Sodium 200mg	8%	Protein 17g	
*Percent Daily Values (DV) are based on a 2,000 calorie diet.	Vitamin A 0%• Vitamin C 0%• Calcium 0% • Iron 6%			

Nutrition Facts

Serving size 1 can (360mL)

Amount Per Serving

Calories 140

	%Daily Value*
Total Fat 0g	0%
Sodium 20mg	1%
Total Carbohydrate 36g	12%
Sugars 36 g	
Protein 0g	0%

*Percent Daily Values are based on a 2,000 calorie diet.

Food labeling

The new food label in place as of 1994 features an improved nutrition panel called "Nutrition Facts." Serving sizes are more consistent than before and are stated in household and metric units, based upon the amount customarily eaten at a given time. Reference amounts are broken down into 139 categories regulated by the FDA and 23 meat and poultry categories (regulated by the USDA). For example, cookies have a reference amount of 30 g; for breads it is 50 g. The top of the food label provides the number of servings per container and the total number of calories, as well as the calories derived from FAT. One of the most useful features is a listing of how much sodium, fat, CHOLESTEROL, fiber, sugar and other nutrients as a percentage of the daily allotment is in a serving.

The new mandatory components (underlined) are listed below in the order in which they must appear, together with certain permitted voluntary components.

- total calories
- calories from fat
- calories from saturated fat
- total fat
- saturated fat
- polyunsaturated fat
- monounsaturated fat
- cholesterol
- sodium
- potassium
- total carbohydrate
- dietary fiber
- soluble fiber
- insoluble fiber
- sugars
- sugar alcohol (for example, the sugar substitutes xylitol, mannitol and sorbitol)
- other carbohydrate (the difference between total carbohydrate and the sum of dietary fiber, sugars and sugar alcohol if declared)
- protein
- vitamin A
- percent vitamin A represented by beta carotene
- vitamin C
- calcium
- iron
- other essential vitamins and minerals may be listed.

If a claim is made about any of the optional components as to health benefits, or if a food is fortified or enriched with them, nutrition information for these components is required.

Amounts in grams are listed both in terms of grams (or milligrams) and as a percent of the Daily Value (DV), based on the amounts supplied by a typical daily diet supplying 2,000 calories. Certain variations of the format are mandatory. For example, to prevent parents from restricting fat intake for young children, the labels for foods for children under two years of age cannot list information on fat or calorie content. (Rules for labeling infant formulas are covered under a separate act, the Infant Formula Act of 1980.) Food labels for children under four such as infant formulas and baby foods cannot list Daily Values or percentages for calories, fat, protein and carbohydrate because they have not been determined for such young children, though Daily Values for vitamins and minerals is permissible.

Packaged foods must list the common (generic) name of the product such as spaghetti or chicken soup; the name and address of manufacturer, distributor or packer, and net contents. standards of identity (standard recipes long in use and approved by the FDA) exist for 300 or so staples like catsup, mayonnaise, ice cream, peanut butter, salt, sweeteners and preservatives, and their contents need not be listed.

Sometimes the daily values are maximum levels; the daily value for fat is 65 grams or less. Other values are minimums; the daily value for carbohydrates is equal to 300 g or more.

Terminology

Certain terms on food labels presently have no legal meaning: "natural," "dietetic," "health food." Others terms are now defined by the FDA and the USDA:

1. High: High indicates a benefit to the consumer by providing more than 20% of the amount of a given nutrient recommended for daily eating (daily value), as in "high protein."
2. Good Source: This term indicates a given food is beneficial in providing 10% to 19% of the amount of the daily value per serving.
3. Light: A food labeled light contains one-third fewer calories than a comparable food. When used otherwise, light must specify its reference to look, taste or smell, as in "light in color."
4. More: Indicates that a food has at least 10% more of the nutrient than a comparable food.
5. Fresh: Raw food. Refers to food that has never been frozen, processed or preserved.
6. Lean: Per 100 g lean, cooked meat or poultry contains less than 10 g of fat (less than 4 g of saturated fat) and less than 95 mg of cholesterol.
7. Extra Lean: Extra-lean cooked meat or poultry contains less than 5 g of fat (and less than 2 g of saturated fat) and less than 95 mg of cholesterol per 100 g.
8. Imitation: Both the FDA and the USDA require that a product be labeled "imitation" if it contains an ingredient making it nutritionally inferior to the product with the traditional ingredient. Taking pizza as an example, the FDA requires that if the product uses less than 100% real cheese, it must be labeled imitation.

The following illustrate definitions for "free," "reduced," "low," and "less" as they pertain to sugar, calories, fat, cholesterol, sodium and fiber—as provided by the FDA Consumer Special Report, "Focus on Food Labeling" (May 1993).

Sugar "Sugar free": less than 0.5 g per serving.
"No added sugar," "Without added sugar," "No sugar added":

1. No sugars added during processing or packing, including ingredients that contain sugars (for example, fruit juices, apple sauce or dried fruit).
2. Processing does not increase the sugar content above the amount naturally present in the ingredients. (A function-

ally insignificant increase in sugars is acceptable from processes used for purposes other than increasing sugar content.)
3. The food that it resembles and for which it substitutes normally contains added sugars.

"Reduced sugar": at least 25% less sugar per serving than reference food.

Calories "Calorie free": fewer than 5 calories per serving.
"Low calorie": 40 calories or less per serving or, if the serving is 30 g or less or 2 tablespoons or less, per 50 g of the food.
"Reduced calories" or "Fewer calories": at least 25% fewer calories per serving than reference food.

Fat "Fat free": less than 0.5 g of fat per serving.
"Saturated fat free": less than 0.5 g per serving and the level of trans-fatty acids does not exceed 1% of total fat.
"Low fat": 3 g or less per serving, or if the serving is 30 g, or less or 2 tablespoons or less, per 50 g of the food.
"Low saturated fat": 1 g or less per serving and not more than 15% of calories from saturated fatty acids.
"Reduced fat" or "Less fat": at least 25% less per serving than reference food.
"Reduced saturated fat" or "Less saturated fat": at least 25% less per serving than reference food.

Cholesterol "Cholesterol free": less than 2 mg of cholesterol and 2 g or less of saturated fat per serving.
"Low cholesterol": 20 mg or less and 2 g or less of saturated fat per serving or, if the serving is 30 g or less or 2 tablespoons or less, per 50 g of the food.
"Reduced cholesterol" or less cholesterol: at least 25% less and 2 g or less of saturated fat per serving than reference food.

Sodium "Sodium free": less than 5 mg per serving.
"Low sodium": 140 mg or less per serving or, if the serving is 30 g or less or 2 tablespoons or less, per 50 g of the food.
"Very low sodium": 35 mg or less per serving or, if the serving is 30 g or less or 2 tablespoons or less, per 50 g of the food.
"Reduced sodium" or "Less sodium": at least 25% less per serving than reference food.

Fiber "High fiber": 5 g or more per serving. (Foods making high-fiber claims must meet the definition for low-fat, or the level of total fat must appear next to the high-fiber claim.)
"Good source of fiber": 2.5 g to 4.9 g per serving.
"More fiber" or "Added fiber": at least 2.5 g more per serving than reference food.

The number of grams of fat and of saturated fat are listed. The phrase "partially hydrogenated" can designate any vegetable oil that is from 5 to 60% saturated. Unfortunately, few foods indicate the percentage of total calories derived from fat. This is vital information in terms of nutritionists' recommendations that fat contribute a maximum of 30% of calories, and that saturated fat contribute no more than 10% of calories.

Health Claims

ADVERTISING contributes significantly to the public awareness of nutrition, and some food ads now list health benefits of nutrients. Current regulations specify that claims on packages cannot be misleading. The FDA permits food manufacturers to produce food labels describing certain health benefits of a particular food if they are well established and if the virtues of a well balanced diet are also emphasized. Food labeling rules permit only seven kinds of health claims for foods. (An eighth, the relationship between folcin [folic acid] deficiency and birth defects is pending.) Information must be consistent with a reasonable diet and FDA-approved summaries of evidence. The following illustrate permissible claims (quoted from the FDA Consumer Special Report, "Focus on Food Labeling" [May 1993]).

Calcium and osteoporosis Nutrient/Food-Disease Link: Low calcium intake is one risk factor for osteoporosis, a condition of lowered bone mass or density. Lifelong adequate calcium intake helps maintain bone health by increasing as much as genetically possible the amount of bone formed in the teens and early adult life and by helping to slow the rate of bone loss that occurs later in life.

Requirements: Food or supplement must be "high" in calcium; must not contain more phosphorus than calcium. Claims must cite other risk factors; state the need for regular exercise and a healthful diet; explain that adequate calcium early in life helps reduce fracture risk later by increasing as much as genetically possible a person's peak bone mass; and indicate that those at greatest risk of developing osteoporosis later in life are white and Asian teenage and young adult women, who are in their bone-forming years. Claims for products with more than 400 mg of calcium per day must state that a daily intake over 2,000 mg offers no known added benefit to bone health.

Sodium and hypertension (high blood pressure) Nutrient/Food-Disease Link: Hypertension is a risk factor for coronary heart disease and stroke deaths. The most common source of sodium is table salt. Diets low in sodium may help lower blood pressure and related risks in many people. Guidelines recommend daily sodium intake of not more than 2,400 mg. Typical U.S. intakes are 3,000 to 6,000 mg.

Requirements: Foods must meet criteria for "low sodium." Claims must use "sodium" and "high blood pressure" in discussing the nutrient-disease link.

Dietary fat and cancer Nutrient/Food-Disease Link: Diets high in fat increase the risk of some types of cancer, such as cancers of the breast, colon and prostate. While scientists don't know how total fat intake affects cancer development, low-fat diets reduce the risk. Experts recommend that Americans consume 30% or less of daily calories as fat. Typical U.S. intakes are 37%.

Requirements: Foods must meet criteria for "low fat." Fish and game meats must meet criteria for "extra lean." Claims may not mention specific types of fats and must use "total fat" or "fat" and "some types of cancer" or "some cancers" in discussing the nutrient-disease link.

Dietary saturated fat and cholesterol and risk of coronary heart disease Nutrient/Food-Disease Link: Diets high in saturated fat and cholesterol increase total and low-density (bad) blood cholesterol levels and, thus, the risk of coronary heart disease. Diets low in saturated fat and cholesterol decrease the risk. Guidelines recommend that American diets contain less than 10% of calories from saturated fat and less than 300 mg cholesterol daily. The average American adult diet has 13% saturated fat and 300 to 400 mg cholesterol a day.

Requirements: Foods must meet criteria for "low saturated fat," "low cholesterol" and "low fat." Fish and game meats must meet criteria for "extra lean." Claims must use "saturated fat and cholesterol" and "coronary heart disease" or "heart disease" in discussing the nutrient-disease link.

Fiber-containing grain products, fruits, and vegetables and cancer Nutrient/Food-Disease Link: Diets low in fat and rich in fiber-containing grain products, fruits and vegetables may reduce the risk of some types of cancer. The exact role of total dietary fiber, fiber components, and other nutrients and substances in these foods is not fully understood.

Requirements: Foods must meet criteria for "low fat" and, without fortification, be a "good source" of dietary fiber. Claims must not specify types of fiber and must use "fiber," "dietary fiber," or "total dietary fiber" and "some types of cancer" or "some cancers" in discussing the nutrient-disease link.

Fruits, vegetables and grain products that contain fiber, particularly soluble fiber, and risk of coronary heart disease Nutrient/Food-Disease Link: Diets low in saturated fat and cholesterol and rich in fruits, vegetables and grain products that contain fiber, particularly soluble fiber, may reduce the risk of coronary heart disease. (It is impossible to adequately distinguish the effects of fiber, including soluble fiber, from those of other food components.)

Requirements: Foods must meet criteria for "low saturated fat," "low fat" and "low cholesterol." They must contain, without fortification, at least 0.6 g of soluble fiber per reference amount, and the soluble fiber content must be listed. Claims must use "fiber," "dietary fiber," "some types of dietary fiber," "some dietary fibers" or "some fibers" and "coronary heart disease" or "heart disease" in discussing the nutrient-disease link. The term "soluble fiber" may be added.

Fruits and vegetables and cancer Nutrient/Food-Disease Link: Diets low in fat and rich in fruits and vegetables may reduce the risk of some cancers. Fruits and vegetables are low-fat foods and may contain fiber or vitamin A (as beta carotene) and vitamin C. (The effects of these vitamins cannot be adequately distinguished from those of other fruit or vegetable components.)

Requirements: Foods must meet criteria for "low fat" and, without fortification, be a "good source" of fiber, vitamin A or vitamin C. Claims must characterize fruits and vegetables as foods that are low in fat and may contain dietary fiber, vitamin A or vitamin C; characterize the food itself as a "good source" of one or more of these nutrients, which must be listed; refrain from specifying types of fatty acids; and use "total fat" or "fat," "some types of cancer" or "some cancers," and "fiber," "dietary fiber," or "total dietary fiber" in discussing the nutrient-disease link.

Tips for Reading a Food Label

If the first ingredient listed on the label is VEGETABLE OIL or SUGAR, the food is very high in calories. If the food label contains several alternative names for refined sugar—DEXTROSE, FRUCTOSE, high FRUCTOSE CORN SYRUP, SUCROSE, malt sugar, maltose, HONEY—it is a high-sugar food. The phrase "made with pure vegetable oil" may mask the fact that the food is made with COCONUT OIL or PALM OILS, vegetable oils that are more saturated than BUTTER and lard. SATURATED FAT is a suspected cause of HEART DISEASE. To minimize intake of a given potential problem ingredient, a rule of thumb is to avoid any product listing that particular ingredient among the first five additives.

Food containers and wrappers often provide other types of information that do not deal with nutrient content, such as food grades, product dating and universal bar codes.

Product dating　Four kinds of dating are used for perishable foods and milk and dairy products. "Pack date" refers to the day the food was manufactured, processed or packaged. "Pull" or "sell date" is the last date on which the product should be sold, assuming proper storage and handling. MILK, YOGURT, ice cream and cold cuts are examples of food with pull dates. "Expiration dates" define the last date the food should be eaten; infant formulas display "use by" dates. A "freshness date" resembles an expiration date, but baked goods can still be used after the freshness date. While safe and wholesome, the food beyond the freshness date might not taste as good as the fresh product. Generally product dating is not regulated by the FDA.

Universal product code (UPC)　A bar code, a block of parallel lines of various widths, with numbers, that appears on most food labels. Each code designation is unique to a given product. Stores equipped with computerized checkout can read these codes and automatically record sales. Together with a computerized system, UPC functions as an automatic inventory system to follow the rate of sales and reordering data. The universal product code is not regulated by the FDA.

(See also FOOD ADDITIVES; FOOD GRADING; PESTICIDES.)

Food and Drug Administration, *Focus on Food Labeling.* Washington, D.C. : Department of Health and Human Services, 1993.

Kurtzweil, Paula, "Answers to Consumer Questions about the Food Label," *FDA Consumer*, 29:5 (June 1995), pp. 6–9.

food and the nervous system

The relationship among food, behavior and emotions. Research over the last two decades has brought a deepened understanding of brain chemistry, together with a renewed interest in the effects of diet on behavior and mental well-being.

One focus is on NEUROTRANSMITTERS, chemicals that carry signals between individual nerve cells. The synthesis of at least five neurotransmitters may be affected by the brain concentrations of certain raw materials. Significantly, diet can influence concentrations of these raw materials. Most research on food and neurotransmitters has focused on SERO-TONIN, which normally induces relaxation, increased tolerance to pain and decreased carbohydrate consumption. It has been proposed that serotonin may inhibit eating behavior because some bulimics (binge-purge eaters) are deficient in serotonin. The brain converts the amino acid TRYPTOPHAN to serotonin, and a high-carbohydrate meal may lead to increased TRYPTOPHAN levels in the brain, increased brain serotonin and sleepiness. On the other hand, a high-protein meal may promote mental alertness temporarily because after protein digestion, relatively more of the amino acid TYROSINE is taken up by the brain. This may lead to a rise in norepinephrine, a neurotransmitter responsible for maintaining a state of alertness. These effects do not seem to extend beyond a single meal, however, and long-term studies of diet suggest that brain tryptophan and serotonin do not function as a brain signal in linking protein consumption to the regulation of protein intake, or presumably to carbohydrate intake. The body generally controls total caloric intake rather precisely, but not protein and carbohydrate intake, which can vary considerably from meal to meal.

A second category of brain chemicals implicated in food and behavior is neuropeptides. These are composed of chains of amino acids (polypeptides), though they are much smaller than proteins. The production of several neuropeptides varies with the time of day (circadian rhythm), which could affect preference for specific foods at different times. Neuropeptides believed to inhibit eating include:

- CHOLECYSTOKININ A polypeptide hormone that suppresses appetite for fat and carbohydrate.
- Cyclo His-Pro (histidyl-proline diketopiperazine) This small molecule is derived from just two amino acids: HISTIDINE and PROLINE. It is released into the bloodstream after a meal and may be present for up to 12 hours afterward.

Other neuropeptides may activate eating behavior:

- Neuropeptide Y (NPY). This brain chemical stimulates APPETITE for carbohydrate within minutes after it appears in the brain of experimental animals. The effect lasts for 24 hours. Levels increase between meals and decrease after eating.
- Galanin. A brain protein that triggers craving of fatty foods and stimulates fat uptake. Experimental animals with a high galanin content in the region of the brain called the HYPOTHALAMUS tend to eat more fat and gain more weight than those with less of this brain protein. The level of galanin rises throughout the day and stimulates appetite for fat at lunch time and at dinner.

Food choices are based on many factors other than HUNGER, including state of physical and emotional health, cultural beliefs, food preferences and economic status, among others. While socioeconomic factors affect which foods are chosen, biochemical mechanisms, including sugar consumption, nutrient deficiencies, exposure to toxic materials and food sensitivities, help regulate the kinds of foods selected, the time of eating and the amount of food consumed.

Sugar and mood　This is a controversial area. A variety of clinical studies suggest that sugar does not generally cause changes in mood or hyperactivity. Other studies and considerable anecdotal evidence suggest that in susceptible people excessive sugar consumption can alter BLOOD SUGAR levels, change brain function and cause mood swings. Blood sugar may temporarily drop several hours after eating. Thus, a heavy lunch tends to exaggerate the afternoon slump, possibly because large meals apparently increase blood flow to the gut, away from the brain. A drop in blood sugar (HYPO-GLYCEMIA) can cause irritability, depression, FATIGUE and moodiness because the brain is exquisitely dependent upon blood sugar to meet most of its energy needs.

Nutrient Deficiencies It is well established that vitamin and mineral deficiencies can have long-term effects on mood. Severe, chronic deficiencies of VITAMIN B$_6$, VITAMIN B$_{12}$, VITAMIN C, FOLIC ACID and NIACIN can cause symptoms resembling SENILITY, DEPRESSION and schizophrenia. However, these are complex illnesses that probably have multiple causes. To the extent that nutritional deficiencies contribute to mental disturbances, supplementing with vitamins can sometimes help alleviate symptoms. Experts stop short of claiming that vitamin supplements can cure mental illness. Indirect evidence links oxidative damage from free radicals to a decline in brain function with aging and with certain degenerative diseases of the nervous system. The implication is that antioxidants are essential for healthy brain function. In experimental animals deficiencies in the above nutrients, as well as in IRON, COPPER and ZINC, impair neurotransmitter synthesis. It is not clear to what extent subclinical deficiencies affect the brain and behavior. Some lines of research suggest that abnormal levels of copper and other minerals may predispose males to violent behavior.

Toxic metals Exposure to HEAVY METALS can have many effects on the nervous system and behavior. As examples, too much CADMIUM can partially block the uptake of the essential trace mineral zinc. LEAD pollution lowers intelligence and scholastic performance, especially in younger children.

Food sensitivities Traditionally, food sensitivities and allergies have not been considered important influences of behavior. However, evidence is accumulating that indicates food allergies can trigger mood swings, anxiety and fatigue in susceptible individuals when the allergic attack focuses on the nervous system. Sensitivities to whole milk and other foods have been implicated in schizophrenia, depression and aggressive behavior in some instances. (See also ALLERGY, FOOD; APPETITE; BULIMIA NERVOSA; FEINGOLD DIET; HUNGER.)

White, J.W. and Wolraich, M., "Effect of Sugar on Behavior and Mental Performance," *American Journal of Clinical Nutrition*, 62: supp. (1995), pp. 242S–49S.

food poisoning Diseases caused by microorganisms and transmitted through food. Estimates of food-borne gastroenteritis (irritational the stomach and intestines often accompanied by vomiting and diarrhea) range from 33 million to 81 million annually, depending upon the estimates of unreported cases. Bacteria, viruses, fungi, worms and protozoa are major causes of food-borne disease throughout the world. Disease-producing (pathogenic) organisms are usually transmitted by the oral-fecal route, generally through contamination of food and water. Most food poisoning in the United States is caused by bacteria. A variety of bacteria may produce toxic materials (toxins) rather than cause infections. Food inherently contains bacteria unless sterilized. Bacteria can also be introduced from external factors, such as soil, dust, poor sanitary habits, inadequate hygiene, household pets and insects.

Microbial contamination causes problems in foods that are not cooked long enough or are handled improperly after cooking. Heating food destroys most viruses and bacteria, however, bacteria can rapidly multiply in food left at room temperature or kept warm. Refrigeration slows bacterial growth, while freezing prevents it. If food is left unattended for a long enough time, certain bacteria will produce very toxic substances that may not be destroyed by heating (or freezing).

The following are prominent examples of possible microbial contamination of food:

Salmonellosis The bacterium SALMONELLA can contaminate raw or undercooked beef or poultry and foods coming into contact with them or their juices, as well as raw or undercooked eggs. Since salmonella is spread by fecal contamination, inadequate hygiene by food handlers increases the risk. Symptoms (nausea, vomiting, cramps, chills) usually begin within 12 to 48 hours. Salmonellosis can be fatal to children, elderly persons and those with low immunity.

Shigellosis The bacterium Shigella can contaminate foods handled by an infected person with poor hygiene, or foods undercooked or stored at room temperature. Symptoms (nausea, bloody stools) appear in one to seven days. Shigellosis can be serious in elderly people, infants and those with lowered immunity.

Infectious hepatitis (type A) The hepatitis virus type A can contaminate food handled by infected food handlers and shellfish contaminated by raw sewage. Symptoms (jaundice, liver damage) appear in 15 to 50 days. This disease can be fatal.

Escherichia coli 0157:H7 Can cause hemmorhagic colitis and hemolytic uremic syndrome. This strain of *E. coli* is linked to contaminated raw or undercooked meat and to contaminated milk. Symptoms include bloody diarrhea, severe abdominal cramping and kidney damage. The disease can cause permanent kidney damage and death in young children.

Staphylococcal food poisoning The bacterium Staphyloccus contaminates food that has been handled under unsanitary conditions and by infected food handlers, especially those with skin infections. It may be present in foods like potato or tuna salad. Symptoms (nausea, diarrhea, abdominal cramping, vomiting) can begin in one to eight hours.

Parahemolytic food poisoning Species of the bacterium Vibrio may contaminate fish and shellfish exposed to raw sewage. Symptoms (abdominal pain, diarrhea, headache, chills, bloody stools) can begin in 15 to 24 hours.

Viral gastroenteritis Intestinal viruses (rotaviruses, enteroviruses, norwalk virus, parvovirus) can contaminate foods processed by infected food handlers. These viruses also occur in shellfish contaminated by raw sewage. Symptoms (vomiting, nausea, diarrhea) occur in 12 to 48 hours.

Campylobacteriosis The bacterium Campylobacter can contaminate meat and poultry and by fecal exposure in packing plants. Typical sources are undercooked or raw beef, poultry, shellfish and untreated water. Symptoms (fever, diarrhea, bloody stools cramps) can begin within two to five days.

Perfringens food poisoning   The bacterium *Clostridium perfringens* can contaminate foods that are slowly cooled or held at room temperature too long. Typically these are meat and poultry dishes that are covered or wrapped with limited exposure to air. Symptoms (diarrhea, abdominal pain, nausea, vomiting) are usually mild and begin in 8 to 24 hours.

Botulism   The bacterium *Clostridium botulinum* can contaminate improperly cooked low-acid foods, like green beans or corn, that are home cooked. It can grow in potatoes covered with butter or oil and left at room temperature for too long a period. This bacterium produces an extremely powerful nerve toxin that causes double vision, difficult breathing and, in extreme cases, death. Symptoms begin within 8 to 36 hours.

Worms   Occur in fish (clonorchiasis, opisthochiasis) and pork (TRICHINOSIS, cysticercosis, balantidiasis), among others.

Seafood Poisoning   Scromboid FISH POISONING is an example of fish poisoning. Shellfish poisoning can be the result of red tide contamination (dinoflagellate).

Suggestions for Preventing Food Poisoning

1. Wash hands with soap before preparing food. Use a fresh dish towel. Many food-borne illnesses are due to fecal contamination.
2. Assume that all raw meat, fish and poultry are contaminated. Do not mix raw meat (especially HAMBURGER, PORK and roast beef) with fresh vegetables. Do not use the same cutting board, sponges or utensils for raw meat and fresh vegetables. Do not use the same utensils or even the same kitchen sponge for both raw meat and cooked meat. This can reintroduce bacteria into the cooked meat.
3. Cook food thoroughly. Meat should not be pink and juice should run gray. Freeze or refrigerate leftovers, particularly any food that is wrapped or coated with breading. Refrigerator temperature should be kept below 40° F. Do not leave food at room temperature for more than one hour.
4. Thaw meat or poultry in the refrigerator, microwave or in cold running water rather than at room temperature.
5. Do not stuff a turkey ahead of roasting time and then refrigerate it. This could allow time for disease-producing bacteria to multiply. Stuff the bird and cook it immediately.
6. Marinate meat and poultry in the refrigerator rather than at room temperature.

Heche, Annabel, "The Unwelcome Dinner Guest: Preventing Food-borne Illness," *FDA Consumer*, (Jan.-Feb., 1991), pp. 16–25.

Roberts, Diane, "Sources of Infection: Food," *Lancet*, 336 (October 6, 1990), pp. 859–61.

Schardt, David and Schmidt, Stephen, "Keeping Food Safe," *Nutrition Action Healthletter*, 22:3 (April 1995), pp. 4–7.

food preservation   Strategies to preserve food and prevent spoilage. Common methods include DEHYDRATION, ANTIOXIDANTS, PRESERVATIVES, FERMENTATION, refrigeration, freezing and heat processing.

Dehydration   This is an ancient method of food preservation. The removal of water from foods deprives microorganisms of an environment suitable for their growth. Heat is used to dehydrate fruit, herbs, milk, meat and fish. To better maintain nutrients, foods may be freeze-dried. In this process, water is removed by evaporation from foods that have been rapidly frozen and maintained at low temperature and low pressure. Restricted exposure to air helps to prevent oxidation of sensitive nutrients in dehydrated foods. Therefore dehydrated foods are sealed against air and moisture.

Antioxidants   To control oxidation, a wide variety of substances can be added to foods. ANTIOXIDANTS prevent the reaction of oxygen with sensitive materials in foods. Thus they reduce rancidity and increase product shelf life. Butylated hydroxytoluene (BHT), butylated hydroxyanisole (BHA) and VITAMIN C (ascorbic acid) delay browning and preserve color and freshness of foods.

Preservatives   Compounds such as CALCIUM PROPIONATE, SODIUM BENZOATE, sodium NITRATE, SODIUM chloride and SULFITES retard microbial growth in many processed foods.

Fermentation   Fermented foods are generally more stable than unfermented ones. Mold and bacteria can produce LACTIC ACID, ethanol or other substances that inhibit microbial degradation. CHEESE, YOGURT, kefir and BUTTERMILK are more stable than fresh milk.

Pickling   Pickling involves the addition of vinegar, salt and spices to vegetables (like cucumbers), fish (pickled herring) or meat.

Refrigeration   Freezing and refrigeration slow the reaction of food constituents with oxygen and with enzymes in foods themselves. Lowered temperatures also retard microbial proliferation and prevent spoilage.

Cooking   Heat processing destroys microorganisms and can destroy endogenous ENZYMES that would alter food quality. BLANCHING destroys surface microorganisms and inactivates enzymes that could change their color, flavor or nutritive value. PASTEURIZATION inactivates a portion of the microorganisms present in MILK and delays spoiling. Sterilization requires heating foods at 100° C to 120° C in order to destroy bacterial spores. Heat will cause the loss of certain nutrients like FOLIC ACID and vitamin C, depending on the temperature and duration of heating.

food processing   Methods used to preserve and to prepare agricultural and livestock products as foods. Historically, food processors have emphasized safety, convenience and acceptability, and there is a growing awareness of nutritive value as a major quality. "Minimally processed" foods are treated by routine kitchen procedures only, including slicing, mixing, chilling, freezing, drying, grinding, mincing, and cooking procedures such as boiling, braising or baking.

Industrial preservation methods include refrigerating, freezing or chilling, drying, fermentation as in pickling, adding chemical preservatives as in salting or curing, and more recent innovations such as freeze-drying. Food technology also incorporates procedures such as blanching (short-term heating), extracting, fractionating (separating into fractions) and extruding (pushing through a small hole).

Advantages of Food Processing

Food processing helps prevent food from spoiling and packaging reduces losses from insects and rodents during storage. Food preservation prevents food from deteriorating quickly and seems essential in order to provide an adequate food supply throughout the year in all regions of America. Some processing procedures improve food safety: Adding preservatives and antioxidants to foods and pasteurizing beverages are examples. Canned goods must be heated rigorously to destroy all microorganisms, though this destroys some vitamins. Sometimes processing destroys antinutrient factors. As an example, heating soybeans and other beans destroys a trypsin inhibitor, a protein that blocks the action of a digestive enzyme. Processed foods may require less meal preparation time, an important consideration for anyone attempting to save time and effort.

CONVENIENCE FOODS are either partially or completely prepared before sale. They need not be low in nutrients if made primarily from basic ingredients. On the other hand, some convenience foods do not equate with home-prepared foods. Certain prepared dinners have been found to be low in THIAMIN, VITAMIN B$_6$ and VITAMIN E. Reheated frozen TV dinners tend to be low in folic acid. The concern among nutritionists is that American children may associate salty, sweet and high-fat foods with good taste and good diet.

Fabricated foods are either imitations or completely new food forms. TEXTURIZED VEGETABLE PROTEIN, fish protein (powder), modified STARCH, corn sweeteners, sodium CASEIN (milk protein), COCONUT OIL and PALM OIL are combined in a myriad of innovative ways to create foods ranging from non-dairy creamer, non-dairy imitation cheese, imitation whipped cream, imitation pecans, breakfast bars and a host of sweets and synthetic drinks. Some fabricated foods are designated "food analogs" designed to imitate a natural food. Meat analogs are made from extruded soy protein or other texturized vegetable protein. In animal feeding experiments engineered foods, which by chemical analysis seem nutritionally equivalent to conventional foods, may be inferior in some cases.

When a food is made to resemble a familiar or conventional food, the U.S. FDA requires that it be labeled "imitation" unless the food is nutritionally equivalent to the original in all respects except fat and caloric content. If the fabricated food contains as much vitamins, minerals and protein as the food it resembles, the food can be given a new descriptive name, though it need not contain real foods such as apples, blueberries or lemon. The term "formulated food" usually applies to food that is designed for a specific need; infant formulas are a well-known example. Such products find use in hospitals for total or supplemental feedings, such as liquid diet formulations.

Disadvantages of Food Processing

Most controversy has centered around highly refined or highly processed foods. Although some food processing methods improve nutritional quality, loss of some nutrients frequently occurs during processing. The degree and type of processing influences the extent of losses. Compare a baked potato with a fabricated potato chip, which has been cooked, mashed, dehydrated, rehydrated, mixed with additives, shaped and fried. The final product is a popular snack food low in nutrient density and high in fat and salt. Additives are commonplace in highly processed foods. Salt is usually used for added flavor, far in excess of the amount used in home cooking. Because consumers become accustomed to the taste of highly salted commercially prepared foods, they may come to view home cooking as bland.

Added sugar sweetens foods, making them more appealing to consumers' sweet tooths, and increases the ease of processing in some instances. The sugar content of commercially processed foods can be needlessly high. Popular dry BREAKFAST CEREALS can be 50% sugar; even canned fruit may be packed in syrup. Furthermore, a product can be high in refined sugar although the word "sugar" does not appear on the food label. Thus DEXTROSE, malto-dextrins, CORN SYRUP, corn syrup solids, high FRUCTOSE CORN SYRUP, HONEY, corn sweeteners and MOLASSES on a food label all indicate that refined sugar has been added to the food. Fat is added to create pleasant textures and taste in cookies, crisp snack foods like CHIPS and CRACKERS, muffins and even granola. The added fat is likely to be saturated or hydrogenated for stability and extended shelf life. (See also FOOD ADDITIVES; FOOD LABELING.)

food sensitivity (FOOD INTOLERANCE)   Any negative physiologic reaction to a food. Food sensitivity is the broadest category of responses to foods and includes both physiological and psychological causes. Food sensitivities include two broad categories: food intolerances, which do not involve the immune system, and food allergies, which reflect reactions of the immune system. Food sensitivities can cause a variety of symptoms such as abdominal pain and alternating diarrhea and constipation resembling IRRITABLE BOWEL SYNDROME. Typical examples include sensitivity to molds or to certain added chemicals in foods; the inability to digest foods; psychological disorders relating to food (such as bulimia and anorexia nervosa); and conditioned responses to food.

The following are considered common food sensitivities:

Lactose intolerance   The most common food intolerance is due to the inability to digest milk sugar (lactose). Though infants and young children produce the enzyme needed to degrade lactose, production declines in many adults, so that mild sugar in dairy products and processed foods can overwhelm the digestive tract. Colonic fermentation produces gas and diarrhea in many Asians, Afro-Americans and people of Mediterranean heritage.

MSG (monosodium glutamate) sensitivity (MSG related syndrome)   Some people react to large amounts of this flavor enhancer added to prepared foods in Chinese and Italian restaurant cooking. MSG related syndrome ("Chinese restaurant syndrome") may involve a burning sensation and chest pain. MSG is a component of hydrolyzed vegetable protein, also used as a flavor enhancer.

Sensitivity to red wine   Susceptible people can get headaches after drinking red, not white, wine. The cause is not clear; possibly tannins, complex pigments from grape skins, may trigger a reaction.

Sensitivities to artifical food coloring and preservatives

People who are sensitive to yellow #5 food coloring are often sensitive to aspirin. Some parents report that reducing these substances in the diet relieves symptoms associated with hyperactivity. Sulfites can trigger reactions in susceptible people. Sulfites are found in certain preserved foods like sauerkraut and dried fruit and wine.

Food allergies may cause a rapid response like asthma, hay fever, swelling and hives or they may cause delayed symptoms, like headache, diarrhea and fatigue. Some food allergies can be life-threatening when the food causes severe shock (anaphylactic shock). The most common foods that produce immediate reactions include eggs, milk, wheat, soybeans, seafood, nuts and peanuts (a legume, not a true nut).

The diagnosis of food sensitivities is the first step; this requires supportive evidence. There are several time-honored strategies to pinpoint cause and effect, including a complete medical history and food or diet diaries. A challenge test involves introducing a suspected food after avoiding it for several weeks and noting any subsequent reactions. Optimally, neither the patient nor the health care provider knows the identity of the challenge substance.

The skin test is a standard diagnostic procedure for non-food allergies. In this procedure minute amounts of suspected allergens are inserted beneath the skin to detect hypersensitivity. A weal and reddening at the application site is an indication of a probable allergy. A variety of laboratory tests are designed to assess specific antibody levels to specific substances in foods. (See also ALLERGY, FOOD; ANOREXIA.)

Young, Elispeth, et al., "A Population Study of Food Intolerance," *Lancet*, 343 (May 7, 1994), pp. 1127–30.

food spoilage   The decay or decomposition of food due to microbial metabolism. Bacteria and molds are always present on foods exposed to air. In an appropriate environment, with suitable temperature and moisture, they will begin to break down constituents in food. Refrigeration slows the process because microbial metabolism is based on chemical reactions that slow at lower temperatures. However, several species of yeasts and molds that can spoil food grow slowly at refrigerator temperatures, and will eventually decompose even refrigerated foods. Unlike bacterial contamination in foods, moldy food (like moldy bread and cheese) is visible. Organisms that cause FOOD POISONING generally cannot grow in the refrigerator; campylobacter (CAMPYLOBACTERIOSIS) is one important exception.

Spoiled or rotten food is usually obvious because it tastes and smells bad. On the other hand, organisms that cause food poisoning cannot be spotted so easily. Use safety precautions in handling and in storing food. Besides microbial attack, food can also be destroyed by insects, endogenous enzymes, spontaneous chemical reactions (such as reaction with oxygen), burning during excessive cooking, and physical changes brought about by freezing, heating and handling. (See also: BOTULISM; SALMONELLA.)

Food Stamp Program (Food Stamp Act of 1977 and Food Stamp Act of 1964)   A federal program designed to maintain health and to raise the level of nutrition of low-income households by enabling those households to buy nutritious food in greater variety and thus improve their diets. Administered by the Department of Agriculture in cooperation with county and state welfare agencies, the program is designed to increase a household's purchasing power. Food stamps are currently given free to families that are certified, as by Aid to Families with Dependent Children.

Specific regulations frequently change; however, in general, eligibility criteria specify limits for monthly net income and financial resources. A household receiving Aid to Families with Dependent Children assistance automatically qualifies for food stamps. Permanent residency is not required. Their net value depends upon the size and resources of the household. Stamps are used like money for buying food (except pet food); beverages (except alcoholic beverages); seeds and plants for growing food. The maximum allotment of stamps is equivalent to the U.S. Department of Agriculture's Thrifty Food Plan. This plan was developed by the Agricultural Research Service to provide adequate quantities of most nutrients, but not all, as a guide to making healthful food choices.

Consumer freedom of food choice means that consumers may purchase foods with low nutrient value. Thus, effectiveness of the program is restricted by the degree of nutrition education, which may be limited. Funding remains a continuing problem. As of March 1993, 27.4 million Americans used food stamps. (See also DIETARY GUIDELINES FOR AMERICANS.)

food toxins   Substances in foods that adversely affect health. Toxins can be classified as CARCINOGENS, pharmacologic agents and agents that block nutrient function.

Carcinogens are natural cancer-causing agents that may occur in the following:

1. moldy grains and nuts (AFLATOXIN)
2. barbequed meat (BENZOPYRENES)
3. CABBAGE (thiourea)
4. certain herbs (ALKALOIDS)
5. certain vegetables and processed meat products (NITRATE and NITRITES, which are converted to NITROSOAMINES)
6. fermentation products (ethyl carbamate) in pickled herring and sauerkraut.

Pharmacologic agents in foods affect organ function and/or cellular metabolism. They include:

1. Certain CHEESES. TYRAMINE affects the nervous system.
2. Nuts and pits—ALMOND, APPLE, APRICOT, cherry, peach, pear, and plum. These products contain cyanogenetic GLYCOSIDES, which release cyanide and block cellular respiration.
3. Mussels and CLAMS. After ingesting the dinoflagellate responsible for red tides, *Gonyaulox*, mussels and clams can cause muscle weakness and paralysis.
4. Certain cheeses, preserved meat and preserved fish. These products may contain nitrosoamines, which cause cancer and liver damage.

5. Legumes. These vegetables contain a family of proteins called hemagglutinins, which can rupture red blood cells and damage intestinal mucosa in susceptible people and slow growth. Cooking inactivates hemagglutinin.

6. Members of the brassica family (including cabbage, KALE, BRUSSELS SPROUTS, CAULIFLOWER, BROCCOLI, TURNIPS and RUTABAGA). These vegetables contain glucosinolates, which produce the inorganic ion thiocyanate. Thiocyanate can cause hyperplasia of the thyroid gland, GOITER, because it blocks iodine assimilation, required for thyroid hormone formation.

7. Certain fish. There are a variety of fish toxins that can poison the nervous system.

8. RHUBARB. An acid in rhubarb called OXALIC ACID binds CALCIUM, and in excess, oxalic acid can contribute to kidney stones.

9. Fungi. A variety of mycotoxins can damage the liver and affect the nervous system.

Certain materials or enzymes in foods interfere with nutrient assimilation or function, but are often inactivated by heating and cooking.

1. Beans and soybeans. Thorough cooking destroys a protein called trypsin inhibitor, which blocks protein digestion; hemagglutinin, which retards growth; and lipoxidase, an enzyme that destroys VITAMIN A.

2. Cottonseed oil. This oil contains sterculic acid, a fatty acid that interferes with reproduction in experimental animals when consumed in large amounts.

3. Fish and clams. Raw seafood contains varying amounts of thiaminase, an enzyme that breaks down the B vitamin THIAMIN.)

4. Milk. Milk contains LACTOSE (milk sugar), which can create diarrhea in individuals who cannot digest this carbohydrate.

5. Cereal grains contain varying amounts of PHYTIC ACID, a phosphate-containing acid that binds calcium and IRON.

6. Vegetables and fruit. Fresh produce contains variable amounts of an enzyme called ascorbic acid oxidase that destroys VITAMIN C when exposed to air.

7. Raw eggs. Raw egg white contains ovamucoid, a protein that blocks protein digestion, and AVIDIN, a protein that binds BIOTIN and blocks its absorption. (See also FOOD POISONING.)

food trends   See EATING PATTERNS.

food wrap   Film plastic wrap and shrink wrapping, used to wrap and package food. Plastic food wrap contains plasticizers that have caused tumors in mice. While their effect in humans are unknown, it is not advisable to wrap plastic around food that is to be cooked. Plasticizers are absorbed by fatty and oily foods, even with refrigeration. Thus fatty foods like cheese should be stored in containers rather than wrapped in plastic sheeting.

Components that leach out of packaging into foods are known as indirect additives. Moist foods, especially those containing alcohol, fat or acids favor migration of organic compounds into a food. The FDA monitors packaging that comes into contact with food, and manufacturers are required to obtain FDA approval for all materials used in food packaging. Migration of package components usually is not a problem if the food is dry. (See also MICROWAVE COOKING.)

formula   See INFANT FORMULA.

fortification   The addition of nutrients to food to increase their nutrient content to levels greater than found in unprocessed foods in the same class. Homogenized MILK is fortified with ERGOSTEROL and VITAMIN D, and fruit juices are sometimes fortified with VITAMIN C. Several juices also contain CALCIUM.

The U.S. FDA has proposed fortifying grain products with folic acid in order to protect women who may become pregnant. As little as 400 mcg of folic acid daily greatly reduces the risk of neural tube defects. Grain products—flour, rolls, beans, bread, corn grits, corn meal, rice and noodles—would be fortified with 140 mcg of folic acid per 3.5 oz serving. (See also ENRICHMENT.)

four food groups   See BASIC FOOD GROUPS.

frame size   An assessment of a person's bone size and musculature. Bone mass correlates with muscle mass, and larger-boned people generally have larger muscles. The breadth of the elbow bones is used as an index of frame sizes for insurance-derived HEIGHT-WEIGHT TABLES. These in turn are used to estimate an optimal body weight. The weight tables also employ heights based on one-inch heels and weights based on fully clothed. (See also DIETING; OBESITY.)

Framingham Study   An early U.S. study of factors associated with HEART DISEASE. This epidemiologic research (population study) was designed to estimate risk factors in the development of heart disease by studying 5,000 men and women, aged 32 to 60, living in Framingham, Massachusetts, between 1949 and 1969. Subjects enrolled in this study initially did not have signs of coronary heart disease. They were examined every two years for signs and symptoms of cardiovascular disease. The risk of heart disease was found to increase with the following:

1. Smoking. All other factors being equal, the risk of heart disease for smokers was 1.5 times higher than for nonsmokers.

2. Obesity. Individuals 20% or more heavier than "optimal" body weight had three times the risk of death due to heart attack.

3. Male gender. Other factors being equal, 45-year-old men were found to be three times more likely to develop heart disease as women.

4. Physical inactivity. Active persons had one-third to one-half the risk of heart attack or angina as sedentary individuals.

5. Elevated blood pressure. People with readings (systolic blood pressure) of 180 or higher were about twice as likely to have heart disease as those who had a systolic pressure of 120, other factors being the same.

6. High blood sugar levels (glucose intolerance). Having a blood sugar level of 120 or greater, or passing sugar in the urine, was associated with a greater risk of heart disease. Thus the risk of angina pectoris or sudden death for obese diabetics was 2.5 times as great as for obese nondiabetics.

7. Elevated blood CHOLESTEROL. This alone accounted for a modest increase in risk of heart disease; but when associated with other risk factors, elevated blood cholesterol increased the risk. (See also: AGING; DIETARY GUIDELINES FOR AMERICANS.)

frankfurter (weiner) A sausage made of BEEF, PORK or VEAL or a combination of these MEATS. Turkey frankfurters are also available. The meat, together with seasonings and nitrates, is placed in casings, then smoked, steamed and finally chilled. Frankfurters are a high-FAT, high-SODIUM food. Most of the fat is saturated. A beef and pork frankfurter provides 145 calories; protein, 5.1 g; carbohydrate, 1.1 g; fat, 13.1 g; iron, 0.52 mg; sodium 504 mg; zinc, 0.83 mg; niacin, 1.2 mg. It contains 23 mg of cholesterol. For comparison, a turkey frankfurter provides 102 calories: protein, 6.4 g; carbohydrate, 0.7 g; fat, 8.3 g; iron, 0.77 mg; sodium, 550 mg; zinc, 1.0 mg; niacin, 1.77 mg; and cholesterol, 44 mg. (See also CONVENIENCE FOOD; DIETARY GUIDELINES FOR AMERICANS; HOT DOG.)

free radicals Highly damaging molecules or ions that often contain oxygen. Free radicals possess a single electron; unlike stable molecules with pairs of electrons, these renegades attack innocent bystander molecules of the cell by removing an electron to make up for their own electron deficiency. Once they have been produced, free radicals can multiply via chain reactions, making them even more dangerous to the cell. Free radicals likely to be encountered in the body include superoxide, NITRIC OXIDE, hydroxyl radicals and lipid radicals (lipid peroxyl radicals). Certain activated forms of oxygen, including singlet oxygen, lipid peroxides and HYDROGEN PEROXIDE, can generate free radicals, though they are not radicals themselves.

Numerous health conditions are possibly linked to free radical damage: CANCER, ATHEROSCLEROSIS, HYPERTENSION (high blood pressure), ALZHEIMER'S DISEASE and SENILITY, weakened immune system, CATARACTS, lung disease, ARTHRITIS, emphysema, Parkinson's disease, and even AGING. Free radicals damage cells by attacking vulnerable sites, the most important being: DNA, the genetic blueprint; ENZYMES that catalyze the reactions for life, and lipids and proteins that make up cell membranes.

Sources of Free Radicals

Exposure to free radicals is unavoidable because the body uses oxygen to derive energy from burning fuel molecules. For example, as mitochondria, the cell's powerhouses, consume oxygen, they produce highly unstable forms of oxygen, including superoxide and hydroxyl radicals, when functioning under par. In addition, hydrogen peroxide, which can break down to form free radicals, is a normal byproduct of many types of cells containing peroxisomes, small bodies within cells that can degrade fatty acids and other substances.

Free radicals are also generated by defensive cells. Phagocytes, cells that engulf foreign invaders, destroy bacteria and virus-infected cells by bursts of toxic chemicals, including superoxide, NITRIC OXIDE (another radical) and hydrogen peroxide. Chronic infection and the ensuing inflammation can create prolonged oxidative stress on the body. Nitric oxide also functions in the body as a nerve chemical (neurotransmitter) and regulatory molecule.

Detoxifying enzymes like CYTOCHROME P450 in the liver, which is responsible for inactivating pollutants and toxic compounds, can yield byproducts that form free radicals. It is ironic that in making some molecules more easily excreted, the body's defense system can create more dangerous substances.

People who are prone to iron storage disease (HEMOCHROMATOSIS) or who consume excessive iron may increase their risk of free radical damage because reduced iron atoms can spontaneously react with oxygen to produce free radicals.

Environmental factors play a key role in free radical damage. Besides being produced by normal physiologic processes, free radicals are generated by ultraviolet light and ionizing radiation such as X-rays, radon and gamma rays. Some environmental pollutants like ozone and nitrogen oxides react within the body to form free radicals.

Consequences of Free Radical Attack

In view of the prevalance of free radicals, it is not surprising that cells experience free radical damage frequently. An estimated 10,000 damaging attacks are made on a cell's genes daily, though nearly all of this damage is normally repaired by enzymes. However, free radicals can damage and inactivate repair enzymes over time. Cumulative damage to repair enzymes can slow the DNA repair so that DNA damage increases with age, as does the risk of mutations and cancer. Besides DNA and protein, lipids can be targets. Free radical attack on polyunsaturated FATTY ACIDS yields oxidixed lipids (lipid peroxides) that can break down to free radicals and toxic fragments.

Materials outside of cells can also be injured by free radicals. LDL (LOW-DENSITY LIPOPROTEIN), which transports CHOLESTEROL to tissues via the bloodstream, is another free radical target. Oxidized LDL is implicated in the development of plaque formation in arteries (atherosclerosis). According to the free radical theory of aging, the body possesses a powerful collection of antioxidant defenses; however, some free radicals inevitably escape and are able to attack cells. Over time the body's defensive mechanisms reach the point at which cellular repair can no longer keep up with oxidative damage and damaged proteins, lipids and DNA accumulate. Ultimately a point is reached at which cells are impaired and consequently organ function declines. Eventually the body's ability to ward off cancer and to maintain itself is compromised.

Antioxidants

Antioxidants are substances that can block the oxidation of target molecules in the cell. Antioxidants can either quench free radicals ("chain breakers") or they can block the initiation of free radical attack ("preventive inhibitors"). Chain breakers include VITAMIN E and VITAMIN C. Preventive inhibitors include defensive enzymes, such as CATALASE, SUPEROXIDE DISMUTASE and GLUTATHIONE PEROXIDASE. Trace mineral nutrients function as antioxidants when they function as cofactors of enzymes. COPPER, MANGANESE and ZINC are cofactors for the enzyme superoxide dismutase, which inactivates superoxide. SELENIUM is a cofactor for glutathione peroxidase, an enzyme that converts peroxides to safe intermediates, while catalase degrades hydrogen peroxide to water and oxygen.

Glutathione, the sulfur-containing antioxidant of the cytoplasm and beta carotene quench active forms of oxygen or bind metal catalysts that could otherwise produce free radicals. These antioxidants complement each other: Vitamin C is a powerful, water soluble antioxidant, while beta carotene and vitamin E are fat-soluble free radical traps. The increased consumption of polyunsaturated vegetable oils increases the requirement for vitamin E. Plant substances called FLAVONOIDS also can act as powerful antioxidants. The long-term health benefits of eating adequate fruits and vegetables is due in part to these important substances.

Much previous research indicates that the consumption of ample amounts of fruits and vegetables helps prevent disease. These foods contain multiple antioxidants including hundreds of carotenoids in addition to beta carotene. Combinations of free radical quenchers as found in foods, rather than a single antioxidant, will best prevent free radical damage in the body. Investigators hypothesize that boosting protection against free radical damage by dietary antioxidants may help people live longer. For example, vitamin E or vitamin E with carotenoids seem to help prevent cancer or heart disease.

Thomas, M.J., "The Role of Free Radicals and Antioxidants: How Do We Know That They Are Working?" *Critical Reviews in Food Science and Nutrition*, 35:1,2, 1995, pp. 21–39.

french fries (french fried potatoes)   A high-fat food and common FAST-FOOD menu item. To make french fries, potatoes are usually sliced into strips and fried. Fast-food french fries are precooked at the factory, then refried immediately before purchase. More fast-food restaurants are using vegetable oil, to avoid cholesterol, rather than lard or beef tallow for frying. Nonetheless, fried potatoes absorb FAT: French fries provide about 50% of their calories as fat. Any food providing more than 30% of its calories as fat can be considered a fatty food. A further problem is the fact that the hydrogenated vegetable oil that is commonly used is more saturated then untreated oils, and contains modified fats called *trans* fats. As a result, french fries may contain as much artery-clogging fat as potatoes fried in beef tallow. A plain baked potato (202 g) contains 220 calories; plus fat, 0.2 g; vitamin C, 26 mg; and sodium, 16 mg. An equivalent amount of french fries (200 g cooked in vegetable oil) provides almost three times as many calories: 632 calories; fat, 33.2 g; sodium, 432 mg; and vitamin C, 20 mg (See also CONVENIENCE FOOD; FRIED FOOD.)

freshness   Product freshness refers to the degree of chemical change in a food due to breakdown by enzymes and chemical processes within the food itself. Oxidation, change in color and texture or flavor of a food, and loss of nutrients like VITAMIN C are possible consequences. In contrast, spoilage represents the action of molds, fungi, yeasts and bacteria growing on the food. (See also FOOD ADDITIVES; FOOD SPOILAGE.)

fried food   Food that has been cooked in fat or oil. Fried foods are both high-FAT and high-CALORIE because of the absorption of cooking fat or oils. Foods cooked with a batter or breading also absorb high levels of fat. This is a concern for two reasons: Excessive fat is linked to an increased risk of clogged arteries (atherosclerosis) and cancer, and a surplus

of calories is a major contributor to OBESITY in the United States. Dietary fat is one of the largest contributors to obesity and to cancer (after cigarette smoking). According to DIETARY GUIDELINES FOR AMERICANS, fat should account for no more than 30% of daily calories.

POLYUNSATURATED VEGETABLE OILS like safflower, corn, sunflower and soybean oil are often used in frying. High temperatures convert these oils to potentially harmful products. Their oxidation products (peroxides and epoxides) yield free radicals and reactive compounds called aldehydes that can damage the LIVER, slow growth and cause chromosomal damage in lab animals. There is less of an oxidation problem in cooking with fresh oil at medium temperatures. However, there is no guarantee that the fried food eaten in restaurants has not been overheated.

It is generally recommended that consumption of fried foods be reduced. Many more healthful options exist, including baked or broiled foods. (See also CHICKEN; CONVENIENCE FOOD, DIETING; EATING PATTERNS; FAST FOOD.)

frozen desserts, fat-free   Frozen desserts made without milk FAT or cream. Several fat-free options are now available that contain no cream and no CHOLESTEROL. Frozen non-fat yogurts, sorbets, sherbets and fruit bars fall into this category. They may contain FRUCTOSE or polydextrose (derived from cornstarch) as sweeteners, cellulose gel and gums as thickeners, non-fat milk or whey and flavors. Calories range from 50 to 90 per half-cup serving and there may be only 1 g of fat. Such desserts are more healthful than standard ice cream, which contains 150 calories and 8 g of fat. Fat substitutes are now being marketed in frozen desserts.

Non-butterfat frozen desserts can be useful in lowering daily fat intake. DIETARY GUIDELINES FOR AMERICANS recommends reducing daily fat consumption to less than 30% of total calories. Cholesterol intake should be reduced to the equivalent of no more than four egg yolks per week. Nonetheless, low-fat, low-cholesterol desserts should not take the place of whole foods like grains, vegetables and fruits. In terms of weight control, there is no substitute for exercise and good eating habits. (See also DAIRY-FREE FROZEN DESSERTS; OBESITY.)

frozen entrees   CONVENIENCE FOODS that often provide excessive CALORIES, FAT and SODIUM. Gourmet and "lite" varieties are increasingly being marketed. To reduce the consumption of fat, food additives and calories from frozen entrees:

1. Read labels. Look for "light, low fat" designations on food labels. As a guideline, eat less than 10 g of fat per meal. If the CALCIUM, VITAMIN and FIBER contents are low, the food is probably processed and contains more fat. Eat fewer foods in which fat contributes more than 30% of the calories. This is the limit recommended in DIETARY GUIDELINES FOR AMERICANS for overall fat consumption.
2. Avoid SULFITE. This preservative is often added to seafood entrees, sauerkraut and other canned vegetables and dried fruit. Sulfite can cause strong reactions in sensitive people.
3. Avoid MONOSODIUM GLUTAMATE (MSG) and its cousin, HYDROLYZED VEGETABLE PROTEIN, which are flavor enhancers. These additives can cause reactions in sensitive people, including migraines and mood swings.

4. Be aware that SURIMI is artificial shellfish. If the food label lists pollack and other fish, ARTIFICIAL FOOD COLORS and other food additives, surimi and not real shellfish is being offered.

5. Notice the sodium content of frozen entrees. Americans consume two to five times more sodium than needed. The maximum recommended sodium intake is 3,000 mg per day. A single frozen dinner may easily supply this much. (See also MSG RELATED SYNDROME; OBESITY.)

fructose (fruit sugar, levulose)   A simple sugar found in HONEY and FRUIT, especially dried fruit. Fructose is three times sweeter than table sugar (SUCROSE). Typically fructose accounts for 10% of the daily CALORIES for the U.S. population; much of it comes from sucrose, which is half fructose. As a refined CARBOHYDRATE, fructose is increasingly used as a FOOD ADDITIVE. In the form of high FRUCTOSE CORN SYRUP, processed from cornstarch, it is added to almost all soft drinks in place of table sugar, and consumption has increased 250% over the last 15 years.

Fructose has been recommended as a sweetener for diabetics because it is slowly converted to BLOOD SUGAR. Consequently, the requirement for insulin, the hormone that increases blood glucose uptake by tissues, is lowered, as compared to an equivalent amount of table sugar. However, if DIABETES isn't controlled, fructose can eventually lead to excessively high blood sugar in susceptible people.

It is estimated that a fructose intake twice the average consumption can increase blood fat (TRIGLYCERIDES), blood CHOLESTEROL and URIC ACID in 10 to 15% of adults with elevated blood fat (triglycerides) and insulin levels. Diets high in fructose and low in copper and magnesium also increase blood lipids and increase the risk of heart disease. There is a risk of CATARACTS and kidney stones in susceptible individuals with long-term high consumption of fructose. High consumption of any kind of sugar depletes the body of CHROMIUM, required with insulin to stimulate cells to absorb and metabolize blood sugar. In individuals with elevated blood insulin and blood sugar, as in a prediabetic condition, excessive fructose consumption can aggravate a chromium deficiency. (See also GLYCEMIC INDEX; NATURAL SWEETENERS.)

Riby, J.E., et al., "Fructose Absorption," *America's Journal of Clinical Nutrition*, 58:5 (Supp) (1993), pp. 748S–53S.

fructose corn syrup (high fructose corn syrup, HFCS)   A major food additive that often replaces table sugar (SUCROSE). It is prepared from CORN SYRUP, which consists mainly of GLUCOSE, by enzymatic treatment. Fructose corn syrup contains 40 to 90% FRUCTOSE. Fructose corn syrup is sweeter than table sugar, so less needs to be added to achieve the equivalent level of sweetness.

While table sugar consumption has declined in recent years, high fructose and fructose corn syrup consumption has more than made up the difference. Thus the total sweetener consumption rose from 118 pounds per person in 1975 to the current annual consumption of about 150 pounds. This is equivalent to eating a cup of sugar daily. On the average, soft drinks represent 65% of fructose corn syrup consumption. It is used in cranberry juice and sauces, fruit sherbet and ice cream, jellies and jams, catsup, MAYONNAISE, spaghetti sauce, sweet pickles, cookies, syrup, bread, peanut butter and wine coolers.

There is a risk of cataracts and kidney stones with long-term use of fructose in susceptible individuals. Large amounts of dietary fructose can increase blood lipids and may increase the risk of HEART DISEASE. (See also DIETARY GUIDELINES FOR AMERICAN; EATING PATTERNS; FOOD ADDITIVES; NATURAL SWEETENERS; TEETH.)

fruit   The pulpy tissue associated with seeds. In botany, the ovary of a plant; according to this definition, EGGPLANT, CUCUMBERS and PUMPKINS are fruits. However, the USDA prefers to define a fruit as a plant food if it is usually eaten as a DESSERT or as a snack between meals, or accompanies breakfast, rather than being a main course of a meal.

Fruits are often classified into the following groups:

- Aggregate fruits consist of many tiny seed-bearing fruits combined in one mass and developed from many ovaries. Strawberries, BLACKBERRIES and RASPBERRIES are examples.
- Berries are fruits from a single ovary but they may contain more than one seed. GRAPES and persimmons belong to this group. According to this classification, BANANA is a berry that has lost the ability to form seeds.
- Drupes are fruits that contain a single seed fruit that develops entirely from a single ovary. CHERRY and PEACH are examples.
- Hesperidium refers to CITRUS FRUITS; they contain a many-seeded, multisectioned fruit enclosed by a tough skin. LEMONS and ORANGES are typical.
- In multiple fruits, ovaries and receptacles derived from a common base become the fruit. PINEAPPLE and FIGS belong to this category.
- False berries are represented by BLUEBERRIES and CRANBERRIES. These fruits are the result of a fusion of an ovary and a receptacle.
- Pomes are represented by APPLES and PEARS. This many-seeded fruit results from the fusion of an ovary and receptacle.

Worldwide, the leading fruit crops are: grapes, bananas and plantains (varieties used before ripening), citrus fruits (oranges, tangerines, lemons, limes, grapefruit and pomelos), followed by apples, melons and mangos. In the United States citrus fruits, grapes and apples are the leading fruit crops. Citrus fruit production is limited primarily to California, Texas and Florida. Because of domestication, many fruit-bearing plants have been altered so extensively that they cannot be grown without human propagation. Fruit production has increased steadily this century because of increased popularity in most countries and the expansion of food processing, which allows fruits to be eaten year-round. In recent years much of the increased consumption in the United States has been in processed fruit, rather than fresh fruit.

Fruits are generally rich sources of VITAMIN C, POTASSIUM, soluble and insoluble FIBER, FLAVONOIDS (plant antioxidants) and simple SUGAR. The most common sugars in fruits are GLUCOSE and FRUCTOSE: The sugar content varies from 6 to 20%. Bananas and figs are among the highest in sugar content. The net caloric content is also a function of processing, because canned fruit is often packed in syrup, which adds extra calories.

Fruit Juice

Common beverages are prepared from fruits such as oranges, grapes, apples or more exotic fruits like guavas or papayas. Fresh fruit juices are excellent sources of vitamin C and potassium. Their caloric content is derived almost exclusively from simple sugars. The vitamin C content may have been depleted in the processing of commercially available juices.

The amount of fruit juice actually put into a juice drink varies, and the U.S. FDA does not require manufacturers to specify how diluted a juice drink is. If the product label specifies "juice" only, the product contains pure fruit juice. If the label says anything else, for example, juice drink, juice cocktail, juice blend or fruit punch, the product is diluted juice. Cranberry "cocktail" is less than one-third cranberry juice. In 1994 federal regulators estimated that 10% of all fruit juice sold in the United States had been adulterated, most often by adding sugar or orange byproducts. Young children drink large quantities of fruit juices, such as apple juice, and this may displace higher calorie, more nutrient-rich foods in their diet, causing malnutrition, diarrhea and tooth decay.

Fruit, Dried

Most commonly apples, APRICOTS, DATES, figs, NECTARINES, peaches, PLUMS, prunes and seedless grapes are commercially dried in the United States. When the water content of a fruit is reduced to about 24% from about 90%, spoilage is reduced. Sulfuring or sulfiting agents, which are used as preservatives in the drying process, can destroy thiamin. Dried fruit is a rich source of fructose, glucose, fiber, iron and potassium. Raw or stewed dried fruit can help with bowel regularity. (See also BALANCED DIET; DEHYDRATION; EXERCISE; PECTIN.)

fruitarian A VEGETARIAN whose diet relies primarily on fruits. (See also LACTO-OVO-VEGETARIAN.)

fruit leather A snack food prepared from fruit pulp and dried as a thin sheet. Fruit leathers are not as nutritious as fresh fruit because they contain lower amounts of vitamins. However, they have less fat and less added sugar than candy. Fruit leathers often contain added sweeteners. (See also CANDY; SULFITES.)

fruit sugar See FRUCTOSE.

fumaric acid An additive used to provide tartness in foods and beverages. Fumaric acid finds use in gelatin desserts, puddings, pie fillings, candy and powdered soft drinks. It is also used as an acidic ingredient in LEAVENING AGENTS (agents used to make dough rise). Fumaric acid is recognized as a safe additive. It is an intermediate of the KREB'S CYCLE, the central energy-producing pathway of metabolism, hence is readily broken down. (See also FOOD ADDITIVES.)

fumigants Gaseous PESTICIDES. A typical example of a fumigant is methyl bromide, a post-harvest fumigant used to control insects in stored GRAINS, nuts, fruits and vegetables. Methyl bromide is also used for macadamia nuts, BROAD (fava) BEANS, SWEET POTATOES and other root crops, kiwi fruit, cereal, FLOUR, spices, LENTILS and leafy vegetables. Direct exposure to this chemical by workers causes toxicity.

functional foods (foods for specific health use) Foods or food ingredients that have been modified so that they provide health benefits above and beyond the levels they traditionally contain. The food can benefit physical performance, overall health and mental well-being in addition to its ability to supply given nutrients. A functional food can be part of a daily diet, and it can enhance specific body functions, such as enhancing the immune system in the prevention of disease, or it can aid in the recovery of a disease. Examples include protein-enriched sports drinks with collagen, soft drinks with fiber and iron, calcium-rich beverages, tea fortified with calcium, bread with soluble fiber, cereals with bran, iron-fortified candy, candy with fructooligosaccharides, sausage with fiber and milk and yogurt with lactobacillus species and bifidobacteria. The judicious use of such foods in the diet could provide a more individualized program tailored to meet specific needs. (See also BIOCHEMICAL INDIVIDUALITY; GENETIC ENGINEERING.)

fungicides PESTICIDES used to prevent molds from developing in produce during shipping and storage. Most fungicides have been shown to cause cancer in experimental animals. A typical example is CAPTAN, used on FRUITS such as APPLES, PEACHES and STRAWBERRIES, and on VEGETABLES such as CORN, GARLIC, CABBAGE, LETTUCE, CARROTS, BEETS, PEAS, BEANS, KALE and SPINACH. Captan is sometimes used in packing boxes for post-harvest treatment. Captan has been found in oils and shortening because it is fat-soluble. This fungicide can cause cancer in experimental animals and is toxic to fish, birds and bees. Chlorothalonil (Bravo), a fungicide used on vegetables, including beans, TOMATOES, ONIONS, BROCCOLI, cabbage, CUCUMBER, lettuce, and on fruit, including watermelon and CANTALOUPE, causes tumor in rats and mice. A family of fungicides called EBDs (Maneb, Mancozeb and Metiran) is now permitted by the EPA on 43 crops including apples, corn, tomatoes, potatoes, cucumbers and onions because it is now believed to cause only a minor cancer risk (one additional cancer patient per million people over a lifetime). (See also CARCINOGENS; DELANEY CLAUSE.)

fungus A member of a broad division of plants lacking the green photosynthetic pigment chlorophyll. Molds, yeasts and MUSHROOMS belong to this plant family. Fungi degrade dead organic materials or living tissue for nutrients. Molds, mushrooms and yeast belong to this class of plants. Edible mushrooms and molds employed in the maturation of CHEESE are useful fungi. Yeasts (ascomycetes) are employed in FERMENTATION for WINE and BEER production. Several antibiotics are fungal products. As pathogens, fungi can cause ringworm, athlete's foot and thrush (mycotic infections). Several species of fungi produce toxic agents (mycotoxins). (See also AFLATOXIN; ASPERGILLUS; CANDIDA ALBICANS.)

furcelleran A natural GUM obtained from seaweed. Furcelleran resembles CARRAGEENAN, also obtained from a seaweed. It is used occasionally as a FOOD ADDITIVE to thicken processed foods and to help puddings gel. Its long-term safety has not been carefully examined.

galactose A simple SUGAR found in the diet in milk sugar (lactose). Galactose is a six-carbon sugar as is the more common GLUCOSE (BLOOD SUGAR). Unlike glucose, however, it does not occur by itself in foods. DIGESTION (hydrolysis) of lactose by the intestinal enzyme LACTASE yields equal amounts of galactose and glucose. Before galactose can be utilized by the body for energy, it must first be transformed into glucose by the LIVER. Certain people have a genetic susceptibility to galactose accumulation. Galactose is a building block of carbohydrate chains associated with carbohydrate-containing lipids (glycolipids) and proteins (GLYCOPROTEINS). (See also CARBOHYDRATE METABOLISM; GALACTOSEMIA.)

galactosemia A rare genetic disease due to an inability to degrade the sugar GALACTOSE normally. The most common defect is the inability to convert galactose to GLUCOSE, an essential preliminary step for galactose to be used for energy production. Because galactose cannot be extensively degraded when the path to glucose is blocked, it accumulates in the blood of galactosemic patients. This leads to severe mental retardation unless special galactose-free (milk-free) diets are administered shortly after birth. The prevalence of galactosemia is about one in 50,000. (See also CARBOHYDRATE METABOLISM.)

gallbladder A dark-green organ that concentrates and stores BILE from the LIVER. Bile is a mixture of powerful emulsifiers needed to digest and absorb FAT and oils and fat-soluble vitamins. When the INTESTINE detects food and fat released by the stomach, the intestine releases the hormone CHOLECYSTOKININ into the bloodstream, which causes the gallbladder to release bile into the DUODENUM, the upper section of the small intestine. (See also DIGESTIVE TRACT.)

gallstones (cholelithiasis) Gravel-like deposits in the gallbladder in which BILE is stored. The gallbladder releases bile during meals to aid fat digestion and absorption. Many people consuming Western diets develop gallstones. The causes of gallstone formation are unknown. Risk factors include high-fat, low-fiber diets, female gender, obesity, aging, CROHN'S DISEASE, cystic fibrosis and alcoholic cirrhosis of the liver.

The more refined and processed the foods in the diet, the greater the risk of developing gallstones. High-fiber diets may increase bile flow, thus preventing stone formation. For example, pre-1950s northern Canadian Inuit populations consuming a traditional diet had no record of gallstones. As a Western diet became more popular, the incidence of gallbladder disease shot up.

Food allergies are also a contributing factor, especially allergies to egg, pork and onion. Hypochlorhydria (low stomach acid) may underlie maldigestion and food allergies, thus contributing to symptoms such as abdominal pain, bloating and gas.

The composition of gallstones ranges from almost pure CHOLESTEROL to mixtures of bile salts, cholesterol, calcium carbonate and BILE PIGMENT (bilirubin). In the United States most stones are of the mixed variety. Frequently, stones are small enough to pass through the duct leading to the intestine. Other stones often remain in the gallbladder without causing discomfort. When large stones become lodged in the common bile duct, a painful gallbladder attack ensues (choledocholithiasis).

It is clear that materials normally dissolved in bile create stones, and that stone formation begins with bile saturation. Bile contains cholesterol emulsified by bile salts and LECITHIN for digestion. Cholesterol will precipitate when there is a decrease in bile acids, water or lecithin content in bile. For example, less bile salt is made with AGING, making cholesterol more insoluble.

Paumgartner, G. and Sauerbruch, T., "Gallstones: Pathogenesis," *Lancet*, 338 (November 2, 1991), pp. 1117–24.

gamma globulins (serum antibodies, immunoglobulins) A family of specialized proteins (antibodies) that are the first line of defense against foreign invaders like bacteria and viruses in the bloodstream. Unlike most serum proteins that are made by the LIVER, gamma globulins are products of B cells and related plasma cells of the IMMUNE SYSTEM. Most antibodies in the blood belong to the IgG class. Together with circulating white blood cells, they constitute "humoral immunity." Gamma globulin shots temporarily boost immunity for protection against diseases such as HEPATITIS. (See also ALLERGEN; ALLERGY, FOOD; ANTIBODIES.)

gamma hydroxybutyric acid A compound that has been promoted by some body builders as a muscle-enhancing agent. It occurs naturally in the central nervous system, and it has been used as a general anesthetic and hypnotic or tranquilizing substance. However, gamma hydroxybutyric acid has caused comas and convulsions in susceptible individuals, and the U.S. FDA has warned consumers against its use because of possible serious adverse side effects.

gamma linolenic acid (GLA) A polyunsaturated FATTY ACID found in seed oils such as borage, evening primrose and blackcurrant. GLA is the raw material for a family of PROSTAGLANDINS, hormone-like lipids that regulate many physiologic processes. GLA forms the PGE$_1$ class of prostaglandins that counterbalance the effects of other prostaglandins (PGE$_2$) by decreasing inflammation, expanding blood vessels (vasodilation), lowering blood pressure and reducing the tendency to form blood clots. This may be the basis for the observation that GLA may help reduce pain associated with rheumatoid arthritis.

GLA is derived from LINOLEIC ACID, the ESSENTIAL FATTY ACID, and belongs to the omega-6 family of fatty acids. GLA possesses 18 carbons. Its three double bonds are located at different points along the chain. The structure of GLA differs from ALPHA LINOLENIC ACID, an omega-3 essential fatty acid. Therefore GLA and alpha linolenic acid are not interchangeable and serve different functions in the body.

Specific nutrients NIACIN, VITAMIN B$_6$, VITAMIN C and ZINC participate in the formation of PGE$_1$. The ability to produce GLA from linoleic acid seems to diminish with age, diabetes, high alcohol consumption and high blood CHOLESTEROL. Therefore supplementation may be helpful in certain situations. GLA is one of the polyunsaturated fatty acids of

BREAST MILK, suggestive of its importance in development and growth.

garbage Waste materials derived from meal preparation and uneaten meals. The FDA estimates that Americans discard about 15% of the food they purchase each year. Ten percent of purchased food never reaches the plate because of spoilage. Garbage disposal is becoming a more critical regional issue as landfill sites fill up.

Recycling is a cheaper alternative than landfills and makes environmental sense. Recycling garbage need not take much time. These important steps can fit into most busy schedules:

1. Use aluminum beverage containers sparingly. Aluminum is much more expensive to produce than glass or cardboard. Squash soft drink cans and store them to bring to a recycling center.
2. Buy paper, glass and cardboard food packaging and recycle those items. Minimize buying plastic and styrofoam food containers. Most cities have programs that recycle #1 and #2 class plastics.
3. Buy bulk food items to reduce packaging expenses; reuse shopping bags.
4. Start a vegetable garden. Even small-scale patio or balcony gardens can be very productive. Compost vegetable garbage (not animal wastes) to recycle mineral nutrients and replace the need for chemical fertilizers.

garlic (*Allium sativum*) This bulbous plant is closely related to ONIONS, leeks and chives. The ancestor of modern garlic grows in Central Asia, and garlic has been cultivated for at least 5,000 years. The underground compound bulb is made up of cloves or sections. Garlic is strong-scented and strong-flavored, and has many culinary applications. Most of the garlic produced in the United States comes from California. Much of the commercially grown garlic is processed to garlic powder.

The healing power of garlic is recognized through Chinese folk traditions dating back thousands of years. Research has shown that garlic can lower blood CHOLESTEROL, especially the undesirable fraction of serum cholesterol (LDL [LOW-DENSITY LIPOPROTEIN]) and serum fat in animals and humans. Eating half a clove of garlic a day may lower blood cholesterol by 9%. Garlic reduces the tendency to form blood clots, though the conjecture that garlic decreases the risk of CARDIOVASCULAR DISEASE has been challenged. The suggestion has also been made that eating garlic and onions on a regular basis may lower the risk of stomach CANCER because materials isolated from garlic inhibit cancer production in experimental animals. Garlic can prevent dietary nitrites, used as a preservative in processed meat, from forming nitrosoamines, which can cause cancer, or can block their action. Garlic boosts the IMMUNE SYSTEM by increasing natural killer cells and phagocytic activity of white cells, and this may explain its anticancer activity.

Garlic contains 0.4% volatile oil containing a variety of unusual organo-sulfur compounds, believed to be responsible for most of the pharmacologic and antimicrobial actions. "Allylsulfides" increase the production of so-called "phase 2" liver detoxification enzymes (glutathione transferases) that increase the water solubility of cancer-causing compounds and toxins, speeding their excretion. Diallylsulfide may protect against lung cancer. Other compounds in garlic seem to limit tumor cell growth. However, garlic yields different active ingredients depending on the way it is prepared. Garlic juice possesses antibacterial activity, antifungal activity and antiviral activity. "Allicin" causes the pungent odor of raw garlic and seems to be partly responsible for antimicrobial activity.

Garlic has been reported to lower blood pressure in experimental animals and in humans and to inhibit blood platelet clumping, a necessary step in clot formation in vessels. Garlic reduces inflammation by blocking the formation of agents that induce it, including PROSTAGLANDINS, thromboxanes and LEUKOTRIENES. Steam distillation of garlic juice produces a sulfur product called ajoene, which inhibits a prostaglandin, PGE_2, which induces pain. Garlic sauteed in oil produces still other sulfur compounds, vinyldithiins, which are bronchial relaxers (they open air passageways in the lungs).

Garlic supplements have yielded mixed results. Though odoriferous, fresh garlic seems to be generally more effective than garlic powders and oils. Certain products carefully prepared from freeze-dried garlic appear to be effective. Garlic usually does not cause side effects, but in sensitive people garlic can cause allergic symptoms. Gastrointestinal upsets can be diminished by mixing crushed fresh garlic in oil and mixing this with food.

Fogarty, M., "Garlic's Potential Role in Reducing Heart Disease," *British Journal of Clinical Practice*, 47:2 (March/April 1993) pp. 64–65.

gas   See FLATULENCE.

gastric acid   See STOMACH ACID.

gastric bubble   A severe treatment for OBESITY that decreases the capacity of the stomach by inflating a plastic balloon in the stomach. The original intention was that the stomach would always feel full, so APPETITE would thus be curbed. About 17,000 patients have received gastric bubbles. About 75% of the patients lose 2 pounds per week, the same as with a well-balanced, calorie-restricted diet plan. The other 25% did not lose weight; some even gained weight.

The bubble is not a solution for rapid weight loss; and, without changing eating patterns and diet, it is not likely the effects will be permanent. The inventors of the bubble stress the need for nutrition counseling and behavior modification. Gastric bubbles increase the risk of ULCERS and intestinal blockage; it is now recommended that the gastric bubble be used for three months at most and only for patients who are 100 pounds overweight. (See also ADIPOSE TISSUE; DIETING.)

gastric juice   Secretions from glands lining the stomach. Up to 700 ml of gastric juice are secreted daily. Different types of secretory cells produce gastric juice. "Chief cells" produce pepsinogen, the inactive form of the stomach's protein-digesting enzyme, PEPSIN. "Parietal cells" produce hydrochloric acid (STOMACH ACID). This very strong acid creates a pH of 1.2 to 3.0, equivalent to 10 to 50 ml of dilute hydrochloric acid. The acid unfolds food PROTEINS, making them more accessible to attack by digestive enzymes. To further aid digestion, acid activates pepsin to initiate protein DIGESTION. The strong acid also helps sterilize ingested food and destroy bacterial toxins.

Gastric juice contains a LIPASE or fat-degrading enzyme that when secreted can liberate BUTYRIC ACID from BUTTERFAT; as well as INTRINSIC FACTOR, a protein that binds vitamin B_{12} and aids vitamin B_{12} absorption by the small intestine. Chloride in gastric juice is efficiently absorbed by the intestine and is recycled. (See also ACHLORHYDRIA.)

gastric ulcer (peptic ulcer)   An open sore in the lining of the stomach. Two major forms of ulcers are duodenal ulcer (in the upper region of the small intestine) and gastric or stomach ulcer. Gastric ulcers are somewhat less common. Most patients with gastric ulcers report abdominal discomfort about an hour after a meal, or during the night. Acid secretion is normal or reduced, rather than excessive. Eating or using ANTACIDS relieves the pain.

There are several causes of gastric ulcer. ASPIRIN, phenylbutazone, indomethacin and other non-steroidal anti-inflammatory agents can cause stomach bleeding and ulcer formation. ALCOHOL, smoking and COFFEE (whether decaffeinated or not) decrease tissue resistance and may play a causative role. ACHLORHYDRIA (the absence of stomach acid) is associated with gastric ulcers. Heredity is a factor. The bacterium HELICOBACTER PYLORI (*H. pylori*) is associated with chronic gastric inflammation and ulcers. High levels of antibodies against *H. pylori* can often be detected in the blood of gastric ulcer patients, and long-term eradication of *H. pylori* often clears up stomach ulcers and inflammation and prevents ulcer recurrence. Ulcer patients have a tendency to suppress emotions. Whether stress is involved in the development of ulcers is controversial.

Conventional medical treatment involves the use of drugs that block stomach acid secretion (cimetidine, ranitidine) or agents that coat ulcers and bowel. Cimetidine (Tagamet) is the second most commonly prescribed drug in the United States. Food sensitivities are implicated in experimental and clinical studies of gastric ulcer, and ELIMINATION DIETS have been used in preventing recurrent ulcers. Calcium carbonate antacids should not be used for gastric ulcer because they trigger excessive stomach acid secretion later (rebound effect). In botanical medicine, a liquorice extract called deglycyrrhizinated liquorice has been used as an anti-ulcer agent, shown to be as effective as cimetidine and ranitidine. Eradication of *H. pylori* requires treatment with antibiotics and bismuth compounds. (See also ACID INDIGESTION.)

Loguercio C. et al., "Glutathione Prevents Ethanol Induced Gastric Mucosal Damage and Depletion of Sulfhydryl Compounds in Humans," *Gut*, 34:2 (1993), pp. 161–65.

gastrin   A hormone formed by pyloric glands in the lower region of the stomach. In response to food, gastrin is released into the bloodstream where it stimulates the secretion of stomach acid by specific cells in the stomach lining called parietal cells. Gastrin also stimulates intestinal peristalsis. (See also DIGESTION.)

gastritis Any inflammation of the stomach lining. Gastritis may be accompanied by nausea and vomiting, or by a sense of fullness after eating a small meal. Gastritis is one of the most common stomach ailments and it increases the risk of stomach cancer. A variety of factors have been implicated as causative agents. Excessive consumption of ALCOHOL, rich food, COFFEE and tea, and other irritating foods can result in this condition.

Among the most common causes of gastritis is ASPIRIN, which may cause stomach bleeding. Other drugs can cause acute symptoms: sulfonamide, certain antibiotics, and quinine. Viral and bacterial infections may be involved. Pernicious ANEMIA (due to vitamin B_{12} deficiency), gastric ulcer and polyps, diabetes and adrenal insufficiency often accompany chronic gastritis. Symptoms are intermittent and variable. They include loss of appetite, mild nausea, a feeling of fullness or abdominal pain, recurrent heartburn or pain in the upper abdominal region, and vomiting. Eliminating the offending irritant and avoiding alcohol, caffeine, smoking and foods that provoke a response may help reduce pain. Symptoms may be relieved by medications (such as cimetidine) that coat the lesions or reduce acid production. Deglycyrrhizinoted licorice has been used to help heal peptic ulcers.

Recurrent, chronic gastritis can indicate an underlying problem. For example, food allergies can cause gastric inflammation and other gastrointestinal symptoms. The bacterium HELICOBACTER PYLORI is frequently associated with chronic stomach inflammation. Elimination of infection by antibiotics and bismuth compound treatments can eliminate recurrent episodes. (See also ACID INDIGESTION.)

Fay, M., Fennerty, M.B., Emerson, J., Larez, M., "Dietary habits and the risk of stomach cancer: a comparison study of patients with and without intestinal metaplasia," *Gastroenterology and Nursing*, 16 (4) 1994, pp. 158–62.

gastroenterology A specialized branch of medicine focusing on the structure, function and pathology of the STOMACH, INTESTINES, ESOPHAGUS and related organs like the LIVER and PANCREAS. (See also GASTROINTESTINAL DISORDERS.)

gastrointestinal Concerning the stomach and intestines. (See also DIGESTION.)

gastrointestinal disorders A wide variety of conditions affecting the gastrointestinal tract (digestive system), including food sensitivities; structural defects; infections by viruses and bacteria (such as *Helicobacter pylori* and *Escherichia coli*) and by organisms causing food poisoning; parasites such as giardia; fungal pathogens like yeast; stress; glandular imbalances, such as HYPOCHLORHYDRIA (low stomach acid). Diet is directly related to problems due to nutritional deficiencies, food allergies, food sensitivities and low fiber intake. LACTOSE INTOLERANCE is an example of a common food sensitivity. In the United States, overall rates of gastrointestinal illness range from 1.5 to 1.9 illnesses per person per year. Diarrheal illnesses are second only to CARDIOVASCULAR DISEASE as a cause of death worldwide, and they are the leading cause of childhood death. The following is a listing of important gastrointestinal disorders:

1. GASTRITIS. Characterized by gastric pain due to a generalized inflammation of the stomach lining.
2. Gastric Ulcers and DUODENAL ULCERS. Open sores in the stomach or intestinal wall. The pitting may be severe enough to cause internal bleeding.
3. Chronic constipation.
4. Chronic DIARRHEA.
5. COLITIS. Characterized by inflammation and/or ulcer of the colon and rectum.
6. ILEITIS. An inflammation and ulceration of the small intestine that causes alternating diarrhea and constipation, occasionally with vomiting.
7. LIVER CIRRHOSIS. Scarring of the liver.
8. HEPATITIS. Inflammation of the liver often due to viral infection.
9. Gastric carcinoma.
10. Hiatus hernia. The bulging of the stomach through the diaphragm.
11. MALABSORPTION. Maldigestion and infection by bacteria and parasites are possible causes.
12. MALDIGESTION. Can lead to secondary nutrient deficiency states. Inadequate pancreatic enzymes, low stomach acid (hypochlorhydria) and carbohydrate intolerance, such as lactose intolerance, may be involved.
13. DIVERTICULITIS.
14. Hemorrhoids.

(See also CELIAC DISEASE; FLATULENCE; INFLAMMATORY BOWEL DISEASE; LACTOSE INTOLERANCE; SPRUE.)

Hartmann, Franz and Jenss Harro, "The gastrointestinal tract," in *Principles and Practice of Environmental Medicine*. Tarcher, A.B., ed. New York: Plenum Medical Book Co., 1992, pp. 121–37.
Nair, Prakash and Mayberry, John F., "Vegetarianism, Dietary Fiber and Gastrointestinal Disease," *Digestive Diseases*, 12 (1994), pp. 177–85.

gastrointestinal tract That part of the DIGESTIVE TRACT represented by the stomach and the intestines and their ancillary glands, including the liver and pancreas. (See also DIGESTION.)

gastroplasty A surgical procedure that reduces the functional size of the stomach by stapling a portion (sealing off). This is a drastic weight reduction strategy used for severely obese individuals. Weight loss ensues because the capacity for food intake is reduced. (See also DIETING; GASTRIC BUBBLE; OBESITY.)

gastrostomy A surgical procedure introducing a passageway from the STOMACH cavity through the abdominal wall (fistula). When the ESOPHAGUS is closed off, for example due to tumors, or when swallowing reflexes are inhibited, as in some stroke patients, food may be introduced into the stomach through such an opening. (See also DIGESTION.)

gavage Liquid feeding that occurs with a tube through the nasal passage to the ESOPHAGUS and the STOMACH (nasal gavage). Gavage also refers to feeding via a stomach tube (gastrogavage).

gelatin A processed form of animal PROTEIN that dissolves when mixed with hot water and gels upon cooling.

Gelatin absorbs 5 to 10 times its weight as water. It is commercially prepared by the breakdown of connective tissue protein, especially COLLAGEN, from the bones of slaughtered animals. Gelatin is a low-quality protein because it is deficient in many essential AMINO ACIDS, including TRYPTOPHAN and METHIONINE.

Gelatin is used as a culinary thickening and stabilizing agent. It is used with flavorings in desserts and pudding mixes, and in candy, jellies and ice cream. Commercial gelatin desserts usually contain high levels of SODIUM, SUCROSE and artificial coloring to make them look and taste like fruit desserts. Despite popular opinion, gelatin neither strengthens nails nor helps cure ulcers. (See also BIOLOGICAL VALUE.)

gemfibrozil   A cholesterol-lowering drug that has been shown to raise HIGH-DENSITY LIPOPROTEIN (HDL), the desirable CHOLESTEROL. (See also CHOLESTEROL-LOWERING DRUGS.)

gene   A unit of heredity that defines a trait or characteristic. A gene represents a region of DNA that codes for the sequence of AMINO ACIDS of a specific protein. Consequently DNA is said to be the "blueprint" of the cell's proteins. The cell nucleus contains a set of chromosomes with many thousands of genes.

MUTAGENS are agents that alter genes by attacking the DNA molecule, changing the genetic structure and causing mutations. Once a mutation has occurred, it is passed from one generation to the next. Mutagens are a diverse group of agents: Certain endogenous chemicals in plants, as well as pollutants, certain PESTICIDES and some synthetic FOOD ADDITIVES, even ultraviolet light, can cause mutations. This is a major concern because most mutagens are cancer-causing agents (CARCINOGENS).

In the nucleus of a human cell, chromosomes occur in pairs. Each member of a pair of genes is called an allele, which may be dominant or recessive. In a simple scenario, one or both genes of a pair of alleles may be dominant; therefore the trait or characteristic determined by the gene is expressed. A recessive trait (autosomal recessive gene) will not be expressed if it is paired with a dominant gene, though it will nonetheless be carried along through inheritance. Individuals who carry the recessive trait possess one normal gene and one modified gene and are classified as heterozygotes (hybrids). A gene coding for a defective protein would be expressed when two recessive genes are inherited (homozygotes), leading to the occurrence of certain rare genetic diseases at birth.

Several genetic diseases are based upon altered metabolism due to mutant enzymes. About 5% of cases with highly elevated blood cholesterol are due to genetic alterations in proteins responsible for cholesterol metabolism or transport. Typical examples are PHENYLKETONURIA, which reflects a defect in the metabolism of the amino acid PHENYLALANINE, and GALACTOSEMIA, the result of a defect in the metabolism of the SUGAR GALACTOSE. The severe effects of PKU can be avoided by strict dietary measures initiated soon after birth to avoid ingesting excessive amounts of phenylalanine. Early detection is the best strategy. Individuals who carry a recessive gene and a normal gene usually do not experience the genetic disease. For example, about one person in a hundred carries the trait for phenylketonuria while those with PKU possess a pair of abnormal genes—a much rarer occurrence (one out of 10,000 births).

Genetic polymorphism refers to the multiple genetic variants for a given protein, such as HEMOGLOBIN, the oxygen carrier protein of red blood cells. Most of the protein variants function more or less normally and do not directly cause disease. On the other hand, it is the slight differences in proteins reflecting differences in genetic makeup that account for individual traits among people. As a consequence, there will be slightly different nutrient requirements for optimal health among different persons. Their levels of liver detoxication enzymes will also vary. This variation partially explains why different individuals vary in their susceptibility to toxins, medications, anesthics and even cigarette smoke. (See also BIOCHEMICAL INDIVIDUALITY; GENETIC ENGINEERING).

general adaptation syndrome   See STRESS.

"generally recognized as safe" (GRAS)   Substances added to foods that are judged as safe because of their long history of usage without apparent harmful effects. The 1958 law regulating food additives exempted about 700 apparently safe chemicals and materials, which were approved by the FDA as food additives without further study. Subsequently developed food additives have had to meet requirements for premarket clearance in the FDA.

The GRAS "grandfather" clause is the source of controversy because the most widely used food additives are on the GRAS list and the safety of some have been questioned. The FDA has reevaluated the GRAS listings. Some materials like SULFITES have been banned or restricted on the basis of new data indicating potential health problems. ARTIFICIAL FOOD COLORS are another class that is being reevaluated and restricted. (See also FOOD, DRUG AND COSMETIC ACT.)

"GRAS: What It's All About," *Health Freedom News*, May 1993, pp. 34–36.

genetic engineering (bioengineering, biotechnology)   The chemical modification of genes of plants, animals and microorganisms. Typically, additional genetic messages are removed from one organism and inserted into chromosomes of another type to create the ability to synthesize new proteins in the recipient (transgenic product). A genetically engineered BOVINE GROWTH HORMONE now being sold in the United States can boost milk production in cows by 10%. Genetic engineering may improve the protein quality of plant foods and feed for livestock. Research is progressing to develop protein-enhanced BEANS, CORN, SOYBEANS (also more oil), WHEAT, ALFALFA, RAPESEED and sunflower. A renewed interest in the disease-prevention and the health-enhancing properties of foods has sparked other efforts to improve these characteristics in foods; for example, breeding carrots with increased levels of the antioxidant BETA CAROTENE. Technology is producing plants resistant to insects to viral diseases and to HERBICIDES. Some of the first experiments with genetically engineered crops have yielded tomato plants that produce animal antibodies against viral infections, conferring disease resistance. Alternatively, infection-resistant genes from other plant species have been inserted into tomatoes, making them resistant to bacterial infection. Planting crops that have herbicide-tolerant genes may help farmers control weeds in crops that would otherwise be damaged. One method is to insert an altered gene for a specific plant enzyme normally targeted or inactivated by a given herbicide. The change can make the enzyme insensitive to the herbicide. Another approach is to insert a gene for a new enzyme that detoxifies the herbicide. For example, a gene from petunia protects soybean plants from herbicides; a bacterial gene inserted into corn protects it against the European corn borer.

Genetic alteration may yield crops that can grow in cooler or warmer, wetter or drier climates. Plants may someday produce drugs such as vaccines and human hormones. Genes from other species can be incorporated in plants to develop products that are more nutritious or are sweeter; have a better flavor or more color for consumer appeal; and/or have a longer shelf life. The first genetically engineered whole food to be approved by the U.S. FDA is a tomato that has an extended shelf life due to an altered tomato gene that makes an enzyme that promotes softening.

Viruses affect many crops, ranging from wheat, corn and POTATOES to TOMATOES and CITRUS FRUIT. By inserting a gene coding for a protein of an attacking virus into a susceptible plant species, the recipient plants tolerate tobacco, alfalfa and cucumber mosaic viruses as well as potato viruses. Virus-resistant potatoes and tomatoes have been field-tested.

A number of concerns have been expressed by food scientists, consumer groups and policymakers. There is concern that plant geneticists may engineer crops to improve processing and yield at the expense of good nutrition. Cosmetic changes could be developed that might mask unripe or overripe foods. Safety is another concern. Genetically engineered plants could make higher levels of known toxic substances. Viral genes that can increase a plant's resistance to a pest could produce altered plant viruses that may harm plants.

Transferring genes could cause allergies. For example, genes from a peanut plant to another plant could make the new variety able to trigger reactions in those with peanut allergies. The FDA does not require special labeling for genetically engineered foods, except to potential allergens. Another possibility is the production of plant toxins in genetically engineered food.

On the other hand, several fears about genetically engineered products have not materialized: Designer plants and bacteria so far produced do not change animals, nor do they appear to spread from the area of use.

Three federal agencies regulate genetically engineered products in the United States. The Department of Agriculture must first approve field tests of transgenic (genetically engineered) plants. The Environmental Protection Agency establishes the tolerance levels of all synthetic pesticides in such food crops. The FDA evaluates all genetically engineered plant foods to determine whether the new genetic trait constitutes a FOOD ADDITIVE or other major plant alteration. The FDA does not require special labeling or review unless alteration of a food changes its nutritional value or produces possible toxins or allergens. (See also DNA; FUNCTIONAL FOODS; GREEN REVOLUTION.)

Hileman, Bette, "Views Differ Sharply Over Benefits, Risks of Agricultural Biotechnology," *Chemistry and Engineering News*, 73:34 (1995), pp. 8–17.

geophagia   The consumption of inedible materials such as clay, dirt and chalk. Famine has been associated with earth and clay eating, but clay eating is not limited to hardship. Clay is consumed around the world in spices, condiments or relishes. The hypothesis that clay eating is a response to deficiencies of minerals like iron or calcium has not been supported by hard evidence, possibly because the minerals in clay may be readily absorbed. Another proposal is that clay eating is a detoxifying strategy allowing people to make wider use of plants as food. In certain cultures pregnant women have traditionally eaten clay to settle their stomach. A common over-the-counter remedy for diarrhea is kaolinate, a major mineral in clay.

germ   The nutrient-rich embryo of seeds or kernels. This area is vitamin-rich and contains VITAMIN E plus THIAMIN, RIBOFLAVIN, NIACIN and plant oils. Wheatgerm is removed during the milling and refining process to obtain white flour. (See also BRAN, WHEAT; ENDOSPERM; GRAIN; WHEAT.)

gestational diabetes   See DIABETES, GESTATIONAL.

ghee   See BUTTER, CLARIFIED.

giardiasis   An intestinal infection caused by the protozoan parasite *Giardia lamblia*. This disease usually is associated with contaminated drinking WATER that may look clean. Water chlorination may not destroy giardia cysts, therefore water treatment may not remove this parasite. In the United States, giardiasis is the most frequent cause of waterborne diarrhea, and an estimated 2 to 5% of adults are infected. The numbers are higher for children; in some counties of western states of the United States, the percentage of infected adults may be as high as 13%. It can be transmitted by fecal contamination, and thus by infected food handlers. Children at day-care centers, and individuals with low stomach acid and compromised immune systems are more likely to acquire giardia.

Symptoms include DIARRHEA, stomach ache, FLATULENCE, ANOREXIA, nausea and vomiting. Giardiasis promotes atrophy of the surface of the small intestine, which can result in LACTOSE INTOLERANCE and MALABSORPTION. However, chronic giardiasis may cause only mild symptoms and people without symptoms are reservoirs of this parasite. In order to minimize the risk of infection, campers are advised to boil water for 10 minutes, or use water purification tablets or a portable water filtration unit. (See also GASTROINTESTINAL DISORDERS; MICROVILLI.)

Di Prisco, Maria C., et al., "Possible Relationship between Allergic Disease and Infection by Giardia lamblia," *Annals of Allergy*, 70 (March 1993), pp. 210–13.

ginger   (*Zingiber officinale*)   A spice originating in the East Indies, now cultivated in many tropical areas including Jamaica, and regions of Nigeria, India and Japan. Ginger is a yellow or reddish-brown underground stem called a rhizome and belongs to a family of reed-like perennials. Several hundred varieties of ginger exist. The characteristic peppery taste of ginger is produced by a compound called gingerin. When harvested at the appropriate time it is not fibrous, nor does it have a bitter aftertaste. Ginger is used fresh or dried, powdered or crystallized, in pickling spices, ginger bread, cakes, puddings, stews and curry bases. Ginger, boiled and preserved in syrup, is known as Canton ginger and is used in desserts.

Dried ginger has been used in folk medicine to treat complaints of the digestive tract, such as gas and bloating, nausea and vomiting, diarrhea and stomach cramps. Ginger also has a long history in treating rheumatism and reducing inflammation.

gingivitis Inflammation of gums (gingiva), a chronic DEGENERATIVE DISEASE. Gingivitis affects 70% of Americans over the age of 65. Inflammation can lead to bleeding gums, recession of gums, destruction of the boney tooth matrix and, eventually, to tooth loss. Gingivitis is associated with vitamin deficiencies and metal poisoning and can be caused by pathogenic organisms associated with dental plaque accumulation. Ill-fitting appliances and dentures can also cause gingivitis. Flossing and prophylactic cleaning by a dental hygienist are the best approaches to prevention. (See also FLUORIDE.)

Donghari, A., McDonnell, H.T. and Langlais, R.P., "Drug Induced Gingival Overgrowth, Adverse Drug Reactions," *Oral Surgery, Oral Medicine, Oral Pathology,* 76:4 (1993), pp. 543–48.

ginkgo (*Ginkgo biloba*) An ancient species of deciduous tree whose leaves have long been used in Oriental medicine. Ginkgo is native to China, and extracts of ginkgo leaves have been used to support heart, brain and lung function for nearly 5,000 years. Ginkgo extracts are standardized in terms of their active components. The leaves contain substances called ginkgolides and bilobalide, complex organic compounds that help fight disease. Ginkgo also contain flavonoids that function as antioxidants, which limit damage due to reactive forms of oxygen and can help reduce inflammation. Furthermore, ginkgo extracts can help maintain normal blood flow in arteries, veins and capillaries and maintain circulation.

Ginkgo leaf extracts can increase and normalize blood flow by relaxing blood vessel walls. They can also improve blood flow to the brain, thereby improving brain function. Ginkgo extracts inhibit the action of a substance called platelet activating factor, which triggers inflammation through the production of oxidized lipids and the migration of attacking white blood cells. They therefore protect areas such as the lungs and intestine against inflammation and tissue damage. Side effects are rare and may include headaches and stomach upsets. (See also SENILITY.)

ginseng (*Panax ginseng*; Chinese ginseng, Korean ginseng) A medicinal herb native to northern China and Korea. Ginseng is widely cultivated in Korea, Russia, China and Japan. It is available as white ginseng, from the dried root, or as red ginseng, which has been steamed. Ginseng is a famous herb of Chinese medicine, long used to restore "yang" energy, specifically to support normal healing processes during infections, to overcome fatigue, and to counter elevated blood pressure and high blood lipids (fat and cholesterol). Ginseng can stimulate the immune system, especially natural killer cells and scavenger immune cells (macrophages) in the liver, spleen and lymph nodes, and

antibody-producing cells. In experimental animals, ginseng has prevented viral infection. However, excessive amounts of ginseng can inhibit the immune response during serious infections. Ginseng may lower the risk of some types of CANCER in experimental animals. Ginseng can also lower elevated BLOOD SUGAR levels and high blood pressure.

Human studies performed in the former Soviet Union support ginseng's role in increasing stamina. Animal studies indicate that it can improve metabolism of the central nervous system and nerves controlling muscles, and spare GLYCOGEN, the glucose reserve, in exercising muscle. A class of plant compounds called saponins appears to be the active ingredient. In terms of adapting to stress, ginseng saponins (ginsenosides) stimulate the adrenal glands by promoting the release of adrenocorticotropin (ACTH) and ENDORPHINS, the brain's own opiates, from the PITUITARY GLAND. The adrenals are responsible for adapting the body to stress by producing hormones such as epinephrine (adrenaline) and cortisol.

Clearly ginseng can affect the body in many ways, and long-term consumption of excessive amounts may have negative consequences. It may depress the central nervous system, cause vaginal bleeding and breast pain in postmenopausal women. Long-term use can lead to "ginseng abuse syndrome," with possible high blood pressure, DIARRHEA, skin eruptions, loss of sleep, edema, nervousness, feminization of males and masculinization of females. One of the problems with ginseng is the wide variation in quality of commercially available products, which range from chewing gum and teas to capsules. Preparations standardized for content of an active ingredient (ginsenoside) and prudent application of ginseng are recommended.

GI tract See DIGESTIVE TRACT.

gland An organ or cell group specialized to secrete products used elsewhere in the body. Simple glands consist of a few cells, while compound glands possess clusters around a lumen or cavity and their secretions leave by a common duct.

Endocrine glands produce HORMONES, and are ductless glands whose secretions directly enter the blood or lymph. Pancreatic islets, the PITUITARY, THYROID, THYMUS and ADRENAL GLANDS are endocrine glands. Major endocrine glands are located in the ovaries, testes, duodenum (upper portion of the small intestine) and stomach.

Exocrine glands export their secretions to other regions via ducts. The exocrine pancreas secretes digestive enzymes, and the LIVER secretes BILE for digestion in the intestine through a duct leading to the small intestine. Mucous glands produce protective materials to coat the surface of the digestive tract and other cavities. Gastric glands in the lining of the stomach secrete GASTRIC JUICE for digestion. The parotoid and salivary glands produce SALIVA. Sudoriferous glands in the skin produce perspiration. (See also ENDOCRINE SYSTEM; PANCREAS.)

gliaden A protein found in wheat, rye and other grains. Together with glutenin, the other major type of GLUTEN protein, gliaden is responsible for the stickiness of dough. The high gluten content of wheat FLOUR creates an elastic, versatile dough for baking. Gliaden contains unusually large amounts of nonessential amino acids, GLUTAMINE and PRO-

LINE. On the other hand, wheat protein and gliaden are low in the essential AMINO ACIDS.

globulins   A group of PROTEINS that are insoluble in pure water but are soluble in salt solutions at neutral pH. An important globulin is serum ALBUMIN, which represents 55% of total soluble protein of blood. Serum albumin helps maintain the osmotic pressure of vessels and appropriate concentration of ELECTROLYTES in blood because it does not cross vessel walls.

Alpha, beta and gamma globulins of blood have different net electrical charges, permitting their separation by an electric field. Alpha globulins include HIGH-DENSITY LIPOPROTEIN (HDL), the lipoprotein that scavenges CHOLESTEROL; ceruloplasmin for COPPER transport; and VERY-LOW-DENSITY LIPOPROTEINS (VLDL), which transport fat synthesized by the liver. Beta globulins include TRANSFERRIN, which transports IRON; LOW-DENSITY LIPOPROTEINS (LDL), which transport cholesterol from the liver to other tissues; and fibrinogen, responsible for blood clotting. The liver also produces inactive enzymes like prothrombin that, when activated, promote clot formation. GAMMA GLOBULINS are circulating ANTIBODIES.

Other globulins occur in plants: edestin (WHEAT); phaseolin (BEANS); legumin (beans, peas); tuberin (POTATO); amadin (ALMONDS); and arachin (peanuts).

glomerular filtration   The first step in the process of urine production. Nephrons, microscopic filtration units of the kidney, permit some substances to pass into the kidney while excluding others. They are composed of a knot of vessels and a microscopic tube called a glomerulus. The filtration rate into the glomerulus is high; for the normal adult the kidneys filter about 48 gallons (180 liters) of fluid per day. Many compounds pass through the pores in the capillary walls, but serum ALBUMIN and most proteins are normally not filtered.

As filtrate passes downstream, tubules allow selective reabsorption of ions like SODIUM and BICARBONATE and small molecules like GLUCOSE, AMINO ACIDS and water. As sodium is transported back into the blood from the tubules, it draws water along with it; therefore most of the water is reabsorbed (taken back up into the bloodstream). Passage of the remaining water is regulated by a pituitary hormone, triggered when the brain (hypothalamus) senses an increase in osmotic pressure (lower water concentration). The tubules also help regulate the pH of the blood. When concentrations of KETONE BODIES, acids produced during severe caloric restriction, or of glucose, produced in uncontrollable diabetes, exceed a point at which they are no longer efficiently reabsorbed, they are also excreted in the urine, causing increased urine production and possible dehydration. (See also ALDOSTERONE; ANGIOTENSIN; ANTIDIURETIC HORMONE.)

glossitis   Tongue inflammation. Acute glossitis is a painful condition in which the tongue is irregularly fissured and ulcerated. Inflammation of the tongue is accompanied by a loss of the rough surface (filliform papillaes) or "bald tongue." The pain associated with glossitis can make eating difficult. Glossitis may be associated with nutritional ANEMIAS and non-tropical SPRUE (a digestive disorder characterized by malabsorption of fat and other nutrients, together with deficiencies of NIACIN, RIBOFLAVIN and VITAMIN B_{12}). (See also AVITAMINOSIS; MALNUTRITION.)

Drinka, Paul J., et al., "Nutritional Correlates of Atrophic Glossitis: Possible Role of Vitamin E and Papillary Atrophy," *Journal of the American College of Nutrition*, 12:1 (1993), pp. 14–20.

glucagon   A HORMONE that increases the levels of BLOOD SUGAR (glucose). Glucagon is produced by alpha cells of the endocrine pancreas and is released into the bloodstream when blood sugar drops. Glucagon has the opposite effect of INSULIN, which is released after a meal to lower blood glucose. Both are constructed of AMINO ACIDS.

To increase blood sugar levels, glucagon stimulates GLYCOGEN breakdown and glucose release by the liver. Glycogen is the glucose polymer for temporary storage. Glucagon also stimulates the liver to convert amino acids to GLUCOSE (a process called GLUCONEOGENESIS). (See also CARBOHYDRATE METABOLISM; ENDOCRINE SYSTEM; EPINEPHRINE.)

glucocorticoid   A hormone produced by the adrenal glands, responsible for maintaining BLOOD SUGAR, limiting inflammation and suppressing the immune response. The principle glucocorticoid is CORTISOL (hydrocortisone). Like other steroid hormones, it is synthesized from cholesterol. Extreme stress can lead to an overproduction of glucocorticoids, which places the body in a "catabolic state," with increased muscle breakdown, decreased antibody production and increased susceptibility to infection and fatigue. Inadequate glucocorticoid production can lead to HYPOGLYCEMIA (low blood sugar) as well as excessive fatigue. (See also ADRENAL GLANDS; ADRENOCORTICOTROPIC HORMONE; HYPOTHALAMUS.)

Demitrack, Mark A., et al., "Evidence for Impaired Activation of the Hypothalamic-pituitary-adrenal Axis in Patients with Chronic Fatigue Syndrome," *Journal of Clinical Endocrinology and Metabolism*, 73:6 (1991), pp. 1224–34.

glucomannan   A form of water-soluble FIBER obtained from Konjac tubers, which originated in Japan. Glucomannan readily absorbs water and swells to form a gel. The increased bulk contributes to a feeling of satiety, and glucomannan has been used as an APPETITE SUPPRESSANT. Like pectin, glucomannan has an effect of lowing cholesterol levels. Glucomannan tablets can lodge in the throat if not pre-dissolved in water. (See also BULKING AGENTS.)

gluconeogenesis   The enzymic system responsible for producing GLUCOSE from non-carbohydrate sources. Gluconeogenesis occurs primarily in the LIVER in response to lowered BLOOD SUGAR. The liver stores surplus glucose as GLYCOGEN, long chains of glucose units, after feeding. Between meals glucose is released from glycogen stores. However, gluconeogenesis becomes important in maintaining blood sugar levels with prolonged fasting. During severe dietary restriction (caloric or carbohydrate restriction) muscle protein is substantially degraded to provide amino acids that the liver readily transforms to glucose. The liver also manufactures glucose from a variety of non-carbohydrate molecules, including from lactic acid during strenuous exercise; from glycerol during fat breakdown; and from PYRUVIC ACID, CITRIC ACID and other intermediates of the KREB'S CYCLE, the central energy-producing pathway of the cell. Gluconeogenesis is lowered in individuals who abuse alcohol or who are susceptible to HYPOGLYCEMIA. (See also CARBOHYDRATE METABOLISM; CORTISOL; GLUCAGON.)

gluconic acid   An ACID derived from glucose and a naturally occurring ingredient in food. Several forms of gluconic acid are also used as FOOD ADDITIVES. Sodium gluconate is used in nonalcoholic beverages and in processed fruit juices to bind (chelate) metal ions that promote spoilage. A derivative of gluconic acid called FERROUS GLUCONATE is used to blacken olives. Another widely used derivative, called gluconolactone, is used in cake mixes, CHEESES, powdered soft drinks, gelatin desserts, processed fruits and vegetables, imitation dairy products and certain cured meats. (See also CHELATE.)

glucosamine (D-glucosamine)   A building block of cartilage. Glucosamine is a raw material for GLYCOSAMINOGLYCANS, structural materials needed for healthy joints. It is also a component of mucins, slippery materials that are part of mucous secretions, and cell coat materials. Glucosamine is normally synthesized from glucose (blood sugar). Apparently, the ability to synthesize and maintain cartilage declines with age. Glucosamine is selectively absorbed and supplementation has been reported to relieve joint pain in OSTEOARTHRITIS by exerting a protective effect on joint tissue and in supporting cartilage repair.

glucose (D-glucose, blood sugar, dextrose)   A simple sugar that is one of the most important CARBOHYDRATES in plant and animal metabolism. As an hexose (six-carbon sugar), glucose has a formula of $C_6H_{12}O_6$. Photosynthesis converts carbon dioxide and water to glucose, which is stored in leaves, stems, fruits, roots, pods and seeds, as glucose, as other sugars or as STARCH, composed of long chains of glucose units. DIGESTION converts starch back to glucose.

Glucose occurs naturally in food. It is a major ingredient of HONEY and SUCROSE (table sugar) and consists of half-glucose and half-fructose, while milk sugar (lactose) contains half-glucose and half-GALACTOSE. Free glucose occurs in fruit (grape sugar). Glucose is a common food additive, listed as DEXTROSE. Glucose from any of these sources is absorbed easily by the small intestine, raising blood glucose levels rapidly.

Glucose is the most important carbohydrate in the body. As BLOOD SUGAR, it is key, supplying about 20% of normal energy needs. Simple sugars such as FRUCTOSE and galactose must first be converted to glucose by the liver to be used for energy. Like all carbohydrate nutrients, glucose yields four calories per gram. Glucose is the major fuel of the brain because it readily crosses the BLOOD-BRAIN BARRIER. The brain accounts for only 3% of total body weight, yet this organ consumes 20% of the glucose in the blood.

The speed at which different sources of starch are digested affects the rate at which glucose is absorbed and blood sugar rises. Slower digestion results in a slower rise in blood sugar and a decreased need for insulin. The rate at which blood sugar rises after a carbohydrate-rich meal depends upon the source and type of carbohydrate, how it has been processed, how it is used after digestion, and whether fat has slowed gastric emptying. Generally the less processed the starchy

food, the slower starch conversion to glucose, the slower the increase in blood sugar, hence less insulin will be required. (See also CARBOHYDRATE METABOLISM; GLYCEMIC INDEX.)

glucose metabolism   Chemical processes by which the body uses the simple sugar GLUCOSE—the most important carbohydrate fuel of the body. It is oxidized by all tissues including RED BLOOD CELLS for ENERGY.

Glucose Degradation

GLYCOLYSIS is the first pathway of carbohydrate utilization, yielding ATP, the energy currency of the cell. Glycolysis converts glucose to a simple three-carbon acid called PYRUVIC ACID. The process is anaerobic: Oxygen does not participate in the reactions. Mitochondria, the "power houses" of the cell, oxidize pyruvic acid to ACETIC ACID, as an activated form called acetyl coenzyme A. Acetyl CoA in turn enters the KREB'S CYCLE, the central energy-yielding pathway, to be oxidized to CARBON DIOXIDE. The complete glucose oxidation traps 40% of the chemical energy in glucose as ATP, a remarkably efficient process.

Glucose is also oxidized anaerobically by the PENTOSE phosphate pathway to ATP and five carbon sugars (pentoses), required for DNA and RNA formation. This pathway also provides NADPH (reduced NICOTINAMIDE ADENINE DINUCLEOTIDE phosphate), the reducing agent for all biosynthetic reduction reactions such as occur in FAT and CHOLESTEROL synthesis. Glucose is the raw material for fat and cholesterol. Surplus glucose yields surplus acetyl coenzyme A, which is converted to saturated FATTY ACIDS and fats by the liver and by adipose (fat) tissue (LIPOGENESIS).

Glycogen Formation

Surplus glucose is stored as GLYCOGEN, long chains of glucose units, in the LIVER and muscle. The liver releases glucose from glycogen into the bloodstream when the blood glucose level drops between meals or in the early stages of fasting in response to hormone signals from the pancreas and adrenal glands. Muscle glycogen supplies muscle cells with glucose for quick energy during strenuous EXERCISE. Muscle glycogen cannot be released from muscle cells as glucose. During vigorous physical activity muscles produce LACTIC ACID as the end product of glycolysis, rather than pyruvic acid, the usual product of glycolysis (see above). Lactic acid accumulation partially accounts for the FATIGUE and cramping associated with vigorous exertion. Lactic acid migrates out of muscle cells into the blood, which transports it to the liver for resynthesis as glucose and eventual storage as glycogen.

Regulation of Blood Sugar

Blood sugar is carefully regulated by homeostatic mechanisms (physiologic processes that tend to keep the body functioning on an even keel). The range is normally maintained between 60 and 100 mg glucose per deciliter of blood by several different hormones. The body must deal with two possible situations: elevated blood sugar and low blood sugar. The hormone INSULIN is released into the bloodstream in response to elevated blood glucose levels after a high carbohydrate meal. Insulin lowers elevated blood sugar by promoting glucose uptake by tissues and stimulating glycogen, fat and protein synthesis. Abnormally high blood glucose (HYPERGLYCEMIA) is a characteristic of diabetes, a severe disease if left untreated.

Abnormally low blood glucose is called HYPOGLYCEMIA. This condition can profoundly affect the nervous system because of its dependency upon glucose for energy. GLUCAGON, CORTISOL and other hormones counterbalance insulin by raising blood glucose levels. Glucagon promotes glycogen breakdown in the liver. Cortisol promotes the conversion of amino acids, released from muscle protein degradation, to glucose by a pathway called GLUCONEOGENESIS. In time of need glucose can also be synthesized from lactic acid, pyruvic acid, products of glycolysis, as well as acidic intermediates of the KREB'S CYCLE, such as CITRIC ACID.

Low-carbohydrate diets are the basis of many fad weight-loss programs. When the diet does not supply enough carbohydrate to maintain blood sugar levels, the body switches over to a starvation mode in order to supply blood glucose. The body adapts to inadequate carbohydrate/calorie intake by breaking down muscle protein into amino acids, to be converted to glucose to supply the brain with energy, as well as by breaking down body fat for more general energy needs. (See also DIET, LOW CARBOHYDRATE; DIET, VERY LOW CALORIE; EXERCISE; GLYCEMIC INDEX.)

glucose oxidase   An enzyme used to degrade GLUCOSE. A product of mold culture, glucose oxidase is used by the food industry to destroy glucose in egg white and whole egg products. Glucose removal facilitates product drying and helps prevent product deterioration. Glucose oxidase helps extend the shelf life of canned soft drinks and is also used to remove traces of oxygen in packaged foods including dehydrated products, mayonnaise and canned foods. This step minimizes changes in color and flavor during storage. (See also FOOD ADDITIVES.)

glucose tolerance   The efficiency with which the body can take up and dispose of glucose, thus lowering elevated blood GLUCOSE. Blood sugar levels higher than normal (HYPERGLYCEMIA) are classified as impaired glucose tolerance. DIABETES MELLITUS is the most common cause of chronically high blood glucose levels. The hormone INSULIN stimulates glucose uptake by tissues; diabetics may produce inadequate insulin, or insulin that is produced may not be able to work effectively at the target tissues. Glucose tolerance can decrease with age, due to decreased tissue responsiveness to insulin. The increased proportion of body fat present in some older people also decreases insulin sensitivity.

Coggan, Andrew and Swanson, Scott, "Nutritional Manipulation Before and During Exercise Affects Performance," *Medicine and Science in Sports and Exercise*, 5 (1992), pp. 331–39.

glucose tolerance factor   An agent that assists the action of INSULIN in lowering BLOOD SUGAR (GLUCOSE). Together with glucose tolerance factor, insulin promotes the cellular uptake of glucose and of amino acids and the increased synthesis of fat and protein. Glucose tolerance factor apparently enhances the effects of insulin; it is inactive unless insulin is present. Glucose tolerance factor may be released into the blood, perhaps by the liver, whenever there is a marked increase in blood glucose or insulin.

Glucose tolerance factor contains the trace mineral nutrient CHROMIUM combined with NIACIN (vitamin B₃) and several amino acids. The factor has been isolated from liver and yeast; one of the best dietary sources of the factor is BREWER'S YEAST. (See also CARBOHYDRATE METABOLISM.)

glucose tolerance test   A diagnostic procedure that measures how effectively a person clears a large dose of glucose from the bloodstream. Typically the patient consumes 100 g of glucose in water before breakfast (after fasting overnight). BLOOD SUGAR levels are subsequently measured at intervals for several hours. In a normal response, the blood sugar level rises sharply during the first hour after ingesting glucose, then returns to the resting or fasting level within three hours as INSULIN is released. If the blood sugar level remains elevated, diabetes or a pre-diabetic condition may be indicated. HYPOGLYCEMIA may be indicated if the blood sugar dips below normal and only slowly returns to the resting level while the patient experiences typical symptoms such as shakiness, sweating and weakness.

The glucose tolerance test may cause significant discomfort in susceptible people. Hypoglycemic individuals can experience blackouts, sleepiness or irritability as their blood sugar plummets. A three-hour test may not be long enough to assess glucose tolerance; five or six hours may be more appropriate. It has been suggested that a more realistic test is a "food tolerance" test, designed to see how the body responds to sugar released by DIGESTION of foods. A diagnosis is strengthened by a simultaneous insulin tolerance test that measures the blood levels of insulin after the glucose challenge. Candidates for a glucose tolerance test include those at risk for diabetes through inheritance, through pregnancy (gestational diabetes) and others. (See also CARBOHYDRATE METABOLISM; DIABETES MELLITUS.)

glucostat   A hypothetical mechanism in the brain by which BLOOD SUGAR levels help regulate APPETITE. According to this proposal, a drop in blood glucose affects the HYPOTHALAMUS, the region of the brain that regulates involuntary activities and integrates response to stress. The hypothalamus responds by activating neural pathways to arouse eating behavior. This seminal concept formed the basis for much of the essential research on brain function and glucose utilization. Evidence continues to accumulate that the hypothalamus contributes to regulating feeding behavior. The fat cell hormone LEPTIN may affect the region of the hypothalamus that regulates satiety. (See also CRAVING; OBESITY.)

glucosuria   The excretion of abnormal amounts of glucose in the urine. Glucosuria often indicates elevated BLOOD GLUCOSE (HYPERGLYCEMIA) caused by DIABETES MELLITUS. Healthy people secrete little glucose in the urine because glucose is rapidly reabsorbed (salvaged) from the filtered fluid by the KIDNEY. However, when blood glucose concentrations reach 300 mg/100 ml, the kidneys' transport maximum absorption rate is exceeded, and glucose is secreted in the urine. Excretion of glucose requires additional water, and DEHYDRATION is a likely consequence due to frequent urination. (See also GLOMERULAR FILTRATION.)

glutamic acid (Glu; glutamate) One of the 20 AMINO ACIDS that are the building blocks of PROTEIN. Glutamic acid is an acidic, nonessential amino acid because the body easily manufactures it as needed from alpha ketoglutaric acid, a common intermediate produced by amino acid degradation and by the KREB'S CYCLE, the pathway central to carbohydrate metabolism. When glutamic acid is neutralized it is called "glutamate." The body converts glutamic acid to GLUTAMINE, another nonessential amino acid. Glutamine formation is a key in the disposal of ammonia for the brain because it crosses the BLOOD-BRAIN BARRIER and transports the nitrogen from ammonia to other tissues for eventual disposal as UREA, a non-toxic end product.

Glutamic acid functions as a NEUROTRANSMITTER, a chemical employed in transmitting signals between nerve cells, and is concentrated in the brain. During a STROKE, glutamic acid is released from cells damaged by the loss of oxygen. It has been proposed that in large amounts, glutamic acid can damage nerve cells; thus a stroke may be related to glutamate-induced damage. Glutamic acid is related to brain function in another way: It is the parent of the inhibitory neurotransmitter gamma aminobutyric acid.

Glutamic acid also appears in supplements and FOOD ADDITIVES. Glutamic acid hydrochloride is a supplement used to increase gastric acidity and to counterbalance a deficiency of hydrochloric acid (STOMACH ACID). MONOSODIUM GLUTAMATE (MSG) is a combination of glutamic acid and sodium. MSG is used as a FLAVOR ENHANCER in prepared and CONVENIENCE FOODS. In susceptible people excessive MSG in food can cause MSG Related Syndrome, including a tingling or burning sensation, heart palpitations, anxiety, urination, thirst or stomach ache. Other food enhancers incorporating glutamate are potassium glutamate and HYDROLYZED VEGETABLE PROTEIN. (See also ACHLORHYDRIA; FOOD LABELING.)

glutamine (Gln, L-glutamine) One of the 20 AMINO ACIDS that serve as raw materials for PROTEINS. The body manufactures this amino acid from GLUTAMIC ACID, therefore it is not classified as an essential amino acid. The brain and muscle synthesize glutamine to dispose of AMMONIA, a toxic metabolic by-product.

Glutamine is released into the bloodstream and transported to the intestine, where it is a preferred fuel. There it is broken down to glutamic acid and ammonia. Ammonia travels directly via the portal vein to the liver, which incorporates it into urea, the end product of nitrogen metabolism. Urea is then released into the bloodstream and excreted by the kidneys.

Though glutamine is normally the most prevalent amino acid in blood, it may be limited in cases of severe trauma such as recovery from surgery or severe burns, and glutamine supplements may be recommended. Glutamine supplements have been used in drug detoxification centers to help minimize the symptoms of drug and alcohol withdrawal. Glutamine may help maintain the integrity of the small intestine. (See also ALCOHOLISM; AMINO ACID METABOLISM.)

Teran, J.C., Mullen, K.D., McCullough, A.J., "Glutamine—A Conditionally Essential Amino Acid in Cirrhosis." *American Journal of Clinical Nutrition*, 62 (1995), pp. 897–900.

glutathione The principal sulfur reducing agent of the cell and a primary ANTIOXIDANT. Glutathione contains three amino acids, including the sulfur amino acid CYSTEINE. Glutathione helps maintain the structure of red blood cell membranes and other cellular proteins and it helps maintain the cytoplasm in a reduced state. Low levels of reduced glutamine are associated with oxidative stress (AGING, toxic exposure, AIDS). As an antioxidant, glutathione assists an enzyme (glutathione peroxidase) that inactivates hydrogen peroxide and oxidized lipids (lipid peroxides), and prevents them from liberating damaging, highly reactive agents. It can also quench free radicals directly.

Glutathione plays an additional, protective role in the liver, where it combines with toxic materials and waste products to permit more efficient excretion. Glutathione also functions as a carrier in the transport of the sulfur-containing amino acids, cysteine and METHIONINE, into cells, and it assists the synthesis of LEUKOTRIENES, extremely potent inflammatory agents. (See also CARBOHYDRATE METABOLISM; DETOXICATION; FREE RADICALS.)

Lenzi, A., et al., "Placebo Controlled, Double-Blind, Cross-over Trial of Glutathione Therapy in Male Infertility," *Human Reproduction*, 8:10 (1993), pp. 1657–62.

glutathione peroxidase A widely distributed ENZYME that functions as an ANTIOXIDANT. Glutathione peroxidase inactivates oxidized lipids (lipid peroxides) and HYDROGEN PEROXIDE, which spontaneously break down to FREE RADICALS, highly reactive chemical species that can damage cells. This enzyme converts hydrogen peroxide to oxygen and water and converts peroxides of polyunsaturated FATTY ACIDS to non-toxic, fatty acids. Glutathione peroxidase requires the trace mineral nutrient SELENIUM as a cofactor. For this reason, selenium is acknowledged as an antioxidant nutrient. (See also BETA CAROTENE; CATALASE; VITAMIN C; VITAMIN E.)

Krinsky, Norman I., et al., "Mechanism of Action of Biological Antioxidants," *Proceedings of the Society of Experimental Biology and Medicine*, 200 (1992), pp. 248–54.

gluten The major PROTEIN fraction of wheat FLOUR. Gluten consists of an equal mixture of two fractions, GLIADEN and glutenin. When moistened, these proteins yield an elastic dough that is easily shaped. The unique rising qualities of WHEAT flour dough are due to its ability to trap carbon dioxide bubbles released by LEAVENING AGENTS. Baking coagulates gluten so that baked goods maintain their shape without crumbling. Hard wheat contains more gluten than soft varieties. The proteins, hordenin from BARLEY, and oryenin from RICE, resemble glutenin.

Gluten-Free Diet

Only the gliaden portion of gluten has been demonstrated to cause severe malabsorption (CELIAC DISEASE) in sensitive people. Although similar proteins occur in other grains including RYE, barley, TRITICALE and OATS, wheat contains by far the largest percentage of gluten; corn and rice contain little gluten-type protein. Individuals with celiac disease need to avoid gluten-containing products, a difficult task because wheat flour is added to a huge variety of foods. Rice, potato, legumes like soybeans and lima beans, or foods classified as grains but belonging to different plant families such as

AMARANTH and QUINOA yield flour that can substitute for wheat in many dishes and baked goods. (See also BREAD.)

Arnason, J.A., et al., "Do Adults with High Gliaden Antibody Concentrations Have Subclinical Gluten Intolerance?" *Gut*, 33:2 (1992), pp. 194–97.

gluten-sensitive enteropathy   See CELIAC DISEASE.

glycemic index

A measure of how rapidly a food or nutrient raises the BLOOD SUGAR level relative to ingestion of a sample of pure sugar, GLUCOSE. Foods with a high glycemic index increase blood sugar almost as rapidly as eating glucose alone. Not all starchy foods are digested and assimilated with equal ease. Those with a low glycemic index are digested slowly and cause a slower rise in blood sugar. Factors influencing the rate of carbohydrate digestion include the type of food and methods of storage, processing and cooking. Furthermore, the presence of one food can affect digestion of another.

A low glycemic index is believed to be generally desirable. When the body digests food more slowly, or converts the food to blood sugar more slowly, less INSULIN is needed to compensate for the increase in blood sugar. For example, FRUCTOSE is slowly converted to glucose by the liver; consequently this refined sugar has a low glycemic index. Foods with a low glycemic index include whole, unprocessed foods like LEGUMES, BEANS, cracked WHEAT, BRAN cereals and bulgar wheat. These foods contain FIBER and minimally processed starch. Foods with a high (less desirable) glycemic index include table sugar and sugar-rich foods, white BREAD, rice puffs, corn flakes, rye crisps, corn CHIPS, some vegetables and instant POTATOES. These foods raise blood sugar almost as rapidly as sugar alone because food processing partially breaks down their starch.

A lower glycemic index for a food may be desirable, especially for diabetics. However, the utility of the glycemic index in meal planning for diabetics is limited. For example, ice cream, a food with a high content of FAT and SUCROSE (table sugar), has a low glycemic index because fat slows stomach emptying and lowers the rate of entry of sugar into the intestine. This does not mean a diabetic should overindulge in ice cream because an excess of fatty foods is potentially hazardous to health. (See also CARDIOVASCULAR DISEASE; DIABETES MELLITUS; DIETARY GUIDELINES FOR AMERICANS.)

Wolever, Thomas and Miller, Janette B., "Sugars and Blood Glucose Control," *American Journal of Clinical Nutrition*, 62:supplement, (July 1995), pp. 212S–21S.

glycerol (glycerin)

A syrupy, clear, odorless liquid with a sweet taste; used as a FOOD ADDITIVE. Glycerol maintains moisture in foods and helps dissolve flavors in prepared foods like MARSHMALLOWS, CANDY, fudge and baked goods. It is used in amounts ranging from 0.5 to 10%. Glycerol is classified as a GRAS (generally recognized as safe) food additive by the U.S. FDA.

As a NUTRIENT, glycerol occurs in chemical combination with FATTY ACIDS in lipids, fat and oils (triglycerides). Glycerol contains three oxygen groups that link up with fatty acids. Glycerol itself is derived from GLUCOSE metabolism and can be converted back to glucose by the liver. (See also CARBOHYDRATE METABOLISM; FAT METABOLISM; GLYCOLYSIS.)

glycine (Gly)

The smallest of the 20 AMINO ACIDS that form PROTEIN. Glycine is the only common amino acid that is symmetrical and therefore no mirror image (D, L) forms. The body converts the amino acid SERINE to glycine; consequently it is not a dietary essential amino acid.

Glycine plays a pivotal role in biosynthesis: Glycine is a building block of HEME, the iron-binding center (porphyrins) of HEMOGLOBIN of RED BLOOD CELLS and oxidation-reduction enzymes (CYTOCHROMES) of the MITOCHONDRIA. It is also a building block of creatine, which is used to replenish ATP in skeletal muscle. Glycine helps form PURINES, nitrogen-containing cyclic compounds that form half the bases of DNA and RNA. The LIVER combines glycine with chemicals to inactivate them and render them water-soluble for excretion. (See also AMINO ACID METABOLISM; DETOXIFICATION; FOLACIN.)

glycocholic acid

An acid in BILE that is important in emulsifying FAT for DIGESTION and absorption. It is synthesized from the amino acid GLYCINE and cholic acid, itself a bile component formed by the oxidation of CHOLESTEROL by the liver. As a FOOD ADDITIVE, glycocholic acid serves as an EMULSIFIER to suspend water-insoluble materials. (See also FAT DIGESTION.)

glycogen

A storage CARBOHYDRATE in animal tissues. Glycogen resembles STARCH, which is the storage form of GLUCOSE in plants. Both are large molecular weight chains composed of glucose building blocks. Unlike starch, glycogen has a very highly branched structure. Because of its high degree of branching, glycogen binds 3 to 5 g of water per gram of glycogen. A normal adult weighing 150 pounds (68 kg) possesses approximately 800 g of glycogen, found predominantly in skeletal muscle and in the LIVER. Muscle accounts for approximately two-thirds of the glycogen in the body.

Liver Glycogen Metabolism

The liver helps regulate BLOOD SUGAR through the synthesis and degradation of glycogen. After a carbohydrate meal, the liver absorbs glucose from the blood and incorporates it into glycogen in response to the pancreatic hormone INSULIN. With low blood glucose, EPINEPHRINE (adrenaline) from the adrenal glands and GLUCAGON from the pancreas signal glycogen breakdown. The liver, alone, can disengage glucose from cellular reactions and release it into the bloodstream.

Muscle Glycogen Metabolism

Insulin, released in response to elevated blood sugar levels, stimulates glucose uptake by skeletal muscle, where it is deposited as glycogen. Muscle glycogen does not form blood sugar. To provide quick energy, epinephrine (adrenaline) activates the enzyme responsible for breaking down muscle glycogen to glucose, which directly enters GLYCOLYSIS for rapid oxidation and conversion to energy.

During vigorous physical EXERCISE muscle cells oxidize a portion of the glucose to LACTIC ACID, which can promote muscle cramping and muscle fatigue. Lactic acid eventually escapes from muscle cells into the bloodstream, where it enters the liver and is converted back to blood glucose.

During recovery from strenuous exercise, muscles take up blood glucose to restore depleted glycogen. The recovery period may last a day or two.

Glycogen in food is not a significant source of carbohydrate. Meat and fish normally contain very little glycogen because their tissues rapidly break down glycogen during slaughter or capture. Oysters, mussels, scallops and clams contain a little glycogen when eaten. (See also CARBOHYDRATE LOADING; CARBOHYDRATE METABOLISM; GLYCOGENOLYSIS.)

Kreitzman, S.N., Coxon, A.Y., Szaz, K.F., "Glycogen Storage: Illusions of Easy Weight Loss, Excessive Weight Regain and Distortions in Estimates of Body Composition," *American Journal of Clinical Nutrition*, 56:supp. 1 (July 1992), pp. 292–93S.

glycogen loading   See CARBOHYDRATE LOADING.

glycogenolysis   The breakdown of glycogen in the LIVER and muscle to glucose. EPINEPHRINE, a hormone of the adrenal glands, signals glycogenolysis in muscle for quick energy and, to a lesser extent, in the liver in response to stress, while GLUCAGON from the endocrine PANCREAS triggers glycogenolysis in the liver to compensate for low blood sugar.

Glycogenolysis is carried out by a specific ENZYME called glycogen phosphorylase, which senses change in blood glucose for the liver. Thus, high blood glucose levels rapidly inactivate the enzyme, because the need for glycogen degradation to supply glucose vanishes. (See also CARBOHYDRATE LOADING; CARBOHYDRATE METABOLISM; GLUCOSE TOLERANCE; GLYCOLYSIS.)

glycolysis   The degradation of GLUCOSE to small, organic acids, such as PYRUVIC ACID or LACTIC ACID, to produce ENERGY without the participation of oxygen (anaerobically). Glycolysis is a primary energy-yielding pathway of carbohydrate metabolism: Ten different kinds of ENZYMES work together, like an assembly line in a factory, to cleave and oxidize glucose in order to produce energy as ATP. To completely release all of the energy locked in the original glucose molecule, pyruvic acid is further oxidized with oxygen-requiring enzymes to CARBON DIOXIDE, yielding more ATP than released simply from glycolysis.

Glycolysis is regulated by enzyme feedback mechanisms and by hormones. In the liver it is increased by INSULIN, a major biosynthetic hormone, and it is inhibited by GLUCAGON, a hormone signaling the liver to increase blood glucose, rather than consuming it. This pathway is inhibited when ATP or CITRIC ACID accumulates in the cell, indicating a saturation of another energy-yielding pathway (the KREB'S CYCLE).

RED BLOOD CELLS and other cells without the mitochondria cannot use oxygen to oxidize fuels and rely strictly on anaerobic glycolysis to produce ATP and lactic acid. Muscles use glycolysis to metabolize glucose for energy, and during vigorous EXERCISE, glucose can be anaerobically converted to lactic acid to provide extra ATP when muscle cells receive limited oxygen to burn fuels. During FERMENTATION to prepare wine and beer, yeast utilize anaerobic glycolysis to convert glucose to ethanol (alcohol). (See also BLOOD SUGAR; CATABOLISM; FEEDBACK INHIBITION; GLUCONEOGENESIS; GLYCOGEN.)

glycoproteins   PROTEINS containing CARBOHYDRATE segments. Glycoproteins represent many classes of proteins including certain ENZYMES, ANTIBODIES, HORMONES and membrane components likely to be involved in cell recognition (for example, that determine blood type) and slippery proteins called mucins. Sugars such as GALACTOSE, MANNOSE and nitrogen derivatives of GLUCOSE and galactose are building blocks as well as acidic sugars. Proteins with very large carbohydrate chains (GLYCOSAMINOGLYCANS) form connective tissue like cartilage while mucins form mucus to protect moist surfaces of tissues. (See also HEPARIN.)

glycosaminoglycans (mucopolysaccharides)   Large carbohydrate chains that support connective tissues such as skin, tendons, cartilage, ligaments and BONE. Glycosaminoglycans also support the structure of ears, auditory tubes and heart valves. Glycosaminoglycans such as chondroitin sulfate are jelly-like substances that help lubricate surfaces of joints and provide resiliency, so that joints resist compression. Other glycosaminoglycans help maintain fluid compartments. For example, hyaluronic acid occurs in the fluid of the eye and joint spaces, while heparin serves as an anticoagulant in veins and arteries. Mucus, secreted to lubricate and protect moist surfaces of the body, is also composed of glycosaminoglycans.

Cells produce glycosaminoglycans from simple sugars or compounds derived from them. For example, amino sugars—GLUCOSAMINE and galactosamine—and the sugar acid, glucuronic acid, come from GLUCOSE (blood sugar). These building blocks are assembled into long chains. SULFUR in the form of sulfate may be attached, and the completed glycosaminoglycans are released into the surrounding (extracellular) space. The synthesis of healthy connective tissue and its repair depend upon adequate supplies of glycosaminoglycan building blocks, including the amino acids GLUTAMINE, METHIONINE and CYSTEINE. Vitamins, such as VITAMIN C, NIACIN and PANTOTHENIC ACID and the trace minerals MANGANESE, COPPER, IRON and ZINC function as enzyme helpers in the process. It is important to note that pain killers, such as non-steroidal antiinflammatory drugs, are often taken to relieve joint pain, although they can interfere with the rebuilding process and slow recovery from joint injury. (See also COLLAGEN; POLYSACCHARIDES.)

Boeve, E.R., et al., "Glycosaminoglycans and Other Sulphated Polysaccharides in Calculogenesis of Urinary Stones," *World Journal of Urology*, 12:1 (1994), pp. 43–48.

glycoside   A compound composed of a simple SUGAR bound to another sugar or other substance. Thus, LACTOSE (milk sugar) is a glycoside of GALACTOSE and GLUCOSE. Plant glycosides contain sugars attached to a variety of other compounds besides sugars. Cyanogenic glycosides found in seeds of apricots and apples yield toxic cyanide upon decomposition. Digitalis (digitoxin) is a glycoside that is a heart stimulant. FLAVONOIDS are a group of plant substances that generally exist bound to sugars and serve as ANTIOXIDANTS and in other useful functions. (See also HESPERIDIN.)

glycyrrhizin (glycyrrhizic acid)   A principal flavor of LICORICE. One of the sweetest natural substances, glycyrrhizin is 50 to 100 times sweeter than SUCROSE. Ammoniated glycyrrhizin is prepared from licorice root extracts and used as a FOOD ADDITIVE. It is used in beverages (root beer), candy, chewing gum and baked goods.

Glycyrrhizin possesses powerful physiologic effects. Excessive ingestion of licorice (several ounces of licorice daily for extended periods) may result in: lowered blood potassium levels, lowered aldosterone levels with sodium and water-retention, HYPERTENSION, fatigue and, in extreme cases, heart failure.

Licorice root has long been used in Chinese medicine in the treatment of lung infections and digestive disorders. Glycyrrhizin has antiviral activity, and in Western medicine it has been used to treat peptic ulcers and Addison's disease. Its anti-inflammatory effects may be the result of an inhibition of the formation of pro-inflammatory PROSTAGLANDINS, derivatives of essential fatty acids.

goat's milk   A MILK sometimes used as a substitute for cow's milk. This milk contains more VITAMIN A and fat than cow's milk, but contains the same amounts of LACTOSE (milk sugar). Goat's milk is low in FOLIC ACID and VITAMIN B_{12}. Although it lacks CASEIN, the major cow's milk protein, goat's milk may cause milk sensitivity, and there is often a crossover allergy between goat's milk and cow's milk. Two-thirds of the children allergic to cow's milk cannot tolerate either goat's milk or cow's milk. (See also ALLERGY, FOOD.)

goiter   An enlargement of the THYROID GLAND often due to IODINE deficiency. Thyroid gland hyperplasia (excessive glandular growth) represents an attempt by the body to compensate for a shortage of the iodine required for synthesizing thyroxine, the thyroid hormone that contains iodine. An iodine deficiency decreases thyroxine production, and lowered thyroxine production leads to increased production of thyroid-stimulating hormone by the pituitary, which stimulates further growth of the thyroid. Excessive consumption of raw soybeans, thiocyanate-containing drugs used to treat high blood pressure, and even excessive iodine can produce goiters.

The first European use of iodine compounds to treat goiter occurred in 1816; however, the ancient Chinese recommended treating goiter with seaweed and burnt sponge, now known to contain large amounts of iodine. They also administered dried animal thyroid glands. Until the early 1920s, goiters were common in the southern United States where the soil contains little iodine. Iodine in the form of sodium iodide was added to SALT in the 1920s. With this addition, goiters disappeared in the United States. People living in certain regions of the world still suffer from iodine deficiency, and goiter is likely to be found inland, where the availability of seafoods is limited, and in areas where the topsoil has negligible iodine, such as the plains of Africa, Asia and South America. (See also FOOD TOXINS; GOITROGENS.)

goitrogens   Plant compounds that can cause thyroid hormone deficiency and GOITER formation. This class of compounds liberates thiocyanate, which can block IODINE uptake and use. CABBAGE, RUTABAGA, TURNIP, KALE, CAULIFLOWER, BROCCOLI, RADISH and KOHLRABI contain low levels of goitrogens. In most cases cooking inactivates goitrogens.

Realistically, goitrogens are a potential problem only if rutabagas and turnips are used as a staple and if the diet is iodine-deficient, an unlikely situation in the United States. A dietary excess of calcium and fluorine enhances the effects of goitrogens. (See also FOOD TOXINS; THYROID GLAND.)

goldenseal (*Hydrastis canadensis*)   A medicinal plant of North America with a long history of Native American use. Goldenseal is now cultivated in the Pacific Northwest. Goldenseal together with barberry (*Berberis vulgaris*) and Oregon grape (*Mahonia aquifolium*) produce alkaloids called berberine, berberastine, canadine and hydrastine, which stimulate the IMMUNE SYSTEM and act as antibiotics. Goldenseal has been used to treat inflammatory conditions such as digestive disorders, ulcers, COLITIS and infections of the digestive tract like traveler's diarrhea, as well as infections of the lungs, throat, sinuses and urinary tract. Goldenseal can also lower fever.

The dried root and underground stem are used as supplements; alternatively, purified berberine can be used. Berberine attacks a wide variety of disease-producing organisms, including parasites, bacteria and yeast and fungi. In addition, it prevents such pathogens from binding to tissues, thus preventing adherence to the host, a first step in the infectious process. Berberine also activates macrophages, cells of the immune system that scavenge bacteria, viruses and tumor cells. It also helps support the spleen, an organ that filters and cleans the blood. Berberine-containing plants are not recommended during pregnancy, and consumption of large amounts can block the utilization of B complex vitamins.

gooseberry (*Ribes grossularia*)   The tart fruit of a prickly shrub, closely related to the currant. Gooseberries grow singly, rather than in clusters. They are usually small, though varieties can be an inch in diameter and they turn amber when they ripen. Gooseberries are native to both the Old World and America. European cultivation probably began in the 10th century. Commercial production began in the 1800s. Gooseberry production in the United States was restricted in the early 1900s when it was discovered that gooseberries were a carrier of a pine blister rust that had caused extensive damage to pine forests by the turn of the century. In the United States gooseberries are grown in Michigan, Oregon and Washington. Different varieties can be either red, white, green or yellow. Raw, 100 g provides 39 calories; carbohydrate, 1.7 g; 1.9 g of fiber; and vitamin C, 33 mg.

Gotu kola (*Centella asiatica*)   A medicinal herb native to China, India, Indonesia and the South Pacific, including Australia. Since prehistoric times Gotu kola has been used for healing wounds and skin conditions. Tradition relates that it promotes longevity. The plant contains triterpenes—including asiaticoside—substances which seem to promote growth of connective tissue and skin. Extracts contain a mixture of substances that are responsible for its multiple effects, ranging from improving mental function to "improving" varicose veins. Although extracts are generally well tolerated, repeated application of isolated asiatoside has been reported to cause skin cancer.

gout A painful joint inflammation, especially of the hands and feet (specifically the big toe of men). Gout may affect the kidneys and the heart as well. Gout is fairly common in America: It occurs in three people per thousand and is 20 times more common in men than in women. This disease is due to abnormal deposits of URIC ACID, the normal end product of PURINE degradation that occurs in the blood and is excreted in the urine. Purines are nitrogen-containing, cyclic compounds that are building blocks of DNA and RNA. Uric acid is borderline soluble at typical blood pH.

The causes of gout are unknown, though OBESITY, inheritance and chronic lead poisoning can contribute to the risk. Elevated uric acid in the blood (hyperuricemia) is associated with gout in susceptible people. Uric acid can accumulate for several reasons. In "primary" gout, uric acid accumulation is the result of certain inherited enzyme deficiencies. In these cases, specific enzyme defects cause excessive purine breakdown or overproduction of purines. In "secondary" gout, uric buildup is associated with cancer, hemolytic ANEMIA, and certain toxic drugs and kidney disease. In the latter situation, the excretion of uric acid is reduced, allowing a buildup to occur. Certain drugs also affect kidney performance and can cause gout: thiazide DIURETICS, salicylates like ASPIRIN, probenecid and ethanibutol.

A high-protein diet and purine-rich foods like caviar, organ meats, YEAST, poultry and anchovies can contribute to the risk of gout in susceptible people. The accumulation of LACTIC ACID, ALCOHOLISM, toxemia of pregnancy, and excessive KETONE BODIES (acidic products of fat metabolism during uncontrolled diabetes) can lead to excessive blood acidity, which can promote uric acid precipitation.

Treatment of gout may involve controlling weight in obese people, avoiding alcohol and reducing consumption of purine-rich foods. Other dietary measures include a liberal intake of liquids (2 quarts of fluid daily) to avoid kidney stones; low-fat, low-protein intake; and increased complex carbohydrate consumption. FISH OIL supplementation has been used to reduce joint inflammation. CHERRIES are claimed to relieve symptoms of gout. Gout can be treated with medications to lower uric acid blood levels, and low doses of the drug colchicine may reduce deposition of uric acid crystals in joints.

Flieger, Ken, "Getting to Know Gout," *FDA Consumer*, 29:2 (March 1995), pp. 19–22.

graded foods Eggs, milk, milk products and meat are graded according to palatability, size, color, texture, appearance and maturity by the U.S. Department of Agriculture. Food packers and processors pay for the grading service. In contrast, food inspection is mandatory for food involved in interstate commerce. Food grading is voluntary and has nothing to do with food safety. (See also FOOD, DRUG AND COSMETIC ACT; FDA.)

grain Cereal grains are members of the grass family. They include WHEAT, MILLET, OATS, RICE, RYE, SORGHUM, TRITICALE and CORN. The development of ancient civilizations relied upon the cultivation of grain, which allowed for more effective food production from the land. Wheat and barley farming began as early as 7,000 B.C. Dried grains store well, and their cultivation spread rapidly in Asia, Africa and Europe. In the New World, corn spread from Mexico into other regions of North America. Much of modern grain production is devoted to livestock feed for meat production.

Cereal grains account for about 40% of the world crop production. Americans eat about 150 pounds of grains per person a year. However, in the early 1900s the average person ate twice as much, 300 pounds a year. This decline correlates with increased consumption of SUGAR and FAT. Grains are dietary STAPLES throughout the world due to their high content of COMPLEX CARBOHYDRATE (STARCH and FIBER), their PROTEIN and the ease of cultivation. Grains generally lack VITAMIN C, VITAMIN D, VITAMIN B$_{12}$ and VITAMIN A. Yellow corn contains small amounts of BETA CAROTENE, the precursor of vitamin A. Grains are low in calcium, and their protein is generally low in the essential AMINO ACIDS such as LYSINE. In modern times cereal grain products and FLOUR have been fortified/enriched with amino acids, vitamins and minerals to increase their nutritional value.

Cereal technology involves modifying starch through malting or sprouting. Seeds are germinated to activate enzymes that partially degrade starch to sugar. This strategy is used in brewing, baking and the production of distilled alcoholic beverages. Milling refers to grinding and/or crushing (rolling) grains to remove fibrous hulls and to produce meal or flour for baking. Products from cereal grains include BREAD and other baked goods, BREAKFAST CEREAL, FLOUR, infant cereal, and popular snack foods like CHIPS and CRACKERS.

Grain substitutes are important alternatives, particularly for those with wheat and GLUTEN sensitivities. AMARANTH, BUCKWHEAT and QUINOA are not related to grains, so cross allergies with wheat are less likely. (See also BRAN; ENRICHMENT.)

Drachman, Linda. *Great Grains*. New York: Simon and Schuster, 1990.

grain alcohol See ALCOHOL.

granola A dry, whole grain BREAKFAST CEREAL and snack food. There are many variations of granola. Typically, commercial varieties contain rolled OATS, HONEY, nuts and dried fruit like DATES. Often COCONUT OIL and PALM OIL are added to make the mixture tastier. These granolas are often high in fat and sugar and may provide more CALORIES than other breakfast cereals.

granulated sugar See TABLE SUGAR.

grape (*Vitus*) A pulpy, smooth-skinned berry, growing in clusters on vines. The grape was domesticated before 5,000 B.C. and is one of the oldest cultivated fruits. The three basic types of grapes are European, North American and hybrids. Seeded and seedless varieties are available. North American grapes are hardy, disease-resistant varieties, including *Vitis abrusca* (Catawba, Concord, Delaware and Niagara are common varieties). Hybrids were developed mainly for wine production. Some are adapted for table use, including Thompson seedless and Tokay/Emperor. Other varieties include Black Beauty, Calmeria (Lady fingers), Cardinal, Champagne (source of dried currants), Flame Seedless, Italia Muscat, Perlette Seedless, Red Globe and Ribier. Raisins are several varieties of sun-dried grapes. European grapes (*Vitus vinifera*) account for about 95% of grapes grown worldwide and represent the common table grape and are used in the production of famous wines. Worldwide grape production is around 67 million metric tons, 60% of which is produced by Europe. The United States accounts for about 7% of the world's production. California produces over 95% of U.S. grapes, mostly the European varieties. American grape varieties are grown primarily in New York, with Pennsylvania, Michigan, Kansas and Washington also contributing.

Grapes are traditionally used in wine making because their high sugar (GLUCOSE) and low acid content make them ideal for fermentation. The best wine-making grapes contain 18 to 24% sugar and 0.5 to 1.5% acidic substances. The acidity decreases and sweetness increases with ripening. Grapes provide low to moderate amounts of vitamins and minerals, but some varieties provide substantial VITAMIN C and FIBER. Red and purple grapes contain anthocyanin, a form of flavonoid that functions as an antioxidant. Food value of 10 seedless grapes (50 g): calories, 35; protein, 0.3 g; carbohydrate, 8.9 g; fiber, 1.0 g; potassium, 105 mg; vitamin C, 5.4 mg; thiamin 0.05 mg; riboflavin, 0.03 mg; niacin, 0.15 mg.

grapefruit (*Citrus paradisi*)   A large yellow-skinned member of the citrus family. A grapefruit can weigh between 2 and 12 pounds, with a diameter ranging from 3 to 6 inches. The yellowish white or pink pulp is juicy and characteristically bitter.

Grapefruit originated in Barbados in the 18th century. Later mutations yielded the Thompson seedless pink variety (1913) and Ruby seedless red variety (1929). The U.S. produces 50% of the world's grapefruit crop. Florida leads in domestic grapefruit production, providing 80% of the U.S. crop. More than half of the domestic crop is processed as grapefruit juice, juice concentrate and canned grapefruit sections. One of the most popular eating varieties is the Marsh Seedless, which yields pink and red grapefruits (Pink Seedless and Ruby Red Seedless). Star Ruby is a newer red variety. Red and pink grapefruit owe their color to small amounts of beta carotene, enough to supply 5 to 12% of the RDA of Vitamin A. Grapefruit is an excellent source of FLAVONOID, a plant material that serves as an antioxidant and anti-inflammatory agent. The flavonoid that contributes most of the bitter taste of grapefruit is called naringin. Grapefruit also provides pectin, a form of soluble fiber that can lower cholesterol levels in blood, in addition to potassium, and VITAMIN C. Grapefruit juice provides vitamin C but not, of course, the fiber of the whole fruit. Food value for half a fruit with peel: calories, 37; protein, 0.8 g; carbohydrate, 9.9 g; fiber, 1.5 g; vitamin C, 47 mg; potassium, 175 mg; thiamin, 0.04 mg; riboflavin, 0.02 mg; niacin, 0.32 mg. One cup of grapefruit juice, sweetened, canned, provides 115 calories; protein, 1.4 g; carbohydrate, 28 g; potassium, 405 mg; vitamin C, 67 mg; thiamin, 0.1 mg; riboflavin, 0.06 mg; niacin, 0.8 mg. (See also CITRUS FRUIT.)

grape juice   One of the sweetest juices. Grape juice is made from crushed grapes. A purple-colored juice indicates that it was prepared from grapes with purple skins, usually Concord grapes. Usually grape juice provides no VITAMIN C unless it has been added by the manufacturer. Because of its high sugar content, an 8-oz glass of grape juice provides 128 to 155 calories, higher than orange juice. If the label specifies "grape juice" it must contain 100% juice. Any other wording such as "drink" or "punch" indicates that the product contains little grape juice and is a mixture of sugar (corn syrup) and water. One cup of grape juice, bottled, provides 155 calories; protein, 1.4 g; carbohydrate, 38 g; fiber, 1.26 g; potassium, 160 mg; thiamin, 0.05 mg; riboflavin, 0.03 mg; niacin, 0.15 mg.

grapeseed oil   An oil extracted from seeds after grapes have been pressed to prepare wine or grape juice. Grapeseed oil is sometimes marketed as an alternative to olive oil. In individuals with elevated serum CHOLESTEROL on low-fat diets, this oil may raise the level of HIGH-DENSITY LIPOPROTEIN (HDL), the desirable form of cholesterol, without affecting overall cholesterol levels. A variety of materials in foods, such as soluble FIBER in OAT bran and PSYLLIUM, can lower LOW-DENSITY LIPOPROTEIN (LDL) cholesterol, but few foods have been shown to raise HDL levels. Moderate alcohol consumption and some cholesterol lowering drugs have been shown to raise HDL. (See also ATHEROSCLEROSIS; DIETARY GUIDELINES FOR AMERICANS.)

grape sugar   See GLUCOSE.

GRAS   See "GENERALLY RECOGNIZED AS SAFE."

green number 3   See ARTIFICIAL FOOD COLORS.

Green Revolution   A period between the late 1960s and early 1970s when high-yield cereal grains and synthetic fertilizers were exported to developing nations with the aim of increasing crop production. Advances in farming technology in the 1960s offered the potential of doubling or even tripling grain production in certain regions in developing countries. This technology, in conjunction with international agricultural research centers that produced new varieties of WHEAT, CORN and RICE, could dramatically improve production per acre of cultivated land. Many special varieties of cereal grains required extra water, fertilizer and PESTICIDES to obtain maximum yields. By the 1970s petrochemical pesticides and fertilizers and widespread irrigation in developing nations permitted massive crop cultivation and high productivity. It is estimated that the Green Revolution was responsible for an extra 50 million tons of grain annually.

More recent advances pose the prospect of a second Green Revolution, and biotechnology is capable of producing new plant strains with desirable qualities. However, the question remains whether technology alone will eradicate HUNGER in the world. The Green Revolution did not address the questions of high birth rates and population growth, illiteracy, disenfranchised small farmers, poverty, inadequate food distribution, civil strife or the increased resistance of insects to pesticides. Malnutrition often occurred as cereal grains displaced legumes in the food supply in some developing countries. In addition to advances in agricultural technology, political and economical solutions are also needed to overcome world hunger.

In a shift of emphasis, 13 international agricultural research centers, working under the Consultative Group on International Agricultural Research, embarked upon a plan to broaden their focus (1990). They emphasize management of natural resources, including forestry, fisheries, irrigation management and farming systems research. (See also GENETIC ENGINEERING.)

Walsh, John, "The Greening of the Green Revolution," *Science*, 252 (April 5, 1991), p, 26.

grits   Coarsely ground cereal grain, from which the outer layer (BRAN) and nutrient-rich germ have been removed. Grits are more finely ground than groats, although both have had their hulls removed. Grits from CORN are known as hominy grits. Grits are also prepared from BUCKWHEAT, RYE, OATS and RICE.

In contrast, groats represent larger fragments of hulled grains. Groats can be prepared from buckwheat, oats, BARLEY, WHEAT, and corn. Cracked wheat refers to either wheat groats or grits. Buckwheat groats, also known as KASHA, are commonly used.

ground beef   See HAMBURGER.

growth hormone (GH, somatotropin)   A hormone that primarily stimulates growth and maturation of tissues, rather than controlling the developmental processes. When growth hormone is administered to elderly men, their short-term and long-term memory improves; their body fat diminishes and their lean body mass (muscle) increases. Growth hormone is the only hormone produced by the anterior pituitary that does not affect other hormone-secreting glands. It increases protein synthesis, as well as fat and carbohydrate utilization, and it increases amino acid uptake in muscles. Growth hormone enhances bone synthesis and the formation of red blood cells.

Growth hormone release follows a circadian rhythm: Blood levels peak during sleep and decline during the day. EXERCISE increases growth hormone production. It is regulated by "growth hormone release inhibiting factor" and "growth hormone releasing factor" from the HYPOTHALAMUS, the part of the brain that regulates the PITUITARY GLAND, the master gland of the ENDOCRINE SYSTEM (hormone secreting glands). (See also AGING; ANABOLISM; BOVINE GROWTH HORMONE.)

Lambert, M.I., et al., "Failure of Commercial Oral Amino Acid Supplements to Increase Serum Growth Hormone Concentrations in Male Body-builders," *International Journal of Sport Nutrition*, 3:3 (September 1993), pp. 298–305.

growth promoters   See ANIMAL DRUGS IN MEAT.

GTF   See GLUCOSE TOLERANCE FACTOR.

guanine   A nitrogen-containing base that is a building block of DNA and RNA. Guanine in one DNA chain pairs with ADENINE in a second (complementary) DNA strand. This specificity between strands of DNA helps direct the replication of DNA and the formation of RNA, which directs protein synthesis. Guanine also forms guanosine triphosphate, GTP, a high-energy compound like ATP, required as an energy source for protein synthesis, activating internal enzymes when regulatory molecules like hormones bind to the outer cell surface, and other processes.

Guanine is not a dietary essential, because it is readily synthesized in the body from three amino acids (ASPARTIC ACID, GLYCINE and GLUTAMINE) together with derivatives of the coenzyme of FOLIC ACID (tetrahydrofolate). It is also salvaged and reused by the body. Guanine occurs in all plant and animal foods, especially organ meats like liver and glandular tissues, and also in seeds. It is degraded by the body to URIC ACID and excreted. (See also DISODIUM GUANYLATE; GOUT; PURINE.)

guar gum   A vegetable GUM used as a thickening agent. Guar gum is obtained from the guar plant, *Composia teragonolobus*, grown in India and the United States. Guar gum is a form of soluble FIBER and contains long chains composed of the sugars MANNOSE and GALACTOSE. Guar gum dissolves in cold water, readily forms gels and is one of the most widely used gum stabilizers in foods. It is used commercially to thicken beverages, ICE CREAM, gravies, salad dressing, doughs and batters, snack foods and even pet foods, and it provides resiliency to dough, batters and artificial whipped cream. Guar gum is considered a safe additive.

Guar gum gel may help lower blood cholesterol. It has been used as an appetite suppressant; because it swells in water, it has also been used as a BULKING AGENT to promote the sensation of being full. It does not help prevent constipation because it slows movement of material through the gastrointestinal tract. Unlike bran, guar gum is broken down in the gut by gut microorganisms.

Groop, Per-Henrik, et al., "Long Term Effects of Guar Gum in Subjects with Non-insulin-dependent Diabetes Mellitus," *American Journal of Clinical Nutrition*, 58:4 (1993), pp. 513–18.

guava (*Psidium guajava*)   A round, yellow to white, aromatic fruit that is a native of the Caribbean. Guavas are cultivated in tropical regions and in California and Florida. Guavas range in size from that of a cherry to that of an apple. The pulp is generally white, though some varieties produce a crimson pulp. The fruit is used in fruit salads and fruit juices, in jam, jelly and pie fillings, and as a condiment for meat dishes. Guavas are an excellent source of soluble fiber (pectin), which can help lower blood cholesterol, and of vitamin C. The nutrient content per 3.5 oz (100 g) serving is 60 calories; protein, 0.77 g; carbohydrate, 14.5 g; fat, 0.57 g; vitamin A, 285 retinol equivalents; vitamin C, 234 mg; niacin, 1.12 mg; thiamin, 0.051 mg; riboflavin, 0.046 mg.

guidelines   See DIETARY GUIDELINES FOR AMERICANS.

gum   A form of fiber used as a FOOD ADDITIVE. Gums form gels and are used by manufacturers to thicken and stabilize many foods, including ice cream, whipping cream, dough, gravies, salad dressing and snack foods. Gums are also used to change food textures and to increase the moisture-holding capacity in canned meats. Several gums have been used as bulking agents to avoid constipation. Because they swell in water and increase the feeling of satiety, some have also been used as APPETITE SUPPRESSANTS. Gums consist of long chains of sugar units, such as glucose, galactose and sugar acids, linked together, thus representing a form of COMPLEX CARBOHYDRATE. Some gums contain repeating units of multiple sugars.

Natural gums occur in microorganisms and in plant cell walls. Gums are often secreted by plants to heal wounds in the bark. Gums from tree extracts include arabic, ghatti, karaya, larch and tragacanth. Certain gums occur in seeds, including guar, locust bean, psyllium and quince. AGAR, algin, CARRAGEENAN and FURCELLERAN represent gums isolated from species of seaweed. Microbial fermentation produces XANTHAN GUM, while beta glucan is derived from OATS and BARLEY. Synthetic gums are made of chemically modified CELLULOSE, microcrystalline cellulose, carboxymethylcellulose and modified starches, such as carboxymethyl starch and hydroxyethyl starch. Chemically modified versions of ALGINATES, PECTIN, locust bean gum, and GUAR GUM are also employed as thickeners.

Gums are classified as water-soluble FIBER, and they exert several important physiologic effects:

1. Increased glucose tolerance. Soluble fibers such as guar gum and pectin reduce the rate at which glucose is absorbed by the intestine when mixed with foods, and they have been used in the diets of diabetics to decrease blood glucose levels after a meal. Guar gum reduces blood glucose levels and insulin responses to an oral glucose load.
2. Slowed lipid absorption. Soluble fiber and gums slow fat digestion.
3. Lowered cholesterol. Guar gum, GUM ARABIC, oat gum and pectin lower blood cholesterol levels. Since gums bind BILE salts, synthesized from cholesterol, it has been proposed that they reduce the reabsorption, and thus reutilization, of cholesterol and bile acids by the liver. According to this theory, cholesterol would be diverted to bile salt synthesis and excretion away from the blood. Gums may therefore indirectly increase the ability of the liver to remove cholesterol from the blood.
4. Colonic fermentation. Gums are degraded by intestinal bacteria to simple sugars that are fermented to short-chain, saturated fatty acids (ACETIC ACID, PROPIONIC ACID, BUTYRIC ACID). These supply substantial fuel for the colonic mucosal cells and the body. (See also GUM GHATTI.)

gum arabic (acacia)   A soluble GUM obtained from the acacia tree in Sudan. Gum-arabic is a form of complex carbohydrate (polysaccharide) containing GALACTOSE and acidic derivatives of GLUCOSE, among other sugars. Gum arabic is used to stabilize buttered syrup and dry mixes (like pancake mixes and powdered drinks), ice cream and the foam in beer. It is used to prevent granulation of candy and helps dissolve oils like flavors in soft drinks. Like other natural gums, it is not digested but is fermented by colon bacteria. Occasionally gum arabic causes an allergic reaction. Gum arabic is considered a safe FOOD ADDITIVE, though few tests to establish long-term safety have been performed.

gum disease   See GINGIVITIS.

gum ghatti   A vegetable GUM produced by a tree found in India (anogeissus). It is a form of complex carbohydrate (polysaccharide) and contains xylose, GALACTOSE, MANNOSE and an acid derivative of GLUCOSE as building blocks. Relatively small amounts are imported for use in salad dressing and butter-flavored syrups. (See also FIBER; FOOD ADDITIVES.)

haddock (*Melanogrammus aeglefinus*)   A lean saltwater FISH related to COD, though smaller. Haddock is an important food fish; its white flesh has a pleasant, somewhat bland taste. Haddock can be prepared in any recipe for cod or FLOUNDER. Smoked haddock is called finnan haddie. Haddock is an excellent source of high-quality PROTEIN; raw, 3.5 oz (100 g) = 79 calories; protein, 18.3 g; fat, 0.66 g; calcium, 23 mg; cholesterol, 60 mg; niacin, 3 mg; thiamin, 0.04 mg; riboflavin, 0.06 mg.

hair analysis   A convenient, reasonably inexpensive, preliminary screening tool for detecting mineral imbalances, to be confirmed by other diagnostic tests. Minerals accumulate in hair as it grows. Hair analysis can be used in the early screening for accumulated toxic metals, including MERCURY, ALUMINUM, COPPER, LEAD and CADMIUM. It has also been used to assess body levels of trace minerals (iron, copper, manganese, zinc) and to compare minerals in populations living in different regions with differing degrees of pollution and soil depletion of minerals. These hair samples are easily obtainable, and analytical methods (atomic absorption spectrometry, X-ray fluorescence spectrometry, among others) are sufficiently sensitive to permit accurate analysis of small samples.

Hair analysis is a controversial test. Some laboratories do not provide reproducible results, and hair is easily contaminated with shampoo, conditioners, dyes and air pollutants. Findings have been overinterpreted: as an example, hair levels of some MINERALS like SODIUM and POTASSIUM do not correlate with body levels. (See also HEAVY METALS.)

halibut (*Hippoglossus*)   A saltwater FISH found in all oceans. Halibut is one of the most important food fish. It is flat and resembles a huge FLOUNDER. The lean flesh is firm with pleasant flavor and texture. Halibut liver oil is an excellent source of VITAMIN A and VITAMIN D, and is a primary commercial source of these vitamins. Food value of 3.5 oz (100 g) raw has: calories, 100; protein, 19.0 g; fat, 1.1 g; calcium, 13 mg; cholesterol, 50 mg; niacin, 8.3 mg.

ham   The rear leg of a hog. Ham is a red MEAT containing 34% of total calories derived from FAT, classified as saturated, and provides high-quality PROTEIN together with many VITAMINS and MINERALS. Dietary guidelines recommend minimizing foods whose fat calories account for more than 30% of the total. The glistening greenish sheen on the surface of sliced ham is a sign of oxidation, not necessarily spoilage.

To minimize SODIUM intake, reduce consumption of all cured pork products, including ham. Roasted ham contains per 3 oz (85 g): calories, 207; protein, 18.3 g; fat, 14.2 g; cholesterol, 53 mg; iron, 0.74 mg; sodium, 1,009 mg; zinc, 1.97 mg; thiamin, 0.51 mg; niacin 3.8 mg; riboflavin, 0.21 mg. For comparison lean, roasted ham contains per 3 oz: calories, 133; protein, 21.3 g; fat, 4.7 g; and sodium, 1,128 mg. Canned ham contains per 3 oz: calories, 140; protein, 17.8 g; fat, 7.2 g; sodium, 908 mg. (See also DIETARY GUIDELINES FOR AMERICANS; FAT, HIDDEN; FATTY ACIDS.)

hamburger   Ground BEEF to which beef fat (beef tallow) can be added to bring the fat content up to 30% by weight.

Hamburger is the most commonly eaten MEAT in the United States, representing a major contributor of total fat and saturated fat to the average diet. The average fat in lean ground beef is 21%, while extra-lean hamburger contains 15% fat. When fat is drained after cooking, both regular hamburger and extra-lean have about the same cooked weight. Hamburger can be prepared from fresh or frozen beef, and seasoning may be added. Water extenders or binders cannot legally be added. Only 12 states presently require that the fat content of ground beef be listed on food labels. DIETARY GUIDELINES FOR AMERICANS recommends that healthy Americans reduce their consumption of saturated fat. Hamburger and ground beef need to be cooked thoroughly to destroy possible disease producing strains of the bacterium E. coli 0157,H7, a leading cause of bloody diarrhea in the United States.

There is no fixed definition of ground beef, which can also contain up to 30% fat by weight. However, fat cannot be added to ground beef. If ground beef is designated on the label as being derived from a particular cut of meat, then the product must consist of beef derived entirely from the cut so identified.

As a lower fat alternative to hamburger, request ground round roast or top round steak. These cuts of meat contain only 6% fat, representing 29% of the total calories. Food value of "lean" hamburger, per 3 oz (85 g) broiled is: calories, 230; protein, 21 g; fat, 16 g; cholesterol, 74 mg; calcium, 9 mg; iron, 1.8 mg; zinc, 3.74 mg; riboflavin, 0.18 mg; niacin, 4.41 mg; thiamin, 0.04 mg; B_6, 0.39 mg. For "regular" hamburger, the value per 3 oz (85 g) broiled is: calories, 245; protein, 20 g; fat 17.8 g; cholesterol, 76 mg. (See also ANTIBIOTICS; CHOLESTEROL.)

hard cider   See CIDER.

hardening of the arteries   See ARTERIOSCLEROSIS.

hard water   See WATER.

hawthorn (*Crataegus oxyacantha*)   A spiny tree or hedge whose berries have medicinal properties. Hawthorn is native to Europe. Folk traditions describe the use of berries and flowers as beneficial supplements for INFLAMMATION ranging from ARTHRITIS to sore throats; for vascular conditions such as angina, hypertension (high blood pressure) and ATHEROSCLEROSIS (clogged arteries). Substances in hawthorn extracts inhibit constriction of blood vessels and strengthen arterial walls, thereby possibly protecting against plaque deposits.

Hawthorn berries and blossoms contain FLAVONOIDS, particularly anthocyanins and proanthocyanins, colored pigments of berries including blueberries, cherries and grapes. These flavonoid compounds stabilize collagen, the primary structural protein of connective tissue, as well as of tendons, cartilage and ligaments. They act as antioxidants, prevent free radical (oxidative) damage, and prevent the release and synthesis of substances that promote inflammation, such as prostaglandins, histamines and leukotrienes.

HCl   See STOMACH ACID.

HDL   See HIGH-DENSITY LIPOPROTEIN.

head cheese   A cold cut prepared from the MEAT of calf and pig heads, including cheeks, snouts, lips and possibly brains, hearts, tongues and feet. Cooked meat, stripped from bones, is ground, seasoned and then pressed to create a single jellied mass. (See also BEEF; FOOD PROCESSING; HAM.)

heart attack (myocardial infarction, MI)   A condition resulting from the blockage of a coronary artery, an artery feeding the heart. When oxygen supplied to the heart muscle becomes limited, the tissue may be irreparably damaged. Symptoms include prolonged pressure or painful tightness at the center of the chest, possibly spreading to the left arm and shoulder and to the neck and jaw. There may also be nausea and vomiting, shortness of breath and sweating. The odds of heart attack increase with well-established risk factors: a family history of heart disease; being male; high blood pressure; obesity; diabetes; increasing age; cigarette smoking; low folic acid; a high intake of saturated fat; a sedentary life-style; and repressed anger/anxiety. A healthful diet, regular exercise, stress management, social and emotional support, maintaining a desirable body weight, avoiding smoking, and a semi-vegetarian type of diet with reduced fat are recommended.

Blood clots are one of the dangers of clogged arteries. When clots lodge in arteries feeding the heart, they block blood flow. The heart requires a constant supply of nutrients and oxygen from the blood, and being deprived of oxygen even briefly will damage the heart muscle.

It is critically important to secure immediate medical care for a heart attack by dialing 911. Many heart attack patients die before they get to the hospital, and delays in summoning help can be costly. (See also ATHEROSCLEROSIS; BLOOD CLOTTING; CHOLESTEROL; CORONARY ARTERY DISEASE; HOMOCYSTEINE; STROKE.)

Morrison H. I., et al, "Serum Folate and Risk of Fatal Coronary Heart Disease," *Journal of the American Medical Association*, 275:24 (June 26, 1996), pp. 1893–96.

U.S. Department of Health, Education and Welfare, *How Doctors Diagnose Heart Disease*. Washington, D.C.: DHEW Publication No. (NIH) 78-753.

heartburn   See ACID INDIGESTION.

heart disease   See ATHEROSCLEROSIS; CARDIOVASCULAR DISEASE; CORONARY ARTERY DISEASE; HEART ATTACK; STROKE.

heart-healthy diet   See CHOLESTEROL; DIETARY GUIDELINES FOR AMERICANS.

heat inactivation   The loss of biological activity of a substance, such as an ENZYME, when heated to sufficiently high temperatures. In the case of enzymes, heat alters structures critical for catalysts. COOKING at high temperatures destroys vitamins such as VITAMIN C, FOLIC ACID and THIAMIN. Through oxidation or other chemical changes, polyunsaturated FATTY ACIDS and even CHOLESTEROL become oxidized when heated at sufficiently high temperature in the presence of air. The essential AMINO ACID, LYSINE, is partially destroyed when grain protein and carbohydrate are heated together. Several processed BREAKFAST CEREALS contain less lysine than present in flour because they have been baked.

heavy metals Industrial chemicals of LEAD, MERCURY, CADMIUM, CHROMIUM, NICKEL, antimony and ARSENIC. These chemicals are general enzyme poisons, and the toxic effects of these industrial wastes is well established. As an example, lead exposure causes ANEMIA by blocking a key step in the synthesis of HEMOGLOBIN, required for the formation of RED BLOOD CELLS.

As a general rule, the greater the exposure to a toxic metal, the greater the risk of poisoning. Widespread pollution has created chronic low-level exposure in many regions of the United States, thus increasing the risk of heavy metal poisoning. Therefore, minimizing heavy metal exposure in air, food and WATER can lead to dramatic, long-term health benefits.

Nutrients like sulfur-containing amino acids, selenium and VITAMIN C seem to have the ability to counteract heavy metals in the body, while diets low in CALCIUM, IRON or ZINC increase lead uptake. The body has several defense mechanisms against toxic exposure. One of these is metallothionens, proteins rich in the sulfur amino acid CYSTEINE that bind heavy metals and speed their removal. Metallothionen synthesis is triggered by exposure to heavy metal ions. The following are specific examples of common toxic metals:

Arsenic, which occurs in PESTICIDES, smog and cigarette smoke, is believed to interfere with neurological development, and high doses increase the risk of some types of cancer. Cadmium may cause high blood pressure and heart abnormalities, bronchitis, lung fibrosis and emphysema. Small amounts are common in consumer items ranging from cigarettes and pesticides to food. Drinking water may be contaminated with cadmium because soft water dissolves the cadmium in galvanized pipes.

Lead exposure leads to distractibility, DIARRHEA, irritability and lethargy. More serious consequences are smaller fetal brain size, increased BIRTH DEFECTS, decreased IQ, anemia, CHRONIC FATIGUE, aching limbs, kidney disease and sometimes coma. Though the U.S. EPA banned leaded paints and has required lowered lead levels in gasoline, Americans still are exposed to lead through drinking water, glazed ceramic dinnerware, old paint and decades of environmental pollution.

Selenium is a water and soil contaminant in some regions of the United States. In trace amounts, the appropriate chemical form of selenium is an essential nutrient. However, the margin of safety of selenium is small, and ingesting only five times the level deemed safe and adequate can cause toxic side effects. (See also BREASTFEEDING.)

height-weight tables Standards of weight and height by age used to assess an appropriate body weight for normal people. Several different tables have been developed. The Metropolitan Life Insurance Company assembled the best-known height-weight table, based upon the heights and weights of policy holders. It was later realized that weight depends upon body build; therefore, values for an "IDEAL BODY WEIGHT" were adjusted by including different values for "small," "medium" and "large" body sizes. Since ideal body weight implies making a judgment and is subjective, a more liberal version of these tables was published in 1983, based on data obtained from 1959 to 1983. The 1983 revision came up with a "desirable body weight" that is 10% greater than that on the older table. This revision suggests that a woman of average frame and average height (5 feet 4 inches) wearing 3 pounds of clothing and wearing one-inch heels would weigh 126 to 138 pounds. For an average male (5 feet 9 inches tall, wearing 5 pounds of clothing), the range is 148 to 160 pounds.

Several limitations of life insurance tables restrict their usefulness. Their weights are based on values that were simply reported, not measured. Insurance policy holders for whom the data were collected do not represent the whole U.S. population. High blood pressure, smoking and diabetes—factors that can affect general health and body weight—are not considered. There is no firm definition of "frame size." Thus, tables of this kind represent a subjective evaluation. The tables would suggest that a wide range of weights (30 to 40 pounds) poses no risk, in contradiction to common experience. Newer information indicates that excess FAT, not weight, is critical. Furthermore, it is important to establish how the fat is distributed in order to assess risks. (See also BODY MASS INDEX; OBESITY.)

Helicobacter pylori (*Campylobacter pylori*) A spiral-shaped bacterium that can infect the stomach and cause GASTRIC ULCERS, duodenal ulcers and symptomatic, as well as atrophic GASTRITIS (stomach inflammation). While stomach acid kills many bacteria, *H. pylori* burrows deep into the mucus layer to the underlying mucosal cell surface, where it is protected from stomach acid. Fifty percent of Americans over the age of 50, and 75% of subjects older than 65 have antibodies against *H. pylori*, suggesting a wide prevalence of infection. While many adults exhibit evidence of antibodies to this bacterium, it is not clear why only a small percentage develop duodenal ulcers. On the other hand, irradication of *H. pylori* with bismuth compounds combined with several antibiotics decreases the risk of ulcer relapse and yields a significant improvement in ulcers and stomach inflammation. Almost 90% of patients with the most common type of stomach CANCER, intestinal-type gastric adenocarcinoma, are infected with *H. pylori*. It is not known whether *H. pylori* actually causes cancer, however. Several population studies support the theory that this bacterium is associated with stomach cancer. (See also GASTROINTESTINAL DISORDERS.)

Graham, D.Y. and Go, M.F., "Helicobacter Pylori: Current Status," *Gastroenterology*, 105 (1993), pp. 279–82.

hematocrit A clinical lab test used to assess the health of red blood cells. The hematocrit represents the volume of packed red blood cells, expressed as the percentage of total blood volume. For men the average hematocrit is 47%, with a range of 40 to 54%, and for women the average is 42%, with a range of 37 to 47%. Children's hematocrit varies depending on the age. Serious fluid loss without cell loss, as in DEHYDRATION, raises the hematocrit, while blood loss or ANEMIA lowers the hematocrit. (See also HEMOGLOBIN.)

heme An IRON-containing red pigment found in red blood cells. HEMOGLOBIN, the oxygen transport protein of blood, requires heme to bind molecular oxygen reversibly. Heme also functions as a helper group of CYTOCHROMES, enzymes responsible for transporting electrons in energy-generating reactions of MITOCHONDRIA.

Heme is synthesized in the bone marrow by the parents of red blood cells (reticulo-endothelial cells). Iron is bound within a complex ring structure, synthesized from small building blocks: GLYCINE, the simplest AMINO ACID, and SUCCINIC ACID, produced from fat and carbohydrate breakdown. Heme synthesis requires VITAMIN B$_6$, and LEAD inhibits the process. Therefore vitamin B$_6$ deficiency and lead poisoning cause ANEMIA. When the spleen removes wornout red blood cells it converts heme to the BILE PIGMENT, bilirubin, and recycles the released iron.

Much of the iron in meat, fish and poultry occurs as heme, which is readily absorbed by the intestine. Absorption of this heme iron is not diminished by PHYTIC ACID, a metal binder occurring in certain plant materials, nor is it increased by VITAMIN C. In contrast, most of the iron in vegetables is not bound to heme and is less readily absorbed. The efficiency of non-heme iron absorption from plant sources is only 10 to 20% that of heme iron. Vitamin C increases the uptake of iron from non-heme sources. Some forms of FIBER bind minerals and lower intestinal absorption of non-heme iron.

hemicellulose   A form of dietary FIBER, plant material resistant to digestive enzymes. Hemicellulose helps form plant cell walls. Annual plants contain 15 to 30% hemicellulose by dry weight in their cell walls, while wood contains 20 to 25% hemicellulose. Dietary sources of hemicellulose include FRUIT, vegetables, LEGUMES, cereal, BRAN, wholegrain flours, nuts and seeds. Dietary hemicelluloses absorb water, provide bulk and soften stools. They are broken down by intestinal bacteria. Excessive amounts of hemicelluloses may interfere with mineral absorption.

Hemicellulose is structurally distinct from water-soluble fibers such as gums and pectin and insoluble fiber like CELLULOSE. Hemicellulose contains long chains of repeating sugar units. Pentosans are chains of PENTOSES, five-carbon sugars like xylose and arabinose. Pentosans form the largest group and occur in cereal grains. Galactosans, chains of the simple sugar GALACTOSE, form a second group. Acidic hemicelluloses also occur in food.

hemochromatosis   A rare condition caused by excessive IRON deposits in tissues, including the LIVER, PANCREAS and skin. Symptoms include liver enlargement, weakness, moderate weight loss, bronzed skin, diabetes and eventually heart failure. Hemochromatosis is 10 times more frequent in men than in women.

Abnormal iron metabolism can be caused by a genetic defect (primary hemochromatosis) characterized by increased accumulation of iron in tissues. The inherited trait for iron storage disease is relatively common among whites, affecting perhaps as many as one person in two hundred. This suggests that the tendency to accumulate dietary iron is a more general problem in the U.S. than generally recognized. Alternatively, excessive iron consumption can lead to abnormally high iron storage (secondary hemochromatosis). This can occur with chronic iron supplementation in men, because they do not usually lose iron, and in alcoholics, because several alcoholic beverages contain iron. (See also FERRITIN.)

Herbert, Victor, "Everyone Should Be Tested for Iron Disorders," *Journal of the American Dietetic Association*, 92:12 (1992), pp. 1502–09.

hemoglobin   The oxygen transport protein of blood and the predominant protein in red blood cells. Hemoglobin is a complex PROTEIN; it contains a total of four individual amino acid chains called globins. Adult hemoglobin contains two alpha globin chains and two beta globin chains. Hemoglobin also contains the iron-containing pigment HEME, which is required to bind oxygen. Heme imparts a red color to hemoglobin and to red blood cells.

Hemoglobin is a dynamic molecule and changes its shape and oxygen-carrying characteristics to help regulate oxygen delivery and blood pH. It binds oxygen when the oxygen concentration is high in blood exposed to air in the lungs. Next, arteries carry oxygen-rich red blood cells from the lungs to capillaries, where hemoglobin responds by releasing more of its bound oxygen (the Bohr effect). The released oxygen then diffuses into cells to enable them to continue the oxidation of fuel molecules. During this process of shedding oxygen molecules hemoglobin binds carbon dioxide and hydrogen ions and returns them to the lungs via the veins. In the lungs hemoglobin picks up more oxygen and simultaneously releases carbon dioxide and hydrogen ions.

An adult normally produces 6.25 g of hemoglobin daily. The hemoglobin blood content of women is 12 to 16 g per 100 ml of blood, and of men, 14 to 18 g. ANEMIA is a deficiency of normal red blood cells. Deficiencies of IRON, VITAMIN A, VITAMIN B$_6$, VITAMIN B$_{12}$, VITAMIN D, VITAMIN E and FOLIC ACID may cause anemia.

Over 400 mutant hemoglobins are known. Most do not alter normal physiological function of hemoglobin. However, certain mutations lead to abnormal hemoglobins that malfunction and produce fragile red blood cells and, consequently, anemia, including sickle cell anemia and thalassemias. Alteration of a single amino acid in a chain of 146 amino acids causes sickle cell anemia.

Environmental factors can decrease hemoglobin function. Carbon monoxide poisons hemoglobin, and cigarette smokers' blood contains much more carbon monoxide than that of non-smokers. Furthermore, babies born to smoking women are smaller than average because they receive less oxygen during fetal development. (See also ERYTHROPOIESIS; HEMATOCRIT.)

Davie, Sarah J., et al., "Effect of Vitamin C on Glycosylation of Proteins," *Diabetes*, 41 (1992), pp. 167–73.

hemolytic anemia   A deficiency of red blood cells caused by their rapid destruction and characterized by chronic fatigue. Typically, hemoglobin breakdown products accumulate, leading to JAUNDICE, the accumulation of yellow pigment in the skin and in the whites of the eyes. Rapid turnover of red blood cells may be caused by genetic diseases that lead to the production of abnormal HEMOGLOBIN, as in sickle cell ANEMIA and thalassemias. Defects in red blood cell enzymes can also cause hemolytic anemia. A deficiency of one such enzyme, glucose-6-phosphate dehydrogenase that helps maintain adequate levels of GLUTATHIONE, a cellular ANTIOXIDANT, is the most common of these defects. Acquired hemolytic anemia can be caused by exposure to potentially damaging chemicals, including certain drugs (antimalarials, pimaquine and Atrabine). (See also IRON.)

hemolytic-uremic syndrome   See ESCHERICHIA COLI.

hemosiderosis   A condition associated with excessive iron deposition, particularly in the LIVER and spleen. Hemosiderin is the insoluble iron complex formed in the liver with iron accumulation. Hemosiderosis can be caused by:

1. excessive red blood breakdown associated with chronic infection, malaria, hemolytic anemias, PERNICIOUS ANEMIA or multiple blood transfusions;
2. excessive uptake of dietary iron;
3. impaired utilization of iron.

Under severe conditions, with extreme accumulation of iron, the resulting disease is called HEMOCHROMATOSIS. This condition in turn causes liver damage and pancreatic damage, which can lead to DIABETES.

heparin   A carbohydrate that is a naturally occurring anticoagulant (prevents blood from clotting). Heparin is produced by mast cells (cells that also contain inflammatory agents like histamine) in connective tissue, the liver and certain white blood cells. Heparin prevents the formation of FIBRIN clots. (Fibrin is the insoluble protein produced when blood clotting is triggered.) In capillaries, heparin also activates the lipoprotein LIPASE, the enzyme that releases FATTY ACIDS from CHYLOMICRONS and VERY-LOW-DENSITY LIPOPROTEINS, particles that transport fat in the blood. (See also FAT METABOLISM; GLYCOSAMINOGLYCANS.)

hepatic   Refers to the LIVER.

hepatitis   Chronic inflammation of the LIVER. Symptoms include JAUNDICE, liver enlargement, fever and gastrointestinal disturbances. Hepatitis can cause a loss of APPETITE, headache and a change in taste sensation. It can interfere with DIGESTION, leading to MALNUTRITION. Hepatitis can be caused by drugs, poisons and viruses.

Infectious hepatitis refers to a family of viral diseases spread orally. Hepatitis A is caused by the hepatitis A virus usually transmitted orally through fecal contamination of food utensils, due to poor hygiene by food workers who have been infected with the virus. Fecal contamination can also spread through drinking WATER. Eating shellfish contaminated by raw sewage is a common cause of infectious hepatitis. The long incubation period, three to six weeks, makes it difficult to associate hepatitis with a specific food. GAMMA GLOBULIN may prevent the disease, provided the shots are administered soon after exposure. Travelers to countries typified by poor sanitation may be advised to receive gamma globulin shots, which will offer protection for up to three or four months. Hepatitis E is an enteric (small intestinal) form of hepatitis that has been associated with waterborne outbreaks of hepatitis in developing countries. Other forms of hepatitis (such as hepatitis B) are spread through blood. (See also FOOD POISONING.)

Fried, M.W., "Therapy of Chronic Viral Hepatitis," *Medical Clinics of North America*, 80:5 (September 1996), pp. 957–72.

herbal medicine (botanical medicine)   The branch of medicine that emphasizes the therapeutic properties of plants. Ancient medical traditions from India (Ayurvedic Medicine) and China (Oriental Medicine) and others emphasize the health benefits of specific plants and plant products, and medicinal plants provided the foundation of the modern pharmaceutical industry. Recent environmental awareness of the diversity of species in threatened tropical rainforests has rekindled research in the pharmacological effects of indigenous plants. Although natural products, they offer the advantage of containing multiple active principles that possess a variety of often complementary properties. Often the active ingredients of herbs correct an underlying problem rather than simply treating a symptom. Most herbal preparations are considered foods by the U.S. FDA and they cannot be labeled with health claims.

Quality control is an issue with herbal preparations. Their potency is affected by the plant's age at the time of harvest, the season of harvest, the type of soil used for cultivation, the climate and the methods of storage and preparation. Producers often measure the amounts of active ingredients in a given herbal preparation or extract and then adjust the strength to a standard level to assure a reproducible activity.

The appropriate amount consumed is a second concern; an amount that is safe for an adult may not be safe for a child. Some herbs are appropriate for short-term use, and not for long periods.

A third concern is safety. According to the U.S. FDA, extracts of the following plants are potentially dangerous: arnica, belladonna (deadly nightshade), Culcana, blood root, Scotch broom, buckeye nuts, heliotrope, hemlock, henbane, jalop root, jimsonweed, lily of the valley, lobelia, mandrake, mistletoe, morning glory, periwinkle, St. John's wort, spindle bean, tonka bean, snakeroot, wormwood (once used to flavor absinthe, a liqueur).

Often foods themselves provide substances that promote health. Beyond the nutrients they contain, ONIONS, GARLIC, CHILI PEPPERS, LICORICE, TURMERIC, CRANBERRY, GINGER, DANDELION, BLUEBERRIES and cherries contain a variety of substances that fight infection, reduce the risk of cancer, stimulate the nervous system or reduce inflammation, (See also ALFALFA; CHAMOMILE; COMFREY; GINSENG; GOLDENSEAL; HAWTHORN; PEPPERMINT; SARSAPARILLA; STRAWBERRY.)

Wehrbach, M.R. and Murray, M.T. *Botanical Influences on Illness.* Tarzana, Calif.: Third Line Press, 1994.

herbicides   A diverse family of chemicals used to kill weeds during cultivation of crops. Many herbicides are suspected of causing CANCER or BIRTH DEFECTS. The health risks of herbicides are greatest for those with chronic exposure, such as farm workers and professional applicators. The following herbicides are examples currently in use:

- Alachor is a widely used herbicide and is among the most dangerous.
- Alrazine accounts for about 10% of PESTICIDE sales in the United States and was restricted by 1991. This herbicide has been found to widely contaminate underground water supplies in the United States.
- Dinoseb was subject to an emergency ban by the EPA in 1986 because of a possible link to birth defects, skin rashes, cancer and sterility in experimental animals. Because a substitute was not developed, the EPA permitted the continued use of Dinoseb on LENTILS, PEAS, CHICKPEAS, green beans and RASPBERRIES.

- Linuron is a common herbicide used on SOYBEANS, carrots, celery, asparagus, corn, potatoes and wheat. It is associated with tumors in experimental animals. Linuron frequently contaminates water supplies.
- Paraquat is used to treat fields before planting or before harvest. It is used extensively in soybean agriculture and in orchards. Paraquat cannot be washed off produce, and direct exposure to this chemical is hazardous. Inhalation of its mist causes lung inflammation and repeated exposure can lead to kidney and lung damage. It is also toxic to fish.
- 2,4-D is widely used by home owners and home gardeners to kill dandelions. It is the toxic agent in over 1,500 pesticide products. Exposure is greatest for children and animals who play in treated areas. Farmers use 2,4-D on CORN, WHEAT and hay. A recent National Cancer Institute study links this weed killer with cancer of lymphoid tissue in experimental animals. (See also DIOXIN; PESTICIDES.)

herbs   The leaves, shoots, stems and seeds of many widely distributed plants. In contrast, SPICES are prepared from the FRUIT, bark or pepper corns from tropical plants. Culinary herbs have appealing aromatic or savory characteristics and make food tasty and flavorful. In addition many herbs affect physiological processes, which is the basis for their medicinal properties. In some cases research has provided deeper insights into the active ingredients.

Culinary herbs that exhibit physiologic effects include:

- ANISE and CARAWAY may relieve gas and stomach cramps. Caraway contains carvacrol, a compound that eases muscle spasms.
- Carrot seed may relax smooth muscles, relieve stomach cramps and lower blood pressure.
- Celery seed contains phthalides, chemicals that are sedatives. Celery seed has antibiotic activity. Celery juice may lower blood pressure.
- CHERVIL contains the mild carcinogen estragole, which is also found in basil and tarragon.
- Coriander (cilantro) may lower BLOOD SUGAR and increase GLUCOSE TOLERANCE. Coriander lowers blood fat. According to folklore, it curbs bad breath.
- Dill oil reduces cramps, lowers blood pressure and slows heartbeat in experimental animals. Dill water reduces colic, according to folklore.
- FENNEL contains sulfur compounds that relieve cramps. According to folklore, it helps with colic and upset stomach.
- LOVAGE seeds, leaf and root can be steeped in boiling water to prepare a tea, used in folk medicine to reduce water retention and ease joint pain. Lovage increases urination and water loss in experimental animals.
- PARSLEY lowers blood pressure and stimulates uterine contractions in experimental animals. Parsley acts as a mild LAXATIVE and also freshens the breath. Parsley oil contains apiol and myristicin, which induce menstruation. Parsley oil can induce miscarriages and should not be administered during pregnancy.

Herbs of the mint family that exhibit physiologic effects:

- BASIL relieves FLATULENCE and gastrointestinal discomfort.

- Lemon balm is an ANTIOXIDANT. Animal studies suggest the oil relieves inflammation.
- MARJORAM may relax smooth muscles and relieve stomach cramps. According to folklore, marjoram tea eases cramps and upset stomach.
- OREGANO can function as an antiseptic. Its oil contains carvacrol, which possesses broad antimicrobial properties. It relieves upset stomach and is a smooth muscle relaxant. According to folklore, chewing oregano reduces toothache pain.
- ROSEMARY and SAGE contain strong antioxidants. Like CLOVES, oregano and GINGER, they have long been used to preserve food. Sage is used commercially to preserve salad oil and potato chips. According to folklore, rosemary aids memory and induces sleep.
- THYME contains thymol, an antiseptic. Thyme is used as a mouth wash. Oil of thyme causes dangerous side effects, however.

Bremness, Lesley. *The Complete Book of Herbs*. London: Dorling Kindersley, 1988.

hermetically sealed   Refers to food containers that do not permit entry of either microorganisms or air. For example, bottled or canned foods are hermetically sealed. (See also FOOD PROCESSING.)

herring (*Clupea harengus*)   A small, saltwater FISH related to the shad and SARDINE. It is silvery and streamlined, reaching a length of 10 in. at maturity. A freshwater variety is known as cisco. Herring is an important food fish that is also processed for animal feed. Intensive fishing practices worldwide have placed this fish in jeopardy.

Herring is an oily fish, and most of the fat is unsaturated. It is available frozen, pickled or smoked. Herring roe is used to prepare CAVIAR. Pickled herring, 3 oz (85 g), provides calories, 190; protein, 17.3 g; fat, 12.8 g; cholesterol, 66 mg; calcium, 31 mg; iron, 1.2 mg; sodium, 138 mg; zinc, 0.85 mg; vitamin A equivalents, 20; niacin, 2 mg; thiamin, 0.04 mg; riboflavin, 0.18 mg.

hesperidin   A substance found in rinds of ORANGES and lemons and in the peels of ripe fruit. A mature orange contains about a gram of hesperidin. Citrus FLAVONOIDS are commercially extracted from the pulp remaining after juicing oranges and lemons. Hesperidin is believed to strengthen capillary walls in conjunction with VITAMIN C. Like most flavonoids, it is also an ANTIOXIDANT and limits oxidative damage. (See also CITRUS FRUIT.)

heterocrine   Refers to tissues that secrete different types of materials. The PANCREAS is a notable example; it combines an endocrine function (secretion of hormones INSULIN and GLUCAGON by islet tissue directly into the blood) and an exocrine function (secretion of digestive enzymes into ducts that lead to a cavity [the intestine]). (See also ENDOCRINE SYSTEM.)

heterocyclic amines (HCAs)   A family of cancer-causing agents that occur in cooked MEAT. HCAs tend to form inside meat with longer cooking times and higher temperatures of barbecuing. They cannot be scraped off and once eaten they can become activated to attack DNA of cells, a possible first step in cancer development. HCAs can also inflame the heart.

There are several ways to minimize the risk of HCAs. Precooking hamburger for a short time before barbecuing seems to eliminate some of the compounds that can form HCAs. On the other hand, green and black tea contain tannins, bitter substances in brewed tea, that can block the ability of HCAs to damage DNA. Garlic and onions behave similarly. The green plant pigment chlorophyll can also block the damaging effects of HCAs. Supplementing with the bifidobacteria can protect the colon against HCAs. (See also CARCINOGEN.)

hexose A large class of simple sugars composed of six carbon atoms. They can serve as an energy source (provide calories). FRUCTOSE and GLUCOSE are the two most important hexoses in the diet. As BLOOD SUGAR, glucose is the most important CARBOHYDRATE fuel in the body. Hexoses also function as building blocks for more complex sugars and for important large molecular weight carbohydrates (polysaccharides). Thus, fructose is linked to glucose in SUCROSE (table sugar), and LACTOSE contains two hexoses, GALACTOSE and glucose. Polymerized MANNOSE is found in glucomannan, a form of fiber. STARCH, GLYCOGEN and CELLULOSE are polysaccharides made from glucose. (See also NATURAL SWEETENERS.)

hiatus hernia (hiatal hernia) The protrusion or bulging of the STOMACH through the esophageal opening (hiatus) of the diaphragm into the chest. Aging or damage of supportive tissue can lead to hiatus hernia and DIVERTICULOSIS, which is the bulging of the large intestine. For Americans there is a 50% chance of having a hiatus hernia after the age of 40. Symptoms resemble DYSPEPSIA, including a burning pain under the breastbone and heartburn in which stomach contents regurgitate into the ESOPHAGUS, causing inflammation. Inability to breathe deeply and frequent belching are also experienced. Symptoms are most noticeable after a large meal, when straining or when stooping.

Hiatus hernia is often a recurrent condition. Several steps can be taken to minimize its effects:

1. Good posture to allow less crowding of organs in abdominal area.
2. Avoid overeating to the point of feeling uncomfortably full. Light meals will be less likely to force the stomach through the diaphragm.
3. Eat in a peaceful environment.
4. Physical manipulation by a skilled therapist may be able to move the stomach down. Bouncing on your heels can create a jarring effect, with gravity moving the stomach down into place.
5. Avoid swallowing air; this inflates the stomach.
6. Licorice extract has been recommended for helping hernias to heal.

hidden fat See FAT.

high blood pressure See HYPERTENSION.

high-calorie foods See FAT, HIDDEN.

high complex carbohydrate diet See DIET, HIGH COMPLEX CARBOHYDRATE.

high-density lipoprotein (HDL) A type of lipid-protein complex or particle in the blood that scavenges CHOLESTEROL from peripheral tissues and transports it to the LIVER for disposal. HDL's function is opposite that of LOW-DENSITY LIPOPROTEIN (LDL), which transports cholesterol to tissues. HDL can transfer cholesterol to another lipid carrier, VERY-LOW-DENSITY LIPOPROTEIN (VLDL), prior to its conversion to LDL.

Because HDL possesses the highest protein content, which is more dense than lipid, HDL is the densest of the various circulating lipoproteins. HDL precursor is synthesized by the liver. HDL_3 is an intermediate form, to which lipids and proteins are added from other lipoproteins in the circulation. The mature, spherical HDL is called HDL_2. Generally speaking, the higher the HDL level, the lower the risk of ATHEROSCLEROSIS. Women have a lower risk of heart disease than men and their HDL levels are higher. Evidence suggests that HDL_3 is inversely linked to the risk of coronary heart disease more strongly than HDL_2.

HDL contains proteins that determine its role. For example, Apoprotein D catalyzes cholesterol transfer between HDL and LDL, and Apoprotein CII is transferred to VLDL and CHYLOMICRONS, enabling these lipoproteins to interact in capillaries to release fatty acids from the fat they carry so that fatty acids can be taken up by cells. HDL salvages Apoprotein CII from chylomicron and VLDL remnants for recycling. Apoprotein AI activates an enzyme that converts cholesterol to a storage form.

Strategies to Raise HDL Levels

Though HDL is not a nutrient and cannot be consumed, a variety of approaches can raise or at least maintain HDL levels while lowering LDL cholesterol:

1. Exercise. Even moderate, regular physical exercise appears to increase HDL levels.
2. Lose weight. Obesity is correlated with decreased HDL levels.
3. Avoid cigarettes; smoking decreases HDL levels.
4. Eat less FAT and oils, especially less saturated fat. The more saturated fats in the diet, the higher the level of LDL, the less desirable form of cholesterol. Substituting OLIVE OIL and other monounsaturates in place of other cooking oils may be beneficial by raising HDL levels.
5. Eat FISH in place of red meat several times a week. Fish and fish oil may help raise HDL while lowering LDL levels.
6. Eat more whole grains, vegetables and legumes.

HDL Measurements

Guidelines suggest that if the serum cholesterol level is about 200, it is worthwhile to have a lipoprotein analysis, which measures HDL, LDL and blood fat levels. Usually HDL levels are expressed as a ratio of total cholesterol/HDL. A ratio of 4.0 correlates with an average risk of heart disease, and a ratio above 4.0 suggests the risk is greater than normal. An even more discriminating analysis involves measurement of Apoprotein B (a specific protein marker for LDL) to

Apoprotein A (a specific marker for HDL). The Apoprotein A to Apoprotein B ratio correlates more reliably with the risk of coronary heart disease than even the ratio of HDL cholesterol to total cholesterol. (See also DIET, HIGH COMPLEX CARBOHYDRATE.)

high-fat foods   See CALORIE; CHEESE; CONVENIENCE FOOD; FAT, HIDDEN; MEAT.

high-fructose corn syrup   See FRUCTOSE CORN SYRUP.

high oleic oils   Vegetable oils that contain a relatively high percentage of the monounsaturated fatty acid, oleic acid. This fatty acid contains one double bond, unlike polyunsaturated fatty acids. OLIVE OIL and certain canola oils are examples.

histamine   A chemical that triggers INFLAMMATION and typical "hay fever" symptoms: itching, sneezing, hives, runny nose, swelling, heat and soreness. Other inflammatory agents are kinins, PROSTAGLANDINS, LEUKOTRIENES and complement. Histamine is synthesized by many cells, especially mast cells, which initiate inflammation in connective tissue. Basophils (a type of white blood cell) and blood platelets (small cell fragments that assist in clot formation in vessels) also synthesize histamine. Histamine release is triggered by scavenger cells attracted to the site of injury. Histamine makes capillaries leaky, allowing water to collect in the affected tissue, thus causing swelling; immediately after injury, blood vessels dilate in the area of injury. The increased permeability permits defensive materials in the blood better access to the injured area.

Antihistamines are drugs that block the action of histamine and relieve hay fever symptoms of allergy attacks, but not of colds. The use of antihistamines poses a number of possible problems. They can worsen ASTHMA, PEPTIC ULCERS, kidney disease and glaucoma and can increase difficulty in urination (enlarged prostate). Newer antihistamines like terfenadine (Seldane) do not by themselves usually cause sleepiness. When taken during pregnancy some antihistamines may cause birth defects.

Antihistamines may also cause blurred vision and drowsiness. They can exaggerate drowsiness when taken with tranquilizers or alcohol, and severe sedation can occur if antihistamines are also taken with antidepressants, sleep inducers, narcotics, cocaine or marijuana. (See also IMMUNE SYSTEM.)

Oken, R.J., "Antihistamines, a Possible Risk Factor for Alzheimer's Disease," *Medical Hypotheses*, 44:1 (1995), pp. 47–48.

histidine (HIS, L-histidine)   An AMINO ACID that serves as a PROTEIN building block. It is a required nutrient in growing children and is classified as a semi-essential or conditionally essential nutrient, which must be supplied in their DIET. Histidine is classified as an aromatic amino acid unique among the common amino acids in its ability to act as a physiological pH BUFFER. A deficiency of histidine can cause ANEMIA because it is a major building block for HEMOGLOBIN, the oxygen transport protein of red blood cells. Other symptoms of histidine deficiency include FATIGUE and scaly dry skin.

Histidine is converted to HISTAMINE, a trigger of inflammation by mast cells, which fight localized infections. MEAT, FISH and POULTRY are rich sources of all essential amino acids, including histidine. (See also AMINO ACID METABOLISM.)

homeostasis   Maintaining the body's internal environment within well-defined limits that support life. Homeostasis refers to an internal environment providing optimal concentrations of WATER, nutrients, ions and oxygen; an optimal temperature; and an optimal osmotic pressure. Homeostatic mechanisms regulate BLOOD SUGAR concentration and pH, body temperature, blood pressure and osmotic pressure. STRESS creates an imbalance within the body. External "stressors" include loud noises and extreme temperatures; internal stressors include pain, mental disturbances and high blood pressure. Stress-induced imbalances are counteracted by the many homeostatic mechanisms that return the body to balance. They dissipate heat and dispose of lactic acid produced during exercise, for example.

Every structure of the body contributes to maintaining a normal internal environment. In particular, homeostatic responses are controlled by the nervous system and the ENDOCRINE SYSTEM (hormone-producing tissues). The regulation and integration of these two systems is accomplished by the PITUITARY GLAND, the HYPOTHALAMUS and the ADRENAL GLANDS. The hypothalamus is the region of the brain that controls the autonomic nervous system, nerves that regulate the pituitary gland, the "master gland" of the endocrine system, smooth muscles such as those around blood vessels, and cardiac muscles. The parasympathetic and sympathetic portions of the autonomic NERVOUS SYSTEM counterbalance each other. The sympathetic division adapts the body to stress, while the parasympathetic division of this system restores energy to tissues and restores the body after stress. (See also ADRENAL GLANDS; FEEDBACK INHIBITION; FIGHT OR FLIGHT RESPONSE.)

homocysteine   An artery-damaging amino acid produced as a normal byproduct of amino acid breakdown. Homocysteine comes from the essential amino acid, METHIONINE, as it is broken down to form CYSTEINE, another sulfur-containing amino acid. Unlike methionine and cysteine, homocysteine is not used by the body as a protein building block. Instead it is usually recycled back to methionine when there are ample B vitamins. Accumulated evidence links high homocysteine levels in the blood to an increased risk of heart attack and stroke. In one U.S. population (the Framingham Heart Study), nearly one-third of adults 67 or older have high blood homocysteine levels. In the Physician's Health Study which followed, approximately 22,000 male doctors found that elevated blood homocysteine levels, even in the range considered normal, correlated with an increased risk of heart attacks. Hypothetically, homocysteine could injure the lining of blood vessels (a vascular toxin), it could increase the production of muscle cells surrounding vessels and it could promote blood clots.

Usually, the amount of homocysteine in the blood is low. However, ENZYMES responsible for amino acid conversions may be deficient in some people, while others may not consume enough of key vitamins that function as enzyme helpers. In the Framingham study, two-thirds of the people with high homocysteine do not consume enough of the B vitamins. Especially inadequate intake of FOLIC ACID. VITAMIN B$_6$, riboflavin and VITAMIN B$_{12}$ can raise blood levels of homocysteine. Theoretically, with vitamin deficiencies, enzymes do not operate efficiently, cellular machinery slows down and homocysteine backs up and accumulates in the blood. Supplementation with folic acid and vitamin B$_{12}$ can help reverse the effects of deficiencies, improve the action of inefficient enzymes and lower blood homocysteine. It is estimated that about 400 mcg of folic acid daily can lower homocysteine levels to safe levels. It is not yet proven that lowering homocysteine prevents heart disease, however. Folic acid occurs in dark-green vegetables including broccoli and spinach, and in fruits, such as oranges and apples and in liver. (See also CARDIOVASCULAR DISEASE; NEURAL TUBE DEFECTS; PROTEIN.)

Motulsky, Arno G., "Nutritional Ecogenetics: Homocysteine-related Arteriosclerotic Vascular Disease, Neural Tube Defects, and Folic Acid," *American Journal of Human Genetics*, 58 (1996), pp. 17–20.

Selhub, Jacob, et al., "Vitamin Status and Intake as Primary Determinants of Homocysteinemia in an Elderly Population," *Journal of the American Medical Association*, 270:22 (December 8, 1993), pp. 2693–98.

homogenized milk   See MILK.

honey   A syrupy, sweet liquid obtained from plant nectar by honey bees. Honey contains the simple sugars FRUCTOSE, GLUCOSE, small amounts of other sugars and traces of MINERALS and VITAMINS, though the quantities are far below the daily requirements. Consider honey a refined CARBOHYDRATE that provides only CALORIES, like other NATURAL SWEETENERS. Honey is sweeter than table sugar and contains more calories; honey contains 65 calories per tablespoon, while table sugar supplies 46 calories.

The color and flavor of honey depends on the proportion of sugars and varies with the source of the nectar. In the United States most honey is produced from ALFALFA and clover. Tupelo honey from the southern United States contains more fructose and seldom granulates. Honey is used in the baking industry to keep breads and cakes moist and to improve the browning quality in baked goods. To substitute honey for table sugar in recipes, reduce liquid by a quarter-cup for each cup of honey used.

Commercial honey is heated to destroy yeasts, then filtered and bottled, while raw honey may be only strained and bottled. Honey has a low pH and a high osmotic pressure and is not a friendly environment for bacteria. Nonetheless, raw honey should not be fed to infants because it may contain enough bacterial spores to cause BOTULISM, a type of FOOD POISONING. This does not occur in older children and adults. Honey from some types of rhododendrons, especially in the Pacific Northwest and Northeast, can cause sudden illness, mimicking a heart attack. Symptoms may last up to 24 hours. The recommendation is to use blended honey from a variety of sources.

honeydew melon   (*Cucum*) A member of the muskmelon family, which includes CANTALOUPE, CASABA and other melons. Honeydews have a smooth, yellowish-white rind and a sweet, green flesh. The nutrient content for half a melon provides: calories, 225; protein, 3.0 g; carbohydrate, 59 g; fiber, 7.0 g; potassium, 1,755 mg; thiamin, 0.5 g; riboflavin, 0.1 mg; niacin, 3.85 mg; vitamin C, 160 mg.

hormone   A chemical messenger sent through the bloodstream to target tissues. The name hormone is derived from the Greek word "*hormon*," which means "to set in motion." The brain and nervous system control hormone release from specialized tissues called endocrine glands, and the ENDOCRINE SYSTEM consists of all the hormone-producing tissues. They include the HYPOTHALAMUS, the PITUITARY GLAND, ADRENAL GLANDS, endocrine PANCREAS, THYROID and PARATHYROID glands, glands of the stomach and intestine, pineal gland, THYMUS, ovaries, testes and placenta. Each endocrine gland secretes a characteristic hormone or set of hormones. Hormones from each source act on a specific target tissue or tissues.

The hypothalamus is a region of the brain that activates the pituitary gland, known as the master gland, by means of "releasing hormones." The hypothalamus also makes two hormones that are released through the pituitary gland: ANTIDIURETIC HORMONE (ADH) decreases the amount of WATER in urine by increasing SODIUM retention in the kidney; OXYTOCIN stimulates lactation and uterine contractions for birth.

The pituitary gland is connected to the brain through the hypothalamus. It regulates many other glands by producing "trophic hormones." A thyroid stimulating hormone (TSH) signals the thyroid gland to produce thyroid hormone. Adrenocorticotropic hormone (ACTH) triggers the adrenal cortex to produce its hormones, especially CORTISOL. Follicle stimulating hormone (FSH) regulates ovulation in females and sperm formation in males. Lutenizing hormone (LH) regulates ovulation with FSH. PROLACTIN promotes breast development and lactation during pregnancy. GROWTH HORMONE (GH) increases general PROTEIN build-up while speeding fat breakdown and maintains the skeleton and skeletal muscles. Melanocyte stimulating hormone (MSH) causes a rapid decrease in the synthesis of melanin in pigmented skin cells.

The adrenal glands produce several hormones. The adrenal medulla (inner region) secretes EPINEPHRINE and norepinephrine for rapid adaptation to stress, and the adrenal cortex (outer layer) secretes cortisol (to compensate for stress) and ALDOSTERONE (to conserve sodium). With decreased cortisol, the body is more sensitive to allergies, inflammation, and BLOOD SUGAR imbalances.

The endocrine pancreas consists of small clusters of cells (islets of Langerhans) embedded in the pancreatic gland. Insulin is produced by beta cells. This hormone stimulates other tissues to remove GLUCOSE and AMINO ACIDS from the blood thus lowering blood sugar. Islet tissue also contains alpha cells that produce GLUCAGON, a hormone that raises blood sugar levels, an effect opposite that of insulin.

The thyroid secretes thyroid hormone (thyroxine), which helps regulate basal metabolism (stimulates oxygen consumption), lipid metabolism and nerve function, and calcitonin, which decreases calcium concentrations in the blood and slows bone breakdown.

The pineal gland is influenced by light entering the eye. It releases melatonin, believed to help regulate body rhythms.

Parathyroid glands secrete parathyroid hormone, which increases blood calcium levels and counterbalances calcitonin.

The thymus produces thymosin, a hormone that helps to develop and maintain the IMMUNE SYSTEM. T cells, an important class of white cells, are produced in bone marrow and migrate to the thymus gland, where they mature.

Testes secrete testosterone, the major male sex hormone. Testosterone promotes secondary male characteristics, such as facial hair, muscular development and genital development.

Ovarian follicles produce ESTROGEN, the feminizing hormone and hormone of growth, and the corpus luteum secretes primarily progesterone. Female sex hormones help regulate the menstrual cycle, maintain pregnancy and regulate ovulation.

The placenta produces human chorionic gonadotropin, which provides a stimulus for the continued production of progesterone, which is required to keep the embryo attached to the uterine lining.

Hormones of the Digestive Tract

Several hormones regulate the activity of the digestive tract. The pyloric mucosa (the lining of the lower region of the stomach) and duodenum (the first section of the small intestine) produce GASTRIN, a hormone that stimulates stomach juice production. Proteins, CAFFEINE, SPICES and ALCOHOL stimulate gastrin production. In addition, the duodenum secretes the hormone enterogastrone in response to CHYME (partially digested food from the stomach) and FAT. This hormone reduces intestinal motility (peristalsis) and reduces secretion of gastric juice. The duodenum also produces CHOLECYSTOKININ, which stimulates the GALLBLADDER to release BILE into the intestine; SECRETIN, which signals duct cells to secrete BICARBONATE to neutralize stomach acid; pancreozymin, which stimulates the release of pancreatic digestive enzymes. Chyme triggers the release of secretin and pancreozymin. (See also ANDROGEN; PROSTAGLANDINS.)

hormone-free meat   See MEAT CONTAMINANTS.

horseradish (*Armoracia rusticana*)   A pungent, bitter HERB and a member of the mustard family. Horseradish has been cultivated in the Near East for at least 2,000 years. The root is ground or grated and used as a CONDIMENT or relish. Freshly grated horseradish releases enzymes that activate substances responsible for its characteristically strong odor and flavor. These components evaporate and will dissipate with time. Adding an acidic ingredient like vinegar or mayonnaise blocks enzyme action and decreases the flavor. Horseradish is served with fatty meats, cocktail sauces, cold cuts and FISH. Horseradish, MUSTARD and certain vegetables contain low levels of GOITROGENS. High levels of these agents block IODINE uptake by the thyroid gland, needed to produce thyroid hormone. However, usual consumption of such vegetables and condiments is not deemed harmful, and they add variety and nutritional value to many dishes. (See also SPICE.)

hospital-induced malnutrition (iatrogenic malnutrition)   Malnutrition occurs during hospitalization after patients have been fed inadequate diets for several weeks. A study reported in the 1970s suggested that 30 to 50% of hospitalized people left the hospital in worse nutritional condition than when they arrived as patients. Hospitals generally have improved their menus since then, though hospitalization still does not guarantee optimal nutrition. A 1996 study of 57 hospitals found that only four routinely offered patients menus that met all federal dietary guidelines: Fewer than 20% kept cholesterol below 300 mg/day, while half kept salt intake below 6 g/day and dietary fiber at more than 20 g/day. (See also DIETARY GUIDELINES FOR AMERICANS; MALNUTRITION.)

Kerstetter, J.E., et al., "Malnutrition in the Institutionalized Older Adult," *Journal of the American Dietetic Association*, 92:9 (September 1992), pp. 1109–16.

hot dog (FRANKFURTER)   A heavily processed meat product resembling a sausage in shape. Though viewed as a PROTEIN source, a typical hot dog contains only about 5 g of protein, the same as an average hot dog bun. Red meat hot dogs are a high-fat food: FAT accounts for 80% of the CALORIES. This is true even when the label indicates hot dogs are "80 percent fat free." The USDA permits the designation of "80 percent fat free" to indicate any hot dog containing less than the standard 30% fat by weight, provided the standard is also listed on the food label. This term refers to fat content by weight and provides no indication of fat calories.

"Lean" hot dogs may contain 20% fat, rather than the usual 30%. Because half of the weight of the hot dog is WATER, the percentage of calories from fat is 71%, higher than 20%. Often CHICKEN and turkey hot dogs contain 8 to 9 g of fat, as much as red meat hot dogs; they are not low-fat foods. TOFU hot dogs are meat-free and contain 30% less fat than regular hot dogs and no CHOLESTEROL.

Manufacturers add nitrates and NITRITES to hot dogs and other cured meat foods to prevent the growth of disease-producing bacteria, to add flavor and to enhance their color.

These preservatives form nitrosoamines in the digestive tract, which may pose a cancer risk. (See also DIETARY GUIDELINES FOR AMERICANS; FAT, HIDDEN; FOOD LABELING.)

humectant   A FOOD ADDITIVE used to maintain moisture, texture and freshness in prepared foods. Humectants attract water in air and tend to retain water. CORN SYRUP, GLYCEROL, glycerol monostearate, propylene glycol and SORBITOL are common examples of humectants. They are used to keep candies, shredded COCONUT and MARSHMALLOWS from drying out. They are generally considered as safe food additives.

hunger   A compelling need to eat caused by food deprivation. Hunger is often accompanied by a painful feeling and weakness and is unpleasant. Energy stores are mobilized with hunger. In contrast, APPETITE is usually associated with pleasure during food consumption. Rhythmic contractions (PERISTALSIS) of an empty stomach are responsible for hunger pangs; these become more frequent the longer a meal is delayed. To a limited extent, stomach contractions are regulated by blood sugar levels and by distension of the stomach when filled. Hunger is regulated primarily by several brain centers, including the hypothalamus, via a "feeding center" and a "satiety center." Normally the hypothalamus functions as an integration center for a variety of signals; possibly brain centers sense a decline in blood sugar levels, for example. Other hypotheses involve the production in the brain of neuropeptides. Some are identical with gut peptides, where they stimulate or inhibit eating. Cholecystokinin, formed in the gut and in the brain, inhibits eating. Long-term control of body weight relies upon mechanisms that are currently being defined. LEPTIN, a protein produced by body fat, signals the brain to stop producing signals that stimulate feeding. Leptin could curtail production of specific brain peptides and it could block norepinephrine and related neurotransmitters that trigger hunger and increase basal metabolism. Overall eating patterns reflect internal regulatory mechanisms; psychological influences such as stress and mood; environmental factors like climate; and diseases such as mental illness, BULIMIA NERVOSA, ANOREXIA NERVOSA. (See also OBESITY.)

hunger, world   HUNGER continues to be an international issue. An estimated 1.3 billion malnourished people will populate the planet by the year 2000. Hunger is common among developing nations as well as among subpopulations of developed nations. Children are the most vulnerable to MALNUTRITION. In developing countries of Asia and Africa BREASTFEEDING assures adequate nutrition until about six months of age. Subsequently, hunger takes a greater toll. Practices such as relying on formula feeding rather than breastfeeding are detrimental when the formula is diluted or cannot be prepared with sterile water or refrigeration. Failure of children to grow at a normal rate indicates chronic, severe problems. Malnourished infants who survive chronic hunger bear the emotional and physical burden, with mental retardation as a possible consequence. Indirect consequences of marginal nutrition include infectious diseases, diarrhea, and parasitic diseases such as malaria. Protein-calorie malnutrition due to severe food restriction is the most prevalent form among children.

Maternal nutrition is often marginal where hunger is endemic, and women in developing countries often bear the brunt of hunger within a family. The mother often feeds her family first and subsists on what is left. Too, these women often provide physical labor required to obtain food for families, even during pregnancies.

Poverty and hunger are linked by a complex web: lack of education, poor health, little political voice, inadequate food distribution and lack of technical information—enforced by those possessing education and political and military power, who control resources and rely on cash crops, and who hold a monopoly on technology. Overpopulation is another pressing concern worldwide. It is projected that human population will reach 6 billion by the year 2000. In another century, it is projected to be 12 billion. However, poverty links hunger and overpopulation.

World food production can provide all people with ample calories, according to the United Nation's FOOD AND AGRICULTURAL ORGANIZATION. Generally, when there has been economic growth and equal distribution of resources among most groups in a population, population growth rates have declined. Land reform in which more people have an input in food production also seems essential. The GREEN REVOLU-

TION of the 1960s failed to achieve its goal of making countries self-sufficient in food production because it generally ignored local culture, traditional agriculture, and economic factors such as dependency on imported chemical fertilizers. Food distribution is a critical factor. The problem of unequal distribution of resources is compounded by the fact that in most countries governments dictate daily life. In addition at least 20% of total food produced yearly is wasted by spoilage and pests, contributing to food shortages.

Multinational corporations involved in exporting plantation crops and a preoccupation with profitability may indirectly contribute to hunger when cultivated land is used for luxury and export crops, rather than for traditional staples, despite starvation and local severe malnutrition. Thus regions of Africa are net exporters of coffee, cocoa, peanuts and cattle, as well as beans and barley, despite having the greatest incidence of severe malnutrition among children.

The Presidential Commission on World Hunger (1980) concluded that nations have the capability of remedying global hunger and that the global demand for food requires political and technical solutions to the above problems, that assistance programs need to focus on self-reliance, and that developing countries need to develop effective food production and distribution systems and to emphasize education. (See also INFANT FORMULA.)

Center on Hunger, Poverty and Nutrition Policy, Tufts University School of Medicine. *Statement on the Link Between Nutrition and Cognitive Development in Children.* 1994.

Mellor, John W. and Gavian, Sarah, "Famine: Causes, Prevention and Relief," *Science*, 235 (January 30, 1987), pp. 539–45.

The United States Conference of Mayors. "A Status Report on Hunger and Homelessness in America's Cities 1991. A 28 City Survey," December 1991. Washington, D.C.: U.S. Conference of Mayors, 1991.

hunger suppressants   See APPETITE SUPPRESSANTS.

HVP   See HYDROLYZED VEGETABLE PROTEIN.

hydrochloric acid   See DIGESTION.

hydrocortisone   See CORTISOL.

hydrogenated vegetable oil   Vegetable oil that has been modified by the addition of hydrogen. Hydrogenation is an industrial process that adds hydrogen atoms to double bonds of oils, polyunsaturated FATTY ACIDS. Hydrogenation creates a more saturated FAT (filled up with hydrogen atoms) and thus hardens or solidifies vegetable oils. Most commercially available polyunsaturated oils (CORN OIL, SOYBEAN oil, SAFFLOWER oil, SUNFLOWER oil and COTTON-SEED OIL) are partially hydrogenated to retard rancidity, to increase shelflife, and to make them thicker and more spreadable.

The degree of hydrogenation varies with the type of product. Solid fats like stick MARGARINE and vegetable SHORTENING are the most hydrogenated. Vegetable shortening is highly hydrogenated vegetable oil, the equivalent to LARD, though less saturated than BEEF TALLOW. Tub margarine is made of partially hydrogenated oils and is 20% saturated. However, it is much less saturated than BUTTER, which is 66%

saturated. Partially hydrogenated vegetable oils are somewhat more saturated than untreated oils. For example, soybean oil is initially 15% saturated and ends up 20% saturated after partial hydrogenation.

During hydrogenation some of the polyunsaturated fatty acid content is converted to monounsaturates with a single double bond instead of multiple double bonds. Also during hydrogenation, a fraction of the polyunsaturated fatty acids are converted to TRANS-FATTY ACIDS, in which some of the existing double bonds straighten. Trans-fatty acids raise cholesterol levels and are associated with an increase in the risk of heart attack. Whether the risk is greater than with saturated fats is unknown. Hydrogenated vegetable oil supplies 80% of the trans-fatty acids Americans ingest. The long-range health effects of these industrial byproducts are unknown.

Partially hydrogenated vegetable oils, including soybean, cottonseed, corn and rapeseed oils, are common food additives to increase the flavor and taste of processed foods. Foods with partially hydrogenated or hydrogenated vegetable oils include foods such as most kinds of CHIPS (potato chips, corn chips and the like), CRACKERS, rye crisps, margarines, shortening, frozen pizzas, salad dressing, low-cholesterol MAYONNAISE and even FROZEN ENTREES. Food labels presently list fat content and often use the term "partially hydrogenated oil" without further explanation, which provides little detailed information. Nonetheless, added oil indicates added calories. The general recommendation is to cut back on all fats and oils to lower the risk of cancer and heart disease. Eating an excess of saturated fat, whether it is animal fat or hydrogenated vegetable oil, increases the risk of CARDIOVASCULAR DISEASE. (See also CONVENIENCE FOOD; DIETARY GUIDELINES FOR AMERICANS; PROCESSED FOOD.)

Longnecker, Matthew P., "Do Trans Fatty Acids in Margarine and Other Foods Increase the Risk of Coronary Heart Disease?" *Epidemiology*, 4:6 (November 1993), pp. 492–95.

hydrogen peroxide   A powerful oxidizer. Solutions of hydrogen peroxide are colorless and have a biting taste. They are used as a bleaching agent, and as a bactericide and a disinfectant for the mouth, nose and throat. Hydrogen peroxide can spontaneously break down into FREE RADICALS, a highly reactive chemical species.

Hydrogen peroxide also is a product of METABOLISM, especially in the LIVER. It is generated in organelles called PEROXISOMES. Additionally, scavenger white blood cells (phagocytic leukocytes) produce a burst of highly reactive forms of oxygen, including hydrogen peroxide, to destroy engulfed microorganisms. The body's antioxidant system generates hydrogen peroxide. SUPEROXIDE DISMUTASE is an enzyme that degrades a free radical called superoxide to hydrogen peroxide. Hydrogen peroxide is decomposed very rapidly by glutathione peroxidase and CATALASE, other ANTIOXIDANT enzymes.

hydrolysis   An important type of chemical reaction that forms the basis of DIGESTION. During hydrolysis, a bond between atoms of a compound is split by incorporating a water molecule, giving rise to the name hydrolysis (hydro = water, lysis = splitting). Hydrolysis creates two smaller molecules (fragments). Digestive enzymes catalyze (speed up) the hydrolysis of food molecules.

LIPASES are enzymes that hydrolyze (break down) FATS and OILS to produce GLYCEROL and FATTY ACIDS. Proteolytic enzymes (PROTEASES) like TRYPSIN and PEPSIN catalyze the degradation of proteins to amino acids. AMYLASE, a pancreatic enzyme, hydrolyzes STARCH to maltose, a sugar containing two glucose units. Intestinal enzymes help complete carbohydrate digestion. Thus MALTASE digests maltose to glucose and LACTASE digests LACTOSE (milk sugar) to glucose and GALACTOSE. (See also CARBOHYDRATE; CARBOHYDRATE METABOLISM; DIGESTIVE TRACT.)

hydrolyzed vegetable protein (HVP)   An additive in PROCESSED FOODS used to enhance the flavor of meat dishes like beef stew, instant soups, sauces and gravy mixes. HVP is no longer added to BABY FOODS. It is prepared by breaking down PROTEIN of SOYBEANS, PEANUTS, WHEAT or CORN into AMINO ACIDS and small fragments. On a food label, HVP can legally be called a "natural flavor" with no further description, though often it contains up to 20% MSG (MONOSODIUM GLUTAMATE) and is a hidden source of this FLAVOR ENHANCER. (See also ARTIFICIAL FLAVORS; FOOD LABELING.)

hydrophilic   Refers to the ability of certain compounds to attract WATER molecules. Ions (electrolytes) like those of SODIUM, POTASSIUM and CHLORIDE are hydrophilic, as are water-soluble organic compounds such as sugars, simple acids (lactic ACID, vitamin C, acetic acid), B VITAMINS (niacin, biotin, riboflavin, thiamin) and AMINO ACIDS. Large molecules can also be hydrophilic, and thus dissolve in water solutions. Many proteins found in blood and the cytoplasm fall into this category. Certain insoluble substances like cellulose, while water-insoluble attract water molecules and form "wettable" surfaces. The surfaces of cells contain carbohydrate structures and phospholipids that attract water and permit the cell to survive in an aqueous medium. Foreign materials that enter the body through water, food and air or are ingested directly like medication may accumulate unless they are chemically modified to make them more water-soluble so they can be secreted. Particularly the liver is well stocked with a large group of "detoxifying" enzymes that increase the hydrophilic properties of these substances. (See also BUFFER; EMULSIFIERS; MICELLE.)

hydrophobic   Refers to the ability of certain compounds to be attracted to organic solvents such as hexane and oils in FAT and to repel water. Hydrophobic substances include lipids, a diverse family of water-insoluble substances like fats, oils, and CHOLESTEROL. When transported in blood, which is primarily water, these hydrophobic substances are enclosed by a layer of proteins and phospholipids as microscopic droplets (micelles) that are water-soluble. These particles are called LIPOPROTEINS and include LDL-cholesterol (so-called "bad" cholesterol) and HDL-cholesterol (a desirable form of cholesterol). Agents such as BILE acids act like detergents to suspend fats and oils as MICELLES in water-based digestive juices. Bile acids and bile salts, as well as phospholipids, possess a hydrophobic end and a hydrophilic (water-attracting) end. They form a ball-shaped shell, in which the attracting portions of the molecules face outward to interact with water, while their hydrophobic regions point inward, embedded in the oily droplet they surround.

Certain amino acids possess hydrophobic regions (side chains): PHENYLALANINE; METHIONINE, TRYPTOPHAN, ALANINE, LEUCINE, ISOLEUCINE and VALINE. When they are building blocks of functional proteins like ENZYMES, serum proteins and antibodies, the hydrophobic amino acids are buried within the interior of the protein molecule away from the surrounding water molecules rather than on the exterior. In contrast, insoluble proteins of skin and hair (keratins) repel water because their hydrophobic amino acids are exposed. (See also EMULSIFIERS; VITAMIN.)

hydroxybutyric acid   See BETA HYDROXYBUTYRIC ACID.

hydroxyproline   An oxidized form of the amino acid PROLINE that is a feature of COLLAGEN, the structural protein of connective tissue. Hydroxyproline is not classified as a dietary essential amino acid, nor is it used to assemble proteins because it is formed from proline after a protein chain is synthesized. Hydroxyproline in collagen stabilizes its fibrous structure. Hydroxyproline is synthesized by the enzyme, proline oxidase, which requires VITAMIN C. Chronic vitamin C deficiency therefore prevents connective tissue maturation, resulting in capillary fragility, susceptibility to bruising and bleeding gums, and joint pain. (See also SCURVY.)

hyperacidity   See HYPOCHLORHYDRIA.

hyperactivity (attention deficit-hyperactivity disorder, ADHD)   Behavior disturbances characterized by overactivity and restlessness, aggressive behavior, poor self control and short attention span. As many as 4% of children suffer from hyperactivity, which affects more boys than girls through adolescence. As many as 30 to 50% of individuals who had ADHD as children continue to have it as adults. Multiple factors have been implicated in hyperactivity and inattentiveness:

1. Artificial FOOD ADDITIVES. It has been hypothesized that synthetic chemicals like ARTIFICIAL FOOD COLORS, PRESERVATIVES and salicylates (compounds related to aspirin) affect the nervous system.
2. Food allergies and FOOD SENSITIVITIES may also affect behavior. Clinical studies indicate that elimination of offending foods from an allergic child's diet can sometimes improve scholastic performance dramatically.
3. Abnormal CARBOHYDRATE METABOLISM. Some people with ADHD may be unable to metabolize SUGAR normally. Behavioral problems have been reported to be linked with excessive sugar consumption in these individuals.
4. Family environment. There is a growing appreciation among counselors that often the hyperactive child acts out emotions that reflect the parent's emotional turmoil.
5. Toxic exposure. Excessive aluminum, lead and copper may be associated with hyperactivity as well.
6. Nutritional deficiencies. Deficiencies of iron, calcium, magnesium, zinc and essential fatty acids have been tied to fidgeting, restlessness and learning difficulties. Occasionally children respond to niacin, vitamin B$_6$ and thiamin supplementation.

Following a Feingold-type diet that limits consumption of artificial colors and preservatives and eliminates sensitive foods from the child's diet can sometimes be beneficial. However, experience has shown that effective treatment involves the entire family in order to create a supportive environment. Conventional treatment to regulate ADHD relies on psychological counseling, behavior modification and drugs (stimulants, tranquilizers and tricylic ANTIDEPRESSANTS). These drugs can have profound side effects; for example, Ritalin (methylphenidate) can retard growth. Specific nutritional recommendations are centered around the following factors. A high protein, low carbohydrate diet with limited refined sugar may be beneficial. The role of sugar in behavior is a controversial area. The DIETARY GUIDELINES FOR AMERICANS state that sugar does not cause hyperactivity. Indeed several clinical trials have not detected an association. On the other hand, excessive dietary sugar leads to nutrient deficiencies that contribute to hormonal imbalances that impact behavior. (See also ADDICTION AND SUGAR; ALLERGY FOOD; FEINGOLD DIET.)

McGuiness, Diane, "Stimulants and Children," *Mothering*, 60 (1991), pp. 1–4.
Rapp, Doris. *Is This Your Child?* New York: William Morrow and Company, 1991.

hyperalimentation   Orally administered liquid diets providing high levels of one or more nutrients. In medicine, intravenous hyperalimentation refers to the administration of a solution containing all essential nutrients, including AMINO ACIDS (3.5%), GLUCOSE (25%), VITAMINS and ELECTROLYTES (ionic substances) required to sustain life. Three liters daily supplies 3,000 CALORIES and 105 g of amino acids. It is usually infused into a major vein leading into the heart (superior vena cava) via a catheter, so that highly concentrated solutions are quickly diluted in the blood. This procedure is usually used in cases of severe illness, including PANCREATITIS, CANCER, severe MALNUTRITION, gastrointestinal blockage, trauma and other medical conditions.

hypercalcemia   An excess of CALCIUM in the blood. Regulatory mechanisms involving calcitonin, a HORMONE from the thyroid gland that lowers blood calcium; parathyroid hormone from the PARATHYROID GLANDS that raises blood calcium; and VITAMIN D help maintain blood calcium levels within very narrow limits, regardless of diet. Hypercalcemia therefore is most often caused by a hormonal abnormality. Possible causes include CANCER, overproduction of calcitonin by the parathyroid glands or excessive ingestion of vitamin D. Symptoms associated with hypercalcemia include vomiting, loss of appetite and possibly kidney stones. (See also ENDOCRINE SYSTEM.)

hyperchlorhydria (hyperacidity)   The excess in secretion of hydrochloric acid in the stomach. In the absence of food, hyperchlorhydria causes a burning sensation after meals. Excessive acid production is associated with strong emotional responses, HUNGER pains and it may aggrevate DUODENAL ULCERS. Emotional disturbances and food sensitivities can cause excessive production of STOMACH ACID. Hormonal imbalance may relate to an increased sensitivity of parietal cells (acid-secreting cells of the stomach) to the

hormone GASTRIN, which stimulates acid production; to hyper-secretion of gastrin after meals; or to a decreased ability to inhibit gastrin release when the acidity of GASTRIC JUICE contents drops.

Pain associated with hyperchlorhydria can be relieved by ANTACIDS. However, the use of calcium carbonate antacids is associated with a rebound in gastric juice (stomach acid) production. (See also DIGESTION.)

hypercholesterolemia Elevated blood CHOLESTEROL. This condition affects an estimated 25% of Americans. This is a concern because elevated cholesterol is a risk factor for ATHEROSCLEROSIS and HEART DISEASE. Opinion varies regarding the level of cholesterol that is considered abnormal. Some guidelines consider that moderate risk of heart disease exists when the cholesterol value is greater than 200 mg/deciliter for people between the ages of 20 and 29 years; or greater than 220 for those between 30 and 39 years; or greater than 240 for those 40 or older. Cholesterol levels that are 20 points greater for any age bracket put the individual into the high risk category (high hypercholesterolemia). In other words, the high risk threshold is 220 for 20 to 29 year olds; 240 for 30 to 39 year olds; and 260 for those 40 or older.

Causes of hypercholesterolemia include long-term unhealthy dietary and life-style choices, diabetes, kidney disease, HYPERTENSION (high blood pressure) and inheritance. Familial hypercholesterolemia (Type IIA HYPERLIPOPROTEINEMIA) refers to an inherited tendency toward high cholesterol values (excessive LOW-DENSITY LIPOPROTEIN, LDL, the less desirable form of cholesterol). Elevated blood cholesterol due to inheritance accounts for only 5% of cases. In this disease, the body's mechanism for the removing of LDL from blood can be defective, allowing cholesterol to accumulate in the blood, where it is more likely to clog arteries.

Individuals with hypercholesterolemia may be advised to lower their FAT intake, especially saturated fat, to less than 10% of fat calories; to restrict cholesterol intake to less than 200 mg daily; to reduce their weight (if overweight); and to stop smoking. Eating a variety of foods, emphasizing whole grains, vegetables, lean meat, fish and poultry helps to lower cholesterol. Eating less fatty red meat and less processed food that contains COCONUT OIL and PALM OIL also helps lower fat consumption. Drug therapy may be recommended when the cholesterol is very high, when the cholesterol value doesn't drop with diet therapy and other life-style changes, and when the risk of cardiovascular disease is high for other reasons, such as heredity. (See also CHOLESTEROL-LOWERING DRUGS.)

hyperglycemia (HYPERINSULINISM) Elevated BLOOD SUGAR (GLUCOSE). Normally, blood sugar rises within 30 to 60 minutes after eating starchy foods, then returns to a baseline level within three to five hours as starch is digested to glucose and is absorbed. If the blood sugar level remains elevated, a prediabetic or a diabetic condition may be indicated. In this case the PANCREAS may not synthesize enough INSULIN or the cellular mechanisms responding to insulin may be defective. Sustained high blood-sugar levels promote the bonding of glucose to proteins, including HEMO-

GLOBIN. The resulting proteins do not function normally. Their gradual accumulation may contribute to altered organ deterioration associated with uncontrolled diabetes mellitus. (See also CARBOHYDRATE; CARBOHYDRATE METABOLISM; DIABETES MELLITUS; GLUCOSE TOLERANCE; HYPOGLYCEMIA.)

Surwit, Richard S. and Schneider, Mark S., "Role of Stress in the Etiology and Treatment of Diabetes Mellitus," *Psychosomatic Medicine*, 55:4 (1993), pp. 380–93.

hyperinsulinism Excessive secretion of INSULIN by the endocrine (hormone-secreting) PANCREAS. Sustained high blood insulin levels can produce unusually low BLOOD SUGAR (HYPOGLYCEMIA). Extreme hyperinsulinism represents a glandular imbalance. On the other hand, a short-term, transient insulin excess may occur when blood glucose rises in response to ingesting a large amount of SUGAR or NATURAL SWEETENERS, causing a subsequent drop in blood sugar. This situation represents an overcompensation by the pancreas called "postprandial" hypoglycemia (low blood sugar after eating). Chronic hyperinsulinism, that is, resistance to the action of insulin for years, is linked to a constellation of signs and symptoms related to noninsulin-dependent DIABETES MELLITUS, such as OBESITY, increased blood pressure, elevated blood sugar, blood triglycerides and LDL-cholesterol, with decreased HDL-cholesterol (SYNDROME X). Chronic stress and elevated adrenal hormone, especially CORTISOL, are also associated with syndrome X. Furthermore, insulin resistance may turn out to be almost as serious a risk factor for CORONARY HEART DISEASE as such well-known-factors as cigarette smoking and high blood pressure. (See also ENDOCRINE SYSTEM; HORMONE.)

hyperkalemia Excessive levels of POTASSIUM in the blood. Normally potassium is concentrated inside cells, where it helps maintain fluid volume. During nerve transmission and muscle contraction, potassium moves out of cells and SODIUM moves in as these ions briefly trade places across the cell membrane. Excessive potassium in the blood causes a serious sodium-potassium imbalance that interferes with muscle contraction and the transmission of nerve impulses. The heart dilates and gradually becomes weaker. Overdosing with potassium supplements or using excessive amounts of SALT SUBSTITUTES can significantly raise blood potassium levels. Hyperkalemia is a serious complication of kidney failure, shock and severe DEHYDRATION. (See also ELECTROLYTES; MINERALS.)

hyperlipemia Excessive lipids in the blood. The accumulated lipids may be cholesterol, fat (triglycerides) or both. (See also HYPERLIPOPROTEINEMIA; HYPERTRIGLYCERIDEMIA.)

Tato F., et al., "Effects of Fish Oil Concentrate on Lipoproteins and Apolipoproteins, in Familial Combined Hyperlipidemia," *Clinical Investigations*, 71:4 (1993), pp. 314–18.

hyperlipoproteinemia (hyperlipidemia) Excessive level of lipid-protein complexes in the blood. LIPOPROTEINS transport CHOLESTEROL and FAT (also known as TRIGLYCERIDES) through the bloodstream. Although these lipids are insoluble in blood, which is mainly water, they become soluble when emulsified, as when bound to certain proteins called apolipoproteins and phospholipid. The levels of lipoproteins are influenced by diet, hormonal balance, age, weight, stress and illness. Severely elevated blood lipids may be due to heredity. Excessive blood cholesterol and excessive blood fat warrant medical attention. The American Heart Association recommends a gradual reduction of total fat, saturated fat and cholesterol as a dietary approach to treating hyperlipoproteinemia. It recommends restriction of total fat intake to less than 30% total calories; restriction of saturated fat consumption to less than 10% of fat calories and restriction of cholesterol to less than 300 mg daily. Weight reduction is also advised, and medication under a doctor's supervision may be appropriate. In a Step 2 program, cholesterol consumption would not exceed 200 mg daily and saturated fat would represent no more than 7% of total daily calories.

There are four major lipoproteins of the blood:

1. VLDL (VERY-LOW-DENSITY LIPOPROTEINS) carries fat synthesized by the liver to tissues.
2. CHYLOMICRONS transport fat from digested food to tissues, first through the lymphatic system, then through the bloodstream.
3. LDL (LOW-DENSITY LIPOPROTEINS) transports cholesterol from the liver to tissues.
4 HDL (HIGH-DENSITY LIPOPROTEINS) carries cholesterol from tissue back to the liver for disposal.

In one of the most widely used classification systems, hyperlipoproteinemias are categorized according to the types of lipoprotein that accumulate:

1. Type I is characterized by elevated chylomicrons (triglycerides plus cholesterol). This rare inherited condition is often caused by a deficiency of lipoprotein lipase, the enzyme in capillaries that releases fatty acids from chylomicrons so they can be taken up by cells. Type I usually appears in childhood.
2. Type IIa is a common inherited disease, characterized by elevated LDL and cholesterol. In severe cases it leads to early ATHEROSCLEROSIS and premature death. Milder forms are not obviously due to family history. Secondary forms of Type IIa may be due to excessive dietary cholesterol, liver disease or hypothyroidism.
3. Type IIb is characterized by elevated LDL, VLDL, cholesterol and triglycerides. Often this is a rare inherited condition; milder forms may be sporadic. Type IIb is usually not detected until adulthood.
4. Type III (relatively uncommon compared to the other types) is characterized by elevated VLDL (which contains cholesterol plus triglycerides), due to an abnormal composition of VLDL. Type III is frequently an inherited condition, usually detected in adulthood.
5. Type IV is a common disease, characterized by elevated VLDL and triglycerides with normal or elevated cholesterol due to an elevated production of normal VLDL. It is probably an inherited condition. Often half of the patients' close adult relatives will also have Type IV. Type IV is worsened by obesity and alcohol consumption and often appears after the age of 20. Secondary causes include diabetes, pregnancy, ALCOHOLISM and kidney disease.

6. Type V (uncommon) is characterized by both elevated chylomicrons and elevated VLDL (triglycerides plus cholesterol), thus representing a "mixed" type hyperlipidemia. When inherited, more than half of a patient's close relatives have Type IV or Type V hyperlipoproteinemia. Clinically, Type V resembles Type I. (Elevated chylomicrons and VLDL may also result from alcoholism, kidney disease or diabetes.)

(See also CHOLESTEROL-LOWERING DRUGS; FAT METABOLISM; HYPERCHOLESTEROLEMIA.)

hyperplasia   The overproduction of tissue mass without the formation of a tumor. Often a gland or organ responds to increased demand, excessive use or nutrient deficiency by increasing tissue mass. GOITER is an overgrowth of the thyroid gland responding to chronic IODINE deficiency. (See also GROWTH HORMONE.)

hypertension (high blood pressure)   Chronically elevated blood pressure. Up to 50 million American adults have abnormally high pressure. Millions more have increased risk because their blood pressure is on the high side of normal. Added together, perhaps as many as 75% of Americans over the age of 35 may face dangerously high blood pressures in their lifetimes. This is a major public health concern because, typically, there are no obvious symptoms for 15 to 20 years, until STROKE, HEART ATTACK, kidney failure and/or blindness strike. Even after reducing hypertension to normal blood pressure, the risk of illness and death (mortality) is greater than in people without a history of hypertension. Adults should know their blood pressure and they should check it yearly.

Blood pressure is a measure of fluid pressure against vessel walls. "Optimal" blood pressure is considered to be 110/70, while a "normal" blood pressure is below 120/80. The larger number (numerator) is the "systolic" pressure due to heart pumping, measured in millimeters of mercury. The smaller number represents the "diastolic" pressure between beats, when the heart rests. Though there are no precisely defined rules regarding abnormal blood pressure, as a general guideline consistent systolic pressures of 150 to 160 or consistent diastolic readings of 99 or greater signal hypertension that requires medical treatment and need to be controlled. The risk of CARDIOVASCULAR DISEASE and kidney disease increases when either systolic or diastolic pressures are consistently high, and the odds increase further when both numbers are high.

Blood pressure values representing mild hypertension vary with age. For young adults 140/90 is considered borderline high, but it may be considered high normal for those over 60. Mild forms of hypertension do not have to be treated with drugs, because diet modification and life-style changes can usually control mild forms of hypertension. A diastolic pressure of 85 to 89 represents borderline hypertension.

Diastolic hypertension is caused by the restriction of small arteries (arterioles) flowing into the capillary bed. Systolic pressure rises temporarily after stress, physical exercise, eating and drinking; thus, there is no single cause for this condition. Hypertension is more common in men than in women and is more common among African Americans than whites.

The risk increases with age, and after the age of 50 it is more common in women. Hypertension also runs in families. Having parents or siblings with hypertension increases the risk. Other causes relate to hormone imbalance, abnormal capillary structure or nervous system–directed constriction of blood vessels. ARTERIOSCLEROSIS causes hypertension in elderly persons. Hypertension can also result from chronic kidney disease, as well as from LEAD and CADMIUM exposure.

The role of diet and environment is illustrated by the observation that blood pressure has increased with age only in industrialized nations. Prevention focuses on education in the following big areas. Several recommendations pertain to diet:

Consume adequate CALCIUM, ZINC and MAGNESIUM. Deficiencies of these minerals increase the risk of hypertension. Studies suggest that hypertensive individuals consume less calcium than people with normal blood pressure, and calcium supplementation seems to help with mild to moderate hypertension. Low cellular magnesium levels correlate with increased blood pressure (hypertensives) and adequate magnesium intake is essential for cardiovascular health. However, there is no guarantee that calcium supplementation will lower blood pressure. Taking calcium supplements daily can lessen hypertension in a majority of patients, while it can worsen hypertension in a minority.

Increase dietary FIBER consumption with whole GRAINS, FRUIT and VEGETABLES. A high-fiber, high complex carbohydrate diet may prevent many forms of cardiovascular disease.

Reduce fat intake. A low-fat diet may lower blood pressure. In particular, vegetable oils rich in essential fatty acids, including LINOLEIC ACID, can decrease hypertension.

Reduce SODIUM (salt) consumption while increasing POTASSIUM from fresh fruit and vegetables. Low potassium intake is linked to hypertension. Americans consume much more salt and other sources of sodium than necessary for body functions. In a survey of 32 countries, people with normal weight but high sodium intake were up to seven times more likely to have high blood pressure than those whose weights were low and whose sodium intake was low. About one-third of hypertensives are sensitive to sodium. In these people, excessive consumption of salt (sodium chloride) together with inadequate dietary potassium seems to induce hypertension. Lowering sodium consumption can often decrease blood pressure in people with normal blood pressure, as well as those with hypertension.

Reduce ALCOHOL consumption. Drinking increases blood pressure due to increased EPINEPHRINE production by ADRENAL GLANDS. More than one or two drinks daily increases the odds for many diseases. An estimated 5 to 7% of hypertensive cases can be accounted for by excessive drinking.

Other Life-style Changes Are Important

- Lose weight. OBESITY increases blood pressure, and those who are overweight face odds that are two to six times greater than people with normal weight. Surplus body weight accounts for 20 to 30% of hypertensive cases.
- Exercise regularly. The exercise and weight management programs need to be tailored to the individual. Aerobic exercise is one of the most effective ways to normalize blood pressure. People who exercise regularly do not generally experience an age-related increase in blood pressure. Daily exercise is most effective; low-intensity (walking) to moderate-intensity (jogging) exercise seem to be as effective in lowering blood pressure as high-intensity exercise (running).
- Reduce stress. Anxiety and the suppression of anger increase the risk of hypertension in middleaged men and in teenagers. Many techniques, including biofeedback, yoga, meditation and selfhypnosis, are effective.
- Treat DIABETES and high blood cholesterol for cardiovascular health. Elevated blood sugar increases the odds of hypertension in middleaged women, and diabetes increases the risk of vascular disease generally.
- Stop smoking. Smoking is a contributing factor in hypertension, independent of all other factors. There are many reasons for stopping smoking, including decreasing the risk of cancer, heart attack and stroke.
- Avoid common DIET PILLS. PHENYLPROPANOLAMINE can raise blood pressure.

In assessing hypertension, a number of risk factors need to be evaluated. Life-style changes and weight reduction may be the first therapeutic strategy, rather than medication. There is an increased emphasis on non-drug therapy because of potentially harmful drug side effects. Consult a health care professional regarding supplements for hypertension. The National Heart, Lung and Blood Institute operates a toll free information line on hypertension at 1-800-575-9355. (See also HEART DISEASE.)

Farley, Dixie, "High Blood Pressure. Controlling the Silent Killer," *FDA Consumer*, 25:10 (1991), pp. 28–33.

Liebman, Bonnie, "One Nation, Under Pressure," *Nutrition Action Healthletter*, 22:6 (July/August 1995), pp. 1, 6–9.

hyperthyroidism   Overactivity of the THYROID GLAND leads to profound systemic changes, due to overproduction of thyroxine, the major thyroid HORMONE. This hormone increases the BASAL METABOLIC RATE, the rate at which energy is consumed to maintain body functions at rest. Symptoms include hyperactivity, weakness and, in extreme cases, weight loss, heat intolerance, excessive sweating, increased heart rate and sexual dysfunction. (See also ENDOCRINE SYSTEM; HYPOTHYROIDISM.)

hypertriglyceridemia   Chronically elevated blood FAT, also called TRIGLYCERIDES.

A normal serum triglyceride value after an overnight fast is around 100 mg per deciliter. Values greater than 500 increase the risk of CARDIOVASCULAR DISEASE, HEART ATTACK and PANCREATITIS. If elevated LDL (LOW-DENSITY LIPOPROTEIN, the undesirable form of cholesterol) accompanies elevated triglycerides, the risk of heart disease doubles. Hypertriglyceridemia is often an inherited disorder. Obesity, consumption of excessive alcohol, use of oral contraceptives, estrogens, thiazide DIURETICS or beta blockers also increases the odds of this condition. Excessive VITAMIN A, CAFFEINE and alcohol consumption and low CHROMIUM intake aggravate this condition. Fatty or sugary foods raise blood fat levels only temporarily after a meal.

Treatment calls for reduction of dietary fat, especially SATURATED FAT, and increased dietary COMPLEX CARBOHYDRATES together with weight reduction. Diabetics on high-fiber, high complex carbohydrate diets need to monitor their serum triglyceride levels, which can rise with such diets. (See also DIET; FAT METABOLISM; FIBER; HYPERLIPOPROTEINEMIA.)

U.S. Department of Health and Human Services. *Treatment of Hypertriglyceridemia*, Washington, D.C.: National Institutes of Health Consensus Development Conference Summary, 4:8.

hyperuricemia   Excessive URIC ACID levels in the blood. Although most people with high uric acid in the blood have no symptoms, this increases the risk factor for GOUT, a painful inflammation of joints due to deposits of uric acid. Elevated uric acid can result from inherited alterations in metabolism, such as the overproduction of the precursors of PURINES, building blocks of DNA, the genetic material, and of RNA, which directs protein synthesis. Factors favoring the precipitation of uric acid include excessive alcohol consumption; accumulation of KETONE BODIES, acids produced during uncontrolled diabetes; and occasionally the use of DIURETICS (water pills). A low purine diet restricts consumption of purine-rich food like anchovies, SARDINES and organ meats. (See also ARTHRITIS.)

hypervitaminosis   Toxicity due to an excessive intake of VITAMINS, especially overdosing with fat-soluble vitamins. Fat-soluble vitamins are not readily excreted and thus accumulate in fatty tissue. In contrast, the water-soluble vitamins are excreted by the kidney and, with the exception of VITAMIN B$_{12}$, are not stored.

Chronic high levels of VITAMIN A (e.g., 25,000 retinol equivalents or more per day) are linked to birth defects. Recent studies indicate that even 10,000 IU of 3,000 retinol equivalents per day are linked to an increased risk of birth defects. The consumption of 50,000 retinol equivalents for several months can cause toxic symptoms in adults such as headache, fatigue, nausea, hair loss and blurred vision. Liver damage is possible. Symptoms disappear when vitamin A intake is restricted. VITAMIN D excess (25,000 to 250,000 IU daily for several months) can cause kidney stones, kidney failure and heart irregularities. Excessive VITAMIN K can also be toxic. Symptoms include liver damage and JAUNDICE. VITAMIN E appears to be the safest of the fat-soluble vitamins.

Rothman, K.J., et al. "Teratogenicity of High Vitamin A Intake," *New England Journal of Medicine*, 333:21 (November 23, 1995) pp. 169–73.

hypoalbuminemia   An abnormally low level of serum ALBUMIN in the blood. Serum albumin represents 55% of the soluble protein of blood and as such it helps maintain the proper water concentration between blood and tissues. When less serum protein is synthesized, fluid tends to accumulate in tissues (EDEMA). Severe protein deficiency (starvation) causes the liver to decrease production of all serum proteins. The result is more readily observed with serum albumin. Thus a starving child may appear fat because of the severe edema. (EMACIATION; MALNUTRITION.)

hypocalcemia   Abnormally low blood CALCIUM. Circulating calcium concentration is maintained within a

very narrow range, in spite of fluctuation in dietary calcium. This condition most frequently represents a kidney abnormality or glandular disturbance, especially a deficiency of the parathyroid hormone, parathormone, the hormone responsible for raising blood calcium levels. (See also GLOMERULAR FILTRATION; PARATHYROID GLANDS; VITAMIN D.)

hypochlorhydria   Inadequate production of hydrochloric acid (STOMACH ACID). Although some free acid is present in gastric juice, it is inadequate to digest PROTEIN efficiently. Because there is inadequate acid to sterilize stomach contents, lowered stomach acid increases susceptibility to chronic infection by pathogenic bacteria, yeast and parasites and increases the likelihood of other gastrointestinal imbalances, including inflammation, maldigestion and nutrient MALABSORPTION. Diabetes, chronic GASTRITIS, FOOD SENSITIVITIES and SPRUE (severe intestinal malabsorption) can lower stomach acid production. Cimetidine (Tagamet and Zantac) are medications that severely reduce gastric juice secretion. (See also ACHLORHYDRIA; ANTACIDS.)

Wright, J.V. *Dr. Wright's Guide to Healing with Nutrition.* New Canaan, Conn.: Keats Publishing, 1990.

hypoglycemia, fasting   Chronic low BLOOD SUGAR that occurs during fasting (between meals). Symptoms are persistent and include headache, FATIGUE, lethargy, confusion and, in extreme cases, amnesia and unconsciousness. Hormonal imbalances, such as HYPOTHYROIDISM, low cortisol production, drug side effects and tumors can cause chronic fasting hypoglycemia. Individuals with disorders of the metabolism of glycogen (the storage form of carbohydrate) are also prone to fasting hypoglycemia. Underlying causes chronic need to be treated to ameliorate this condition. (See also HYPOGLYCEMIA; POSTPRANDIAL.)

Anderson, Richard A., "Chromium, Glucose Tolerance and Diabetes," *Biological Trace Element Research*, 32 (1992), pp. 19–24.

hypoglycemia, postprandial (reactive hypoglycemia, alimentary hypoglycemia)   A marked decline in BLOOD SUGAR within two to five hours after a meal, typically to less than 60 mg of glucose per deciliter. Postprandial hypoglycemia may be an early signal of non-insulin dependent DIABETES in middle-aged individuals. Normally, blood sugar is maintained between 70 and 110 mg per deciliter in order to supply the brain with glucose, its primary energy source. After eating a carbohydrate meal, the PANCREAS may overreact by releasing too much INSULIN, causing blood sugar to plummet below normal, baseline levels. Other mechanisms more slowly respond to raise blood sugar levels. The adrenal gland secretes EPINEPHRINE and GLUCOCORTICOIDS; the pancreas secretes GLUCAGON and the pituitary produces GROWTH HORMONE to increase blood sugar levels.

Hypoglycemia typically causes the mid-morning and mid-afternoon slumps. Any of the following may be observed during hypoglycemic episodes: sweating, anxiety, intense heartbeat, trembling, craving for food, hunger pangs, feeling lightheaded, inability to concentrate. However, the symptoms are transient. The feelings and perceptions of a patient undergoing a test to measure blood sugar levels after eating carbohydrate, need to be monitored.

Note that some symptoms resembling postprandial hypoglycemia occur with several serious disorders not involving hypoglycemia, and medical expertise is recommended to rule them out.

A variety of factors affect the level of blood sugar after a meal:

1. The rate of glucose uptake. The nutrient composition of the meal can prevent a precipitous drop in blood sugar due to an insulin overshoot. Certain types of carbohydrate (unrefined complex carbohydrates) are digested more slowly to glucose than others. Fat and fiber slow the rate of carbohydrate digestion and sugar absorption.
2. High blood insulin. Secretion by the pancreas may be excessive. This is more likely to occur in response to a sudden, high rise in blood sugar. Alternatively, excessive insulin medication can cause high insulin levels. In either case, excessive insulin promotes a dramatic decline in blood sugar.
3. Altered carbohydrate metabolism, especially by the liver. A key to maintaining blood sugar levels between meals is the ability of the liver to synthesize glucose (GLUCONEOGENESIS) and to liberate glucose from stores (GLYCOGEN).

Frequent causes of postprandial hypoglycemia include:

1. ALCOHOLISM. Consuming alcohol while eating may cause hypoglycemia if too much insulin is released and if glucose formation is blocked after drinking. A more serious situation can develop if liver glycogen stores are minimal, as occurs during chronic alcoholism. In this case, 3 to 10 drinks can prevent the liver from manufacturing enough blood glucose to fuel the brain, and a crisis can occur between 6 and 36 hours after drinking, sometimes leading to unconsciousness and death. Alcohol-induced hypoglycemia is particularly treacherous because symptoms resemble intoxication and glucose may not be administered in time to prevent unconsciousness.
2. Chronic, severe stress and adrenal exhaustion. The adrenal glands may not produce enough CORTISOL to promote protein breakdown and thus supply inadequate AMINO ACIDS for gluconeogenesis. This condition can also be the result of chronic starvation, and disease with fever.
3. Dietary factors. Excessive consumption of refined carbohydrate and natural sweeteners can cause erratic blood sugar due to a rapid rise in blood sugar followed by overcompensation by the pancreas, liberating excessive insulin.
4. Starvation. Too little carbohydrate is consumed to maintain normal blood sugar.
5. Carbohydrate maldigestion. This can lead to inadequate carbohydrate assimilation, even when carbohydrate intake is normal.
6. Liver disease. This can diminish the ability to produce glucose from amino acids and other non-carbohydrate building blocks of glucose.
7. Strenuous exercise can temporarily deplete blood sugar.

Treatment of postprandial hypoglycemia often involves:

1. Eating small, frequent meals, high in PROTEIN (20% of total calories) and COMPLEX CARBOHYDRATES (35 to 45% of calories) to maintain a slow, steady liberation and uptake of glucose.
2. Avoiding SUGAR, refined sweeteners (CORN SYRUP, high FRUCTOSE CORN SYRUP, DEXTROSE, FRUCTOSE) and sweets to minimize sudden increases in blood sugar levels and over-reaction by the pancreas.
3. Consuming less CONVENIENCE FOODS and high-calorie foods that generally have a high sugar and highly refined carbohydrate content.
4. Avoiding COFFEE and alcohol. They can accentuate the symptoms of hypoglycemia.
5. Reducing stress with meditation or yoga to normalize endocrine function. Many individuals can manage stress effectively if they eat properly and exercise.
6. Controlling FOOD SENSITIVITIES, which may accentuate blood sugar variations.

hypokalemia   Low blood POTASSIUM. Typically this accompanies severe DIARRHEA because potassium in secretions is lost. Hypokalemia can occur during treatment for diabetes (ketoacidosis) involving the accumulation of ketone bodies, acidic products of fat metabolism. In addition, certain DIURETICS (water pills) cause excessive potassium excretion. Symptoms of hypokalemia include muscle weakness and muscle cramps. (See also HYPERKALEMIA.)

hypothalamic-pituitary-adrenal axis (HPA axis)   A pivotal integration of the nervous system and the hormonal (endocrine) system. The HPA axis integrates fundamental physiological and metabolic processes, including circadian (daily) rhythms. The hypothalamus monitors the autonomic nervous system. The autonomic nervous system regulates visceral activities such as dilation of blood vessels, blood pressure and rate of heartbeat, movement of the gastrointestinal tract, and most glandular secretions (sweat glands, salivary glands, gastric and intestinal glands, and the pancreas). Most changes occur involuntarily and automatically. The sympathetic division stimulates activity of an organ, whereas the parasympathetic division decreases activity.

The hypothalamus in turn regulates the pituitary, the master hormone-secreting gland. In particular the pituitary regulates ENDOCRINE glands such as the adrenal cortex, which is triggered to release CORTISOL into the bloodstream. In turn, cortisol regulates many metabolic processes including protein breakdown, fat turnover and blood sugar formation. Subsequently, elevated blood cortisol binds to receptors in the HYPOTHALAMUS and the PITUITARY, which limits further adrenal stimulation. Such finely timed feedback loops assure precise integration of these regulatory processes. (See also HOMEOSTASIS.)

hypothalamus   An array of nerve cells and fibers, located near the upper region of the brain stem, that regulate body temperature, water and ELECTROLYTE balance, blood pressure, reproduction, APPETITE and possibly body weight and HUNGER. The hypothalamus is classified as a neuroendocrine gland because it is made up of nerves and at the same time it produces HORMONES. The hypothalamus processes emotions like embarrassment, anger and fright, and at the same time it integrates the autonomic nervous system, responsible for regulating many involuntary functions like heartbeat, blood pressure, peristalsis (contraction of smooth muscles of the DIGESTIVE TRACT) and the secretion of most glands, including sweat glands, glands producing digestive juices (salivary glands, pancreas, stomach and intestinal glands) and even a portion of the ADRENAL GLAND (adrenal medulla), which releases the stress hormone EPINEPHRINE (adrenaline).

The hypothalamus produces two hormones, transported to and secreted by the posterior lobe of the pituitary: ANTIDIURETIC HORMONE (ADH), which accelerates reabsorption of WATER into blood from the urine in kidney tubules, and OXYTOCIN, which stimulates contractions of the uterus at the termination of pregnancy and stimulates milk release. The hypothalamus regulates the PITUITARY GLAND, the master gland of the ENDOCRINE SYSTEM, by means of a battery of hormones. Thyrotropin-releasing hormone directs the pituitary gland to release thyroid stimulating hormone. Corticotropin-releasing factor directs the pituitary to release ACTH, which activates the adrenal glands. The hypothalamus also secretes growth hormone releasing hormone, and growth hormone inhibiting hormone (somatostatin), which regulate pituitary secretion of growth hormone; luteinizing hormone releasing hormone, which directs the pituitary to release luteinizing hormone to help regulate the menstrual cycle; and prolactin releasing hormone, which directs the pituitary to release prolactin, a hormone that helps control breast development and milk formation during pregnancy. Finally, the hypothalamus produces follicle stimulating-hormone releasing hormone which directs the pituitary to release follicle stimulating hormone to help regulate the menstrual cycle.

Body fat signals the brain (hypothalamus) to stop feeding by secreting a protein called LEPTIN into the bloodstream. Leptin is believed to direct the brain to curtail eating (satiety), by shutting down production of hunger signals, for example, by altering the production of neuropeptides or the release of neurotransmitters that stimulate feeding. Hunger, craving and satiety are complex phenomena involving the integration of a vast amount of information by the brain and central nervous system. The hypothalamus plays a central role in this integration. (See also HOMEOSTASIS; HYPOTHALAMIC-PITUITARY-ADRENAL AXIS.)

Chrousos, J.S., "The Hypothalamic-pituitary-adrenal Axis and Immune-mediated Inflammation," *New England Journal of Medicine*, 332:20 (May 18, 1995), pp. 1351–62.

hypothyroidism   The condition resulting from inadequate production of thyroid HORMONES. Thyroid hormones, THYROXINE and triiodothyronine, helps regulate metabolism throughout the body; any decrease in the production or utilization of those hormones would be expected to affect major processes like energy production. FATIGUE and low body temperatures may indicate the THYROID GLAND is not working with maximum efficiency, and thyroid hormone production may be low. In some cases the pituitary gland may produce inadequate thyroid stimulating hormone (TSH) Clinical laboratory tests frequently measure levels of thyroid hormones as well as TSH and thyroid releasing hormone (TRH). Severe adult hypothyroidism is called myxedema and is characterized by a puffy, bloated face with dry, rough skin and hair loss.

The thyroid gland helps regulate the body's temperature and metabolic rate, and hypothyroidism can lower the BASAL METABOLIC RATE by 35 to 40%, which in turn causes reduced muscle tone, depression, sluggishness, low body temperature and excessive fatigue. Motivation declines. In children hypothyroidism can delay growth and mental development. In women there may be heavy menstrual bleeding. Metabolic processes are affected; the efficiency of using protein, carbohydrate and fat as fuels declines, and blood CHOLESTEROL and FAT levels generally increase, increasing the risk of CARDIOVASCULAR DISEASE.

Mild hypothyroidism is common in the Great Lakes region, possibly due to low iodine content in midwestern soils. Other conditions can cause fatigue, including low adrenal steroid hormones, infection, ALLERGY and MALNUTRITION. There have been reports of childbirth correcting mild hypothyroidism. Chronic hypothyroidism warrants medical attention. Clinical laboratory tests can measure serum thyroid hormone levels (T_3 and T_4), as well as thyroid stimulating hormone from the pituitary, to help uncover underlying imbalances. (See also CHRONIC FATIGUE; CORTISOL; ENDOCRINE SYSTEM; HYPOGLYCEMIA.)

Singer, Peter A., et al., "Treatment Guidelines for Patients with Hyperthyroidism and Hypothyroidism," *Journal of the American Medical Association*, 273:10 (1995), pp. 808–12.

iatrogenic malnutrition See HOSPITAL-INDUCED MAL-NUTRITION.

IBD See INFLAMMATORY BOWEL DISEASE.

IBS See IRRITABLE BOWEL SYNDROME.

ice cream A frozen DESSERT containing flavored, sweetened frozen cream and MILK products like CASEIN and SUGAR. Frozen desserts based on EGGS, cream and milk were apparently invented in the 1600s, though frozen blends of fruits were served in ancient China, where salt mixtures were used to lower the temperature below freezing. Ice cream is a favorite dessert; Americans eat an average of 15 quarts a year per person.

Ice cream is a high-CALORIE, high-FAT and high-sugar food. Unless it is homemade, ice cream will usually contain artificial coloring, flavorings and stabilizers such as LOCUST BEAN GUM, GUAR GUM, CARRAGEENAN, GELATIN, and alginic acid or cellulose derivatives. Federal law requires that ice cream contain at least 10% fat (BUTTERFAT), and most regular ice creams provide 10 to 12% butterfat. Super-premium vanilla ice cream contains 16 to 20% butterfat. In contrast, ice milk contains 2 to 7% fat, while sherbet contains 1 to 2% fat. Ice cream usually contains SUCROSE (table sugar) or other sweeteners. Emulsifiers like POLYSORBATES and MONOGLYC-ERIDES stabilize ice cream during processing. Non-dairy frozen desserts resembling ice cream have no legally defined butterfat content, and though they are low-fat options, some-times these desserts have more total calories per serving than traditional ice cream due to their high sweetener content.

One cup of rich vanilla-flavored ice cream with about 16% fat provides: 349 calories; protein, 4.1 g; carbohydrate, 32 g; fat 23.7 g; cholesterol, 88 mg; calcium 151 mg; vitamin A, 219 retinol equivalents; thiamin, 0.04 mg; riboflavin, 0.28 mg; niacin, 0.12 mg.

One cup of regular vanilla ice cream with about 11% fat provides: 269 calories; protein, 4.8 g; carbohydrate, 31.7 g; fat, 14.3 g; cholesterol, 59 mg; calcium, 176 mg; vitamin A, 133 retinol equivalents; and similar amounts of thiamin, riboflavin and niacin to those found in rich vanilla ice cream.

One cup of vanilla-flavored ice milk with about 4% fat provides: 184 calories; protein, 5.2 g; carbohydrate, 29 g; fat, 5.6 g; cholesterol, 18 mg; calcium, 176 mg; vitamin A, 52 retinol equivalents; and similar amounts of other vitamins. (See also DAIRY-FREE FROZEN DESSERTS; DIETARY GUIDELINES FOR AMERICANS.)

ideal body weight An outmoded standard for body weight that originated from data collected by U.S. life insurance companies from their policy holders who lived the longest. Ideal body weight was listed as the average weight for a given age, height, body or "frame" size. From these data grew the classic definition for OBESITY as a weight 20% greater than the ideal body weight. Part of the problem with this standard of ideal body weight lies in the nature of HEIGHT-WEIGHT TABLES. Weight charts and tables do not take into account individual variations in body structure (muscles and bone mass); consequently, there is no standard for measuring small, medium or large body frames.

There is no single ideal body weight for a group of people because every person has an individual, desirable weight. Selecting a realistic body weight as a goal has proven to be far more useful than striving for a rigidly defined standard. A realistic body weight is one that can be readily maintained without intermittent DIETING.

A measure of body FAT is more useful than total body weight because body weight may not correlate with the amount of fat on a lean person. Furthermore, ideal body weight provides no indication of fat distribution. Some fat deposits are riskier for heart disease than others. Methods of accurately measuring body fat at clinics include buoyancy testing with underwater weighing (requiring a special tank) and skin fold thickness measured by skin calipers or by skin resistance measurements.

Suggestions for estimating an optimal body weight include: For males, take 106 pounds for the first 5 ft of height, then add 6 lbs for each additional inch of height. For females, take 100 pounds for the first 5 ft, then add 5 lbs for each additional inch (See also BODY MASS INDEX; FATFOLD TEST.)

idiopathic   A medical term that is applied to a disease or condition arising spontaneously from an unknown cause. Idiopathic GOUT and high blood pressure are examples.

ileitis   See CROHN'S DISEASE.

ileum   The last three-fifths of the small INTESTINE that joins the large intestine (COLON). The length of the ileum varies among individuals, ranging from 15 to 30 ft in adult males. Flow of material between the ileum and colon is regulated by the ileocecal valve. The ileum absorbs FAT, fat-soluble vitamins, CALCIUM, MAGNESIUM, VITAMIN B$_{12}$ and AMINO ACIDS. BILE salts, which act as the detergents in bile required for fat DIGESTION, are also absorbed in the ileum and are recycled by the liver to be released once again in bile. (See also ENTEROHEPATIC CIRCULATION.)

illness   (sickness)   Ill health or disease. This condition is the opposite of wellness; illness reflects imbalanced body functions and can thus be regarded as a change away from the healthy state, in which all systems function within normal limits (HOMEOSTASIS).

An illness may be localized, in which a limited region of the body is affected, or it may be systemic, in which several parts of the body or the whole body are affected. Pain is often associated with illness, though pain is not equivalent to disease. Pain generally indicates that an imbalance exists in the body. The imbalance could reflect an unhealthy life-style, such as dietary excess or deficiency, or it could be associated with infection and inflammation.

Most illnesses are self-limiting, meaning that the body generally can cure itself when given the opportunity. It is now clear that the body's systems work together to maintain health. Particularly important are the IMMUNE SYSTEM, the NERVOUS SYSTEM and the ENDOCRINE SYSTEM (hormone-producing system). An imbalanced immune system affects the brain, and the brain alters immunity and hormone production. Hormones in turn affect nerve function. As an example, perceived STRESS can trigger a FIGHT OR FLIGHT RESPONSE by the brain. The stress response is modified by hormones, and sustained, elevated adrenal hormones due to prolonged stress affect the immune system and decrease the immune response to foreign invaders.

Whether or not an individual becomes ill depends on a complex interplay of many factors, broadly categorized according to medical history and environmental influences. Family history reflects patterns of inheritance, over which one has no control. Genetic predisposition thus increases the risk of many chronic, degenerative diseases of AGING, such as OSTEOPOROSIS, heart disease and STROKE, high blood pressure and DIABETES. Health history can have a profound effect on susceptibility to illness. Thus prior injury, deficiency or illness can set the stage for a subsequent illness. As examples, arthritis can begin at the site of a former injury, and prolonged treatment with a broad-spectrum antibiotic can destroy beneficial gut bacteria and promote a yeast infection. Prior drug treatment can alter the body's ability to destroy alcohol, and pretreatment with alcohol can alter the body's ability to degrade many drugs. In terms of public health, immunization against polio, flu or tetanus reduces the risk of these diseases. At the beginning of the 20th century niacin deficiency caused widespread pellagra and associated mental illness in the South. The enrichment of bread and grain products with the B vitamin NIACIN in the 1920s essentially eliminated pellagra as a public health issue in the United States.

Due to differences in inheritance and environment, toxic exposure, nutritional status and medical history, each person is biochemically unique. As a result of distinctive genetic makeup (genetic polymorphism), certain people synthesize different levels of specific enzymes (biological catalysts) and other aspects of defensive physiologic systems. Thus, individuals vary in their ability to protect themselves against damaging effects of oxidizing agents (free radicals), and to detoxify potentially dangerous chemicals that they eat or drink or breathe at home or in the workplace.

Although neither a family history nor a medical history can be altered, life-style choices can profoundly impact susceptibility to illness. The most frequently cited RISK factors for illness and premature death include the use of tobacco and alcohol, accidental injury, unwanted pregnancy, drug abuse and inadequate nutrition. The growing awareness that prevention is the most cost-effective and permanent solution to many health issues has lead many physicians to work with their patients as partners in health to empower them in making healthful choices for themselves and their families.

This approach could possibly decrease American deaths before the age of 65 by two-thirds, even without further breakthroughs in medicine and nutrition.

Prevention and Personal Responsibility

The health-conscious individual can focus on four essential steps in maintaining health and preventing illness: positive attitude, a healthy diet, regular exercise and minimizing toxic exposures. Humanistic psychology emphasizes the importance of a positive mental attitude in preventing illness and maintaining health. The immune system and the repair mechanisms of tissues are well designed to ward off infection, to cure disease and to repair injury. DEPRESSION seems to diminish this capacity. For example, depression causes a drop in the production of interleukin, proteins that help regulate the immune response and help activate cancer-killing lymphocytes. Clinical statistics in the United States suggest psychological stress can harm the heart, increasing the risk of re-hospitalization among patients with cardiac problems. Group therapy, meditation and other practices may improve cardiovascular health in patients with clogged arteries by modifying their response to psychological stress.

Susceptibility to disease reflects nutritional status; the nutritional environment affects the expression of inherited traits. Either overnutrition or UNDERNUTRITION can set the stage for chronic illness. Excessive fat consumption increases the risk of cancer and obesity, while inadequate amounts of most nutrients eventually lower the body's defense against disease, including cancer. On the other hand, a healthy diet provides optimal amounts of all nutrients to assure health, while avoiding detrimental food constituents.

Probably the best strategies to avoid chronic illness associated with aging are regular physical exercise coupled with wise food choices. A sedentary life-style is linked to an estimated 250,000 deaths annually in the United States. Exercise decreases the risk of heart disease, stroke, high blood pressure (hypertension), adult onset diabetes, osteoporosis (thin bone disease) and colon and breast cancer.

Minimizing exposure to potentially damaging agents such as solvents, pollutants and cigarette smoke is also important. The amount, type and length of exposure to a toxic material at home or in the workplace affects health. Only recently have studies been undertaken to determine additive, long-term effects on health of continued low level-exposure to pesticides and industrial pollutants in food and water and air. (See also ANTIOXIDANT; BIOCHEMICAL INDIVIDUALITY; DEGENERATIVE DISEASES; DETOXIFICATION.)

imitation fat   See FAT SUBSTITUTE; OLESTRA; SIMPLESSE.

imitation flour   See FLOUR SUBSTITUTE.

imitation food   A processed food that is nutritionally inferior to the real food. The designation "nutritionally inferior" on a food label means that the food contains 10% less of one or more nutrients than the food for which it substitutes. The food industry has devoted considerable financial resources toward producing imitation food, most often substitutes for MEAT, FISH, dairy products and FRUIT. For example, SURIMI is imitation seafood. Compared to real foods, imitation foods often have a longer shelf life and often are tastier. Food additives are carefully selected for this purpose. Imitation foods are often less expensive than the real foods. Imitation foods are generally less nutritious than the foods they replace because processing destroys or removes important nutrients. Relatively few nutrients are added back.

Current regulations specify that food labels must list ingredients in descending order according to weight, meaning that the first ingredient listed is the most predominant. If the first item listed on the food label is one of the following, the food is likely to be fabricated or highly processed: any natural sweetener such as corn sweetener, high FRUCTOSE CORN SYRUP, HONEY, DEXTROSE, SUCROSE or corn syrup solids; TEXTURIZED VEGETABLE PROTEIN; and sodium caseinate. The presence of artificial food colors, MSG (MONOSODIUM GLUTAMATE), COCONUT OIL, palm or palm kernel oil and PRESERVATIVES also indicates that the food is imitation or highly processed. (See also CONVENIENCE FOOD; FOOD ADDITIVES; FOOD LABELING.)

immune system   An elaborate, finely tuned defense system to destroy and counter the effects of viruses, bacteria, yeasts and foreign substances that operate within tissues and cells and in the bloodstream. The immune system recognizes "self" from "non-self," substances not part of the body. Another feature of the immune system is memory. It can remember previous invaders and mount a rapid response to them when they reappear. When the immune system is healthy it destroys foreign elements without causing symptoms, but an imbalanced immune system can set the stage for disease. Foreign substances and microorganisms may not be recognized or destroyed, resulting in chronic infection or even CANCER and AIDS. An imbalanced immune system can attack the body's own tissues, creating AUTOIMMUNE DISEASES, or it can overrespond to common substances, creating allergies, such as food allergies.

Organization of the Immune System

The two branches of the immune system are "cellular immunity" and "humoral immunity." The first depends on the active participation of different types of cells. Cellular immunity includes macrophages, cells that engulf foreign invaders. These scavengers are amoebalike cells that surround and digest foreign particles, viruses and bacteria. Macrophages live in tissues like the spleen (splenocytes), the LIVER (Kupffer cells), the lymph (wandering macrophages), the spinal cord, the brain (microglia) and connective tissue.

Lymphocytes are an important type of white blood cell. T cells are highly specialized lymphocytes that attack viruses, tumors and transplanted cells and regulate the immune system. T cells are processed by the THYMUS GLAND. They work with B cells, which produce defensive proteins called ANTIBODIES. In a typical scenario, macrophages first engulf foreign materials called ANTIGENS and transform fragments of the antigens for display on their cell surfaces. Certain T "helper" cells, acting as "generals," "read" these antigens and in turn stimulate the production of specialized T "killer" cells, foot soldiers that destroy abnormal cells or foreign materials.

The different types of immune cells communicate with each other via protein messengers called LYMPHOKINES. For example, macrophages produce a lymphokine called interleukin-1 to activate T helper cells, which in turn produce interleukin-2, to stimulate the production of the killer T cells. Helper T cells also produce gamma INTERFERON, which activates killer T cells.

Mast cells are a type of T cell that lives in tissues and fights local infection. When they contact foreign materials and cells, mast cells destroy them. Mast cells also release special chemicals like HISTAMINE, as well as certain lymphokines that trigger inflammation marked by swelling (EDEMA), redness, itching, sneezing and runny nose. Lymphokines also trigger phagocytes (macrophages) to destroy foreigners and dispose of signal proteins once they have done their work.

Humoral immunity pertains to blood and lymph. It relies on cells that release defensive PROTEINS called complement and antibodies into the bloodstream to fight infection. Antibodies (gamma globulins) are Y-shaped proteins designed to target a particular antigen, by which a substance is recognized as being foreign. An antibody can neutralize the enemy either by binding to it or by targeting it for attack by other cells and chemicals. After antibodies bind foreign cells, complement ruptures them. Complement also triggers localized inflammatory reactions, leading to common symptoms of pain, redness and swelling, as well as to an increased concentration of defensive cells at the point of injury or infection.

B cells, which originate in bone marrow, are a type of lymphocyte that yield plasma cells, specialized to produce antibodies when exposed to foreign invaders. B cell proliferation, maturation and antibody production are stimulated by T helper infected cells. Another type of T cell, called T suppressor cells, gear down the immune system by turning off B cell production. Thus T suppressor cells limit allergic attacks and auto-immune reactions.

Immunity

Immunity is a hallmark of the immune system. The recovery from an infection renders the individual immune to subsequent attack by the particular pathogen (disease-causing agent). Immunity to chicken pox is a common example. The underlying mechanism relies on memory T and memory B cells in the bloodstream, which signal a red alert for a quick attack the next time a conquered virus invades again. These memory cells multiply rapidly when they again encounter any antigen they remember.

Nutrients that May Benefit the Immune System

The immune system requires a rich array of nutrients, including protein, FATTY ACIDS, VITAMINS and MINERALS, for normal function. A JUNK FOOD diet can lead to overnutrition (too many calories and fat) and malnutrition, (too little trace minerals and vitamins) that weaken the immune system. Malnourished individuals lacking adequate protein or calories are prone to disease. Low-level deficiencies of many nutrients seem to lower the effectiveness of the immune system. Supplements can boost immunity, especially in elderly people. It seems clear that a wise approach to support the immune system nutritionally includes a varied diet—reducing fat to less than 30% of daily calories and emphasizing whole foods, FRUITS and VEGETABLES, especially those rich in VITAMIN C, BETA CAROTENE and other carotenoids. Supplementing the diet with 100% of the RDA (RECOMMENDED DIETARY ALLOWANCE) of B vitamins and trace minerals for insurance may also be prudent when a diet is compromised by junk food or when the diet provides fewer than 1,600 calories.

ANTIOXIDANT nutrients such as vitamin C, VITAMIN E, SELENIUM, COPPER, MANGANESE and beta carotene may enhance immune responses by lowering the burden of FREE RADICALS, thus protecting immune cells against the cumulative oxidation and free radical attack due to the release of powerful oxidizing agents as superoxide, hydrogen peroxide and hydroxyl radicals.

Vitamin C deficiency lowers the immune response in animal models. Adequate vitamin C increases T and B cell production and helps attacking cells migrate to sites of infection while making viruses and bacteria more sensitive to destruction. Furthermore, vitamin C acts as an antioxidant, and it protects cells against reactive chemicals produced by mast cells used to destroy foreigners.

Vitamin E enhances both humoral and cell-mediated immunity, while vitamin E deficiency contributes to reduce T cells, killer cells and macrophage function. Vitamin E supplementation boosts the immune system in elderly men and women consuming a typical diet, suggesting that older people require more vitamin E than specified by the adult Recommended Dietary Allowance to assure a fully functional immune system.

Selenium is a cofactor for an important antioxidant enzyme, glutathione peroxidase, which neutralizes lipid peroxide that could damage the immune cells. Selenium works with vitamin E to stimulate the immune response to infection in experimental animals. Together they may help protect against cancer. Selenium increases T helper cells and increases antibody production in experimental animals. However, excessive selenium depresses the immune system.

Other specific nutrients support the function of the immune system:

FOLIC ACID is required for immunity and lymphocyte production. Folic acid is often deficient in the American diet.

IRON is required to produce T and B cells. Iron deficiency is associated with increased incidence of common infection among children.

MAGNESIUM is needed by the complement system to activate phagocytes. It is also required for antibody production. Americans typically do not consume enough magnesium.

PANTOTHENIC ACID and VITAMIN B_6 help keep the lymphatic system and thymus gland healthy.

VITAMIN A and beta carotene help maintain thymus gland function during stress. Overproduction of cortisol, a stress-induced hormone from the adrenal glands, tends to shrink the thymus gland, which is critical for fully functioning T cells. Beta carotene is the precursor of vitamin A. Limited studies suggest that beta carotene may also stimulate helper T cells. Studies of children in developing nations indicate that there is a direct relationship between vitamin A deficiency and decreased resistance to infection. On the other hand, excessive vitamin A can decrease immune system function.

Vitamin B_6 plays an important role in maintaining optimal immunity, including antibody production and phagocytic activity. Vitamin B_6 deficiency impairs the immune system in a number of ways. It lowers cell-directed immune responses, described earlier, and leads to decreased thymus function. Vitamin B_6 deficiency during gestation in experimental animals impairs immune functioning even in first and second generation offspring.

ZINC helps maintain lymph glands and the thymus gland, thereby helping to fight chronic infection. Zinc is required for many important enzymes, and it is not surprising that zinc deficiency decreases T cell and B cell function and macrophage activity. However, too much zinc (for example, 20 times the RDA) can depress immunity. Zinc, in combination with other trace minerals including copper, iron and manganese, appears to improve B and T cell function in older people.

Copper deficiency is associated with an increased risk of infection. Copper deficiency diminishes the effectiveness of the humoral system in lab animals. Copper is an essential component of SUPEROXIDE DISMUTASE, an antioxidant system, and CYTOCHROME C oxidase, an enzyme system required for energy production.

Immunity, Stress and Exercise

Stress, whether physical or emotional, can alter hormonal output and immune response. A high level of stress increases the risk of illness and injury in the following year and shortens the life span.

Emotional well-being is supported by proper diet and regular physical EXERCISE. Moderately intense exercise increases the production of ENDORPHINS, the brain's own opiates, which can bolster parts of the immune system. Studies indicate that interleukin-1 and interferon, which help the body respond to infection or injury, increase after moderate exercise. Moderate exercise also increases killer cell activity.

Strenuous aerobic exercise may decrease efficiency of the immune system and temporarily increase susceptibility to illness by increasing the production of adrenal stress hormones. Among the hormones produced is cortisol, which limits inflammation by blocking the immune system. With continued stress, production of protective antibodies (such as secreted IgA, the antibody that protects the intestine and other body cavities against invasion by foreign substances). Chronic stress also decreases killer cell activity, increasing a person's susceptibility to disease. (See also AGING; B COMPLEX; ENDOCRINE SYSTEM; MALNUTRITION; NERVOUS SYSTEM; PSYCHONEUROIMMUNOLOGY.)

Shronts, Eva P., "Basic Concepts of Immunology and Its Application to Clinical Nutrition," *Immunology and Clinical Nutrition*, 8:4 (1993), pp. 177–83.

inborn errors of metabolism Abnormal gene products can cause metabolic imbalances, resulting in disease. Generally the inherited defect leads to the inadequate formation of an enzyme. Occasionally, inadequate formation of a COENZYME (enzyme helper) limits enzyme function or the protein-based signaling system that regulates a given enzyme's function. Most genetic defects are classified as autosomal recessive, meaning that they are not sex-linked. Full expression of the imbalance can occur only when both chromosomes contain the defective gene coding for a given enzyme and normal genes coding for that enzyme are absent. Examples of genetic diseases related to nutrients include familial HYPERCHOLESTEROLEMIA (high blood CHOLESTEROL), sickle cell anemia, GALACTOSEMIA and PHENYLKETONURIA. PKU is an inherited inability to metabolize the essential AMINO ACID, PHENYLALANINE. PKU responds to nutritional intervention. During infancy and childhood PKU patients receive carefully balanced diets that provide only enough phenylalanine to support growth. Labels for foods containing the artificial sweetener ASPARTAME must warn phenylketonurics because of its phenylalanine content. (See also DNA; FOOD LABELING; MUTATION.)

Brusilow, S.W., and Maestri, N.E., "Urea Cycle Disorders: Diagnosis, Pathophysiology and Therapy," *Advance in Pediatrics* 43 (1996), pp. 127–70.

indigestion See GASTROINTESTINAL DISORDERS.

individuality See BIOCHEMICAL INDIVIDUALITY.

induction (enzyme induction) The increased production of an ENZYME in response to external stimuli. Enzymes function as biological catalysts of cellular chemical reactions. The body can adapt to a limited extent to changes in the diet and to environmental influences by altering the levels of enzymes in a given tissue. For example, a high carbohydrate diet leads to increased production of AMYLASE, the starch-digesting enzyme of the pancreas. Starvation decreases levels of digestive enzymes and enzymes responsible for fat and glycogen synthesis but induces enzymes required for fat and carbohydrate degradation. Enzymes that synthesize BLOOD SUGAR (glucose) from amino acids are also induced by starvation.

Excessive alcohol consumption induces liver alcohol oxidizing systems so that alcohol will be cleared from the blood more efficiently. Similarly, many medications induce liver enzymes responsible for drug degradation. Certain cellular enzyme levels increase in response to hormones and to growth promoters. Examples include the hormones ESTROGEN (female sex hormone), CORTISOL (adrenal hormone regulating energy metabolism and degradation) and GROWTH HORMONE (a pituitary hormone involved both in growth and maintenance of tissues, especially muscles). INSULIN provides the broad impetus for increased enzyme production in many tissues. Insulin from the PANCREAS is perhaps the most general anabolic hormone; that is, it promotes enzymes leading to the accumulation of protein, fat and carbohydrates. (See also DETOXIFICATION.)

infant formula A manufactured food designed to nurture the infant during the first year of life, until weaning. Commercial infant formulas are either non-fat cow's MILK-based or soybean-based. Common formulas are available in powdered form, as concentrates, or as ready-to-feed liquid with no prior preparation. No formula exactly reproduces human milk; on the other hand, formulas can provide adequate nutrition for babies.

In the late 1970s production of chloride-deficient formulas caused delayed speech, slowed growth and poor muscle control in babies who had consumed the products. Partially in response to this disaster, Congress passed the Infant Formula Act of 1980, which mandates the U.S. FDA to see that this synthetic food meets nutrient standards based upon the American Academy of Pediatrics' recommendations to assure infant growth and development.

In 1982 the U.S. FDA adapted quality-control procedures to monitor the production of this food. As a result, infant formulas are nutritionally similar though not identical to breast milk in total protein, total fat, calcium to phosphorus ratio, energy content (calories/100 ml), content of the essential fatty acid linoleic acid, and electrolytes (sodium, potassium, chloride).

There are advantages to infant formulas. There is no limit to the supply, and a mother has greater freedom to care for other children or to return to work. Other family members can participate in feeding sessions, developing the warmth of that association. The mother of a formula-fed infant can offer the same closeness and stimulation as the BREASTFEEDING mother.

The number of nursing mothers in the United States has been declining since 1982. In 1992 an estimated 53% of women in the United States breastfed their infants one week after leaving the hospital (*New York Times*, October 10, 1993). Several weeks of breastfeeding assures that the mother's antibodies will be present in the infant.

Cow's milk formula resembles its source in terms of type of milk protein, total fat, and calcium to phosphorus ratio. It has been adjusted so that the total protein content, carbohydrate, fat, major minerals, linoleic acid and vitamins are similar to breast milk. The La Leche League International does not recommend substituting formula or breast milk with straight cow's milk until the baby is a year old or older (eating the equivalent of three baby food jars of solid food per day). Unprocessed cow's milk is not a suitable food for infants for many reasons.

Cow's milk contains three times as much protein as human milk, and this protein is more difficult for babies to digest. Manufacturers either pre-soften or pre-digest this protein, or they add whey to adjust the protein ratio. Butterfat is also poorly digested by infants; therefore it is replaced by vegetable oils. Because the higher concentration of phosphate and other dissolved minerals in cow's milk increases the burden on immature kidneys, minerals are adjusted to resemble breastmilk. Lactose or corn syrup solids are used to adjust the carbohydrate content. Bovine milk protein contains much more of the essential amino acid phenylalanine than human milk protein. This situation could affect infants who cannot tolerate high phenylalanine for genetic reasons (see PHENYLKETONURIA).

Cow's milk in infant formulas sometimes triggers an ALLERGY, especially if there is a family history of allergies. Cow's milk-based formula as a supplement to breastfeeding is less of a problem when the baby is six months or older.

For infants who are sensitive to cow's milk, liquid formulas containing soy protein fortified with the essential amino acid methionine and with soybean oil are available. A variety of formulas are prepared from coconut oil and corn oil, but these oils contain very little alpha linolenic acid, an essential fatty acid. Human milk contains substantial amounts of a large fatty acid called DOCOSAHEXAENOIC ACID (DHA). DHA, which is necessary for normal brain and eye development, is not added to formula. There is a consensus that formula should at least contain linolenic acid, the precursor of DHA, which the infant's body may convert to DHA.

A wide variety of infant formulas is available to meet special needs. Infants with lactose intolerance can drink formulas in which lactose is replaced by other carbohydrates. Formulas can be adapted to adjust protein ratio, linoleic acid content or to lower sodium content. Special formulas are available for pre-term babies.

Ready-to-use formula, as well as powdered formula, sometimes contains ALUMINUM. This is not a problem for babies with normal kidneys; however, premature babies may tolerate it poorly. CARRAGEENAN-containing formula should not be given to premature infants. This seaweed product is used to stabilize fat by forming gels in milk.

The infant formula industry employed questionable marketing practices in developing countries, which led to a 1977 consumer boycott against the Swiss-based Nestlé company. For example, they dressed staff in hospital garb while introducing infant formula to new mothers, and used misleading ads. In 1979, Nestlé, which accounted for 50% of formula sales to the Third World, and the U.S. government formally agreed to voluntary guidelines that banned marketing abuses in developing nations.

In 1981 the United Nations World Health Organization voted overwhelmingly to approve an international code of conduct to restrict advertising and marketing of baby formula, usually powdered, which can lead to infant malnutrition and death when improperly used. Though not binding, the new guidelines apply to infant formula promotion in industrialized nations as well as developing nations. Proper use of infant formula is often impossible in poorer areas of the world, where the water used to mix the formula is often contaminated. (See also BABY FOOD.)

Lonnerdal, B., "Nutritional Aspects of Soy Formula," *Acta Paediatric Supplementation*, 402 (1994), pp. 105–08.

inflammation (inflammatory response) A defensive response to irritation, injury or infection usually characterized by heat, redness, swelling and pain at the injury site. This response is triggered by physical agents, chemical agents or disease-producing organisms. Swelling is due to increased blood vessel leakage of fluids, and redness is due to vasodilation, the increase in diameter of blood vessels, especially capillaries so that they carry more blood. With increased vessel leakage (permeability), substances normally retained in blood such as water, antibodies (defensive proteins), phagocytic cells and clot-forming components, migrate into tissues at the site of injury.

Cellular Materials that Promote Inflammation

HISTAMINE, kinins, PROSTAGLANDINS, LEUKOTRIENES and complement contribute to inflammation. Histamine, derived from the amino acid HISTIDINE, is released from white cells (basophils), mast cells and other cells when injured. Kinins are proteins that induce vasodilation, increase vessel leakiness, attract phagocytic cells and cause pain. Prostaglandins are hormone-like materials that function in the immediate area where they are produced. They play many roles, including intensifying pain and promoting fever, which helps combat infections. Leukotrienes are extremely powerful inflammatory agents. Complement is a group of blood proteins that stimulate histamine release, destroy bacteria and promote phagocytosis (engulfing other cells and fragments). Pain can result from injured nerves or from irritation by released microbial products.

Non-steroidal anti-inflammatory drugs (NSAIDS) are often used to combat inflammation. These drugs, which are often non-prescriptions items, can themselves cause damage to the stomach or intestinal lining; in some instances they may harm the liver when used in excess. (See also ASPIRIN; IMMUNE SYSTEM.)

inflammatory bowel disease (IBD) A chronic inflammation of the intestinal wall involving painful swelling and open sores. Eventually the intestinal wall becomes scarred, which narrows the intestinal opening. IBD affects 1 to 2 million Americans. It differs from CELIAC DISEASE, a grain (especially wheat) intolerance, and from

IRRITABLE BOWEL SYNDROME (spastic colon), a much more common, less serious condition involving muscle contractions, rather than chronic inflammation. Two distinct disorders are classified as inflammatory bowel disease: CROHN'S DISEASE and ulcerative COLITIS. Crack-like ulcers and abnormal granular growths in the intestine often accompany Crohn's disease, while ulcerative colitis occurs only in the large intestine and involves inflammation and ulceration.

IBD symptoms include persistent (sometimes bloody) DIARRHEA, flatulence, cramps, low-grade fever and weight loss, as well as problems such as ARTHRITIS and inflamed eyes or skin. Children may be affected by retarded growth and retarded sexual development. IBD increases the risk of colon CANCER.

IBD is reported mainly in developed countries, where it is most common between the ages of 12 and 40. The causes of IBD are unknown. It does not seem to be caused by stress. One theory is that IBD is an AUTOIMMUNE DISEASE in which the person's own immune system attacks the intestine. Clearly, immune imbalances seem to play a part. Another view is that bacteria, viruses or toxic chemicals initiate IBD. Dietary factors have also been implicated.

Conventional medical treatment involves drugs and/or surgery. Drugs reduce inflammation and can lead to a remission. However, steroids have side effects like high blood pressure, diabetes and thinning of bones. Typical treatment recommendations include:

- Eating a well-balanced diet that provides adequate nutrients to maintain and repair the intestinal tract.
- Eating several small meals throughout the day. This may be more effective for good digestion and assimilation than eating three big meals.
- Avoiding irritating foods that could increase inflammation. These differ from person to person, though seeds, nuts and corn, lactose and dairy products, fried or greasy foods and coffee are often the culprits.
- Getting enough exercise and managing stress. Severe stress suppresses the immune system and encourages inflammation.
- Seeking expert medical advice. The National Foundation for Ileitis and Colitis provides important information to patients and their families.

Gross, V., et al., "Free Radicals in Inflammatory Bowel Diseases—Pathophysiology and Therapeutic Implications," *Hepato-Gastroenterology*, 41 (1994), pp. 320–27.

Podolsky, Daniel K., "Inflammatory Bowel Disease," *New England Journal of Medicine*, 325:14 (October 3, 1991), pp. 1008–16.

inhibition   Restricting the activity of a cellular or physiologic process. Several different mechanisms are involved in inhibition.

Hormones   Hormones may serve as inhibiting agents because they can inhibit the release of other hormones. Thus, the ovaries produce inhibin (a hormone that inhibits the secretion of the ovarian hormones), follicle stimulating hormone and lutenizing hormone, at the end of the menstrual cycle. Elevated CORTISOL from the adrenal glands inhibits the release of ADRENOCORTICOTROPIN (ACTH) from the PITUITARY GLAND. ACTH stimulates the release of cortisol.

Enzymes   Enzymes are protein catalysts. Characteristically, they lose activity when blocked by inhibitors. Enzyme inhibitors can be distinguished by their action on an enzyme:

"Competitive enzyme inhibitors" are compounds that mimic the chemical that the enzyme usually alters (the substrate). Competitive inhibitors masquerade as the usual substrate, thus tricking the enzyme and combining with it. Since the enzyme is unable to chemically alter the competitive inhibitor, the inhibitor simply "sits" on the enzyme, blocking access of incoming molecules that should be transformed.

Enzyme poisons like toxic heavy metals—LEAD, MERCURY and CADMIUM—can bind to enzymes without competing with substrates and can permanently inactivate enzymes.

Certain key regulatory enzymes may be reversibly inhibited by the accumulation of key products of metabolism. One example is the feedback inhibition of a METABOLIC PATHWAY, a sequence of functionally linked enzymes. In this type of inhibition, a surplus of the final product of the pathway can inhibit the pathway. For example, the buildup of ATP, the energy currency of the cell, can inhibit enzyme systems like GLYCOLYSIS that generate ATP. Such feedback mechanisms help the cell avoid wasteful overproduction of products. (See also ENDOCRINE SYSTEM; INDUCTION.)

inositol (myoinositol)   An essential building block of cell membrane LIPIDS. Chemically, inositol is a cyclic ALCOHOL with six hydroxyl groups, one per carbon atom. Inositol is a constituent of the inositol-containing phospholipid, phosphatidylinositol, a component of inner-cell membranes. Derivatives of inositol function as HORMONE relay signals in cells. Diverse hormones such as VASOPRESSIN (from the pituitary gland), EPINEPHRINE (from the adrenal gland) and releasing factors from the HYPOTHALAMUS stimulate the release of inositol triphosphate from phosphatidylinositol.

Animal studies show that inositol may protect against ATHEROSCLEROSIS and against hair loss. Inositol is also supposed to help reverse nerve damage caused by diabetes in animals. Oral supplementation in human diabetics has not verified this result. Diabetics should consult their health care providers before taking inositol supplements. Inositol has a low toxicity.

Nutritionists have not yet established the optimum amount of inositol in the diet. It is widely distributed in food and is also manufactured in the body. Sources include CITRUS FRUIT (except lemons), CANTALOUPE, whole grain bread, cooked beans, green beans and nuts. Inositol occurs in grains such as PHYTIC ACID, in which six phosphate groups are attached to the inositol molecule. Phytic acid can bind minerals and limit their uptake. (See also VITAMIN.)

Shamsuddin, Abulkalaman M., "Inositol Phosphates Have Novel Anti-cancer Function," *Journal of Nutrition*, 125 (supp. 3; 1995), pp. 725S–32S.

insect infestation of food   A variety of insects can infest food storage as well as food processing facilities and their output. Several of these insects pose health hazards. High standards have been established to assure wholesome food produced under sanitary conditions.

The warehouse beetle is native to California. Its larvae are covered with tiny, sharp hairs. When eaten, these beetles can irritate the GASTROINTESTINAL TRACT, causing nausea and vomiting. Cockroaches carry potential pathogenic bacteria, including SALMONELLA. The cigarette beetle can chew holes through styrofoam, cardboard and even aluminum food packaging. This opens up the product to other sources of contamination. Flour beetles feed on food residues left from inadequate cleaning of facilities.

Whole wheat and whole grains attract moths and other insects, which are attracted to the oily ingredients that are removed from white flour. Grain products may become infected at home through improper storage, while flour and mixes can become infected once the package is opened. They also may be infected between processing and packaging of the final product. The U.S. FDA allows 25 insect fragments per ounce of flour (up to that amount, they are not considered a health hazard). To avoid lengthy storage at home, buy small amounts of whole grain flour and store flour in sealed containers. If the flour becomes infected, freeze it for 24 hours to kill insects. Freezing is also an appropriate method of storing whole grains. Flour and cereal, nuts, raisins and the like should be stored in sealed containers to prevent insect and larva from contaminating these foods. (See also FOOD, DRUG AND COSMETIC ACT.)

insulin A protein HORMONE, secreted by beta cells in the PANCREAS, that stimulates the uptake of BLOOD SUGAR by many tissues. Insulin counteracts the effects of GLUCAGON, the pancreatic hormone responsible for raising blood sugar. Insulin is used therapeutically to treat DIABETES MELLITUS and is either purified from pork or beef pancreas or is genetically engineered of human origin. Insulin is produced by small cell clusters in the pancreas called the islets of Langerhans. Insulin itself is hormonally regulated. An increase in blood sugar levels stimulates insulin release. PANCREOZYMIN, an intestinal hormone, also stimulates insulin release. The trace mineral CHROMIUM, which appears in the form of GLUCOSE TOLERANCE FACTOR, is required for optimal insulin activity.

Insulin exerts a profound effect on glucose HOMEOSTASIS. Once glucose is absorbed it can be oxidized for energy production or it can be converted to triglycerides (fat). More generally this hormone favors the formation of GLYCOGEN, LIPIDS and PROTEIN (anabolic activity). Muscle and fat cells require insulin to absorb surplus glucose from the blood after a meal. On the other hand, the brain utilizes blood glucose independently of insulin. In ADIPOSE TISSUE, insulin activates fat synthesis from glucose, while in MUSCLE, insulin promotes the storage of glucose as glycogen, the polymer that functions as the storage form of glucose. Insulin also promotes amino acid uptake and increased muscle protein synthesis. In the liver, insulin stimulates the formation of triglycerides and glycogen from glucose while blocking glucose formation and glycogen breakdown.

Excessive insulin can lead to low blood sugar (HYPOGLYCEMIA). In postprandial HYPOGLYCEMIA, blood sugar drops after eating carbohydrates. One reason for this is that the pancreas overreacts to the sudden rush of glucose by releasing excessive insulin. The subsequent drop in blood sugar may cause fatigue, irritability and other symptoms.

The mechanism of insulin action is still not completely understood, although the hormone was discovered over 70 years ago. Insulin increases glucose transport into cells, activates or inactivates certain enzymes responsible for glucose metabolism and storage, and changes the level of protein synthesis at the gene level. Initially, insulin binds to specific binding sites (hormone receptors) on the cell surfaces of target tissues. Binding causes the release of one or more intracellular messengers that lead to altered metabolism. The nature of the signal mechanism is under active investigation. Insulin may activate certain enzymes called protein kinases, regulatory enzymes that in turn modulate enzymes required for energy utilization. One outcome is the activation of enzymes for glycogen synthesis.

Insulin Resistance

A low response to insulin is called insulin resistance, which typically elevates blood sugar levels. Up to 25% of non-obese Americans are estimated to have an inherited inefficient response to insulin. European and American research implicates insulin resistance and elevated blood sugar in the development of some forms of CORONARY ARTERY DISEASE. The mechanism by which insulin resistance might cause heart disease remains unknown.

The most extreme case of insulin resistance is diabetes. Most diabetic patients exhibit a degree of insulin resistance. In non-insulin dependent diabetes (Type II diabetes), there is a loss of insulin sensitivity and a decline in the maximal response elicited by insulin. According to one scenario the problem may reflect the inability to use insulin effectively because of too few insulin binding sites on target cells. Thus, insulin resistance can be caused by defective insulin receptors or other defective proteins, and it can provoke a decline in insulin production.

Secondary factors that can affect insulin resistance in target cells include: STRESS, fever, FASTING and STARVATION, as well as liver CIRRHOSIS, KETOSIS, OBESITY, puberty, high blood sugar and AGING. Also, the excessive production of hormones like CORTISOL, glucagon, EPINEPHRINE and GROWTH HORMONE can induce insulin resistance. With obesity there is a loss of insulin sensitivity by peripheral tissues, also due to a decrease in relative amounts of hormone receptors. (See also AMINO ACID METABOLISM; CARBOHYDRATE METABOLISM; DIABETES MELLITUS; ENDOCRINE SYSTEM.)

Gerstin, H.C., and Yusuf, Salim. "Dysglycaemia and Risk of Cardiovascular Disease," *Lancet*, 347 (April 1996), pp. 949–50.

Orci, L., Vassalli, J-D., Perrelet, A., "The Insulin Factory," *Scientific American* (September 1988), pp. 85–94.

insulin-dependent diabetes See DIABETES MELLITUS.

interferon A family of proteins secreted by virus-infected cells that function as the body's first line of defense against a wide variety of viruses. Three basic types of interferon have been identified: White blood cells secrete leukocyte interferon; connective tissue cells produce fibroblast interferon; and immune system cells produce lymphocyte interferon. Most interferons can block viral proliferation in infected cells by binding to adjacent cells, converting them to a virus-resistant state. Lymphocyte interferon also modulates the immune system on T cells, a class of immune cells derived from the THYMUS GLAND. The interferon also acts as a growth factor and stimulates T cell proliferation, also stimulating the killing action of certain T cells. Consequently, interferon has been used on a limited basis as an anticancer agent. Note that interferon differs from ANTIBODIES, which are proteins synthesized by specialized cells of the IMMUNE SYSTEM to combat a specific foreigner. Antibodies can attack bacteria as well as viruses in the bloodstream but do not fortify cells against viral attack.

international unit (IU) A standardized amount of physiologically active material such as a HORMONE, an ENZYME or a VITAMIN. International units are based on measurements of biological effects, such as increased growth rate in experimental animals.

The weight of active material represented by an international unit varies with the specific material. For example, fat-soluble vitamins are sometimes listed on supplement labels in terms of IU. The REFERENCE DAILY INTAKE (RDI) for VITAMIN D is 400 IU, equivalent to 10 mcg, based on experiments with rats and chicks, while the RDI for VITAMIN E (alpha-tocopherol) is 30 IU, equivalent to 20 mg. For VITAMIN A (retinol), the RDI is 5,000 IU, representing 1,500 retinol equivalents or 1,500 mcg. (See also RECOMMENDED DIETARY ALLOWANCES.)

interstitial fluid (intercellular fluid) Fluid that bathes cells and tissues. Interstitial fluid serves important functions. It buffers cells against extreme pH, delivers oxygen and nutrients to cells, removes wastes and serves as an avenue for defensive cells of the immune system. Interstitial fluid contains white BLOOD cells (LEUKOCYTES). Leukocytes also enter tissue fluid from the bloodstream by squeezing through capillary walls and migrating to the site of infection and inflammation. Interstitial fluid, together with blood and lymph, help maintain the internal environment within normal limits. When interstitial fluid flows through lymphatic vessels, it is called LYMPH.

Cell-free constituents of blood and fluid normally penetrate capillaries. Whole blood does not penetrate vessel walls unless they are injured. These materials include water, ions like SODIUM and CHLORIDE, GLUCOSE and other nutrients, as well as small proteins. PLATELETS, small cell fragments that promote clotting, together with serum proteins, blood and RED BLOOD CELLS, are retained within vessels and do not appear in the interstial fluid. (See also BUFFER; ELECTROLYTES; HOMEOSTASIS.)

intestinal flora Microorganisms, chiefly bacteria, that normally occupy the latter part of the small intestine and extensively colonize the COLON. Intestinal bacteria are more numerous than all of the cells of the body. Bacteria living in the intestine weigh several pounds and represent one-third of the dry fecal weight. An estimated 400 different bacterial species inhabit the digestive tract, and the concentration in the colon far exceeds the level in the small intestine. Twenty species comprise 75% of the total number of bacterial colonies, and anaerobic (oxygen-sensitive) bacteria greatly outnumber aerobic bacteria. Many types of gut bacteria have established a symbiotic relationship through evolution. Most

are anaerobic and thrive without oxygen, while others can live under both aerobic and anaerobic conditions.

Bacteria implant in the infant's intestine shortly after birth. *Bifidobacterium infantis* is promoted by breastfeeding. Later in life, a full complement of bacteria is normally in place. Different bacteria favor different regions of the intestine. *Bifidobacterium bifidum* is a major component of the large intestine in adults, while LACTOBACILLUS ACIDOPHILUS inhabits both the small and large intestine. *Streptococcus faecalis* and *Escherichia coli* are normal inhabitants of the intestine. However, if E. coli spreads to the urinary tract, it can cause bladder infections. Virulent species of E. coli produce enterotoxins that cause diarrhea.

Beneficial Effects of Gut Flora

The normal gut flora degrade toxins and foreign compounds. They break down food constituents such as fiber and undigested starch into short-chain fatty acids like ACETIC ACID, PROPIONIC ACID and BUTYRIC ACID, which serve as major fuels. Butyrate is a preferred energy source for cells lining the colon. Intestinal bacteria enhance bowel function, such as PERISTALSIS, increasing the time required for material to pass through the digestive system. Intestinal bacteria also provide B vitamins like biotin and fat-soluble vitamin K. By occupying an important biological niche, beneficial bacteria control the spread of undesirable microorganisms. They produce factors that limit growth of potential pathogens and create an acidic, anaerobic environment that also limits the growth of undesirable species. Some strains of normal gut bacteria produce substances that suppress potential pathogens. Yeasts are generally present in very low numbers, if at all, because they are held in check by beneficial bacteria like the acid-producing varieties.

Imbalanced Gut Flora (Gut Dysbiosis)

An unhealthy gastrointestinal tract can alter gut flora. Thus imbalanced intestinal flora can be caused by low stomach acid (hydrocholoric acid), diarrhea or constipation or by malnutrition. Broad-spectrum antibiotics can wipe out entire populations of beneficial bacteria. When stomach acid is low, food is not sterilized; surviving microorganisms can proliferate in the warm, moist and nutrient-rich intestine, thus setting the stage for intestinal disease due to yeast, parasites and pathogenic bacteria. Low stomach acid also increases the probability of maldigestion.

Altered gut flora can in turn cause intestinal damage, maldigestion and MALABSORPTION. Incompletely digested foods can provide unusual substrates for gut bacteria, which they can convert to harmful substances. For example, a high meat diet induces certain bacteria to break down amino acids to amines and phenols, compounds that can damage intestinal cells.

Endotoxins, poisonous materials released by bacterial overgrowth, can inflame the gut. This increases intestinal permeability or leakiness, permitting further toxin uptake. Alternatively, bacterial enzymes can break down BILE salts and estrogens, altering LIVER regulation of these materials. Maldigestion can occur when intestinal inflammation causes decreased production of intestinal digestive enzymes. For example, atrophy of the intestinal lining accompanies infestation by giardia, a common intestinal parasite. Likewise, poor absorption of nutrients will occur under these conditions.

Gut flora can be normalized by taking lactobacillus and bifidobacteria supplements, as well as supplementing other beneficial bacteria, by drinking plenty of clean water, by eating fewer refined foods and less fat and meat, and by eating more whole (minimally processed) foods and more fiber from vegetables and fruits. Nutrients that support the immune system and stress reduction also help balance gut microorganisms. (See also CANCER; HYPOCHLORHYDRIA;)

Gorbach, Sherwood L., "Lactic Acid Bacteria and Human Health," *Annals of Medicine*, 22 (1990), pp. 37–41.

Roberfroid, M.B., et al., "Colonic Microflora: Nutrition and Health," *Nutrition Reviews*, 53:5 (1995), pp. 127–30.

intestine   The long tube connecting the stomach and anus. It is divided into two segments, each with different functions.

Small Intestine

The small intestine leads to the large intestine or colon. It is narrower and longer than the colon. The small intestine is the major site of digestion and uptake of nutrients, including CARBOHYDRATE, AMINO ACIDS, FATTY ACIDS, WATER, MINERALS and VITAMINS released by stomach and intestinal secretions.

The small intestine begins at the valve regulating the opening of the stomach (pyloric sphincter) and coils its way through the abdominal cavity before joining the large intestine. The average diameter of the small intestine is 1 inch (2.5 cm) and the length is about 20 feet (6 m) in an adult. The surface of the small intestine is like a wrinkled shag rug. This surface structure increases the efficiency of nutrient absorption. The highly convoluted surface is coated with fuzzy, microscopic projections called VILLI. There are 10 to 40 villi per square millimeter. Cells lining the small intestine possess microscopic hairlike projections called MICROVILLI, which further increase the surface area so that the total surface area of the inner surface of the small intestine is about the size of a tennis court. The small intestine secretes important digestive enzymes that complete the process of DIGESTION. They include LACTASE, MALTASE and SUCRASE, which break down carbohydrate to simple sugars together with enzymes capable of digesting protein fragments to amino acids (aminopeptidases). Once nutrients like sugars, vitamins, minerals and amino acids are absorbed by cells lining the intestine (mucosal cells), they pass into CAPILLARIES and enter the bloodstream or pass into the LYMPHATIC SYSTEM if they are fat soluble.

Because of its huge surface area and daily exposure to many foreign materials and microorganisms, the intestinal tract is subject to disease. The intestine protects itself against the onslaught of bacteria, bacterial cell wall fragments and products of bacterial metabolism, and against food antigens (foreign materials) by several mechanisms. The lining secretes MUCUS, a thick viscous fluid that creates a physical barrier, and lysozyme, an enzyme that attacks certain bacteria. The intestine also secretes a major ANTIBODY called secretory IgA. This antibody binds to specific organisms and keeps them from attacking the mucosal cells, often a prerequisite for infection. It also binds specific antigens like food proteins and prevents their penetration. Stress can lower secretory IgA production, increasing the likelihood of intestinal imbalance and infection.

Colon (Large Intestine)

The large intestine is about one-quarter of the length of the small intestine and averages 2.5 inches (6.5 cm) in diameter. The opening between the terminal portion of the small intestine (ILEUM) and the large intestine is regulated by the ileocecal valve. Digestive enzymes are not secreted in the colon, which is the site of the last stage of food breakdown. Colonic bacteria degrade much of the undigested material received from the small intestine (CHYME). FIBER and undigested carbohydrates are metabolized to CARBON DIOXIDE, hydrogen, methane and simple saturated acids like ACETIC ACID and BUTYRIC ACID, which are absorbed and used as fuels. Colonic bacteria also degrade certain amino acids to smelly compounds (skatole and indoles), responsible for fecal odor. BILE PIGMENT (bilirubin) is converted to brown pigments. B vitamins and VITAMIN K synthesized by bacterial action are absorbed in the large intestine, as are SODIUM, CHLORIDE and other minerals. The large intestine also absorbs water from fecal material, creating a formed stool.

Different types of bacteria occupy different regions of the intestine. *Bifidobacterium bifidium* is a major component of the large intestine in adults, while LACTOBACILLUS ACIDOPHILUS favors the small intestine. Strains of ESCHERICHIA COLI are normal inhabitants of the intestine. Yeasts are generally in very low numbers, if present at all. However, reduction in beneficial bacterial populations can permit yeast and other potential pathogens to proliferate. INFLAMMATORY BOWEL DISEASE, DIARRHEA, IRRITABLE BOWEL SYNDROME, CONSTIPATION, ILEITIS, LEAKY GUT syndrome, several types of FOOD POISONING, and parasitic diseases like giardia are a few of the more common intestinal disorders. (See also ACIDOPHILUS; BIFIDUS FACTOR; CANDIDA ALBICANS; DIGESTIVE DISORDERS; DIGESTIVE TRACT.)

Evans, Mary Ann and Shronts, Eva P., "Intestinal Fuels: Glutamine, Short-chain Fatty Acids and Dietary Fiber," *Journal of the American Dietetic Association*, 92:10 (October 1992), pp. 1239–6.

intoxication   See ALCOHOL.

intracellular fluid (ICF)   Refers to the total amount of WATER contained within cells. This fluid accounts for twice as much water as outside of cells and represents nearly 40% of the total body weight. EXTRACELLULAR FLUID refers to water excluded from cells. Because water readily diffuses across cell membranes, the intracellular and the extracellular compartments are linked. Consequently, massive water losses will draw water out of cells and eventually alter cell function. Physiologic processes ranging from regulation of body temperature, waste removal and kidney function to the function of the central nervous system and distribution of oxygen and nutrients, rely upon water balance. (See also CYTOPLASM; DEHYDRATION; ELECTROLYTES.)

intrinsic factor   A protein produced by the stomach lining and required for intestinal absorption of VITAMIN B_{12}. Gastric PARIETAL CELLS normally secrete intrinsic factor during digestion. Intrinsic factor binds tightly vitamin B$_{12}$ released from food during intestinal digestion. The resulting B$_{12}$-intrinsic factor complex is selectively absorbed by the epithelial cells lining the ILEUM, the latter portion of the small intestine. If the stomach does not secrete enough STOMACH ACID (a condition called HYPOCHLORHYDRIA), it probably does not make enough intrinsic factor either. With too little intrinsic factor, vitamin B$_{12}$ cannot be assimilated by the body, leading to a chronic deficiency. This causes PERNICIOUS ANE-MIA, as well as neurological symptoms. Vitamin B$_{12}$ is required for DNA synthesis and cell proliferation. Restricted vitamin B$_{12}$ uptake due to a lack of intrinsic factor leads to ANEMIA because the BONE marrow cannot produce adequate red blood cells without adequate vitamin B$_{12}$. The linkage between vitamin B$_{12}$ deficiency and neurological damage is poorly understood.

Abnormal intrinsic factor production is genetically linked; susceptibility runs in families. Vitamin B$_{12}$ injections, and possibly oral supplementation of massive amounts of vitamin B$_{12}$ (1,000 mcg or more per day), may permit adequate vitamin B$_{12}$ assimilation when intrinsic factor and stomach acid production are low. Because FOLIC ACID also supports cell proliferation similar to vitamin B$_{12}$, folic acid is usually administered with vitamin B$_{12}$. (See also ACHLORHY-DRIA; AGING; SENILITY.)

inulin   A POLYSACCHARIDE that is a polymer composed primarily of the simple sugar FRUCTOSE. Inulin plays a minor role in the diet; it is common to only a few foods, including ARTICHOKES, ONIONS and GARLIC. Fresh foods contain higher levels of inulin than stored foods because most of the inulin might be broken down to fructose during storage. Inulin is poorly digested, but once it is absorbed it is filtered by the glomerulus, the KIDNEY structure that removes materials from the blood during urine formation. Since inulin is excreted in urine by the kidney, its rate of appearance in urine is a measure of GLOMERULAR FILTRATION rate, the rate at which the kidney can remove soluble materials from blood.

invert sugar   A mixture of GLUCOSE and FRUCTOSE, the two simple sugars that make up table sugar (SUCROSE). Sucrose hydrolysis by acid or by the enzyme invertase yields a 50/50 mixture of these two sugars that is both sweeter and more soluble than table sugar. Invert sugar is an additive in the manufacture of candy because it prevents the sugar in candy from crystallizing. Like all sugar sweeteners, it contributes only calories to the diet. (See also FOOD ADDITIVES; NATURAL SWEETENERS.)

iodine (iodide)   An essential trace mineral nutrient required to produce thyroid hormones. The element iodine occurs in food and in the body as the ionized or chemical form called iodide. The THYROID GLAND combines iodide with the AMINO ACID, TYROSINE, to produce thyroxine and tri-iodothyronine. These hormones control the body's idling speed (BASAL METABOLIC RATE) and support normal growth and development.

Symptoms of iodine deficiency include sluggishness (HYPOTHYROIDISM), weight gain and, in extreme cases, an enlarged thyroid gland (GOITER). During pregnancy, iodine deficiency can cause severe mental retardation (cretinism) in children. Before salt was iodized in the 1920s, goiters were common in areas of the United States, especially the South, with iodine-deficient soils. Though rare, goiter sometimes occurs in women and children in certain areas of California, Texas and the South, and in Manitoba and Saskatchewan, Canada. Goiter is still common in parts of Africa. Certain substances called GOITROGENS in vegetables like CASSAVA and rutabagas block iodine uptake and may contribute to the occurrence of goiter when excessive amounts of these foods are consumed.

Sources of iodide include SEAWEED, shellfish like shrimp, clams and oysters, marine fish and iodized salt. Iodine occurs in food in other chemical forms besides iodide. SODIUM iodate, a commercial dough oxidizer, occurs in some commercially baked goods. Milk and milk products may contain traces of free iodine, used as a disinfectant for milk cows and in milk production.

The typical diet supplies more than twice the U.S. REFER-ENCE DAILY INTAKE (RDI) of 150 mcg. Consuming 2 mg per day is generally considered safe for healthy adults. Breast milk contains iodine to provide for the infant's requirements, and lactating women require extra iodide in their diets. An additional 50 mcg of iodine per day is recommended. Iodine as supersaturated potassium iodide has been used clinically in the treatment of asthma, slow lymphatic drainage, sebaceous cysts, fibrocystic breast disease and to promote desirable balance of estrogens. Iodine, as a water purifier, possesses antiviral and antibacterial activity. Excessive amounts of iodide can cause iodine-induced goiter. Other side effects include rash and allergies.

Iodized Salt

In the United States, sodium iodide has been added to table salt (sodium chloride) to create "iodized salt" since 1924. It provides 76 mcg of iodine per gram of salt. With this ENRICH-MENT, goiter virtually disappeared in America. Small amounts of additives stabilize iodine in iodized salt and prevent caking: They include GLUCOSE, sodium thiocyanate, sodium aluminum silicate or sodium BICARBONATE. SEA SALT is not a good source of iodine. Although sea water is rich in iodide, iodide is lost during purification. Note that sea salt and iodized salt contribute the same amount of sodium as standard table salt. (See also FORTIFICATION; HYPERTENSION; TRACE MINERALS.)

Hetzel, Basil S., "The Control of Iodine Deficiency," *American Journal of Public Health*, 83:4 (April 1993), pp. 494–95.

iron   A versatile trace mineral nutrient that performs essential functions in the body. The presence of iron is responsible for the red color of BLOOD. Red blood cells contain vast amounts of HEMOGLOBIN, the red oxygen transport protein of blood. Hemoglobin is red because it contains HEME, the red, iron-rich pigment that actually binds oxygen and transports it to tissues. Iron deficiency leads to decreased red blood cells (ANEMIA). Muscles contain a red, iron-containing protein called myoglobin, which stores oxygen for muscle contraction. The body contains a total of 3 to 5 g of iron. Hemoglobin represents 65% of this iron; about 30% occurs as FERRITIN, the iron storage complex found in the LIVER, spleen and BONE marrow.

Iron plays many roles. It is required to oxidize fuels to produce energy needed to maintain tissue functioning. Iron functions in CYTOCHROMES and other mitochondrial enzymes that burn CARBOHYDRATE and FAT to form ATP, the cell's chemical energy currency. In this context, it is noteworthy that iron promotes the formation of CARNITINE, a compound required to transport fatty acids into mitochondria to be burned.

Connective Tissue   This is the matrix that holds cells and tissues together. Iron-containing enzymes are involved in the formation of structural proteins COLLAGEN and ELASTIN, required to form connective tissue.

Defensive cells   The bacteria-killing white blood cells (neutrophils) depend upon iron to help generate highly reactive forms of oxygen (superoxide) that function as bacteriocides (bacteria destroying agents). Inadequate iron reduces the effectiveness of the immune system. The production of T-lymphocytes and red blood cells requires rapid DNA synthesis. An iron-dependent enzyme synthesizes DEOXYRIBOSE, the carbohydrate building block of DNA. Iron deficiency slows DNA synthesis.

Nervous system   Iron is required in the synthesis of neurotransmitters, DOPAMINE, SEROTONIN and norepinephrine. Neurotransmitters are chemicals that help conduct impulses between nerve cells.

Liver   Glucose (BLOOD SUGAR) formation from amino acids requires iron. CYTOCHROME P450 is an iron-dependent enzyme system that helps the liver destroy toxic chemicals and waste products.

Antioxidant enzyme   Iron assists the action of CATALASE, a ubiquitous enzyme that degrades HYDROGEN PEROXIDE to water and oxygen. Hydrogen peroxide is a by-product of cellular reactions and it is a powerful oxidizing agent unless inactivated.

Iron Deficiency

Iron deficiency is one of the most prevalent nutritional problems worldwide. Perhaps 1 billion people are to some extent iron-deficient. Half the world's inner city and rural poor may not be getting enough iron. Iron deficiency is the major nutritional deficiency among children, notably 1-to 2-year-olds and older children from low-income households. This is a concern in developing nations where the diet is inadequate (predominantly vegetarian) and parasitic diseases like schistosomiasis and malaria are common. As indicated by iron depletion data, as many as 60% of the U.S. population may not get enough iron. Teenagers who rely on a junk food diet, dieters and pregnant or lactating women, individuals with liver disorders or blood loss, and low-income elderly persons may develop iron deficiency. An estimated 10 to 20% of women of childbearing age in the United States, Japan and England may be anemic (severely iron deficient) due to poor eating habits and blood loss through menstruation. Inadequate iron absorption among the elderly, due to use of antacids and low stomach acidity, frequently causes iron deficiency.

Subclinical (mild) iron deficiency, due to diminished iron storage without full-blown symptoms of iron deficiency, occurs long before anemia develops. Symptoms include FATIGUE, decreased alertness and learning problems in chil-

dren, muscle weakness, susceptibility to chronic infections and frequent colds, low stomach acid and poor digestion, slow growth, dizziness and rapid heartbeat. Iron deficiency impairs work capacity and endurance.

Anemia represents the final stage of chronic, severe iron deficiency. Depleted iron reserves cause excessive fatigue due to inadequate oxygen delivery to tissues. Iron supplementation will cure anemia due to iron deficiency, but it will not cure pernicious anemia, which is due to VITAMIN B_{12} deficiency, nor will iron cure anemias based on other nutritional deficiencies such as vitamin B_6.

A variety of laboratory tests are used to evaluate iron deficiency. The most sensitive clinical test for mild iron deficiency measures serum ferritin. Serum ferritin may decline to 12 mcg/liter without visible symptoms. With serious iron deficiencies, the level of the iron-transport protein in the blood, transferrin, is elevated, but it contains less iron than usual (less than 16% saturation). With severe deficiency hemoglobin levels decline and small red blood cells appear, a condition called microcytic anemia, and the packed volume of red blood cells, the HEMATOCRIT, declines.

Sources of Iron

Animal sources are the best food sources of iron because the iron in flesh (heme) is highly absorbable. These include MEAT, especially liver, POULTRY and FISH, as well as iron-fortified flour, egg yolk, BREAD and cereals. Iron uptake is increased by cooking acidic foods in an iron skillet. Red wines often contain iron. Non-heme iron, as found in vegetables and iron-fortified foods, is often poorly absorbed. Non-heme iron also occurs in meat. Only 1.4% of the iron in spinach and of the iron in soybeans is absorbed because it is tightly bound to plant materials that resist the action of digestive enzymes. Absorption is increased by the addition of VITAMIN C and small amounts of animal protein. Iron uptake is blocked by substances in grains called PHYTIC ACID, by the TANNINS in tea, ANTACIDS, ASPIRIN, the fiber in wheat BRAN, as well as excessive use of zinc supplements. The iron content in typical foods (milligrams per 100 g) is as follows: almonds, 4.7; dried beans, 2.4–2.7; beef, 3.0; blackstrap molasses, 16.1; bread, 2.2–2.4; milk chocolate, 1.0; caviar, 11.8; chicken, 1.3–1.8; eggs, 2.3; liver, 8.8–14.2; oyster, 8.1; peanut butter, 2.0; popcorn, 2.1; pork, 2.6; sardines, 2.9; shrimp, 2.0; tofu, 1.9. Organically complexed iron, for example with CITRIC ACID, SUCCINIC ACID or with vitamin C, is well absorbed. Oxidized iron (ferric, Fe^{3+}) is not as well absorbed as reduced iron (ferrous, Fe^{2+}).

Requirements

The body hoards iron and efficiently recycles it; only small amounts (1.0 mg per day for adults) are excreted. The RECOMMENDED DIETARY ALLOWANCE (RDA) for pre-menopausal women (15 mg/day) is higher than for men (10 mg/day) to compensate for blood losses.

The RDA for iron varies with age, and the RDA during pregnancy and lactation is greater. The recommended daily intake during pregnancy is 60 mg per day. Iron supplements are required to achieve this level and are usually prescribed for pregnant women in the United States. Treatment of iron deficiency anemia calls for increased dietary iron, under pro-

fessional guidance. A chronic iron deficiency may set the stage for excessive menstrual blood loss, thus causing a vicious cycle. Iron supplementation can remedy this situation. Iron supplements should be taken at a different time than vitamin E because iron rapidly oxidizes vitamin E. Iron supplements often contain chelated iron, that is, iron bound to organic compounds in order to facilitate absorption. Examples include iron gluconate and iron aspartate.

Safety

Iron supplements may cause stomachache, diarrhea, constipation and dark stools, though iron complexed with protein may cause fewer side effects.

Iron overload can occur with inherited iron storage disease (HEMOCHROMATOSIS), a common trait. Particularly men who are susceptible to hemochromatosis and who take high iron supplements for long periods may develop iron overload. They should probably avoid iron supplements. Iron supplements should probably be avoided by healthy, nondeficient people for additional reasons: Excessive iron suppresses the immune system. High blood levels of iron are associated with increased risk of free radical damage and cancer. Stored iron (ferritin) can be a risk factor for coronary diseases. U.S. men with high blood concentrations of ferritin (more than 200 mcg per liter) are more likely to suffer heart attacks as men with lower ferritin values. It is postulated that too much iron can promote the formation of highly reactive forms of oxygen (FREE RADICALS) that can attack LOW-DENSITY LIPOPROTEIN (LDL), a particularly dangerous type of CHOLESTEROL. Oxidized LDL is more likely to stick to arterial walls and trigger fatty plaque buildup, which can clog arteries. Scientists also speculate that free radicals themselves damage arterial walls and heart muscle tissue. Do not exceed 18 mg of iron per day unless advised to do so by a physician.

Several thousand children are poisoned each year by iron supplements. As few as six iron supplement tablets can kill a child. Get the child to a hospital immediately if consumption of iron supplements is suspected. (See also CATABOLISM; ERYTHROPOIESIS; GLUCONEOGENESIS; MITOCHONDRIA; TRACE MINERALS.)

Pollitt, E., "Iron Deficiency and Cognitive Function," *Annual Review of Nutrition*, 13 (1993), pp. 521–37.

irradiated food   See FOOD IRRADIATION.

irritable bowel syndrome (IBS, spastic colon, irritable colon, mucous colitis)   A common intestinal disorder characterized by spasms (irregular contractions) of the COLON or large intestine, with alternating CONSTIPATION and DIARRHEA with heartburn, cramps and gas. In this situation food does not move normally downstream through the intestine and cramps result. Excessive STOMACH ACID is a secondary problem. IBS accounts for half of all gastro-intestinal problems among Americans, and it is more common than HEPATITIS or ulcerative COLITIS. Women are the most susceptible to IBS. The disease often begins between the ages of 20 and 40. Symptoms may resemble CROHN'S DISEASE, peptic ulcer or gynecological problems. LACTOSE INTOLERANCE can mimic symptoms of IBS, as can reaction to excessive fructose or sorbitol used as sweeteners. Reactions to CORN, WHEAT, CITRUS FRUIT, TEA and COFFEE have been implicated in IBS. Recent research suggests that the

IMMUNE SYSTEM overreacts, imbalancing the control of inflammation. Gut microflora may also be imbalanced; parasitic or bacterial infection can adversely affect the health of the intestine and cause symptoms resembling IBS.

Extra FIBER may be beneficial in the treatment of constipation; food sources include whole GRAINS, whole fruits, PEARS, berries, PEAS, prunes and BRUSSELS SPROUTS. PSYLLIUM seed powder, various fiber supplements and fiber cookies are other options. However, a health care provider should be consulted before beginning a high fiber diet in the presence of digestive disease. Avoid coffee and fatty, gas-provoking and irritating foods. Stress reduction and gut-directed hypnotherapy can help in some cases. If pain is associated with a bowel movement, consult a physician to rule out identifiable causes such as diverticulosis, tumor or intestinal blockage. (See also ALLERGY; CAFFEINE; DIGESTION; DIGESTIVE DISORDERS; DIGESTIVE TRACT; INFLAMMATORY BOWEL DISEASE.)

Thompson, W. Grant, "Irritable Bowel Syndrome: Pathogenesis and Management," *Lancet*, 341 (June 19, 1993), pp. 1569–72.

irritable colon   See IRRITABLE BOWEL SYNDROME.

ischemia   The reduction of oxygen supply to the heart so that cardiac muscle cells are weakened. Ischemia is often caused by the narrowing of arteries such as in ATHEROSCLEROSIS or by blood clot formation. Angina pectoris or chest pain is due to ischemia of the heart muscle. (See also CARDIOVASCULAR DISEASE; CHOLESTEROL; HEART ATTACK.)

isoflavone   A class of non-nutrient plant substances with potential anticancer effects. Isoflavones occur in relatively high concentrations in soy products and in varying amounts in several hundred other plants. The content varies with the variety, time of harvest and geographic location. Isoflavones belong to the general class of FLAVONOIDS; they possess complex ring structures with oxygen atoms attached. Genistein and daidzein are two examples of isoflavones. Their general shape resembles the steroid hormone estrogen, a major female hormone. It is possible that isoflavones block estrogen from binding to targets, a needed step in hormone-dependent cancers like cancers of the breast, ovary and endometrium. They could also stimulate the production of an estrogen-binding protein in the blood, or they could block liver enzymes that activate compounds to become cancer-causing agents (carcinogens). Vegetarians whose diets are enriched in soy products and tofu have a lower risk of cancer.

Clarkson, T.B., et al., "Estrogenic Soybean Isoflavones and Chronic Disease," *Trends in Endocrinology and Metabolism*, 6:1 (1995), pp. 11–16.

Isoleucine (Ile, L-isolucine)   A dietary essential AMINO ACID. Isoleucine is classified as a non-polar (water-repelling) amino acid. It possesses a side chain resembling a lipid and does not attract water molecules. The side chain of isoleucine is branched, and like LEUCINE and VALINE, the other BRANCHED CHAIN AMINO ACIDS, it cannot be assembled by the body. These amino acids are largely degraded in the MUSCLE, rather than by the LIVER. Infants require an estimated 70 mg per kilogram of body weight daily, children (2 to 12 years) about 30 mg per kilogram daily, while adults require 10 mg per kilogram daily.

These figures reflect the high growth rates of children. The total amount of high-quality PROTEIN needed daily to support growth and maintenance increases from about 13 g per day for infants to 46 to 63 g per day for adults due to their increased body weight. (See also AMINO ACID METABOLISM; BIOLOGICAL VALUE.)

isothiocyanate   A family of sulfur-containing plant substances with potential anticancer effects. Isothiocyanates and related thiocyanates occur in high levels in vegetables of the cabbage family (cruciferous vegetables). Isothiocyanates seem to block the reactions of cancer-causing agents at sensitive sites within the cell, and they also seem to suppress the expression of cancer after cancer has been initiated. Animal studies indicate that isothiocyanates can inhibit dangerous chemical changes to DNA in the cancer-generating stages. Possibly these substances increase liver production of protective "phase II" enzymes. These detoxication enzymes attach innocent molecules to potentially harmful compounds to help flush them out of the body (glutathione transferase is an example).

Zhang, Yuesheng and Talalay, Paul, "Anticarcinogenic Activities of Organic Isothiocyanates: Chemistry and Mechanism," *Cancer Research*, 54: supp. (April 1, 1994), pp. 1976S–81S.

IU   See INTERNATIONAL UNIT.

jam A preservative prepared from boiled SUGAR syrup and crushed or pureed FRUIT. Jams need a single cooking step. Fruits like ripe APPLES, QUINCES, currants, CRANBERRIES, GOOSEBERRIES and PLUMS contain PECTIN, a complex carbohydrate that will gel upon cooling. Low pectin fruit like BLUEBERRIES, APRICOTS, CHERRIES, BLACKBERRIES, GRAPES and PINEAPPLE or stalks of RHUBARB have to be mixed with pectin—or pectin-containing fruits—to obtain a thicker consistency. Jam flavor reflects the amount of sugar used in syrup. The less sugar, the more pronounced the fruity flavor. Jam, like jelly, is a high-calorie, refined CARBOHYDRATE food: A quart of jam typically contains 2 to 2.5 cups of sugar. (See also NATURAL SWEETENER.)

jaundice A yellowing of skin, mucous membranes and whites of the eyes (scleroe) due to the buildup of BILE PIGMENT (bilirubin) in the body. Jaundice itself is not a disease, but indicates an underlying problem.

Three conditions promote jaundice (bilirubin accumulation):

1. Prehepatic jaundice reflects the excessive breakdown of red blood cells. Bilirubin is produced during the degradation of the red pigment of the oxygen-carrying protein HEMOGLOBIN during disposal of aged red blood cells. Bilirubin travels to the LIVER, where it is processed for excretion. In prehepatic jaundice the rate of bilirubin production exceeds the liver's ability to process incoming bilirubin, for example in hemolytic ANEMIA.

2. Hepatic jaundice reflects abnormal liver function. HEPATITIS, liver CIRRHOSIS and certain liver diseases imbalance liver metabolism and decrease the liver's ability to process bilirubin.

3. Extrahepatic jaundice occurs when interference with BILE release from the GALLBLADDER forces bilirubin to back into the liver. Bile duct obstructions commonly include GALLSTONES.

(See also DIGESTION; HEME.)

jejunum The middle segment of the small intestine. The jejunum is about 8 ft (2.5 m) long and lies between the DUODENUM (the first 10 in) and the ILEUM, the last 12 ft of small intestine. Like other regions of the small intestine, the jejunum possesses a large surface area due to its highly wrinkled surface. It is covered by numerous hair-like protrusions called VILLI. Furthermore each villus cell surface is covered with microscopic projections called MICROVILLI. These physiologic features dramatically increase the absorptive area and aid nutrient absorption and assimilation. (See also DIGESTION; DIGESTIVE TRACT.)

jelly A sweet, thickened spread composed of boiled FRUIT juice. Jellies are used on toast and in biscuits and pastry. Commercial jelly contains at least 55% fruit. Home-prepared jellies can contain as much as 60% sugar. Jelly is therefore a source of refined CARBOHYDRATE and a high-calorie food with few nutrients other than sugar. Jelly requires two cooking steps. In the first, JUICE is extracted from the fruit and filtered. The clear juice is then cooked with sugar until a gel forms. Often juices are extracted by pressure cooking. However, high temperatures destroy PECTIN, a form of fiber required for gel formation. Pectin is added back in this case. (See also EMPTY CALORIES; NATURAL SWEETENER.)

joule The international scientific standard unit for ENERGY measurement used for all branches of science. Recommended by the International Organization for Standardization, the joule was adopted by the U.S. Bureau of Standards in 1964. One joule is equal to 4.184 calories and is a measure of mechanical energy while the calorie is based on heat (thermal energy). Nutrition references still use KILO-CALORIES as a measure of energy in foods. For example, caloric values (in kilocalories) of foods are published in the USDA's *Handbook 8*; they can be converted to kilojoules (thousands of joules, abbreviated kJ.) by multiplying the listed calories by 4.184.

juice The liquid extract of FRUITS and VEGETABLES. Juices typically contain only small amounts of FIBER and pulp, which are removed by filtration. Juices can be freshly prepared, concentrated and frozen, canned or bottled. Juices contain sugars, soluble minerals and vitamins that can be released when plant tissues are crushed or pulverized. Plant leaves yield green, chlorophyll-rich juices.

Preparing juices at home with juicers is popular in the United States. On the other hand consumers spend more than $9 billion on prepared fruit juices and fruit drinks annually. These preparations are subject to food labeling regulations. The U.S. FDA does not require manufacturers to specify the amount of fruit juice used in a given juice. Manufacturers must list ingredients in order of predominance, but not by percentages. Listing percentages of ingredients would indicate the actual ratios of the more expensive juices such as kiwi, strawberry or peach. If the product label specifies "juice" only, then the product contains only pure fruit juice. Any other designation indicates a diluted juice. Apple juice and white grape juice are among the least expensive juices to produce and are frequently used in mixtures. Proposals by the U.S. FDA would require manufacturers to reveal how much juice is actually in "juice cocktail" or "juice drink."

A juicer/juice extractor is a popular mechanical device that extracts juices from vegetables and fruits. Juicers pulverize the vegetable or fruit by rotary blades. The pulp, seeds and skin care separated from the juice by centrifugal filtration. In contrast, blenders combine pulp and juice.

Fresh juices provide a convenient way of increasing consumption of vegetables and fruits while cutting back on soft drinks as part of a healthful diet that includes lower fat, more whole grains, vegetables and fresh fruit. Eating whole fruits and vegetables can provide essential nutrients and lower the risk of cancer and help reduce the risk of diseases associated with deficiencies and aging. No juice is a panacea. Juicing removes most fiber and pulp, which retain significant amounts of vitamins, minerals and perhaps as yet unknown materials that promote health. Fiber may have

beneficial effects, including lowering the risk of colon cancer. There are few studies on the stability of vitamins in juices or on the efficacy of vitamins in the extracts.

Fresh juices served immediately are better than those stored because oxidation begins to change the color, flavor and nutritional quality after the juice is made. Juice combinations of vegetables may begin to separate soon after they are made. The juice is only as good as the produce used; therefore, using organically grown produce and cleaning produce before juicing make sense when whole produce is to be juiced. Ginger and mint can improve the flavor of many juice mixtures. (See also AGING; BALANCED DIET.)

Calbon, Cherie and Keane, Maureen. *Juicing for Life*. Garden City Park, N.Y.: Avery Publishing Group, 1992.

junk food A highly processed FOOD. Compared to unprocessed foods, junk foods generally contain less nutritive value beyond their caloric content due to added sugar, refined starch, fat or oils. Junk food therefore represents a major source of "empty calories" in the typical American diet. Junk food is often based on refined grains, such as white flour. Obvious examples include CHIPS, CRACKERS, doughnuts, cookies, packaged sweet snacks and sugar-laden BREAKFAST CEREALS. Gelatin desserts, soft ice cream, candy and soft drinks fit into this category as well.

Potential Problems with Junk Food Diets

Individual foods are neither "good" nor "bad." Whether a food is appropriate depends on how much and how often it is eaten, as well as on the health and nutritional status of the individual consuming it. Reliance on junk food is often a direct cause of nutrient-deficient diets in the U.S. Food manufacturing removes many nutrients; consequently, junk foods contain less FIBER; less trace minerals like ZINC, MANGANESE, SELENIUM, CALCIUM, CHROMIUM, COPPER and IRON; and less vitamins like VITAMIN A, VITAMIN B_6, VITAMIN C and FOLIC ACID than usually found in unprocessed or minimally processed foods. Simultaneously, food manufacturing adds many materials not present in the original whole food, including: salt, SUGAR, SATURATED FAT and OIL, synthetic preservatives like BHA and BHT, artificial colorings and flavors. To partially correct for nutrient losses in processing, FLOUR and grain products (like processed breakfast cereals) are enriched with NIACIN, THIAMIN and RIBOFLAVIN to bring them up to the levels found in whole grain. However, enrichment replaces few of the vitamins and trace minerals, and none of the fiber lost during food manufacture.

Overnutrition is a second consequence of diets relying on junk foods. Junk food is a major source of surplus calories and saturated fat in the typical U.S. diet, and a high fat intake is directly tied to a higher risk of CANCER and coronary heart disease. Excessive junk food is a major cause of OBESITY, a critical health problem in the United States. Saturated fats—such as HYDROGENATED VEGETABLE OIL, COCONUT OIL or palm kernel oil, LARD and BUTTER—generally increase blood CHOLESTEROL levels, perhaps setting the stage for clogged arteries. Characteristically, junk food contains large amounts of refined sweeteners such as high FRUCTOSE CORN SYRUP, DEXTROSE, maltose malt sugar, corn sweetener and HONEY, as well as SUCROSE.

Who eats junk food? On any given day 46 million Americans eat FAST FOOD, which now shapes many children's eating habits. Studies suggest that children between the ages of 6 and 11 are more likely to eat cookies than fruit for snacks. Children between 1 and 5 are just as likely to drink powdered and carbonated soft drinks as they are to drink orange juice. (See also CONVENIENCE FOOD; FOOD PROCESSING.)

Bandini, L.G. and Dietz, W.H., "Myths about Childhood Obesity," *Pediatric Annals*, 21:10 (October 1992), pp. 647–52.

juvenile diabetes   See DIABETES MELLITUS.

kabob (kebab)   Chunks of seasoned meat grilled or roasted on skewers. The name comes from the Turkish "sis kebab," meaning skewered, roasted meat. Traditionally, marinated mutton or lamb is skewered with pork fat or mutton fat. American variations of ingredients include veal, meatballs and vegetables like onions, peppers, mushrooms and tomatoes. (See also BARBECUED MEAT.)

kale (*Brassica oleracea acephala*)   A dark-green leafy vegetable of the cabbage family. Kale is closely related to the European wild CABBAGE. There are many different leaf forms of kale, from curly to plain, and colors range from bluish-green to red-brown and purple. Kale withstands the stress of cold weather and severe frosts, and gardens can provide fresh greens into autumn.

Kale holds its texture when cooked, making it a useful ingredient in soups, meat loafs, stews and the like. Eaten raw it can be used in mixed salads. Kale can be blanched, steamed, sauteed or microwaved. Like other leafy greens, kale contains high levels of BETA CAROTENE (provitamin A). One cup, cooked (130 g), provides: 42 calories; protein, 3.5 g; carbohydrate, 7.3 g; fiber, 3.7 g; calcium, 94 mg; potassium, 296 mg; vitamin A, 962 retinol equivalents; thiamin, 0.07 mg; riboflavin, 0.009 mg; niacin, 0.70 mg; vitamin C, 53 mg. (See also CHARD; SPINACH.)

karaya gum   A FOOD ADDITIVE that serves as a thickening agent and is not absorbed by the INTESTINE. Karaya GUM, obtained exclusively from the sterculia tree in India, pre-vents fats and oils from separating in whipped products and salad dressing and in the meat juices in sausages. It also improves the texture of ice cream and has been used as a LAXATIVE. Karaya gum is unique in that it expands to up to 100 times its dry volume when wet. Some individuals are allergic to karaya gum, but it is presumably safer than other thickening agents since little of it is absorbed. However, long-term safety studies have not been performed. The question of whether this gum binds nutrients and prevents their absorption has not been resolved. (See also BULKING AGENTS.)

kasha   Roasted BUCKWHEAT; a coarse or finely ground, hulled GRAIN that can be cooked like RICE. The roasting process conveys a nutlike flavor. Buckwheat is not a grass, therefore it is not related to the cereal grains. Individuals who are allergic to wheat protein (GLUTEN) can often tolerate buckwheat. In the United States buckwheat is most commonly eaten as an ingredient in pancakes. Kasha is also an Eastern European dish. Russian kasha refers to small buckwheat pancakes. Polish kasha is a sweet pudding prepared either with BARLEY or with SEMOLINA.

kefir   Fermented milk. A traditional beverage of the Middle East and southern Russia. Originally kefir was prepared from camel's MILK; now cow's milk is fermented instead of camel's milk. The fermentation process produces LACTIC ACID, which gives kefir its tangy flavor. Fermentation also produces a low level of *alcohol* (generally about 1%). One cup provides 150 calories; protein, 9.3 g; carbohydrate, 8.8 g;

fat, 4.5 g; calcium, 350 mg; potassium, 205 mg; vitamin A, 155 mg; thiamin, 0.45 mg; riboflavin, 0.44 mg; niacin, 0.30 mg. (See also YOGURT.)

keratin   A PROTEIN that is the major constituent of skin, hair, nails and the protein matrix of tooth enamel. Keratin is a highly insoluble protein, classified as a structural protein. Its role in protecting the body is passive only. Alpha keratin occurs in mammals and consists of highly coiled protein chains that form insoluble fibers. This protein contains high levels of the sulfur-containing AMINO ACID, CYSTEINE. The cysteine sulfur atoms of adjacent keratin chains cross-link with each other, making keratin resistant to stretching and contributing to water-insolubility and strength of hair. For this reason, keratin also resists digestion. Keratin in skin is softer than in hair and nails because it has less sulfur content, and therefore less cross-linking. Toxic HEAVY METALS bind to keratin in hair, and mineral analysis of hair samples can reveal the accumulation of toxic elements like LEAD, CADMIUM or MERCURY. (See also HAIR ANALYSIS.)

ketchup (catsup)   In North America, a thick tomato sauce used to flavor MEAT, FISH, HAMBURGERS, FRENCH FRIES and HOT DOGS. Ketchup is made of tomato puree, SALT, VINEGAR and a variety of spices. Typical ketchup contains 25% SUGAR and represents one of the hidden sources of this sweetener, though it is not considered sweet. Ketchup is also a hidden source of SODIUM. One tablespoon (17 g) contains 18 calories; protein, 0.3 g; carbohydrate, 4.3 g; sodium, 156 mg; and trace levels of vitamins. (See also CONDIMENT; FOOD PROCESSING.)

keto acid   A class of weak ACIDS with a carbon atom skeleton. The keto acids are more highly oxidized acids than FATTY ACIDS and appear as intermediates in metabolic pathways of the body, which oxidize fatty acids and CARBOHYDRATES for energy production. Keto acids contain a keto group, an oxidized carbon atom found in a class of organic compounds called ketones.

Typical keto acids of cellular METABOLISM include: PYRUVIC ACID (three carbon atoms), produced from the single sugar GLUCOSE by GLYCOLYSIS, the major pathway of glucose degradation. Alpha ketoglutaric acid (five carbon atoms) and OXALOACETIC ACID (four carbon atoms) are intermediates of the KREB'S CYCLE, the central energy-producing pathway of the cell. Oxaloacetic acid is important for several reasons. It is both the starting point and the end point of the Kreb's cycle. Furthermore, oxaloacetic acid can be converted to glucose for BLOOD SUGAR.

Keto acids are produced in the degradation of certain AMINO ACIDS by removal of their amino groups (nitrogen-containing groups). Thus, the amino acid ALANINE yields pyruvic acid; ASPARTIC ACID yields oxaloacetic acid; and GLUTAMIC ACID yields alpha ketoglutaric acid. The process is reversible so that an addition of an amino group to pyruvic acid forms alanine; to oxaloacetic acid, forms aspartic acid; an addition to alpha ketoglutaric acid forms glutamic acid. Because these amino acids are readily synthesized by the body from common keto acids, they are not essential to the diet. (See also AMINO ACID METABOLISM; CARBOHYDRATE METABOLISM; GLUCONEOGENESIS.)

ketogenic   Refers to compounds converted to KETONE BODIES, a kind of metabolic acid, during their chemical breakdown for energy production. Ketogenic compounds include free FATTY ACIDS and the amino acid LEUCINE. Most amino acids are both ketogenic and "glycogenic"; that is, their complex structures are broken down into both ketone bodies and the sugar GLUCOSE. Excessive accumulation of ketone bodies may acidify the body, leading to imbalances. (See also ACIDOSIS; AMINO ACID METABOLISM.)

ketone bodies   The water-soluble products of excessive fat breakdown. Ketone bodies represent ACETOACETIC ACID, BETA HYDROXYBUTYRIC ACID and ACETONE, which are synthesized by the liver. They accumulate in the blood during prolonged fasting, STARVATION, crash DIETING and ALCOHOLISM. Each of these conditions promotes high rates of fat degradation. Fatty acids cannot be completely oxidized for energy under these conditions and are instead converted to ketone bodies. The accumulation of ketone bodies in the blood and their excretion in the urine indicates a potentially hazardous metabolic imbalance. (See also ACIDOSIS; FAT METABOLISM; KETOSIS.)

ketosis   The accumulation of KETONE BODIES in the blood due to incomplete oxidation of FATTY ACIDS. Excessive fat breakdown can occur during uncontrolled diabetes, ALCOHOLISM, crash DIETING and with high-fat, low-carbohydrate diets. Prolonged high levels of ketone bodies (ACETOACETIC ACID and BETA HYDROXYBUTYRIC ACID), can acidify the blood (ACIDOSIS). Furthermore, ketone body excretion in the urine can lead to excessive water loss (starvation diuresis). DEHYDRATION is potentially hazardous. Ketosis causes disturbances in ELECTROLYTES (dissolved minerals like SODIUM, POTASSIUM and CHLORIDE) in body fluids. Imbalanced electrolytes can alter heart function and nervous system responses. Severe ketosis can cause coma and, ultimately, death.

kidneys   Organs that regulate the amounts of key ingredients in blood, including WATER, the pH (acidity) and the levels of minerals (ELECTROLYTES), and in excreted waste products. By regulating water excretion in urine, kidneys also regulate the BLOOD PRESSURE. There are two kidneys, located close to the backbone at the back of the abdomen. Each is about 4 in (10 cm) long and each contains approximately one million filtering units called NEPHRONS, resembling small tubes. The nephrons filter a huge amount of fluid; about 425 gallons (1,930 l) per day for adults. However, only a very small fraction, 2 liters, leaves as urine, because most of the water, and most of the other useful blood constituents, are reabsorbed and recycled.

Nephrons are supplied with blood from the kidney artery, and a small cluster or "tuft" of capillaries (glomerulus) feeds each nephron. The glomerulus acts as a filter under pressure. The filtrate, the fluid emerging form the glomerulus, contains small molecules like water, salts (dissolved minerals, SODIUM, POTASSIUM, CHLORIDE), GLUCOSE, UREA (the end product of protein degradation) and creatinine (the waste product of muscle metabolism). Larger particles like proteins and cells are retained in the blood by the glomerulus.

The filtrate passes through the convoluted tubules of the nephron, where most of the sodium chloride is reabsorbed into the blood. The tubules help regulate the sodium content and the pH of the blood by exchanging electrolytes like AMMONIA, potassium and chloride. The final product is urine.

Glucose at normal blood concentrations is completely reabsorbed by the kidneys into the blood. In DIABETES MELLITUS the blood sugar concentration may be so high that more glucose appears in the filtrate than can be reabsorbed, and thus it passes into the urine (glucosuria). Because water follows the glucose, frequent urination accompanies glucose in the urine and may cause DEHYDRATION. Certain metabolic acids called KETONE BODIES may accumulate in the bloodstream with ALCOHOLISM, untreated diabetes, crash DIETING and other situations. Once their levels exceed the kidney threshold, ketone bodies are excreted in the urine. This, too, can cause dehydration and electrolyte imbalances that further compromise the patient's health.

Urine represents the concentrated waste; 99% of the water has been reabsorbed by the time urine reaches the ureters, which are tubes that drain into the bladder. The kidneys regulate water balance. If there is too much fluid in the body, the kidneys excrete more water as urine. When there is too little fluid, they retain more water and urine becomes more concentrated. Environmental temperature also affects kidney function because sweating increases water losses, prompting the kidneys to retain more water. Kidneys add potassium and hydrogen ions, ammonia, and bicarbonate to the filtrate to control blood pH.

HORMONES regulate kidney function. Water retention can be regulated by a pituitary hormone, ANTIDIURETIC HORMONE (ADH). Release of this hormone is stimulated when the brain (HYPOTHALAMUS) detects a low blood-water concentration. ADH increases water loss from cells, allowing more water to pass back into the blood. ALDOSTERONE, a hormone from the adrenal glands, regulates sodium excretion. If the sodium level drops, for example from sweating or DIARRHEA, aldosterone levels increase, salt reabsorption from the filtrate increases and water is retained.

The kidneys also process hormones. VITAMIN D is activated by the kidneys; they convert calcidiol (25-hydroxyvitamin D) to the hormone calcitriol (1,25 dihydroxyvitamin D). They also produce erythropoietin, a hormone that stimulates BONE marrow to produce RED BLOOD CELLS, and renin, a hormone that controls blood pressure. (See also BLADDER INFECTIONS; GLOMERULAR FILTRATION; KIDNEY STONES.)

kidney stones Mineralized particles occurring in the kidney and upper urinary tract. In the United States, they are more prevalent than stone formation in the gallbladder. Most kidney stones contain CALCIUM as carbonate, phosphate or oxalate. Kidney stones are quite common in the United States. An estimated 10% of men and 15% of women over 30 years of age will eventually experience this disease. A kidney stone is formed when the concentration of mineral salts in urine increases to the point of saturation, at which time the mineral will spontaneously crystallize. DEHYDRATION and increased calcium in urine favor stone formation. High urinary calcium can reflect a high intake of VITAMIN D, excessive consumption of ALUMINUM or MILK, overactive THYROID (hyperthyroidism), lengthy immobilization or kidney disease. Calcium oxalate stones are more likely with vitamin B$_6$ deficiency; with high consumption of foods like SPINACH rich in the organic acid OXALIC ACID; intestinal disease (particularly of the ileum); fatty stools; and abnormal metabolism of certain organic acids.

Possible Causes

Certain metabolic diseases, such as parathyroid malfunction and certain diseases of the bone, cause kidney stones. MILK ALKALI SYNDROME is associated with an increased risk. Many toxic metals, especially CADMIUM, increase the risk of stone formation. In addition, several dietary factors are often linked. Inadequate water intake prompts the formation of insoluble salts. Inadequate VITAMIN K could promote stone formation because the vitamin assists in the synthesis of a protein that inhibits stone formation. INSULIN insensitivity and OBESITY increase the risk of stone formation. Certain foods contain high oxalic acid levels; therefore, reduced intake of COCOA, tea, spinach, chard beet leaves, RHUBARB and PARSLEY decreases the risk. Consuming more FIBER-rich foods, like fruit and vegetables, is likely to decrease the risk of kidney stones. VITAMIN B$_6$ deficiency is also linked to oxalate-stone formation. URIC ACID occasionally forms stones, a process favored by the excessive consumption of nucleic acid-rich foods like yeast and organ meats, and by certain anti-cancer drugs.

The prevention of kidney stones relies on dietary changes:

- Drink plenty of water. Adequate water is needed to keep salts dissolved.
- Avoid sugar, refined carbohydrate, and excessive animal protein, salt and caffeine. These tend to increase the level of calcium in urine.
- Avoid cola soft drinks. These contain phosphate, which promotes stone formation.
- Avoid over-consumption of aluminum containing antacids.
- Minimize alcohol consumption. High alcohol consumption favors dehydration.
- Emphasize magnesium rich foods. Magnesium deficiency is linked to kidney stone formation, so eating foods with a high magnesium content—barley, wheat bran and other whole grains, avocados, bananas and lima beans—or supplements can reduce the risk.
- Citric acid keeps calcium solubilized, and citric acid supplementation has been used to reduce the incidence of kidney stones.

(See also GALLSTONES.)

Burtis, William J., et al., "Dietary Hypercalciuria in Patients with Calcium Oxalate Kidney Stones," *American Journal of Clinical Nutrition*, 60:3 (September 1994), pp. 424–29.

kilocalorie A measure of ENERGY content frequently used in nutrition. The term CALORIE is frequently used synonymously with kilocalorie although strictly speaking it should be capitalized (Calorie). The prefix "kilo" means 1,000. Thus, one kilocalorie (abbreviated kC.) is the amount of heat required to increase the temperature of 1,000 g (1 l) of water by 1° C (from 15.5° C to 16.5° C), while a calorie (small c.) refers to heating 1 g of water by 1° C. The caloric content of foods and daily energy requirements are given in kilocalories. A small calorie is one-thousandth of a kilocalorie. However, the international standard for energy content is based on the JOULE; 1 kilocalorie equals 4.18 kilojoules.

kiwi fruit (*Actinidia chinensis*) An egg-sized fruit that originated in China and is now cultivated in New Zealand, France, Israel and California. Kiwi fruit has a thin, brown, hairy skin. The fruit is pale green with a tangy taste and is eaten raw, used in fruit salads and tarts or as a garnish with meat and fish. Each raw fruit (46 g, peeled) provides 46 calories; protein, 0.8 g; carbohydrate, 11.3 g; fiber, 1.16 g; calcium, 15 mg; potassium, 80 mg; vitamin C, 31 mg; thiamin, 0.02 mg; riboflavin, 0.01 mg; niacin, 0.06 mg.

kohlrabi (*Brassica oleracea, var. caulorapo*) A stem vegetable of the CABBAGE family. Its bulbous stalk (resembling a turnip) distinguishes its appearance from other members of the cabbage family. Kohlrabi was popular in the Middle Ages in central and eastern Europe. Currently, kohlrabi is grown in California. Kohlrabi is a source of VITAMIN C, CALCIUM and IRON. Small stems are more tender than the more mature vegetable. It is cooked like a turnip or celery root. Cooked, sliced kohlrabi (1 cup, 165 g) provides 48 calories; protein, 3 g; carbohydrate, 11.4 g; fiber, 2.3 g; calcium, 50 mg; iron, 0.66 mg; potassium, 561 mg; vitamin C, 89 mg; thiamin, 0.07 mg; riboflavin, 0.03 mg; niacin, 0.64 mg. (See also CELERIAC.)

konjac (*Amorphophallus konjac*) A tuber cultivated in the Far East that is a traditional ingredient in Japanese cooking. The tuber is processed to yield a light-colored flour. Konjac has been used to make noodles (shiritaki noodles) and heat-stable gels such as mitsumame, a fruit dessert. The flour is used in food processing as a thickener for soups, sauces and desserts. Konjac flour provides a form of FIBER, a complex carbohydrate called GLUCOMANNAN that forms viscous solutions in water. When added to processed foods, konjac helps other plant-based thickeners like CARRAGEENAN, XANTHAN GUM and CORNSTARCH work more efficiently. (See also FOOD ADDITIVES; PASTA; THICKENING AGENTS.)

kosher Foods permitted by Jewish law. Jewish dietary laws, known as kashruth, define the fitness and appropriateness of foods. Acceptable and unacceptable foods fall into three food groups: "Milchig" refers to dairy products and MILK; "fleishig" refers to MEAT, fowl and products derived from them; and "pareve" refers to foods that can be eaten with either milk or meat. These neutral foods are FRUITS, VEGETABLES, GRAINS, FISH and EGGS. Acceptable fish have fins and scales; SHELLFISH are excluded. Domestic fowl are permitted, as are animals with a split hoof who chew their cud, a group that includes cattle, goats, sheep and deer. Pigs (pork) are not acceptable. CONVENIENCE FOOD is not kosher unless certified by rabbinical authority, signified by the name and insignia on the package. BREAD must be baked by observant Jews under rabinnical supervision. Bread is normally a pareve food.

All meat and fowl must be killed according to prescribed methods. Kosher slaughter involves the use of a sharp knife to quickly sever the carotid arteries, jugular bone and windpipe of a live animal by a trained slaughterer (schochet).

Kosher slaughter of poultry must also be done by hand. Some Jews follow a stricter interpretation of rules concerning acceptability. "Glatt kosher" meat means the organs, especially the lungs of kosher-killed animals, have been inspected for blemishes or defects. Glatt kosher meat must be soaked and salted within 72 hours of slaughter.

GRAPE JUICE and WINE, traditionally used in religious ceremonies, must be prepared by observant Jews. To be kosher, grape juice must be properly separated and heated. If grape-flavored sodas with real fruit juice are not prepared in this way, the soda is not kosher. The Union of Orthodox Jewish Congregations of America has published guidelines regarding the kosher status of food and beverage ingredients.

Jews who keep kosher may not eat insects. This poses a problem for fresh produce, especially green, leafy vegetables, which may require inspection. Aphids are a common problem, and fresh produce from health food stores and roadside outlets requires inspection.

The Passover holiday has additional kosher requirements extending over an eight-day period. Many products, kosher for the rest of the year, are not kosher for Passover. Leavened grain and related materials are avoided to commemorate the departure of the Jews from Egypt. Legumes, corn, rice and mustard are not eaten during Passover by Jews of European ancestry.

To separate meat and dairy, the kosher kitchen employs two sets of pots, pans, dishes, utensils and table linen to be used separately for dairy and meat. Pareve foods can be prepared and eaten with either set. The utensils are washed and stored separately. Currently, an estimated 500,000 families in the United States and perhaps 50,000 families in Canada abide by kosher dietary laws. Some non-Jewish groups, such as Seventh Day Adventists and Moslems, sometimes purchase specific kosher foods to meet their religious needs, and some consumers consider the kosher seal an indicator of quality. (See also EATING PATTERNS.)

Regenstein, Joe M. and Regenstein, Carrie, "The Kosher Dietary Laws and Their Implementation in the Food Industry," *Food Technology*, 42, (June 1988), pp. 86–94.

Kreb's cycle (citric acid cycle, tricarboxylic acid cycle) A branch of metabolism consisting of a coordinated sequence of enzymes that operate in a cyclic fashion to oxidize the major fuels of the body to produce ENERGY. The Kreb's cycle is a major METABOLIC PATHWAY and produces approximately 90% of the body's energy production by oxidizing FATTY ACIDS, AMINO ACIDS and CARBOHYDRATES to carbon dioxide. The Kreb's cycle occurs in MITOCHONDRIA, particles in the cell's cytoplasm that function as cellular powerhouses.

Prior to entering the Kreb's cycle, fuel molecules are broken down to ACETIC ACID, a two-carbon molecule that is attached to a carrier molecule called COENZYME A. The product, ACETYL COENZYME, feeds into the Kreb's cycle. The acetic acid unit (two carbon atoms) combines with a simple acid with four carbon atoms, OXALOACETIC ACID, to create CITRIC ACID (six carbon atoms), the first true product of the Kreb's cycle. Subsequent oxidations release carbon dioxide and regenerate oxaloacetic acid, which can again react with incoming acetyl COA to continue the cycle.

Certain B complex VITAMINS support energy production from food in part because they assist the Kreb's cycle. They include NIACIN, RIBOFLAVIN, PANTOTHENIC ACID and THIAMIN. B vitamins must first be converted to a COENZYME or enzyme helper to catalyze chemical reactions performed by the cycle. Thus coenzyme A is the coenzyme form of pantothenic acid.

The Kreb's cycle is coupled with other pathways supporting energy production by mitochondria, the cell's powerhouses. Coenzymes of niacin and riboflavin, as well as COENZYME Q, carry electrons from the oxidations of the Kreb's cycle to the terminal ELECTRON TRANSPORT CHAIN, which reduces OXYGEN to form WATER and simultaneously forms ATP, the cell's energy currency. When the Kreb's cycle slows down, this slowdown inhibits glucose oxidation, allowing it to be shunted to storage mechanisms by the liver. (See also CARBOHYDRATE METABOLISM; FAT METABOLISM.)

Barron, John T., Kopp, Stephen J., Tow, June, "Fatty Acid, Tricarboxylic Acid Cycle Metabolites and Energy Metabolism in Vascular Smooth Muscle," *American Journal of Physiology*, 267 (August 1994), Part 2, H764–69.

kudzu (*Pueraria lobata*)   A fibrous root vegetable, native to subtropical Asia; kudzu is used as a source of complex carbohydrate. It is chopped into cubes and cooked with soups in order to thicken them, and is available in Oriental food markets. The food value, in 100 g (raw) is: calories, 120; protein, 2.1 g; carbohydrate, 27.8 g; fiber, 0.7 g; and essentially no fat. (See also STARCH.)

kumquat (*Fortunella spp.*)   A small CITRUS FRUIT, with a sweet rind and a sour pulp. Kumquats are about the size of a quail's egg and have a thin, orange-red skin that is eaten with the fruit. Kumquats originated in China and are now cultivated in Australia, the Far East, Florida and California. Kumquats can be eaten raw with skins, in jam and in baked goods like cakes. Nutrient content of one fruit (raw, 20 g) provides 12 calories; Protein, 0.17 g; carbohydrate, 3.1 g; fiber, 0.7 g; vitamin C, 7.1 mg; thiamin, 0.02 mg; riboflavin, 0.02 mg.

kwashiorkor   A severe malnutrition disease caused by a chronic protein-deficient diet. Kwashiorkor is the classic protein deficiency disease in which caloric intake may be adequate, but consumption of too little PROTEIN causes serious MALNUTRITION. Protein and ENERGY are required for growth and maintenance of the body. People consuming too little food to supply either will degrade their own body protein and fat. Thus, protein malnutrition and energy malnutrition overlap. Symptoms include EDEMA, apathy, decreased resistance to disease, delayed development, de-pigmented hair and scaly skin. Symptoms in children include bloated belly, DIARRHEA, fatty liver and ANEMIA.

Kwashiorkor is more common in developing tropical and subtropical nations. In low socioeconomic regions of Africa, the Near East, Asia and Central and South America, the disease often begins with the birth of a second child. The weaned, first-born child must then rely on cereals, often a protein deficient diet within the community. This does not supply enough amino acids to maintain a child, nor to support growth. It can be prevented by diets providing adequate protein and energy to meet the child's growth requirements. (See also BALANCED DIET; HUNGER, WORLD; STARVATION.)

Subotzky Eve, et al., "Plasma Zinc, Copper, Selenium, Ferritin and Whole Blood Manganese Concentrations in Children with Kwashiorkor in the Acute Stages during Refeeding," *Annals of Tropical Pediatrics*, 12 (1992), pp. 13–22.

label See FOOD LABELING.

labile Refers to the chemical alteration of molecules, often leading to the loss of biological function. Cells are composed of a huge array of molecules ranging from ultra-stable, very simple minerals like SODIUM chloride to complex molecules assembled from carbon atoms (organic compounds). Very large molecules (macromolecules) such as PROTEINS, and nucleic acids like DNA and RNA, are among the most complex organic molecules in the body. Macromolecules are hundreds to many thousands of times larger than simple sugar molecules. Such huge molecules tend to be fragile: They are easily altered with heat, cooking or by acidic or alkaline conditions.

Certain nutrients are labile as well. Dissolved VITAMIN C is readily oxidized by air, while excessive cooking destroys the B complex vitamins THIAMIN and FOLIC ACID. Baking dough at high temperatures can destroy the essential amino acid LYSINE in wheat protein. Polyunsaturated FATTY ACIDS, major constituents of fats and oils, are readily oxidized when exposed to air, light and heat; fat RANCIDITY (decomposition) is the culmination of this process. Internal processes can destroy biomolecules as well. Certain hormone-like derivatives of ESSENTIAL FATTY ACIDS, PROSTAGLANDINS and LEUKOTRIENES, are exceedingly labile and break down in a matter of seconds. The chemical currency of the cells, ATP, survives only minutes in cells before being broken down (hydrolyzed). (See also FREE RADICALS.)

lactalbumin The major protein of whey, which is the soluble protein fraction remaining after MILK has curdled. Untreated cow's milk contains 20% lactalbumin and 80% CASEIN. Lactalbumin occurs in two forms, alpha-lactalbumin and betalactalbumin. Alpha-lactalbumin is a constituent of lactose synthetase, the enzyme that synthesizes LACTOSE (milk sugar). In a milk allergy, the immune system recognizes as foreign a milk protein such as lactalbumin. It will mount an allergic response when exposed to this food constituent. (See also ALLERGY, FOOD; ANTIGEN.)

lactase The intestinal enzyme that digests LACTOSE (milk sugar). Lactase breaks down lactose to its simple sugar building blocks, GLUCOSE and FRUCTOSE. This is an essential step in digestion because lactose itself cannot be absorbed by the intestine into the bloodstream, while glucose and fructose are readily absorbed. No other digestive enzyme can perform this task.

Intestinal lactase levels are high during infancy and early childhood, until the age of 5 to 6. Whether lactase activity persists into adulthood is genetically determined. In most populations of the world, lactase activity and the ability to digest milk drop dramatically after weaning ("primary lactase deficiency"). In contrast, northern and western Europeans and their descendants often maintain high lactase levels throughout adulthood. Secondary lactase deficiency can occur as a result of intestinal disease. For example, infection by an intestinal parasite giardia (GIARDIASIS) correlates with and often causes gut inflammation and lactase deficiency. (See also FOOD SENSITIVITY; LACTOSE INTOLERANCE.)

lactase deficiency   See LACTOSE INTOLERANCE.

lactic acid (lactate)   A common acidic food additive. Lactic acid is used as an acidifier in CHEESE, carbonated fruit, beverages, frozen desserts and green olives. It prevents discoloration of fruit and vegetables. Calcium lactate, the calcium salt of lactic acid, is used in condensed milk and powdered milk. Certain bacteria like lactobacillus degrade carbohydrate to lactic acid. Commercial lactic acid is produced by fermenting CORNSTARCH, MOLASSES, potato starch or whey. Lactic acid bacteria ferment milk sugar (LACTOSE) in the formation of cottage cheese, YOGURT and sour milk. Fermentation in SAUERKRAUT and related food processing yields lactic acid, which acts as a preservative. Lactic acid is naturally produced in the body by glycolysis, the enzyme system in the body that degrades the simple sugar GLUCOSE to provide energy without the participation of oxygen. Lactic acid is produced by muscles during strenuous exercise, when oxygen availability is limited. Lactic acid buildup is partially responsible for muscle cramps and FATIGUE related to vigorous EXERCISE. Lactic acid migrates out of muscle cells into the bloodstream. It is carried to the liver, where it changes back to glucose. The liver releases glucose to be returned to muscles and again broken down to lactic acid.

Madl, C., et al., "Lactic Acidosis in Thiamin Deficiency," *Clinical Nutrition*, 12 (1993), pp. 108–11.

Lactobacillus acidophilus   A beneficial, acid-producing bacterium that is normally found in the healthy intestine. Lactobacillus species, which tend to occupy the lower portion of the gut, are considered "friendly bacteria" because they produce nutrients like vitamins (BIOTIN, VITAMIN K) and short-chain fatty acids, especially BUTYRIC ACID, used as fuels by the intestinal lining. These bacteria help combat disease-causing microorganisms; they produce factors that inhibit the growth of undesirable organisms and, by filling an ecological niche, they prevent them from proliferating. Many potential pathogens do not thrive in an acidic, anaerobic environment that is created by beneficial bacteria. Extensive exposure to "broad-spectrum" antibiotics like penicillin and tetracycline destroys beneficial intestinal bacteria as well as the disease-producing bacteria, leaving the intestine prone to overgrowth by yeast and other species. (See ACIDOPHILUS; CANDIDA ALBICANS; INTESTINAL FLORA.)

lactoferrin   An IRON-binding protein in breast MILK. Lactoferrin helps block the growth of potentially pathogenic bacteria that require iron for growth in the infant's intestine. Lactoferrin secretion varies among healthy women for unknown reasons. (See also LACTALBUMIN.)

lacto-ovo-vegetarian   A person who eats no red MEAT, FISH or fowl. The diet consists of FRUIT, VEGETABLES, seeds, nuts, MILK, EGGS and their products. (See also VEGETARIAN.)

lactose (milk sugar)   The major carbohydrate of MILK. This sugar is a primary energy source for infants. It also improves intestinal absorption of CALCIUM and other minerals. Because the human INTESTINE does not absorb lactose, it must be digested to be used. Lactose digestion occurs in the intestine of infants, growing children and some adults. The enzyme LACTASE breaks down lactose to its simple sugar constituents GALACTOSE and GLUCOSE, which are easily absorbed into the bloodstream by the intestine. Glucose is used directly; galactose is converted to glucose by the liver. A deficiency of lactase in adults leads to LACTOSE INTOLERANCE (lactose maldigestion).

Lactose is a very common, safe FOOD ADDITIVE. It enhances flavors and helps in the browning of baked goods such as BREAD, waffles, biscuits and brownies. Lactose may also be found in frozen VEGETABLES, soups, salad dressing, cereals, breakfast drinks, sauces, hot chocolate, gravies, sherbet, processed meat and cake mixes. Lactose is also used to manufacture pills because it makes firm tablets when compressed. It is included in 20% of prescription pills and 5% of non-prescription pills.

lactose intolerance (lactose maldigestion)   An adverse reaction to MILK and dairy products due to the inability to digest milk sugar (lactose). Lactose is the primary carbohydrate in cow and human milk. Lactose intolerance is the result of a deficiency of lactase, the intestinal enzyme responsible for lactose digestion. Lactose intolerance represents a FOOD SENSITIVITY, not a food ALLERGY, and the IMMUNE SYSTEM is not involved. Lactase is normally produced until early childhood. In adults, production of this enzyme is genetically controlled. Large populations are deficient in lactase. In the United States lactose intolerance occurs in 79% of Native Americans, 75% of African Americans, 51% of Hispanics and 21% of whites. In Asia, Africa and Latin America the prevalence ranges from 15 to 100% of the population. A secondary lactase enzyme deficiency, parastic infections like giardiasis intestinal damage from prolonged use of non-steroidal antiinflammatory drugs can also lead to lactose intolerance.

When undigested lactose reaches the COLON it is fermented by bacteria to produce acids and gases: methane, hydrogen and carbon dioxide. In excess, these fermentation products can cause symptoms such as abdominal bloating, DIARRHEA and stomach cramps. Lactose intolerance covers a range of sensitivities. Some individuals who maldigest lactose may be able to consume a small amount of lactose, such as a cup of milk (8 g of lactose), without symptoms. The type of dairy product also determines symptoms. Yogurt containing viable cultures of bacteria used in its preparation, such as *Lactobacillus bulgaricus*, contains less lactose and may be tolerated. Aged cheese also contains less lactose, and it may not cause symptoms, especially if aged for six months or more. Cheese manufacture discards most of the lactose as whey; aging of cheeses converts the remaining lactose to lactic acid. Enzyme-treated milk can help reduce symptoms. Commer-cially prepared lactase drops can be added to milk to lower the lactose content by 70% after 24 hours in the refrigerator. Alternatively, lactase tablets can be ingested before eating dairy foods to lower lactose burden.

Lactose intolerance can be confirmed by medical diagnosis. The test involves ingesting 50 g of lactose in water (for fasting adults). After ingestion, the extent to which lactose is digested can be measured indirectly by assessing an increase in the level of blood glucose, or by measuring hydrogen produced by intestinal fermentation by breath testing.

Johnson, Abiodun, et al., "Correlation of lactose maldigestion, lactose intolerance and milk intolerance," *American Journal of Clinical Nutrition*, 57 (1993), pp. 399–401.

laetrile (amygdalen, "vitamin B$_{15}$") A compound composed of GLUCOSE, hydrogen cyanide and benzaldehyde (the flavor of bitter ALMONDS). Laetrile occurs in apricot pits and certain seeds of fruits. Although sometimes referred to as a vitamin, laetrile is not a true vitamin because the body does not rely upon it for physiologic processes. On the other hand, laetrile has been used in medical treatment. Advocates have claimed that laetrile prevented and/or controlled CANCER. By 1980 nearly half of the states in the United States had legalized laetrile for cancer treatment. To examine the validity of treatment, a large clinical study was performed at the Mayo Clinic. This study did not find any beneficial effects of laetrile treatment on patients with advanced cancer. Laetrile can be toxic because of its ability to form cyanide in the body. In this study, some patients even developed symptoms of cyanide poisoning. Laetrile is not approved by the FDA for the treatment of cancer.

lamb The flesh of young sheep; considered a source of red MEAT. In practice lambs or yearlings fall into the lamb category, while mutton refers to adult sheep. Mutton is much darker muscle meat than lamb meat and has a stronger flavor. Mutton is eaten in other parts of the world. Lamb is preferred in North America because of its juiciness, tenderness and flavor. The fat is highly saturated, like beef tallow. Lamb accounts for only about 1% of the total meat production in the United States, and Americans generally eat less than 2 lbs per person per year on average. Lamb chops (cooked, 2.2 oz, 63 g) provide 220 calories; protein, 20 g; fat, 15 g; cholesterol, 7.7 mg; calcium, 16 mg; iron, 1.5 mg; thiamin, 0.04 mg; riboflavin, 0.16 mg; niacin, 4.4 mg (See also PORK.)

lamina propria The layer of connective tissue lying beneath the lining of the gastrointestinal tract. This layer surrounds the DIGESTIVE TRACT and contains lymph vessels and lymph nodes, masses of lymphatic tissue, and blood vessels. Blood and lymph vessels transport absorbed nutrients to other parts of the body. The lamina propria protects the body against disease because it releases an ANTIBODY called secretory IgA to help neutralize the huge load of foreign materials to which the digestive tract is subjected with each meal. Secretory IgA binds potentially pathogenic organisms to prevent them from attaching to the mucosal lining; it also binds food proteins and other foreign materials and limits their penetration into the body. (See also ANTIGEN; INTESTINE.)

La Pacho (*Tabebuia avellanedae*; pau d'Arco, taheebo) A tree from South America that produces bark with medicinal properties. La Pacho has a long history of folk use in treating infections. The tree produces a complex mixture of quinones, compounds with complex, oxygen-containing ring structures, including lapachol. Extracts possess strong antimicrobial activity, including versus the yeast CANDIDA ALBICANS, staphylococcus and other disease-producing bacteria, as well as against certain parasitic infections. Extracts of La Pacho bark have been used to reduce inflammation and vaginitis. A beverage is prepared by boiling the whole bark in water. In South America La Pacho is used to treat for certain forms of cancer, in addition to infections. Although isolated ingredients in high amounts may produce anemia and increase blood clotting in animals after long-term usage, there have been no reports of human toxicity using brewed whole bark preparations. In moderation, La Pacho seems relatively safe.

lard FAT released from cooking and processing of PORK. One of the highest grades of lard is kettle-rendered lard, prepared from fat trimmings. Refined lard is bleached and purified and has a mild flavor. Commercial lard contains added hydrogenated fat to increase its melting point to make it firmer. The antioxidants—BHA, BHT, VITAMIN E and PROPYL GALLATE—retard RANCIDITY. Lard is considered a saturated fat.

Like all fat, lard provides 9 calories per gram. Lard consumption in the United States has steadily declined since 1950 from a yearly per capita consumption of 13 pounds to less than 2 pounds. Lard is used commercially in processed foods such as baked beans, chili, baked goods like muffins, and refried beans. VEGETABLE SHORTENING has largely replaced home use. Shortening is prepared from hydrogenated COTTONSEED OIL, PEANUT oil, SOYBEAN oil or COCONUT OIL, and mixtures of vegetable oils and animal fat. (See also BEEF TALLOW; HYDROGENATED VEGETABLE OIL.)

lasagne A PASTA or dried wheat dough cut in wide ribbons. The flat ribbons are usually cooked with alternating layers of minced meat topped with Parmesan cheese. Green lasagne is flavored with SPINACH and pink lasagne is flavored with tomatoes. Typical of pasta, hard glutinous wheat is used to make flour for lasagne. To prepare this form of pasta, paste made from moistened flour is shaped by pressing it through extruders; then it is dried. (See also MACARONI; STARCH.)

lathrogen A toxic substance found in certain members of the pea family that can cause lathyrism, a condition characterized by muscular weakness and spastic paralysis of the legs. CHICKPEAS, the flat podded vetch (*Lathyrus cicera*) and the Spanish vetchling (*L. clymenum*) possess an amino acid (beta N-oxayl.L-alpha beta diaminopropionic acid) that is toxic to nerve cells. Outbreaks of lathyrism have occurred in certain regions of North Africa and Asia after poor wheat crops and famine when seeds of the Lathyrus family were harvested for food. (See also FOOD SENSITIVITY.)

lauric acid A saturated FATTY ACID occurring in MEDIUM-CHAIN TRIGLYCERIDES, a readily absorbable and easily metabolized oil. Lauric acid occurs in small amounts in BUTTER, COCONUT OIL, PALM OIL and several other vegetable oils. Because it contains 12 carbon atoms it is classified as a medium-chain fatty acid. The more common long-chain saturated fatty acids in the body possess 16 carbons (PALMITIC ACID) or 18 carbons (STEARIC ACID). All of these fatty acids are "saturated", that is, they are filled up with hydrogen atoms. (See also FAT; SHORT-CHAIN FATTY ACIDS; TRIGLYCERIDES.)

laxative A material or drug that induces bowel movements to relieve CONSTIPATION. Laxatives can be classified as BULKING AGENTS, which increase the water content of the stool; as agents that increase bowel contraction; and as lubricating agents.

Bulking agents are the safest laxatives. BRAN, and other vegetable-based natural FIBERS, such as flaxseed, and fiber-rich foods will soften the stool by absorbing water and encouraging rapid transit through the digestive tract. Bulking agents can interfere with absorption of some vitamins and medications (aspirin, digitalis, antibiotics, anticoagulants) and should be taken between doses of medications.

Certain medications increase water content by drawing water into the intestine, thus softening the stool. MAGNESIUM salts, Epsom salts and milk of magnesia all have this effect. Lubricants include mineral oil and glycerin suppositories. The prolonged use of mineral oil blocks the uptake of minerals (ZINC, CALCIUM and POTASSIUM) and of vitamins A, D, E and K, and excessive use can promote OSTEOMALACIA, a soft bone disease. In general, laxatives should not be used extensively without medical supervision because they can mask root causes of persistent constipation such as colon cancer, kidney disease, underactive thyroid gland, mental depression, improper diet or lack of exercise. (See also PSYLLIUM.)

LDL See LOW-DENSITY LIPOPROTEIN.

lead A toxic HEAVY METAL and widespread industrial pollutant. People have a thousand times more lead in their bones than did their prehistoric forbears. By 1980 almost one-third of urban Americans had seriously high levels of lead in their blood. This led the EPA to ban leaded gasoline and leaded paints; subsequently, the percentage of Americans with high lead levels has fallen to 2% of the population. However, lead poisoning remains an epidemic for children. The health of an estimated 400,000 babies born each year in the United States may be compromised to some extent by their mother's lead contamination. Pregnant women, young children and elderly persons are most sensitive to lead. Persistent lead exposure among children remains a concern because the average amount detected is enough to cause subtle lead poisoning. The United States Public Health Service estimates between 3 and 4 million children under the age of five may suffer delayed development due to lead toxicity, and some children 1 to 3 years old who are exposed to lead may suffer permanent damage (lowered IQ). About 1.5 million schoolchildren have high enough lead levels in their blood to cause serious health problems.

Symptoms of subacute lead poisoning include distractibility, diarrhea, irritability and lethargy. More serious consequences are smaller fetal brain size, increased birth defects, hearing difficulties, impaired memory and decreased IQ. These may lead to an individual being stigmatized as a slow learner or underachiever. Balance is affected at a lead level of 18 mg/dL, a level well below that of 25 mg/dL, which is designated as safe by the CDC (Centers for Disease Control). Lead hinders children's growth. Lead may affect the pituitary gland, or it may inhibit growth factors guiding bone growth. Growth hormone and insulin-like growth factor production diminish with lead exposure, as does another pituitary hormone, thyroid stimulating hormone. Adults run an increased risk of high blood pressure and decreased male fertility with lead exposure.

Symptoms of acute lead poisoning include severe ANEMIA, hair loss, CHRONIC FATIGUE, pallor, headache, CONSTIPATION, aching limbs, kidney disease, high blood pressure, nerve damage (hearing loss and mental retardation), GOUT and sometimes coma. Diets low in CALCIUM, IRON and ZINC increase lead absorption, while increased calcium absorption blocks lead uptake.

Sources of Lead Contamination

Glazed ceramics Glazed dinnerware can be deadly because the pigments often contain lead. Poorly glazed pottery or pottery fired at low temperatures is often a problem with homemade or tourist goods. The lead soaks out of this pottery into acidic foods like fruit juices and tomatoes.

Canned milk or canned seafood containers Soldered seals can contribute high lead levels to the contents.

Bone meal This is not a recommended calcium supplement because animal bones often contain high levels of lead.

Dust from remodeling of older homes Pre-1950 houses in the United States usually incorporated lead-based white paint. Pregnant women must avoid paint dust during remodeling.

Wine bottle stoppers Wine bottles sealed with lead foil can leach lead into the stopper, thus contaminating the contents.

Drinking water Lead leaches out of soldered joints and any lead plumbing. Recent checks show that many building water coolers contaminate water with lead because of soldered joints and lead alloys in fixtures. The EPA estimates that one out of every five people obtains excessive lead from home drinking water due to soldered joints of copper pipes and leaded water pipes in houses 80 years or more old. To minimize the risk, run the water five minutes before drinking. (Charcoal filters don't remove lead from drinking water.) When in doubt, have your water tested for its lead content. (See also INHIBITION.)

Chao, Jason and Kikano, George E., "Lead Poisoning in Children," *American Family Physician*, 47:1 (January 1993) pp. 113–20.

leaky gut (leaky gut syndrome) A condition characterized by the increased intestinal uptake of potentially harmful materials. Leaky gut is caused by conditions that create intestinal inflammation, including excessive alcohol; the prolonged use of certain medications, especially nonsteroidal antiinflammatory drugs or broad-spectrum antibiotics; chronic intestinal infections due to viruses, parasites, yeast or bacteria; maldigestion; or nutritional deficiencies, such as IRON deficiency in children. Bacterial toxins (endotoxins) and ingested toxic materials can also injure the intestine, rendering it more permeable (porous). Leaky gut is associated with compromised immunity and with INFLAMMATORY BOWEL DISEASE like Crohn's disease. Depletion of beneficial bacteria and growth of potentially dangerous bacteria (a situation termed dysbiosis) increase the likelihood of leaky gut. FIBROMYALGIA and CHRONIC FATIGUE are linked to leaky gut as well. Note that the intestine can become so damaged in certain disease states that nutrient uptake slows down and maldigestion of protein and carbohydrate and MALNUTRITION can occur. For example, CELIAC DISEASE (severe wheat protein sensitivity) is associated with decreased gut permeability.

As a result of increased intestinal uptake, partially digested food proteins can be absorbed, which promotes multiple food allergies. Damaging toxins may also find their way into the body. These materials may overburden the liver so that its ability to dispose of toxic materials may be compromised. The influx of foreign substances may also overtax the immune system, creating a long-term drain on the body's reserves. Circulating immune complexes, aggregates of antibodies and toxic materials, can lodge at different locations and can trigger autoimmune reactions, in which the body's defenses attack tissues; RHEUMATOID ARTHRITIS and lupus are possible outcomes.

Treatment involves removing the underlying condition, whether it is the infectious agent, alcohol or medication overuse. Cleaning up the diet to avoid excessive amounts of foods with low nutrient content, such as highly processed, fatty convenience foods, is an important consideration. Specific nutrients become important with a leaky gut. Antioxidants help curb inflammation; BETA CAROTENE, VITAMIN C, folic acid, VITAMIN A, VITAMIN E, and trace minerals such as ZINC are special keys to intestinal health. These nutrients also boost the immune system and the intestinal immune cells to ward off attack. Other nutrients specifically promote intestinal health, including fiber and the amino acid glutamine. (See also ACIDOPHILUS; FATIGUE.) STRESS is known to lower immunity, including decreased production of the major antibody of the intestine, secretory IgA. Correcting dysbosis (imbalanced gut flora) with lactobacillus and bifidobacteria species and fructose-containing fiber may help normalize gut function. Therefore, stress reduction and exercise may be beneficial.

Olaison, Gunnar, "Abnormal Intestinal Permeability in Crohn's Disease: a Possible Pathogenic Factor," *Scandinavian Journal of Gastroenterology*, 25 (1990), pp. 321–28.

lean body mass   A term used to indicate fat-free weight, representing primarily MUSCLE weight. The concept of lean body mass is important in terms of the effectiveness of weight loss and weight management programs. Optimally, weight loss programs that incorporate exercise and gradual weight loss (no more than 1 to 2 pounds per week) facilitate fat loss while minimizing potentially damaging losses of muscle protein. On the other hand, severe caloric restriction and crash DIETING programs will cause loss of both fat and muscle. Often the lean body mass lost with such programs is replaced by fat when previous diet and lifestyle are resumed at the end of a weight loss program. (See also OBESITY.)

lean meat   See MEAT.

leavening agents   Materials added to dough that make it rise prior to baking. The most common examples of leavening agents are BAKING SODA (sodium bicarbonate), BAKING POWDER and BAKER'S YEAST. All of these agents generate carbon dioxide, which is trapped as tiny bubbles in the dough; heat and steam expand the air pockets. Sodium bicarbonate) breaks down to carbon dioxide in the presence of acidic ingredients like sour milk or cream of tartar. Baking powder is a blend of

calcium acid phosphate, cream of tartar or other acids and sodium bicarbonate, which together generate gas when moistened. Baking (heating) releases more carbon dioxide from baking powder. Yeast contains enzymes that ferment glucose, a starch breakdown product, to carbon dioxide and alcohol. Heat evaporates alcohol and inactivates yeast enzymes. Leavening agents are generally considered safe food additives. Baking soda and baking powder add considerable sodium to breads, rolls and crackers. Together these foods contribute 25% of the sodium in the American diet. Only 2% of the sodium comes from salty snack foods like potato chips.

lecithin (phosphatidyl choline)   The best-known phosphorus-containing lipid related to triglycerides (fats and oils). As an important building block of cell membranes, lecithin builds healthy cells. Lecithin helps carry fat and CHOLESTEROL as a part of the lipid transport particles of blood: LDL (LOW-DENSITY LIPOPROTEIN), HDL (HIGH-DENSITY LIPOPROTEIN), VLDL (VERY-LOW-DENSITY LIPOPROTEIN) and CHYLOMICRONS. In BILE, lecithin acts like a soap to dissolve fats and soluble VITAMINS for digestion and absorption.

Lecithin contains GLYCEROL, a product of glucose metabolism, CHOLINE, a nitrogen-containing base, and two long-chain FATTY ACIDS. Lecithin is synthesized by the body, but it also occurs in a wide variety of foods. Good sources include SOYBEANS, liver, CAULIFLOWER, egg yolks and CABBAGE. (The name lecithin is taken from the Greek word for egg yolk.) Commercially, soybeans are the predominant source. As a food additive, lecithin acts as a stabilizer and EMULSIFIER in MARGARINE, CHOCOLATE, frozen desserts, salad dressings and baked goods.

Lecithin Supplements

Using lecithin supplements, together with cutting down on saturated fat, may lower blood cholesterol for some people, and it may raise HDL (high-density lipoprotein, the desirable form of cholesterol), thus protecting against heart disease. Lecithin seems to protect experimental lab animals from developing liver CIRRHOSIS with an alcohol-laden diet, although the details are unknown. Patients taking certain antipsychotic drugs may eventually develop TARDIVE DYSKINESIA, marked by involuntary facial movements; choline and lecithin supplements can suppress such symptoms in some patients. Lecithin may help with short-term memory in certain elderly patients, but it has not been shown to prevent or cure ALZHEIMER'S DISEASE or other age-related dementia. Purified lecithin works best to lower blood choline levels and to help with memory loss. Most lecithin supplements are impure and may contain only 30% lecithin; it is questionable whether typical health food store pills will help with memory. Side effects can occur with large doses of lecithin; some people experience an upset stomach, sweating and a loss of appetite.

Canty, D.J. and Zeisel, S.H., "Lecithin and Choline in Human Health and Disease," *Nutrition Reviews*, 52:10 (1994), pp. 327–39.

leek (*Allium porrum*)   A close relative of the ONION. Leeks are native to Central Asia and have been an important vegetable in Europe since the Middle Ages. The leaves and stem are eaten, rather than the small, narrow bulb. Served raw, leeks can be chopped and mixed with cream cheese or COTTAGE CHEESE. They add flavor to soups and stews and are an important ingredient of quiche and vichyssoise, a creamy potato soup served cold. Leeks are also braised or broiled and served with butter or cheese sauces. Leeks are milder than onions and remain crunchy when cooked. They provide more nutrients than an equivalent serving of onions. In folk traditions leeks have been used to stimulate appetite, protect against infection and limit EDEMA (swelling due to water retention). Leeks (1 cup, 124 g) provide 76 calories; protein, 1.9 g; carbohydrate, 17.5 g; fiber, 1.9 g; calcium, 73 mg; iron, 2.6 mg; vitamin C, 14.9 mg; thiamin, 0.074 mg; riboflavin, 0.037 mg; niacin, 0.50 mg.

legumes (pulse family, pea family)   A very large plant family characterized by seed-bearing pods. Common members are eaten as dried seeds: LENTILS, BEANS (kidney, fava or broad, navy, bush, string, lima, Windsor, SOYBEANS), PEAS, including CHICKPEAS or garbanzos, and PEANUTS. The roots of most legumes harbor bacteria that convert nitrogen in air to nitrogen compounds used by their hosts; therefore, legumes often grow well in depleted soils.

It is believed that legumes were among the earliest plants to be cultivated. This occurred around 10,000 B.C. in Southwest Asia, around 8000 B.C. in the Middle East, and 4000 B.C. in the New World. About 13,000 species are classified as legumes, and many are cultivated for food. Chickpeas, fava beans and lentils probably originated in the Middle East. Soybeans represent roughly 55% of the world's legume production; peanuts, 12%; dry peas, 9%; dry beans, 7%; and chickpeas, 5%. More than one-third of the world legume production is supplied by the United States. Washington, Idaho, Michigan and California are the major producers.

Legumes supply the same calories as grains, but they provide two to four times as much protein. This protein is low in calories and is both fat and cholesterol free. Legume protein is deficient in the essential sulfur-containing amino acid METHIONINE while containing adequate amounts of another essential amino acid, LYSINE. The amino acid composition of legume protein complements that of cereal grains, which are low in lysine but contain adequate methionine. Thus the combination of both foods provides dietary protein that more closely meets protein requirements than either food eaten alone. As an example, a three-quarter-cup serving of cooked legumes provides 11 to 13 g of protein, which would need to be supplemented with 1.5 cups of cooked cereal and three to four slices of whole-grain BREAD to provide adequate, balanced protein. Other foods also complement legume protein; nuts and small amounts of fish or poultry or egg white overcome amino acid deficiency. Soybean is the most complete protein and does not require complementing. Because legumes are less rich protein sources than meat or dairy products, strict vegetarians would need to eat relatively more legumes than people who eat animal foods.

Lentils, beans and peas contain relatively large amounts of FIBER, non-digested carbohydrate. They lower the rate at which BLOOD SUGAR rises, decrease the need for the hormone INSULIN and therefore increase GLUCOSE TOLERANCE. These legumes also contain substances that protect against breast, colon and prostate CANCER. Several of these substances are classified as protease inhibitors; they block certain enzymes that seem to promote cancer. Soybeans contain a group of compounds called isoflavones that are modified in the body

and transformed into substances that may block the entry of the female hormone estrogen into cells. This may decrease the risk of breast and ovarian cancer.

Dried legumes are softened during cooking. Soaking legumes overnight speeds the cooking process. As an alternative, dry beans can be placed in water, heated to boiling for two minutes, and allowed to soak for an hour. Boiling softens the seed coating, allowing water to penetrate more rapidly. (See also COMPLETE PROTEIN; FOOD COMBINING; FOOD COMPLEMENTING; GLYCEMIC INDEX.)

Kleiner, Susan M., "A Hill of Beans: the Latest on Legumes," *The Physician and Sports Medicine*, 23:6 (June 1995), pp. 13–14.

lemon (*Citrus limon*)   A yellow, sour citrus fruit. Lemons originated in Southeast Asia between China and India. The Romans grew lemons in southern Italy, and citrus trees were cultivated by the Persians and the Arabs. Lemons rank among the top 12 fruit crops in the world and are the sixth leading fruit crop in the United States. Lemons and limes were established in Florida by the 1700s. California, Arizona and Florida contribute most of the U.S. lemon crop because of the lemon's sensitivity to frost.

Lemons are an excellent source of VITAMIN C. Lemons and LIMES were recognized for their anti-SCURVY properties by European seamen in the 17th century. However, issuance of lemon juice to sailors was not decreed in the British Navy until the latter 18th century.

The most common varieties of lemons are Eurekas and Lisbons. Lemons are usually picked before they are mature and have a yellow to green color. Ripening is accelerated by exposing the unripened fruit to ethylene, a non-toxic gas produced by many ripening fruit. At least half of the U.S. lemon crop is processed to lemon juice, frozen juice concentrate and lemon-flavored soft drinks. Lemon pulp and rind are used to prepare lemon oil. PECTIN (a water-soluble FIBER) and (plant-based pigments that enhance the effects of vitamin C). Lemon and lime peels and citrus oil contain limonene, an oil that can cause skin irritation. This poses a problem because some commercial lemon-flavored beverages contain peel and peel extracts. They also contain psoralens, which can make the skin sensitive to sunlight and cause inflammation. In addition, lemons contain limonin, the bitter chemical found in the white, spongy part of the rind, which, together with other compounds, can activate defensive enzyme systems in the liver to defend against foreign compounds. Fresh lemon juice (1 cup) provides 60 calories; protein, 0.9 g; carbohydrate, 21.1 g; fiber, 0.85 g; potassium, 303 mg; vitamin C, 31 mg; thiamin, 0.07 mg; riboflavin, 0.02 mg; niacin, 0.24 mg. (See also ALLERGY, FOOD.)

lentil (*Lens esculenta*)   A small, disc-shaped legume. Lentils are one of the oldest cultivated plants; archaeological evidence indicates that they were cultivated in the Near East about 8000 B.C. Lentils are now widely cultivated in the cool season in the tropics and subtropical regions and in the summer season of mild temperate regions. Leading producers of lentils are India, Turkey and Syria. Varieties range from orange to green.

Lentils contain 7.4% PROTEIN, more than cereal grains. Lentil protein is deficient in the sulfur-containing AMINO ACIDS: METHIONINE and CYSTEINE. Methionine is a dietary essential amino acid. Protein from cereal grains supplies ample sulfur amino acids. Therefore the amino acid patterns of lentils and grains complement each other; mixtures of the two foods contain a higher quality protein than either by itself. Lentils are a low-fat food. Only 4% of calories comes from fat.

Cooked lentils are frequently served with other vegetables in casseroles, soups and stews. Lentils contain soluble FIBER, non-digestible plant carbohydrate that causes starches to be digested slowly. Slow digestion produces a smaller rise in BLOOD SUGAR than simple sugars or highly refined carbohydrates; therefore lentils are said to have a low GLYCEMIC INDEX. Lentils in Indian cuisine (dahl) are prepared without the skin of the seed, and therefore contain much less fiber.

Cooked lentils, 1 cup (200 g), provide 215 calories; protein, 16 g; carbohydrate, 38 g; fiber, 10 g; fat, 1 g; calcium, 50 mg; iron, 4.2 mg; potassium, 498 mg; thiamin, 0.14 mg; riboflavin, 0.12 mg; niacin, 1.12 mg. (See also BIOLOGICAL VALUE; COMPLETE PROTEIN.)

leptin   A hormone produced by fat cells that helps regulate fat storage. Leptin is a newly discovered protein that acts on the brain to decrease food intake in obese mice that have a genetic defect in their ability to make this hormone. Although the detailed steps by which this protein acts on the brain have not yet been worked out, it appears to be a key part of the body's weight control system. Administering the genetically engineered hormone to the brains of mice that cannot make leptin regulates their eating behavior and overall body fat. Even lean animals can be forced to lose the fat they possess. Leptin is made by humans, and its effect in the body is being actively investigated. The discovery of this hormone supports the proposal that in some people, OBESITY represents a defect in the body's metabolism and may eventually be treated to correct imbalanced body chemistry. This new research may eventually have a large impact on the health of Americans, because an estimated 50 million people in the United States are overweight. (See also DIET; FAT METABOLISM; WEIGHT MANAGEMENT.)

lettuce (*Lactuca sativa*)   A green VEGETABLE with a leafy head that may be compact or loose. Lettuce belongs to the sunflower family, and it may have been cultivated in ancient Egypt or Persia. Lettuce is a popular salad vegetable in the United States. California is the leading lettuce-producing state, followed by Arizona, Florida, Colorado, Texas and New Mexico. Lettuce is the major salad vegetable produced in the United States; about 30 pounds of lettuce are consumed per person annually. Although tomato production far exceeds that of lettuce, less than 20% of tomatoes are consumed fresh, as in salads.

Crisp-headed lettuce, also known as iceberg lettuce, constitutes the majority of long-distance, commercially produced lettuce. Butterhead (Bibb, Big Boston or White Boston) varieties bruise easily and are more likely to be grown for local markets. Romaine lettuce (cos lettuce) has long, dark-green leaves and is broad-ribbed, with a narrow head. Romaine is flavorful and crisp and has a higher nutrient value than iceberg lettuce. The more dark-green the leaves, the more nutritious the salad green. Thus Romaine lettuce contains six times as much vitamin C and 5 to 10 times as much beta carotene as iceberg lettuce. Browning of lettuce at salad bars was once retarded with sulfite preservatives. Now sulfites are forbidden on fresh produce. VITAMIN C derivatives and other products are now used to keep salad lettuce fresh-looking and crisp.

All types of lettuce have a high water content (94 to 96%). The nutrient content of one head of Boston lettuce (163 g) is 21 calories; protein, 2.1 g; carbohydrate, 3.8 g; fiber, 2.7 g; calcium, 52 mg; iron, 0.49 mg; potassium, 419 mg; vitamin A, 158 retinol equivalents; thiamin, 0.1 mg; riboflavin, 0.1 mg; niacin, 0.49 mg. (See also SULFITES.)

leucine (Leu, L-leucine)   A dietary essential AMINO ACID. Leucine is one of the 20 amino acids required to build proteins. Leucine is classified as a branched-chain amino acid. This group of amino acids possesses hydrophobic (water-repelling) carbon chains that cannot be synthesized by animals. Adults require 14 mg per kilogram body weight daily of leucine in the diet. In the body leucine stimulates protein synthesis in muscles, and it may stimulate the release of insulin to trigger glucose and amino acid uptake from the bloodstream.

Leucine and other branched-chain amino acids are degraded by skeletal muscle in order to produce energy. Unlike many other amino acids, leucine cannot be converted to GLUCOSE by the LIVER and is therefore considered a "ketogenic" amino acid. During excessive fat breakdown that accompanies starvation, branched-chain amino acids including leucine yield KETONE BODIES, acidic by-products. A rare genetic defect in the ability to break down branched-chain amino acids leads to maple syrup urine disease, characterized by mental retardation, convulsions and coma. This condition is treated by limiting the dietary intake of branched-chain amino acids. (See also ISOLEUCINE; KETOSIS; VALINE.)

leukocytes (polymorphonuclear leukocytes, white blood cells)   Cells in the blood that are products of the IMMUNE SYSTEM. Leukocytes differ significantly from the more numerous red blood cells. White blood cells possess nuclei and lack HEMOGLOBIN (the red oxygen transport protein of blood) unlike red blood cells, which lack nuclei but contain large amounts of hemoglobin.

There are several types of leukocytes: white cells with cytoplasmic particles (granular leukocytes) and those without grains (agranular leukocytes). Among granular leukocytes are three subclasses called neutrophils, eosinophils and basophils according to how they react to certain stains under the microscope.

Nearly 60% of leukocytes are neutrophils. They help defend the body against disease-causing bacteria, yeast, fungi and viruses. Neutrophils can enter tissues by passing through capillaries, so that they can engulf invaders. Eosinophils stain orange-red easily; these cells play a role in allergic reactions, and high levels are often associated with allergic attacks and with some parasitic infections. Basophils stain blue-black. They represent less than 1% of the leukocytes.

Agranular leukocytes represent the largest population of white cells and originate from lymphatic tissue and bone marrow. Lymphocytes represent 20 to 40% of leukocytes, and they both regulate the immune system and carry out key defensive roles. Lymphocytes consist of B cells, T cells and natural killer cells. B cells lead to antibody production. Antibodies are proteins released into the bloodstream to help bind and destroy foreign substances. T cells attack virus-infected cells, transplanted tissue and cancer cells. One class of T cells (T helper cells) helps increase the immune response, while another class of T cells (T suppressor cells) helps limit the immune response. Natural killer cells destroy virus-infected cells and cancer cells by engulfing them and by producing chemicals that help destroy these altered cells. Monocytes also belong to the family of lymphocytes and function as scavengers; they mature into macrophages, a type of cell that cleans up infected areas of the body. (See also LYMPH.)

leukotrienes   Powerful inflammatory agents. Leukotrienes are products of ESSENTIAL FATTY ACIDS that increase inflammation and mucus secretion and contract the muscles surrounding blood vessels and the intestines. Extremely powerful substances, leukotrienes are about 10,000 times more potent than HISTAMINE, a noted stimulant of INFLAMMATION. Leukotrienes play a role in immediate allergy attacks (immediate hypersensitivity) and in heart attacks. They constrict lung air passageways, especially the BRONCHI, in asthma attacks. They constrict coronary arteries, which deliver blood to the heart. Leukotrienes are synthesized by various white blood cells; by mast cells (cells found in connective tissue that participate in inflammation and immune reactions); and by brain, heart, lung and spleen. Leukotrienes (C_4, D_4, E_4) contain the sulfur amino acid CYSTEINE. Another leukotriene called LTB_4 attaches white cells to the site of infection or inflammation. LTB_4 is implicated in such diseases as RHEUMATOID ARTHRITIS.

Leukotrienes are linear compounds synthesized from a polyunsaturated FATTY ACID called ARACHIDONIC ACID, itself derived from the essential fatty acid, LINOLEIC ACID. The conversion of arachidonic acid to leukotrienes is not inhibited by ASPIRIN or other non-steroidal antiinflammatory drugs. Therefore, these pain relievers do not remedy asthma attacks. (See also IMMUNE SYSTEM.)

levulose   See FRUCTOSE.

licorice (*Glycyrrhiza glabra*)   A small shrub used to produce natural licorice flavoring. The roots and runners of the licorice plant are used in botanical medicine. Licorice extracts contain a steroid-like molecule, GLYCYRRHIZIN or glycyrrhizic acid. This material is 50 to 100 times sweeter than table sugar. It has been used in mouthwashes and toothpastes because it inhibits plaque growth and because of its pleasing flavor. Licorice has been used for thousands of years in both Western and Eastern medical traditions. In Chinese medicine it has been used to treat stomach ulcers, asthma and upper respiratory (lung) infections among other conditions. Licorice inhibits inflammation due to allergic reactions and reactions to bacterial toxins. Licorice stimulates mucus secretion, which partially explains its utility in treating stomach and intestinal ulcers. It also supports the health of intestinal cells. Glycyrrhizin has also been used to treat viral hepatitis.

Licorice flavoring is used in beverages, candy and baked goods. Most commercial licorice in the United States contains anise as a flavoring agent. If natural licorice is eaten as a steady diet, it often causes salt retention, water retention (EDEMA), swollen ankles and puffy eyes—and thus weight (though not fat) gain. In children, excessive licorice consumption can result in hormone imbalance, diarrhea, vomiting, high blood pressure, low potassium levels and water retention. The regular use of licorice also interferes with certain medications such as DIURETICS, vasodilators and digitalis. The active agent of licorice, glycyrrhizin, can mimic the adrenal hormone aldosterone and slow the disposal of this hormone by the liver. Glycyrrhizin raises blood pressure. Licorice extract, from which glycyrrhizin has been removed (deglycyrrhizinated licorice), can help heal ulcers, apparently without side effects. Licorice should not be used by patients with high blood pressure, kidney failure or those who are taking medications for heart conditions.

life expectancy   The number of years the average person can be expected to live. Wise life-style choices, appropriate nutrition and exercise favor a longer, more productive and satisfying life. (See also AGING.)

life extension   Refers to the hypothesis that VITAMINS and other supplements can extend the life span. The eternal quest for youth leads to the question of whether supplements can help people live longer. There is no complete answer to this question. It is clear that there are no secret formulas, no "magic bullets" and no fountain of youth. Perhaps the more basic question is, how can a person's health, the sense of well-being and happiness, be improved, given his or hers unique inheritance and environmental challenges of living in the 21st century?

Optimal nutrition can minimize the impact of DEGENERATIVE DISEASES. Studies of groups of people throughout the world who are reported to have longer life spans, such as the Masai tribesmen of Africa, Mormons, Seventh Day Adventists and the Chinese, suggest that the healthiest people in the world:

- eat fresh fruit, fresh vegetables and minimally processed foods regularly and drink unpolluted water;
- limit consumption of caffeinated beverages, fatty foods, refined starches like white flour, sugar, strong alcoholic beverages, and potentially harmful drugs;
- avoid excess calories and obesity;
- avoid smoking;
- engage in regular, moderate to vigorous physical EXERCISE;
- live harmoniously with their families and social groups.

(See also AGING; ANTIOXIDANTS; ILLNESS; STRESS.)

Lee, I.M, et al., "Exercise Intensity and Longevity in Men: the Harvard Alumni Health Study," *Journal of the American Medical Association*, 273:15 (April 19, 1995), pp. 1179–84.

light foods (lite foods)   "Light" or "lite" designation on a FOOD LABEL. The U.S. FDA food label regulations that took effect in August 1994 allow food manufacturers to use new terms, each with a specific definition of a food. "Light" or "lite" can be used to describe foods containing one-third fewer calories or half the FAT of a reference food. Alternatively, if the food contains 50% or more of its calories as fat, then the reduction in fat must be 50%. "Light" or "lite" can also refer to a low calorie–low sodium food in which the sodium content has been reduced by 50% of the reference food. All other uses of the term light must specify the sensory quality it describes; for example, its color or texture. (See also ADVERTISING; FOOD LABELING.)

lignin A non-carbohydrate constituent of FIBER that forms protective and structural components of plant cell walls. Lignin is a complex plastic-like material (polymer) that is very insoluble and resistant to chemical breakdown. Crude fiber that remains after acid digestion of plant materials is primarily lignin. Unlike carbohydrate-based fiber, lignin is not degraded by digestive enzymes or gut microbes but passes through the digestive tract intact. It does, however, have important effects on the digestive tract: Lignin decreases the risk of CONSTIPATION by increasing the movement of stools, and it binds BILE salts. This is believed to minimize microbial degradation of these substances and hence decrease exposure of the intestine to toxic derivatives. Decreased exposure is believed to lower the risk of colon CANCER. By binding both bile salts and CHOLESTEROL and moving them out of the body as feces, blood cholesterol levels may be lowered, decreasing the risk of heart disease. Excessive fiber, including lignin, can block mineral absorption. Certain lignin constituents released by the intestine are modified in the body. Such "animal lignins" apparently interact with tissues, weakly mimicking the effects of ESTROGEN, the female sex hormone. Lignin may have a therapeutic role in lowering the risk of breast CANCER. (See also CELLULOSE; PECTIN.)

lima bean (*Phaseolus lunatus*; butter bean) One of the most common BEANS in the U.S. diet. This legume is believed to have originated in Peru between 7,000 and 8,000 years ago. Spanish and Portuguese traders took beans to the Philippines, Africa and other warm regions. Lima beans grow well in the tropics and are an important crop in Africa and Asia. Most U.S. production is in California. Green lima beans grown in the United States are mainly processed (canned and frozen). The common varieties of green lima bean are butter beans (Fordhooks) and baby limas. Green lima beans are cooked the same way as green peas. Dry lima beans are used in soups, casseroles and bean salads. Certain varieties of lima beans, especially colored varieties native to the Caribbean, contain harmful substances (cyanoglycosides). Enzymes produced by intestinal microorganisms release cyanide, a potential poison, from these materials. However, the varieties of lima bean grown in the United States contain negligible amounts of these toxins.

Uncooked beans in general contain a TRYPSIN inhibitory protein that can block the action of this digestive enzyme. They also contain hemagglutinins, proteins that coagulate red blood cells. These proteins are generally inactivated during cooking. Furthermore, soaking dried beans, followed by cooking, renders these agents inactive. Mature beans contain oligosaccharides, short chains of sugars that are not digested but instead are degraded by colon bacteria and may cause gas and bloating. Soaking beans before cooking, and discarding the soak water, lessens the problem.

Thick-seeded lima beans (cooked from frozen beans; 1 cup, 171 g) contain 225 calories; protein, 15 g; carbohydrate,

41 g ; fiber, 15.4 g; fat, 0.8 g; calcium, 47 mg; iron, 2.9 mg; potassium, 608 mg; thiamin, 0.43 mg; riboflavin, 0.05 mg; niacin, 0.9 mg. (See also CYANOGEN.)

lime (*Citrus aurantifolia*) A green-colored citrus fruit, smaller than a lemon. Limes originated in Southeast Asia. Arabs introduced limes into Egypt in 900 A.D., and into Spain by 1200 A.D. With the settlement of the New World, limes were introduced rapidly in the Caribbean Islands, the Florida Keys and Mexico. Today Florida supplies about 10% of the world's lime crop. A cold-resistant variety is grown in India, Mexico, Egypt, the West Indies and other tropical regions. Nearly 50% of the U.S. lime crop is processed as lime juice, lime-based beverages, marmalades, syrups and lime oil. As with lemon, some people are allergic to lime peel. The oil of lime peel (oil of bergamot) can cause skin to blister when exposed to sunlight. The active ingredient, psoralens, occurs in lemon peel and to a lesser degree in carrots, celery, figs, parsley, fennel and anise. Lime juice or beverages flavored by limes may contain lime peel and extracts. Limes are excellent sources of vitamin C. This explains their use by 18th-century navies to prevent scurvy on long voyages.

Lime juice (fresh, 1 cup) contains 65 calories; protein, 1.1 g; carbohydrate, 22.2 g; fiber, 1.0 g; potassium, 268 mg; vitamin C, 72 mg; thiamin, 0.05 mg; riboflavin, 0.03 mg; niacin, 0.25 mg.

linoleic acid A dietary ESSENTIAL FATTY ACID. Polyunsaturated fatty acids like linoleic acid help maintain the flexibility of cell membranes, which is essential for their normal function. Therefore linoleic acid is essential for normal growth and development. Certain details of the molecular structure are important in order to understand its role. This 18-carbon acid contains two double bonds in which pairs of carbons are deficient in hydrogen atoms. Therefore, it is classified as a polyunsaturated FATTY ACID. It belongs to the omega-6 family of fatty acids because the first double bond begins six carbon atoms from the end of the fatty acid. Linoleic acid is classified as a dietary essential because the body is unable to insert double bonds in fatty acids at the sixth carbon of this long chain fatty acid. While the body cannot manufacture linoleic acid, it can convert linoleic acid to longer, more complex fatty acids, especially ARACHIDONIC ACID. In turn the body transforms arachidonic acid to a class of PROSTAGLANDINS of the PG$_2$ series, hormone-like substances that stimulate inflammation, pain, BLOOD CLOTTING, smooth muscle contraction, elevated blood pressure and other physiological processes. Other derivatives of arachidonic acid, hence of linoleic acid, are called LEUKOTRIENES. These are extremely powerful inflammatory agents.

Linoleic acid is the raw material for more complex lipids. The body converts linoleic acid to a close relative called gamma linolenic acid by an enzyme (delta 6 desaturase) as the first step in the synthesis of longer fatty acids from which regulatory substances like prostaglandins are made. This critical step is slowed by AGING, hormonal imbalance, and dietary factors such as zinc deficiency, ALCOHOLISM, excessive sugar consumption and conditions like DIABETES.

Symptoms of essential fatty acid deficiency include severe, resistant ECZEMA, hair loss and impaired wound healing. Deficient animals reveal retarded growth and development. Deficiencies have been reported in infants fed non-fat milk, which lacks linoleic acid.

Many polyunsaturated seed oils supply linoleic acid in the typical American diet. SAFFLOWER oil, SOYBEAN oil, SUN-FLOWER oil, CORN OIL and MARGARINE prepared from these oils are typical sources. Linoleic acid consumption typically ranges from 5 to 10% of calories when American diets supply 25 to 50% of the daily calories as fat. Dietary recommendations generally specify that for a healthy adult the total polyunsaturated fat intake should be about 6 to 7% of daily calories, not to exceed 10%. Research suggests that linoleic acid should represent 5% of calories or 14 g/day. There is no RECOMMENDED DIETARY ALLOWANCE for this or any other polyunsaturated fatty acid, yet. Note that a high intake of polyunsaturated oils increases the need for a fat-soluble ANTIOXIDANT like VITAMIN E because polyunsaturates are more susceptible to oxidation and destruction.

A modified form of linoleic acid, called conjugated linoleic acid, can offer protection against breast cancer in lab animals. Conjugated linoleic acid occurs in animal products like meat and dairy products. However, it should be noted that these animal products contain large amounts of saturated fat and cholesterol, which are risk factors for heart disease. (See also ALPHA LINOLENIC ACID; FAT METABOLISM.)

Roberts, T.L., et al., "Linoleic Acid and Risk of Sudden Cardiac Death," *British Health Journal*, 70 (1993), pp. 524–29.

linseed oil   See FLAXSEED OIL.

lipase   A family of ENZYMES that degrade fats and oils to release free FATTY ACIDS. Three classes of lipase are important.

Pancreatic lipase   The PANCREAS secretes lipase in addition to other digestive enzymes. The free fatty acids are absorbed by intestinal cells, where they are resynthesized back into fat molecules, then packaged in fat transport particles called CHYLOMICRONS, released into the LYMPH and ultimately enter the bloodstream.

Lipoprotein lipase   This lipase occurs in capillary walls, where it breaks down fat being transported in the bloodstream by chylomicrons. Lipoprotein lipase also releases fatty acids from VLDL (VERY-LOW-DENSITY LIPOPROTEIN), a particle that transports fat synthesized by the liver. Free fatty acids migrate into ADIPOCYTES (fat cells), to be stored as fat. They are also absorbed by muscle cells to be burned for energy.

Hormone-sensitive lipase   This lipase occurs in fat cells. In response to EPINEPHRINE (adrenaline), a stress hormone from the adrenal glands, hormone-sensitive lipase rapidly breaks down stored fat to release fatty acids into the bloodstream. Muscle cells can then absorb the fatty acids from the blood and burn them for energy. (See also DIGESTION; FAT METABOLISM.)

lipectomy   See LIPOSUCTION.

lipids   Fat-like, waxy or oily chemicals that repel water and dissolve chemical solvents like petroleum, oils, ether and benzene. The only property all lipids have in common is their insolubility in water (hydrophobicity). Common lipids

in the body include CHOLESTEROL, FAT and oils (collectively called TRIGLYCERIDES), waxes, phosphorus-containing lipids (PHOSPHOLIPIDS) like LECITHIN, as well as VITAMIN A, VITAMIN D, VITAMIN E, VITAMIN K and BETA CAROTENE. Lipids tend to be stored in fat tissue. Certain pollutants are also lipids: industrial chemicals like PBB, PCB; solvents like benzene, toluene, methylene chloride; cleaning solvents; and PESTICIDES like DDT.

Fat is not cholesterol. Confusion arises because these lipids occur together in MEAT and cholesterol dissolves in the fat released during cooking because it is fat-soluble. Therefore removal of fat from meat decreases the cholesterol content. Generally a low cholesterol diet will also be a low saturated fat diet. A high saturated fat diet can increase BLOOD cholesterol in susceptible people due to an effect on cholesterol formation by the liver.

Serum Lipids

Fat and cholesterol are transported by the blood. However, for simplicity in diagnostic lab testing, serum, the cell-free fluid remaining after blood clots, is usually used for analysis. Thus serum lipids consist of fat (serum triglyceride) and serum cholesterol. Following a meal, serum triglyceride levels rise for a short time only, as blood distributes fat absorbed from digested food. High serum triglyceride levels between meals may increase the risk of CARDIOVASCULAR DISEASE for people with high serum cholesterol. To evaluate the risk of heart disease it is often more meaningful to analyze individual forms of serum cholesterol, rather than simply determining total cholesterol. This more detailed analysis measures the amounts of LDL (LOW-DENSITY LIPOPROTEIN), the undesirable form of cholesterol, HDL ("desirable cholesterol," HIGH-DENSITY LIPOPROTEIN) and serum triglycerides separately. Elevated LDL levels and depressed HDL levels may increase the risk of ATHEROSCLEROSIS (clogged arteries).

Lipids including cholesterol and unsaturated fatty acids are sensitive to oxidation. Highly reactive forms of oxygen called FREE RADICALS can extract electrons from these cell constituents to make up for their own deficiency, and in the process they leave behind damaged molecules called lipid peroxides. These in turn are unstable and break down to products yielding more free radicals, as well as chemicals that cause mutations (mutagens) and cytotoxic (cell-killing) agents. Some of these decomposition products are responsible for the smell of rancid fat. Oxidized LDL is implicated in the origin of plaques that can clog arteries and cause heart disease. (See also CHLORINATED HYDROCARBONS; FAT METABOLISM; HYPERTRIGLYCERIDEMIA.)

lipogenesis   The synthesis of fat in the body, chiefly by the LIVER and by ADIPOSE TISSUE (fat tissue). Lipogenesis occurs primarily after a high carbohydrate meal. Fat is formed from smaller building blocks, three FATTY ACIDS and GLYCEROL, an alcohol from glucose metabolism. The process requires ATP, the energy currency of the cell, and BIOTIN. The hormone INSULIN signals lipogenesis in fat tissue, which converts surplus calories to stored fats. Unlike adipose tissue, the liver cannot store fat and must package it in order to transport it to fat cells. To accomplish this task, the liver releases newly formed fat packaged as submicroscopic particles called VERY-LOW-DENSITY LIPOPROTEINS (VLDL) into the bloodstream. This represents emulsified fat, which can be distributed in blood. (See also ANABOLISM; CATABOLISM; FAT DIGESTION; FAT METABOLISM; LIPASE; LIPOLYSIS.)

"Lipogenesis in Diabetes and Obesity," *Nutrition Reviews*, 49:8 (1991), pp. 255–56.

lipoic acid (α-lipoic acid, thioctic acid) A sulfur-containing enzyme helper involved in CARBOHYDRATE degradation. The body synthesizes this fat-soluble COENZYME; consequently it is not classified as a dietary essential. Lipoic acid is not a VITAMIN, nor is it derived from a vitamin. Nonetheless, it plays a critical metabolic role. Lipoic acid functions in the oxidation of carbohydrate by the MITOCHONDRIA, subcellular particles devoted to energy production.

Key chemical transformations require lipoic acid: the oxidation of pyruvic acid (a small acid from GLUCOSE breakdown) to an activated form of ACETIC ACID called acetyl coenzyme A and the oxidation of alpha ketoglutaric acid, a product of the KREB'S CYCLE, which is the central energy-yielding pathway of the cell. CARBON DIOXIDE released in both oxidations represents a major portion of the carbon dioxide expired by the lungs as a metabolic waste product. To accomplish such oxidations, lipoic acid must work together with four vitamin-related coenzymes: thiamin pyrophosphate, derived from THIAMIN (vitamin B_1); FAD (FLAVIN ADENINE DINUCLEOTIDE), derived from RIBOFLAVIN (vitamin B_2); NAD (NICOTINAMIDE ADENINE DINUCLEOTIDE), derived from NIACIN (vitamin B_3); and COENZYME A, derived from PANTOTHENIC ACID (vitamin B_5). Lipoic acid is emerging as a versatile antioxidant. In the reduced form it is able to protect lipids from oxidation due to free radical attack and may protect vitamin E. It quenches superoxide and reactive oxygen compounds generated in the body during inflammation and it may play a role in regulating oxidation-reduction balance of cells. (See also CARBOHYDRATE METABOLISM.)

lipolysis The degradation of fat to its building blocks, FATTY ACIDS and GLYCEROL. In fats and oils, three long-chain fatty acids are normally attached to glycerol, an alcohol derived from glucose breakdown. Lipolysis occurs when stored fat is degraded in response to specific hormone signals that food is not supplying enough energy, or when a stress response is triggered: EPINEPHRINE (adrenaline) from adrenal glands, GLUCAGON from the islet tissue of the PANCREAS, and CORTISOL from the adrenal glands. Skipping meals, as well as exercise, long-term FASTING, surgery, physical trauma, STARVATION, low-calorie diets and ALCOHOLISM, favor lipolysis.

Fat is degraded by a family of enzymes called LIPASES. Epinephrine signals a hormone-sensitive lipase within adipose cells to attack stored fat and release free fatty acids and glycerol into the bloodstream. There, fatty acids bind to serum ALBUMIN, a major blood protein, for transport to tissues like muscles to be oxidized for energy production. Glycerol travels to the liver, where it is converted to BLOOD SUGAR. (See also FAT METABOLISM; GLUCONEOGENESIS; LIPOGENESIS.)

lipoprotein A submicroscopic particle composed of LIPIDS and proteins that transports lipids, water-insoluble materials, through the BLOOD and LYMPH. These fluids are essentially water, yet FAT, CHOLESTEROL and fat-soluble vitamins like VITAMIN A repel water. The problem is fundamental: Water and oils do not mix. To accomplish the difficult task of distributing lipids in water, cells package lipids as tiny droplets of PROTEIN and PHOSPHOLIPID called MICELLES for transport in the bloodstream.

There are four major classes of serum lipoproteins:

Chylomicrons Manufactured by the intestine to transport absorbed fat to tissues. The intestine releases chylomicrons to the lymph, which drains into the blood for general distribution. Chylomicrons carry a protein called apolipoprotein CII (Apo CII) that activates LIPASE, a fat-splitting enzyme located in CAPILLARIES. The released fatty acids are readily absorbed by fat cells and reincorporated into fat for storage; they are also taken up by muscle cells to be burned for energy.

VLDL (very-low-density lipoprotein) Produced by the liver to transport newly synthesized fat to ADIPOSE TISSUE for storage. VLDL deposits its fatty acids on fat cells as described for chylomicrons, above. VLDL remnants are processed to become a cholesterol carrier, LDL (LOW-DENSITY LIPOPROTEIN); surplus lipid and protein are removed and cholesterol is added. Excessive VLDL is indirectly linked to an increased risk of cardiovascular disease.

LDL (low-density lipoprotein) Transports cholesterol out of the liver to other tissues. It is derived from VLDL as described above. LDL contains a single protein called apolipoprotein B (ApoB). This protein is a recognition key that allows LDL to attach to specific docking sites (receptors) on cells. Once LDL binds to the cell surface, it is engulfed, and its cholesterol is deposited within the cell.

Excessive LDL-cholesterol appears to be linked to cardiovascular diseases through oxidation and free radical damage. When LDL-cholesterol becomes oxidized, it can deposit in arterial walls, a process that can eventually clog arteries. Therefore LDL is sometimes referred to as "bad" cholesterol.

HDL (high-density lipoprotein) Manufactured by the liver to scavenge cholesterol from tissues and carry it back to the liver for disposal. It is sometimes called "good" cholesterol because high levels correlate with a reduced risk of HEART DISEASE. A marker protein, apolipoprotein A (Apo A), characterizes this particle. Its name is derived from the fact that HDL is the most dense lipoprotein due to its high protein content. HDL is involved in the processing of other types of lipoprotein particles. It shuttles Apo CII from spent chylomicrons and spent VLDL to newly formed chylomicrons, and VLDL and HDL transfer cholesterol between different lipoproteins. (See also DIGESTION; FAT METABOLISM; PLAQUE.)

Ridker, P.M., Hennekens, C.H., Stampfer, M.J., "A Prospective Study of Lipoprotein(a) and the Risk of Myocardial Infarction," *Journal of the American Medical Association*, 270:18 (November 10, 1993), pp. 2195–2199.

liposuction (lipectomy) A surgical procedure that removes fatty tissue from the belly, thighs, chin and buttocks. It is one of the most popular forms of cosmetic surgery. Because it vacuums out tissue, liposuction is effective for small fatty areas, not large areas. The procedure can remove

1 to 2 pounds of FAT per area, but it cannot transform a fat person into a thin one. Liposuction works best if the patient is in good physical condition and has elastic skin.

Liposuction carries specific risks, including numbness, bruising, blood clots, infections, skin dents, discolorations and kidney problems, skin peeling and prolonged drainage from the wounded tissue. The long-term success rate is not known, nor is it known whether fat will eventually return to the treated area. Liposuction is neither a safe nor an effective weight control strategy; it does not substitute for eating right and for exercising, nor can it cure chronic weight problems. (See also DIETING; EXERCISE; OBESITY.)

lipotrope (lipotropic factor)   Nutrients that may help prevent fat accumulation in the liver. The most commonly studied are METHIONINE, an essential AMINO ACID containing sulfur; CHOLINE, a nitrogen-containing building block of the phospholipid LECITHIN; the B vitamins; FOLIC ACID and VITAMIN B$_{12}$; and INOSITOL, a complex alcohol related to GLUCOSE. Those nutrients promote the synthesis of phospholipids, building blocks of lipoproteins, to transport lipids out of the liver.

A change in liver metabolism during STARVATION can lead to fat deposition. Abnormal fat buildup occurs in the LIVER after damage by viral HEPATITIS, ALCOHOL, solvents, PESTICIDES, HERBICIDES, drugs, steroid hormones and even oral contraceptives. Over time, this leads to permanent liver scarring (CIRRHOSIS). Lipotropes have been shown to be effective in preventing fatty liver in experimental animals; however, they do not prevent fatty liver due to ALCOHOLISM. (See also FAT METABOLISM.)

liquid diets   DIETS that range from clear liquids to complete liquefied foods. Whatever their formulation, the use of liquid diets requires medical supervision.

Clear liquid diets entail only clear liquids such as carbonated beverages; COFFEE and coffee substitutes; flavored gelatins; strained fruit juices; fat-free broths of MEAT, FISH and POULTRY; BOUILLON; consomme and the like. They are used prior to intestinal surgery or X rays of the gastrointestinal tract; and for oral feeding of critically ill patients. They also help maintain FLUID BALANCE.

ELEMENTAL DIETS, also called semi-synthetic diets, are free of FIBER and contain easily absorbed, refined carbohydrates such as simple SUGARS; VEGETABLE OIL as a source of FAT; AMINO ACIDS supplied as purified powders or as hydrolyzed CASEIN (milk protein) or hydrolyzed ALBUMIN (egg protein); and purified MINERALS and VITAMINS. Elemental diets aid DIGESTION and minimize food residues in the colon. They are used prior to surgery of the GASTROINTESTINAL TRACT, and in cases of intestinal disease, severe malnourishment and critical illnesses.

Full liquid diets provide liquefied foods, including meat, fish, MILK and strained cottage cheese; custard and pudding rather than whole EGGS; as well as strained vegetables, strained juices and pureed fruits. Berries with small seeds are excluded, as are strongly flavored vegetables; dry cereals, bread, high fat, chunky soup stews, desserts (with nuts or other solid foods) and strongly flavored seasonings, condiments and spices. These diets are used for patients who cannot chew and/or swallow whole foods; as meal replacements when incorporated into a weight loss program; or as supplemental feeding programs. Liquid diets are usually deficient in certain nutrients; hence supplements may be recommended. They are deficient in fiber, for example.

INFANT FORMULAS are commercially produced and can replace breastfeeding of young infants. They are usually based on cow's milk or a milk substitute such as soy protein that contains added minerals, vitamins, vegetable oil and LACTOSE (milk sugar) to meet specific FDA requirements to assure adequate infant nutrition.

liquid protein diets   See DIETS: VERY LOW CALORIE.

listeriosis   An increasingly common form of FOOD POISONING. Listeriosis gained notoriety in 1985 as the cause of the U.S. outbreak of food poisoning from tainted Jalisco cheese. The culprit is the bacterium *Listeria monocytogenes*. Sources of contamination are usually raw milk cheeses. Many types of soft, ripened cheese like Brie have been recalled by the U.S. FDA in recent years. Besides dairy products, Listeria hides in raw meat, such as uncooked hot dogs. Perhaps as much as one-third of all meat is contaminated. Listeria may also occur in some pre-cooked meats and can contaminate SHELLFISH and even VEGETABLES. Normal cooking temperatures kill Listeria.

Symptoms are flu-like: fever, headache and DIARRHEA. Serious infections resemble blood poisoning. Encephalitis and meningitis can occur in susceptible people as a result of infection. Though most people are resistant to infection by Listeria, particularly sensitive are pregnant women and newborn infants, the elderly and those with a weakened immune system. Listeriosis can cause birth defects.

Listeria survives refrigeration, pasteurization and salt treatment in salt-cured meats. Therefore, consumers rely upon the U.S. FDA for protection with commercially prepared foods. For protection at home, wash all utensils, cutting boards and your hands after touching raw meat and poultry to avoid cross-contamination.

To minimize exposure, scrub raw vegetables well before eating them. Cook meat like HOT DOGS and CHICKEN thoroughly to kill this bacteria. (See also COOKING.)

Skinner, K.J., "Listeria. Battling Back Against One 'Tough Bug,' " *FDA Consumer*, 22 (July–August 1988), pp. 12–17.

lite   See FOOD LABELING.

lite salt   See SODIUM.

lithiasis   The formation of stones in the body. GALLSTONES and KIDNEY STONES are the most common examples. (See also CALCIUM.)

lithium   A nonessential mineral used in the treatment of pathologic manic states. Lithium is closely related to sodium and to potassium. Studies of animals maintained in controlled environments and on very restricted dietary lithium have revealed slowed growth and decreased reproduction. If there is a nutritional requirement for lithium, it seems likely to be easily satisfied by widespread occurrences of lithium in water and plant foods.

In therapeutic doses lithium is used to normalize mood swings in manic-depressive people, individuals with certain personality disorders and alcoholics. Lithium can also affect the THYROID GLAND. Overdose can cause DIARRHEA, nausea, vomiting, muscle weakness and, in extreme cases, convulsions and coma. Excessive lithium can block hormonal control of kidneys, leading to excessive water loss (DIABETES INSIPIDUS). Nonsteroidal and anti-inflammatory agents increase lithium toxicity. (See also MINERALS; TRACE MINERALS.)

liver The largest organ of the body and a metabolite that performs many physiologic processes. The adult liver weighs 3 to 5 pounds. Blood from the intestines carries nutrients absorbed after DIGESTION directly to the liver via the portal vein. Certain nutrients like fat-soluble vitamins and vitamin B12 are absorbed in the liver. Other nutrients are sent on to other parts of the body. Toxic materials are normally inactivated and then excreted.

The liver performs many vital functions:

Produces bile Bile contains BILE ACIDS, synthesized from CHOLESTEROL; they act as detergents to dissolve dietary FAT and facilitate fat digestion.

Maintains blood sugar The liver functions as a "glucostat" to maintain BLOOD SUGAR within a normal range. For example, it absorbs excess blood sugar (GLUCOSE) after a carbohydrate meal when blood sugar is high and converts it to a storage substance called GLYCOGEN. Conversely, the liver breaks down glycogen back to glucose when the blood sugar level drops too low. When the need for glucose is very high, as during fasting and crash dieting, the liver can manufacture it from non-carbohydrate substances, including most AMINO ACIDS, LACTIC ACID, PYRUVIC ACID and several acids derived from the central pathways for energy production from fat and carbohydrate oxidation (KREB'S CYCLE).

Synthesizes lipids The liver synthesizes cholesterol and fat from glucose under conditions of glucose excess. It forms particles, VLDL (VERY-LOW DENSITY LIPOPROTEIN) and HDL (HIGH-DENSITY LIPOPROTEIN) and, indirectly, LDL (LOW-DENSITY LIPOPROTEIN), which permit transporting these LIPIDS in the bloodstream.

Detoxifies products of metabolism, as well as many foreign substances The liver converts toxic AMMONIA, a by-product of protein (amino acid) breakdown, to the safe, excretable end product, UREA. Steroid hormones are often oxidized and attached to sulfate to increase their water solubility and thus may facilitate excretion. Some by-products are excreted in bile; the BILE PIGMENT, biliburin, is an example. Poisons, environmental pollutants and medications such as birth control drugs can be oxidized or degraded by Phase I enzymes, including CYTOCHROME P450 enzymes. A second set of enzymes called transferases (Phase II enzymes) attach amino acids (GLYCINE, TAURINE), sugar derivatives (glucuronic acid) or other, highly water-soluble compounds like glutathione to further increase the water solubility of the modified toxins and ease their excretion by the kidneys and bile.

Synthesizes blood plasma proteins The liver synthesizes most of the soluble proteins that occur with blood: serum ALBUMIN, the major soluble protein of blood; blood-clotting factors; transport proteins, such as TRANSFERRIN (used for iron transport); in addition VLDL, HDL and LDL mentioned above.

Oxidizes alcohol The liver is the major site for disposing of ALCOHOL. The enzymes are called ethanol oxidizing systems.

Activates vitamins The liver converts BETA CAROTENE, the precursor of vitamin A that occurs in plants, to VITAMIN A as needed.

Stores many essential nutrients The liver stores fat-soluble nutrients like VITAMIN A, VITAMIN D and VITAMIN K, as well as non-lipid nutrients like IRON and VITAMIN B12.

Plays a role in the disposal of aged red blood cells While the liver serves as a major "garbage disposal unit" of the body, the risk of liver damage increases with excessive exposure to PESTICIDES, alcohol, hydrocarbons, toxic heavy metals like LEAD and MERCURY, solvents like carbon tetrachloride, spray paints and degreasers. Liver diseases such as hepatitis (liver inflammation) and CIRRHOSIS (liver scarring) can profoundly affect metabolic processes.

Calf liver is an excellent source of B complex vitamins, including vitamin B12, vitamin B6, folic acid and riboflavin; trace minerals like iron and zinc, and vitamin A. It contains little calcium like most meat; the cholesterol content is high. Fried beef liver (3 oz, 85 g) provides 185 calories; protein, 23 g; carbohydrate, 7 g; fat, 7 g; cholesterol, 410 mg; calcium, 9 mg; iron, 5.3 mg; vitamin A, 9,120 retinol equivalents; thiamin, 0.18 mg; riboflavin, 3.52 mg; niacin, 12.3 mg. (See also CARBOHYDRATE METABOLISM; DETOXIFICATION; GLUCONEOGENESIS; HOMEOSTASIS.)

liver cirrhosis See CIRRHOSIS.

lobster (*Homarus*) A crustacean belonging to the same family as crabs and shrimp. Crustaceans have rigid exoskeletons or shells with jointed bodies and legs. Lobsters are the largest shellfish. The European lobster is found off the coast of Norway and Britain. Its color is violet blue and green. The Northern lobster is found in coastal waters of the east coast of Canada and the United States. Most lobster is harvested in the summer and fall in Canada, Massachusetts and Maine.

The average lobster is a foot long (30 cm) and weighs up to 3 pounds (450–1,250 g). Its claws and tail are full of meat. Its abdomen is in seven sections; it terminates in a fan-shaped tail that is also full of meat. Spring (rock) lobsters come from the Southeastern United States and Pacific waters. These lack the large pincer claw of the Northern species, and most of the meat is in the tail. Cooked lobster tails are usually imported from Australia, New Zealand and South Africa. A live lobster can be identified by a reflex action of the eyes as opposed to a dead animal. Lobsters can be killed humanely by placing them below −10° C for two hours; they can then be plunged into boiling water. When cooked, lobster turns red. They should be cooked to 165°. The small legs should pull off easily. There are many lobster dishes: Newburg, Thermidor, grilled and roasted lobster. Souffles and mousses are also popular.

Shellfish generally are low in calories and in both total fat and saturated fat. A 3-oz (85 g) serving of lobster provides 77 calories; protein, 16 g; fat, 0.76 g; calcium, 26 g; sodium, 272 mg; cholesterol, 81 mg; thiamin, 0.37 mg; riboflavin, 0.04 mg; niacin, 1.23 mg. (See also SEAFOOD.)

locust bean gum (carob bean gum)   A GUM obtained from the bean of the carob tree. Produced in Greece, Italy, Portugal and Spain, carob bean gum is used as a thickening agent and texturizer for ICE CREAM, salad dressing, pie filling and barbecue sauce. When added to dough, it makes baked goods like cakes retain their shape. It improves the consistency and palatability of gels and other thickeners (CARAGEENAN). In large amounts, locust bean gum acts as a mild LAXATIVE. Locust bean gum is considered a safe FOOD ADDITIVE.

lopid   See CHOLESTEROL-LOWERING DRUGS.

lovage (*Levisticum officinale*)   A perennial aromatic HERB related to PARSLEY and CELERY. Lovage originated in Persia. It grows to a height of 5 to 7 feet; its leaves resemble celery and the greens have a celery-like flavor. Leaves and seeds can flavor many types of dishes, such as meats, salads and soups. The dried root is sometimes used as a condiment. Lovage seeds are used as a flavoring in candy manufacturing. (See also SPICE.)

low-density lipoprotein (LDL)   The lipid-protein particle that transports CHOLESTEROL from the LIVER to other tissues via the bloodstream. LDL carries 60 to 80% of the cholesterol found in serum (the clear fluid remaining after blood has clotted and blood cells are removed). LDL consists of an envelope of PHOSPHOLIPID, a fat-like substance that acts like a detergent to surround and dissolve oily cholesterol droplets. LDL is absorbed by muscle and fat cells, where it is captured by specific docking sites on cell surfaces. A unique protein called apolipoprotein B on the LDL provides a recognition site or "zip code" for docking sites on target cells. Once absorbed by cells, LDL is destroyed and its cholesterol is either incorporated in cell membranes or is stored. Interference with LDL uptake causes blood cholesterol levels to rise, increasing the risk of ATHEROSCLEROSIS.

Elevated LDL is considered to be an approximate or rough index of cardiovascular risk among U.S. men. Because elevated LDL is believed to increase the risk of heart disease, LDL has often been called "bad" or "undesirable" cholesterol. Even borderline-high LDL cholesterol levels (130 to 159 mg per 100 ml [dl] of serum) have been linked to an increased risk of clogged arteries and of heart attacks among American men. Accordingly, a target level for LDL-cholesterol is less than 130 mg/dL; for people with heart disease, the levels of cholesterol-LDL should be 100 mg/dL or less.

A second important form of blood cholesterol is called HDL (HIGH-DENSITY LIPOPROTEIN). HDL can be thought of as a scavenger, transporting cholesterol from tissues like muscle back to the liver for disposal. Both LDL cholesterol and HDL cholesterol can be measured by routine lab tests. In general, a lowered LDL and an elevated HDL are desirable. HDL cholesterol should be greater than 35, for men (or 50 for women) and values greater than 65 can protect against diseased arteries. More accurate assessments of cardiovascular risk are based on measurements of LDL and HDL and LDL/HDL ratio. The most specific way of assessing LDL/HDL ratios relies on laboratory tests that measure apolipoprotein B (Apo B), the marker substance for LDL, and apolipoprotein A (Apo A), the specific protein marker for HDL.

The level of LDL-cholesterol and the associated risk of heart disease depend upon many factors including inheritance, the amount of fat in the diet and how a person chooses to live. Factors that raise LDL (and lower HDL) levels include: a high saturated fat diet; cigarette smoking; a lack of exercise; obesity; excessive alcohol consumption; and a family history of high blood cholesterol. Factors that lower LDL include: regular aerobic exercise; POLYUNSATURATED OILS and MONOUNSATURATED OILS substituted for saturated fat in the diet; adequate fiber in the diet, including soluble FIBER such as PECTIN and oat BRAN; and weight management and stress management.

Oxidized LDL represents a dangerous form of cholesterol and it is the most active blood lipid in promoting atherosclerosis. Oxidized LDL is present in clogged arteries as deposits called PLAQUE. Macrophages, scavenger cells in artery walls, may oxidize excessive LDL, or they may selectively take up oxidized LDL to become cholesterol-filled "foam" cells in arteries. Foam cells seem to set the stage for plaque buildup. Other lines of evidence support this hypothesis. Antibodies against oxidized LDL appear in patients with advanced atherosclerosis. Oxidized LDL attracts more cells (monocytes) from the blood to enter the artery wall and become resident macrophages. Furthermore, oxidized LDL helps immobilize those macrophages, thus trapping them inside arteries. Oxidized LDL can itself damage cells and possibly injure arterial walls. It is thought that the resulting damage to the arterial lining causes the release of growth factors that stimulate the migration and growth of muscle cells at the damaged area in the arterial wall. These processes may continue over years, leading eventually to plaque buildup, narrowed arteries and, ultimately, to blocked arteries and heart attack or stroke.

The exact mechanisms by which LDL is oxidized and a definition of the details of plaque formation are being actively investigated. It is known that oxidative damage in the body occurs by FREE RADICALS and other reactive forms of oxygen. These highly reactive molecules readily attack sensitive molecules in the cell, such as DNA, lipids and protein. Antioxidant drugs can inhibit atherosclerosis in lab animals with elevated blood cholesterol levels that are susceptible to this disease. A growing body of evidence links the protective effects of antioxidant nutrients such as VITAMIN E, vitamin C, beta carotene and carotenoids, selenium and zinc to decreased lipid oxidation and lowered risk of CARDIOVASCULAR DISEASE. (See also HYPERCHOLESTEROLEMIA; LIPOPROTEINS.)

Jailal, I. and Grundy, S.M., "Effect of Combined Supplementation with Alpha Tocopherol, Ascorbate and Beta Carotene on Low-density Lipoprotein Oxidation," *Circulation*, 88:6 (1993), pp. 2760–86.

Steinberg, Daniel and Witztum, Joseph L., "Lipoproteins and Atherogenesis," *Journal of the American Medical Association*, 264:23 (December 19, 1990), pp. 3047–52.

low-fat cheese   See CHEESE.

low-fat diets   Diets that drastically reduce the consumption of fats, oils and fatty foods. The unmodified PRITIKIN DIET limits fat intake to approximately 10% of total calories, while the MACROBIOTIC DIET, based on grains, vegetables, legumes and condiments, also entails a similar low-fat intake. A life-style change program has been developed for patients with heart disease that offers an alternative to bypass surgery to stop the progression of the disease. The program involves a vegetarian diet providing 10% fat, together with moderate exercise, stress management and group support.

Ultra-low-fat diets are more difficult to follow than other diets because fats and oils satisfy hunger both by slowing the emptying of the stomach after a meal and by providing pleasing flavors ("mouth feel"). People generally are more successful in reducing their fat calories to 20% than any lower. Heredity may determine how people will respond to low-fat diets. Those who inherit small, dense versions of LDL ("bad CHOLESTEROL") and who also have low levels of HDL ("good cholesterol") may respond better to low-fat diets. Sharply reducing saturated fat intake may cause a drop in HDL. This can be minimized by losing excess weight or by regular aerobic exercise.

Current federal guidelines and the American Heart Association recommend lowering fat intake to less than 30% of calories because excessive fat is linked to heart disease, cancer and obesity. Other experts are recommending reduction to 20 or 25% of calories to obtain a greater benefit and decreased risk. (See also HEART DISEASE; FAT METABOLISM.)

luncheon meats (cold cuts)   Highly processed meat typically served for sandwiches and hors d'oeuvres. Luncheon meats are prepackaged and pre-sliced. BOLOGNA and salami are typical examples. Characteristically, luncheon meats contain significant FAT, saturated fat, SALT and NITRITE. Nutrition information on the food label is based upon the size of the slice. As with any food listing ingredients by the serving size, multiply the nutrient content per serving (provided by the food label) by the number of servings you actually eat to determine calories, fat and so on.

Beef and pork luncheon meats are often highest in calories and fat. However, turkey salami, turkey bologna and chicken may contain as many calories as cold cuts made from beef or pork, due to fat, for example, from added skin. Most luncheon meats provide about 20 mg of cholesterol per slice. Sodium nitrite is used to cure meats and to preserve their color. The sodium content can range from a low of 80 mg to a high of 400 mg of sodium per slice. DIETARY GUIDELINES FOR AMERICANS recommends choosing a diet low in fat, sodium and cholesterol. Fat should be less than 30% of calories.

To reduce sodium and fat consumption when eating luncheon meats, try turkey breast, turkey ham and chicken breast as reasonable alternatives to any bologna, meat loaf or salami, which are high-fat fare. In contrast, skinless turkey or chicken breast is considered lean meat. Substitute mustard and onions for mayonnaise in sandwiches. Pickles and olives increase sodium substantially. Adding vegetables like sprouts, cucumbers, lettuce and tomatoes increases the fiber content considerably. (See also FOOD PROCESSING.)

Lupus erythematosus (systemic lupus erythematosus, SLE)   An inflammatory disease in which defense proteins of the IMMUNE SYSTEM (ANTIBODIES) form complexes with tissue proteins, leading to tissue damage. A disease in which the body attacks itself is classified as an AUTOIMMUNE DISEASE. Lupus symptoms include a red facial rash, intermittent fever, severe joint pain and bouts of extreme fatigue. The disease may affect different regions of the body, including the skin, the joints, the heart and blood vessels, the lungs, the brain and the kidneys. Women are ten times more prone than men; lupus affects two U.S. women per thousand. This serious disease is sometimes fatal. Common signs and symptoms include fever, arthritis damage to the nervous system, weight loss, sensitivity to light and possibly heart disease and kidney failure. A lab test (ANA, antinuclear antibody tests) is used to monitor SLE.

Early intervention can control lupus and reduce the risk of irreversible kidney damage. Standard treatment involves the use of drugs (corticosteroids) and immune suppressants to limit INFLAMMATION. Lupus is associated with low stomach acid production (HYPOCHLORHYDRIA). Food allergies may be correlated with the incidence of SLE and should be checked. The relationship between SLE and candida yeast overgrowth remains controversial. Two steroid hormones, DHEA and testosterone, may help normalize immune function and they have been used to treat autoimmune disease. Gotu kola (*Centilla asiatica*), a medicinal herb long used in China and India, has been reported to alleviate lupus. Vitamin B_6 sometimes relieves symptoms. FISH OILS may play a role in treating a variety of autoimmune diseases, including lupus; possible benefits of fish oil for lupus are derived from animal studies and anecdotal reports. Omega-6 fatty acids, as found in black current, borage and evening primrose oils can help out immune disorders. (See also MAST CELL.)

Mills, John A., "Systemic Lupus Erythematosus," *New England Journal of Medicine*, 330:26 (1994), pp. 1871–77.

lycopene   The principal pigment responsible for the color of TOMATOES, PAPRIKA and pink GRAPEFRUIT. Structurally, this red plant pigment resembles BETA CAROTENE and belongs to the carotene family of yellow-orange plant pigments (carotenoids). Unlike beta carotene, however, lycopene lacks VITAMIN A activity; the body cannot transform it to the vitamin. Lycopene is prevalent in the testes and in the plasma, where it occurs at a greater concentration than beta carotene. Consuming foods rich in carotenoids can lower the risk of colon and bladder cancer and reduce tumor growth in mice. Lycopene and related carotenoids can function as antioxidants to quench free radicals. These highly reactive molecules are generated in the body and can damage tissues and promote aging and disease. Carotenoids complement the antioxidant activity of beta carotene, and together they help reduce inflammation, maintain healthy cell membranes and modulate the synthesis of families of prostaglandins and leukotrienes, fatty acid derivatives that stimulate inflammation. (See also CAROTENOIDS.)

lymph   The protein-rich fluid that escapes from blood vessels (capillaries) and flows between cells. Lymph has a composition resembling blood PLASMA, the fluid remaining after blood has clotted. While lymph contains ELECTROLYTES (dissolved minerals), GLUCOSE and other nutrients and certain proteins from blood, it also contains fat from digestion when it drains the intestinal tract. Lymph flows into lymphatic ducts leading to major ducts (the thoracic duct and the right lymphatic duct) that drain into large blood veins above the heart.

lymphatic system (lymph system)   A system of vessels and organs that helps defend against infection. The lymph system consists of lymphatic vessels, narrow tubes that transport a watery colorless fluid through tissues to the bloodstream. Unlike the CIRCULATORY SYSTEM (the heart and blood vessels), the lymphatic system is not a "closed loop" because it is a network of one-way roads, consisting of increasingly larger ducts (channels) and ultimately draining into the bloodstream. Diffuse lymphatic tissue and lymph nodules occur in the tissue lining passageways of the body, especially the gastrointestinal tract.

The lymphatic system can be considered a specialized connective tissue that contains defensive cells of the IMMUNE SYSTEM. Cells in lymphatic tissue, lymphocytes, help protect the body against foreign cells and cancer cells. Lymph nodes are checkpoints along the lymphatic highway; they filter the lymph and destroy foreign materials and microorganisms. The infection-fighting cells are called lymphocytes. Certain nodules such as tonsils, Peyers patches in the ileum of the small intestine, and nodules in the appendix consist of large aggregates of lymphatic tissue. (See also ALLERGY, FOOD.)

lymphocyte   See IMMUNE SYSTEM.

lymphokines (cytokines)   A large family of specialized proteins that regulate the immune system. Lymphokines are chemical signals mainly produced by T cells, white blood cells that help regulate the immune response, especially to combat infection by viruses, fungus, parasites and certain cancers. Lymphokines activate antibody-producing cells (B cells). Certain lymphokines called interleukins act as growth promoters to stimulate the growth of T cells, while others destroy targeted diseased cells (tumor necrosis factor) or they can activate macrophages. Another type of lymphokine called interferon acts as a defensive protein to inhibit the production of viruses.

Lymphokines can direct lymphocytes, sensitized to a foreign invader, to destroy invading agents according to the following scenario. In the first stage, defensive cells called macrophages engulf foreigners and in turn release a lymphokine called interleukin-1, when they meet a foreign substance (ANTIGEN). If the antigen is a food, interleukin-1 may help trigger a food allergy. Interleukin-1 then stimulates T cell production. In the next stage, activated T cells release a second lymphokine, interleukin-2, which further stimulates T-cell formation and the production of cytotoxic T cells, specialized in destroying invaders. (See also ALLERGY, FOOD; AUTOIMMUNE DISEASE; INFLAMMATION.)

lysine (Lys, L-lysine)   A dietary essential AMINO ACID and a required building block of proteins. Lysine cannot be fabricated in the body and must be supplied by the diet. It is the only essential amino acid with two amino groups (nitrogen bearing groups). It is positively charged in body fluids and is classified as a basic amino acid because it can function chemically as an alkaline substance.

Sources of lysine (high lysine/arginine content) include red meat, fish, poultry, eggs, peanuts, soybeans, milk, brewer's yeast and potatoes. Of the various essential amino acids in grain proteins, lysine is usually present in limited amounts; consequently, plant breeding programs have developed high lysine strains of BARLEY, SORGHUM and CORN. Food processing and baking at high temperatures tend to destroy lysine because during extensive heating or prolonged storage lysine in cereal protein reacts with carbohydrate, yielding an inactive complex. About a third of the lysine in dry breakfast cereals is unusable by the body for this reason. The adult daily requirement is 12 mg per kilogram of body weight per day.

Some evidence suggests that lysine supplements lessen outbreaks of herpes virus infection and diminish related symptoms, especially when supplemented with VITAMIN B_6 and MAGNESIUM. It may be beneficial to restrict consumption of ARGININE, another basic amino acid required for protein synthesis that may be a dietary essential in serious disease states and liver damage. Excessive lysine supplements may antagonize arginine. (See also AMINO ACID METABOLISM.)

lysosome   A small particle, found in the cytoplasm of many types of cells, that is responsible for degrading cellular debris. Lysosomes contain powerful degradative enzymes to completely break down proteins, as well as bacteria that are engulfed by cells. Lysosomes also recycle components of worn-out organelles and cellular structures so that amino acids, cholesterol and fatty acids can be reused. A typical LIVER cell can recycle about half of its contents per week. LDL (LOW-DENSITY LIPOPROTEIN), the cholesterol transport particle in the blood, is absorbed by muscle and fat tissue and degraded by their lysosomes. This is the way cholesterol is deposited within cells.

Normally, lysosomal enzymes are confined within lysosomes to prevent indiscriminate DIGESTION of the cell. However, during tissue repair, lysosomal enzymes released from damaged cells help digest any cellular debris and prepare the area for repair and wound healing.

macaroni   A form of PASTA in which pieces of wheat dough are formed into various shapes and dried. Macaroni may be strands (like spaghetti), shells (conchiglie) or tubes (cannelloni; elbow macaroni), among others, and it can be bent, corrugated, straight or take the form of spirals. Macaroni is composed of flour from durum wheat (a "hard wheat" rich in protein), farina (a coarsely ground endosperm of other wheats) and SEMOLINA, the coarsely milled, starchy endosperm of durum wheat after bran and germ have been removed. Semolina, farina and durum wheat flour can be used in any combination or they can be used separately. Semolina is high in protein, which gives dough the strength to hold up to the mechanical processing needed to make pasta. A small amount of disodium phosphate is added to make pasta cook more quickly. Products marked "enriched" must contain specific amounts of certain vitamins and minerals: 4 to 5 mg of THIAMIN; 1.7 to 2.2 mg of RIBOFLAVIN; 27 to 34 mg of NIACIN; and 13 to 16.5 mg of IRON per pound. Eggs may be an optional ingredient for macaroni. Other pasta variations include whole wheat, beet, spinach, and soy macaroni products. (See also BREAD; COMPLEX CARBOHYDRATE.)

mackerel (*Scomber scombrus*)   A saltwater predatory fish related to tuna, with a very streamlined body. This important food fish is typically 14 in (35 cm) in length. The Atlantic mackerel ranges from Labrador to Cape Hatteras. The king mackerel, *Scomber omovus cuvalia*, is found in coastal waters from the Carolinas to Brazil. Mackerel is an oily fish and represents one of the richest sources of marine oils, EICOSAPENTAENOIC ACID and other omega-3 fatty acids. These fatty acids lower blood lipids and may reduce the risk of ATHEROSCLEROSIS, and they help reduce symptoms of autoimmune diseases like RHEUMATOID ARTHRITIS. By decreasing the tendency of blood clot formation, they lower the risk of STROKE and HEART ATTACK. The outer layers of mackerel meat are red; the interior layers are lighter in color. Most commercial mackerel is canned. Fresh mackerel is very perishable. The nutrient content of 3 oz (85 g) provides 174 calories; protein, 15.8 g; fat, 11.8 g; cholesterol, 60 mg; calcium, 10 mg; thiamin, 0.15 mg; riboflavin, 0.265 mg; niacin, 7.72 mg. (See also OMEGA-3 FATTY ACIDS; SALMON; SEAFOOD.)

macrobiotic diet   A DIET emphasizing plant foods and complex carbohydrates (STARCH and FIBER). The macrobiotic diet was introduced by George Ohsawa in the 1960s in California and it continues to be a popular diet. The macrobiotic diet encompasses more than foods; the belief that DIGESTION and assimilation are aided by eating slowly in a peaceful, harmonious atmosphere is fundamental. In its earliest form as put forth by advocates, the macrobiotic diet was an imbalanced diet emphasizing RICE and GRAINS. Brown rice was considered an optimal balance of "yin" and "yang" forces. The rigorous application of macrobiotic principles frequently caused MALNUTRITION, with ANEMIA, slowed growth, RICKETS, even kidney damage, especially in children. The modified macrobiotic diet used today, which can vary with personal needs, is wholesome and tasty and includes locally produced foods and whole grains. Animal products are used as condiments, rather than as main dishes. The diet varies with the climate and season, to minimize use of chemical preservation and unnecessary food processing. Meals consist of 50 to 60% whole grains. The macrobiotic diet supplies about 73% of total carbohydrate; only 15 to 20% of the CALORIES are fats and oils (from whole grains and vegetable oils). Brown rice, MILLET, OATS, RYE, BUCKWHEAT, cous cous, whole WHEAT, LEGUMES, VEGETABLES, FRUITS, NUTS and seeds complete the foundation. Legumes supply 5 to 10% of calories in the form of adzuki, lima, kidney, navy, mung, pinto and soy beans. Bean sprouts are useful adjuncts. Sea vegetables like arame, hijiki, kombu, nori and wakame provide texture, flavor and essential nutrients. Seafood and poultry are incorporated according to dietary goals or preferences. (See also HIGH COMPLEX CARBOHYDRATE DIET; VEGETARIAN.)

Schneede, J., et al., "Methylmalonic Acid and Homocysteine in Plasma as Indicators of Functional Cobalamin Deficiency in Infants on Macrobiotic Diets," *Pediatric Research*, 36:2 (1994), pp. 194–202.

macronutrient Nutrients required by the DIET in amounts ranging from a fraction of a gram to more than a gram. The major minerals, CALCIUM, MAGNESIUM, SODIUM, POTASSIUM, CHLORIDE and PHOSPHORUS are considered macronutrients. These balance body fluids and build bones and teeth. CARBOHYDRATE, FAT, OIL and PROTEIN, together with WATER, are considered other macronutrients. Together they make up the bulk of food. Fat and carbohydrate must be eaten in large amounts daily because they provide the fuel that keeps the body's machinery operating. Proteins supply building blocks to replace worn out and damaged proteins. The recommended distribution of calories looks like this: For an adult requiring 2,000 calories daily, less than 600 calories (less than 30% of the total) should come from fat (67 grams or 4 tablespoons). How much less than 30% is debatable. Fifty grams of protein (1.75 oz) supplies 200 calories (20% of the total). The remaining 1,200 calories (60%) would come from carbohydrates, preferably COMPLEX CARBOHYDRATES as found in whole grains, LEGUMES and VEGETABLES (roughly 300 g or two-thirds of a pound).

Fat is a concentrated form of ENERGY because it provides more than twice as many calories per gram as do carbohydrate or protein. The typical American diet provides about 40% of total calories as fat. Fifteen to 25% of calories as fat and oils may be more appropriate to reduce the risk of CANCER, HEART DISEASE and OBESITY. Current dietary guidelines recommend choosing a diet reduced in total fat, saturated fat and cholesterol, with oils and fats to be used sparingly.

For the average American, carbohydrate supplies about 40 to 45% of the total calories, with sweeteners like SUCROSE, FRUCTOSE and CORN SYRUP representing about half of this (about 130 to 150 pounds per year per person.) U.S. dietary goals publicized in the 1970s called for cutting SUGAR consumption by two-thirds while doubling STARCH intake with whole vegetables and grains. Current guidelines are less specific. They call for eating ample amounts of vegetables, fruit and grain products daily: with six to eleven servings of bread and grain products; three to five servings of vegetables; and two to four servings of fruits with sweets to be used sparingly.

Food supplies amino acids for building the thousands of proteins of the body. An adult needs to eat only 40 to 50 grams of protein a day, though the typical diet supplies twice this amount. The body treats surplus amino acids as excess fuel: They are either converted to fat or they are burned for energy.

Drinking the equivalent of two quarts of water each day replaces water lost due to waste disposal, urine and feces, and to perspiration. Water is essential as a coolant and as the fluid of cells and tissues needed for their normal operation. (See also DIETARY GUIDELINES FOR AMERICANS; ELECTROLYTES.)

macrophage See IMMUNE SYSTEM.

macular degeneration (age-related macular degeneration [AMD]) A progressive impairment of the macula, a cluster of cells at the center of the retina responsible for central vision. Exudative AMD is caused by scarring and hemorrhaging of the macula, which is the most harmful form of AMD. This disease is the leading cause of irreversible blindness in the United States. Approximately one quarter of people aged 65 or older have AMD; so far there is no cure. The cause of AMD is not certain, though recent evidence implicates oxidation and free-radical damage. Older men and women with exudative AMD who consumed most dark green leafy vegetables were 43% less likely to develop AMD, compared to those who ate the least amounts of those vegetables and CAROTENOIDS, a group of red, orange and yellow plant pigments that includes BETA CAROTENE. Primarily two pigments, lutein and zeaxanthin, accounted for this reduction in risk of advanced AMD. It is possible that these carotenoids protect the retina by filtering out damaging light, and they may act as free radical scavengers. Spinach and chard are good sources of zeaxanthin and lutein. Data from the Baltimore Longitudinal Study of Aging suggests that VITAMIN E helps lower the risk of AMD. These studies have not determined the appropriate level of a given ANTIOXIDANT in protecting against AMD, nor have they indicated the optimal duration of consumption. Animal studies have suggested that VITAMIN C can protect the retina against oxidative damage. While excessive copper may damage the retina, ZINC is an essential nutrient for the retina, and supplementation may benefit patients with inadequate dietary zinc. GINKGO BILOBA can help normalize circulation in the retina. (See also CATARACT.)

mad cow disease (bovine spongiform encephalopathy, BSE) A fatal brain disease in cattle. BSE was first diagnosed in Britain in 1986. After an incubation period of three to five years with normal behavior, BSE-infected cattle begin to stagger and become aggressive. The brains of such animals at autopsy look spongy and under the microscope nerve cells reveal protein fiber buildup. BSE is a member of a group of brain disorders characterized by chronic wasting that seem to be caused by a rogue protein or prion, a self-replicating protein. A slow virus could be involved. Prions appear to multiply in the brain, spinal cord, spleen and thymus; they do not trigger an immune response in host animals.

The cause of the bovine epidemic begins with the fact that a related disease, scrapie, infects sheep in Britain. Sheep carcasses were processed for animal feed as a protein supplement. Apparently the diet can transmit the infection from sheep to cows. Since the discovery of BSE, the practice of feeding rendered sheep to cattle has ceased and infected cattle have been destroyed. BSE does not seem communicable among calves of afflicted cows and the epidemic has declined.

The possibility that the infection can be transmitted to other species raised the concern that beef or milk products from infected animals could transmit the disease to humans. In 1996 a possible link between BSE and a new variant of a very rare human disease, Creutzfeldt-Jakob disease, was reported in Britain. Most cases of Creutzfeldt-Jakob disease appear to be randomly distributed with an annual incidence of one person in a million. Tracing the disease has been difficult because the incubation period may last between 5 and 30 years. The prions are very resistant to heat treatment and resist cooking temperatures, and they resist degradation by digestive enzymes. Therefore it is possible that prions ingested in food could be absorbed.

No ruminants and ruminant products have been imported into the U.S. from countries known to have BSE and mad cow disease has not been detected here. The World Health Organization has recommended that all countries ban the use of ruminant tissues in ruminant feed. A voluntary ban was instituted in this country in 1996. A variety of marketed drugs are derived from cattle tissue and many contain fractions of cows blood. Gelatin is believed safe due to processing. (See also EPIDEMIOLOGY.)

magnesium A major mineral nutrient. The body contains 20 to 28 g of magnesium; 40% is found in tissues like MUSCLE and 60% occurs in BONE and teeth, where it is combined with phosphate. Among soft tissues the liver and muscles contain the highest levels. Within cells magnesium is the second most prevalent type of positively charged ion (cation) after potassium. Magnesium is required for all major metabolic processes involving ATP, the chemical energy currency of the cell. More than 300 enzymes are activated by magnesium and magnesium-ATP complexes. It functions in energy-consuming processes like biosynthesis of protein and of DNA and RNA; sugar breakdown (GYLCOLYSIS); and ATP-dependent transport of materials into the cell. Magnesium is essential for the transmission of nerve impulses; for electrical potentials of cell membranes; muscle contraction; ATP formation; and maintenance of blood vessels.

Possible Roles in Maintaining Health

Magnesium is essential for normal calcium metabolism. In muscle contraction, magnesium balances the effects of calcium, which stimulates contraction. Thus magnesium regulates calcium uptake by cells to activate functions like heartbeat. Magnesium may also:

- protect against CARDIOVASCULAR DISEASE. It can help reduce high BLOOD PRESSURE, lower CHOLESTEROL as LOW-DENSITY LIPOPROTEIN (LDL) and increase HDL (HIGH-DENSITY LIPOPROTEIN) cholesterol;
- protect against lead poisoning;
- protect against migraine and DEPRESSION;
- help maintain normal heart function and prevent irregular heartbeat (cardiac dysrhythmia). The imbalance between calcium and magnesium may increase the risk of cardiovascular disease, and magnesium deficiency increases the risk of severe disruptions of cardiac rhythm;

- help alleviate PREMENSTRUAL SYNDROME, when used with ZINC and VITAMIN B_6 in certain cases;
- prevent KIDNEY STONES;
- alleviate preeclampsia and ECLAMPSIA, a syndrome in pregnancy characterized by high blood pressure and protein in the urine. In serious cases eclampsia can lead to convulsions and coma.

Sources

Magnesium is found in MEAT (especially liver); POULTRY; FISH and SEAFOOD; green vegetables like BROCCOLI; dairy products; hard water; TOFU; AMARANTH; wheat germ; pumpkin seeds; instant coffee; PEANUTS, CASHEWS, BRAZIL NUTS; BREAKFAST CEREALS; cocoa powder; BLACKSTRAP MOLASSES; and YEAST. Magnesium is lost during FOOD PROCESSING.

Requirements

The adult Recommended Dietary Allowance (RDA) for magnesium is 350 mg per day for men and 280 mg for women. The typical American diet provides about 120 mg per 1,000 calories. Thus a person consuming 1,500 calories or less is likely to be magnesium deficient. Factors that increase the need for magnesium due to limited uptake or increased losses include high dietary FIBER; too much phosphate (as soft drinks) and alcoholic beverages; high psychological stress; some DIURETICS (water pills) and regular, strenuous EXERCISE. Excessive calcium in supplements may compete with magnesium. Disease and conditions that cause magnesium depletion include MALABSORPTION, MALNUTRITION, ALCOHOLISM and intravenous feeding using nutrient mixtures that do not contain enough magnesium. Marginal deficiency is very common among teenagers and people who diet; diabetics; pregnant and lactating women; those who drink heavily; elderly persons with poor eating habits; those taking diuretics and digitalis; athletes; women with osteoporosis; and individuals with severe kidney disease and severe DIARRHEA.

Early symptoms of magnesium deficiency, including a loss of appetite, upset stomach and diarrhea, are vague, making diagnosis of a mild deficiency difficult. Symptoms of long-term deficiency relate to the nervous system: confusion, apathy, depression, irritability, irregular heartbeat, muscle weakness, tremors, convulsions and poor coordination, as well as a lack of APPETITE, listlessness, nausea and vomiting. Measurement of white blood cell magnesium can be used to help assess the nutritional status of this mineral.

Safety

Excessive use of the home remedies Epsom salts and milk of magnesia leads to deficiencies of other minerals, even toxicity. Overdose with magnesium antacids (1,500 mg or more daily) is indicated by low blood pressure, drowsiness, nausea, slurred speech and unsteadiness. Magnesium toxicity can occur when the kidneys cannot clear large overloads. While magnesium appears to be safe, it should not be taken by patients with kidney disease or by those with heart problems (atrioventricular blocks). A physician should be consulted prior to using supplements. (See also TRACE MINERALS.)

Altura, Burton M., "Magnesium: Growing in Clinical Importance," *Patient Care* 28:1 (January 15, 1994), pp. 130–36.

malabsorption Symptoms related to long-term inadequate nutrient absorption. A person can eat a BALANCED DIET and still be malnourished if the intestine cannot absorb nutrients or if DIGESTION is incomplete. The most common nutritional deficiencies involve minerals like CALCIUM and IRON, and vitamins such as FOLIC ACID, VITAMIN B_6 or VITAMIN A.

Symptoms are varied, depending on the kind of nutrient that is deficient. Fatigue and lowered resistance to infection are common indicators. Vitamin and mineral deficiencies alter metabolism and lower immunity. Vitamin and iron deficiencies can cause ANEMIA, "tired blood." Chronic suboptimal calcium intake leads to OSTEOPOROSIS. B complex vitamin deficiency leads to a sore tongue.

Causes of Malabsorption Include the Following

- rapid transit time (diarrhea);
- inadequate chewing;
- inadequate digestion caused by low stomach acid production (HYPOCHLORHYDRIA). This is one of the consequences of aging.
- impaired absorption due to an unhealthy intestinal lining. Severe food allergies, sensitivities and inflammation (like CELIAC DISEASE and Crohn's disease) injure the absorptive surface of the intestine (MICROVILLI);
- inadequate intestinal digestive enzymes. Enteropeptidase is required to activate pancreatic enzymes. Disaccharidases are required to break down sugars like lactose (milk sugar) and sucrose (table sugar). Parasitic infection can damage the intestinal lining and decrease production of these enzymes. Lactose deficiency is age-related among most adults worldwide. Those of Northern European extraction often continue to make ample lactase enzyme throughout their lives;
- bacterial overgrowth of the small intestine, which can block absorption and limit digestion;
- impaired pancreatic output. Low stomach acid or more serious conditions like pancreatitis can decrease the output of digestive enzymes;
- lowered bile production, which reduces fat digestion and the uptake of fat-soluble vitamins (A, D, K and E);
- materials that absorb minerals and may prevent their uptake by the intestine. FIBER, PHYTIC ACID and OXALIC ACID in VEGETABLES, GRAINS and LEGUMES are examples;
- competition by drugs. Certain drugs can block the absorption of minerals and vitamins;
- excessive minerals in the diet: for example, too much ZINC blocks copper uptake;
- inadequate INTRINSIC FACTOR. Paralleling low stomach acid production, the stomach may produce too little intrinsic factor to facilitate vitamin B_{12} uptake.

(See also BIOAVAILABILITY; DEFICIENCY, SUBCLINICAL; DRUG-NUTRIENT INTERACTION; GLOSSITIS.)

Kuroki, Fumitoshi, et al., "Multiple Vitamin Status in Crohn's Disease. Correlation with Disease Activity," *Digestive Diseases and Sciences*, 38:9 (September 1993), pp. 1614–18.

maladaptation See TOLERANCE TO TOXIC MATERIALS.

malnutrition Impaired health due to imbalanced diet or to abnormal physiologic processes required to absorb and use optimal amounts of nutrients. Thus malnutrition can reflect not obtaining enough nutrients (undernutrition), or it may mean excessive amounts of nutrients (overnutrition), or both. Reliance on highly processed foods can lead to simultaneous overnutrition and undernutrition.

Overnutrition The major dietary problems in the Western World reflect excessive food, rather than a lack. Excessive CALORIES, refined CARBOHYDRATE, FAT, saturated fat and sodium set the stage for modern diseases such as CANCER, CARDIOVASCULAR DISEASE, DIABETES, HYPERTENSION and OBESITY.

Undernutrition Primary undernutrition refers to ingesting inadequate amounts of nutrients to sustain normal growth, to maintain freedom from illness or even to achieve optimal health. Populations in developing nations often suffer from chronic undernutrition. Being significantly underweight shortens the life span and takes an immense toll in human suffering. STARVATION represents severe undernutrition; the diet does not provide enough major nutrients (protein, carbohydrate and fat) to maintain the body. The physiological results are the same as for prolonged fasting. Other symptoms include dry skin, sores that do not heal, edema, inflamed tongue, flabby muscles, slow growth and development, and FATIGUE and apathy. Prolonged starvation wastes the body because it must literally consume itself to survive. ANEMIA and a failure to grow are severe consequences. Inadequate body stores of vitamins and minerals generally lead to a decreased immunity and a greater risk of infection.

Other symptoms are common: slowed knee reflexes; abnormal pigmentation of eye membranes (conjunctiva), redness of eyes and eyelids; dull, brittle hair that is easily plucked and sometimes lighter in color than normal; swollen, bleeding gums; receded gum line; swollen parotid glands and THYROID GLANDS; chapped, red or cracked lips; brittle, rigid nails; rapid heartbeat; high blood pressure and enlarged liver in children.

Secondary undernutrition refers to the body's inability to efficiently use nutrients. This situation can be caused by poor digestion, inadequate uptake due to an unhealthy intestine, or by competition of nutrients with each other or with drugs. Mild (subclinical) malnutrition without major deficiency symptoms is much more common than severe undernutrition in the United States, but it is much harder to detect. The most common symptom is fatigue.

Twenty to 25% of elderly Americans are undernourished. As of 1992, there were 30 million people in this group; 6 million are considered at high risk of malnutrition, and one million are outright malnourished. The elderly are the least nutrition conscious Americans of any age group. The Nutrition Screening Initiative is a national project to promote routine nutrition screening and better nutrition among older people.

The elderly are prone to malnutrition because of poverty; isolation; loss of sense of TASTE; loss of teeth and GINGIVITIS; multiple medications that cause loss of sense of taste; constipation and MALABSORPTION of nutrients; poor eating habits; reliance on PROCESSED FOODS; tendency to skip meals; a high prevalence of chronic disease and physical impairments that limit the ability to shop for or cook food; and a lack of concern about nutrition.

Malnutrition in Children

Poverty and malnutrition go hand in hand, and children suffer the most worldwide. Mild undernutrition is much more common worldwide than starvation, although famine is endemic in certain regions of Africa. Marginal intake of vitamins, minerals and/or amino acids in a child's diet can lead to lowered immunity and a decreased ability of white cells to fight off infections, as well as slowed mental and physical development.

The failure of babies to thrive most often results from an inadequate diet. MARASMUS refers to the form of starvation occurring when the diet does not supply enough calories. The skeletal image usually associated with starvation reflects marasmus. Muscle wasting supplies the body with energy. Children with marasmus adapt by slowing their growth rates, which can have severe, long-term effects on mental and physical development. KWASHIORKOR is the form of starvation occurring when the diet supplies enough carbohydrate to meet daily calorie needs, but lacks adequate PROTEIN. The starving child may appear puffy and swollen because of severe edema. In reality the starving child receives too little protein, carbohydrate, fat, vitamins, minerals and emotional warmth.

Malnutrition among children of affluent, well-educated parents is a recent phenomenon in the United States. Some well-intentioned, well-educated parents apply their low-fat diets to their children to decrease the risk of childhood obesity and of heart disease later. Children grow rapidly, and low-calorie, low-fat diets can retard their growth and development. Consult a specialist before putting a child on a diet. (See also BIOAVAILABILITY; CHOLESTEROL; DEFICIENCY, SUBCLINICAL.)

"When Bacterial Overgrowth Causes Malnutrition," *Emergency Medicine*, 26:1 (January 1994), pp. 45–46.

malt A product of germinated BARLEY used in brewing beer. To prepare malt, germinated barley is bleached and dried to prevent further sprouting. During germination, seed enzymes cleave STARCH to the sugar, maltose, and split cell wall FIBER (hemicelluloses) into fermentable simple sugars. Other GRAINS such as RYE and WHEAT can also be malted. Malted milk is prepared by combining whole milk with the filtrate from a mixture of barley milk and wheat flour.

Malt is fermented by yeast to ALCOHOL when beer is brewed. Malting and brewing were among the earliest discoveries of civilization. Egyptians have brewed beer since 5,000 B.C. Beer is prepared by first warming malt and non-malted grains (a mixture called a "mash"). Mash is then filtered to obtain a sugar-rich liquid, which is boiled with hops, then fermented by adding yeasts. Whisky manufacture depends upon fermentation of mashes without filtration, then distilling the alcohol and other volatile materials.

maltase The ENZYME that digests maltose, a sugar from starch DIGESTION. The small intestine produces maltase to degrade maltose. This sugar is produced by the action of AMYLASE, the starch digestion enzyme found in saliva and in pancreatic secretions. Because maltose is too large to be absorbed by the intestine, it must be degraded to its building block, the simple sugar GLUCOSE, which is readily absorbed. Therefore maltase plays a critical role in carbohydrate digestion. (See also CARBOHYDRATE METABOLISM; LACTASE; SUCRASE.)

maltol A FOOD ADDITIVE used as a FLAVOR ENHANCER. Maltol accentuates the flavor of CHOCOLATE, VANILLA and fruit-flavored beverages and foods. A closely related compound, ethyl maltol, is a more powerful flavor enhancer. Both are used in gelatin desserts, ICE CREAM, jams and baked goods with fruit flavors. Because ethyl maltol tastes sweet, its use allows the sugar content of a food to be reduced by 15%. Ethyl maltol masks the bitter taste of the artificial sweetener saccharin. Levels of maltol added to foods range from 15 to 250 mcg per gram (parts per million); ethyl maltol is added at considerably lower levels. Small amounts of maltol occur naturally in bread, coffee, cereals, soybeans and malt products. Heated condensed milk, whey and soy sauce also produce maltol. Maltol and ethyl maltol are considered safe food additives. (See also ARTIFICIAL SWEETENERS; NATURAL SWEETENERS.)

mandarin orange (*Citrus reticulata*; tangerine) A citrus fruit with a unique sweet flavor related to the sweet orange. Mandarin oranges have a loose skin that is easily peeled. Certain red varieties are called TANGERINES, though the term tangerine is not a botanical classification. Apparently mandarin oranges originated in Southeast Asia. Many varieties may have been developed in India, China and Japan. Mandarin and hybrid strains are grown in most subtropical and even tropical regions throughout the world. Florida is the major domestic producer of tangerines. The original strains have been improved and crossbred with other citrus fruit. (For nutrient content see ORANGE.)

manganese A trace mineral nutrient. Manganese is needed for normal brain and muscle function, building bones, BLOOD CLOTTING, CHOLESTEROL synthesis, fat synthesis, and DNA and RNA synthesis. Manganese activates the enzyme responsible for the formation of urea, the waste product of protein degradation. In carbohydrate metabolism manganese is required for the synthesis of glucose from non-carbohydrate substances (GLUCONEOGENESIS). Manganese assists the action of SUPEROXIDE DISMUTASE, which degrades superoxide, a free radical and a highly damaging form of oxygen. In addition, manganese is required to synthesize components of mucopolysaccharides (GLYCOSAMINOGLYCANS), components of connective tissue. A manganese-dependent enzyme of the brain synthesizes the AMINO ACID, GLUTAMINE, as a way of removing AMMONIA, a toxic product of nitrogen metabolism. Conditions possibly associated with manganese deficiency include OSTEOPOROSIS, RHEUMATOID ARTHRITIS, LUPUS ERYTHEMATOSUS, allergies, ALCOHOLISM and diabetes.

Sources

Good sources of manganese are NUTS, TEA, whole grains, BRAN, dried fruit and leafy green vegetables. Their manganese content varies, depending on the manganese content of the soil. Eighty-six percent of manganese is lost in prepared white flour. Dairy products, FISH, MEAT (other than organ meats) and POULTRY are poor sources of manganese. Inadequate absorption of manganese from plant sources may be a problem because digestion of plant food releases only a small fraction of the manganese it contains. Manganese supplements are best taken as a balanced multi-mineral preparation.

Requirements

The body contains low levels of manganese, and only minute amounts are required each day to maintain this level. The manganese concentration in tissues is stable primarily due to carefully controlled excretion.

There is no RECOMMENDED DIETARY ALLOWANCE for manganese. Instead the Food and Nutrition Board has estimated a safe and adequate daily intake as 2.0 to 5.0 mg for adults. Symptoms of manganese deficiency in experimental animals include pancreatic pathology and diabetes-like symptoms, impaired growth, reproductive abnormalities, skeletal abnormalities, convulsions and ataxia (abnormal muscle movements). Certain groups might be deficient in manganese: women, especially those on weight loss diets; anyone on a calorie-restricted diet; aged people; and VEGETARIANS.

Safety

While manganese is relatively non-toxic, too much manganese can interfere with the absorption of other minerals like IRON. High manganese intake can cause nerve damage, immune system malfunction, and damage to PANCREAS, LIVER and KIDNEY. Excessive calcium supplements can interfere with manganese and iron uptake because they all use the same entry mechanism into intestinal cells. (See also ALLERGY, IMMEDIATE FAT METABOLISM.)

Freeland-Graves, Jeanne, "Manganese: an Essential Nutrient for Humans," *Nutrition Today*, (November-December 1988), pp. 13–19.

mango (*Mangifera indica*)   A tropical FRUIT with an oval shape, produced by a tropical evergreen. Mangoes are green when unripe. The ripened fruit is yellow-orange and the juicy pulp is sweet and somewhat sour. Though not a popular fruit in North America, mangoes are an important fruit crop in the tropics, and they rank seventh among the most popular fruit crop worldwide. Mangoes seem to have originated in the broad region between Thailand and India, and they have been cultivated since 5000 B.C. They are now grown in most tropical countries. India remains the largest producer of mangoes.

The ripe fruit is eaten raw or used in jams, preserves and juices; unripened fruit is used in chutneys, a popular condiment in India. Mangoes can be seasoned with turmeric for this purpose. Nutrient content of one mango, raw (207 g), is 135 calories; protein, 1.1 g; carbohydrate, 35.2 g; fiber, 2.9 g; folic acid, 0.6 g; potassium, 323 mg; vitamin A, 806 retinol equivalents; vitamin C, 57 mg; thiamin, 0.12 mg; riboflavin, 0.12 mg; niacin, 1.21 mg.

manioc   See CASSAVA.

mannitol   A NATURAL SWEETENER, mannitol is used in chewing gum, soft candy, BREAKFAST CEREALS, frosting and sugarless diet foods. It is also used as an anti-sticking agent for chewing gum because it does not absorb moisture. It occurs naturally in ASPARAGUS, OLIVES, PINEAPPLES and seaweed. Commercially it is synthesized from the simple, common sugar GLUCOSE. Mannitol is classified as a sugar alcohol but is not a sugar. Mannitol is not used efficiently by the body, nor does it raise blood sugar rapidly. Mannitol supplies only about half the calories of glucose and has about 70% of the sweetness of table sugar. Mannitol is considered a safe FOOD ADDITIVE. It is not metabolized to acids by oral bacteria. Tooth decay is caused by these organic acids and therefore this additive may help prevent tooth decay.

Mannitol's rather poor absorption by the intestine results in osmotic DIARRHEA when large amounts are ingested. It is a LAXATIVE at a dose of 10 to 20 g daily. Such huge doses can worsen kidney disease. The U.S. FDA requires that the ingredient label warn of the laxative effect with excess consumption when daily ingestion of mannitol could reach 20 g. Mannitol may increase urination because much of it is eliminated unchanged by the kidneys. It has been used to prevent the kidneys from shutting down during major surgery. (See also ARTIFICIAL SWEETENERS; DENTAL CARIES; SORBITOL.)

mannose   A simple SUGAR found in CARBOHYDRATE-containing proteins. In the body mannose is formed from glucose and is used in the formation of short chains of sugars (oligosaccharides) that are attached to certain proteins (GLYCOPROTEINS). When attached to certain proteins, mannose may function as a recognition marker that governs the cellular distribution of the protein and its metabolic rate within tissues. Mannose is much less common than glucose (BLOOD SUGAR) and does not occur free in foods. Mannose contains six carbon atoms and belongs to an important family of sugars (the aldohexoses) of which glucose is a member. (See also MANNITOL.)

MAO inhibitors (monoamine oxidase inhibitors) Drugs used to treat psychological depression and high blood pressure. Examples include Marpian, Nardil and Parnate. They block a key enzyme required to form DOPAMINE and norepinephrine, synthesized by nerve cells to conduct nerve impulses between cells.

Foods containing TYRAMINE, a degradation product found in fermented foods, are dangerous when taking MAO inhibitors because tyramine in the presence of MAO inhibitors drastically increases blood pressure. This effect may be severe enough to cause a STROKE or a HEART ATTACK. Symptoms of tyramine–MAO inhibitor interactions include vomiting, severe headaches and nosebleed. Tyramine-containing foods to avoid include; aged CHEESES (like Brie, Camembert, cheddar, processed American), cured MEAT (like pastrami), anchovies, AVOCADOS, BANANAS, BEETS, caffeinated beverages, chicken liver, CHOCOLATE, canned FIGS, MUSHROOMS, pickled herring, RAISINS, sausages, sour cream, chianti wine, sherry and yeast extract. (See also DRUG-NUTRIENT INTERACTION; NEUROTRANSMITTER.)

maple syrup   A syrup prepared from the sap of the sugar maple tree (*Acer saccharum*), native to eastern North America. This sweetener contains sugars like SUCROSE, glucose, FRUCTOSE and a distinctive flavor. During winter, starch is converted to sugar in tree roots, and it is carried up the trunk in the spring. Spring sap contains 4 to 10% sugar. It is collected in spring when the sap begins to flow and before buds open. The collected sap is concentrated by boiling down, which develops the characteristic flavor of maple syrup. The maple flavor is not present in the sap itself. The province of Quebec remains the largest producer of maple syrup (over 20 million gallons yearly). U.S. production is about 5% that of Quebec. In the U.S., Vermont and New York produce the most maple syrup. Commercial maple syrups are often blends of maple syrup and other less expensive syrups.

Consider maple syrup a REFINED CARBOHYDRATE with little nutrient content other than CALORIES. It contains only traces of CALCIUM and POTASSIUM. To prevent crystallization and molds, refrigerate maple syrup but do not freeze. Maple syrup can be contaminated with LEAD if it is collected in or stored in metal containers with soldered seams. Be sure the supplier has used stainless steel during preparation. (See also NATURAL SWEETENERS.)

marasmus A progressive wasting and emaciation due to chronic deprivation of PROTEIN and CALORIES. Symptoms include wasting of MUSCLES and body fat, dry skin, low body weight, lethargy, sunken eyes, severe DIARRHEA, MALABSORPTION, and low body temperature. Diarrhea causes DEHYDRATION and losses of minerals like SODIUM, POTASSIUM and CHLORIDE, causing ELECTROLYTE imbalance. This in turn leads to brain, kidney and heart disorders. If left untreated, death may result. Decreased immunity promotes disease. In adapting to STARVATION, the body consumes tissue, protein and FAT, accompanied by reduced protein synthesis and retarded growth in many tissues. All muscles, including the heart, atrophy.

Causes of marasmus include inadequate food intake; prolonged malabsorption, caused, for instance, by severe diarrhea in infants; and child neglect. Marasmus occurs in infants and children in regions of the world where low-income populations are prone to undernutrition due to an inadequate supply of protein-rich foods, especially animal protein. Dietary protein may be deficient in essential AMINO ACIDS, or the total food intake may be inadequate. In either case consumed protein is used for energy rather than being used to supply essential amino acids for protein synthesis and maintenance.

Marasmatic children need physical and emotional warmth as well as improved nutrition. Treatment is based upon an easily digested diet with meals supplemented with 1 gram of high-quality protein and 50 to 60 calories per pound of body weight. (See also IMMUNE SYSTEM; KWASHIORKOR; MALNUTRITION.)

margarine A non-dairy product resembling BUTTER and prepared from hydrogenated (hardened) VEGETABLE OIL. Since 1950 Americans have eaten more margarine per person a year as butter consumption has declined.

Margarine is usually manufactured from CORN OIL, SAFFLOWER oil, SOYBEAN oil, COTTONSEED OIL, PALM OIL and PEANUT oil, and the amount of saturated fat that margarines contain varies. Small amounts of animal FAT may be added by manufacturers. Unless animal fat is added, margarine does not contain cholesterol. Margarine incorporates partially HYDROGENATED VEGETABLE OIL. Most vegetable oils contain polyunsaturated fats, which are deficient in hydrogen atoms and which are liquid at room temperature. Hydrogenation, a

chemical process, adds variable amounts of hydrogen to polyunsaturates, making them more saturated and harder at room temperature. In the last steps oil is emulsified with emulsifying agents and chilled to solidify the oil and trap water. Additives include salt, yellow coloring (BETA CAROTENE), VITAMIN A, preservatives and butter flavoring.

It is believed that saturated fat, rather than polyunsaturated fat, promotes clogged arteries. Though margarine is more saturated than vegetable oils like corn, safflower and soybean oils, it is much less saturated than coconut, palm or palm kernel oils.

Margarine contains more TRANS-FATTY ACID than butter. Trans-fatty acids are by-products of hydrogenation. The molecular shape of normal unsaturated fatty acids is bent, while saturated fats are straight molecules. Trans-fatty acids are also straight. Like saturated fatty acids, they can pack together more closely, making them more solid at room temperature. Trans-fatty acids raise cholesterol and therefore increase the risk of heart disease. Fried foods, such as french fries and doughnuts from fast food chains, are often cooked with vegetable shortening. Vegetable shortening is laden with trans-fatty acids. Food labels do not list the amount of trans-fatty acids in foods. Margarine and partially hydrogenated vegetable oils contribute more than 80% of the trans-fatty acids Americans consume.

Types of Margarine

Liquid margarine is the least hydrogenated and contains a high fraction of unsaturated oil. Whipped margarine contains air to increase volume and to make the product spread more evenly; the air reduces calories by 40%. Stick margarine is higher in saturated fat than tub margarine or liquid margarine and may contain animal fat (BEEF TALLOW). "Diet" (low-cal) margarine contains one-half to one-third the calories of regular margarine because it contains much more water. Due to the high water content, it cannot be substituted for stick margarine or butter in recipes. Salt-free margarine is available for individuals on sodium-restricted diets.

How does margarine compare with butter? Both contain the same number of calories and salt. Margarine is usually colored with beta carotene to make it look like butter, which derives its color naturally from beta carotene. Margarine contains no cholesterol; butter contains 32 milligrams/tsp. Margarine has 2 g of saturated fat/tsp; butter has 7.5 g. Margarine has 4 g of polyunsaturated fat/tsp.; butter has a half-gram. The PROTEIN, fat, CALCIUM, SODIUM and VITAMIN A contents are comparable. Stick margarine contains 47% monounsaturated fatty acids, 53% polyunsaturated fatty acids and 30% saturated fatty acids. And margarine contains high levels of trans-fatty acids; per tablespoon margarines contain 1 to 3 g.

The American Heart Association recommends selecting a tub margarine that lists as the first ingredient liquid oil, which is less saturated than partially hydrogenated oil. The label may list the P:S ratio. This useful index is a measure of the relative amount of polyunsaturated fat to saturated fat. The American Heart Association recommends a P:S ratio of 2:1 or more.

The American Cancer Society recommends eating less fat of all kinds—margarine, butter, cooking oils, vegetable shortening or lard—to lower the risk of cancer and heart disease. Avoid margarines that do not list liquid vegetable oil first on the label. Avoid those listing coconut oil, palm or palm kernel oil or lard as ingredients in order to reduce consumption of saturated fat. Buy margarines with higher levels of polyunsaturates and choose diet ("light") margarine to reduce the intake of trans-fatty acids. Margarine labels list saturated fat content but do not include trans-fatty acids. Therefore, they reveal only a portion of the content of the LDL-cholesterol raising fat.

Nutrient content of 1 tbsp (14 g) of regular 80%-fat margarine 100 calories; protein, 1.1 g; fat, 11.4 g; sodium, 153 mg; vitamin A, 140 retinol equivalents; and no water-soluble vitamins.

Raloff, J., "Margarine Is Anything but a Marginal Fat," *Science News*, 145 (May 21, 1994), p. 325.

marjoram (*Origanum Majorana hortensis*; sweet marjoram)   An HERB of the mint family. Marjoram is related to OREGANO. It has light-green oval leaves with a mild sage-like flavor. It is used in salads, meat, game, poultry and vegetables, and with tomato-based dishes, including lentils and beans. Marjoram has been used in folk medicine to ease cramps and stomach upsets. Wild marjoram is more commonly known as oregano. (See also SPICES.)

marshmallow   A spongy confection. Marshmallows are a common sweet in the United States. They are prepared with whipped GELATIN or GUM ARABIC, corn syrup, flavoring and table sugar. Marshmallows are used in frosting and in sauces.

Marshmallow is also a medicinal plant, *Althaea officinalis*, that has sweet roots. The root mucilage was formerly used to make marshmallows. In folk medicine it has been used externally to help heal wounds. It is used in ointments for chapped skin. Marshmallow helps decrease inflammation associated with intestinal infections of the urinary tract and genital tissues, and with respiratory infections and asthma. It is also used in cough syrup and cough lozenges. (See also CANDY; EMPTY CALORIES; SUCROSE.)

mast cell   Immune cells in connective tissue that release inflammatory agents when stimulated. Mast cells contain SEROTONIN and HISTAMINE, which cause tiny blood vessels, CAPILLARIES, to dilate and become porous. In the inflammatory response, fluid and defensive cells leak into the tissue and the increased blood flow leads to heat, redness and swelling (more fluid). Defensive substances in the blood like antibodies, defensive cells, and clot-forming substances can then enter the injured area. In particular, scavenger (phagocytic) white blood cells pass more easily to the site of injury. Mast cells are also abundant along blood vessels, where they produce HEPARIN, a substance that acts as an anticoagulant (prevents blood from clotting). FLAVONOIDS, plant antioxidants, can decrease inflammation by desensitizing mast cells. (See also IMMUNE SYSTEM; INFLAMMATION.)

mastication   The act of chewing. Food is ingested through the mouth, where it is pulverized. Teeth grind food particles and mix them with saliva for lubrication and to initiate digestion. The tongue moves chewed food to the pharynx (throat) in order for it to be swallowed. Adequate chewing prepares food for efficient DIGESTION in the stomach and intestine.

Chewing sends signals to the brain to prepare the gastrointestinal tract to release digestive enzymes. Inadequate chewing can cause choking, and gulping food can lead to HEARTBURN. (See also DEGLUTITION; DIGESTIVE TRACT.)

mayonnaise   A spread prepared from egg yolks and oil. Mayonnaise is used in salads, vegetables, a variety of recipes and as a sandwich spread. Mayonnaise is generally prepared from SOYBEAN oil and VINEGAR. Other ingredients include lemon or lime juice, SALT, NATURAL SWEETENER (usually sugar), MUSTARD and other spices, and MONOSODIUM GLUTAMATE. LECITHIN, a fatty substance in egg yolk, suspends (emulsifies) the vegetable oil. Emulsification is not a chemical treatment nor does it alter the nature of the oil. One tablespoon of mayonnaise contains 9 to 10 mg of cholesterol (from egg yolk) and 100 calories.

Imitation mayonnaise contains about one-third the calories and four times the amount of water as regular mayonnaise. Although homemade mayonnaise is considered a risk for food poisoning, food poisoning is not usually the result of mayonnaise spoilage because the acidic contents retard bacterial growth. To reduce fat calories, several strategies seem prudent: Instead of mayonnaise, substitute YOGURT or low-fat COTTAGE CHEESE and BUTTERMILK, seasoned with lemon juice, mustard powder, horseradish, ginger, garlic and herbs.

meal planning   See BASIC FOOD GROUPS; EXCHANGE LISTS; FOOD GUIDE PYRAMID.

meal timing   See DIETING.

measures (metric to English)   The 8-oz cup and the tablespoon are standard measures for recipes. The problem is that nutrition uses the metric system, a scientific notation with liters (close to a quart) and milliliters (ml, 1/1,000 of a liter). It uses grams and milligrams (mg) instead of ounces.

The table below offers metric equivalents for common household measures.

Household Measure	Metric Measure
1 cup (8 oz or 16 tsp)	224 grams or 240 ml
1/8 cup (1 oz or 2 tsp)	28 grams
1 tsp	14 grams or 5 ml
1 tbsp	4 grams or 15 ml
1/4 tbsp	1 gram
1 pound (16 oz)	454 grams
1 quart	0.95 liter
1 fluid ounce	30 milliliters

meat   The edible flesh of animals used as food. BEEF, VEAL, LAMB and PORK are standard fare in the United States; in 1991, the average person ate 63 pounds of beef, 47 pounds of pork and 1.1 pounds of lamb. However, beef's popularity has steadily declined since the late 1970s as CHICKEN and FISH have become more popular. In 1991 Americans consumed 43.9 pounds of chicken. Much of this change in taste is due to consumer concerns about CHOLESTEROL and FAT. Nonetheless meat production has a large economic and environmental impact. Livestock graze on one-third of the land of North America. Half of U.S. crops such as corn go to livestock feed, especially for cattle. Directly and indirectly, through fodder irrigation, farm animals account for a major part of the water consumed in the United States. Half the antibiotics produced are used for livestock.

Meat contains 20 to 23% PROTEIN, variable amounts of fat and approximately 60% water. The fat content depends upon the type of meat, the nutritional state of the animal, the degree of trimming and the method of preparation. Meat and dairy products supply half of the total fat, all of the cholesterol and 75% of the saturated FATTY ACIDS of the standard American diet. Lean meat and fat meat contain about the same cholesterol, 70 to 80 mg per 3-oz serving of lamb, beef, chicken or pork. Although beef and chicken contain about the same amount of cholesterol, beef fat is much more saturated than chicken fat.

Meat is an excellent source of protein, B complex vitamins and certain trace minerals like ZINC and IRON. Meat supplies about 90% of VITAMIN B_{12} in the U.S. diet, 70% of protein, 66% of RIBOFLAVIN, 54% of VITAMIN B_6, 46% of NIACIN and 36% of iron, but only 3% of calcium. Therefore meat is not a very good source of calcium. Meat protein is "high quality," that is, it provides ample amounts of all of the essential AMINO ACIDS that cannot be synthesized by the body. A little animal protein with a meal increases iron uptake from plant food. Fish, poultry and shellfish are flesh and constitute the rest of the meat group, one of the four basic food groups developed in the 1950s to help design a balanced diet. In the food guide pyramid, they represent the protein group with meat, poultry, fish, dried beans, eggs and nuts. Two to three servings of this group is recommended daily.

There are several concerns with a high meat diet:

1. Meat contributes about 35% of the saturated fat to the typical American diet. In particular, red meat contributes about 49 grams of fat per person per day and accounts for about 30% of total fat consumption. Excessive fat is associated with an increased risk of OBESITY, elevated blood cholesterol and increased risk of heart disease and of CANCER. In contrast, POULTRY and fish, provided they are not breaded and fried, add little to the total fat consumption.
2. Excessive protein consumption is generally a bigger problem in the United States than inadequate dietary protein. Protein quality is not generally an issue except in the case of a VEGETARIAN who does not eat a variety of plant protein sources. Too much protein causes calcium loss and promotes bone loss (OSTEOPOROSIS).
3. A high-protein diet may interfere with kidney function, especially in diabetics.
4. Meat is often contaminated with traces of PESTICIDES, growth promoters, drugs and antibiotics. Their long-term effects on health are not known.

Grading Meat

The USDA has defined various grades of beef according to fat content. The type of cut of meat is more important than the grade of meat, which depends on the texture and the amount of visible fat. For example, top round is leaner than rib roast. Regulations apply to beef, mutton, lamb, calf, veal and pork. Government grading of meat is not compulsory. Over half the beef is graded. The grades are U.S. Prime, U.S. Choice, U.S. Select, U.S. Standard, U.S. Commercial, U.S. Utility, U.S. Cutter and U.S. Canner for beef. Pork is graded U.S. No. 1, U.S. No. 2, U.S. No. 3, U.S. No. 4 and U.S. Utility.

Light or "Lite" meat refers to cuts of meat that have at least 25% less fat than standard cuts for that grade of meat. USDA nutritional beef, also known as Natural Beef, refers to meat that has been minimally processed. Growth stimulants, antibiotics and other additives to fatten the animals have been avoided. USDA Light Select, Light Choice and Light Prime contain 25% less fat than the corresponding cuts.

The order in going from least-fat to most-fat grades is as follows: Light Select (or Good), Select (or Good), Light Choice, Choice, Light Prime and Prime. Most ungraded meat is Select (Good); it corresponds to supermarket brands of lean beef. "Extra lean" meat contains less than 5% fat. About half the USDA Select meat cuts fall in this category. NFF1 refers to meat containing less than 3.5% fat. FEF2 refers to cuts of meat with less than 6% fat.

Pork is the flesh of hogs; ham refers to the rear leg muscle or rear quarter. Ninety-five percent "fat-free ham" refers to ham containing 5% of the weight of the ham as fat. Calorie-wise, 20 to 30% of the calories in these hams can be derived from saturated fat, so they are not free of fat. Pork is a high-fat food, although some cuts of pork, trimmed of visible fat, have less fat. For example, center loin provides 8.9 g of fat per 3-oz serving. The same cut untrimmed contains 19 g of fat. Only a small fraction of pork is graded.

Meat Labeling

Labels for processed meat and poultry products are required to provide the nutrient content, amount of fat and number of calories. The listing of fat composition, sodium content and other nutritional information is voluntary. This information can be made available in notebooks or on placards in grocery stores. Ground beef can be called "lean" only if a 3.5-oz serving contains less than 10 g of fat, less than 4.5 g of saturated fat and less than 95 mg of cholesterol.

Ground beef can be labeled "extra lean" if it contains less than 5 g of fat, less than 2 g of saturated fat and less than 95 mg of cholesterol.

Safety

Federal inspection of animal products relies on the Food, Safety and Quality Service of the USDA. The inspection program involves evaluating the quality, characteristics, yield or proportion of important cuts of meat. Freedom from damage, proper labeling, absence of adulteration and disease are key aims of meat inspection. The Wholesome Meat Act of 1967 assures consumers that all meat sold in the United States is either inspected by the federal program or by an equivalent state cooperative program.

Safe handling instructions are available for ground meat and all raw meat products as a measure to combat food poisoning linked to uncooked or partially cooked meat, especially due to a strain of the bacterium ESCHERICHIA COLI 0157:H7. The safe handling instructions notify the consumer that food products may contain bacteria that can cause illness if mishandled or improperly cooked. Keep product refrigerated or frozen. Thaw in microwave or refrigerator. Keep raw meat and poultry separate from other foods. Wash working surfaces (including cutting boards), utensils and hands after touching raw meat or poultry. Cook thoroughly. Keep cooked foods hot and refrigerate leftovers or discard them (rather than eating them after they have been at room temperature).

Cooking meat can create several classes of cancer-causing agents. Charring meat, poultry or fish produces polycyclic aromatic compounds, especially when fat drippings deposit soot on charcoal-broiled food. Scraping off the charred portion can remove these materials. Another class is called heterocyclic amines (HCAs). A combination of longer cooking time and high temperature determines the extent of formation; HCAs tend to form within meat and cannot be scraped off. Once eaten, the liver activates HCAs, which can alter DNA, a first step in cancer development. Pre-cooking hamburger for two minutes drives off some of the raw materials for HCAs, and when barbecued such hamburger produces much less cancer causing material than hamburger exclusively grilled.

Red meat need not be excluded for a fat restricted diet to reduce fat consumption. Eat small portions of lean cuts of meat and trim visible fat before cooking. Roasted meat contains less fat than broiled or braised meat. To avoid producing cancer-causing agents during cooking, don't overcook or char meat. For low-fat meat (5 to 15% fat), buy Light Select (Good), Select (Good) or Light Choice grades.

Meat in Prepared Foods

Food producers are required to meet U.S. FDA standards for meat content in a variety of prepared foods. The amount of meat actually permitted in different foods varies immensely. This is important to keep in mind if meat or protein content is a concern.

The following is a partial listing of FDA standards for meat contents:

Meat Product	Percent Meat
meatballs	65
beef enchiladas	15
beef tacos	15
chili con carne	40
gravy with beef	35
ham salad	35
pizza with meat	15
spaghetti and meatballs	12
chicken with broth	43

Fat and cholesterol in meat and non-meat products are summarized on page 287.

(See also DIETARY GUIDELINES FOR AMERICANS; HAMBURGER; HOT DOG; MEAT, PROCESSED; MEAT CONTAMINANTS; MEAT SUBSTITUTES; STANDARDS OF IDENTITY; TOXOPLASMOSIS.)

Lachelier, Paul, "Systematic Problems in Meat Regulation Need Attention," *Nutrition Week*, 13 (April 8, 1994), pp. 4–5.

meat, processed   Meat that has been modified by chemical treatment and extensive manipulation. This category includes BACON, pastrami, salami, liverwurst, HAM, HOT DOGS, hot SAUSAGES, LUNCHEON MEATS, cold cuts, BOLOGNA and Polish sausage. Sausages and processed meats are some of the fattest foods available. Salami, bologna and liver sausage contain especially large amounts of FAT, and up to 80% of their calories can come from fat. This level is equivalent to a huge 15 to 17 g per 2-oz serving. Processed meats often contain high levels of SODIUM (500 to 1,000 mg per serving). Furthermore, sodium NITRITE is sometimes added as a preservative, or it is added to enhance the color or flavor of the product.

For low-fat processed meat, look for foods providing 2 to 3 g of fat per slice, a reasonably low value for a processed meat. Chicken or turkey breast and products made only from these are leaner than red meat. Read the label carefully. Generally the serving size is one ounce (28 g). If a smaller serving size is used it will have fewer calories. (See also CONVENIENCE FOOD; PROCESSED FOOD.)

meat alternatives   Non-meat or non-animal protein foods. Consumers choose MEAT alternatives to lower animal protein intake, to decrease FAT and consumption and to better utilize plant protein sources. All LEGUMES, whether BEANS, LENTILS or PEAS, contain high levels of protein. No plant source contains cholesterol unless animal fat has been added. "High quality" protein is found in most animal protein and in several plant sources such as soybean and AMARANTH. Such protein provides AMINO ACIDS that cannot be manufactured by the body in appropriate ratios to provide enough protein building blocks to support growth and maintain health.

Non-meat products can be prepared from eggs or egg whites and grain protein. GLUTEN, the protein fraction of wheat, may also be used regardless of its source. Though tofu and soybean protein are low-fat foods, their conversion to meatless burgers, hot dogs and sausages requires extensive processing. Food additives are frequently added along the way. Non-meat alternatives often contain high levels of fat, though most of this is polyunsaturated rather than saturated, as found in red meat. Deep-fat-fried products will be highest in fat; SODIUM is often high as well.

Soybean protein is a widely used meat alternative because it provides a favorable balance of essential amino acids. Soy protein can easily be processed to resemble meat in texture and taste. Two forms, TEMPEH and TOFU, have long been used in traditional diets in Japan, Indonesia and China. They easily absorb flavors and require little cooking. Tempeh utilizes whole soy beans, including FIBER, and contains somewhat less fat than tofu. A typical 4-oz serving of tofu provides 5 to 7 g of fat and 80 to 100 calories, and tempeh provides 4 to 5 g of fat and 150 calories. By comparison, 4 oz of uncooked, extra lean ground beef provide about 18 g of fat and 290 calories.

(See also FATTY ACIDS; FOOD PROCESSING.)

Comparison of Fat and Cholesterol in Meat and Non-Meat Products

Protein Item (grams)	Fat (grams)	Calories	Percent Cals as Fat	Cholesterol
Meat products:				
(28 g) beef & pork bologna	8	89	81	16 mg
(45 g) beef & pork hot dog	13.1	145	81	23 mg
(85 g) hamburger (regular)	17.8	245	65	76 mg
(13 g) pork sausage	4	50	72	11 mg
Typical non-meat (soy-based) products:				
(18 g) non-meat bologna	21	320	60	none
(30 g) non-meat hot dog	18	345	47	none
(17.5 g) non-meat burger	16	219	56	none
(10 g) non-meat sausage	8	175	41	none
(14 g) non-meat turkey	1	80	11	none

meat contaminants Foreign substances, tissue contaminants or excessive amounts of growth-promoting compounds that are present in MEAT. Antibiotics, growth promoters, PESTICIDES and THYROID gland are examples of substances that may contaminate meat and POULTRY. More than 20,000 animal drugs are in use and, according to the U.S. FDA, 500 to 600 synthetic chemicals are present in beef alone; most are probably harmless. However, 42 are suspected of causing cancer and another 20 are suspected of causing birth defects. Some of these chemicals have been found to be present in meat at levels higher than those set by the FDA. Since January 1989, European nations have banned U.S. beef grown with growth-promoting hormones. In the United States there is no way to know which meats, poultry or animal products are even slightly contaminated. U.S. consumers frequently have a choice of buying organic beef and organic poultry, supposedly grown without growth promoters and excessive drugs.

Growth Promoters as Meat Contaminants

Hormones and growth promoters are often given to animals to speed weight gain; occasionally these are misused. Steroid growth promoters can increase the risk of cancer. DIETHYL-STILBESTROL (DES) is an example of a HORMONE-like drug once used to promote growth in beef. It is now banned in the United States, though residues occasionally show up in spot checks of meat. The degree of risk of long-term exposure to low levels of hormone analogs and other drugs in meat is unknown.

Antibiotics as Meat Contaminants

Antibiotics are used as feed additives promoting growth in livestock, which is a boon to livestock growers. However, their use in feed can lead to drug-resistant bacteria, which theoretically could infect people who eat the contaminated meat or dairy products. Antibiotic residues may contaminate meat. As an example, sulfamethazine, a sulfa drug used to treat bacterial infections in cattle, pigs, sheep and poultry, is used as a growth promoter for pigs. Research indicates it causes cancer in lab animals. This drug cannot be given to livestock close to the time of slaughter and cannot be given to milk cows because it is a forbidden contaminant in milk. Nonetheless, there may be significant meat and milk contamination; spot checks have found sulfa drugs in veal and pork and milk from various metropolitan areas in the United States.

Pesticides as Meat Contaminants

Livestock are generally contaminated with trace amounts of a variety of pesticides. Fortunately, the levels are generally very low. Cow's milk is likewise contaminated. Herbicide contamination occurs when animals graze on land contaminated with dioxin-containing herbicides (such as Silvet and 2-4-5T).

Thyroid Gland Contamination

Occasionally meat is contaminated by thyroid glands from carcasses improperly trimmed by meat packers. This could be a problem for patients with heart disease. Symptoms (insomnia, DIARRHEA, nervousness) disappear when the contaminated meat is no longer eaten.

Animal Drugs as Meat Contaminants

Drugs like clorsulon administered to prevent liver flukes in cattle are potential cancer-causing agents. Gentian violet causes cancer, but it is still permitted in animal feed to prevent it from molding. Traces of these chemicals show up in meat, eggs and poultry. (See also ANTIBIOTIC-RESISTANT BACTERIA IN FOOD; CARCINOGEN; MAD COW DISEASE; TOXOPLASMOSIS.)

meat curing A treatment designed to preserve and to add flavor to meat. In the United States this term pertains primarily to pork. Salt (sodium chloride) has been used since ancient times to preserve meat. It is added to processed meats as a preservative and a flavoring agent; it is also added to cause meat particles in products like bologna and hot dogs to stick together. The salt content is high enough to make salted meat products unsuitable for persons restricted to low-salt diets.

Sodium NITRITE, sodium NITRATE and potassium nitrate help prevent a particularly deadly form of food poisoning called BOTULISM. Nitrite is the primary preservative. Nitrites and nitrates also help develop the flavor and texture of cured meats. However, nitrite can combine with AMINES, common nitrogen-containing compounds in food, to form NITROSOAMINES, which are potential cancer-causing agents (CARCINOGEN). As a partial solution to this problem, sodium nitrite can be combined with sodium and potassium ascorbate (VITAMIN C) to inhibit nitrosoamine formation. Garlic also limits nitrosoamine formation.

Smoked meat and fish have been prepared since ancient times. Smoking dries meat, adds materials that act as preservatives and adds characteristic flavor. Smoking may introduce trace amounts of carcinogens (cancer-causing agents), however. Meat packers often use liquid smoke or synthetic smoke for flavoring. "Liquid smoke" is made from wood smoke treated to remove certain dangerous constituents; "synthetic smoke" is a synthetic mixture of chemicals that create a pleasing flavor.

Phosphate is among the most common food additives in cured meat products. Phosphate promotes water uptake by meat, increasing its juiciness. Federal regulations specify that the phosphate level cannot exceed 0.5% and the amount must be listed on the label.

meatless meat See MEAT SUBSTITUTES.

meat packing The slaughter of livestock and preparation of meat for transport and sale. Following slaughter, dressed beef carcasses are chilled at 32° F in a humid atmosphere for a week or so to permit enzymatic breakdown of muscle tissue. Bacteria within the carcass provide a characteristic flavor to beef. (Lamb is not aged.) Beef can be tenderized by injecting cattle with a mixture of plant-derived, protein-degrading enzymes (PROTEOLYTIC ENZYMES) minutes before slaughter. Less tender cuts may be tenderized by blade insertion. Electrically shocked meat is more tender than unshocked meat. Applying an electrical current to the carcass after slaughter prevents rigor mortis and muscle contraction. Consequently, less chilling and less aging time are required.

Mechanical deboning salvages meat left on bones after hand trimming. Ground bones are pressed through a screen to separate bone fragments from tissue. Mechanically deboned meat finds use in SAUSAGE, BOLOGNA and other luncheon meat products. Deboned meat need not be indicated on a food label. Because it contains bone fragments the calcium content is significantly higher than regular meat. The amount of calcium per serving must be shown on the label in order to provide the consumer with an estimate of the bone content.

meat substitutes (meatless meat, meat analogs) Fabricated foods that resemble MEAT in texture and amino acid (PROTEIN) content but are essentially devoid of meat or POULTRY. The most common meat substitutes are primarily either single cell protein or soy protein based. Meat substitutes offer several advantages over meat: They are less expensive; they are convenient to use; they meet dietary restrictions, such as in low-cholesterol diets. Certain meat substitutes approach beef in fat content, however; the fat ranges from 6 g of fat per serving for meatless chicken (36% calories from fat) to 16 g of fat per serving for meatless bologna (51% calories from fat).

Single-cell Protein (SCP)

Protein that is obtained from single-celled organisms such as YEAST, bacteria or algae can be used as food. Brewer's yeast and torula yeast, produced from fermenting wood residues and other cellulose sources, are used as animal feed. Industry is developing an inexpensive, wholesome protein from yeast, and yeast protein is being test marketed. FUNGUS is the source of a protein produced in Britain. This product is high in FIBER and low in fat and CHOLESTEROL. Its texture and flavor are easily changed to resemble beef or poultry and it is used in frozen meatless pies. The potential for single-cell protein production is huge. One thousand pounds of single-cell organisms can produce 50 tons of protein per day, while a thousand-pound steer produces only 1 pound of protein a day and an equal weight of SOYBEANS can produce 80 pounds of protein a day. Among problems in converting single-cell protein to food are: PALATABILITY, protein quality (balanced amino acid content) and digestibility, as well as a high content of NUCLEIC ACID and possible toxins.

Soybean Protein

Soybean protein is the most common vegetable meat substitute, marketed as grits, flour, soy protein concentrate (which contains 70% or more soybean as protein) and isolated soy protein (90% protein). These basic forms can be extruded or spun. Spun soy protein is most often used as meat analogs, simulated (meatless) bacon bits, ham chunks, chicken chunks, hamburger patties, sausages, bacon slices and turkey chunks, which look and taste like the authentic food but with a different texture. Soy protein meal analogs generally contain fat (partially hydrogenated vegetable oils), artificial coloring and flavoring (possibly monosodium glutamate), soy sauce and salt. They may be enriched with several vitamins. Soy protein is a nutritious source of protein without cholesterol. It is low in trace minerals like IRON and ZINC, however. (See also TEXTURIZED VEGETABLE PROTEIN.)

meat tenderizer Mixtures of powdered protein-digesting ENZYMES used to make tough MEAT more tender. The enzymes may come from PAPAYA (papain), PINEAPPLE (bromelain), FIGS (ficin), bacteria (subtilisin) and FUNGI. These powerful enzymes degrade fibrous protein of connective tissue and MUSCLE and are destroyed during cooking. Most commercial tenderizers include seasonings, SALT and MSG (MONOSODIUM GLUTAMATE). Meat tenderizers are considered safe additives. (See also FOOD ADDITIVES.)

medications See ALCOHOL/DRUG INTERACTIONS; DRUG/ NUTRIENT INTERACTION.

medicinal plants   It is likely that all cultural groups have used plants as therapeutic agents since prehistoric times. China and India have recorded descriptions of medicinal plants as early as 2700 B.C. Egyptian, Greek, Roman and Arab physicians described medicinal properties of plants. Indigenous people of Central America, South America and North America and of Africa have further contributed to the knowledge of medicinal plants.

Research led to the isolation and characterization of the active principles of many botanical medicines now manufactured or isolated by pharmaceutical firms. Among them are morphine (from poppy); reserpine (a tranquilizer from snakeroot); curare (a muscle relaxant from the curare vine); quinine (the first malarial treatment, from the bark of the cinchona tree); digitalis (heart stimulant from foxglove); atropine (pupil-dilating drug from deadly nightshade); and others. Medicinal plants are currently being screened for anticancer and antiviral constituents upon which to base new drugs. With the appearance of antibiotic-resistant bacteria, medicinal plants offer the promise of new treatment.

A set of terms describing the use of plant remedies and ailments for which they are employed predates pharmacology. The following is a brief description of key terms used in botanical medicine.

Alteratives   Produce a gradual change in the body, normalizing body functions. Examples include DANDELION, ECHINACEA, GINSENG.

Anodynes   Relieve pain. Examples include hops and wintergreen.

Appetite stimulants   Examples include ALFALFA, ANISE, CHAMOMILE, CELERY, dandelion, ginseng, mint, PARSLEY, ROSEMARY, savory.

Astringents   Contract certain tissues and decrease mucous discharge. Examples include bayberry; BLACKBERRY; witch hazel.

Carminatives   Reduce FLATULENCE (gas). Examples include aniseed, CAPSICUM, CARDAMOM, CUMIN, FENNEL seed, GINGER root, LOVAGE root, NUTMEG, PEPPERMINT, spearmint, valerian root.

Cathartics   Relieve CONSTIPATION. Examples include CHICORY, dandelion.

Demulcents   Oily or mucilaginous materials that soothe digestive upsets. Examples include BORAGE, chamomile, ginger root, sassafras.

Diaphoretics   Induce sweating. Examples include borage, chamomile, ginger root, sassafras.

Diuretics   Induce frequent urination. Examples include alfalfa, buchu leaves, celery, chicory, corn silk, dandelion, horehound, parsley (root), wild carrot.

Expectorants   Loosen phlegm, mucous secretion from lungs and wind pipe. Examples include angelica, GARLIC, horehound, LICORICE.

Febrifungis   Antipyretics that lower body temperature during episodes of fever. Examples include angelica, BALM, borage, dandelion.

Nervines   Counterbalance stress and fatigue by calming, soothing the body. Examples include chamomile, hops, passion flower, valerian root.

Stimulants   Examples include angelica, bayberry leaves, capsicum, cardamom, sarsaparilla root, wintergreen.

Tonics   Stimulate appetite, invigorate. Examples include celery seed, ginseng, goldenseal, hops.

There are several caveats in using medicinal plants:

- A number of plant species may be harmful (e.g., comfrey, lobelia, sassafras root).
- Allergic reactions may occur in susceptible people.
- Safe and adequate doses depend upon many variables. Often it is difficult to standardize herbal preparations because of variation in harvesting, storage and growth conditions. Furthermore, doses tolerated in adults may be harmful to children.
- Often claims like "blood purifier" are used without definition. Professional medical advice is prudent for any chronic symptoms.

(See also HERBS.)

Mediterranean Diet Pyramid   A food guide based on the traditional diet of Greece, Crete and southern Italy. These areas are noted for their low incidence of heart disease, cancer and other chronic diseases, possibly due to the low consumption of saturated fat during the 1960s or earlier. The Mediterranean Diet Pyramid was publicized in 1994 by the Oldways Preservation and Exchange Trust, the Harvard School of Public Health, and the World Health Organization Regional Office for Europe.

The foundation of the Mediterranean Diet Pyramid is the daily consumption of bread, pasta, rice, couscous, bulgar and other grains, potatoes, large amounts of fruits and vegetables, with beans, legumes and nuts as a source of protein. The Mediterrean diet also recommends small daily servings of yogurt and low-fat cheese, as well as olive oil in place of butter and other oils, cheese, pastries and meat. Cheese and yogurt are limited to one half-ounce (1 tablespoon) of cheese and one cup daily, respectively. Sweets and eggs can be eaten once or twice a week; poultry and fish are limited to two or three servings weekly. Red meat is limited to a few times a month. Unlike other guides, this food guide allows for wine in moderation (one glass per day for women, two glasses for men). It also calls for regular physical exercise.

There are several points to consider when using this food guide. Eating more fats and oil regardless of source can increase the risk of weight gain, especially for overweight diabetics. Healthy southern Italian men in the 1960s consumed 30% of their calories as fats and oils. The pyramid cautions that consuming more than 35% of calories as fat may be satisfactory for active individuals without weight problems. It is not recommended to drink alcohol to decrease the risk of heart disease, because there are safer ways, such as increasing the exercise level and stopping tobacco use. (See also CARDIOVASCULAR DISEASE, FOOD PYRAMID.)

Willett, W.C., et al., "Mediterranean Diet Pyramid: a Cultural Model for Healthy Eating," *American Journal of Clinical Nutrition*, 61:6, supp. (1995), pp. 1402S–06S.

medium-chain triglycerides (MCTs)   Fats derived from COCONUT OIL and palm kernel oil. Coconut oil contains 60% MCT. MCTs are prepared commercially by synthesis using saturated fatty acids containing 6 to 12 carbon atoms. In contrast, the fatty acids commonly found in fats and oils contain carbon chains with 16 or 18 carbon atoms. Saturated fats are filled up with hydrogen atoms. MCTs provide 8.3 calories per gram while fat provides 9 calories per gram; therefore, MCTs cannot be classified as "diet" foods.

MCTs are more easily absorbed than the usual animal fats and vegetable oils. They are broken down to free fatty acids and directly enter the bloodstream, where they can be used immediately for energy production by the LIVER and MUSCLE. They are not as readily stored in fat. In contrast, the usual dietary fats and oils must be packaged as particles called CHYLOMICRONS by intestinal cells, released into the lymphatic system, and subsequently broken down in capillaries before their fatty acids can be taken up by tissues.

MCTs are used in oral and intravenous feeding formulas as a quick source of energy for patients requiring nutritional support, such as premature infants and patients with fat maldigestion (such as CELIAC DISEASE and CROHN'S DISEASE) or severe trauma. They have also been used in a variety of nutritional supplements as a source of quick energy and to aid in weight control by increasing heat production (thermogenesis). However, research has yielded mixed results on this last point. MCTs tend to lower serum cholesterol levels more than unsaturated vegetable oils. They may cause abdominal cramping and bloating. In excess they can be converted to KETONE BODIES, acids that accumulate in the blood and disrupt acid-base balance. (See also FAT DIGESTION: FAT METABOLISM.)

Megremis, C.J., "Medium-Chain Triglycerides: a Nonconventional Fat," *Food Technology*, 45:2 (1991), pp. 108, 110, 114.

megadose   A relatively large amount of a nutrient not easily obtainable by eating food. There is no fixed definition for the megadose of a VITAMIN or MINERAL. As a rule of thumb, a megadose can be defined as being greater than ten times the RECOMMENDED DIETARY ALLOWANCE (RDA). Megadoses of nutrients can therefore range from milligram to gram quantities, depending upon the particular nutrient. The extent to which vitamin and mineral supplements taken in excess of the RDA have a beneficial effect on health remains controversial. There is a consensus that supplements even at high levels can help remedy conditions due to obvious nutrient deficiencies. Subtle deficiencies that do not cause deficiency diseases are less well recognized, more common and less often treated. Complicating the picture is the fact that individual nutrient requirements are a function of inherited tendencies toward disease, health history and environmental factors at home and work, as well as life-style choices. Thus the level of supplements effective for one individual may be ineffective for another.

Certain nutrients taken in excess can cause side effects; the levels of vitamins causing toxicity vary considerably among individuals. Certain trace minerals may cause adverse effects at levels only five to ten times the RDAs, and fat-soluble vitamins such as VITAMIN A and VITAMIN D accumulate in the body with excessive consumption and cause toxic symptoms. On the other hand, vitamins in reasonable amounts are generally far safer than most prescription drugs and even over-the-counter medications like aspirin or cortisone creams. (See also BIOCHEMICAL INDIVIDUALITY; HYPERVITAMINOSIS; ORTHOMOLECULAR MEDICINE.)

Lamm, D.L., et al., "Megadose Vitamins in Bladder Cancer: a Double-blind Clinical Trial," *Journal of Urology*, 151:1 (January 1994), pp. 21–26.

megaloblastic anemia   A condition resulting from a deficiency of normal RED BLOOD CELLS in which the blood contains primitive red blood cells called megaloblasts. These large nucleated cells are found in the bone marrow as parents to normal, mature red blood cells, which lack nuclei. Megaloblastic anemia occurs in cases of severe deficiencies of B vitamins VITAMIN B_{12} and FOLIC ACID, which are required to produce new cells, including red blood cells.

megavitamin therapy   See ORTHOMOLECULAR MEDICINE.

melatonin   A hormone produced by the pineal gland, which lies deep within the brain. During the day, light enters the eye and triggers nerve signals that shut down melatonin production. In the dark, melatonin is released into the bloodstream where it helps coordinate hormonal activity with the NERVOUS SYSTEM. It may even help regulate the sleep cycle and help overcome jet lag. Melatonin may regulate complex processes including fertility.

There are hints that melatonin influences AGING. Melatonin production declines with age. In experimental animals, melatonin has been shown to increase the life span, though long-term effects in humans are unknown. Two possible mechanisms may come into play. Melatonin may slow down wear and tear throughout life. It can act as an ANTIOXIDANT to help clear the body of oxidative damage accumulated during the daytime due to normal metabolism, as well as exposure to pollutants like cigarette smoke and ozone. Several degenerative diseases, including heart disease and cancer, have been linked to oxidative damage. In addition, melatonin can increase immunity and delay the age-dependent shrinkage of the thymus gland in lab animals. The thymus is the home of T cells, key white blood cells that fight infection. Though synthetic melatonin is available in health food stores, this supplement is clearly a hormone, and it is not a nutrient in the sense of a vitamin or other building block for the body, and it should be used judiciously. (See also ENDOCRINE SYSTEM; FREE RADICAL; IMMUNE SYSTEM.)

Reiter, R.J., et al., "Melatonin: Its Intracellular and Genomic Actions," *Trends in Endochronology Metabolism*, 7:1 (1996), pp. 22–27.

melon   The sweet, juicy FRUIT of several plants of the cucurbit (gourd) family, which includes SQUASH and CUCUMBERS. CANTALOUPE, CASABA, HONEYDEW, musk crenshaw, Persian, and WATERMELON are typical representatives. Most melons originated in the Middle East and were cultivated by the ancient Egyptians and the Romans. Watermelon originated in Africa and in North America. Various types of melons are imported from Central America. Chile and New Zealand. Florida, Texas, Georgia, California and Arizona supply the domestic market of cantaloupes, watermelons, honeydew melons and the like.

Melons are round or oblong fruit grown from either climbing or trailing vines. The pulp may be white, green, yellow, pink or red. All melons are about 90% water. They are good sources of POTASSIUM and VITAMIN C. When the pulp is deep orange, they are an excellent source of vitamin A, in the form of BETA CAROTENE.

menadione   A synthetic form of VITAMIN K used as a supplement. Unlike natural vitamin K, this analog is smaller and has no side chain attached. It is processed by the LIVER. Vitamin K is required in the formation of certain clotting proteins of the BLOOD and in the formation of several proteins found in BONE, blood and the kidneys. While large amounts of vitamin K are not generally toxic, excessive menadione can cause hemolytic ANEMIA and excessive production of BILE PIGMENT and JAUNDICE in newborn infants.

Menke's syndrome   A rare genetic disease caused by the inability of the intestine to absorb COPPER adequately. Copper is an essential TRACE MINERAL nutrient, and copper malabsorption leads to progressive mental retardation, low body temperature, skeletal abnormalities, abnormal hair development and degeneration of connective tissue structures such as the aorta and other vessel walls. A copper-dependent ENZYME (lysyloxidase) stabilizes collagen fibers incorporated in vessel walls. Progressive nerve damage associated with Menke's syndrome often causes death at a very early age. (See also COLLAGEN; LYSINE.)

mental retardation   See BIRTH DEFECTS.

mercury   A toxic HEAVY METAL and an environmental pollutant. Chemically combined mercury, (mercury ions) is a widespread industrial waste; combustion pollutants may be a primary cause of mercury pollution. Once released into the environment mercury can combine with carbon to create a more toxic form of mercury called methylmercury, which accumulates in the FOOD CHAIN because it is fat-soluble and concentrates in fatty tissues. Predatory fish, at the top of the aquatic food chain, possess the highest levels. The average American adult consumes 2 to 3 mcg of mercury daily. TUNA, shark and swordfish are generally contaminated with mercury. One bite of a tuna fish sandwich may be equivalent to the amount of mercury released in the average person's fillings in a day.

Because many rivers and lakes are polluted by industrial wastes, domestic freshwater fish are often contaminated with mercury. The high levels of methylmercury in fish has triggered health advisories for many lakes in the United States and Canada. Native Americans subsisting on locally caught fish or on game animals eating those fish, are also at risk. In communities relying on fish for food, people can be consuming 200 times the federally designated tolerable level. Health departments in at least 21 states, including Michigan, Minnesota and Wisconsin, have established advisories for mercury contaminated freshwater fish.

Methylmercury acts as a nerve poison and the brain is susceptible to mercury toxicity. Adults eating fish containing substantial amounts of methylmercury can suffer irreversible nerve and brain damage. The fetus is extremely sensitive to methylmercury. Low doses can lead to retardation due to severe brain damage.

To minimize consumption of mercury, avoid tuna and swordfish if pregnant. Eat saltwater fish like salmon, rather than freshwater fish harvested from polluted water; do not eat freshwater fish from polluted waters more than two to four times a month. (See also AMALGAM FILLINGS; BIRTH DEFECTS; BREASTFEEDING.)

Foulke, Judithe, "Mercury in Fish," *FDA Consumer* (September 1994), pp. 5–8.

Lorscheider, Fritz L., et al., "Mercury Exposure from 'Silver' Tooth Fillings: Emerging Evidence Questions a Traditional Dental Paradigm," *FASEB Journal*, 917 (April 1995), pp. 504–08.

metabolic acidosis   Excessive acid in body fluids, especially the blood. This condition may be the result of the production of acids like KETONE BODIES during excessive fat breakdown; the loss of BICARBONATE, a blood BUFFER; or the loss of essential ELECTROLYTES due to kidney disease. The accumulation of ketone bodies accompanies STARVATION, FASTING, crash DIETING, uncontrolled diabetes and chronic ALCOHOLISM. Aspirin poisoning can contribute to ACIDOSIS. Excessive acid production can cause severe mineral loss and DEHYDRATION due to increased urine volume. (See also FAT METABOLISM.)

metabolic alkalosis   See ALKALOSIS.

metabolic pathway   A series of ENZYMES (protein catalysts) that function together like an assembly line to degrade larger molecules or to manufacture larger molecules from raw materials. The final product of a metabolic pathway is thus the result of many chemical modifications, mostly carried out one step at a time.

Pathways can be synthetic (anabolic) when larger cell constituents are synthesized from smaller building blocks. Such pathways require energy. Degradative (catabolic) pathways break down compounds, often with the release of ENERGY that can be trapped as ATP, the "energy currency of the cell." ATP supplies energy for biosynthetic reactions and other energy-consuming processes like muscle contractions and nerve transmissions.

Metabolic pathways may exist in the cytoplasm as water-soluble enzymes. GLYCOLYSIS, the pathway that breaks down glucose, the most common sugar in the body, is carried out by a cytoplasmic pathway. On the other hand, enzymes may be bound together; such multi-enzyme complexes operate as a cohesive unit. The formation of fatty acids occurs in this fashion. Alternatively, enzymes may be membrane-bound. Enzymes transporting electrons from cellular oxidations to oxygen to form water and ATP by mitochondria (the ELECTRON TRANSPORT CHAIN) represent such a membrane-bound system.

Pathways may be linear or they may be circular (cyclic), in which case a final product participates in the initial step of the pathway by acting as an acceptor for an incoming molecule that will be modified as it moves down the pathway. The UREA CYCLE, which converts ammonia, the toxic nitrogen waste product of amino acids, to non-toxic urea, operates in this manner.

Metabolic pathways are often integrated with cellular functions through changes in the cytoplasmic environment.

Certain enzymes are bottlenecks, limiting the flow of material through the pathway. They may be turned on or off by compounds produced by other pathways. FEEDBACK INHIBITION represents a slight variation of this theme. In this scenario the accumulation of the final product of a pathway inhibits the bottleneck enzyme, and thus the pathway balances supply with demand. As an example, excessive CITRIC ACID inhibits glycolysis, and the accumulation of ATP, the energy currency of the cell, inhibits both glycolysis and the Kreb's cycle, major energy-producing pathways of the cell.

Many hormones regulate metabolic pathways. GLUCAGON and EPINEPHRINE (adrenaline) are hormones that make fuel available for tissues. They raise blood sugar levels by activating enzymes that break down liver GLYCOGEN, the storage form of glucose, to release glucose and raise blood sugar. In addition, epinephrine stimulates enzymes that break down body fat to release fatty acids, thus raising blood fatty acid levels. (See also ANABOLISM; CATABOLISM; INHIBITION; METABOLISM.)

metabolic water WATER produced by reactions carried out in the cell. An average of 13 ml of water is formed for every 100 calories of food completely oxidized to carbon dioxide. The complete oxidation of 100 g of carbohydrate to carbon dioxide yields 60 ml of water; 100 g of protein yields 40 ml and 100 g of fat yields 110 ml. Consequently a typical American diet produces about 200 ml of water daily. However, this is still only a fraction of the water needed to replenish water lost in urine, feces and respiration. About 2 liters per day are required to replenish water losses. (See also DEHYDRATION; ENERGY; METABOLISM; OXIDATION.)

metabolism The sum of chemical reactions performed by cells. In metabolism, ENZYMES, the protein catalysts of cells, work together like assembly lines. Such functional systems are called METABOLIC PATHWAYS. Metabolism is conveniently broken down into two categories: CATABOLISM and ANABOLISM.

Catabolism

Catabolism refers to enzyme systems that oxidize fuel nutrients (carbohydrates, amino acids and fat) to ENERGY and to waste products, CARBON DIOXIDE and WATER. Catabolism traps chemical energy as ATP in the MITOCHONDRIA, the cell's powerhouse. Catabolism also includes the degradation of nutrients and more complex structures to provide smaller, simpler molecules for cellular building blocks for the cell.

Catabolic pathways include:

1. UREA CYCLE, which produces the major nitrogenous waste, UREA, excreted in urine.
2. KREB'S CYCLE, the central energy-yielding pathway of the cells, producing carbon dioxide by degrading fat, amino acids and carbohydrate.
3. GLYCOLYSIS, which breaks down GLUCOSE (blood sugar) and smaller oxidation products (pyruvic acid, lactic acid) while delivering energy to the cell independently of oxygen.
4. OXIDATIVE PHOSPHORYLATION, the formation of ATP accompanying a sequential series of oxidation-reduction reactions leading ultimately to the reduction of oxygen to water.

Anabolism

Anabolism refers to enzyme pathways that build up cellular components, rather than tear them down. Anabolism produces all of the machinery to operate and reproduce cells. Anabolic precursors require chemical energy, most of which is provided in the form of ATP, the energy currency of the cell produced by catabolism.

Anabolism is stimulated by INSULIN after meals containing carbohydrates. This HORMONE stimulates cells to store surplus chemical energy as fat (from fatty acids) and glycogen (from glucose). Over a longer period of time, anabolism occurs when the body is growing, as during pregnancy, childhood, adolescence, body building and fat accumulation.

Anabolic pathways include:

1. Fatty acid and fat synthesis, for energy storage.
2. Cholesterol synthesis; cholesterol functions in membranes and serves as a hormone precursor.
3. DNA and RNA synthesis; DNA stores information while RNA functions in guiding the synthesis of proteins.
4. Protein synthesis, which includes synthesizing enzymes and certain non-steroid hormones.
5. Glycogen synthesis, the formation of the storage carbohydrate glycogen by muscle and liver.
6. Amino acid synthesis; formation of 10 of the 20 amino acids.

Health and maintenance of body weight require a balance between the opposing processes of anabolism and catabolism. When anabolism exceeds catabolism, synthetic processes prevail. In this situation the body's overall metabolism shifts to building protein and to storing energy as fat and glycogen. When the body requires more energy than is provided by food, catabolism exceeds anabolism, breakdown and degradation exceed synthesis, and the body burns carbohydrate, fat and protein. The body switches to a CATABOLIC STATE during illness, surgery and starvation. (See also AMINO ACID METABOLISM; BASAL METABOLIC RATE; CARBOHYDRATE METABOLISM; FATTY ACIDS.)

Forster, R.E. and Estrabrook, R.W., "Is Oxygen an Essential Nutrient?" *Annual Review of Nutrition*, 13 (1993), pp. 383–403.

metabolite A chemical produced by enzyme-catalyzed reactions. Metabolites may be products of degradation: Metabolites of GLUCOSE degradation include simple acids like LACTIC ACID, PYRUVIC ACID and ACETIC ACID coupled to a carrier molecule called COENZYME A. Metabolites of amino breakdown include AMMONIA and UREA as nitrogen-containing waste products, and acids like alpha ketoglutaric acid and OXALOACETIC ACID. Bilirubin or BILE PIGMENT is a primary metabolite of hemoglobin, the oxygen-transporter of red blood cells. Metabolites are also products of synthetic reactions of the cell. For example, the brain chemicals (NEUROTRANSMITTERS) DOPAMINE and norepinephrine are metabolites of the amino acid TYROSINE. Bile acids for fat digestion are metabolites of CHOLESTEROL. Drugs and medications are metabolized (altered chemically) by the liver so they can be inactivated and excreted.

metalloenzyme An ENZYME or protein catalyst that requires a metal ion to complete its catalytic site where reactions occur. Many trace mineral nutrients function as enzyme helpers:

Copper A variety of enzymes require COPPER: Lysyloxidase helps assemble connective tissue; cytochromic oxidase transfers electrons to reduce oxygen to water in the final step of oxidation of fuels; and a type of SUPEROXIDE DISMUTASE destroys superoxide, a potentially damaging form of oxygen.

Iron Most IRON-containing enzymes are involved in oxidations and reductions: CYTOCHROMES transport electrons in the oxidation of fuel molecules to liberate energy and in the oxidation of potentially damaging materials to increase their water solubility, hence decrease their toxicity. A variety of oxidases perform one-step oxidations.

Zinc Over a hundred different enzymes require ZINC, including DNA polymerase, the enzyme that synthesizes DNA chains, and RNA polymerase, which synthesizes RNA. DNA and RNA synthesis is required for cell multiplication. Zinc is required by superoxide dismutase, and CARBOXYPEPTIDASE, a digestive enzyme.

Magnesium Many enzymes that utilize ATP, the cellular form of chemical energy, are activated by MAGNESIUM-ATP combinations.

Manganese Superoxide dismutase and pyruvate carboxylase require MANGANESE. The enzyme that initiates liver synthesis of glucose from amino acids during fasting requires manganese.

Selenium GLUTATHIONE PEROXIDASE, a SELENIUM-containing enzyme, destroys two types of potentially damaging compounds: HYDROGEN PEROXIDE and LIPID peroxides, produced when lipids are attacked by oxygen.

Molybdenum Two important enzymes require MOLYBDENUM: Xanthine oxidase is involved in the synthesis of the waste product URIC ACID; sulfite oxidase destroys SULFITES.

Cobalt The only known role for COBALT is its function as part of an enzyme helper derived from vitamin B_{12}. It is required by at least two different human enzymes. (See also COENZYME; TRACE MINERALS.)

methanol (wood alcohol; methyl alcohol) The simplest type of ALCOHOL. Methanol is derived from wood processing and, unlike ETHANOL, which comes from the fermentation of grains, is highly toxic. As little as 20 milliliters can cause permanent blindness or even death. Treatment of methanol poisoning involves administering ethanol. Ethanol competes with liver enzymes and prevents them from converting methanol to a toxic by-product, formaldehyde. Most cases of methanol poisoning are due to ingestion of methanol in lieu of alcoholic beverages and liquors. (See also INHIBITION.)

methionine (Met, L-methionine) An essential AMINO ACID that contains sulfur. The body cannot manufacture methionine; therefore it must be supplied by digesting food PROTEIN. Methionine is a critical building block for cellular proteins, and this versatile amino acid plays many roles. It functions as the raw material for the sulfur-containing amino acid CYSTEINE; for the formation of acetylcholine, a NEURO-

TRANSMITTER (chemical synthesized by the nervous system for transmitting impulses between cells); for the hormone EPINEPHRINE (adrenaline); and for CHOLINE, required to form LECITHIN, a FAT lipid substance containing phosphorus. Lecithin functions as a building block of the lipid carriers in the bloodstream, like LDL (LOW-DENSITY LIPOPROTEIN) and VLDL (VERY-LOW-DENSITY LIPOPROTEIN) to transport fat and CHOLESTEROL. Methionine is converted to sulfate, used by the LIVER to solubilize toxic chemicals and waste products so they can be excreted. TAURINE, a compound used to form BILE salts for fat digestion, is a non-protein amino acid derived from methionine. Methionine is converted to HOMOCYSTEINE, a simplified sulfur amino acid that eventually is transformed to CYSTEINE, a sulfur amino acid commonly used by the body, via vitamin B_6 dependent steps. Methionine can be regenerated from homocysteine via steps dependent on FOLIC ACID. With folic acid and vitamin B_6 deficient diets, blood levels of homocysteine rise. Population studies have demonstrated that elevated homocysteine levels increase the risk of CARDIOVASCULAR DISEASE.

Sources of methionine include: MEAT, FISH, POULTRY, GARLIC, ONIONS, BEANS and legumes. Grains are generally low in sulfur amino acids. Infants require 58 mg of sulfur amino acids per kilogram of body weight daily; adults require 13 mg. A chronic protein deficiency leads to inadequate intake of dietary essential amino acids, including methionine, and produces stunted growth, EDEMA, fragile hair, loss of muscle mass and hormonal irregularities. Homocystinuria, an inherited disease due to incomplete breakdown of methionine, can lead to CARDIOVASCULAR DISEASE. One person in 200 carries this genetic trait. (See also DETOXIFICATION; KWASHIORKOR; LIPOPROTEIN; LIPOTROPE.)

Ghoshal, Amiya and Farber, Emmanuel, "Biology of Disease. Choline Deficiency, Lipotrope Deficiency and the Development of Liver Disease Including Liver Cancer: a New Perspective," *Laboratory Investigations*, 68:3 (1993), pp. 255–60.

methylene chloride An organic solvent sometimes used to manufacture decaffeinated COFFEE. Methylene chloride is classified as a chlorinated hydrocarbon because it contains chlorine and carbon. Such compounds have been linked to CANCER. Although the U.S. FDA concluded this solvent causes cancer, it considers the level remaining in decaffeinated coffee so low that the health risk of exposure is negligible. Habitually drinking large amounts of decaffeinated coffee could pose a problem, however. Other manufacturers use ethyl acetate, a non-toxic solvent, or water extraction to remove most of the caffeine from roasted coffee. (See also CARCINOGEN; FOOD ADDITIVES.)

micelle A microscopic particle that permits the suspension of insoluble liquids in water. Micelles require detergent-like molecules (dispersing agents), which possess a characteristic molecular structure. They have a fat-soluble (hydrophobic) region at one end of the molecule to interact with the lipid-soluble material being dispersed, and a water-attracting (hydrophilic) region to interact with water at the opposite end. The result of combining dispersing agents and lipids is a stable suspension of microscopic droplets. The body forms a variety of micelles to transport lipids via the lymph and blood. Typical examples include CHYLOMICRONS, which transport dietary fat from the intestine to other tissues, and LOW-DENSITY LIPOPROTEIN (LDL), which transports CHOLESTEROL from the liver to peripheral tissues. (See also HIGH-DENSITY LIPOPROTEIN; VERY-LOW-DENSITY LIPOPROTEIN.)

microgram   A very small metric unit of weight, abbreviated mcg. One microgram is one-millionth of a gram, or one-thousandth of a milligram. Certain trace nutrients are required daily in only microgram amounts, as illustrated by the following adult RDAs (RECOMMENDED DIETARY ALLOWANCES): VITAMIN B$_{12}$, 1.6–2.0 mcg; VITAMIN D, 5 mcg; VITAMIN K, 65 to 80 mcg; FOLIC ACID, 180 to 200 mcg; and IODINE, 150 mcg. (See also MEASURES; TRACE MINERALS; VITAMIN).

micronutrients   Nutrients that are required by the body in trace amounts—milligrams (thousandths of a gram) or micrograms (millionths of a gram). Though only tiny amounts of certain VITAMINS and MINERALS are required, they nonetheless serve extremely important roles. Inadequate trace nutrients is a major health issue for certain populations both in the United States and throughout the world, for several reasons. Micronutrients are most likely to be lost or destroyed because of their instability in highly processed foods; thus refined foods and synthetic foods are likely to be deficient in many micronutrients. Only a few micronutrients are added to processed foods by enrichment programs.

Vitamins   The weight of all B vitamins needed by the average person daily amounts to no more than 10 staples. The reason such small amounts are required is that they serve as enzyme helpers (coenzymes). Enzymes function as chemical catalysts; they are used repeatedly before wearing out and are needed in only small amounts. In contrast with B vitamins, vitamin C does not function as an enzyme helper. While trace amounts of this vitamin will prevent the vitamin C deficiency disease of scurvy, much more is needed for tissue repair, wound healing, toxic chemical disposal and to maintain a strong immune system. Low amounts of fat-soluble vitamins are required daily and their functions are diverse: VITAMIN A forms a visual pigment and is needed for normal tissue development; VITAMIN K assists blood clotting; VITAMIN E is an ANTIOXIDANT; and VITAMIN D forms a hormone.

Trace minerals   Together the quantities of minerals like ZINC, IRON, CHROMIUM, COPPER, IODINE, MANGANESE and MOLYBDENUM required daily would be a pill weighing a fraction of a gram. These micronutrients generally serve as enzyme helpers (cofactors). Iodine is required in the formation of thyroid hormones and chromium supports the blood-lowering effects of INSULIN. The daily requirements of major minerals (CALCIUM, PHOSPHORUS, SODIUM, CHLORIDE and POTASSIUM) are thousands of times larger. (See also JUNK FOOD; NUTRIENT DENSITY.)

microvilli   Minute, hair-like extensions of the surface of cells lining the small INTESTINE and used to absorb nutrients. The inside of the small intestine resembles a wrinkled shag carpet. VILLI are analogous to the shag and make up the "brush border" of the intestinal surface. Cells that make up the villi are themselves covered with still thinner fibers called microvilli, visible only through an electron microscope. The villi and microvilli provide the intestine with a huge surface area: If its fuzzy inner surface were flattened out, the total surface area of the intestine would be the size of a baseball diamond.

AGING, health, diet history and FOOD SENSITIVITIES can lead to a flattening of microvilli and villi. Loss of this rough surface drastically reduces the amount of nutrients that can be absorbed by the body during DIGESTION. Thus aging and food sensitivities can lead to MALNUTRITION even when consuming a BALANCED DIET. An extreme example of food sensitivity is CELIAC DISEASE, a severe sensitivity to grain protein that destroys intestinal villi. Celiac disease may cause severe malnutrition and retard growth of children. (See also DIGESTIVE TRACT; MALABSORPTION.)

microwave cooking   A rapid heating technique that generally requires one-quarter to one-half the cooking time of an electric oven. Microwave COOKING entails heating foods by means of electromagnetic energy; microwaves are like FM radiowaves. Microwaves cook by causing water molecules in food to vibrate rapidly, which creates heat in the interior of food quickly. Early versions of microwave ovens leaked microwave radiation; however, newer models of microwave ovens are much safer, and the amount of radiation leakage is extremely low. Furthermore, the radiation is non-ionizing radiation, less harmful than the ionizing radiation of X rays. Leakage can occur if the door seal is damaged.

To avoid microwave exposure: Make sure the door of the microwave oven *closes* properly and that the seal on the door is not damaged. Keep seals clean and do not operate these ovens with an object caught in the door. Any oven can leak radiation if the interlocking system does not work. Avoid standing in front of a microwave oven when it is running. Newer pacemakers have shields that protect against microwave interference. People with pacemakers from 1990 or earlier should stand at least 5 feet away from a working microwave oven. Metal twist ties, leaded glass or metal-trimmed porcelain can create arcing and cause fires.

More food is being prepared with microwave ovens than ever before: 80% of U.S. households now use microwave ovens and they are the best-selling appliance in the United States. Because foods cooked in microwave ovens require less time and less water, microwave cooking removes fewer minerals and vitamins than conventional cooking, especially when food is reheated. Microwave cooking does not brown food. Cooking at high temperatures, like baking, produces compounds that can cause cancer in experimental animals; microwaving food virtually eliminates this hazard. Microwave cooking generally does not heat MEAT hotter than boiling water.

It is important to stir foods during microwave cooking. Microwaves may not penetrate a roast or CHICKEN uniformly; consequently uncooked portions of meat may contain bacteria such as SALMONELLA, which can cause FOOD POISONING, and in PORK, parasites causing TRICHINOSIS. Therefore, when microwaving POULTRY be sure to turn or rearrange the pieces at least once during the cooking interval to ensure even and complete cooking. Microwaved bacon contains much less NITRITE than fried bacon, and therefore produces much less NITROSOAMINE than fried bacon. Nitrosoamine is a cancer-causing agent formed when the preservative sodium nitrite is heated with meat.

To avoid overheating foods and causing injury from exploding foods, pierce the skins of tomatoes, potatoes and hot dogs to release steam. Never cook eggs in the shell. Remove lids or caps from containers and cover with a pyrex, microwavable ceramic lid or with vented plastic wrap. Baby foods and formula should not be microwaved because of the danger of overheating. Allow pastries with jelly fillings to cool—hot fillings can cause burns. It is recommended to microwave meat on paper, not on a platter because meat touching a ceramic surface can become hot enough to create materials that can cause DNA damage (mutagens). (See also FOOD IRRADIATION.)

Farley, Dixie, "Keeping up with the Microwave Revolution," *FDA Consumer* (March 1990), pp. 17–22.

microwave popcorn   Microwave popcorn accounts for two-thirds of the popcorn market. Microwaving is a quick and easy method of making popcorn, though it may not be as nutritious as air-blown popcorn. Microwavable popcorn can contain 50 to 60% of its calories as added FAT. Partially hydrogenated VEGETABLE OIL, COCONUT OIL or PALM OIL can double the calories. Another disadvantage: Microwavable popcorn contains excessive amounts of SALT. Check the label of microwave popcorn to determine whether a brand contains added salt, ARTIFICIAL FLAVOR or coloring or synthetic ANTIOXIDANTS (BHA and BHT). As an alternative, try air-blown popcorn; one cup is equivalent to just 90 calories. Garlic powder, yeast, chili powder or Parmesan CHEESE will stick to the popcorn if misted with a spray bottle of water first. Do not microwave popcorn in a brown paper bag; it could catch fire. (See also COOKING.)

migraine headache   A severe form of recurrent headache that causes throbbing pain, light sensitivity, vomiting, diarrhea and altered visual perception. The cause of migraines are not entirely understood. TYRAMINE-containing foods and beverages are implicated in perhaps 10% of cases. These foods include CHOCOLATE, aged cheeses and red wine, and avoiding these may be helpful. Eliminating offending foods can also alleviate symptoms. Magnesium deficiency is associated with migraines. Intravenous treatment with MAGNESIUM and VITAMIN B_6 can also be beneficial. Magnesium counters muscle spasm, and it acts like certain calcium-channel blockers used in conventional treatment to reduce symptoms. (See also ALLERGY, FOOD.)

milk   Liquid secreted by mammals to nourish their young. Milk from goats, sheep, buffalo and cows is consumed in different parts of the world and is converted into a diverse group of products, including BUTTER, CHEESE, dried milk, YOGURT, KEFIR and ICE CREAM. Goat's milk accounts for about 3% of the world milk supply, yet in Asia and Africa goat's milk represents an important part of the diet. Goat's milk resembles cow's milk in composition, though its droplets are smaller and remain suspended during storage. In contrast cow's milk will separate upon standing, and in the United States most cow's milk is homogenized. Milk and milk products comprise one of the basic four food groups, a system long used in meal preparation guidelines in the United States. Dairy products contribute a substantial part of the typical American diet (15 to 20%).

Whole cow's milk is prominent in European and North American diets, although many other adult populations of the world cannot tolerate it because they have lost the childhood ability to digest milk sugar (LACTOSE INTOLERANCE). Cow's milk contains about 88% water. Solids include CARBOHYDRATE, PROTEIN, MINERALS and VITAMINS; the exact composition is affected by the season, the type of feed, the environmental temperature and the breed of dairy cattle. In the typical American diet milk provides about 10% of the daily allowances of ENERGY, 11% of fat intake, 20% of the protein, 72% of CALCIUM, 30% of PHOSPHORUS and 12% of VITAMIN A. In the United States all milk except raw milk is fortified with vitamins A and D. Typically the amounts are relatively small: One cup of milk contains 20% of the DAILY REFERENCE INTAKE (RDI) of vitamin D and 10% of the RDI of vitamin A. Milk typically provides 36% of the RDA of RIBOFLAVIN. However, when milk is stored in plastic bottles, fluorescent lighting can destroy riboflavin and vitamin A within a day. Riboflavin in milk packaged in cardboard containers is stable.

Whole milk contains 4% fat because most of milk is water. Milk fat represents about 48% of the calories in milk, far above the 30% fat calories recommended for daily consumption by dietary guidelines. Milk fat is considered saturated fat. Whole milk contains 22 mg of CHOLESTEROL per cup. Reduced cholesterol milk contains about 25% of the original cholesterol content.

Whole milk contains 3.3% protein in the form of whey and CASEIN. Casein accounts for about 80% of the milk protein and gives milk its white color. Whey protein remains after casein and fat have been removed from milk for cheese manufacture. The proteins in milk enhance the uptake of the B vitamin FOLIC ACID in the INTESTINE.

Potential Problems with Cow's Milk

As a food for children   Cow's milk evolved to support the growth of a calf, and it differs from human milk in important ways. Cow's milk is low in CARNITINE, an amino acid used in energy production that is very high in human milk. Manufacturers of INFANT FORMULAS now add carnitine. Cow's milk contains little IRON. Infants fed cow's milk alone can become iron-deficient and grow slowly. Once the baby's body has become iron deficient, mental development slows even after iron supplements have been given to remedy the iron deficiency.

Do not substitute breast milk or formula with straight cow's milk until the baby is a year old. Though breast milk and formula contain plenty of fat to support the infant's growth, cow's milk does not supply enough fat for the infant. Finally, there is a potential for allergies and milk intolerance when cow's milk is given to young children too early in their development. Although skim milk is lower in fat than whole milk and is a desirable option for adults, a baby's kidneys may not be able to handle skim milk's very concentrated protein.

As a food for adults   Humans are the only species that drink milk as adults. Milk is an excellent source of calcium and vitamins; however, it is a high-fat food. Butterfat is a highly saturated fat, and high consumption of saturated fat promotes clogged arteries. Milk may contain a variety of low-level contaminants because grain-fed cattle can be exposed to pesticides and environmental pollutants like PCB and PBB, which cattle eliminate through their milk. As an example, the pesticide heptachlor extensively contaminated milk produced in Hawaii in 1982. ANTIBIOTICS and growth promoters added to livestock feed are also eliminated through milk. The levels of contaminants are generally quite low, though amounts vary. Rarely, the antibiotic penicillin has been detected in milk at high enough levels to cause a reaction in sensitive people. The veterinary antibiotic sulfamethazine is not approved for use in dairy cattle feed. This drug causes tumors in lab animals. Nonetheless, this substance has periodically been found to contaminate milk. U.S. FDA intervention has decreased this occurrence. Milk boosts the production of stomach acid so it is no longer recommended for ulcers. Recent studies suggest that milk partially blocks the anti-ulcer medication cimetidine.

Milk Processing

To prevent cream from separating from fresh milk, butterfat is broken up into tiny droplets, too small to rise to the top of a milk carton. This homogenization is accomplished by forcing the milk through a nozzle at high pressure. No law requires milk to be homogenized.

Milk is heated, or pasteurized, to kill certain disease-producing bacteria. Besides killing harmful bacteria, pasteurization kills the lactic acid bacteria responsible for souring milk. Pasteurized milk will nonetheless eventually spoil, since not all bacteria are killed. Ultra-high temperatures used to sterilize milk are normally reserved for canned milk or packaged milk stored at room temperature. Pasteurization does not destroy nutrients.

Comparison of Nutrient Contents

Whole milk (1 cup, 8 oz) provides 210 calories; protein, 7.9 g; carbohydrate, 11.4 g; fat, 8.2 g; cholesterol, 33 mg; calcium, 290 mg; vitamin A, 76 retinol equivalents; thiamin, 0.09 mg; riboflavin, 0.41 mg; niacin, 0.22 mg. Other milk preparations contain similar amounts of protein, carbohydrate, calcium, thiamin, riboflavin and niacin. Vitamin D and vitamin A are added.

Low-fat milk (2% fat) contains half the fat content of whole milk. However, it is not a low-fat food. Though it contains 2% fat by weight, this amount is equivalent to 30% of the total calories. Sometimes low-fat milk is fortified with non-fat dry milk solids. One cup of 2% milk provides 121 calories; protein, 8.1 g; carbohydrate, 11.7 g; calcium, 297 mg; fat, 4.8 g; cholesterol, 22 mg; vitamin A, 140 retinol equivalents; thiamin, 0.1 mg; riboflavin, 0.4 mg; niacin, 0.21 mg. One percent milk supplies 1% fat by weight. Only 21% of its calories come from fat. One cup provides 105 calories; protein, 8 g; carbohydrate, 11.7 g; fat 2.5 g; cholesterol, 10 mg; calcium, 300 mg; vitamin A, 145 retinol equivalents; thiamin, 0.1 mg; riboflavin, 0.42 mg; niacin, 0.21 mg. Skim milk contains less than 0.2% fat but is also homogenized. A cup contains 86 calories; protein, 8.3 g; carbohydrate, 11.9 g; fat 0.44 g; cholesterol, 4 mg; calcium, 302 mg; vitamin A, 149 retinol equivalents; thiamin, 0.09 mg; riboflavin, 0.34 mg; niacin, 0.22 mg.

Powdered whole milk. To remove water, milk is sprayed in a drying oven to dry milk droplets. The exposure to hot air can oxidize fat and cholesterol. Oxidized forms of these lipids are potentially harmful; oxidized cholesterol is thought to contribute to ATHEROSCLEROSIS. Powdered skim milk contains very little fat or cholesterol and lacks the oxidized lipids prevalent in powdered whole milk. A cup of powdered non-fat milk provides 244 calories; protein, 23.9 g; carbohydrate, 35.5 g; fat, 0.51 g; cholesterol, 12 mg; calcium, 837 mg; vitamin A, 483 retinol equivalents; thiamin, 0.28 mg; riboflavin, 1.19 mg; niacin, 0.61 mg.

Skim Milk and Children's Diets, Raw Milk

Malnourished young children have been observed in American families whose parents restricted their fat consumption, including substituting skim milk or non-fat milk for whole milk out of fear of childhood OBESITY. Baby obesity is probably a function of total calorie intake, not just fat intake. Adequate fat is essential to support the rapid growth and development required by young children. Use caution when decreasing a child's caloric intake and seek medical advice about fat restrictions for children.

Certified raw milk—commercially available, unprocessed milk that has not been heated—is certified by states that assure strict sanitary conditions have been met in its production. Consumers selecting this type of milk believe it is more nutritious than homogenized, pasteurized milk. Nonetheless, there is a very real risk of developing food poisoning (SALMONELLA) unless milk is pasteurized, and the FDA has banned interstate sales of raw milk. Raw milk production is tightly controlled through state certification procedures. Many first-time users of raw milk develop gastrointestinal disease. Infants and elderly persons are especially at risk. People who habitually drink raw milk develop immunity to at least some of the disease-causing bacteria in raw milk. (See also ALLERGY, FOOD DIETARY GUIDELINES FOR AMERICANS; MILK ALLERGY.)

Gern, J.E., et al., "Allergic Reactions to Milk-contaminated 'non-dairy' products," *New England Journal of Medicine*, 324:14 (1991), pp. 976–78.

milk-alkali syndrome A condition resulting from high calcium levels in the BLOOD. Milk-alkali syndrome can occur during long-term high consumption of MILK together with alkaline substances such as ANTACIDS. Excessive calcium may contribute to kidney stones, or it may be deposited in soft tissue and harden them. Symptoms include vomiting, gastrointestinal bleeding and hypertension. (See also ACIDOSIS; ALKALOSIS)

milk allergy A reaction of the immune system to milk and milk products. The immune system recognizes milk proteins as foreign and overreacts by triggering an allergic attack. Allergies to COW'S MILK and to milk products are among the most common food allergies in the United States. A milk ALLERGY may show up quickly, with symptoms such as hives and asthma or more severe symptoms (immediate hypersensitivity), or it may show up hours after contact (delayed hypersensitivity), with symptoms ranging from ringing ears to joint pain.

The best way to avoid an allergic attack is to avoid milk and milk products. Examine food labels carefully to see whether the milk protein products CASEIN or whey have been added. For delayed reactions, milk and milk products should be avoided long enough for the body to recover (up to several weeks). Once symptoms have declined, try eating the suspected food and monitor carefully how your body responds. Depending upon the response, you may be able to eat dairy products occasionally (perhaps once a week or two) after the IMMUNE SYSTEM recovers. (See also BREAST-FEEDING; ELIMINATION DIET; LACTOSE INTOLERANCE; ROTATION DIET.)

milk intolerance   See LACTOSE INTOLERANCE.

milk thistle (*Silybum marianum*)   A thistle used in botanical medicine to treat liver disorders. Milk thistle grows in Europe and in the United States. Extracts of leaves, seeds and fruit have been used in folk medicine to assist milk production in nursing mothers and for jaundice. Extracts of milk thistle are now used in pharmaceutical preparations to prevent liver damage and increase liver function. Silymarin extract is a mixture of complex substances that prevent liver damage due to FREE RADICALS by acting as ANTIOXIDANTS. Free radicals are highly reactive molecules that can attack cells and damage their membranes and their DNA. Silymarin helps the liver detoxify foreign substances by increasing the production of GLUTATHIONE, the cells' own antioxidant. Glutathione also aids in the detoxication of many substances, ranging from hormones to toxic chemicals. A third way that silymarin helps the liver is by blocking the production of LEUKOTRIENES, very potent agents that trigger inflammation. Silymarin may help improve symptoms of CIRRHOSIS, hepatitis, and alcohol and diabetes-induced liver damage, as well as psoriasis. (See also HERBAL MEDICINE; MEDICINAL PLANTS.)

millet (*Panicum miliaceum*)   A cereal GRAIN that is a food STAPLE in parts of India, Africa, China and elsewhere. Millet has been cultivated since prehistoric times in regions of North Africa and Central Asia, though its origin is obscure. Most millet is produced in Asia and Africa. In Europe and the United States millet is grown mainly as forage for poultry and as a bird feeder. Pearle millet, the major type produced for human consumption, is sold as whole grain and can be cooked like other grains.

Millet contains an average of 10 to 12% PROTEIN. While its protein is superior to that of WHEAT or CORN in terms of content of essential AMINO ACIDS, it nonetheless contains less than half the amount of the essential amino acid LYSINE that is found in high-quality protein sources such as meat. Millet lacks GLUTEN, the wheat protein that makes dough prepared from wheat flour elastic; thus millet flour is not suitable for leavened breads. Millet flour is used in making flat cakes and breads. The whole grain is used in soups, stews or as a cooked cereal; millet is also popped, roasted or sprouted. It is used in steamed dishes and deep-fried doughs. Millet (cooked, 1/2 cup, 95 g) provides 54 calories; protein, 1.4 g; carbohydrate, 10.8 g; fiber, 1.3 g; iron, 1.1 g; thiamin, 0.1 mg; riboflavin, 0.06 mg; niacin, 0.4 mg. (See also AMARANTH; BUCKWHEAT; QUINOA; RICE; SORGHUM.)

milligram   A metric measure of weight equivalent to one one-thousandth of a gram; 28 grams equal one ounce. (See also MEASURES.)

milliliter   A metric measure of volume, equivalent to one one-thousandth liter, which is roughly one quart. A milliliter is about one-thirtieth of an ounce. (See also MEASURES.)

mineralocorticoids   Hormones of the ADRENAL GLANDS (adrenal cortex) that regulate WATER and SODIUM excretion in urine. ALDOSTERONE is the primary mineralocorticoid: It increases the recovery of sodium in KIDNEY tubules while losing POTASSIUM. An increase in blood potassium level and a large increase in blood sodium stimulate mineralocorticoid release. The pituitary regulates mineralocorticoid release from the adrenals via the hormone corticotropin. Mineralocorticoid deficiency leads to excessively dilute urine (DIABETES INSIPIDUS), severe dehydration and fluid imbalances, because of the body's inability to concentrate urine. Diabetes insipidus causes the danger of severe DEHYDRATION and ELECTROLYTE imbalance.

Symptoms of mineralocorticoid insufficiency include muscle weakness, abnormal cardiac function and hypertension. LICORICE root has MINERAL corticoid activity; licorice extract is used in some licorice candy and chewing tobacco. (See also FLUID BALANCE; GLUCOCORTICOID.)

mineral oil   See LAXATIVE.

minerals   Inorganic (non-carbon containing) NUTRIENTS. Minerals are elements remaining after a food is burned completely to ash. Minerals cannot be formed in the body and must be obtained from the diet. Mineral nutrients are either positively charged (cations) or negatively charged (ANIONS). Cations are derived from metals, including CALCIUM, cobalt, CHROMIUM, COPPER, IRON, MAGNESIUM, MANGANESE, MOLYBDENUM (as molybdate), POTASSIUM, SELENIUM (as selenate), SODIUM and ZINC. Non-metallic elements yield anions: IODINE as iodide; sulfur as sulfate; phosphorus as phosphate; chlorine as CHLORIDE; and fluorine as FLUORIDE. Combinations of anions and cations yield salts such as sodium chloride, calcium phosphate and sodium iodide.

Minerals serve diverse functions. They provide the building blocks of teeth and bones and are components of connective tissue. They activate enzymes and are responsible for the transmission of nerve impulses and muscle contraction. They help regulate physiologic processes like the pH (hydrogen ion concentration) and blood volume.

The body requires at least 21 different minerals. Seven of these are required in large amounts and are classified as "major" minerals, or macrominerals. The amounts of macrominerals required daily range from a fraction of a gram to several grams. Calcium, phosphate and magnesium are bone builders and metabolic helpers. Potassium, sodium, sulfate and chloride are the major electrolytes (ions) in body fluids. These ions help regulate the acid-base balance of body fluids and balance charged chemicals in the blood. They are partially responsible for osmotic pressure in blood vessels and cells.

TRACE MINERALS, or microminerals, are needed in much smaller amounts. The levels needed per day vary from micrograms (millionths of a gram) to milligrams (thousandths of a gram). Trace minerals include cobalt, iron, manganese, copper, selenium, molybdenum and zinc, which assist the action of enzymes. Chromium and iodine play roles in hormone function, while fluoride helps build teeth and bones. Other trace minerals, including BORON, SILICON and VANADIUM, play unspecified roles.

Macrominerals and trace minerals originate in soil and water. Essential minerals can be depleted by intensive cultivation of a single crop year after year. On the other hand, over-fertilizing can kill microorganisms needed to make soil minerals soluble for crop uptake or alter the chemical composition of the soil so that certain minerals become insoluble and cannot be taken up readily. Soils may be naturally deficient in cobalt, copper, molybdenum and phosphorus; other soils contain excessive amounts of selenium, yielding high-selenium grains and forage. Water supplies contain minerals. "Hard" water contains calcium, magnesium and sometimes iron and fluoride, and "soft" water contains more sodium and potassium and less calcium, magnesium and iron. Drinking water can therefore provide significant amounts of minerals.

Mineral Antagonists in Food

Excessive plant FIBER can bind minerals in food, thus limiting their efficient absorption. CELLULOSE and HEMICELLULOSE, from BRAN, fruits and vegetables, and LIGNIN may increase excretion of calcium, potassium, zinc and other minerals. PHYTIC ACID, a phosphorus-containing compound present in the outer layers of grains, binds calcium, iron and zinc. In terms of supplementation, excessive amounts of one mineral can inhibit the uptake or upset the metabolism of another; zinc and copper, calcium and phosphorous, magnesium and calcium, iron and copper are examples of minerals that can compete with each other. (See also MALABSORPTION.)

minimal daily requirement (MDR)   An outdated reference for judging the adequacy of nutrient intake that is now seldom used. The MDR is based on a model developed in the 1940s that a minimal amount of a vitamin is required to prevent a full-blown vitamin deficiency disease. The MDR is not suitable for either meal planning or DIET analysis.

The MDR is not equivalent to the RDA (RECOMMENDED DIETARY ALLOWANCE), which correlates with the amount of a nutrient estimated to be necessary to maintain the health of most Americans. The RDA was developed to replace the MDR and is used in diet planning and analysis of groups of people. (See also RECOMMENDED DAILY INTAKE; USRDA.)

mitochondria   Small particles that function as the cell's powerhouse to produce energy. Most cells (except red blood cells) contain between 50 and several thousand mitochondria. Mitochondria oxidize nutrients with molecular oxygen and trap ENERGY as chemical energy, ATP, in a process called cellular RESPIRATION. Mitochondria provide more than 95% of ATP required by cells. ATP is a "high energy" compound universally used by organisms to drive biosynthetic reactions and energy-requiring processes like muscle contraction, conduction of nerve impulses, cell division and the transport of nutrients into cells. Fuel molecules are oxidized in a sequence of chemical reaction to carbon dioxide and water. These oxidation steps account for more than 90% of the oxygen used by cells.

Mitochondria contain complex enzyme systems to extract usable energy from fat, carbohydrate and protein. The KREB'S CYCLE is the central oxidation pathway to completely degrade fat (FATTY ACIDS) and the simple sugar GLUCOSE from STARCH to carbon dioxide. Electrons derived from the oxidation reactions pass through the mitochondrial ELECTRON TRANSPORT CHAIN (also called the terminal respiratory chain) to generate ATP. Cytochromes ultimately donate the electrons to oxygen, a process yielding metabolic water.

Mitochondria also provide the cell with raw materials for other molecules. For example, a metabolic acid, OXALOACETIC ACID, from the Kreb's cycle can be used to manufacture glucose when needed by the liver (GLUCONEOGENESIS). Part of urea synthesis also occurs in mitochondria. Urea is the end-product of protein metabolism. Breakdown products of glucose oxidation (acetyl coenzyme A) can be shunted from mitochondria to the CYTOPLASM to be used for fatty acid and cholesterol synthesis.

Mitochondria possess protein-synthesizing machinery of their own. Mitochondria contain their own DNA as well. Certain rare defects in mitochondrial DNA can cause defects in energy metabolism of muscles (myopathies). Mitochondria are susceptible to sustained free radical damage; mitochondrial DNA exhibits tenfold higher oxidative damage than nuclear DNA. This correlates with a higher mutation rate of mitochondrial DNA. Furthermore there is an estimated 25-fold increase in mitochondrial DNA damage in the brain with age. Hypothetically, such change could be linked to neurodegenerative disease. Because mitochondria represent the major energy production sites of cells, mitochondrial damage and decreased ATP production could compromise homeostatic mechanisms that keep the body functioning normally, limiting its adaptation to stress. This could be a factor in chronic fatigue. (See also AMINO ACID METABOLISM; CARBOHYDRATE METABOLISM; OXIDATIVE PHOSPHORYLATION; PEROXISOME.)

Shigenaga, M.K. and Ames, B.N., "Oxidants and Mitochondrial Decay in Aging, in *Natural Antioxidants in Human Health and Disease*, Frei, Balz, ed. San Diego: Academic Press, 1994. pp. 63–106.

modified cornstarch (*derivatized starch*)   A FOOD ADDITIVE used as a thickener. Cornstarch has traditionally been used, but chemically modified cornstarch is more stable and is often used in processed and frozen foods. Short-term safety studies with lab animals have indicated no harmful effects of derivatized starches, and the effects of lifetime exposures are unknown. Before 1985 modified starch was used extensively in baby foods. Much of the industry has reformulated its products without any added starches. (See also INFANT FORMULAS.)

molasses   A thick syrup that is a by-product of cane or beet sugar manufacture. Molasses contains high levels of table sugar (SUCROSE). Because it is less pure than table sugar it contains small amounts of other materials such as TRACE MINERALS and VITAMINS. Nonetheless molasses is classified as a refined SWEETENER and provides primarily CARBOHYDRATE-TYPE CALORIES. Blackstrap molasses, the least refined type of molasses, provides variable amounts of iron and chromium. When cane juice is evaporated to remove excess water, sugar crystallizes and solid sugar can be removed. Blackstrap molasses is the molasses remaining after repeated boilings and removal of crystallized sugar. Most molasses produced in the United States is used in animal feed, in yeast production and in fermentation processes such as rum production. The baking industry uses molasses to impart flavor and to maintain freshness in baked goods. It is also used to flavor caramel candy. In home cooking molasses is also used in baked beans and in glazes on sweet potatoes and HAM. Nutrient contents of 100 g. of medium molasses is 250 calories; protein, 2.4 g; carbohydrate, 60 g; calcium, 290 mg; potassium, 1,063 mg; iron, 6 mg; thiamin, 0.10 mg; riboflavin, 0.10 mg; niacin, 1.2 mg. (See also NATURAL SWEETENERS.)

mold   A type of fungi that degrades stored food and causes spoilage. Molds in the home or workplace may cause environmental sensitivity. Molds characteristically form a network of filaments or threads (mycelium) and spore masses. Some molds produce toxic materials called mycotoxins. Moldy grain can be hazardous because of the production of such toxins, which are linked to cancer and have caused death in many livestock who have ingested moldy corn. Moldy wheat contains toxins called trichothecenes that apparently weaken the immune system and increase susceptibility to disease. One of these (deoxynivalenol) has been studied extensively. Low levels have been reported in common U.S. foods such as BREAKFAST CEREAL, BREAD and even baby food. The U.S. FDA has suggested limiting the level to one part per million in wheat; Canada, Rumania and Russia have set limits for this type of mycotoxin in grain.

The most widely studied mycotoxin is AFLATOXIN, a toxin that causes liver cancer in animals. It is produced by a storage mold that infests damp grains. Aflatoxin is formed by peanuts and corn contaminated by the mold ASPERGILLUS. Aflatoxin does not contaminate sweetcorn, such as frozen corn. Among PEANUT butters, aflatoxin contamination is found to be highest in the fresh, ground varieties. Animal feed ingredients are major sources of aflatoxin in other foods. The amount of aflatoxin permitted by the U.S. FDA in foods is 20 parts per billion, although levels as low as one part per billion cause cancer in experimental animals. Its toxicity in humans is less well established. Still other molds produce the toxin ochratoxin A, which is linked to kidney cancer in lab animals. Surveys have found low levels in a tiny percent of wheat samples. The United States and Canada have not set legal limits for this toxin.

To limit exposure to moldy foods, do not eat any moldy, shriveled or discolored nuts or any nuts that taste bad. In general, discard moldy food, rather than cutting out the moldy section. Molds and fungi send out filaments beyond the immediately obvious moldy area; thus toxins may remain in the food. Aflatoxin is not destroyed by cooking. (See also CANDIDA ALBICANS; FUNGUS.)

molecule   A stable assembly of atoms, tightly bonded together in a predictable fashion. Most NUTRIENTS and components of cells are either molecules or groups of molecules. A few simple molecules play key roles. Thus WATER, which possesses only three atoms, is the most common molecule of the body. OXYGEN (with two atoms) is required to burn fuels in the body for energy production. Somewhat larger molecules include fuels like sugars (GLUCOSE with 24 atoms) and FATTY ACIDS (56 atoms for stearic acid). Vitamins are somewhat more complex molecules, roughly 10 to 30 times larger than water molecules. The most complex molecules are very long chains (polymers) of simple molecules bound together. Thus 20 AMINO ACIDS, the building blocks of protein, are linked together like beads on a chain; proteins are typically chains of 50 to 1,000 amino acids. Thousands of glucose molecules are linked to form STARCH. RNA and DNA, the cellular machinery for manufacturing protein and for storing genetic information, are chains of simple molecular building blocks composed of phosphate, simple sugars called ribose or deoxyribose, and just four nitrogen-containing ring compounds. Lipids such as CHOLESTEROL and fat are other common molecules constructed from simple raw materials, in this case the simple acid, ACETIC ACID. Inorganic compounds formed by MINERALS are not classified as molecules because they separate into separate charged fragments called ions when dissolved in body fluids. (See also CYTOPLASM; METABOLITE.)

molybdenum   A trace mineral NUTRIENT present in all body tissues. Only minute amounts of this mineral are required for health. Molybdenum possibly helps to retard DEGENERATIVE DISEASES, CANCER and AGING. A molybdenum-containing enzyme of the liver (sulfite oxidase) destroys SULFITE, used as a preservative in foods and drugs. In this role molybdenum acts as a detoxification agent. The production of URIC ACID from the degradation of purines (building blocks of RNA and DNA) requires molybdenum.

Good sources of molybdenum include LIVER, whole GRAINS, green leafy vegetables and LEGUMES. A recommended dietary allowance has not been determined for molybdenum, and the requirement for optimal health is not known. A safe and adequate daily intake for adults is estimated to be 75 to 250 mcg. People who rely on a diet of refined and processed foods, who have high levels of uric acid and are prone to GOUT-like symptoms, or who are copper deficient can potentially be deficient in this TRACE MINERAL. High copper intake antagonizes molybdenum uptake; very high levels of molybdenum increase copper losses. (See also MINERALS.)

monoglycerides   Food additive oils used to improve the taste of margarine. Monoglycerides are normal products of fat digestion and occur in foods, where they comprise about 1% of normal fat intake. PEANUT butter contains small amounts of monoglycerides (and the related diglycerides), which contain zero fatty acids rather than a single fatty acid chain. Monoglyceride is also used to make cakes fluffier by trapping air bubbles and helps prevent BREAD from becoming stale.

Monoglyceride derivatives are also used in processed foods. Ethoxylated monoglyceride is a dough conditioner. Acetylated monoglyceride, a waxy substance, is used as a coating on jelly beans and in chocolate coatings on frozen desserts. (See also FOOD ADDITIVES; LIPIDS.)

monosodium glutamate (MSG)   A flavor enhancer for MEAT, POULTRY, SEAFOOD and VEGETABLES, especially in Oriental foods, restaurant foods and processed foods. MSG is a form of the common amino acid glutamic acid, which the body synthesizes and obtains from the diet. Glutamic acid is a product of digestion of food proteins. The body uses glutamic acid as a fine-tuner of brain function, as well as a protein building block.

Producers frequently add MSG to seasoned salt, soy sauce, BOUILLON, gravy mixes, meat bases, cheese dips, CRACKERS, dried and canned soups, pre-cooked and frozen packaged foods, mayonnaise and salad dressing. MSG is frequently added to processed foods like frozen entrees, FRANKFURTERS and canned meat. Present labeling laws require manufacturers to list monosodium glutamate when it is added to foods. Although HYDROLYZED VEGETABLE PROTEIN can contain from 8 to 40% MSG, when added to foods, the label can simply note "natural flavor" or "natural flavoring," without mentioning the MSG content. The U.S. FDA has proposed that the phrase "contains glutamate" be added to labels following hydrolyzed protein in ingredient lists.

Side Effects

This is a controversial area. MSG has long been considered a safe food additive. However, the long-term effects of consuming many grams of MSG are unknown. The amount of MSG in a bowl of won ton soup (3 g) can cause a reaction in sensitive people. Excessive MSG may cause MSG RELATED SYNDROME (Chinese restaurant syndrome) with transient symptoms like numbness of chest, back and neck, worsening of ASTHMA, tingling or burning sensation, heart palpitations, anxiety, frequent urination, thirst, stomach ache or vomiting. MSG reactions generally pass shortly after they are induced. (See also FLAVOR ENHANCERS; FOOD ADDITIVES; FOOD PROCESSING.)

Blaylock, Russell L. *Excitotoxins, the Taste That Kills.* Santa Fe, N.M.: Health Press, 1994.

monounsaturated oils (*monounsaturates*, oleic oils)
A type of plant oil that is more healthful than saturated FATS. The most common monounsaturates include OLIVE OIL, AVOCADO oil, ALMOND oil, CANOLA OIL (a form of rapeseed oil) and certain SUNFLOWER oils. The latter two oils come from hybrid plants whose oils closely resemble olive oil. In terms of their chemical makeup, monounsaturated oils contain predominantly monounsaturated FATTY ACIDS, which simply lack a pair of hydrogen atoms and contain one double bond. These oils contain comparatively less polyunsaturated fatty acids and saturated fatty acids than other oils. As an example, olive oil contains 72% monounsaturated and 9% polyunsaturated fatty acids, while avocado oil and almond oil contain 69% and 68% monounsaturated fatty acids, respectively.

Monounsaturated oils have been recommended as safer and more healthful cooking oils than other oils and fats. They help lower blood CHOLESTEROL, LDL-cholesterol (LOW-DENSITY LIPOPROTEIN, the less desirable kind of cholesterol), while maintaining—or slightly increasing—HDL-cholesterol (HIGH-DENSITY LIPOPROTEIN, the desirable kind of cholesterol). Monounsaturates resist rancidity. When heated during cooking, monounsaturates form fewer FREE RADICALS, highlyreactive chemical fragments, than do POLYUNSATURATED OILS like safflower oil or corn oil. When reading food labels, look for the words "oleic oil, monounsaturated" and "unrefined" as a guide to those oils resembling olive oil. (See also HYDROGENATED VEGETABLE OIL; VEGETABLE OIL.)

mood   See FOOD AND THE NERVOUS SYSTEM.

mouth   The oral cavity. The mouth is defined by four structures: the hard palate, the boney structure that is the roof of the mouth; the soft palate, the arch-shaped structure at the back of the mouth composed of muscle; the uvula, the cone-shaped structure hanging down from the soft palate; and the tongue and its muscles, which form the floor of the mouth.

The teeth and the tongue are accessory structures of the mouth. The tongue functions to move chewed food to the back of the mouth. It has a characteristic rough surface due to small structures called papillae. Taste buds are microscopic nerve endings within the papillae.

Teeth are locked into the socket of the lower and upper jaw. By the time a person reaches the age of 17 to 24 he or she will usually have a full set of 32 teeth. The function of biting off pieces of food and pulverizing it during chewing is aided by saliva, fluid secreted by glands in or around the mouth. Up to a liter of saliva is secreted daily to lubricate food particles and to initiate starch digestion. (See also: DIGESTIVE TRACK; ESOPHAGUS; STOMACH.)

MSG Related Syndrome (Chinese restaurant syndrome)   A reaction to food seasoned with MONOSODIUM GLUTAMATE (MSG). MSG is widely used as a FLAVOR ENHANCER in processed foods, meat, poultry, seafood and vegetables, especially in Oriental cooking. Excessive MSG can be associated with symptoms in susceptible people: a tingling or burning sensation (face, upper back, neck or arms); heart palpitations; anxiety, excessive urination and thirst, stomachache, vomiting; attacks mimicking epileptic seizures in children; asthma and possibly depression. Migraine headaches can result from consumption of food treated with MSG. Generally the symptoms are transitory and do not occur when MSG is avoided. Women are more likely to experience this syndrome than men.

The details of how MSG causes these effects are not known. Caffeine and vitamin B$_6$ may counteract the effects in some people. Some research suggests that MSG related syndrome is the result of histamines found in shrimp paste, soy sauce and other fermented flavorings. It is very important for individuals who develop tightness of the chest should seek medical advice, to be certain more serious problems are not overlooked. (See also FOOD ADDITIVES.)

Tarasoff L. and Kelly M. F., "Monosodium L-glutamate: a Double-blind Study and Review," *Food and Chemical Toxicology*, 31:12 (1993), pp. 1019–1035.

mucopolysaccharide   See GLYCOSAMINOGLYCANS.

mucous membrane   The tissue lining the tubular surfaces within the body such as the lungs, digestive tract, urinary tract and reproductive tract. The mucous membrane includes a supporting, connective tissue layer (*Lamina propria*) and layers of smooth muscle. Frequently it is covered by a layer of MUCUS to form a front-line defense against potential toxic agents. Mucous membranes of the digestive tract both protect the body against foreign intruders and selectively absorb nutrients. They provide a capillary network and a network of lymphatic vessels to distribute the absorbed nutri-

ents. Certain regions of mucous membranes are further specialized with GLANDS that secrete mucus, DIGESTIVE ENZYMES and MINERALS, and binding factors for nutrient assimilation and hormones. The mucosal surface of the small intestine is highly folded to provide an extensive surface area to increase nutrient absorption. (See also DIGESTION; MICROVILLI; VILLI.)

mucus A slippery, sticky secretion from the mucous glands of moist surfaces within the body. Mucus also lubricates food particles, assisting in their smooth movement through the digestive tract. Mucus forms a thick barrier and protects the lining of the stomach from strong stomach acid, and protects the INTESTINE from toxic materials and disease-causing microorganisms. (See also DIGESTIVE TRACT; SALIVA.)

muffin A small, round bread traditionally eaten at breakfast. Muffins are now eaten for lunch, dinner and for snacks. They are frequently high-CALORIE, high-FAT foods, however, and the fat content can range from less than 0.5 g to 16 g. The percentage of calories from fat can range from less than 2% to more than 50%. A majority of commercially available muffins incorporate HYDROGENATED VEGETABLE OIL. Such oils are "saturated"; excessive saturated fat is linked to an increased risk of CARDIOVASCULAR DISEASE. Diet guidelines call for Americans to decrease their consumption of saturated fat from all sources. CHOLESTEROL in muffins comes from whole MILK, whole eggs and lard (when used). A muffin made from whole eggs may contain 20 mg of cholesterol. Fat-free muffins are usually made with egg whites and non-fat milk or skim milk in place of whole eggs and whole milk.

To minimize fat, sodium and cholesterol contributed by muffins:

- Do not eat muffins listing sugar or fat (oil or shortening) as the first or second ingredient. Cheese and chocolate additions increase calories.
- Select fat-free muffins. Muffins using CANOLA OIL, SUN-FLOWER oil and the like are preferable to hydrogenated fat.
- Muffins made from whole grain flour, BRAN, FRUIT and vegetables are generally more healthful.

Nutrient contents for a commercial blueberry muffin (45 g) are 140 calories; protein, 2.7 g; carbohydrate, 22 g; fiber, 1.25 g; fat, 4.9 g; cholesterol, 45 mg; sodium, 225 g; thiamin, 0.11 mg; riboflavin, 0.13 mg; niacin, 1.17 mg (See also BISCUIT; CRACKER.)

multiple sclerosis See AUTOIMMUNE DISEASES.

mung bean (*Phaseolus aureus*) A LEGUME usually consumed in America as bean sprouts. Mung beans probably originated in India and were cultivated in China and Southeast Asia for centuries. More recently, mung beans were introduced into Africa, the West Indies and the United States. India and Pakistan account for most of the world production. In India and Pakistan mung bean flour is prepared from dried beans. For sprouting, moistened beans are allowed to begin growing (germinate) in the dark for four to seven days. A pound (0.45 kg) of mung beans yields 6 to 8 pounds of sprouts (2.7 to 3.6 kg). Sprouts are used in salads or can be stir-fried with CELERY, green PEPPER, beans, ONIONS,

MEAT, FISH or POULTRY. Sprouts can be used in quiches, chow mein and chop suey. Nutrient content of 1 cup of mung beans (104 g) is: 32 calories; protein, 3 g; carbohydrate, 6 g; fiber, 0.84 g; vitamin A, 22 retinol equivalents; thiamin, 0.09 mg; riboflavin, 0.13 mg; niacin, 0.78 mg; vitamin C, 14 mg.

muscle Tissues of the body whose cells have the ability to contract, and therefore to perform physical work. Muscles contract or relax in response to nerve impulses.

Muscle cells shorten their elongated form through the action of contractile proteins called MYOSIN and actin. This complex process utilizes ATP as the energy source; actin interacts with myosin, CALCIUM and ATP. Myosin is the major component of muscle filaments. ATP supplies the energy for contraction of actin-myosin filaments. Energy liberated from ATP is responsible for work and the generation of heat associated with chemical work.

The three basic muscle types are the smooth muscles (found in the walls of internal organs) like the digestive tract and blood vessels; cardiac muscles of the walls of the heart; and skeletal muscles, which are attached to bones.

Smooth muscles surround most internal organs such as the gastrointestinal tract and even blood vessels. Neither smooth muscles nor cardiac muscles can be consciously controlled.

Skeletal muscles are attached to the 206 bones of the body. Their contraction and relaxation determine the movement of the body. They are voluntary; that is, they are consciously controlled. Under the microscope skeletal muscles are banded; hence they are also called striated muscles. Nerve impulses stimulate skeletal cells to contract. Muscles require a rich supply of nutrients and oxygen from the bloodstream; they also require efficient waste elimination and an efficient cooling system. An abundant supply of blood to muscle cells meets both requirements.

The amount of ATP in skeletal muscle available at a given moment permits vigorous physical activity lasting only a few seconds. Therefore ATP must be regenerated within the muscle cell. Unlike other tissues of the body, skeletal muscles alternate between periods of inactivity and great activity. To help meet these needs, they contain a high energy molecule called phosphocreatine, which is used to supplement ATP for a few more seconds. Phosphocreatine and ATP combined provide enough energy for muscles to contract maximally for only about 15 seconds. Therefore ATP must be replenished by the oxidation of fuels. One of these fuels is the simple sugar GLUCOSE, which is available from blood glucose or it is released from muscle GLYCOGEN, the storage form of glucose. During strenuous EXERCISE, when the need for ATP exceeds the oxidative capacity of the muscle, muscles break down glucose to LACTIC ACID to produce ATP without the participation of oxygen. Lactic acid diffuses out of muscle cells to be absorbed by the bloodstream. During starvation skeleton muscle is degraded to amino acids, which are converted to glucose by the liver to fuel the brain.

Fatty acids absorbed from the bloodstream represent the second major energy source. During low to moderate exercise, fatty acids supply half the energy required by skeletal muscles. Fat becomes the major fuel during medium to intense exercise, lasting more than 1.5 hours; thus fat can supply as much as 70% of the calories needed during moderate exercise lasting four to six hours. (See also AEROBIC; CARBOHYDRATE METABOLISM; GLYCOLYSIS; OXYGEN DEBT; STARVATION.)

mushroom (Basidiomycetes, Ascomycetes) A diverse family of fungi sometimes used as food. Basidiomycetes represent certain club fungi characterized by fleshy fruiting bodies (toadstools). They grow in soil containing organic matter and also can grow on living trees or on dead wood. Cup fungi (Ascomycetes) such as truffles are also often classified as mushrooms.

Together Basidiomycetes and Ascomycetes represent about 10,000 species of mushrooms. Currently about 30,000 tons of mushrooms are harvested commercially each year in the United States. The five most popular cultivated mushrooms are: *Agaricus bisporus*, which is the light-colored, mild mushroom most common to Americans. Oyster mushrooms (*Pleurotus ostreatus*) resemble oysters in shape and color. The oyster mushroom is common in the Far East and in Europe. Padi straw mushrooms (*Volvariella volvaeae*) are produced in the Orient where they are grown in rice paddies and are usually sold dried. Truffles (*Tuber melanosporum*) are the most expensive mushrooms. This cup FUNGUS grows underground in association with beech and oak trees. Truffles are produced primarily in France and Italy.

Shiitake (*Letinus edodes*) has a smoky flavor and grows on hardwood logs. It is grown mainly in China and Japan and is exported in canned, dried or pickled forms. Shirtake is also currently grown in California. These mushrooms can be stir-fried or sauteed with onions. Other popular types of mushroom include wood ears and portabellos.

Several wild mushrooms are popular. Chanterelles are deep yellow-orange. A versatile mushroom, chanterelles are used in soups, casseroles and stews. The Morel has a nutty flavor. This mushroom is shaped like a pine cone. Use it in soups, casseroles, stews and sauteed dishes.

Raw mushrooms contain hydrazines, substances shown to cause cancer in experimental animals. Many hydrazines can be eliminated or destroyed by cooking or drying.

Poisonous mushrooms There is no completely foolproof way of distinguishing safe from unsafe wild mushrooms; many wild varieties are poisonous. The severity of mushroom poisoning varies with the amount and the type of mushroom eaten, as well as with the season. As a rule of thumb, if symptoms appear within two hours after eating the mushroom, the illness probably will not be severe. If symptoms develop more than two hours after eating the mushroom, emergency treatment may be required.

Nutrient content of common mushrooms (1/2 cup, cooked from raw, 78 g) is 21 calories; protein, 1.7 g; carbohydrate, 1.6 g; fiber, 0.77 g; potassium, 278 mg; thiamin, 0.06 mg; riboflavin, 0.23 mg; niacin, 3.5 mg. (See also AMANITA; MOLD.)

Leibenstein, Margaret. *The Edible Mushroom.* Old Saybrook, Conn.: Globe Pequot, 1993.

mustard A popular condiment prepared from ground mustard seeds. White mustard (*Brassica hirta*), brown mustard (*Brassica nigra*) and Ethiopian mustard (*Brassica carinata*) are used in the United States. Brown mustard is also known as Indian mustard; it is grown for its leaves as well as for its seeds. These species originated in different regions of Eurasia: White mustard apparently came from the eastern Mediterranean; brown mustard from India; black mustard from Asia Minor; Ethiopian mustard is a hybrid. Brown mustard has been used for at least 5,000 years. Mustard powder is ground mustard seed; it is also marketed as a paste.

The hot ingredients are liberated by enzymatic action when mustard powder is moistened. The typical condiment is a mixture of mustard seed powder, salt, vinegar and SPICES, and it may contain wine and acidic preservatives (tartaric acid and CITRIC ACID). Though low in CALORIES, the commercial product is high in SODIUM. In folk medicine mustard is used in a poultice to relieve lung congestion due to colds and to relieve the pain associated with arthritis. Mustard can irritate the skin of some people.

mustard greens (*Brasicca juncea*) A dark-green leafy vegetable. These cooking greens belong to the cabbage family and resemble kale. Oriental mustard greens are a milder tasting variety. Mustard greens are cooked before eating; steaming and sauteeing are common methods of preparation. The greens can be served with cheese or white sauce. Alternatively, the greens can be included in casseroles, omelets or soups. Mustard greens provide (cooked, 1 cup) 21 calories; protein, 3.2 g; carbohydrate, 2.9 g; fiber, 2.9 g; calcium, 104 mg; iron, 1.7 mg; vitamin A, 424 retinol equivalents; thiamin, 0.06 mg; riboflavin, 0.09 mg; niacin, 0.61 mg.

mutagen Agents that produce permanent changes in gene structure. Mutagens alter genes by chemically altering the structure of DNA, the genetic material of cells. They produce new traits, passed from one generation to the next. Most mutagens are also CANCER-causing agents (CARCINOGENS). Sample mutagens include tobacco smoke, asbestos, PESTICIDES, industrial chemicals like formaldehyde and vinylchloride, and solvents like benzene. Some mutagens occur in food naturally. Examples include hydrazines in mushrooms. Grilled, fried or broiled fish, poultry and meat contain mutagens. Other types of mutagenic agents include ultraviolet light, X rays, gamma rays and radiation from radon seepage into basements from soil.

Certain substances are not themselves mutagens; rather they are converted to mutagens in the body. NITRITE, a food preservative, is converted in the stomach to NITROSOAMINES, reactive nitrogen-containing compounds that are mutagens and carcinogens. Benzopyrene in soot deposited on BARBECUED MEAT and certain pesticides are activated by the liver to highly reactive compounds that can attack DNA and cause mutations.

Bruger, M.P.M., et al., "Cigarette Smoking and Human Papillomavirus in Patients with Reported Cervical Cytological Abnormality," *British Journal of Medicine*, 306 (March 20, 1993), pp. 749–52.

mutation A permanent alteration in the structure of DNA, the genetic material of a cell. The alterations in DNA can be passed on from one generation to the next unless repaired. Cells possess elaborate mechanisms to repair damaged DNA by environmental influences (mutagens) as well as within cells by wear and tear. One theory of AGING proposes that, over time, an individual's DNA repair system becomes less capable of performing its task and DNA damage accumulates, leading ultimately to CANCER. Appropriate nutrition can support DNA synthesis and repair, as well as minimizing the impact of agents that can cause mutations. Key to countering the latter agents are ANTIOXIDANTS, compounds that either destroy highly reactive chemicals called FREE RADICALS or prevent further oxidative damage. Antioxidant nutrients include VITAMIN C, VITAMIN E and BETA CAROTENE (pro-vitamin A), as well as SELENIUM and other TRACE MINERALS. (See CANCER PREVENTION DIET; GENE.)

myelin (myelin sheath)   The fatty material that covers certain nerve fibers and acts as an insulator. Many axons (cytoplasmic extensions of nerve cells) lying beyond the brain and spinal cord are surrounded by this multiple-layered, lipid-rich segmented covering. Myelin increases the speed of nerve impulse conduction and helps maintain the integrity of the axon. Myelin is responsible for the white color of nerve tissue. Myelin contains complex lipids called sphingomyelin as well as PHOSPHOLIPIDS such as LECITHIN. Vitamin B_{12} is essential for healthy myelin; severe vitamin B_{12} deficiency can lead to irreversible nerve damage. Diseases like multiple sclerosis are related to myelin destruction. (See also AUTOIMMUNE DISEASES; NERVOUS SYSTEM; NEUROTRANSMITTER.)

myosin   The major protein responsible for muscle contraction. It comprises about 65% of the total muscle protein. Myosin chains combine to form thick filaments (myofilaments). ATP is degraded by myosin; in the presence of CALCIUM, myosin shifts to a bent, low-energy configuration. This pulls along the attached actin chain (an intracellular protein chain), thus contracting muscle fibers. (See also EXERCISE.)

myxedema   A condition resulting from low THYROID function. Myxedema is characterized by a low basal metabolic rate (low rate of metabolism) and decreased heat production. The symptoms include apathy; exhaustion and chronic FATIGUE; drowsiness; sensitivity to cold; coarse, thickened skin; and EDEMA (swelling due to fluid accumulation). Myxedema can be caused by a deficiency of IODINE, atrophy of thyroid gland, or excessive use of anti-thyroid drugs. Depressed thyroid function can be due to autoimmune attack in the thyroid gland. (See also HYPOTHYROIDISM.)

naphthoquinone   See VITAMIN K.

narcotics   See ADDICTION.

National Cholesterol Education Program   See CHO-LESTEROL.

National Research Council (NRC)   The branch of the National Academy of Sciences that has as its mission to promote the effective use of scientific information and to advise the federal government on scientific and technical matters. The NRC provides services for following policies set by both the National Academy of Sciences and the National Academy of Engineering in meeting the needs of government, the public and scientists. It is administered by these academies, as well as by the Institute of Medicine.

Among the many responsibilities of the NRC is the development and evaluation of nutrient standards for good health. The Food and Nutrition Board of the NRC appointed a committee to draft the first RECOMMENDED DIETARY ALLOWANCES (RDAs) in 1941 and the first edition was published in 1943. Revised editions of the RDAs have generally appeared every five years. The most recent version (the 10th edition) was published in 1989. Dietary patterns emphasizing varieties of foods from different food groups are described in the Food and Nutrition Board's "Diet and Health," published as a basis for planning meals that especially meet the RDAs. (See also DIETARY GUIDELINES FOR AMERICANS; NUTRIENT; VITAMIN.)

National School Lunch Program   See SCHOOL LUNCH PROGRAM.

natural flavors   See FLAVORS.

natural food   Foods that have been minimally processed and grown without the use of synthetic fertilizers and pesticides. Other than for meat and poultry, the term "natural" has not been defined legally and therefore has many interpretations. The "natural" food label is a strong selling point, and food producers have capitalized on consumer interest. Thus the word "natural" may be used to describe PROCESSED FOODS and synthetic food and beverages, which sometimes are highly processed and contain preservatives and artificial coloring. A beverage labeled "natural" might be completely synthetic, with only the lemon flavor as a non-synthetic ingredient; a product labeled "Natural Juice Apple Pie" may indicate only the juice is natural. Read the fine print to determine what is behind the use of the word natural on a food label. Natural food also has the connotation of being free from additives like PRESERVATIVES, EMULSIFIERS and thickeners. Under current U.S. FDA regulations, an entire food cannot be labeled natural if it contains synthetic ingredients, ARTIFICIAL FLAVORS or ARTIFICIAL FOOD COLORS.

Natural Meat

According to the USDA, MEAT or poultry labeled "natural" has not been processed more than in usual kitchen practice. This refers to procedures that can be performed in the kitchen: washing, shredding, chipping, grating, grinding, chopping, mixing and cooking. Natural meat must come from animals raised without hormones or at least not exposed to feedlot growth stimulants (such as antibiotics) to fatten live-stock later than 60 days before slaughter. The "natural beef" label doesn't guarantee the meat is absolutely free of antibiotics and growth factors because some producers feed hormones and antibiotics up to 60 days before slaughter. This time may be inadequate to completely clear chemical residues from some animals. Natural beef represents perhaps 5% of all beef sold in the United States (1991). (See also FOOD ADDITIVES; ORGANIC FOODS.)

Steteville, Robert, "Organic Foods Find Growing Shelf Space," *Business*, May/June 1992, pp. 40–43.

natural sweeteners   Naturally occurring CARBOHY-DRATES or compounds related to SUGARS that are used as sweeteners. Carbohydrate sweeteners contribute 4 CALORIES per gram (less than half as much as fat). The most common are the simple sugars or materials that are primarily sugars: FRUCTOSE and high fructose corn syrup; GLUCOSE (known in the food industry as DEXTROSE); CORN SYRUP; various forms of SUCROSE, including MOLASSES, brown sugar, table sugar, turbinado sugar and cane sugar; BARLEY MALT; HONEY; fruit concentrates; and ground dates (date sugar). Amasake is a sweetener prepared from fermented rice. Each provides carbohydrate with only a few other nutrients; therefore the content of VITAMINS, minerals and FIBER, as compared to that found in whole foods, is low (EMPTY CALORIES).

Sugar alcohols taste sweet and are not as easily metabolized as sugars. MANNITOL, related to the sugar mannose, is poorly utilized. XYLITOL, derived from the sugar xylose, while degraded, contributes fewer calories than sugar. SORBITOL, related to sorbose, is the most widely used sugar alcohol and is only slowly absorbed by the intestine. Relative to table sugar, fructose is 1.7 times as sweet; glucose, 0.7; mannitol, 0.7; and sorbitol, 0.6.

Potential Problems with High Sugar Consumption

Undernutrition   Sugars supply empty calories because they provide low or negligible amounts of key nutrients. CARBOHYDRATE METABOLISM requires B vitamins like THIAMIN and minerals like ZINC, CHROMIUM and MAGNESIUM. Excessive concentrated sweeteners displace more nutritious food and increase the body's burden for these nutrients. Few people relying on a junk food diet increase their consumption of high-quality foods to make up the difference.

Overnutrition   Excessive consumption of sugar and refined carbohydrate represents excessive calories. Surplus calories are converted to FAT, regardless of their source. It should be noted that starches and sugars are not in themselves inherently fattening unless they represent excess calories.

Blood sugar imbalances   The excessive consumption of simple sugars and sucrose can cause BLOOD SUGAR levels to fluctuate. In contrast STARCHES in vegetables and legumes are often slowly digested and glucose is absorbed slowly, permitting a more balanced control of blood sugar.

Cavities   Excessive sugar consumption leads to more cavities and contributes to soaring dental costs.

U.S. DIETARY GUIDELINES FOR AMERICANS call for eating less sugar and more complex carbohydrate, starch and fiber (whole foods) as vegetables, fruits and legumes. The FOOD GUIDE PYRAMID, the most recent meal planning guideline, specifies eating sweets sparingly. (See also ADDICTION AND SUGAR; INVERT SUGAR; MAPLE SYRUP; NUTRIENT DENSITY; TEETH.)

Anderson, G.H. "Sugars, sweetness and food intake," *American Journal of Clinical Nutrition*, 62 (supp. 1; 1995), pp 195S–202S.
Wolever, T.M., Miller, J.B. "Sugars and blood glucose control," *American Journal of Clinical Nutrition*, 62 (supp. 1; 1995), pp. 212S–221S.

natural vitamins   See VITAMIN.

nectar   A FRUIT drink made with fruit juice and fruit pulp. Typical nectars are made from APRICOT, GUAVA, MANGO, PEACH and other fruit. Ingredients are specified by the STANDARDS OF IDENTITY established by the U.S. FDA. These are standard recipes long used by the food industry. Nectars include various combinations of fruit juice, SUGAR and other natural sweeteners, together with fruit puree, fruit pulp, VITAMIN C and CITRIC ACID. The term nectar also refers to a sweet, syrupy fluid secreted by flowers and collected by bees to produce HONEY.

nectarine (*Prunus persica*)   A subspecies of PEACH with a smooth skin and a distinctive flavor. The close similarity between nectarines and peaches is demonstrated by the fact that nectarines occasionally mutate to peaches and vice versa. Nectarines and peaches are believed to have originated in China. There are more than 150 different varieties of nectarine, differing slightly in taste, shape, size and skin coloring. Fantasia, Summer Grand, Royal Giant and May Grand are popular varieties. Presently the United States is a major producer, and California produces most of the domestic crop. Hard nectarines can be softened by storing them in a paper bag at room temperature for several days. The mature fruit does not get very much sweeter, but it can become softer and juicier.

Nutrient contents of one raw nectarine, without pit, is 67 calories; protein, 1.3 g; carbohydrate, 16 g; fiber, 3.13 g; fat, 0.6 g; potassium, 288 mg; vitamin A, 100 retinol equivalents; vitamin C, 7 mg; thiamin, 0.02 mg; riboflavin, 0.06 mg; niacin, 1.35 mg.

nephron   The functional unit of kidneys that filters the blood. The nephron further modifies filtered fluid from the blood to produce urine. Nephrons are composed of two structures: renal tubules and the glomerulus, a cluster of CAPILLARIES. WATER, MINERALS, GLUCOSE, VITAMINS, AMINO ACIDS, very small proteins, nitrogenous wastes and small molecules migrate from the capillaries of the glomerulus and enter the renal tubule, which draws urine from the kidneys.

As the filtrate moves down the tubules, nearly 99% of the water is reabsorbed into the blood. Only 1.5 liters (1%) leaves as urine daily. By reabsorbing most of the materials, the body can retain essential nutrients, while disposing of wastes like UREA. For example, normally all of the glucose filtered by the glomerulus is reabsorbed, thus maintaining blood glucose levels. So much liquid is filtered by the kidney that if nutrients were not reabsorbed back into the bloodstream, the blood would be drained of these materials within half an hour.

The region of the tubule adjacent to the capsule (proximal tubule) reabsorbs glucose, amino acids, SODIUM, CHLORIDE, BICARBONATE, POTASSIUM and water. Farther down the tubule, sodium, chloride, urea and water are reabsorbed. Sodium and water are controlled by the hormone ALDOSTERONE. The kidney releases potassium and AMMONIA to maintain ELECTROLYTE balance and water balance of the blood. In order to maintain blood pH close to 7.4 (neutral pH) and to maintain acid-base balance, sodium is reabsorbed while hydrogen ions are released.

The kidney plays a role in vitamin D metabolism as well. Tubules of the kidney activate VITAMIN D by converting a partially modified form (called hydroxycholecalciferol) to the fully active hormone, called calciferol. (See also GLOMERULAR FILTRATION.)

nervous system   A primary communication system consisting of the brain, spinal cord and nerve fibers radiating to all parts of the body. The brain and spinal cord occupy a central position in the body and are called the "central nervous system" (CNS). The nervous system transmits information via electrical nerve impulses conducted between nerve cells. Impulses are generated by changes in the body's internal or external environment.

Specialized cells of the nervous system are called neurons and neuroglia. Neuroglia are connective tissue cells supporting the neurons, while neurons are specialized cells of the nervous system that conduct nerve impulses. The nervous system is composed of billions of neurons. With age, neurons are progressively and irreversibly lost.

Sensory neurons transmit impulses to the spinal cord and brain from all regions of the body, while motoneurons transmit impulses away from the brain and spinal cord to muscles and glands. Interneurons lie within the gray matter of either the brain or spinal cord and conduct impulses from sensory neurons to motoneurons. A fatty layer called MYELIN insulates nerve fibers, bundles of neurons.

Neurons contain a cell body with nucleus, CYTOPLASM and MITOCHONDRIA. Each neuron possesses many dendrites, highly branched extensions of the cell body that are the "receiving" parts of neurons and conduct a nerve impulse toward the cell body; and an AXON, a single, long cytoplasmic extension that conducts nerve impulses away from the cell body to another cell. Axons contain mitochondria but no protein synthesizing machinery; they vary in length from a few millimeters up to a meter or more. The ends of axons terminate in bulb-like structures that store NEUROTRANSMITTERS. These chemicals determine whether an impulse will pass onto the next cell. Nerve fiber refers to any process projecting from the cell body. Typically, sensory neurons transmit impulses from the skin, sense organs, muscle joints and viscera to the spinal cord and the brain. Motoneurons convey impulses from the brain and spinal cord to either muscles or glands. Connecting neurons (intraneurons) carry impulses from sensory neurons to motor neurons and occur in the brain and spinal cord.

Many nutrients support nerve function, and the following minerals are critical. CALCIUM is required for nerve transmission; when blood calcium levels fall, nerves become hypersensitive, and the result is frozen muscles (tetany). High calcium concentrations depress nerve irritability. The amount of neurotransmitters (serotonin, acetylcholine, norepinephrine) released is proportional to the calcium concentration in the nerve terminus. POTASSIUM and SODIUM are important in nerve transmission. Stimulation of a nerve causes potassium to migrate out of the neuron and sodium to migrate inward, altering the membrane potential (electrical current) and conducting a nerve impulse down the axon.

Individual nerve cells communicate at specialized gaps called synapses by means of chemical messages called neurotransmitters. When a nerve impulse reaches the end of an axon it triggers the release of neurotransmitters that migrate across the gap and stimulate a nerve impulse or other response in the receiving cell. Neurotransmitters are often derived from AMINO ACIDS. Dopamine and norepinephrine are derived from the amino acid TYROSINE, while TRYPTOPHAN supplies SEROTONIN. Cholinergic nerve fibers release the neurotransmitter ACETYLCHOLINE and are derived from the nitrogen-containing nutrient CHOLINE.

The peripheral nervous system contains sensory nerves. These carry information from organs like the skin to the brain. Efferent (motor) nerve fibers carry impulses from the brain to specific regions such as skeletal muscles.

The autonomic nervous system adapts the body to change. It consists of two functional parts. The sympathetic nervous system responds to stress, and adaptations include dilation of bronchi and increased heart rate. The PARASYMPATHETIC NERVOUS SYSTEM returns the body to the normal, unstressed state, counterbalancing the sympathetic nervous system. It restores energy during rest and recuperation.

The average human brain weighs about 3 lbs (1.4 kg) and contains 11 billion cells. Although it represents only 2% of the total body weight, it consumes 20% to 30% of the GLUCOSE from digestion and CARBOHYDRATE METABOLISM. The thalamus of the forebrain is an egg-shaped mass that relays sensory information to other regions of the brain. It seems to help with concentration. Lying beneath the thalamus is the HYPOTHALAMUS, which regulates eating, drinking, sexual behavior, heat production and emotions. It also controls the ENDOCRINE SYSTEM, a system of hormone-secreting glands located throughout the body.

Twelve pairs of nerves are attached at the under surface of the brain. Several are important in regulating eating and digestion. Their fibers conduct pulses between the brain and the head, neck, thorax and abdominal cavity. The olfactory nerve is responsible for the sense of SMELL. The trigeminal nerve functions in the sensations involving the face, teeth and chewing (MASTICATION). The facial nerve is responsible for TASTE. The glossopharyngeal nerve controls taste, swallowing, salivation and sensations in the throat region. The vagus nerve also regulates swallowing, sensations of throat and larynx, and of the abdominal regions; for example, it regulates PERISTALSIS. The hypoglossal nerve regulates tongue movements (swallowing).

It is now known that brain peptides, such as ENDORPHINS, are synthesized in the intestine, while hormones bind to targets in the brain and affect its function. The nervous system can activate the immune system, while chemicals released by the immune response can affect the central nervous system. The gastrointestinal tract is surrounded by an elaborate network of nerves so that the stomach and intestines are directly linked to the brain. The ability of the digestive system to monitor food has important ramifications for WEIGHT MANAGEMENT, SATIETY and hunger. With the discovery that the hormonal system (endocrine system) as well as the immune system can affect the brain and alter behavior and mood, and that the nervous system can alter the immune response and hormone balance, has come a new appreciation of the interdependency of these three systems in maintaining a balance among all systems of the body (HOMEOSTASIS). This synthesis has spawned a new scientific discipline, psychoneuroimmunology.

In addition to supplying energy, primarily as glucose, food can alter the nervous system in important ways. One focus has been in the formation of neurotransmitters, chemicals manufactured by nerves to help transit nerve impulses. Two amino acids that serve as the raw materials for the manufacture of neurotransmitters are tryptophan and tyrosine. Tryptophan forms the neurotransmitter serotonin, used to regulate relaxation and sleepiness. Low blood levels of tryptophan are linked to depression, and some clinical studies suggest that tryptophan supplementation can lessen depression. Tryptophan tends to make normal people drowsy, and it has been sold as a mild sleep inducer. However, the U.S. FDA has banned its sale because of deaths associated with contaminated tryptophan. Foods low in protein and rich in carbohydrate can raise brain levels of tryptophan, probably because they stimulate the release of insulin, which lowers the blood levels of most amino acids, except for tryptophan. According to one hypothesis, tryptophan in the blood competes with more abundant, branched chain amino acids, which also possess lipid-like properties, for entry into the brain. The amount of tryptophan reaching the brain increases after eating starchy or sweet foods. On the other hand the more numerous amino acids can displace tryptophan for entry into the brain after eating a protein-rich meal. As a result, brain tryptophan levels may drop. The observation is that normal healthy adults can feel relaxed, sleepy or more calm or lethargic within two hours following a high-carbohydrate meal. Another possibility is that glucose from carbohydrate digestion can affect the brain's activity.

The amino acid tyrosine is converted to the neurotransmitter norepinephrine, which helps maintain mental alertness. The brain level of norepinephrine drops with stress. Tyrosine supplements may help combat fatigue and improve the ability to perform mental tasks. A light lunch or snack increases mental functioning and decreases the error rate in tasks, and seems to sharpen the mind.

Certain B vitamins help in the manufacture of serotonin and norepinephrine: vitamin B_6, vitamin B_{12} and folic acid. Deficiencies of any of these vitamins can promote depression, senility and decreased ability to concentrate. Correction of the B vitamin deficiency can ease these symptoms. Even in healthy elderly people without obvious deficiency symptoms, a lower level of folacin and vitamin B_{12} has corresponded to lower scores on reasoning tests. Surveys have shown that between 20 and 66% of healthy people over the age of 65 possess low levels of vitamin B_6, vitamin B_{12} and folic acid. (See also ADDICTION; DIGESTIVE TRACT; FOOD AND THE NERVOUS SYSTEM; MOUTH.)

Morgane, Peter J., et al., "Prenatal Malnutrition and Development of the Brain," *Neuroscience and Behavioral Reviews*, 17 (1993), pp. 91–128.

net protein utilization (NPU) An index used to estimate the ability of a food PROTEIN to supply indispensable AMINO ACIDS. Only retained nitrogen is measured. The NPU is based upon the ratio of the amount of dietary protein converted to body protein divided by the amount of protein eaten. Thus, a poorly digested protein would have a low NPU score. In this respect, it differs from the BIOLOGICAL VALUE, which does not account for digestibility of food. Frequently proteins are measured for their growth-promoting effect on young animals or for their ability to maintain nitrogen equilibrium, a balance between protein nitrogen consumed and the amount lost daily (NITROGEN BALANCE). Since only retained nitrogen is measured, NPU does not specifically assess the inefficiency of digestion. Thus a poorly digested protein would have a low NPU score. (See also CHEMICAL SCORE.)

neural tube defects (NTD) Congenital disorders related to the incomplete development of the neural tube. Neural tube defects contribute to infant mortality throughout the world. Anencephalus is the absence of brain and spinal cord. In spina bifida, the spinal cord is pushed through the wall of the spinal canal between vertebrae. Encephalocele refers to the protrusion of the brain through a cranial opening. Both genetic and environmental factors are implicated. The B vitamin FOLIC ACID prevents the recurrence of NTD and seems likely to reduce the prevalence of NTD in general when supplementation is initiated before conception or carried out through the first weeks of pregnancy. Women who are considering pregnancy are advised to consult a qualified physician for their nutrient needs.(See also BIRTH DEFECTS; HOMOCYSTEINE; VITAMIN.)

"Prevention of neural tube defects: results of the Medical Research Council Vitamin Study," MRC Vitamin Study Reseach Group. *Lancet*, 338 (1991), pp. 131–37.

neuron See NERVOUS SYSTEM.

neuropathy, peripheral Disease of the peripheral nerves (the nerves feeding into the spinal column and brain). Nutritional deficiencies can cause peripheral nerve degeneration. Severe deficiency of the B vitamin THIAMIN, a disease whose chief characteristic is BERIBERI, also leads to neuropathy. Certain toxic chemicals like plasticizers and several medications such as Isoniazid also cause neuropathy. Diseases affecting the entire body like diabetes, certain AUTOIMMUNE DISEASES like Guillain-Barre syndrome, and a variety of rare hereditary diseases are associated with peripheral neuropathy. Neuropathy can be caused by HEPATITIS, infectious mononucleosis, ALCOHOLISM and lead poisoning. (See also DEFICIENCY DISEASE; HEAVY METALS; NERVOUS SYSTEM.)

"Megadoses of Vitamin B_6 Produce Disorders," *The Nutrition Report*, 10:12 (December 1992).

neurotransmitter A chemical required to transmit nerve impulses between nerve cells. Unlike an electrical network, nerves are not continuous; the end of a nerve cell does not touch its target. Instead, individual nerve cells are separated by a microscopic gap called a synapse. In response to a nerve impulse traveling down the nerve cell, the nerve ending releases neurotransmitter molecules, which then diffuse across the gap and bind to the adjacent cell. Depending upon the nature of the receiving cells, this contact can stimulate or inhibit the target cell.

At least three classes of neurotransmitters respond to diet: Catecholamines (DOPAMINE and norepinephrine) come from the AMINO ACID, TYROSINE. Eating a protein-rich meal can increase blood tyrosine levels and increase levels of this amino acid in the brain. Elevated brain tyrosine increases dopamine and norepinephrine production, promoting wakefulness and alertness.

On the other hand, SEROTONIN tends to induce relaxation and sleep. Serotonin comes from the essential amino acid-TRYPTOPHAN. Eating a meal high in carbohydrates is believed to increase indirectly brain tryptophan levels. Elevated blood sugar stimulates insulin release; this hormone stimulates the uptake by muscle of amino acids that compete with tryptophan for uptake by the brain, allowing more tryptophan into the brain. This in turn leads to higher serotonin formation in the brain, promoting a state of relaxation. Amino acid research in humans is still considered preliminary.

ACETYLCHOLINE is manufactured from CHOLINE, a nitrogen-containing nutrient and raw material for neurotransmitter synthesis. The body can synthesize choline, and it comes also from dietary lipids, particularly LECITHIN, a common phosphate-bearing lipid found in most foods. Acetylcholine participates in many brain functions, including memory. Victims of ALZHEIMER'S DISEASE have low levels of acetylcholine in their brains. (See also ENDORPHINS; NERVOUS SYSTEM.)

neutral fats   See FAT; VEGETABLE OIL.

NHANES (National Health and Nutrition Examination Survey)   A survey designed to evaluate the nutritional status of Americans. Between 1971 and 1974 (NHANES 1) and again from 1977 to 1979 (NHANES II), the U.S. National Center for Health Statistics conducted single-day diet surveys of more than 20,000 Americans in a wide variety of geographical locations to obtain representative dietary data.

NHANES I concluded that PROTEIN, CALCIUM, VITAMIN A and IRON were generally deficient in the American diet. Most women and many infants did not consume enough iron. NHANES II extended the findings, collecting biochemical data to see whether low nutrient status would reflect low nutrient intake. Low protein and low vitamin A were found in 3% of the people surveyed. Low THIAMIN was found in 29% of black and 14% of white subjects, while low iron was found in 5 to 15% of white and 18 to 27% of black subjects. Later USDA food consumption surveys indicated that about 50% of the U.S. population after the age of one consumed less than 70% of the RDA for vitamin B_6. The average zinc intake among American women was estimated to be 60% of the recommended amount, while surveys consistently reveal that magnesium is a problem nutrient; perhaps as many as 40% of the U.S. population may consume less than 70% of the RDA. FOLIC ACID deficiency is probably the most com-

mon vitamin deficiency in the United States because of the low consumption of dark-green leafy vegetables.

To complement NHANES I and II, the Nationwide Food Consumption Survey was conducted in 1977–78 to examine the types of foods eaten at home and away from home. This survey indicated a trend toward higher weight among Americans, without increased food consumption, reflecting a trend toward less physical activity among Americans.

The most recent nutrition food survey (1987–1988) was seriously flawed. The response rate was poor, raising the contention that results may not represent the nation, and some nutritionists have questioned the utility of the data. (See also EATING PATTERNS.)

niacin (nicotinic acid, vitamin B_3)   A heat-stable member of the B VITAMIN complex needed by the body to extract ENERGY from FAT, CARBOHYDRATE and PROTEIN. Tissues convert niacin to two closely related COENZYMES (enzyme helpers): NICOTINAMIDE ADENINE DINUCLEOTIDE (NAD) and nicotinamide adenine dinucleotide phosphate (NADP). NAD functions as an oxidizing agent used in processes that "burn" fuels to produce energy in the cell. These include the oxidation of GLUCOSE (GLYCOLYSIS) and of FATTY ACIDS. NAD transfers electrons to the mitochondrial ELECTRON TRANSPORT CHAIN, which ultimately reduces OXYGEN to water. This process liberates vast amounts of chemical energy trapped as ATP as well as releasing heat. NADP is generated from the oxidation of glucose (pentose phosphate pathway). The reduced form of NADP, NADPH, is used as a reducing agent in biosynthetic reactions rather than for energy production. CHOLESTEROL, fatty acids and other important compounds require NADPH for their synthesis. NADPH is also the basis of a powerful antioxidant system (GLUTATHIONE) to protect most cells from the damaging effects of highly reactive molecules called FREE RADICALS. NADPH also functions in the synthesis of DEOXYRIBOSE, the sugar building block of DNA.

Possible Roles of Niacin in Disease

PELLAGRA is a severe niacin deficiency disease that mimics schizophrenia. Skin rashes, DIARRHEA and mouth sores are prevalent in pellagra. At the turn of the century pellagra was epidemic in the southern United States among people whose diet was based on corn. By 1937 research demonstrated that niacin cured pellagra-like symptoms in dogs and, shortly thereafter, that niacin treatment cured pellagra. Niacin has been used in food fortification since 1941.

The use of niacin to treat schizophrenia and DEPRESSION is controversial. Generally negative results have been reported for patients with long-standing schizophrenia. Some clinicians reported improvement in patients with schizophrenia using megavitamin treatment with niacin or niacinamide, vitamin B_6 and vitamin C and in patients with depression using niacinamide and tryptophan, together with taking steps to improve the diet. The American Psychological Association disapproved the use of niacin in the treatment of mental disorders in 1979.

Niacin may prevent HEART ATTACKS (a conclusion of the Coronary Drug Project Research Group). MEGADOSES of niacin (1 to 6 g daily) have been used to dramatically lower blood cholesterol and blood fat (triglyceride) levels, while increasing HDL (HIGH-DENSITY LIPOPROTEIN, the desirable form of cholesterol) in patients with heart disease. Niacin reduces the risk of heart attacks for these reasons, and possibly niacin can reverse ATHEROSCLEROSIS. Niacin seems to increase the production of PROSTAGLANDINS. These hormone-like chemicals are produced locally within tissues to help control many physiologic processes such as BLOOD CLOTTING and INFLAMMATION.

Large doses of niacin may alleviate non-inflammatory ARTHRITIS, while low doses of niacin can relieve migraine headaches. Niacin supplements may help normalize blood sugar in patients with hypoglycemia. Large doses of niacin may prevent harmful effects of chemical pollutants, drugs and alcohol, and may help during recovery and drug rehabilitation (the mechanism is not known). This is a promising area of research, but presently niacin cannot be claimed to be a broad-spectrum detoxification agent.

Sources

Good sources of niacin are EGGS, MEAT (especially liver), fish, POULTRY and unprocessed food, including peanuts and potatoes. Coffee provides about 3 mg per cup. Niacin is one of the commonly fortified nutrients; consequently, enriched flour and cereals are good sources. MILK and CHEESE are good sources because they contain large amounts of the essential AMINO ACID, TRYPTOPHAN, which is partially converted by the body to niacin. Protein-deficient diets are often related to pellagra. This explains why diets incorporating milk can prevent or cure pellagra.

The form available from animal foods is NIACINAMIDE, a derivative of niacin; plant foods provide niacin itself. Niacin is one of the most stable of the B vitamins: It resists most cooking procedures and can be stored in the dry state indefinitely without loss. Canning, DEHYDRATION and exposure to air or light cause little destruction.

Up to 70% of the niacin in most cereal grains, including corn, is present as a bound form called niacytin. It is not released during digestion and therefore is poorly absorbed. Traditionally, corn tortillas are prepared from corn pretreated with lime water to improve dough consistency, a treatment that also frees niacin. Pellagra is uncommon in Mexico, Central and South America, where corn is soaked in lime. Presently niacin deficiency and pellagra are common only in certain regions of Africa and Asia, where corn is a major source of protein. Because niacin is so prevalent in high-quality protein, only alcoholics and heavy drinkers are likely to be deficient in the United States. Symptoms of mild deficiency include apathy, headache, irritability and memory loss.

Requirements

The RECOMMENDED DIETARY ALLOWANCE for healthy adult men is 19 mg; for non-pregnant, non-lactating women it is 15 mg. The daily niacin requirement varies with the number of calories burned daily (the energy expenditure) and the protein intake. One niacin equivalent equals 1 mg of preformed niacin or 60 mg of dietary tryptophan.

Niacin can be synthesized in the body from the essential amino acid tryptophan. Tissues can form an average of 1 mg of niacin from 60 mg of tryptophan provided by dietary protein. Consequently a high-quality protein diet supplies substantial tryptophan for niacin synthesis. On the other hand, a protein-deficient diet or a diet relying on low tryptophan protein increases the dietary requirement for niacin. Most animal protein contains 1.4% tryptophan; vegetable protein, 1%; and corn protein, only 0.6%.

Safety

Niacin (but not closely related niacinamide) expands CAPILLARIES and can lead to itching and flushing at doses commonly used in multivitamin supplements (100 mg or more). While nausea, diarrhea and flushing may accompany niacin usage, these side effects are not considered dangerous. Excessive niacin can cause irregular heartbeat, cramps, headache and liver inflammation. "Sustained release" niacin may cause less flushing, but some preparations may be more toxic to the liver. Other forms, such as inositol hexaniacinate, may improve niacin therapy. Large doses of niacin can increase BLOOD SUGAR in diabetics, increase the risk of GOUT and aggravate ulcers. Niacin supplements are not recommended for those with PEPTIC ULCERS, COLITIS, ASTHMA, liver disease, GOUT or erratic heartbeat. Using niacin therapeutically (1,000 mg or more per day) requires medical supervision; liver function and blood sugar need to be monitored. (See also CARBOHYDRATE METABOLISM; CHOLESTEROL-LOWERING DRUGS; FAT METABOLISM; FORTIFICATION.)

Di Palma, J.R. and Thayer, W.S., "Use of Niacin as a Drug," *Annual Review of Nutrition*, 11 (1991), pp. 169–87.

niacinamide (nicotinamide)   A derivative of the water-soluble vitamin NIACIN. Niacinamide is readily formed in the body from niacin and incorporated into two important COENZYMES (enzyme helpers): NICOTINAMIDE ADENINE DINUCLEOTIDE (NAD) and its phosphate-containing analog, nicotinamide adenine dinucleotide phosphate (NADP). By assisting in oxidation-reduction reactions, NAD performs an essential role in energy production from nutrients. NAD is required by all cells in many aspects of metabolism, including CARBOHYDRATE, FATTY ACID and AMINO ACID degradation. The reduced form of NADP, NADPH, participates in reductions required for biosynthesis.

Niacinamide is the most prevalent form of this vitamin in animal products and MEAT, although niacin is more prevalent in plant foods. Niacinamide lacks the capillary-expanding (skin-flushing) activity of niacin and is somewhat safer than niacin; hence it is more often used when large amounts of the vitamin are required. Side effects of niacinamide include nausea, headache, fatigue, sore mouth. Large amounts can injure the liver (jaundice). (See also ANABOLISM; B COMPLEX; DETOXIFICATION; GLUTATHIONE.)

nickel   A possible TRACE MINERAL nutrient. Nickel is now known to be an essential trace mineral nutrient of all higher plants, including cereal grains and legumes, which require nickel for seeds to grow (germinate). Nickel helps plants liberate nitrogen from soil and absorb IRON. Nickel also seems to be a trace mineral nutrient for some animal species, though its function is unknown. Diets that exclude nickel slow growth in sheep, goats, cows and rats. Nickel deficiency decreases red blood cell production in these animals as well. Nickel-deficient chickens develop abnormally. Human requirements, if any, are unknown. A typical American diet supplies an estimated 0.3 to 0.6 mg of nickel daily.

Like many trace minerals, minute amounts may be essential nutrients, though high-level exposure is hazardous. Because nickel is an industrial waste, it has emerged as an environmental pollutant. The toxicity of high doses of nickel is well documented; for example, nickel carbonyl is a hazardous industrial chemical, and exposure in the workplace is regulated. Nickel allergies are linked to jewelry; once a person is sensitized, nickel allergies are long-lasting.

nicotinamide   See NIACINAMIDE.

nicotinamide adenine dinucleotide (NAD, NADH)
An enzyme helper (COENZYME) that functions in oxidation/reduction reactions of cells. NAD contains the B vitamin NIACIN. NAD assists dehydrogenases, a family of enzymes that remove hydrogen atoms from substances (oxidation). Lactate dehydrogenase is a typical dehydrogenase: This enzyme oxidizes LACTIC ACID to PYRUVIC ACID as an intermediate step in the formation of GLUCOSE, the dominant sugar used by the body. Other dehydrogenases oxidize fatty acids and perform oxidation steps in the KREB'S CYCLE, the central energy yielding pathway of the cell.

Nicotinamide Adenine Dinucleotide Phosphate (NADP, NADPH)

NADP closely resembles NAD in structure and function. As the second coenzyme based on niacin it contains an additional phosphate group. The reduced form, NADPH, is used in biosynthetic pathways, including fatty acid and cholesterol synthesis. NADPH is produced by the oxidation of glucose (the pentose phosphate pathway). NADPH supports GLUTATHIONE PEROXIDASE, an important ANTIOXIDANT system for neutralizing oxidative damage to lipids and membranes. (See also B COMPLEX; CARBOHYDRATE METABOLISM; FATTY ACID; OXIDATIVE PHOSPHORYLATION.)

nicotinic acid   See NIACIN.

night blindness (nyctalopia)   A condition resulting from a chronic deficiency of VITAMIN A. Vitamin A is required to form "visual purple," the pigment required for vision in dim light. With vitamin A deficiency, inadequate pigment causes an abnormally slow adaptation in going from vision in strong light to dim light. Hereditary factors may contribute to night blindness as well.

nightshade family   A plant family that includes TOMATOES, POTATOES, EGGPLANT, PEPPERS and tobacco. Anecdotal reports have been interpreted by some to suggest that eating vegetables from this family may promote joint inflammation in susceptible people. However, no carefully controlled studies have been conducted, and the hyptothesis remains unproven. Arthritic symptoms may diminish by avoiding contact with foods that cause reactions. (See also ARTHRITIS; FOOD SENSITIVITY.)

nitrate   An inorganic, nitrogen-containing ion used as a FOOD ADDITIVE for processed MEAT and meat products. Meat can legally contain 91 mg added sodium or potassium nitrate

per pound. Chopped meat can contain 778 mg per pound, and dry, cured meat can contain 991 mg per pound. Its role in meat is not clear, though nitrate seems to provide a reservoir for bacterial conversion to nitrite, which acts as an antimicrobial agent. Nitrite can be converted to a potential cancer-causing agent called NITROSOAMINE.

Nitrate occurs naturally in food. Green VEGETABLES are a major source of nitrates and BEETS, SPINACH and LETTUCE are likely sources. The level depends upon the plant species and variety, the part of the plant consumed, the stage of maturity, levels of fertilizers in the soil, and the rate of plant growth. The estimated-typical daily intake of nitrate is 6 mg from vegetables; 9.4 mg from cured meats; 2 mg from bread; and 1.4 mg from FRUIT and fruit juices. Drinking water supplies an average of 0.7 mg daily. High levels of nitrate can occur in well water in rural areas, due to contamination from feed lots and run-off from fertilizer-affected fields. A limit of 10 mg of nitrate per liter has been set by the U.S. Public Health Service. Nitrate in well water used to prepare formula can be a hazard for infants. Up to six months after birth, stomach acid production in infants is low, which permits bacteria in the intestine to convert nitrate to nitrite. Nitrite can disable infants' hemoglobin and induce a condition called methenoglobinemia, in which nitrite-modified hemoglobin cannot transport adequate oxygen. In older children nitrate is absorbed in the stomach before it can reach intestinal bacteria that could reduce it to nitrite. Infants drink proportionately much more water (in formula) than adults do, and their hemoglobin is also more sensitive to nitrite attack. Formula prepared from distilled water is safer. (See also PROCESSED FOOD.)

nitric oxide (NO)   A small, potentially toxic, compound of oxygen and nitrogen that is also a free radical. Nitric oxide is different from laughing gas, nitrous oxide, N_2O. Nitric oxide serves multiple functions in the body as a freely diffusible messenger molecule. Nitric oxide is synthesized by specific enzymes, nitric oxide synthases, from the amino acid ARGININE.

Nitric oxide serves as a NEUROTRANSMITTER in the brain and other parts of the nervous system and perhaps plays a key role in memory. Neurotransmitters are chemicals that transmit nerve impulses between the gaps that exist between cells. When MACROPHAGES, phagocytic cells of the immune system, are stimulated to respond to foreign invaders and immune activators, they produce large amounts of nitric oxide to wage chemical warfare against viruses and bacteria. Nitric oxide is produced by endothelial cells lining blood vessels where it relaxes blood vessels and helps maintain blood pressure. Too little nitric oxide may play a role in hypertension and angina. It also is involved in penile erection and may be a factor in impotence. Nitric oxide also interacts with blood platelets to decrease platelet aggregation, thus lowing the risk of blood clots. Red blood cells rapidly inactivate nitric oxide by converting it to nitrate for excretion. Excesses of nitric oxide may be a factor in strokes and inflammatory bowel disease. In stroke, too much calcium can enter cells, causing nitric oxide overproduction to toxic levels when oxygen supply is restored. Nitric oxide combines with SUPEROXIDE, another free radical produced in the body, to form peroxynitrite. This powerful oxidizing agent may account for some of the cellular damage that occurs with prolonged inflammation and could contribute to tissue damage in colitis and other conditions.

nitrite (potassium nitrite, sodium nitrite)   A common food additive to processed meat. Nitrites are added to cure MEATS, like LUNCHEON MEATS, liverwurst, salami, BACON, BOLOGNA, HAM and HOT DOGS to prevent them from turning gray and to create a meaty flavor. Cured white meat does not need a pink color, so nitrite is not usually added to it. Nitrite decomposes to nitric oxide, which reacts with pigments in meat to form an appealing pink color. Nitrites can inhibit bacterial growth, and one argument for continuing to use sodium nitrite is that it prevents spoilage and BOTULISM. Dry cured meat may contain 283 mg of nitrite per pound, while chopped meat can contain 71 mg per pound. Dietary vegetables supply 0.20 mg daily, while cured meats supply several milligrams daily. Until the late 1970s, nitrite was needlessly added to BABY FOOD. Yielding to consumer pressure, baby food manufacturers have stopped this practice. Bacterial action on nitrate in saliva and in the intestine can produce several milligrams of nitrite daily.

Safety

Nitrite-containing bacon, when fried, yields NITROSOAMINES, a family of nitrogen-containing, cancer-causing chemicals. Furthermore, significant levels of nitrosoamines appear in cooked SAUSAGE and cured meats. Specific nitrosoamines have caused CANCER in all animals tested. Under conditions present in the stomach, nitrite also can react with AMINES found in protein-containing foods to form nitrosoamines. Population studies have linked nitrite intake and cancer. Though nitrites and nitrates come from vegetables, this does not necessarily lead to nitrosoamines because VITAMIN C and similar chemicals in the food block nitrosoamine formation. The FDA has approved the use of nitrites since they themselves do not cause cancer. Furthermore vitamin C (ascorbic acid) or similar agents must be added to cured meats in order to reduce the risk of nitrosoamines. Nitrite is now listed on food labels. Nitrite-free meat is increasingly available. (See also CARCINOGEN; NITROGEN CYCLE; PRESERVATIVE.)

nitrogen   One of the four major elements used to assemble the carbon-based molecules of life. The other three building blocks are hydrogen, carbon and OXYGEN. Nitrogen is a key constituent of AMINES, alkaline substances found in cells. In all cells, nitrogen appears in the amino acids, which are incorporated into protein, including enzymes; in purines and pyrimidines, the building blocks of DNA and RNA, the information molecules of the cell; in PHOSPHOLIPIDS, the structural elements of membranes; in certain HORMONES; and in brain chemicals (NEUROTRANSMITTERS) synthesized by nerve cells to carry nerve impulses. Nitrogen contributes to the function of HEME (the oxygen-binding pigment of the oxygen-transport protein, HEMOGLOBIN); THIAMIN (vitamin B_1); RIBOFLAVIN (vitamin B_2); NIACIN (vitamin B_3); VITAMIN B_6; and VITAMIN B_{12}. The nitrogen-containing waste product of protein metabolism is urea, excreted in the urine.

In the NITROGEN CYCLE, atmospheric nitrogen is reduced to ammonia by bacteria residing in the roots of legumes like beans or alfalfa. The ammonia is readily taken up by the plant and can be used to fabricate all nitrogen-containing cell building blocks, including chlorophyll. Animals eat these plant materials primarily as amino acids in food proteins. Cells are generally able to adapt this nitrogen source to their own nitrogen-containing compounds. Thus, ultimately plants are the source of nitrogen in animal cells. Lightning can oxidize atmospheric nitrogen to NITRATE, which leaches into soil as rainfall. Alternatively, nitrate, ammonia or urea fertilizers are applied during crop cultivation. Nitrate is rapidly absorbed by plants, while urea breaks down to ammonia. Plant tissues can reduce nitrate to ammonia, which is more readily used. When plant or animal tissue decomposes, bacteria can oxidize nitrogen to nitrate, which can then be reabsorbed by plants to reinitiate the cycle. Denitrifying bacteria are able to transform nitrate back to atmospheric nitrogen (N_2).

nitrogen balance   A measure of the nutritional state of an individual that pertains to PROTEIN and AMINO ACID consumption. Nitrogen balance compares the level of dietary nitrogen, as represented by amino acids of food protein, with the amount of their nitrogen waste products, lost in urine, feces and perspiration.

Proteins of every tissue are constantly being replaced, as they wear out due to chemical changes and are degraded to amino acids. The released amino acids may be reused, or they may be degraded for energy, their nitrogen excreted primarily as UREA. If incoming protein just balances the need for amino acids to compensate for wear and tear, the individual is considered to be in "nitrogen equilibrium." Healthy adults maintaining a steady body weight are generally in this state.

Negative nitrogen balance   When the diet lacks adequate amino acids for growth and maintenance, demand exceeds supply. To compensate, the body breaks down its own protein to supply amino acids. FASTING, ILLNESS, diabetes, fever, surgery, STARVATION, ALCOHOLISM, severe weight loss programs and crash DIETING place the individual in negative nitrogen balance.

Positive nitrogen balance   When the body accumulates protein and new tissue is being built, more nitrogen is stored as protein than is lost as waste. Positive nitrogen balance occurs during rapid periods of growth during childhood, adolescence and pregnancy.

nitrogen cycle   The movement of nitrogen from the atmosphere through organisms. Nitrogen (N_2) as a gas represents about 80% of the atmosphere. Though very abundant, it cannot be used by higher organisms and must be chemically modified to be a nutrient for plants and animals. Bacteria that live symbiotically in the roots of legumes such as PEAS, BEANS and ALFALFA initiate the process. They convert atmospheric nitrogen to the simplest nitrogen compound, AMMONIA (NH_3), via a process called nitrogen fixation. Alternatively, lightning bolts energize nitrogen to react with oxygen in the air to create NITRATE. Plants incorporate both ammonia and nitrate into AMINO ACIDS, which form PROTEIN. When ingested by animals, plant proteins are broken down to amino acids and incorporated into animal protein. The most useful dietary form of nitrogen for humans is protein: It is digested to release amino acids. Most other nitrogen-containing cell components, like DNA and RNA, can be constructed from amino acids. Animals excrete nitrogenous wastes like UREA, the end product of protein metabolism. Soil bacteria can convert waste nitrogen compounds back to atmospheric nitrogen and ammonia, to be reincorporated into plants. Bacteria, fungi and molds decay plant and animal tissues to help recycle key nutrients. (See also GREEN REVOLUTION; HUNGER; LEGUMES; NITROGEN BALANCE.)

nitrosoamine   A cancer-causing agent formed from the common FOOD ADDITIVE, NITRITE. Nitrite is a common additive in highly processed meat products and cured meats. Mice, rats, hamsters, pigs, dogs, monkeys and fish develop CANCER when exposed to several nitrosoamines, which can modify DNA in test tube experiments. In the stomach and intestine they can react with amines, nitrogen-containing compounds present in many foods. Nitrosoamines have been detected in cooked SAUSAGE and BACON, tobacco smoke, cured meats, PESTICIDES, smoked fish, powdered milk, alcoholic beverages and several types of industrial plants, as well as new car interiors. The level of exposure constituting a health hazard to humans is unknown. Vitamin C and garlic inhibit nitrosoamine formation. (See also FOOD PRESERVATION.)

non-dairy creamer (non-dairy whitener)   A synthetic, non-dairy coffee whitener. Consumers usually choose a non-dairy creamer to avoid the calories, CHOLESTEROL and FAT of cream. However, cream replacements contain 0.7 g of fat per teaspoon in the form of emulsified COCONUT OIL, palm kernel oil or partially HYDROGENATED VEGETABLE OIL. Not only does a non-dairy creamer contain as many fat calories as cream, coconut oil is the most saturated fat available, and a high intake of saturated fat promotes elevated blood fat and cholesterol levels. Non-dairy creamers do not contain cholesterol because vegetable oils do not contain cholesterol. On the other hand they may contain CORN SYRUP as a sweetener, whey and sodium caseinate as protein emulsifiers, sodium aluminosilicate as a stabilizer, as well as artificial flavoring and coloring. Non-dairy creamers are nutritionally inferior to milk and are not a milk substitute for children. (See also IMITATION FOOD.)

non-fat dry milk   See MILK.

non-heme iron   See IRON.

non-protein nitrogen   NITROGEN sources other than protein that can be used to build proteins of the body. Though dietary protein supplies most of the nitrogen for protein synthesis as amino acids, other nitrogen sources can contribute nitrogen. AMMONIA can be reincorporated into amino acids and hence proteins. Individuals on low-protein diets utilize alternative sources of nitrogen more effectively than those who are well fed.

noodles   A common form of pasta. The U.S. FDA defines all pastas as either noodles or MACARONI. Noodles must contain one or more of the following: milled durum WHEAT flour, farina (coarsely ground wheat endosperm from less-hard wheat) or semolina (a granular product of milled durum wheat), together with 5.5% egg. (Macaroni need not contain egg.) Noodles are strings or ribbons of unleavened baked dough. Noodles have been a mainstay of Asian cookery since ancient times. RICE flour and MUNG BEAN flour are popular in Southeast Asia. Today noodles are stir-fried, pan-fried or used in soups and sauces. Specific examples include:

- Mung bean thread noodles (transparent noodles or jelly noodles) resemble silver threads. They soften rapidly in water and are a staple in China, Indonesia, Malaysia and Japan.
- Rice noodles are thin and wiry when dry. When soaked in water and cooked, they soften and form the basis of many dishes. Rice noodles are popular in Burma, Cambodia, Indonesia and Vietnam.
- Soba noodles are made from BUCKWHEAT.
- Udon noodles are thick noodles prepared from wheat flour without eggs. They can be either flat or round.
- Bean curd noodles, also called soy noodles, resemble typical egg noodles except they are somewhat thicker and may be grayish in color.

(See also SOYBEAN.)

nucleic acids   Substances that function as the genetic material and the PROTEIN synthesizing machinery of all cells. DNA is the genetic blueprint. Each species possesses a unique DNA that guides all of a cell's structure and functions; it has been called the cell's "master plan." Alterations in DNA lead to altered inheritance.

RNA is considerably smaller than DNA and does not function as a genetic blueprint of the body. RNA serves as a messenger by which information for building proteins can be translated in the cytoplasm. Thus RNA directs the assembly of proteins from amino acid raw materials. Special types of RNA form ribosomes, upon which proteins are constructed, and messenger and transfer RNA to translate genetic codewords into amino acids. Both DNA and RNA are assembled from building blocks: a simple sugar, DEOXYRIBOSE, phosphate, and nitrogen-containing cyclic bases called purines and pyrimidines.

The overall composition of RNA is similar to DNA. Each contains a phosphate, a simple sugar—ribose in RNA and deoxyribose in DNA. RNA and DNA contain four nitrogen-containing ring compounds. Three of these are identical: ADENINE, GUANINE and cytosine. In addition RNA contains uracil, while DNA contains thymin. (See also FREE RADICALS; MUTAGEN; MUTATION.)

"nursing bottle" syndrome   Extensive dental decay in young children due to sucking sweetened beverages for a long period of time. When a baby falls asleep with a JUICE-filled bottle or a bottle filled with a sweet drink, even milk, in its mouth, reduced active sucking and reduced saliva flow allow sugar to bathe the upper teeth and lower back TEETH. This favors bacterial growth, cavity formation and, eventually, extensive dental decay. This syndrome can be avoided by not allowing the infant or young child to fall asleep with a bottle of juice or milk in its mouth. (See also BREASTFEEDING; INFANT FORMULA.)

nut   A seed typically enclosed by a tough woody shell. Nuts are products of trees; ALMONDS, CHESTNUTS and hazelnuts are typical examples. The PEANUT is an example of a nut that is usually the pod of a LEGUME (member of the pea family). Certain varieties of almonds and pecans may have soft as well as hard shells. The COCONUT is the leading nut crop worldwide, followed by peanuts; together they account for 94% of the world nut production. Nonetheless, nut production is small when compared with the yield of GRAINS and LEGUMES, which are major food items.

Nuts have been a staple in hunter-gatherer societies since prehistoric times. Ancient civilizations cultivated almonds, pistachio nuts and WALNUTS in Asia. BRAZIL NUTS, peanuts and cashews originated in South America. Acorns were eaten by Native Americans, who soaked the crushed nuts in water to remove toxic, bitter materials (TANNINS). Though nuts are still harvested in America from wild trees, often nut tree orchards permit more efficient means of production, including mechanical harvesting.

Nuts contain high levels of FAT, CARBOHYDRATE and PROTEIN to nurture the sprouted seedling until it can perform PHOTOSYNTHESIS. Typically, one ounce (1/8 cup) of most nuts contains 13 to 18 g of fat, representing an average of 160 fat calories, and 70 to 90% of calories come from fat. Because of their high fat content, nuts contain 140 more calories per ounce than grains and legumes. On the other hand, the fat in unroasted nuts is unsaturated and unprocessed, an advantage over vegetable shortening or animal fat, which are saturated fats. Brazil nuts, hazelnuts, hickory nuts, peanuts, pecans, pistachios and walnuts provide 4.7 to 10 g of the ESSENTIAL FATTY ACID, LINOLEIC ACID, per ounce (28 g). Americans who eat nuts frequently seem to have a lower risk of heart attack and coronary disease.

Comparison of Unsaturated Fatty Acid Content in Typical Nuts

Calories/oz	Monounsaturated Fat	Polyunsaturated Fat
almonds (167)	68%	22%
pecans (187)	66%	26%
pistachios (162)	71%	16%
peanuts (164)	52%	33%
walnuts (182)	24%	70%

COCONUT OIL has the highest percentage of saturated fatty acid of the common vegetable oils and resists rancidity. Snack nuts (roasted nuts) are usually roasted in palm kernel oil or coconut oil, increasing their saturated fat content. They are also often heavily salted. A cup of roasted peanuts contains 1,000 mg of sodium, one-third of the suggested daily intake. Dry roasted nuts are not cooked in oil, though they may be salted. Nut butters, such as almond butter or peanut butter, can be used as snacks. If unsweetened and if no additives are used, nut butters are equivalent to a typical nut snack. Although usually eaten as a snack food, chopped nuts can be added to fruit salads, yogurt, pancakes, pilaf and baked goods for a pleasing variety.

Macadamia nuts contain 72% fat; they are fried in deep fat and sold as high-calorie snacks or used for confections. Pecans contain a similar high fat level. Chestnuts differ from other nuts in that they contain three to four times more carbohydrate and less fat and protein than other nuts, and their overall nutrient profile resembles that of dry corn or rice products.

In general, shelled nuts are sold vacuum-packed to increase their shelf life; they should be refrigerated or frozen to slow rancidity due to their high unsaturated oil content. Nuts typically contain 20% protein by weight, similar to that found in legumes and about twice as much as found in GRAINS. Peanuts contain 26% protein, the highest protein content among commonly available nuts. Defatted nut meal such as almond meal and peanut flour is used as a protein-rich flour. Nut protein contains higher amounts of most essential AMINO ACIDS when compared to grains, but less than legumes. Nuts contain less LYSINE, an essential amino acid. Mixtures of grains and cereals with nuts provide a complementary mixture of essential amino acids that more nearly matches dietary requirements than either alone.

Nuts are generally good sources of the B complex vitamins (like NIACIN, RIBOFLAVIN and THIAMIN), VITAMIN E, PHOSPHORUS and MAGNESIUM. Roasting destroys thiamin. Most nuts provide other important trace minerals, including CHROMIUM, MANGANESE, ZINC and SELENIUM. Typically, nuts contain up to seven times the amounts of these minerals as found in other unprocessed foods. Nuts also provide CHOLINE, a nutrient required for fat transport and nerve function. (See also COMPLETE PROTEIN; PROTEIN QUALITY.)

Sabaté, J., "Does Nut Consumption Protect Against Ischemic Heart Disease?" *European Journal of Clinical Nutrition*, 47:supp. 1 (1993), pp. S71–S75.

nutmeg (*Myristica fragrans*) A SPICE. The seed of an apricot-like fruit of the nutmeg tree. A tropical evergreen, the outer covering of the seed is removed and dried to produce mace, a close relative of nutmeg. Nutmeg is an important spice for puddings, custards and cakes. Nutmeg can subtly flavor cheese dishes, spinach dishes, white sauces and meat fillings.

Nutrasweet See ASPARTAME.

nutraceutical Foods or food-derived ingredients that have the potential of treating or preventing chronic disease. Many ingredients in foods, particularly those derived from plants, possess the ability to benefit health. Vegetables, fruits, nuts, legumes, spices and teas contain substances that possibly help prevent many of the chronic, degenerative diseases that characterize aging in populations of developed nations. In terms of anticancer effects the various chemicals in foods could affect the two stages of development of cancer. They could prevent damage to healthy cells' DNA, that is, prevent mutations. These agents may block the activation of carcinogens, stimulate the levels of protective enzymes that detoxify carcinogens, or trap carcinogens.

FLAVONOIDS are complex substances widely distributed in vegetables and fruits, often associated with pigments (such as anthocyanins). They are strong antioxidants, linked with cancer prevention, increased immunity and lowered risk of cardiovascular disease. Common sources include red wine, apples, onions and tea. ISOFLAVONES (such as genistein) from soy possess weak estrogen activity and apparently lower the risk of breast cancer. Organo-sulfur compounds in GARLIC and ONION, including allicin, dially disulfide and ajoene, in addition to saponins and flavonoids, possess strong antibacterial and antiviral properties as well as anticancer properties. Vegetables of the cabbage family (cruciferous vegetables) produce SULFORAPHANE and ISOTHIOCYANATES, sulfur-containing chemicals, as well as indoles that can protect against cancer by selectively raising the levels of liver detoxifying enzymes so that the liver can rid the body of potentially mutagenic substances more readily. Many dark green leafy vegetables and orange fruits and vegetables contain orange pigments called carotenoids that enhance the immune system and function as antioxidants, preserve vision and inhibit tumor growth. Ellagic acid from grapes and strawberries deactivates potential carcinogens. Turmeric provides curcuminoids that also inhibit the growth of cancer cells. Regardless of the source, food-derived preparations need to be standardized, that is, the identities and levels of key active ingredients should be known. (See also PHYTOCHEMICALS.)

nutrient   An ingredient of foods that can be used by the body for growth and maintenance of health. Foods are mixtures of nutrients, and the relative amounts of the various nutrients in a given food depend upon conditions of growth, storage, degree of processing and method of cooking. DIGESTION releases nutrients from foods, which can then be absorbed by the intestinal tract. Certain nutrients must be supplied by the diet because the body cannot manufacture them. More than 50 different kinds of nutrients have been identified; 40 are definitely required for human growth, development and health. They include WATER, CARBOHYDRATE, 10 AMINO ACIDS, two types of ESSENTIAL FATTY ACIDS from OILS and FAT, 13 VITAMINS and 15 MINERALS. These nutrients are used for energy, to supply building blocks to replace worn out cell constituents, and for normal cell and tissue function.

Carbohydrates, fat and PROTEIN, together, represent hundreds of grams (approximately a pound) in the adult diet. Distribution of calories among these three MACRONUTRIENTS varies with the culture and the sub-population. Fat and carbohydrate are the major fuels. Dietary protein is the primary source of amino acids used to fashion the body's own proteins. Major minerals like SODIUM chloride; plant structural materials like FIBER; and WATER are also classified as macronutrients because large quantities are needed. Minerals represent ELECTROLYTES and bony, hard structures. The body represents about 65% water; weight-wise, the diet must supply more water than any other nutrient.

Vitamins and trace minerals are classified as MICRONUTRIENTS because they are needed in only minute amounts, ranging from micrograms (1/1,000 gram) to milligrams (1/1,000,000 of a gram). They can form enzyme helpers (the B COMPLEX, trace minerals like ZINC and COPPER); they may build hormones (like VITAMIN D or IODINE); or they may serve a protective role as an ANTIOXIDANT to reduce chemical damage to cells (vitamin C, selenium, among others).

Requirements

A majority of essential nutrients are sufficiently well characterized to warrant recommendations for daily allowances, whatever their source. Nutrient allowances need to provide a reasonable margin of safety to account for factors such as age, STRESS, life-style habits, gender, pregnancy and lactation. The Food and Nutrition Board of the National Research Council formulated RECOMMENDED DIETARY ALLOWANCES (RDA) estimated to meet the needs of 95% of healthy Americans. Nutrient recommendations rely upon biochemical research, clinical case histories of nutrient-deficient individuals, human experimentation with suboptimal diets, animal growth experiments and examination of nutrient intake of healthy people. Reduced nutrient intake as well as excessive nutrient consumption can lead to MALNUTRITION. A BALANCED DIET supplies all nutrients in adequate amounts to maintain health. Reliance on foods containing high levels of fat or calories—as sweets, fatty snack foods and many highly processed foods—crowds out micronutrients like vitamins and trace minerals. (See also COENZYME; COFACTOR; DIETARY GUIDELINES FOR AMERICANS; FOOD PROCESSING; VITAMIN E.)

Department of Health and Human Services, "Surgeon General's Report on Nutrition and Health. Summary and recommendations," Public Health Service Publication 88-50211. Washington, D.C., 1988.

nutrient density   The relative concentration of nutrients in a food as compared to the calories found in wholesome, unprocessed food. Fruit has a higher nutrient density than fruit juice because fruit contains higher proportions of nutrients like VITAMINS, MINERALS, PROTEIN and FIBER, and fruit juice has a higher nutrient density than soda pop. This concept is especially useful in evaluating PROCESSED FOODS. The higher the nutrient density, the closer the food is to the initial unprocessed food and the more key nutrients it has. Thus JUNK FOOD and many highly processed food products made from bleached FLOUR, and manufactured meal products, often have a low nutrient density. Excessive calories contribute significantly to the problem of overweight facing many Americans. The ENRICHMENT and fortification of foods and beverages, the addition of vitamins and minerals, especially to cereal grain products like BREAKFAST CEREALS, flour and BREAD, together with MILK, attempts to improve the nutrient density of these popular foods. (See DIETARY GUIDELINES FOR AMERICANS; FAST FOOD; FOOD ADDITIVES; FOOD PROCESSING; OBESITY.)

nutrition   The science of FOODS, NUTRIENTS and their relationship to health and disease. (See also NUTRITIONIST.)

Goodman, Sandra et al., "Nutrition and Lifestyle Guidelines for People with Cancer," *Journal of Nutritional Medicine*, 4 (1994), pp. 199–214.
Kretchmer, Norman, "Nutrition Is the Keystone of Prevention," *American Journal of Clinical Nutrition*, 60 (1994), p. 1.

nutritional equivalency   Characteristic of a substitute or manufactured food, simulating a basic food and containing as much of the essential nutrients, as defined by the U.S. recommended daily allowances (USRDA), as the basic food. Thus a food can be considered nutritionally equivalent if it is not nutritionally inferior. There are important limitations to the U.S. FDA's definition of nutritional equivalency. A product can be declared nutritionally equivalent though it contains excessive amounts of any of the 20 nutrients for which USRDAs exist or if it contains different nutrient-to-calorie ratios. A food that provides fewer fat calories but equal levels of essential nutrients can be regarded as nutritionally superior. A substitute food can be classified nutritionally equivalent to its traditional counterpart even though it does not contain essential nutrients such as vitamin K and many minerals—CHROMIUM, SELENIUM, MOLYBDENUM, MANGANESE, FLUORIDE—as well as MACRONUTRIENTS, SODIUM, POTASSIUM and CHLORIDE.

The legal definition excludes other factors in foods. For example, dietary FIBER is not considered a component of nutritional equivalency, and uncharacterized materials in vegetables apparently reduce the risk of some forms of cancer and are excluded. Finally, the definition of nutritional equivalency does not generally deal with BIOAVAILABILITY, that is, the degree to which nutrients in food can be absorbed and used. Digestibility, nutrient uptake and interrelationships among nutrients influence nutrient availability in fabricated foods. Functional laboratory tests measure an attribute that reflects nutrient use. As an example, PROTEIN EFFICIENCY RATIO (PER) is a standardized functional test that accesses protein utilization of foods. (See also FOOD LABELING; IMITATION FOOD.)

nutritional supplements See VITAMIN.

nutritional status An assessment of the adequacy of the diet in meeting individual nutrient needs. Nutritional assessment entails a comprehensive health evaluation: Medical history, diet analysis, physical exam, and measurement of height and weight can reflect nutrient status. This evaluation may require laboratory tests to determine the tissue and fluid levels of specific VITAMINS and MINERALS, or measurement of biochemical markers of nutrient adequacy, such as serum FERRITIN, to assess IRON status.

Many factors can influence a person's nutrient status, and sorting them out can be a challenge. An illness can cause appetite loss or difficulty in swallowing or chewing; it can interfere with DIGESTION or assimilation of food or alter nutrient usage or excretion of wastes. An elderly patient may not be able to purchase or prepare adequate food because of physical limitations. Diminished taste with aging may lead to the selection of salty foods. Dentures can make chewing difficult, while diminished stomach acid output can decrease VITAMIN B_{12} absorption as well as mineral absorption and digestion in general. A lack of EXERCISE can contribute to problems of excessive weight. Overmedication can lead to DEPRESSION and disinterest in food, MALNUTRITION and weight loss. (See also ASSESSMENT, NUTRITION; DIET RECORD; DIETITIAN; MALABSORPTION; OBESITY.)

nutritional yeast See BAKER'S YEAST; BREWER'S YEAST; CANDIDA ALBICANS.

nutritionist A professional who specializes in nutritional counseling. Currently, training is not uniform from state to state. Nutritionists' backgrounds range from mail order credentials to Ph.D.s from accredited universities. Most nutrition programs require training in food science and the biological sciences. A number of states have legislation that licenses nutritionists if they are registered DIETITIANS or if they have an advanced degree from a recognized college or university. A graduate of a program in nutrition, nutrition education or dietetics is likely to be qualified. A number of professional organizations offer certification programs that assure high standards and are open to qualified health care professionals, such as the International and American Associations of Clinical Nutritionists and the Certification Board of Nutrition Specialists.

nutrition labeling See FOOD LABELING.

oats (*Avena sativa*)   A common cereal GRAIN grown in temperate regions, particularly in North America and northern Europe. There are six species, including common oats and cultivated red oats, that are grown in the Americas. Oats are classified as winter and spring varieties, according to their planting time. Only about 5% percent of the U.S. crop is used as a food crop; most ends up as livestock feed. An inedible, loose, pithy hull surrounds the kernel, or groat, and must be removed for human consumption.

Pure oats and pure oat BRAN are the least processed form of oats. Oat flakes, prepared by steaming and flaking whole kernels, are the basis for porridge. Oatmeal is prepared by cutting kernels to small granules with a mealy texture. Consumption of old-fashioned oatmeal as a BREAKFAST CEREAL has declined with the increased popularity of ready-cooked oatmeal cereals. Rolled oats, prepared by crushing oats with still rollers, are used in breakfast food, cookies, breads and GRANOLA, which is a mixture of rolled oats, honey, nuts, raisins or dates. Milling produces oat flour. Oat flour contains a natural ANTIOXIDANT that increases the stability of oat flour in storage.

Oat Bran

Oat Bran is derived from an outer layer of oat kernels by milling. It is a good source of SILICON, a trace mineral needed for healthy joints, and a form of FIBER called beta glucan. The fiber in oat bran is water-soluble and differs from water-insoluble WHEAT bran, the kind usually found in bran-enriched breakfast cereals. Eating oat bran daily in muffins and a bowl of hot oatmeal—together with daily exercise and eating less animal FAT as found in red MEAT and BUTTER—can lower blood fat and CHOLESTEROL even in diabetics. Oat bran alone has a modest effect in lowering elevated levels of the less desirable LDL-cholesterol (LOW-DENSITY LIPOPROTEIN). Oat bran has been used as a fat substitute to reduce fat in beef and pork sausage products. A mixture of oatmeal and oat flour has been developed by the USDA as a fat substitute called Oatrim or "hydrolyzed oat flour." Oatrim contains 1 calorie per gram, as compared with 9 calories per gram of fat and 4 calories per gram of STARCH. This fat substitute is being used in baked goods and processed meats, and other products are under development.

Oatmeal

Hot oatmeal is a traditional breakfast, and its emergence as an important source of fiber has caused a resurgence in popularity. Steel cut, rolled or quick cooking oats all contain the same amount of fiber. However, processed, cold oat breakfast cereals contain much less fiber (about 2 g per serving). Dry oatmeal contains about 14% protein, but cooked oatmeal is only about 2% protein. When purchasing oat-based cereals, read the label carefully. Oats should be the first ingredient listed, not sugar.

Nutrient content of regular cooked oatmeal or rolled oats, (1 cup fortified) is: 145 calories; protein, 6 g; carbohydrate, 25.2 g; fiber, 9.23 g; fat, 2.3 g; iron, 1.6 mg; sodium, 285 mg;

vitamin A, 453 retinol equivalents; thiamin, 0.53 mg; riboflavin, 0.29 mg; niacin, 5.9 mg.

obesity   An excessive accumulation of body fat for a given body size based on muscle and bone (frame size). Obesity is considered to be a condition in which fat represents more than 25% of total body weight for men or greater than 30% for women: Weighing 20% or more than "ideal" weight was previously used as a standard for obesity. Americans are gradually gaining more weight. Harris polls conducted in 1983 found 58% as being overweight, in 1990 the figure was 64%; in 1994 it was 69%, and in 1995, 71% of Americans 25 or older were found to be overweight. In 1994 the Institute of Medicine of the National Academy of Sciences concluded that one third of Americans can be considered obese. More than 10% are at least 30% overweight and more than 20% are between 20% and 30% overweight. The prevalence varies among groups. The average American adult gains a pound a year through middle age. Childhood obesity has increased dramatically since 1965 in the United States, reflecting an increased prevalence of obesity among children in Western countries. Twenty-five percent of teenagers and children in the U.S. are believed to be obese.

A key problem is in defining ideal weight because there is no single established standard of ideal body weight. Instead, "desired" or "optimal" body weights are now used as a reference. Obesity is not synonymous with being overweight: overweight refers to an excess of total body weight including muscle mass. A person could have above normal body weight due to muscle accumulation associated with weight lifting or strenuous exercise, for instance.

A variety of methods are used to measure body fat and to establish an optimal body weight, including weight determinations, comparison of body circumferences or diameters, skinfold thickness and bioimpedence (electrical resistance) measurements. A convenient method of judging whether you are too fat (or too thin) is to compare your *body mass index* with recommended standards. The body mass index is calculated by dividing your weight (in kilograms) by your height (in meters) squared. (Weight is determined without clothes and height is measured without shoes.) The most desirable body mass depends upon age. A body mass index greater than 28 is considered medically obese.

The number of obese Americans has increased, despite a national preoccupation with dieting. The fear of being fat has become an American obsession. U.S. society places a premium on being slender and most women and some men have dieted at least once. Being obese or overweight often brings a profound social stigma affecting personal life, life insurance premiums and employment opportunities. Nevertheless, in the 1980s the renewed interest in healthy life-styles in America apparently affected a limited number of people. Sedentary lifestyles continue to prevail.

Types of Obesity

Hyperblastic obesity is characterized by an excessive number of fat cells. Increased fat cell size is classified as hypertrophic obesity, and individuals with hyperblastic-hypertrophic obesity have increased numbers of enlarged fat cells in their adipose tissue. Hyperblastic obesity is usually associated with childhood, while hypertrophic obesity develops later in life and is associated with diabetes and other aspects of metabolic imbalance.

Obesity as a Health Hazard

The National Institutes of Health considers obesity to be a national disease. It has been noted that the death rate increases 2% for each pound over the healthy weight. For persons who are 40 pounds overweight, the death rate is estimated to be 80% higher during the next 25 years of their life. Lean men survive longer than overweight men in the United States. Obesity increases the risk of HEART DISEASE, diabetes, GOUT, ARTHRITIS, CANCER of the liver and esophagus, GALLSTONES, hernia, intestinal blockage, kidney disease and TOXEMIA of pregnancy. In the United States obesity increases the risk of angina, high blood pressure (HYPERTENSION), high blood fat, elevated LDL (LOW-DENSITY LIPOPROTEIN) and sudden death from heart disease. One clue to understanding the relationship between obesity and elevated blood fat is the observation that obese people have higher insulin levels, which seems to promote higher blood lipids.

The location of fat accumulation makes a difference in health risks. Male-patterned obesity, with fat deposited primarily in the abdomen and trunk, is called android obesity (the "spare tire" or "apple" profile). Android obesity in men or women is associated with an increased risk for CARDIOVASCULAR DISEASE, hypertension, elevated BLOOD SUGAR and gallstones. The greater the proportion of abdominal fat, the greater the risk. Abdominal fat may be more readily converted to cholesterol than fat deposited elsewhere. Pear-shaped people, with fat accumulation around the hips, do not experience as much diabetes or high blood pressure or as many heart attacks as those whose fat is around the middle.

Possible Mechanisms for Regulating Body Weight

Complex mechanisms involving the NERVOUS SYSTEM, the ENDOCRINE SYSTEM and the DIGESTIVE SYSTEM, and adipose tissue regulate eating, energy balance and thus obesity. Regions of the brain, such as the HYPOTHALAMUS and the brain stem, help regulate food intake, body weight, body size and body fat content. The hypothalamus plays a critical role in eating and balancing energy requirements with intake. The lateral hypothalamus controls eating activity; the paraventricular nucleus regulates nutrient balance and the ventromedial hypothalamus regulates energy balance by regulating the sympathetic nervous system, which helps the body adapt to stress. The hypothalamus regulates the ENDOCRINE SYSTEM (hormone secreting system). It activates the PITUITARY GLAND, which signals the adrenal gland to release GLUCOCORTICOIDS. In turn, these STEROID hormones regulate the nervous system, appetite and fat metabolism. Obesity is linked to altered function of the brainstem and hypothalamus and to changes in the autonomic nervous system, which regulates energy expenditure and regulates thermogenesis. At the molecular level, altered production of NEUROTRANSMITTERS, chemicals required to transmit nerve impulses, brain peptides and brain hormones, may alter critical control and feedback mechanisms that maintain body weight.

Several hypotheses link food intake and energy balance to regulate body weight through an interplay between the endocrine system and the nervous system. A hypothetical very general control system involves the following components: A proposed "controller" resides in the brain. Signals leaving the brain regulate heat production, physical activity, food intake, energy storage as fat, and metabolism for doing work and producing heat. These factors stimulate the release of hormones. Nutrients and hormones from various glands and fat cells are then carried back to brain centers that in turn generate signals that are interpreted by the hypothalamus to diminish eating. Stomach distension triggers the nervous system to create a feeling of fullness. The action of GLUCOSE (blood sugar) on tissue receptors could also send signals back to the brain to diminish eating behavior.

One hypothesis predicts a "set point" that tends to keep body weight at a constant level. According to the "set point" hypothesis for body weight, each person has a biologically determined body weight, believed to be inherited. In some obese individuals the set point may be set too high. When fat cells decrease in size, for example after DIETING, they could indirectly signal the brain to increase food consumption. Thus an obese person with large numbers of fat cells could crave food, leading to excessive eating after dieting. According to a related hypothesis, some obese people earlier in their lives, perhaps during early childhood, ate much more than their bodies needed during their formative years. According to this proposal, this event patterned the body for burning energy and storing fat. Once overweight, obesity in these individuals could be sustained even when consuming an average amount of food.

Insulin insensitivity correlates with obesity; increasing tissue sensitivity to insulin is hypothesized to lower the body's set point. Very recent discoveries shed light on the relationships among obesity, satiety and noninsulin dependent diabetes. Fat cells normally secrete a protein called LEPTIN that induces satiety. Leptin signals the brain to reduce consumption of fatty foods and possibly to increase the basal metabolism of fat cells. Therefore leptin helps regulate body weight by limiting body fat accumulation. Mice with mutations on the gene coding for leptin become obese. Researchers now believe obese people often make more than enough leptin, but the brain does not respond effectively to shut down eating because its binding sites or cell signaling mechanisms are defective. A region of the brain likely to be affected by leptin is the HYPOTHALAMUS, which integrates many functions of the body. Specifically, the region known as ventromedial nucleus, which regulates satiety, may be involved. Leptin could shut off signals in the brain that direct feeding (hunger signals), including neuropeptides. One possibility is neuropeptide Y, which induces lab animals to eat more carbohydrate and fat. In the set point model, leptin could act like a thermometer: when the body gets too thin, less leptin is made, more food is eaten and less energy is consumed. When the body gets too fat, more leptin is made, less food is consumed and more energy is burned.

A variety of mutations in other genes link obesity and diabetes. As an example, mutations in a protein called beta$_3$-adrenergic receptor, an attachment site which binds a NEUROTRANSMITTER (norepinephrine), increase the risk of middle-age weight gain and diabetes. Under normal condi-

tions norepinephrine produced by the sympathetic nervous system stimulates fat cells to burn stored fats. The implication is that with a faulty neurotransmitter attachment site in fat tissue, the body burns less fat efficiently and calories accumulate. As an alternative to the setpoint hypothesis, the "settling point" theory proposes that body weight is not fixed, but that it is maintained according to feedback loops that are determined by an interplay between genes and environment. Systems controlling hunger and satiety respond rapidly to dietary protein and carbohydrate, but the feedback from a fatty meal may be too slow to prevent overconsumption. Thus increased dietary fat could alter the body's equilibrium and shift body fat upward. The number of fat cells in the body is a determining factor. Fat cells are added during childhood and it could very well be that how much fatty food is consumed and how many calories are burned before adulthood has a major impact for the risk of obesity.

Human obesity is a complex phenomenon with many causes. Inheritance as well as diet and medical history can contribute to excessive weight gain and many questions about the detailed interrelationships remain unanswered. Apparently many genes interact to control weight, it is therefore unlikely that any single pharmacologic agent related to a gene product will substitute for changing the diet and exercising regularly to maintain desired weight. In any event, very extensive clinical experience suggests that diets—that improve insulin sensitivity and glucose tolerance by emphasizing VEGETABLES and LEGUMES and minimizing sugary or high fat foods—together with regular physical exercise can support long-term weight loss and reduce the risk of cardiovascular disease.

Causes of Obesity

Many adults achieve an energy balance in which caloric intake matches energy expenditure. Body fat does not change very much under these conditions. Excessive body fat could be related to eating more calories or to small energy expenditure, or both. Energy expenditure refers to the calories spent for body functions, physical activity, digestion, and food metabolism. Both heredity and the environment play a part in obesity and therefore there is no single approach to treatment. Overeating, differences in metabolism, AGING, genetic predisposition and excessive food consumption during early childhood have been implicated.

Overeating Clearly the prolonged consumption of excessive calories, when energy intake exceeds energy expenditure, leads to obesity. Energy expenditure refers to the calories spent for body functions, physical activity, digestion and food metabolism. Body fat can be reduced only when energy expenditure exceeds caloric intake. The body adapts to excessive food consumption—whether excessive PROTEIN, CARBOHYDRATE, fat or ALCOHOL—by storing the surplus calories as body fat. Many reports have suggested that obese people eat the same, or sometimes less than non-obese people. Using new research methods based on ingesting double-labeled water, that is, water containing a "heavy" form of oxygen (O^{18}) and "heavy" hydrogen (deuterium), investigators have demonstrated that, on the average, obese people generally eat more, but they habitually underreport their food consumption.

Differences in energy expenditure   Generally, though obese people are less active than non-obese people, they tend to use the same amounts of energy because they weigh more. Sedentary life-styles contribute to obesity. More than two-thirds of adult Americans fail to exercise 20 minutes or more three times a week as recommended. Most people will lose weight if such an exercise program is coupled with consuming no more than 1,500 calories daily. Individuals who exercise regularly, or who exercise before and after a high-calorie meal, lose more energy as heat after eating than those who do not exercise.

Differences in metabolism   This picture is unclear. Very rarely do glandular imbalances lead to obesity. Cushing's syndrome, excessive production of glucocorticoids, a form of adrenal hormone, is an example of hormone imbalance that can promote obesity. Obese people do not have unusually slow metabolisms. When resting metabolic rates are compared based upon the muscle/bone mass, there is not a significant difference between metabolic rates of non-obese and obese individuals. Formerly obese individuals preferentially store fat rather than burning it, and studies suggest that overweight and obese people tend to eat more fat and less carbohydrate. In general the body consumes calories more slowly after weight is lost, and it burns calories more rapidly when weight is gained, for fat as well as for thin people. One hypothesis contends that people adjust their metabolism to maintain a "set point" weight. Thus someone who has lost significant amounts of fat (10% of their body weight) will burn fewer calories when exercising than someone who has maintained his or her weight without a weight-loss program. Apparently the body adjusts its metabolism by altering the efficiency of muscles in burning calories. Recently a type of prostaglandin has been shown to act as a hormone to trigger the production of fat cells from immature cells.

Aging   In the United States both men and women tend to become fatter with increasing age. This could be due to a decreased metabolic rate (a lower BASAL METABOLIC RATE) and a sedentary life-style coupled with an easy access to high-calorie food.

Meal frequency   The frequency of meals and meal composition may be a factor in obesity. Eating fewer meals may increase fat deposition, while smaller, more frequent meals, with more food at breakfast and less at supper, may promote weight loss.

TV watching   Excessive TV watching correlates with overeating. Reduced physical activity, lowered metabolic rates, as well as visual cues to eating high-fat snack foods and drinking alcoholic beverages, contribute to the increased prevalence of overweight. Dietary fat, which provides 9 calories per gram, is more fattening than either protein or carbohydrate, which provide 4 calories per gram. Fat calories in food differ from calories in carbohydrate: Fat in food is more easily converted to body fat than is carbohydrate.

Inheritance   One broad generalization can be made: Obesity persists over a life span. Fat children tend to become fat adults, suggesting a predisposition to being overweight. Early adulthood is an important period for the development of life-long patterns. The question remains, to what degree is obesity the product of genetics? Studies with twins suggest that between 50 and 70% of the variability in relative body weight represents genetic variability. Current research focuses on locating specific obesity genes. Genes influence both metabolism and behavior. Many genes regulate hunger and satiety. A flurry of recent research has yielded impartial genetic discoveries: gene *OB* causes fat cells to produce a satiety protein called leptin. A gene then codes for the receptor of this hormone in the brain. Still another gene codes for a hormone-producing enzyme (carboxypeptidase E). A gene that codes for a neurotransmitter receptor (binding site; Beta$_3$-adrenergic receptor) for norepinephrine is also implicated in maintaining weight. Mutations of these genes can increase the risk of obesity and diabetes in lab animals and possibly in people. There will be more to add to this unfinished story as more discoveries are made.

What Characterizes Those Who Successfully Lose Fat and Keep It Off?

A willingness to change   Therapeutic approaches to obesity and weight management have met with only modest success. Only 2 to 10% of Americans who diet to lose weight and participate in weight loss programs will keep the pounds off more than several years. Most of the lost fat is regained within a few months after the dieter discontinues the diet regimen. Dieting without a long-term commitment to changing daily habits is destined to fail.

Attitude is perhaps the most prominent factor in changing behavior. Regarding overeating, understanding underlying feelings for which overeating compensates seems essential for permanent weight loss. Eating can provide immediate gratification, but this seldom resolves deep-seated emotional issues. After short-term sensory satisfaction, emotional pain or longing often returns. For example, responding to feelings of low self-esteem by crash dieting does not solve the underlying issue, and too often the dieter returns to old eating habits. Counselors recommend beginning with an inventory of talents and qualities that fill your life with the most satisfaction and choosing activities and relationships that bring satisfaction and a sense of well-being. These are the well-spring of inner peace.

Slow weight loss   Successful long-term weight control requires the slow loss of body fat without cyclic, on-again, off-again dieting (YO-YO DIETING). Losing a pound a week helps maintain muscle (LEAN BODY MASS) while preferentially losing fat.

Exercise   Exercising for life helps keep the body engine "revved up," so that more calories are burned by muscle and less insulin is required to dispose of elevated blood sugar following meals.

Improved diet   A high-fat, high-calorie, low-fiber diet is thought to be the major dietary factor in obesity in the United States. Therefore the recommended diet might be low in fat, high in fiber and complex carbohydrates (60 to 70% of calories), with adequate protein (10 to 15% of calories). Emphasis on natural, whole foods simplifies this task of avoiding the pervasive high-calorie foods that fill the American food landscape. Another approach to obesity and overweight focuses on helping people through advocacy and social support with the premise that being overweight can be part of an enjoyable, fulfilling life: The Association for the Health Enhancement of Large People and the National Association to Advance Fat Acceptance are two such groups.

Weight Loss Drugs

Drugs that act as APPETITE SUPPRESSANTS, usually by increasing SEROTONIN and dopamine, which act as hormones and as neurotransmitters, may be prescribed for obese patients. Like diets, anti-obesity drugs tend to be effective only as long as the patient follows the prescription. When drugs are withdrawn, weight lost usually returns unless permanent behavior changes have been made. Amphetamines have adverse side effects: They have the potential for addiction and tolerance (more drug is required to get the same effect with chronic use). A newly approved third generation drug, fenfluramine, increases the levels of serotonin, a brain chemical that decreases appetite. However, the long-term safety has been questioned. Another class of drug promotes nutrient malabsorption so that patients taking these drugs do not absorb calories efficiently. However, no present drug is both entirely safe and effective for weight loss, nor is it certain that taking current medications for many years is better than being fat. Drugs that suppress appetite are not recommended for those who wish to lose only 5 to 10 pounds of fat.

Childhood Obesity

An estimated 25 to 30% of U.S. children are overweight. Obesity is recognized as a U.S. epidemic affecting children. The number of obese youngsters increased by more than 50% among children between the ages of 6 and 11 since 1963, and it increased 34% among children between 12 and 17. Low-income minority children face even higher rates of obesity. As many as 80% of obese teenagers will become obese adults.

Childhood obesity is linked to many of the factors that cause adult obesity:

Heredity As in adult obesity, genes play a role. Children born to obese mothers are more likely to be obese. If both parents are obese, the probability of their children becoming obese is very high.

Overfeeding Some babies have more fat cells than usual. If they are also overfed, they are more likely to become obese children. In addition, overfeeding a child may lead to larger, not more, fat cells. This may make controlling weight more difficult as an adult. (It should be pointed out that plump babies do not necessarily become obese adults.)

Lower metabolism Infants who become overweight during their first year have a lower basal metabolic rate than usual. Their mechanism for regulating body weight might be lower than average.

Eating too much fatty food The more JUNK FOOD is consumed, the more likely the child will be obese. The 1988 Surgeon General's report, confirmed by USDA dietary recommendations of 1992, concluded that the standard American diet is too high in fat, especially saturated fat. The Bogalusa Heart Study is an ongoing population study to examine risk factors for cardiovascular disease in children.

Results from this study reveal that children who consume more than 30% of their calories from fat were more likely to eat less CALCIUM, IRON, MAGNESIUM and vitamins like RIBOFLAVIN, NIACIN, THIAMIN, VITAMIN B_6, VITAMIN B_{12} and VITAMIN E.

Too much TV and not enough exercise The odds of becoming obese increase with the number of hours of TV viewed each day. Children's basal metabolic rate decreases, and they get less physical activity. Children who watch TV eat more of the high-calorie, highly processed food they see advertised, and parents fill the role of food "gate keepers." Children eat what is available to them, whether it is candy, soft drinks or fatty convenience foods, or fruit, low-fat foods and sugar-free beverages.

The home environment and parents present the model for a child's eating habits. A child's shift to a more healthful life-style needs to be nurtured by parents to become permanent. As with overweight adults, regular exercise is extremely important in children's health and maintaining a desirable weight. Overzealous dietary restrictions by parents can encourage self-imposed dieting and eating disorders, a prevalent problem among children and adolescents in the United States. As many as 80% of 10-year-old girls suffer from a fear of body fat; some already show signs of dieting, bingeing, overeating and anorexia. The message they are receiving is that any accumulation of body fat is socially unacceptable. However, among white, middle-class, healthy girls in the United States, weight before and during puberty does not seem to be a predictor of weight gain at middle age (50). On the other hand, weight gained after puberty, during early adolescence, has correlated with weight gain as adults. For boys, prepuberty weight appears to be a good predictor of adult obesity. A physician should be consulted before talking to children about weight. Periodic increases in fat, especially among girls, are a normal occurrence. Weight maintenance, after the child has grown into his or her own weight, is preferable to dieting. Generally children can be taught to prefer lower fat foods by exposure and availability. (See also MALNUTRITION; WEIGHT MANAGEMENT.)

Allison, D.B., and Pi-Sunyer F.X., "Fleshing Out Obesity," *The Sciences*, 34 (May–June 1994), pp. 38–43.

Martin, R.J., White, B.D., Hulsey, M.G., "The Regulation of Body Weight," *American Scientist*, 79 (1991), pp. 528–41.

Williams, Christine L. and Kimm, Sue Y.S., eds., "Prevention and Treatment of Childhood Obesity," *Annals of the New York Academy of Sciences*, 699 (1993).

octacosanol A complex alcohol that is a normal constituent of wheat germ and wheat germ oil. Other sources include whole grain cereals, seeds and nuts, and many plant oils and WAXES. Persistent claims that octacosanol supplementation has a positive effect on physical endurance and muscular strength have not been substantiated by research. The Federal Trade Commission concluded that wheatgerm oil did not improve endurance or stamina. Octacosanol seems to improve reaction time. (See also ERGOGENIC SUPPLEMENTS.)

oil See VEGETABLE OIL.

oil palm (*Elaeis guineensis*)   A palm that is a major source of edible oil. The oil palm yields more oil per acre than any other plant. It originated in West Africa, and plantations now exist in Malaysia, China and Indonesia, as well as Tanzania, the Ivory Coast, Nigeria and other regions. Palm oil is prepared from fibrous pulp of the fruit, and palm kernel oil is obtained from the seed or kernel, which contains about 50% oil. Palm kernel oil is used for margarine production and food manufacture. It is among the most SATURATED FATS, containing 86.7% saturated FATTY ACIDS, 1.6% polyunsaturated fatty acids and 11.7% monounsaturated fatty acids. (See also COCONUT OIL; TROPICAL OILS.)

okra (*Hibiscus esculentus; Abelmoschus esculentus*)   A vegetable that bears seeds in edible pods. Okra ancestors may have been widely distributed from Africa to India. Okra now grows in regions with a moderate climate, including the southern states of the United States. Much of the U.S. okra crop is frozen or canned. Okra contains a mucilage that acts as a thickener in soups and stews. Because okra changes to an unappetizing color when cooked in utensils containing iron, copper or brass, glass or stainless steel containers are used. Okra's slippery mucilage is balanced by acidic foods like tomatoes and lemons and by vinegar. Okra, long considered part of Deep South cuisine, is also part of Indian, Caribbean, South American and African recipes.

Nutrient content of okra (8 pods, 85 g, cooked) is: 27 calories; protein, 1.6 g; carbohydrate, 6.1 g; fiber, 2.75 g; calcium, 54 g; iron, 0.38 mg; potassium, 274 mg; vitamin C, 14 mg; thiamin, 0.11 mg; riboflavin, 0.05 mg; niacin, 0.74 mg.

oleic acid   A non-essential FATTY ACID and a common constituent of FATS and OILS found in foods and fat synthesized by the body. Oleic acid is distinguished from the other common fatty acids, the energy-rich building blocks of fats and oils. It contains 18 carbon atoms and a single double bond, is deficient in hydrogen atoms, and thus is classified as a monounsaturated fatty acid. In contrast, saturated fatty acids are building blocks filled up with hydrogen atoms and polyunsaturated fatty acids possessing two or more double bonds and are more unsaturated than oleic acid. Oils rich in oleic acid are called monounsaturated oils. VEGETABLE OILS like olive oil, AVOCADO oil and CANOLA OIL contain high amounts of oleic acid. Oleic acid–rich vegetable oils seem to lower the less desirable forms of blood CHOLESTEROL, LOW-DENSITY LIPOPROTEIN (LDL) with high fat intake, and to increase more desirable forms of cholesterol, HIGH-DENSITY LIPOPROTEIN (HDL). Olive oil is more stable to oxidation than polyunsaturates like safflower oil or corn oil. The recommendation is to decrease fat and oil consumption generally, and to use more monounsaturates in cooking, rather than saturates (butter, lard, shortening, coconut oil or palm oil) or polyunsaturates (such as CORN OIL, SAFFLOWER oil and SOYBEAN oil).

Olestra (sucrose polyester, imitation fat [Olean])   A new non-caloric fat substitute recently approved for use in snack foods such as crackers, potato chips and other chips. Olestra tastes like LARD and VEGETABLE OILS; it is neither digested nor absorbed by the body. By comparison, FAT and oils contain 126 calories per tablespoon. Olestra resembles the structure of fat, except that it has a molecule of sucrose at its core to which are attached eight fatty acids, rather than three. Because it possesses a new substance, sucrose polyester had to be approved by the U.S. FDA. All products containing Olestra will be labeled to notify the consumer that Olestra may cause abdominal cramping and loose stools and that it inhibits the uptake of certain nutrients. Vitamins A, D, E and K have been added. The question of malabsorption of CAROTENOIDS has not been addressed.

In addition to these potential safety problems, animal studies suggest Olestra can cause liver damage, birth defects and cancer. More complete studies are needed to establish its safety. Regardless of their source, fat substitutes cannot replace the need to eat less high-fat food and to change eating habits. (See also WEIGHT MANAGEMENT.)

olive (*Olea europaea*)   The oil-rich fruit of a semitropical evergreen adapted to hot, dry climates. Olives were probably first cultivated in the Eastern Mediterranean region as early as 6000 B.C. There are now over 60 varieties. Mediterranean countries remain major producers; together Italy and Spain produce over half of the world's olives and 60% of world olive oil production. Olives are also grown in Australia, China, Greece, Turkey and France, as well as in the United States. Spanish colonists introduced olives to California in the 18th century; that state continues to be a major domestic supplier. At maturity, ripened olives contain 15 to 35% oil, and OLIVE OIL is a major cooking oil. The oil content varies according to soil conditions, climate and time of harvest.

Olives must be processed for consumption. In the Spanish method, green (unripe) olives are first treated with alkali, then fermented, and canned or bottled. The alkali destroys a bitter constituent called oleuropein. In the American method, half-ripe, reddish fruit are cured in lye (strong alkali). Olives darken as pigments oxidize. They are rinsed and then placed in fermentation tanks containing BRINE. In the Greek method, fully mature olives are harvested and soaked in brine to remove the bitter components. Ripe, pitted olives (10, 47 g) provide 50 calories; protein, 0.4 g; carbohydrate, 2.9 g; fiber, 1.4 g; fat, 4.5 g; calcium, 42 mg; iron, 1.5 mg; sodium, 410 mg; and traces of B vitamins.

olive oil   An oil extracted from ground olives. Spain is currently the world's leading producer of bulk olive oil; Italy is a leading producer of bottled olive oil. The International Oil Agreement was negotiated through the U.N. to ensure olive cultivation and olive oil production in the Mediterranean region.

To produce olive oil, crushed olives are mechanically pressed several times. The temperature for olive oil extraction can be 50° to 110° F. There is no legal definition of "cold-pressed" oil. The hotter the pressing, the more oil is extracted. Olive oil is classified as a monounsaturated fat because it contains large amounts of OLEIC ACID, a monounsaturated FATTY ACID with one double bond and lacking two hydrogen atoms—in contrast with polyunsaturates, containing polyunsaturated fatty acids with two or more double bonds and lacking several pairs of hydrogen atoms, and saturates, containing predominantly saturated fatty acids (no double bonds and completely filled up with hydrogen atoms). Because olive oil is more stable to oxidation and rancidity, olive oil is not chemically stabilized (partially hydrogenated). Olive oil, like all oils, provides 14 g of fat per tablespoon, equivalent to 120 calories.

Proposed Grades of Oil

An independent U.S. FDA analysis of 30 imported olive oils revealed that five were not olive oil and 18 were mislabeled as "extra virgin" oil.

"Extra virgin olive oil" is prepared from mechanical pressing and is filtered without refining. "Virgin olive oil" is not highly refined and has a golden color and a unique flavor and taste. The acid content is no more than 1%. Virgin olive oil is filtered after pressing and is unrefined; the oil has a rather fruity flavor, and its acid content is less than 2%. Oil labeled "olive oil" is usually listed as being "100 percent pure." It is actually a blend of refined and unrefined olive oil and accounts for about 70% of U.S. olive oil consumption. Refining involves extraction at high temperatures and with solvents, neutralization of acids, and bleaching.

Potential Health Benefits of Olive Oil

People who eat predominantly olive oil have lower blood fat and cholesterol and a reduced risk of clogged arteries. Olive oil seems to lower blood levels of the less desirable form of CHOLESTEROL, LDL (LOW-DENSITY LIPOPROTEIN), while raising the level of HDL (HIGH-DENSITY LIPOPROTEIN), the more desirable kind of cholesterol. If the intake of polyunsaturates increases substantially above 7% of daily calories, the current average, polyunsaturated oils lower LDL (a desirable effect) but also lower HDL (an undesirable effect). By following current dietary guidelines that call for eating less fat (less than 30% of total calories) and less saturated fat (less than 10% of calories), people necessarily increase their consumption of unsaturates. Substituting monounsaturated oils for saturates and polyunsaturated fats and oils may be desirable while decreasing total fat consumption because high consumption of polyunsaturates is more likely to promote the oxidation of LDL cholesterol, the less desirable form, thus increasing the probability that oxidized LDL will be taken up by blood vessels and create plaque in arteries. Furthermore, animal studies suggest polyunsaturates can increase the risk of some forms of cancer. Cooking with olive oil instead of polyunsaturated vegetable oils (safflower oil, corn oil, etc.) may be advantageous because olive oil does not break down as readily when heated. (See also ATHEROSCLEROSIS; CARDIOVASCULAR DISEASE; FAT METABOLISM.)

"Special report: olive oil," *UC Berkeley Wellness Letter*, 11:9 (June, 1995), p. 6.

omega-3 fatty acids   See ESSENTIAL FATTY ACIDS; FLAXSEED OIL.

omega-6 fatty acids   See ESSENTIAL FATTY ACIDS.

onion (*Allium cepa*; common onion)   A vegetable with an underground bulb. Onions are closely related to GARLIC and leeks and belong to the lily family. Onions apparently originated in central Asia and were harvested in prehistoric times. Onions were grown in ancient Egypt, Greece and Rome, as well as China. There are more than 500 varieties; all of the edible species possess a pungent bulb. Europeans introduced onions to the Americas. Today China, the United States and India produce the largest yields, and onions rank sixth among vegetable crops worldwide.

Green onions may be harvested before the onion has matured. Alternatively, mature onion bulbs can be harvested. The length of time that dried bulbs can be stored ranges from several days to months, depending upon the variety, their stage of maturity and temperature and humidity during storage.

There are two types of dry onion. Flat onions, elongated Spanish onions and Bermuda onions are usually mild flavored. They do not store as well as globe or late crop onions, which frequently possess a stronger flavor. The latter store well and can be marketed throughout the year. Onions can be canned, dehydrated, frozen or pickled.

Onions and their relatives possess a complex family of sulfur compounds related to the sulfur-containing amino acid cysteine. Once their layers are cut, the sulfur-containing compounds come into contact with an enzyme called allinase that releases volatile (gaseous) compounds that can irritate eyes. Cooking onions and garlic modifies these sulfur compounds, and they are not so irritating after cooking.

The medicinal properties of onions and garlic have been known for thousands of years, and recorded use includes treatment of wounds and infections, tumors, worms and parasites, weakness, FATIGUE and asthma. Onions resemble garlic in terms of active ingredients and therapeutic effects. The consumption of garlic and onions correlates with lowered blood cholesterol levels. Generally the higher the dose of garlic and onions, the greater the reduction. Onions seem to lower blood CHOLESTEROL by helping to block cholesterol synthesis. Onions and garlic contain a variety of pungent, sulfur-containing compounds. One of these lowers BLOOD SUGAR; another counteracts blood platelet stickiness and reduces the tendency for blood to clot and, at the same time, raises HDL (HIGH-DENSITY LIPOPROTEIN), the desirable form of cholesterol that protects against cardiovascular disease. Onions help decrease elevated blood sugar levels in diabetics, possibly by slowing the breakdown of insulin, the hormone responsible for stimulating sugar uptake from the blood. They may also increase insulin secretion.

Onions as well as garlic possess anti-inflammatory effects. They contain compounds that block the production of inflammatory agents. For example, onions contain the FLAVONOID, QUERCETIN, a plant pigment known to reduce INFLAMMATION.

Both onions and garlic have antibiotic properties and have been shown to be effective against fungi, bacteria and parasites. Furthermore, onions and garlic contain substances that block tumor growth in animals. Sulfur compounds apparently induce enzyme systems in the LIVER that detoxify potentially harmful compounds. Flavonoids are ANTIOXIDANTS that block damage due to free radical attack. Free radicals are highly reactive molecules that avidly attack cells. Flavonoids play a role in the anticancer properties of onions and garlic because free radical damage is linked to cancer.

Raw, chopped onions (1 cup, 160 g) provide 54 calories; protein, 1.9 g; carbohydrate, 11.7 g; fiber, 2.64 g; iron, 0.59

mg; potassium, 248 mg; vitamin C, 13 mg; thiamin, 0.1 mg; riboflavin, 0.02 mg; and niacin, 0.16 mg. (See also CARCINOGEN; HEART ATTACK.)

orange (*Citrus sinensis*; sweet orange, common orange, China orange) A popular orange-colored CITRUS FRUIT. Oranges are the most popular fruit crop in the United States. Orange trees grow in semi-tropical regions and probably originated in Southeast Asia and Southern China. The Chinese cultivated oranges in ancient times. Spanish explorers and colonists brought the orange to the New World in the 16th century. In the United States oranges are cultivated in Arizona, California, Texas and Florida, the latter the most important domestic source. The three principal varieties of orange include the sweet (common, China orange), *C. sinensis*; the loose-skinned orange, *C. mobilis*; and the sour, bitter Seville orange, *C. aurantium*. Sweet oranges are represented by the blood orange, the navel orange and the Valencia (Spanish) orange, in addition to the Hamlin, Jaffa and Pineapple varieties. Only sweet oranges are grown commercially in the United States. The color of the orange peel does not necessarily indicate maturity because most oranges are picked green and exposed to ethylene gas at warm temperatures to enhance the orange color. Sour oranges, such as the Seville, are grown in Spain for marmalade and orange liqueurs.

Three quarters of U.S. orange production is processed and 80% of this ends up as frozen orange juice concentrate. Oranges and orange juice contain large amounts of VITAMIN C, and this contributes a substantial percentage of the vitamin C intake in the typical U.S. diet. The white inner portion of the peel is a good source of FLAVONOIDS, plant substances that act as antioxidants to prevent oxidative damage.

Certain individuals may be allergic to components in the orange peel and neither the peel nor products made from it should be eaten by such people. Citrus peel also contains citral, a compound that blocks the action of vitamin A. Organic orange peels have not been sprayed with pesticides. One orange (131 g) provides 60 calories; protein, 1.2 g; carbohydrate, 15.4 g; fiber, 2.97 g; potassium, 237 mg; vitamin C, 70 mg; thiamin 0.11 mg; riboflavin, 0.05 mg; and niacin, 0.37 mg.

Orange Juice

Fifteen percent of the domestic orange crop is used for fresh orange juice. Commercial orange juice may contain up to 10% mandarin orange juice and up to 5% sour orange juice. Frozen orange juice concentrate contains up to four times higher concentrations of nutrients than fresh juice. Orange juice can be used to enhance the flavor of root vegetables and can be added to jams and marmalades. Orange juice is a good source of vitamin C and POTASSIUM. Most 100% orange juices provide 60 mg of vitamin C or more and 80 to 100 calories per cup. The current Reference Daily Intake (formerly the USRDA) for vitamin C is 60 mg. Vitamin C is readily oxidized upon exposure to the air to an inactive form. Fresh-squeezed orange juice loses 60% of its vitamin C when stored for 24 hours at room temperature, or 20% when orange juice is refrigerated.

Once prepared, orange juice should be kept chilled in a sealed container to reduce losses of vitamin C. In comparison with fresh orange juice, canned orange juice has been heated, reducing the levels of vitamin C. Up to 10% of U.S. frozen orange juice concentrate was estimated to be adulterated with sugar, orange solids or chemical extenders in 1993. Some of the modifications have been subtle and difficult to detect. One cup of freshly squeezed orange juice provides 111 calories; 1.7 g protein; carbohydrate, 25.8 g; fiber, 0.5 g; potassium, 496 mg; vitamin C, 124 mg; thiamin, 0.22 mg; riboflavin, 0.07 mg; niacin, 0.78 mg.

Orange Drinks

Orange drinks and sodas are not orange juice. Their orange color is due to ARTIFICIAL FOOD COLORS. They represent empty calories because they are usually low in vitamin C and potassium and contain added SUCROSE, high FRUCTOSE CORN SYRUP or ASPARTAME as SWEETENERS.

oregano (*Origanum vulgare*; wild marjoram) An herb used in cooking. The flavor of oregano's dark-green leaves resembles that of THYME and sweet MARJORAM, but is more pungent. The dried herb possesses a stronger flavor than fresh leaves. Oregano is often used to season Mexican and Italian dishes (PASTA and PIZZA), beans, meat such as lamb, poultry and tomato soups. Before refrigeration, oregano was used to retard food spoilage. The essential oils of oregano possess a wide range of antifungal and bacterial activities.

organelle A subcellular particle or membrane component within cells that possesses a specialized metabolic function. Examples include MITOCHONDRIA, the nucleus, LYSOSOMES and ENDOPLASMIC RETICULUM.

Each type of cell, with the exception of RED BLOOD CELLS, contains up to several hundred small, bean-shaped structures known as mitochondria. They are about the size of bacteria and contain their own DNA and protein synthesizing machinery. Mitochondria are called the powerhouses of the cell because they provide the enzymes that convert fuels such as FAT and CARBOHYDRATE to ENERGY, yielding metabolic end products, WATER and CARBON DIOXIDE. In the typical cell, mitochondria produce more than 90% of the cell's chemical energy in the form of ATP.

Most cells except red blood cells contain a nucleus that houses DNA, the genetic blueprint of the cell, together with the machinery for synthesizing (replicating) DNA. The nucleus also contains enzymes needed to repair damage to DNA. DNA directs the formation of RNA molecules, which guide protein synthesis in the cytoplasm.

Lysosomes function as the cell's garbage disposal units. They degrade worn-out, damaged structures and PROTEIN whose components will be recycled. Endoplasmic reticulum is a complex membrane that houses enzymes that deactivate drugs and chemicals; that activate the B vitamin FOLIC ACID; elongate fatty acids; and synthesize specialized products for secretion, like digestive enzymes of the PANCREAS. (See also DNA; GENE; LIVER; METABOLISM.)

organic foods Foods that have been grown without chemical fertilizers and synthetic PESTICIDES. In the case of

MEAT and dairy products, organic refers to animals raised without the use of growth promoters like hormones, antibiotics and other substances that are added to animal feed. Any packaging or processing has been carried out without the use of synthetic compounds.

In 1990 the U.S. Congress passed the Organic Foods Production Act to establish uniform standards of organic food production as well as organic farming management. Organic farmers and organic food handlers seeking to be recognized as "organic" and to use the "organic" label must meet national standards through certification procedures. A federal advisory board, the National Organic Standards Board (NOSB), was established to implement the act.

The act imposes registration requirements and standards for what may be labeled "organic." The aim is to have all organic products sold in the United States certified. Nearly all produce contains at least traces of pesticides because very stable pesticides were used throughout the country for decades and traces often contaminate soil and water supplies. Certified organic food contains significantly fewer pesticides at lower levels than non-organic produce. Documentation will be required for organic claims that will detail the location where produce was grown and pest control methods employed. Organic farming emphasizes animal manure, cultivation of legumes (plants that add nitrogen back to the soil) and biological pest control. According to NOSB recommendations, a product can be "certified organic" if it contains at least 95% organic ingredients. The manufacturer needs to list the percentage of organic ingredients on the food label, or on the information panel, unless the food is 100% organic. In the latter case, the designation "organic" can be placed on the front of the product.

In the past individual markets have employed different standards for classifying a product as "organic." Certification of organic food by an independent third party addresses this issue. Organic food certification programs entail testing sample foods to verify low tolerances of pesticides, farm inspection, and inspection of records of pest control and the type of fertilizer used. Approximately half the states now have certification programs. One of the goals of the Organic Food Production Act is to define a uniform national certification criteria for organic growers and producers. This plan requires the accreditation of individual organic certifiers, to be defined by the NOSB. There are about 40 certification agencies in the United States and Canada, including the CALIFORNIA CERTIFIED ORGANIC FARMERS (CCOF) and the Farm Verified Organic (FVO).

Some states currently certify "transition" produce, that is, produce from farms that formerly used pesticides that have since been withdrawn from use. The period of transition to organic may require one to three years without the use of synthetic fertilizers and pesticides. This time period permits organic matter in soil to accumulate, to establish a balance with pests, and to allow pesticides previously applied to soils to decay or dissipate.

Crop standards, an organic handling plan that specifies certification requirements for organic food processors, and a national list of approved synthetic ingredients and prohibited substances fall under the developmental tasks of the board. Also to be resolved how NOSB standards can be streamlined with international organizations so growers will not pay for two certification fees; how government and state certifiers will cooperate in certification programs; and the type of seal for organic produce—either a generic government seal or seals of individual certifiers.

Present recommendations are to prohibit the use of antibiotics in animals that will be consumed for meat, and to restrict their use in breeder animals. As of spring 1996 the USDA had not completed its final version of the long-awaited national organic standards and they are not likely to be completed until the end of fiscal year 1996. Final recommendations for national organic standards will be reviewed by the USDA, the EPA and the FDA.

Organic foods may be more costly, depending upon the season, because more hand labor is involved when synthetic pesticides are omitted, and organic farming carries greater business risks. Organic food may not look as attractive as non-organic produce because some chemicals that create a cosmetic effect have not been used. Nutrient-depleted soils will produce crops with decreased levels of trace nutrients, and good soils increase the nutritional quality of produce. There is evidence that organic produce may be more nutritious than produce from conventional farms, in terms of boron, calcium, chromium, copper, iodine, iron, magnesium, manganese, potassium, silicon, selenium and zinc. For example, comparisons of trace minerals in organic and conventionally grown apples, corn, peas, potatoes and wheat purchased over a two-year period suggested that the average nutrient content of organic foods can average twofold greater than that of conventional commercial produce. One explanation is that synthetic fertilizers of nitrate, phosphates and other minerals do not enrich soils with a broad spectrum of nutrient minerals. Commercially grown food contained more aluminum, lead and mercury.

Organic farming provides environmental dividends as well. It requires less energy, minimizes groundwater pollution and reduces soil erosion. Manure benefits the soil by building loam and increasing water holding capacity. Legumes increase soil nitrogen for crops. Farm worker safety is also a consideration because synthetic pesticides pose the greatest risk to farm workers. The high crop yields of modern agriculture result partially from the use of chemical fertilizers and synthetic pesticides. The tonnage of pesticides applied to U.S. farms has grown 33-fold since World War II, and pesticide toxicity has increased tenfold. The decreased use of synthetic pesticides, together with crop rotation and biological pest control, in combination with organic farming methods and judicious use of certain synthetic pesticides and fertilizers and conservation, seems a realistic approach to preserve resources. (See also CERTIFIED ORGANIC VEGETABLES; NATURAL FOOD.)

Clark, J.B., "Interim Assessment of the National Organic Standards Process at USDA," *Pesticides and You*, 13:1 (Spring 1993), pp. 6–20.

National Organic Directory: A Guide to Organic Information and Resources. Davis, Calif.: Community Alliance with Family Farmers, 1995.

organic meat   MEAT grown without growth promoters like hormones, antibiotics and other substances that are added to animal feed. (See also ANTIBIOTIC-RESISTANT BACTERIA IN FOOD.)

organ meat   MEAT that represents internal organs such as the LIVER, kidney, heart and brains. In contrast, non-organ meat is comprised primarily of muscle and connective tissue. Sweetbreads are derived from the thymus gland of young cattle. (See also PROCESSED FOOD.)

ornithine   A non-essential AMINO ACID required in the formation of UREA, the end product of PROTEIN metabolism. Ornithine is made by the body. Though not incorporated into proteins, ornithine helps the LIVER convert the toxic nitrogen waste AMMONIA to urea via the UREA CYCLE, the enzyme system responsible for urea formation. Urea is eliminated by the KIDNEYS in urine. Ornithine is converted by the body to ARGININE, an amino acid that functions as a protein building block. Ornithine also forms polyamines, a family of nitrogen-containing chemicals that play a role in cell differentiation and growth.

Ornithine Supplements

Ornithine, as well as arginine, has found its way into health food stores. Body builders and athletes use ornithine out of the belief that it stimulates the production of GROWTH HORMONE.

Growth hormone causes muscle growth in normal animals. Moderate amounts of arginine and ornithine do not seem to affect growth hormone levels. Very large oral doses of ornithine may stimulate the release of growth hormone; however, the evidence that it can selectively burn fat and build muscle remains skimpy. Ornithine's beneficial effects for athletes may be partially due to its role in eliminating nitrogen waste products. In addition, in lab animals ornithine seems to stimulate the THYMUS GLAND, thus boosting immunity. Consumption of large amounts of single amino acids over time may cause potentially dangerous side effects. Seizures have been reported to occur with high doses of ornithine, and the long-term effects of a high dosage of ornithine are not known. Ornithine supplements are not recommended for patients with kidney or liver conditions. (See also AMINO ACID METABOLISM; EXERCISE; LYSINE.)

orthomolecular medicine   The use of NUTRIENTS and naturally occurring materials to treat illness and disease due to inherited enzyme deficiencies. Human nutrition has moved beyond treating disease to preventing illness and improving the quality of life and using large amounts of VITAMINS. Magavitamin therapy is one strategy to treat deficiencies that are the result of increased needs due to inheritance, though it continues to be controversial. The basis for this approach is the variability in enzyme levels and efficiencies among individuals. Mutant enzymes can require much larger amounts of vitamins than usual in order to function optimally. Vitamin and mineral therapy has successfully been used to treat disease and to improve health in some cases. Furthermore, evidence points to a biochemical imbalance in neurological disorders and learning disabilities, among others. Psychological disorders can be viewed in some instances as early symptoms of subclinical vitamin deficiencies. On the other hand, megavitamin treatment is not considered a successful treatment for schizophrenia by the American Psychiatric Association.

There is a growing awareness that mild deficiencies of minerals and vitamins play a role in chronic diseases. Deficiencies of antioxidant vitamins are linked to CARDIOVASCULAR DISEASE and certain forms of CANCER, for example. Nutrient malabsorption can lead to deficiencies with aging and therapeutic doses of vitamins and minerals may be required to prevent such common conditions as osteoporosis. Environmental stress in the form of air pollutants, drugs and viral infections and reliance on convenience foods increases vitamin needs, and supplementation can be an effective strategy in these situations.

Conditions where large amounts of vitamins (more than ten times the Recommended Dietary Allowance) are well recognized clinically include treatment of elevated blood cholesterol with B vitamin niacin, and of skin disorders with vitamin A derivatives. On the other hand, the use of vitamins to treat conditions other than well-established deficiency diseases is still considered unorthodox in some medical circles. Megavitamin treatment is not always effective. The literature on megavitamin therapy also contains exaggerated claims of cure based on misinterpretations of data from case studies of treated individuals. Vitamins are generally safer than most synthetic drugs and they are less expensive. There is a consensus that supplements do not substitute for a wholesome diet. Excessive amounts of any nutrient can lead to possible side effects and toxicity. Seek the advice of a qualified health care professional before launching a nutrient supplementation program. (See also MALABSORPTION.)

Kodama M. and Kodvama T., "Is Linus Pauling, a Vitamin C Advocate, Just Making Much Ado About Nothing?" *In Vivo*, 8:3 (May–June 1994), pp. 391–400.

ossification   The process of bone formation. Ossification requires CALCIUM, MAGNESIUM and PHOSPHORUS as primary building blocks. Many trace nutrients are needed for bone building: MANGANESE, BORON, VITAMIN D, VITAMIN K, VITAMIN C, VITAMIN A, FLUORIDE, COPPER, ZINC and SILICON. The rate of bone growth is controlled by hormones such as GROWTH HORMONE from the PITUITARY GLAND and steroid hormones produced by the ovaries and testes. The growth of the SKELETON requires increased intake of calcium over the amount lost (positive calcium balance) until adult size is reached, usually by the late teens or early twenties. Lengthwise bone growth in women is generally completed earlier than in men.

Osteoblasts are cells that form calcified deposits to make up bony structure. They secrete the connective tissue protein COLLAGEN, which forms filaments that in turn form a matrix. Osteoblasts connect with another type of cell called osteocytes, which are bone cells that are surrounded by crystallized minerals and lie deep within bone. Thus osteocytes and osteoblasts remain connected with each other and maintain bone structure. Throughout life, bone is constantly being reabsorbed and reformed. Adult bone replacement amounts to about 18% per year. (See also OSTEOMALACIA; OSTEOPOROSIS; RICKETS.)

osteoarthritis   A chronic, degenerative joint disease and the most common form of ARTHRITIS. Cartilage may be destroyed and bone spur formation can limit joint function. Weight-bearing joints such as ankles, hips, spine and knees are often affected. A point is reached at which repair mechanisms can no longer keep up with wear and tear. Joints may be stiff and sore due to damage through prolonged usage. Most Americans over the age of 50 experience a degree of osteoarthritis. Osteoarthritis may follow infections or joint injury. STRESS, excessive weight, poor posture, imbalanced musculoskeletal system, even poor muscle tone aggravate the condition. Physical therapy, structural alignments and exercise may aid in treating early degenerative joint disease.

It is important to curtail INFLAMMATION. Scavenger cells, MACROPHAGES, summoned to the damaged area, release substances that destroy cell debris and can damage surrounding healthy tissue. In addition, FREE RADICALS, extremely reactive oxidants, cause chronic inflammation when produced at joints. ANTIOXIDANTS like vitamin E, VITAMIN C, BETA CAROTENE and related carotenoids and FLAVONOIDS can quash free radicals and reduce inflammation. Flavonoids are natural antioxidants found in the pulp of citrus fruit, most vegetables and fruits. High levels of fish and fish oil and seed oils from flax, borage and black currant lessen pain and may help arthritic patients. These oils belong to the omega-3 class of fatty acids, known to blunt inflammation. They give rise to a family of PROSTAGLANDINS (PG₃) fat-derived hormones that control inflammation. Food allergy and food sensitivity can aggravate inflammation in degenerative joint disease. A diet that eliminates food allergens may minimize overreaction of the immune system in food-sensitive people. Niacinamide has been used to improve the range of joint motion and to help lessen pain and swelling. Glucosamine, a building block of joint cartilage, and chondroitin sulfates, a type of GLYCOSAMINOGLYCAN found in cartilage may help repair aging joints. Animal studies have indicated that purified chondroitin sulfates can stimulate cells responsible for synthesizing connective tissue. Manganese is required by enzymes manufacturing chondroitin sulfate as well. (See also ESSENTIAL FATTY ACIDS; OSTEOPOROSIS; RHEUMATOID ARTHRITIS.)

Berkson, D.L., "Osteoarthritis, Chiropractic and Nutrition," *Medical Hypotheses*, 36:4 (December 1991), pp. 356–67.

osteomalacia (adult rickets)   An adult bone disease caused by chronic vitamin D deficiency or by a deficiency of CALCIUM or PHOSPHORUS. In osteomalacia bones do not calcify properly; they become soft and flexible, leading to a distortion of the pelvis, spine and rib cage. Symptoms include pain in these regions and progressive weakness. When the diet contains adequate calcium and phosphorus, osteomalacia can easily be prevented with extra VITAMIN D during the winter months. Vitamin D is manufactured in the skin when exposed to sunshine; it has been commonly added to milk and milk products since the 1940s. (See also OSTEOPOROSIS.)

osteoporosis   A chronic, *degenerative disease* due to the loss of bone mass or increased bone porosity. The term "osteoporosis" means, literally, porous bones. The affected bones are deficient in CALCIUM, phosphorus and other minerals, and they contain less structural protein. In contrast, another bone disease, OSTEOMALACIA, results from soft bones due to altered mineral ratios. Osteoporosis is the most common bone disorder in America. It occurs much more frequently in women than in men. Men have larger bones, eat more calcium and get more exercise than women, though

alcoholic men are an exception. Mineral loss from bones typically begins in the twenties, and 50% of the bone loss in women occurs before menopause. Postmenopausal osteoporosis (type I) is the most common form; type II osteoporosis occurs with AGING. In both men and women, symptoms include curved spine, loss of height, and brittle, accident-prone bones, particularly the spine and hip. Calcium is preferentially lost from the long bones of the legs, the spine, the jaw bone, the wrists and the ankles when there is not enough calcium in the diet, or when it is poorly absorbed. Loss of bone of the spine can lead to compression fractures and a loss in weight frequently associated with aging. With reduced bone support, gums may be damaged and teeth may be lost.

The social and economic impact of osteoporosis is enormous. An estimated 20 to 45 million Americans have this disease. About 1.3 million fractures due to weakened bones occur each year in the United States. With osteoporosis fractured bones mend slowly. Complications from broken bones cause 40,000 deaths per year in women, more than either breast or cervical CANCER. In the United States 22% of all women over the age of 60 have spinal compression fractures that may cause pain, loss of appetite, heartburn or difficulty in breathing. More than 250,000 osteoporosis-related hip fractures occur yearly, and the lifetime risk for U.S. women for hip fractures is 15%. Complications of hip fractures decrease survival by 5 to 20%. As many as half of the patients with hip fractures are unable to walk afterward.

The rate at which bone is lost also affects the risk of osteoporosis. Contrary to common belief, bone is a dynamic tissue; it is constantly being formed and broken down. Until the early twenties, more bone is made than broken down as growth progresses. Bone mineral content of the spine and wrist reaches a maximum density in the late 30s and early 40s. After peak bone loss has been reached, there is little change until the forties, when the balance between synthesis and degradation shifts to favor degradation. Bone loss accelerates at menopause and continues at a high rate for about 10 years. Afterward, bone is lost at a rate of 0.2 to 0.5% per year. Typically a U.S. female will lose between 30 and 50% of her cortical bone (the spongy interior bone structure). It has often been assumed that menopause triggers bone loss. However, the rate of bone loss increases rapidly between the ages of 40 and 44, much earlier than menopause, which in the United States occurs at an average age of 52.

Osteoporosis is a complex disease involving both genetic and environmental factors, including such non-modifiable factors as gender, ethnic background, body build, family history of osteoporosis and age. Nevertheless, osteoporosis is one of the most preventable of the degenerative diseases.

Medical history affects the risk of osteoporosis as follows:

- Hormone imbalance. Because hormones maintain bone structure, hormonal imbalances can lead to osteoporosis. Examples include deficiencies of estrogen due to surgical removal of ovaries, and to postmenopause; Cushing's syndrome (excessive production of GLUCOCORTICOIDS by the adrenal glands); conditions that lead to excessive glucocorticoids, as chronic stress or overmedication with hydrocortisone; and overproduction of hormones from the pituitary gland; and cortisone and thyroid medications;

- Certain rare genetic diseases (Marfan's syndrome, homo-cystinuria);
- RHEUMATOID ARTHRITIS;
- Conditions that promote ACIDOSIS, such as chronic obstructive lung disease and possibly diabetes;
- Milk sensitivity or milk allergy;
- Anorexia nervosa;
- Conditions that lead to severe calcium malabsorption. These include excessive use of medications, such as certain anticonvulsant drugs and anticancer drugs that block calcium uptake; low stomach acid production (hypochlorhydria, achlorhydria); stomach surgery; and anti-ulcer drugs, like cimetidine, which blocks stomach acid production and limits calcium digestion).

Life-style factors play a major role in determining the risk of osteoporosis, including:

- A lack of physical, weight-bearing exercise (sedentary life-style, being bedridden). Exercise such as walking, jogging and dancing increases bone density and delays bone loss at all ages. On the other hand, strenuous exercise such as running a marathon can disrupt hormone balance and increase bone loss.
- Excessive alcohol consumption contributes to malnutrition and increased bone loss.
- Cigarette smoking increases bone degradation and limits bone rebuilding.
- Stress, both emotional and physical—fear, trauma, dehydration, surgery and the like—can lead to bone loss in many elderly persons, depending upon the degree of calcium malabsorption, the absorbability of dietary calcium and other life-style influences.

Various dietary factors affect bone strength and bone turnover. These include a deficiency of calcium, trace minerals and vitamin D. High bone density is a major factor in decreasing the risk of bone loss, and strong bones require adequate dietary calcium. Bones can be thought of as a bank account: The larger the bone and the more calcium it has, the more it can tolerate slow withdrawal as the body ages. With age, the ability to absorb calcium declines; this difference is made up by increased production of hormones that promote mineral loss from bone. Calcium deficiency is linked to osteoporosis.

The RECOMMENDED DIETARY ALLOWANCE (RDA) for calcium in the United States is 800 mg for adult women. The RDA for girls and young women between the ages of 12 and 19 is 1,200 mg; they generally get only 900 mg of calcium daily. American women generally consume less than 500 mg of calcium daily after menopause, which increases the risk of osteoporosis. The National Institutes of Health recommends that postmenopausal women not taking estrogen, and men over 65, consume 1,000 to 1,500 mg of calcium daily. The extra 1,000 mg they need to add could come from any one of the following: supplementation with about 1,000 mg of calcium; consuming 3 cups of milk, 2 cups of nonfat yogurt, 4 oz of cheese, 9 oz of sardines, or 4 to 5 cups of cooked broccoli or kale daily. These portions of canned fish and vegetables are much more of these foods than most people want in a day. Furthermore, many women decrease their intake of dairy products due to milk sensitivity and lactose intolerance, therefore many may opt for calcium supplements.

MAGNESIUM is also quite important in maintaining bone strength. Supplementation with magnesium together with calcium may help prevent bone thinning and actually help rebuild bone in post-menopausal women with osteoporosis. A mild magnesium deficiency increases the risk of osteoporosis. Magnesium deficiency is associated with lowered levels of calcitriol, the active form of VITAMIN D (see below). Magnesium may help the secretion of PARATHYROID hormone, required for the formation of adequate calcitriol.

In addition to major mineral nutrients, calcium, and magnesium, many trace mineral nutrients support calcium uptake and contribute to bone strength. BORON deprivation increases urinary excretion of calcium, and adequate dietary boron may cut the bone loss associated with menopause. Boron may affect parathyroid hormone and the activation of estrogen and vitamin D to calcitriol. Adequate boron seems to diminish bone losses associated with menopause. COPPER plays a role in calcium assimilation; it is required to stabilize COLLAGEN, the structural proteins that help form the matrix for calcification. Osteoporosis occurs with copper deficiency; the bones of copper-deficient animals are fragile.

FLUORIDE is associated with increased bone mass and with a reduced risk of osteoporosis. However, the appropriate levels in treating osteoporosis have not been defined. Current research is exploring the use of parathyroid hormone and the use of fluoride with calcium citrate to stimulate bone building. Sodium fluoride with calcium may help prevent bone fractures; however, fluoride must be administered carefully because of possible side effects.

Vitamins

Vitamin D is required for calcium absorption. It is converted to the hormone calcitriol, which stimulates the production of calcium uptake proteins. Vitamin D is formed in the skin and is also obtained from the diet, though milk and fortified cereals are the only major sources. The liver and kidneys process the vitamin to calcitriol. This activated form of Vitamin D is ten times more effective in stimulating calcium absorption than vitamin D. Studies show that elderly patients who remain indoors during the winter without exposure to sunlight or its equivalent run the risk of decreased calcium uptake.

VITAMIN C is required for normal collagen fiber formation, and presumably for normal calcification. Low VITAMIN B$_6$, FOLIC ACID and VITAMIN B$_{12}$ deficiencies may contribute to the risk of osteoporosis. These vitamins play a role in the metabolism of sulfur-containing AMINO ACIDS, METHIONINE and CYSTEINE. The accumulation of a by-product of methionine degradation, HOMOCYSTEINE, may occur with deficiencies, and this build-up is implicated in osteoporosis as well as other degenerative diseases. VITAMIN K plays a role in the formation of a calcium-binding protein, osteocalcin. Proper mineralization requires adequate levels of this protein. Vitamin K is abundant in green leafy VEGETABLES, a possible factor in the protection against osteoporosis afforded by a vegetarian diet.

Other dietary factors increase the risk of osteoporosis. Crash dieting or severe caloric restriction leads to mineral malnutrition, including calcium deficiency. Close examination of the typical American diet reveals a high protein intake but frequent deficiencies of trace minerals required for bone building. Urinary calcium losses appear to increase with high-protein diets, irrespective of dietary calcium. High-protein diets are also high-phosphate diets, and excessive phosphate also increases calcium excretion.

Vegetarian diets correlate with decreased prevalence of osteoporosis, though initial bone mass of vegetarians may be equivalent to that of meat eaters. Vegetarian diets provide less protein and phosphorus but more boron. Each of the following factors increases bone loss.

- Excessive sugar consumption increases calcium excretion.
- Excessive coffee and caffeine intake appear to increase calcium excretion. Generally, the more coffee that is consumed, the less milk. Women who drink milk throughout their adult lives may be able to counter the bone-thinning effects of coffee.
- Excessive soft drinks containing phosphate. A high phosphate diet with limited calcium limits calcium absorption and increases bone degradation.
- Excessive sodium has been linked to increased risk of osteoporosis and increased urinary losses of calcium.
- Decreased estrogen production after menopause increases bone loss. Theoretically, estrogen stimulates vitamin D to increase calcium intake; it slows calcium loss by the kidneys; and it increases production of a hormone to store calcium in bone. With estrogen deficiency, osteoclasts, cells that break down bone, are more sensitive to parathyroid hormone, causing increased bone breakdown. While estrogen therapy for elderly women stops further bone loss and decreases the risk of fractures of thinned bones after menopause, alone it may not prevent osteoporosis.

Recommendations

1. Consume enough calcium and magnesium. Girls and young women can take calcium supplements and eat calcium-rich foods to build up their bone density during their growth years. A daily consumption of up to 1,000 mg of calcium before menopause and 1,500 mg daily after menopause is recommended. People who are susceptible to kidney stones need to consult their physician before calcium supplementation. Several hundred mg of magnesium are generally well tolerated; more can lead to diarrhea.
2. Obtain enough vitamin D from fortified milk and milk products to deposit calcium into bones. Adequate sunshine enables the skin to make vitamin D.
3. Obtain enough, manganese, copper and zinc. These minerals help with calcium utilization for bone building.
4. Avoid excessive fiber supplements, high-protein diets, and soft drinks with phosphate.
5. Drink fluoridated water. Fluoride assists bone building. Routine use of fluoride in treating osteoporosis awaits controlled clinical studies.
6. Stop smoking.
7. Exercise regularly throughout life. Walking daily, cycling, dancing, bike riding and similar exercises are most beneficial in retaining calcium in bone.

8. Avoid excessive amounts of antacids that contain aluminum. Aluminum can interfere with normal calcium absorption and assimilation.
9. Consult a specialist regarding estrogen replacement therapy after menopause. For calcium to reverse osteoporosis after menopause, a woman may need to take low doses of estrogen and to exercise daily in addition to calcium supplementation. Who should not take estrogen? Women who are obese, who have a history of breast cancer or blood clotting problems. Estrogen therapy requires medical supervision because of potential side effects. (See also OSTEOARTHRITIS.)

Avioli, Louis V., "Significance of Osteoporosis: a Growing National Health Care Problem," *Orthopaedic Review* (September 1992), pp. 1126–29.

Gaby, Alan R., *Preventing and Reversing Osteoporosis*. Rocklin, Calif.: *Prima Publishing*, 1993.

ovalbumin   The major egg PROTEIN. Ovalbumin represents about 25% of the total protein of EGG white.

Overeaters Anonymous (OA)   An organization that provides support groups based upon the Twelve Step Program of Alcoholics Anonymous. These groups can help people deal with issues surrounding compulsive eating, bingeing and purging. There are no dues, and participation is voluntary. It is run entirely by volunteers.

Members of OA focus on getting control of their own lives and identifying underlying emotional issues, not on DIETING, nor on losing weight, nor even on food. There are no weigh-ins and no guarantees of weight loss. Eating disorder programs managed by hospitals and clinics often send their participants to OA to strengthen their own behavior modification strategies. A recent national survey of OA membership found that the average member had lost 31 pounds, and one in five members has maintained a stable weight loss over five years. This is much higher than most standard weight loss programs. (See also OBESITY; WEIGHT MANAGEMENT.)

overweight   The state of being at least 10 to 20% over optimal body weight. About 70% of Americans are overweight (1996). OBESITY, on the other hand, is defined as being 25% more than optimal body weight (men) or more than 30% (women). (See also DIETING; FAT; IDEAL BODY WEIGHT; WEIGHT MANAGEMENT.)

ovo-vegetarian   One who eats plant-derived foods and eggs. An ovo-lacto-vegetarian is one who eats only plant-derived foods. (See also VEGETARIAN.)

oxalic acid/oxalate   An acid found in a variety of vegetables that binds CALCIUM very tightly. Oxalic acid forms salts called oxalates with minerals, making them less available for absorption. SPINACH, beet greens, CHIVES, RHUBARB and PARSLEY contain significant amounts of calcium, but they also contain high levels of oxalic acid. However, oxalic acid does not block calcium uptake of IRON or of the calcium in other foods. It is not clear whether cooking greens makes calcium more available. Even with oxalates, these green leafy vegetables will supply significant TRACE MINERALS, plus VITAMINS and FIBER, and should be part of a BALANCED DIET.

Oxalic acid may be a potential by-product of excessive vitamin C consumption in excess of amounts achievable from dietary sources in cases of kidney disease and of those prone to the formation of calcium oxalate KIDNEY STONES, based on anecdotal reports in a small number of cases.

Oxalic acid consumption may be a problem for people who are prone to kidney stones, or those who eat a lot of BRAN for fiber and whose diets are high in oxalates and low in calcium. MAGNESIUM increases the solubility of calcium oxalate and decreases the probability of kidney stones, and VITAMIN B₆ reduces oxalate production. Getting enough VITAMIN K is also important: Vitamin K assists in the formation of a urinary protein that inhibits calcium oxalate precipitation and helps inhibit kidney stone formation. (See also MALABSORPTION.)

oxaloacetic acid   An acid that is both the starting point and final product of the KREB'S CYCLE. This cycle plays a central role in the oxidation of FAT, CARBOHYDRATES and AMINO ACIDS for energy production by the body. Oxaloacetic acid receives incoming carbon atoms to form CITRIC ACID. Sequential oxidation steps release these carbon atoms as CARBON DIOXIDE, the ultimate end product, while regenerating oxaloacetic acid. Oxaloacetic acid serves a second role: It can accept nitrogen to generate the acidic AMINO ACID, ASPARTIC ACID. It is also required to synthesize GLUCOSE (BLOOD SUGAR) from amino acids to fuel the brain during STARVATION. (See also CARBOHYDRATE METABOLISM; GLUCONEOGENESIS.)

oxidation   The primary chemical reaction by which chemical ENERGY is released from food for use by cells. The oxidation of fuel molecules in foods involves the addition of oxygen atoms to carbon atoms and the removal of hydrogen atoms. The ultimate oxidation product of carbon compounds is CARBON DIOXIDE. Indeed, carbon dioxide in expired air comes from the direct oxidation of FAT, CARBOHYDRATE, PROTEIN and other fuel molecules by cells in the body.

Most oxidation takes place in small particles in the cytoplasm known as mitochondria. These cellular powerhouses consume more than 90% of the oxygen that the cells use. They oxidize most of the fuels to carbon dioxide, while producing ATP. This form of chemical energy is readily used to power energy-requiring operations of the cell. The total energy released by oxidations occurring in cells is the same as when substances are burned in a test tube. The difference lies in the fact that within cells oxidation proceeds in small steps, speeded up by ENZYMES, in order to capture chemical energy efficiently. About 40% of the potential energy trapped in the simple sugar GLUCOSE, for example, is captured as ATP.

Cellular oxidations require electron carriers called COENZYMES as enzyme helpers. The most important are NICOTINAMIDE ADENINE DINUCLEOTIDE (NAD), derived from the B vitamin NIACIN, and FLAVIN ADENINE DINUCLEOTIDE (FAD), derived from the B vitamin RIBOFLAVIN. In this process oxygen is reduced to water (metabolic water), also produced by mitochondria, which generate about 200 ml daily.

Many degradative enzymes function together as METABOLIC PATHWAYS. Important energy-yielding pathways oxidize glucose (GLYCOLYSIS) and carbohydrate, fatty acids and amino acids (KREB'S CYCLE). Most ATP formation occurs in mitochondria via a pathway called OXIDATIVE PHOSPHORYLATION. (See also AMINO ACID METABOLISM; CARBOHYDRATE METABOLISM; FAT METABOLISM.)

oxidative phosphorylation   The oxygen-dependent process of trapping chemical ENERGY released by the OXIDATION of fuel molecules. Oxidative phosphorylation occurs in MITOCHONDRIA, small particles in cells that function as powerhouses. Cellular oxidations in mitochondria release electrons that are transported to oxygen. Their passage to oxygen is performed by a sequence of electron carriers and enzymes known collectively as the ELECTRON TRANSPORT CHAIN. When electrons are transported from one electron carrier to the next and ultimately to oxygen, a portion of the released energy is trapped as ATP; the remainder is lost as heat. ATP is a chemical form of energy universally used by cells to drive energy-requiring processes, from the contraction of muscle fibers and the transport of nutrients into cells to the biosynthesis of cellular constituents for cell growth and maintenance. Only mitochondria possess the enzyme machinery for coupling the flow of electrons to the reduction of oxygen to water, and simultaneously to synthesize ATP.

Electron transport and ATP production can be uncoupled, that is, oxidations can occur with decreased ATP production. Various chemicals alter the structure of mitochondria and act as uncouplers; certain environmental pollutants, poisons and drugs can interfere with ATP production, with potentially disastrous effects on cellular metabolism. Poisons like cyanide block electron transport, hence ATP production, in cells. The drug dinitrophenol was once marketed as a weight loss aid because it allowed more fuel to be burned with less ATP production. But the use of dinitrophenol led to excessive heat production, and it was banned. Even large amounts of normal products such as BILE PIGMENT, bilirubin and fatty acids can act as uncouplers. Certain patches of body fat called brown fat possess mitochondria that can be hormonally uncoupled to produce heat to protect newborn mammals, including infants. Thyroid hormone and the nervous system can regulate the efficiency of ATP production to a limited extent.

oxygen (molecular oxygen)   The element that accounts for approximately 21% of Earth's atmosphere and is essential for aerobic organisms. Animals require ample oxygen to oxidize food to ENERGY. Carbon atoms are oxidized to CARBON DIOXIDE, the first metabolic waste product. Oxygen acts as the ultimate oxidizing agent of fuel molecules, and it is reduced to WATER, the second waste product.

Oxygen taken up from air in the lungs must be distributed throughout the body to all cells via the circulatory system. Thus oxygen is absorbed into the bloodstream at the lungs, where it binds to the oxygen carrier protein in RED BLOOD CELLS called HEMOGLOBIN. Oxygenated red blood cells are pumped to tissues and oxygen is released in capillaries in response to acidic waste products and carbon dioxide from cellular metabolism, and to a low oxygen concentration. Oxygen molecules simply diffuse (migrate) into cells to participate in cellular oxidations.

Oxygen can be partially reduced by enzymes to form highly reactive molecules. Thus, activated phagocytic cells (neutrophils, macrophages) produce the FREE RADICAL superoxide, which can destroy invading microorganisms. Overproduction of superoxide during chronic INFLAMMATION can readily damage cellular components like proteins, lipids and DNA. Cells possess defense mechanisms to combat such agents. COPPER, MANGANESE and ZINC activate the enzyme SUPEROXIDE DISMUTASE, which neutralizes superoxide. (See also ANTIOXIDANT.)

oxygen debt . The amount of OXYGEN required to support the physiologic response to strenuous physical activity. Oxygen debt is characterized by rapid or labored breathing (hyperventilation) and increased metabolic rate that continues when EXERCISE ceases. During mild physical exercise, oxygen delivered by the bloodstream is adequate for muscles to oxidize GLUCOSE (BLOOD SUGAR) completely to CARBON DIOXIDE. The liberated energy powers muscle contraction. However, during vigorous exercise, oxygen delivery to muscle cells becomes too slow to produce enough ATP from the oxidation of glucose and fatty acids to meet the increased demand of muscle contraction. In this case additional ATP can be generated by the incomplete oxidation of glucose through a process called anaerobic GLYCOLYSIS.

Glycolysis is the initial stage of carbohydrate oxidation, which oxidizes glucose to a fragment called PYRUVIC ACID and produces ATP without the participation of oxygen. In muscle cells, the increased need for ATP outstrips the cells' ability to oxidize pyruvic acid during strenuous exercise. In this case pyruvic acid is converted to LACTIC ACID, which diffuses into the bloodstream to be processed to glucose by the liver. Panting at the end of strenuous exercise provides additional oxygen, which is used to replenish cellular ATP and to rebuild GLYCOGEN (stored glucose) in muscle fibers. Lactic acid accumulation may be partially responsible for the fatigue and stress that accompany strenuous exercise. During the recovery period the oxygen debt is repaid, lactic acid buildup is disposed of, energy stores are replenished, and the breathing rate normalizes. (See also ANAEROBIC; CARHOHYDRATE METABOLISM.)

oxytocin A HORMONE that induces lactation and stimulates milk ejection. Oxytocin causes mammary ducts to contract to eject milk. It also induces maternal behavior in females (sexual arousal) in many animal species. Oxytocin induces labor by causing vigorous contractions of the uterus to expel the fetus, and it is released in large quantities just before delivery.

Oxytocin is synthesized by the HYPOTHALAMUS, a part of the limbic system of the brain that is the center of emotions and motivation. Oxytocin is stored and released from the PITUITARY GLAND, the master gland that regulates the hormonal endocrine system. Alcohol suppresses oxytocin release. Chemically, oxytocin belongs to the family of peptides, small chains of amino acids. (See also BREASTFEEDING.)

oyster (*Ostrea spp.*) A saltwater shellfish belonging to the family of bivalve mollusks. Though indigenous to many parts of the world, oysters are now farmed to avoid depletion and to minimize their contamination from polluted water. East Coast and West Coast varieties are available in the United States. In oyster cultivation small seed oysters are first attached to a stationary support. As they grow in size they are transferred to beds, where their growth can be supervised. Traditionally it was recommended that oysters and clams be harvested only in months containing an "r" (September through April) to avoid contamination by blooms of "red tide" microorganisms. These organisms produce a poison that accumulates in oysters and mussels and can cause food poisoning. State health departments monitor shellfish and may restrict harvest in other months. A marine bacterium, *Vibrio vulnificus*, can infect warm brackish waters and infest shellfish such as oysters. The bacterium can cause blood poisoning in compromised individuals with a weakened immune system.

Fresh oysters are traditionally eaten raw with lemon juice or sauce. However, the consumption of raw or partially and cooked shellfish substantially increases the risk of food poisoning and of diseases transmitted by sewage, such as hepatitis A and Norwalk virus. Cooked oysters are far safer. They can be poached, browned, cooked on skewers or used in soups and sauces. Oysters canned in oil contain more calories than fresh oysters. Oysters are an excellent source of ZINC, though different varieties contain differing amounts. One oyster, cooked (100 g), provides 90 calories; protein, 5 g; carbohydrate, 5 g; fat, 5 g; cholesterol, 35 mg; calcium, 49 mg; iron, 3 mg; zinc, 9 mg; thiamin, 0.15 mg; riboflavin, 0.29 mg; niacin, 2.1 mg.

oyster shell A common CALCIUM supplement. Oyster shell calcium is not a recommended calcium source because it contains variable amounts of LEAD, a widespread environmental pollutant. Lead resembles calcium and is incorporated into the bone and shells of many organisms. (See also HEAVY METALS; SEAFOOD.)

PABA (para-aminobenzoic acid) A bacterial growth promoter. Bacteria use PABA to manufacture FOLIC ACID. In humans and animals folacin is a B VITAMIN required for cell multiplication and growth; humans cannot convert PABA to folacin, so PABA is not a vitamin. In animals like rats and mice, PABA can stimulate intestinal bacteria to produce enough folic acid to meet the animals' needs. This explains why PABA was once considered a vitamin. PABA is widespread in foods; GRAINS, wheat germ and organ meats are noteworthy.

Personal accounts attesting to the efficacy of the effect of oral doses of PABA in reducing hair loss and symptoms of ARTHRITIS have been reported. However, if taken orally, PABA may cause nausea and diarrhea. PABA can accumulate in tissues and damage the liver. Until recently PABA was a common ingredient in sunscreen to block ultraviolet radiation, which ages the SKIN. Applied to the skin, PABA can cause rash in susceptible people. When taken orally PABA may make the skin more sensitive to sunburn and increase the risk of skin cancer, and it can increase bacterial resistance to sulfa drugs. PABA has been used as a pharmaceutical agent to treat rickettsial infections. Rickettsia are microorganisms lying between viruses and bacteria in their complexity that cause diseases such as typhus and Rocky Mountain spotted fever. (See also ANTIMETABOLITE; ULTRAVIOLET LIGHT.)

packaging The container used to store and display food items. In addition to storing a food safely, in the context of marketing, packaging refers to the visual impact of a packaged food, an important factor in sales. Many brands of food must compete with similar products on a store shelf in order to catch the consumer's eye. Food choices in U.S. SUPERMARKETS have more than doubled during the last 20 years, yet consumers spend an average of 30 minutes per visit to a supermarket, the same length of time as earlier.

The shapes, sizes, colors, designs, letters and pictures, even the information on the food labels, can prompt a shopper to buy one product over the next. For example, brown and gold and country scenes can be used to promote more wholesome products like wholewheat bread. Packages can also project a calculated image to target a specific consumer group. Thus, children are targeted for pre-sweetened cold BREAKFAST CEREALS. The packing image may reflect a health consciousness or it may play upon consumer fears, desires for acceptance, success, romance or even a desirable life-style.

Plastic Food Containers

Plastics generally decompose very slowly because they are resistant to microbial attack, oxidation and light degradation. Newer types of plastics are less resistant to environmental exposure. Starch can be added to produce biodegradable plastics, making them more easily broken down by soil organisms. Photodegradable plastics break down when exposed to the ultraviolet light in sunlight. PVC food containers are made with polyvinyl chloride: they release minute amounts of cancer-causing vinyl chloride used to make this plastic. After reviewing the safety of PVC, the U.S. FDA approved the use of PVC food packaging while setting a limit for vinyl chloride. Manufacturers responded by minimizing vinyl chloride in containers. (See also ADVERTISING; PRODUCT PLACEMENT.)

pagophagia   The medical term for an insatiable desire for ice cubes. Often other crunchy materials like celery stalks, raw carrots and seeds are craved. The cause of this behavior is not known for certain; pagophagia may be a symptom of a mineral deficiency. Pagophagia can be distinguished from PICA, a CRAVING for materials not considered food, such as clay, dirt, plaster and starch.

palatability   The degree to which FOODS are pleasing or acceptable, based upon physical characteristics. Foods can be rejected or accepted on the basis of their sensory properties; visual appearance, flavor and aroma contribute to food preferences. The social environment plays a role, and acceptance of foods can be a learned response. Certain ingredients can make a food more acceptable. FAT contributes to the palatability and popularity of many foods: MEAT; fried foods, including stir-fried foods; baked goods like chips, CRACKERS and pastry; and CONVENIENCE FOODS.

The palatability of a food also relates to physiologic responses including SMELL, texture in the mouth ("mouth feel"), temperature of the food and TASTE sensations of sweet, sour, salty and bitter. Taste sensitivity diminishes with age, with smoking and with certain diseases. As an example, cancer patients often experience a metallic, bitter taste that alters their acceptability of red meat. Smell and taste of foods are closely linked. When a substance is smelled, olfactory organs in the nose interact directly with odor molecules. (Merging olfactory sensations with taste sensations gives rise to the distinctive flavors of foods.)

palm   See OIL PALM.

palmitic acid   A saturated FATTY ACID that is a common constituent of FAT and coconut oil. Palmitic and related fatty acids are classified as saturated because their carbon atom building blocks are fully occupied by hydrogen atoms. The body produces palmitic acid, consequently it is not a dietary essential fatty acid. Palmitic acid containing 16 carbon atoms is readily converted to other common fatty acids—stearic acid, and a saturated fatty acid with 18 carbons, and OLEIC ACID, the most common monounsaturated fatty acid. Oleic is formed from stearic acid by the removal of two hydrogen atoms to create one double bond.

Palmitic acid is a predominant component of dietary saturated fat, including COCONUT OIL and BUTTERFAT. High consumption of saturated fats, especially those containing large amounts of palmitic acid, correlates with elevated serum CHOLESTEROL and an increased risk of CARDIOVASCULAR DISEASE among American men. Saturated fats seem to promote the formation of blood clots; possibly palmitic acid reduces the formation of substances that reduce the stickiness of blood PLATELETS, particles that promote clot formation.

Recent dietary recommendations to lower the risk of cardiovascular disease suggest reducing overall fat consumption to less than 30% of daily calories. Some experts recommend a more drastic reduction to less than 25% and a decreased consumption of saturated fats (less than 7% of calories) and modest increases in consumption of polyunsaturated fats and monounsaturated fats. (See also ATHEROSCLEROSIS; DIETARY GUIDELINES FOR AMERICANS; FAT METABOLISM.)

palm oil (palm kernel oil, palm oil)   Oil obtained from a variety of palm used in cooking and in food processing. Palm oils are among the most common FOOD ADDITIVES because they are inexpensive and contribute a satisfying taste in processed foods like potato and corn chips, cookies and CRACKERS, as well as popcorn sold at movie theaters. As food additives they contribute surplus calories to convenience foods.

Palm oils are a source of SATURATED FAT. Saturated fats are fats whose carbon atoms are filled up (saturated) with hydrogen atoms. This distinction is important because of the link between increased saturated fat consumption and an increased risk of high blood CHOLESTEROL and heart disease in susceptible people. Palm oil is more saturated (49%) than LARD (41%), though less saturated than BUTTERFAT (62%). At 82% saturated FATTY ACIDS, palm kernel oil is second only to COCONUT OIL, the most saturated fat. Excessive consumption of palm oil by Americans is believed to carry the same risks of HEART DISEASE for susceptible people as does animal fat. (See also FATTY ACIDS; OIL PALM; TROPICAL OILS.)

pancreas   An elongated, tapered gland that functions both as a source of hormones (endocrine function) and as a source of digestive ENZYMES (exocrine function). The pancreas is about 8 in long (12.5 cm) and lies adjacent to the stomach within the first bend of the small intestine. The tail of this gland extends to the spleen. Its ducts drain into the upper reaches of the intestine (DUODENUM).

Endocrine Function

Nestled within pancreatic tissue are about a million small clusters of cells called pancreatic islets (islets of Langerhans). The clusters are composed of three kinds of cells: alpha cells, which secrete GLUCAGON, a hormone that raises BLOOD SUGAR; beta cells, which secrete INSULIN, the hormone that lowers blood sugar; and delta cells, which secrete somatostatin, a hormone that blocks the release of insulin and glucagon. Capillaries surrounding each islet take up these hormones for distribution by the bloodstream. The release of glucagon and insulin is regulated by feedback systems. When blood sugar falls below a threshold level, chemical sensors in alpha cells stimulate glucagon release. When blood sugar rises above normal, sensors in beta cells stimulate insulin release. In juvenile DIABETES MELLITUS (insulin-dependent diabetes melitus) the insulin producing cells are destroyed and the patient must rely on insulin injections.

Exocrine Function

The bulk of cells in the pancreas are devoted to producing digestive enzymes. Digestive enzymes are secreted by specialized clusters of cells called acinar cells into small ducts that drain into larger ducts and on into the intestine. Pancreatic duct cells secrete BICARBONATE to neutralize STOMACH ACID. Ultimately secretions leave the organ via large ducts that empty into the SMALL INTESTINE.

The pancreas secretes between 1.2 and 1.5 liters of pancreatic juice daily. This fluid contains digestive enzymes capable of degrading all major fuel nutrients in foods, together with bicarbonate, electrolytes (ions) like CHLORIDE and SODIUM, and water. Pancreatic enzymes include PROTEASES, which digest PROTEIN; LIPASE, which digests fat; phospholipase, which degrades PHOSPHOLIPIDS; and AMYLASE, which digests starch. Proteases and phospholipase are synthesized and released as inactive precursors (ZYMOGEN) to prevent these powerful enzymes from degrading pancreatic tissue. Premature activation, as in PANCREATITIS, leads to painful inflammation and, ultimately, to tissue damage. When pancreatic zymogens reach the intestine, they are converted to active enzymes. An intestinal enzyme called ENTEROPEPTIDASE first activates TRYPSIN, itself a powerful protein-degrading enzyme. Trypsin in turn activates other protein-degrading enzymes, in a cascade of activations. Most digestive enzymes are themselves broken down to constituent amino acids, which are absorbed and recycled. This represents a considerable savings because the pancreas secretes 20 to 30 g of protein daily that otherwise would be lost.

Pancreatic enzyme secretion is regulated by the PARASYMPATHETIC NERVOUS SYSTEM via the vagus nerve, the branch of the nervous system regulating involuntary actions, and by hormones. SECRETIN, released by the intestine when it contacts partially digested food (CHYME) from the stomach, regulates bicarbonate secretion. Secretion of digestive enzymes is signaled by CHOLECYSTOKININ, a hormone secreted when the small intestine contacts fat or protein released by the stomach. (See also DIGESTION; ENDOCRINE SYSTEM.)

pancreatin   A digestive aid generally prepared from hog pancreas. Pancreatin contains major pancreatic enzymes, chiefly AMYLASE for starch digestion, proteolytic enzymes for protein digestion and LIPASES for fat digestion. The potency of a given preparation varies depending upon the producer. Pancreatic enzymes are inactivated by the strong acidic environment of the stomach; therefore, coated tablets can permit active enzymes to reach the intestine, where the protective coating dissolves and the enzymes digest food at the relatively neutral pH of the intestine. Alternatively, pancreatin can be protected by taking sodium bicarbonate simultaneously to neutralize stomach acid. (See also DIGESTION; DIGESTIVE ENZYMES.)

pancreatitis   Inflammation of the PANCREAS. There is a spectrum of symptoms ranging from mild to severe. Acute (severe, rapidly developing) pancreatitis may lead to tissue damage, characterized by sudden, intense abdominal pain, vomiting and shock, and can be life-threatening. About 0.2% of U.S. general hospital admissions represent acute pancreatic necrosis (tissue death). Acute pancreatitis usually occurs at midlife and is generally caused by ALCOHOLISM or by bile duct obstruction (GALLSTONES). The damage appears to be caused by premature activation of DIGESTIVE ENZYMES, either due to release within pancreas cells or leakage of enzymes out of blocked duct systems. Free radical damage has been linked to pancreatitis. Chronic alcohol consumption is believed to lead to obstruction of pancreatic ducts. When it is necessary to minimize pancreatic secretion during medical treatment, oral intake of food is stopped and the patient is fed intravenously.

Mild (subclinical) pancreatitis can lead to progressive tissue damage but is not usually preceded by a severe attack. Recurrent pain may occur at intervals for years. Attacks can be precipitated by alcohol abuse, overeating or by the use of prescription drugs. Again, the most likely cause of mild pancreatitis is alcoholism, and typically MALNUTRITION plays a role. Diagnosis is difficult because of the wide range of clinical manifestations and because patients may not exhibit symptoms early in the disease process. (See also CIRRHOSIS.)

Scott, P., et al., "Vitamin C Status in Patients with Acute Pancreatitis," *British Journal of Surgery*, 80 (June 1993), pp. 750–54.

pancreozymin   See CHOLECYSTOKININ.

pangamic acid (calcium pangamate, "Vitamin B$_{15}$")   Generally a mixture of chemicals including a compound called dimethylglycine, claimed to increase athletic performance. Pangamic acid is not really a VITAMIN, and it has no known essential function in animals or humans. However, manufacturers are able to bottle a variety of substances under the name of vitamin B$_{15}$. The material is widely distributed in foods ranging from BREWER'S YEAST to LIVER. Dimethylglycine is itself formed from the essential AMINO ACID methionine and is related to the simple amino acid glycine.

Very few studies outside the former Soviet Union have shown any beneficial effect in athletic performance. There, pangamic acid was used to treat ALCOHOLISM, FATIGUE, diabetes, heart disease, HEPATITIS and AGING. Available evidence indicates pangamic acid does not increase oxygen utilization, or cardiovascular response to EXERCISE.

Pangamic acid could potentially serve as a source of methyl groups to help reuse METHIONINE. It could also help protect against fatty liver in experimental animals, and it may help the body use fat. CHOLINE is a safer alternative, however. Evidence for the effectiveness of pangamic acid in cancer treatment is mixed: Pangamic acid may cause CANCER in some experimental animals, while inhibiting cancer in others. Its use is considered experimental. Dimethylglycine has been used to treat cataracts and epilepsy. (See also ERGOGENIC SUPPLEMENTS.)

pantothenic acid   A widely distributed water-soluble VITAMIN and a member of the B complex. The name is derived from the Greek word *pantothen*, meaning "everywhere." Indeed, pantothenic acid is present in all cells, whether plant or animal. The commercially available form is the calcium salt, calcium pantothenate. Pantothenic acid plays a pivotal role in energy production from FAT, CARBOHYDRATE and PROTEIN. Pantothenic acid forms the core of COENZYME A, the enzyme helper that carries FATTY ACIDS throughout metabolism, including fat synthesis and fat degradation. The oxidation of carbohydrates, fatty acids and amino acids eventually yields the very simple acid, ACETIC ACID, bound to coenzyme A as acetyl coenzyme A. In turn, acetyl coenzyme A feeds the metabolic machinery (KREB'S CYCLE) of the cell's powerhouse, the MITOCHONDRIA, where the carbons of acetic acid are oxidized to CARBON DIOXIDE to produce useful chemical ENERGY in the form of ATP. Furthermore, coenzyme A helps synthesize certain important compounds like CITRIC ACID; most LIPIDS, including CHOLESTEROL; STEROID hormones; and KETONE BODIES, fat derivatives made during starvation. Coenzyme A is required in the synthesis of the important NEUROTRANSMITTER, ACETYLCHOLINE, a chemical required for nerve transmission. Other functions of coenzyme A include the synthesis of HEME for the formation of the red blood cell protein HEMOGLOBIN.

Pantotheine (pantothine) a daughter molecule of pantothenic acid, contains the additional sulfur amino acid CYSTEINE. It may lower serum cholesterol and TRIGLYCERIDES in those with elevated levels, while pantothenic acid has little effect. Animal studies indicate that heart levels of pantotheine decline when oxygen supply is limited. It may be easier to convert pantotheine to coenzyme A than pantothenic acid, and therefore pantotheine may be a more effective therapeutic material in certain instances.

Good sources of pantothenic acid include LIVER, dried BEANS and PEAS, whole GRAINS, wheat germ, dark-green VEGETABLES, NUTS like peanuts, EGGS and YEAST. Lesser amounts occur in MILK and other vegetables. Refined, heavily processed foods and fruits contain little pantothenic acid, and pantothenic acid is partially destroyed by food processing. Beneficial INTESTINAL FLORA contribute pantothenic acid.

Possible Roles in Maintaining Health

Anecdotal reports attest to the claim that pantothenic acid can increase athletic performance. However, studies have yielded mixed results. Pantothenic acid blood levels are significantly lower in patients with RHEUMATOID ARTHRITIS, and preliminary clinical trials suggest that pantothenic acid may alleviate pain and joint stiffness in such patients. Pantothenic acid supplementation speeds wound healing in experimental animals; whether this occurs in humans remains to be seen. Preliminary evidence suggests that pantothenic acid can boost the liver's ability to oxidize alcohol. Studies with experimental animals suggest antibody production decreases with pantothenic acid deficiency, and pantothine supplementation may stimulate the IMMUNE SYSTEM. Pantothenic acid deficiency causes gray hair in animals, but supplements apparently do not reduce graying hair in people.

The levels of pantothenic acid required for optimal health remain unknown, and there is no RDA (RECOMMENDED DIETARY ALLOWANCE). It is estimated that 4 to 7 mg per day is safe and adequate for healthy people. The REFERENCE DAILY INTAKE is 10 mg per day. Deficiencies are rare, though anyone relying on a diet of highly processed foods can be at risk.

Outright deficiency symptoms have rarely been reported and occur only among severely malnourished people. However, pantothenic acid deficiencies have been produced in experimental animals. Symptoms of prolonged pantothenic acid deficiency include sore feet, burning pain in heels, vomiting, cramps, fatigue, insomnia and respiratory infections.

Advocates believe that daily supplements in moderate amounts are reasonable as a preventive measure for healthy people. Pantothenic acid as well as vitamin C have been recommended to support adrenal glands during stress. Side effects of megadoses (10 to 20 g) include diarrhea, sleepiness,

depression or nausea. There is no known toxicity for this versatile vitamin. However, long-term safety research has been inadequate. (See also AGING; CARBOHYDRATE METABOLISM; FAT METABOLISM.)

papain A protein-degrading enzyme obtained from PAPAYA leaves and from the sap of the green fruit. Commercially, papain powder is used as a MEAT TENDERIZER. To be effective, it must penetrate the meat; sprinkling the surface of MEAT with tenderizer should be followed by piercing with a fork. Papain is sometimes injected into cattle before slaughter to tenderize meat and during meat packing. When added to beverages it breaks down protein particles that create cloudiness. As a food supplement, papain is used as a digestive aid. Cooking destroys papain, though it resists stomach acid. In medicine papain digests dead tissue, and it has been used as a "biological scalpel" in the treatment of herniated lumbar disks. Papain preparations have also been used to treat stomach problems. (See also CARBOHYDRATE METABOLISM; DIGESTION; FAT METABOLISM; FOOD ADDITIVES.)

papaya (*Carica papaya*) The melon-like fruit of a small, palm-like evergreen that probably originated in Central America. Papaya is now cultivated in tropical regions worldwide. India, Indonesia, Chile, Mexico and Zaire rank among the top producers. Papayas also come from Hawaii, Florida, Puerto Rico and Central and South America. The fruit may weigh up to 20 lb (9.1 kg). Ripe papaya is yellow-orange on the outside, with a sweet, red-orange pulp. It may be round or elongated depending on the variety. The most common variety in U.S. markets is the Solo. Mexican papayas are much larger. Papaya are usually eaten fresh, in salads and in sherbets. Papayas are also juiced, pickled and candied. Papaya leaves and fruit contain PAPAIN and chymopapain, powerful protein-degrading enzymes that are used as digestive acids and MEAT TENDERIZERS. Papaya is a good source of potassium and vitamin C. Nutrient content of whole fruit (304 g, edible portion) is: 117 calories; protein, 1.9 g; carbohydrate, 29.8 g; fiber, 5.2 g; potassium, 780 mg; vitamin A, 612 retinol equivalents; vitamin C, 188 mg; thiamin, 0.08 mg; riboflavin, 0.10 mg; niacin, 1.03 mg. (See also PROTEASE.)

paprika A red seasoning prepared from grinding a sweet red PEPPER into a powder. Paprika has a high VITAMIN C content. Paprika's flavor is enhanced when cooking with onions and is often used in stews, chilis, lentil and curry dishes. Nutrient content of 1 tsp (2.1 g) is: 6 calories; protein, 0.3 g; carbohydrate, 1.3 g; fiber, 0.5 g; fat, 0.3 g; vitamin C, 1.4 mg; thiamin, 0.01 mg; riboflavin, 0.04 mg; niacin, 10.35 mg. (See also CONDIMENT.)

parasites in food and water Potentially harmful microorganisms that capture their nourishment from their host. Many parasites that infect the gastrointestinal tract are single-cell animals (protozoa). They often involve complex life cycles, such as maturation in different parts of the body and in different hosts. They may form very stable cysts that persist in the environment. Among protozoa that have been recently associated with contaminated water or food are *Giardia lamblia, Cryptosporidium parvum, Cyclospora cayetanen-*

sis, *Dientamoeba fragilis* and *Entamoeba histolytica*. Raw fish may be contaminated with roundworms, tapeworms and flukes.

Giardia is a flagellated organism with worldwide distribution and it is among the most commonly diagnosed intestinal parasites. Giardia causes diarrhea, abdominal pain, flatulence, diarrhea and weight loss (GIARDIASIS). Giardia may become dormant, with no obvious symptoms, though the patients can transmit the disease; that is, they are carriers. Giardia contaminates water supplies in many parts of the United States and giardiasis is often linked to poor sanitation. People drinking untreated water from streams and wells are most likely to get this intestinal infection. Outbreaks have been attributed to contaminated municipal water supplies in regions of Oregon, Colorado, Utah, Washington, New Hampshire and New York. Patients who have immunodeficiency syndromes are at risk for giardiasis, and in persons with AIDS, giardia might be an important pathogen. People living in close quarters, children and campers can become infected with this parasite.

Cryptosporidium causes cryptosporidiosis with watery diarrhea, cramping and anorexia. If diarrhea has persisted for more than two weeks, patients may require fluid and electrolyte replacement. The parasite is common in the environment, and animal-to-person and waterborne transmission have been observed. Person-to-person transmission occurs through fecal contamination, especially in day-care centers and hospital settings. An outbreak in 1993 in Milwaukee due to contaminated municipal water supply caused diarrhea in some 400,000 people. Drinking apple cider and exposure to contaminated water at water parks have also been linked to outbreaks. Ingesting as few as 30 cysts can cause infection. For people with AIDS and others whose immune systems are compromised, such as children and the elderly, cryptosporidiosis can be life threatening. Neither usual filtration systems nor chlorination destroy cryptosporidium, thus most water treatment facilities do not eliminate the parasite.

Cyclospora has only recently become a public health concern in the U.S., although the distribution of this parasite is worldwide. Travel to developing countries increases the risk of infection. Cyclospora infects the intestine causing cramps, vomiting, weight loss and explosive diarrhea lasting one to three weeks. It was first identified in the United States in 1990 and it possibly infected fresh fruit, causing 1,000 cases in 14 states in 1996.

D. fragilis is widely distributed in the United States and surveys have detected an incidence of 1.4% to 19% for a given population. Institutionalized people and children in day-care centers are commonly infected. The mode of transmission is not known. *D. fragilis* causes intermittent diarrhea, abdominal pain, nausea, fatigue, and elevated white cell counts. Symptoms may persist over long periods until treatment is begun.

E. histolytica causes amoebic dysentery and is most prevalent in the tropics and subtropics. The usual mode of transmission is through the oral-fecal route, although disease can be transmitted sexually. *E. histolytica* infection is common in many areas, however, few individuals develop clinical symptoms, which include persistent bloody diarrhea with pain and cramping. Symptoms can mimic ulcerative colitis.

The parasite can become dormant and the patient may not exhibit any symptoms. On the other hand, in 2% to 8% of cases the parasite penetrates the intestinal wall and invades other organs such as the liver, possibly causing jaundice. The severity of the disease is related to the strain of the infecting organism and the patient's immune status. Symptoms may last indefinitely until treated.

Specific antiparasitic drugs are typically used to eradicate these parasites. Boiling water at least one minute or using a filtration device that removes particles less than one micron in diameter can remove parasites. Bottled water that has been distilled or purified by reverse osmosis is the safest type. A high standard of personal hygiene is warranted to avoid cross-infection among family members and those living in close quarters. (See also FOOD POISONING.)

parasympathetic nervous system   A division of the autonomic NERVOUS SYSTEM that regulates involuntary processes to conserve energy, balance systems of the body and return the body to normal operation after it has responded to an injury or threatening situation. The autonomic nervous system regulates activities of smooth muscles of internal organs (viscera), heart muscle and certain glands. It is composed of two divisions that complement each other. The parasympathetic portion counterbalances the sympathetic nervous system, which responds to stressful events and expends energy.

The parasympathetic nervous system originates from nerves in the brain stem and in the lower (sacral) portion of the spinal cord. It contracts the pupil, iris, ciliary muscles (which results in clear vision), lungs, salivary glands, the heart, INTESTINE, LIVER, STOMACH, KIDNEY, PANCREAS and spleen, bladder, rectum and reproductive organs. Parasympathetic nerve impulses to digestive glands and to the gastrointestinal tract stimulate DIGESTION and absorption of nutrients, for example. (See also HOMEOSTASIS; STRESS.)

parathyroid glands   Small HORMONE-secreting glands embedded in the THYROID GLAND. Usually two parathyroids are attached to each side of the thyroid gland. They release a single hormone called parathyroid hormone (parathormone, PTH) into the bloodstream; the hormone increases blood levels of CALCIUM and MAGNESIUM. It is noteworthy that parathormone secretion is regulated without participation of the PITUITARY GLAND, the master endocrine gland. When the level of calcium in the blood drops, more PTH is released. When the calcium level of the blood rises, less PTH is secreted, and CALCITONIN is released by the thyroid gland to lower blood calcium levels.

PTH stimulates the uptake of calcium, phosphate and magnesium by the intestine when adequate levels of VITAMIN D are present. It does this by stimulating the activation of vitamin D to calcitriol D_3 and by activating BONE-degrading cells (osteoclasts) and stimulating their production. Osteoclasts then release calcium and phosphate in the blood. In addition, PTH directs the kidneys to excrete phosphate in the urine. (See also ENDOCRINE SYSTEM.)

parenteral nutrition   Introducing nutrients into the body by means other than the mouth when patients cannot eat or drink. Parenteral nutrition is used to bypass the INTES-

TINE and DIGESTION by feeding nutrients intravenously, by injection under the skin or into muscles (parenteral hyperalimentation). Nutrients adequate to meet caloric requirements can be delivered intravenously. Solutions containing water, ELECTROLYTES and sugar GLUCOSE (dextrose) as an energy source are commonly administered via a peripheral vein on the arm or leg. Other nutrients like VITAMINS, minerals and fats may be included.

Peripheral parenteral nutrition provides about 2,500 calories per day, with 90 g of AMINO ACIDS. Patients who might receive this form of nutrition include those who need short-term support (one to two weeks), those with normal energy needs and normal kidney function, those who need additional nutrients beyond the amounts from oral or tube feeding, and patients for whom insertion of a catheter into a central vein could be a problem.

Total parenteral nutrition (TPN) refers to administering high-concentration nutrients in adequate concentrations to meet total caloric needs via a catheter into a large, rapidly flowing vein, typically flowing into the heart to assure rapid mixing and dilution with blood. Even so, it is much easier to maintain nutrient status by TPN than it is to replenish depleted nutrient stores by TPN. TPN is the most expensive method of feeding. In either peripheral parenteral nutrition or TPN, the patient's response to parenteral formulas needs to be carefully monitored, particularly in terms of caloric needs and nitrogen balance.

TPN is indicated when long-term parenteral nutrition is required, when nutrient requirements are high or when patients are starved or severely malnourished. Typical conditions that may warrant TPN by the central veins include extensive surgery, burns or physical trauma; prolonged vomiting or diarrhea; ANOREXIA NERVOSA; CANCER; and severe digestive conditions like pancreatitis (inflamed pancreas), INFLAMMATORY BOWEL DISEASE, kidney failure, liver failure and others.

Complete parenteral solutions include all essential amino acids, electrolytes, vitamins, MINERALS, and energy sources such as glucose, the traditional energy source, and emulsified FAT. Fatty acids may be combined with LECITHIN, a natural emulsifier, to increase their solubility, or MEDIUM-CHAIN TRIGLYCERIDES may be used directly for energy by cells. Fat emulsions are a concentrated form of energy, and a 10% solution provides 1 calorie per milliliter or 1,000 calories per liter. Fat does not irritate veins as easily as amino acids and glucose. Fat emulsions also provide essential fatty acids. Potential problems with intravenous fat emulsions include backaches, allergic reactions, excessive lymphocytes, blurred vision or other symptoms. Historically, inadequate parenteral nutrition has produced deficiency symptoms and revealed the necessity of essential fatty acids and certain trace minerals. (See also CATABOLIC STATE.)

Klein, G.L. and Coburn, J.W., "Parenteral Nutrition: Effect on Bone and Mineral Homeostasis," *Annual Review of Nutrition*, 11 (1991), pp. 93–119.

parietal cells (oxyntic cell) Stomach cells that secrete both hydrochloric acid (STOMACH ACID) and INTRINSIC FACTOR, a protein needed to bind VITAMIN B_{12} and absorb this vitamin in the INTESTINE. Hydrochloric acid activates the protein-digesting enzyme pepsin. Low stomach acid production contributes to maldigestion, while low production of intrinsic factor correlates with vitamin B_{12} deficiencies ranging from subclinical (mild) deficiencies with no obvious symptoms to severe illness with PERNICIOUS ANEMIA. (See also ACHLORHYDRIA; DIGESTION.)

Parkinson's disease (PD) An incurable neurological disorder leading to muscle rigidity, muscle weakness, slowed movements, tremors and a characteristic halting gait and loss of balance. Parkinson's disease often develops slowly over years and currently affects up to 1 million U.S. citizens, most 50 or older. There is a progressive loss of brain cells that produce DOPAMINE, a type of NEUROTRANSMITTER or brain chemical that helps nerves communicate. Perhaps as many as 30% of children and adolescents who take antipsychotic (neuroleptic) drugs develop Parkinson symptoms (secondary Parkinsonism). These drugs are often prescribed for childhood conduct disorders and to control aggression and violent behavior. The symptoms can persist for months after treatment has stopped.

The cause of cell death associated with Parkinson's disease is unknown, though environmental toxins and an inherited inability to deal with toxins are hypothetical factors. The use of an herbicide (paraquat) correlated with the development of Parkinson's disease in Quebec. Viral infection has not been ruled out, though viruses have not been identified with the disease. There are hints that nutrition can play a role in the development of Parkinson's disease. This disease could be the result of FREE RADICAL damage in some cases. Free radicals are chemical fragments produced in the body that can be very destructive. Antioxidant nutrients prevent free radical damage; whether VITAMIN C and VITAMIN E supplementation may lessen the effects of this disease remains to be proven.

Drugs can control symptoms of Parkinson's disease in some cases. However, their effectiveness becomes sporadic upon prolonged treatment, and the drugs currently employed can cause severe side effects, including mental disturbances and loss of balance. Levodopa (L-dopa) was introduced in the 1960s; this raw material can be taken up by the brain and converted to dopamine. In combination with a synthetic compound called carbidopa to inhibit levodopa breakdown, it is possible to use less of the drug, reducing its side effects. Often there are problems dealing with long-term use of levodopa medication, such as involuntary movements. Presently no anti-Parkinsonian drug slows the natural progression of the underlying disease. Deprenyl, a monoamine oxidase inhibitor, may offer protection against nerve damage. TRYPTOPHAN and TYROSINE are amino acids that have been used with imapramine, an anti-Parkinsonian drug. Consult your health care adviser before using amino acids therapeutically. Tryptophan was withdrawn from the market by the U.S. FDA in 1989.

Digesting PROTEIN yields both tyrosine and PHENYLALANINE, amino acids that compete with anti-Parkinson's drugs for admission through the brain's protective barrier (BLOOD-BRAIN BARRIER); many patients may become immobilized for several hours after eating protein. To reduce this competition, protein can be limited to dinner, although this may limit the drug's effectiveness in the evening. An alternative strategy calls for eating carbohydrate and protein in a ratio of seven to one in meals throughout the day. This is more balanced than a high-carbohydrate/low-protein diet. Legumes, especially broad beans (fava beans), contain L-dopa. Inform your doctor if you add this food to your diet when you are on medication. Taking smaller drug doses every two to three hours and just before meals may be effective; controlled-release formulations may also help maintain constant blood levels during the day. (See also AMINO ACID METABOLISM; MAO INHIBITORS; NERVOUS SYSTEM.)

Fahn, Stanley and Cohen, Gerald, "The Oxidant Stress Hypothesis and Parkinson's Disease, Evidence Supporting It," *Annals of Neurology*, 32:6 (December 1992), pp. 804–12.

parsley (*Petroselinum crispum*)　A biennial HERB used as a seasoning. There are more than 30 varieties, and it is the most common herb in the United States. The parsley family of vegetables includes CARROTS, CELERY and parsnips, as well as other herbs (angelica, CARAWAY, CHERVIL, coriander, CUMIN, DILL, FENNEL, LOVAGE). Parsley originated in the Mediterranean region and has been cultivated for at least 2,000 years. It was apparently first used as an herbal medicine and later as a food. Parsley leaves are used as a flavoring and as a garnish, either dried or fresh, in soups, meat dishes, poultry, fish and stuffing, as well as in vegetable dishes and salads. Parsley can be added to spreads and to butter. Parsley has been used in herbal medicine as a laxative and as a diuretic agent (to increase urination), and it has antimicrobial properties. Folk medicine has a tradition of using parsley to treat jaundice and liver conditions.

parsnip (*Pastinaca sativa*)　A root vegetable that resembles CARROT, to which it is related. Parsnips were developed in the Middle Ages from wild plants growing in the Mediterranean area and for centuries was a staple in Europe until it was displaced by potatoes. It is not a major vegetable crop in the United States. Parsnips are white to yellow, while carrots are orange and possess a distinctive nutty taste. The flavor becomes sweeter after exposure to frost and when stored starch is broken down to sugar. Parsnips can be used in place of turnips. Cooked parsnips can be pureed or mashed with potatoes and can be fried, candied, roasted with meat or baked.

Nutrient content of 1 cup of cooked parsnips (156 g) is: 125 calories; protein, 2.1 g; carbohydrate, 30.4 g; fiber, 4.36 g; fat, 1.4 g; potassium, 573 mg; thiamin, 0.13 mg; riboflavin, 0.08 mg; niacin, 0.15 mg.

pasta　A basic food made from a dried paste of wheat flour. Pasta comes in hundreds of forms and is used in recipes from Asia to America. Pasta is the Italian word for paste. To prepare pasta, flour and water are mixed and the dough is extruded through die plates to shape it, then cut into ribbons, tubes and strings, which are dried. Most commercially available pasta is prepared from SEMOLINA, a refined flour from durum WHEAT. Durum wheat contains a high percentage of GLUTEN, the sticky protein that holds the dough together. Pasta can be prepared from whole wheat flour as well as white flour. Pastas from whole wheat contain about 5 g of fiber per 3.5-oz serving. Japanese pasta is prepared from soft whole wheat with a lower gluten content than semolina. In this case, dough is generally rolled into flat sheets, then cut.

Although various shapes of pasta bear Italian names, the U.S. FDA defines pasta as either MACARONI or NOODLES. Macaroni is made without eggs and contains three basic ingredients: semolina; farina, a coarsely ground starchy flour that contains less protein than durum wheat; and/or flour from durum wheat. Noodles contain in addition a minimum of 5.5% egg (by weight). Consequently, noodles provide fat and cholesterol. Rather than being a fattening, calorie-rich food, pasta is a good source of COMPLEX CARBOHYDRATE. For example, 82% of the calories in spaghetti comes from carbohydrate, the rest from protein. Pastas can be fattening when oil, CHEESE, BUTTER, heavy cream or fatty meats are added. These contain far more calories. Corn, quinoa and rice pasta are also available; they are as healthful as wheat pasta. They must be labeled "pasta substitutes" on the food label because they do not conform to federal definitions for pasta. (See also BREAD.)

O'Neill, Molly, "So It May Be True After All: Eating Pasta Makes You Fat," *New York Times Science Times*, (February 8, 1995), pp. B1, B7.

pasteurization　A method of FOOD PROCESSING that involves heat to destroy harmful microorganisms and microorganisms that cause spoilage. Louis Pasteur discovered the process that bears his name when he found that WINE and BEER could be preserved by heating above 57.2° C (135° F). Now MILK, CHEESE, egg products, wine, beer and fruit juices are generally pasteurized at temperatures between 60° C and 100° C (212° F). Products are cooled rapidly after the heat treatment to prevent being cooked.

Milk is pasteurized by heating at 62° C for 30 minutes or by flash heating, a process that involves heating at high temperatures for a short time. These processes kill 97 to 99% of non-spore-forming, pathogenic bacteria, including tuberculosis bacteria, salmonella and streptococcus. Pasteurization does not kill all microorganisms in a food or beverage, however. The growth of surviving organisms may be retarded by additional procedures such as chilling. Pasteurization can kill microorganisms that would otherwise compete with a pure starter strain of a bacterium or yeast used in food processing. Cheese making is an example where pasteurization is important. Pasteurization is effective in destroying certain pathogens (disease-producing microorganisms) in milk without altering the overall quality of the product; this process is appropriate to destroy heat-susceptible organisms such as yeasts in fruit juices. (See also FOOD PRESERVATION.)

pau d'arco　See LA PACHO.

PCBs　See POLYCHLORINATED BIPHENYLS.

pea (*Pisum arvense* and *P. sativum*)　A LEGUME that ranks among the 10 most important VEGETABLE crops worldwide. Peas were cultivated by the Chinese in 2000 B.C., and dried peas have been uncovered in Egyptian tombs. In modern times peas were scientifically studied to produce new varieties. Garden peas are treated as fresh vegetables, while dried peas, like chickpeas and split peas, require long cooking times. Dry green peas are the main pea crop in the United States; Idaho and Washington produce most of the domestic dry peas. Dried peas are used in canned soups and dehydrated pea soup. Dried split peas cook in about 25 minutes while quick-cooking peas can be cooked within 15 minutes because they have been pre-treated with enzymes and steamed. The United States produces more fresh green peas than any other country. Most of the U.S. crop is either frozen or canned; frozen green peas represent the leading frozen vegetable in America. They retain their flavor and color. Most canned peas contain added salt and sugar. Snow peas are meant to be eaten with the pod intact.

Peas provide FIBER, IRON and the B COMPLEX vitamins. As a source of minerals, peas contain much less calcium and phosphorus than BEANS. Like other legumes, peas contain substantial protein, However, pea protein is deficient in the sulfur amino acids CYSTEINE and L-METHIONINE, and it contains sufficient amounts of another dietary essential amino acid, LYSINE, to complement the low lysine content in grain protein, so that combining legume protein with grain protein (cereal products) yields a mixed protein with a higher quality than that obtained by eating either alone.

P. arvense is the field pea, grown for its seeds. It grows wild in the Republic of Georgia and probably originated in central Asia and Europe. Its seeds are gray-brown, while the garden pea produces green seeds. Field peas are not used for food in the United States. Generally they are grown to fertilize fields and to provide animal fodder. Like other legumes, this vegetable can grow in nitrogen-depleted soils because its roots possess nodules that contain bacteria that convert atmospheric NITROGEN to nitrogen compounds readily absorbed by the plant.

Nutrient content of cooked green peas (1/2 cup from frozen peas, 80 g) is: 63 calories; protein, 4.1 g; carbohydrate, 11.4 g; fiber, 7.7 g; iron, 1.25 mg; potassium, 134 mg; thiamin, 0.23 mg; riboflavin, 0.14 mg; niacin, 1.18 mg. (See also FOOD COMPLEMENTING.)

peach (*Prunus persica*)   A juicy, sweet FRUIT produced by a tree related to APRICOT, CHERRY and PLUM. The peach is classified as a drupe, that is, a fruit whose hard seed or pit is enclosed by a soft pulp with a thin skin. The peach probably originated in China, where it is described in writings from 2000 B.C. Colonists brought the peach to North America, and now it is grown in 32 states and in Canada. The United States and Italy are the world's major producers of peaches and the related NECTARINE. California produces over 60% of the domestic peach crop, and peaches are the third most popular fruit grown domestically. There are thousands of varieties, though relatively few are important commercially. Peaches can be classified as either cling peaches, if the stone is difficult to remove from the flesh (e.g., Fortuna, Gaume, Johnson, Paloro and Sims), or freestone, if the pit comes free easily (e.g., Elberta, J.H. Hale, Redhaven, Hiley and Golden Jubilee). Peach fuzz is removed mechanically after harvest. U.S. peaches are sold fresh, frozen or canned. The fresh fruit contains modest amounts of potassium and vitamin C. Nutrient contents of one whole peach, fresh, peeled and pitted (87 g), is: 37 calories; protein, 0.6 g; carbohydrate, 9.6 g; fiber, 2.0 g; potassium, 171 mg; vitamin C, 6 mg; thiamin, 0.01 mg.; riboflavin, 0.04 mg; niacin, 0.86 mg.

peanut (Arachis hypogaea; ground nut, goober, ground pea, earth nut)   An annual legume that produces an underground pod with two or more edible kernels.

Peanuts are not true NUTS. Peanuts were cultivated by ancient peoples of Mexico and South America. Colonists took peanuts to Africa and other countries, and they are now a major crop in India, the People's Republic of China, the United States, Africa (Sudan, South Africa, Senegal), the Far East (Indonesia) and South America (Argentina, Brazil). Southern states such as Georgia, Alabama, the Carolinas, Virginia, Florida and Mississippi lead the United States in peanut production.

Peanuts are dried after harvesting and stored until processing. Most nuts sold in pods represent a variety called large-seeded Virginias. Small seeded varieties or runners are used primarily to make PEANUT BUTTER. Spanish peanuts are used in candies, peanut butter and salted nuts. During processing, unshelled peanuts are cleaned, whitened and polished before marketing. Shelling reduces the shelf life by about 70%. The skin and seed coat are removed by blanching. Peanuts are dry-roasted for candy, peanut butter and baked goods. Nuts may also be roasted in oil and served as a snack food. Roasted whole peanuts are soaked in saltwater, dried and then roasted in the shell. Roasting increases the flavor of peanuts by increasing the amounts of free AMINO ACIDS and SUGAR in kernels. Raw peanuts are cooked like beans. Peanuts can be defatted by roasting them in VEGETABLE OIL under pressure to remove 60 to 80% of the oil. Worldwide, peanuts are mainly processed for their oil or converted to peanut flour. The protein content is 26% and, like most legumes, peanut protein is somewhat low in the essential amino acid LYSINE. In developing nations peanut flour is mixed with other protein sources like fish, flour, sesame and millet to increase the overall protein quality. Nutrient contents of 1 cup (oil roasted, salted, 145 g) provide: 841 calories; protein, 38.8 g; carbohydrate, 26.8 g; fiber, 11.7 g; fat, 71.3 g; calcium, 125 mg; iron, 2.7 mg; potassium, 1,020 mg; sodium, 626 mg; thiamin, 0.42 mg; riboflavin, 0.15 mg; niacin, 2.15 mg.

Peanut Oil

Nearly 70% of the world peanut crop is used for oil product, and peanut oil accounts for 20% of the total vegetable oil consumption. Peanuts are rich in oil: 100 pounds of whole nuts yields 32 pounds of oil, and small podded varieties contain 50% oil. The oil contains 76 to 82% unsaturated FATTY ACIDS, that is, fatty acids with double bonds. Monounsaturated fatty acids represent 48.4% of the total; polyunsaturated fatty acids, 33.6%; and saturated fatty acids, 18%. Peanut oil is used as a cooking oil because it has a high smoke point (that is, it produces smoke only at high temperatures). The oil is also used in salad dressing, vegetable shortening and MARGARINE. (See also AFLATOXIN.)

peanut butter   Due to its popularity, half the U.S. peanut crop ends up as peanut butter. The annual U.S. consumption of peanut BUTTER is about 3 lbs per person. Peanut butter is prepared by grinding dry roasted peanuts and may contain added SALT, SUGAR, flavors, HYDROGENATED VEGETABLE OIL and ANTIOXIDANTS to retard spoilage. By law, at least 90% of the content must be peanuts in order for a product to be labeled as "peanut butter." Peanut butter is an excellent source of protein; however, it is also a high-FAT food. About 80% of its calories come from fat. One tablespoon contains about 95 calories.

Peanut butter often contains traces of a mold toxin, AFLA-TOXIN, which is produced by a storage mold called ASPERGILLUS that often infests damp nuts and grains. In experimental animals aflatoxin is a very powerful liver CARCINOGEN (cancer-causing agent). Industry monitors aflatoxin levels in peanut butter carefully, and spot-checks have rarely detected levels higher than the legal limit of 15 parts per billion. Levels as low as 1 part per billion can cause cancer in certain species. There is little compelling evidence that eating peanut butter with traces of aflatoxin in amounts usually encountered in the Western diet causes cancer. However, it seems prudent not to eat peanut butter as a steady diet. When making your own peanut butter, avoid stale, discolored or shriveled peanuts, which may be contaminated by mold. Keep freshly ground peanut butter refrigerated to retard spoilage. Nutrient contents of peanut butter (one tablespoon, 16 g) is: 95 calories; protein, 4.6 g; carbohydrate, 2.5 g; fiber, 1.2 g; fat, 8.2 g; iron, 0.29 mg; sodium, 75 mg; thiamin, 0.02 mg; riboflavin, 0.02 mg; niacin, 2.15 mg. (See also SATURATED FAT.)

Hoffman, Donald R. and Collins-Williams, Cecil, "Cold Pressed Oils May Contain Peanut Allergen," *Journal of Allergy and Clinical Immunology*, 93:4 (1994), pp. 801–02.

pear (*Pyrus spp.*)   A popular, juicy FRUIT related to the APPLE and QUINCE. Pears originated in Asia and were cultivated as early as 1000 B.C. They are now grown in temperate zones worldwide. Thousands of varieties of pears have been developed. Pears are round or bell-shaped; the neck may be long or practically indistinguishable. The flesh has a sandy texture due to "grit" cells. The taste ranges from sweet to acidic. Pears grown in North America are the common European pear, *P. communis* (Bartlett, Bosc, Comice, for example); and the Oriental pear, *P. pyrifolia*. Crosses between the two species are blight-resistant and possess a desirable texture and taste. Hybrid varieties include Kieffer, LeConte and Garber. The Anjou is the most popular winter pair; the Bartlett is the leading summer pear. Italy, the United States and China are leaders in pear production. Pears are grown in most U.S. states; California, Washington, Oregon, New York and Michigan are among the top producers.

Over 60% of the pear crop is processed (canned or dried). Pears are picked green because the immature fruit is firm and can be transported more easily without bruising. As pears ripen, starch is converted to sugar and the flesh softens. Pears stored in sealed plastic bags will turn brown due to limited oxygen. Lemon juice spread on freshly sliced pears will prevent their darkening. Much of the carbohydrate content is simple sugars (fructose, GLUCOSE and others). When eaten with the skin pears are a good source of fiber. Most vitamin C is also concentrated in the skin. One Bartlett pear (raw, 166 g) provides 98 calories; protein, 0.7 g; carbohydrate, 25.1 g; fiber, 5.0 g; fat, 0.7 g; potassium, 208 mg; vitamin C, 7 mg; thiamin, 0.07 mg; riboflavin, 0.17 mg; niacin, 0.17 mg.

pecan (*Carya illinoensis*)   The seed of the pecan tree, a species of hickory. Pecans are native to the southern United States and the Mississippi River Basin. Georgia alone produces about 40% of the U.S. crop. Nearly 90% of pecans are sold as shelled nuts. Pecans contain 70% oil, a fat content higher than peanuts and most other nuts. Shelled pecans

should be refrigerated or stored in the freezer to minimize rancidity. When frozen, nuts in the shell can be kept for two years. Pecans are used in baked goods, ice cream, candy, salads, desserts and vegetable dishes. The nutrient value of dried pecans (1 cup, unsalted, shelled, 108 g) is: 720 calories; protein, 8.4 g; carbohydrate, 19.7 g; fiber, 6.5 g; fat, 73.1 g; calcium, 39 mg; iron, 2.3 mg; potassium, 423 mg; thiamin, 0.92 mg; riboflavin, 0.14 mg; niacin, 0.96 mg.

pectin   An important type of water-soluble FIBER. Dietary fiber represents the non-digested carbohydrate that strengthens plant cells and acts as an intercellular "cement." Pectin differs from BRAN, which is a common form of insoluble fiber. Pectin is composed of branched carbohydrate chains containing an acidic sugar (galacturonic acid), together with the simple sugars (galactose or arabinose).

Pectin affects health in several ways. Pectin, not bran, lowers BLOOD PRESSURE and blood CHOLESTEROL, and regularly eating soluble fiber as fruit, oat bran and legumes may significantly lower blood cholesterol. Pectin also helps maintain normal BLOOD SUGAR. Pectin softens stools to help prevent bulges in the colon (DIVERTICULOSIS) and hemorrhoids and helps reduce the risk of colon CANCER. Pectin heals COLITIS in experimental animals. A possible explanation is that pectin is broken down by gut bacteria to SHORT-CHAIN FATTY ACIDS, which promote healthy epithelial cell lining of the intestine.

Good sources of pectin include many fruits like APPLES and berries, VEGETABLES, seeds, BEANS, split peas, LENTILS, SQUASH, CARROTS and OAT bran. Pectin is virtually absent from whole grains. Apple peel contains 15% pectin, while onion skins are 11 to 12% pectin. When extracted from plant material, pectin is a white powder that readily forms gels when dissolved in water. Lemon, lime, grapefruit and orange rinds contain up to 30% pectin and are a commercial source of pectin. As a FOOD ADDITIVE, pectin is used for jellies and jams because it gels in the presence of sugar and acid. It is used to thicken barbecue sauces, YOGURT, cranberry sauce and canned frosting. Pectin is classified as a safe additive. (See also COMPLEX CARBOHYDRATE.)

pectinase   A family of enzymes occurring in plants and microorganisms that degrade PECTIN, a form of dietary fiber that causes gel formation. Pectinase softens plant tissue and FRUIT and destroys the gelling capability of many fruit JUICES. Commercially, pectinase is extracted from certain bacteria and plant products and is added by the food industry to clarify fruit juice concentrates, WINE, VINEGAR, syrup and JELLY. (See also FOOD ADDITIVES.)

pellagra   A disease due to a chronic deficiency of the B vitamin NIACIN. In the early 1900s pellagra was widespread in the southern United States when people relied on CORN as their main PROTEIN source. With niacin and RIBOFLAVIN enrichment of grain products and flour in the 1920s, pellagra practically disappeared in Europe and North America. It is associated with chronic ALCOHOLISM and still occurs in other parts of the world in populations with nutritionally inadequate diets relying on corn. The body converts about 2% of the daily intake of the essential amino acid TRYPTOPHAN to niacin. Therefore, diets that provide minimal animal protein and are low in tryptophan, promote pellagra. Niacin deficiency leads to sore tongue (GLOSSITIS), skin disorders like DERMATITIS, bloody DIARRHEA and inflammation of the GASTROINTESTINAL TRACT. Pellagra affects the NERVOUS SYSTEM, causing DEPRESSION, anxiety and psychosis. Pellagra readily responds to treatment with niacin or its counterpart, NIACINAMIDE. (See also ENRICHMENT; FORTIFICATION; MALNUTRITION.)

pentose   A family of simple sugars that are key building blocks of DNA, the genetic material, and RNA, the mechanism guiding protein synthesis. Unlike hexoses like glucose, which contain six carbon atoms, pentoses contain five carbon atoms; ribose and DEOXYRIBOSE are the most common. Both ribose and deoxyribose are synthesized from GLUCOSE (BLOOD SUGAR) and are not required nutrients. Pentoses do not occur free in foods but instead are building blocks of many plant polysaccharides (sugar polymers) as FIBER. For example, D-xylose and L-arabinose are common constituents in fruits and root vegetables. (See also CARBOHYDRATE.)

pepper (*Capsicum spp.*)   A green or red VEGETABLE belonging to the capsicum family. Peppers are native to the New World, where they were harvested in Mexico before 5000 B.C. and were domesticated independently along the Peruvian coast. European explorers introduced peppers to the Old World, where they spread rapidly. Peppers are customarily classified as CHILI PEPPERS (*C. frutescens*) when they possess a strong flavor, and as sweet peppers (*C. annum*) when their large fruit possesses a mild flavor. Peppers now rank among the top 20 important vegetable crops, with China, Nigeria, Spain, Italy, Turkey and Mexico among the leading pepper-producing nations. Florida and California produce most domestic sweet peppers. Much of the U.S. crop is sold as a fresh vegetable. However, peppers may be canned, pickled, dehydrated or frozen. In addition to salads, fresh as well as processed peppers can be used in relishes and garnishes for fish, meats and poultry. Sweet peppers can be stuffed and baked. They add zest to omelets, pizzas and stews. Sweet peppers are an excellent source of vitamin C, and the red varieties contribute vitamin A. Peppers belong to the nightshade family, which includes EGGPLANT, TOMATOES and POTATOES.

The most popular pepper in the United States is bell pepper, a sweet pepper. Bell peppers can be green, yellow-orange or red, depending upon their stage of ripeness. Bell peppers lack the ingredient in chili peppers that gives hot peppers their bite; instead they have a mild flavor. Other types of sweet peppers include banana, Cubanelle and pimento.

Hot peppers contain CAPSAICIN as the active ingredient. This material affects digestion by stimulating salivation, stomach acid production and perhaps PERISTALSIS. Capsaicin also kills bacteria. Capsaicin may also help prevent blood clot formation. Hot chili peppers may contain sufficiently high levels of capsaicin to burn mucous membranes, and irritating, volatile oil may be released during frying. Leading varieties are marketed fresh, dried or canned: Anaheim, ancho, cascabel, cayenne, cherry, habanero, jalapeño, poblano and serrano.

Hot peppers provide important seasonings. These include:

- Cayenne pepper—a hot seasoning prepared from dried chili peppers.
- Chile powder—a hot seasoning prepared from ground red chili peppers. Chili powder often contains cumin, salt, oregano and garlic powder as well.
- Paprika—a mild seasoning prepared from ground, mild-flavored types of sweet pepper.
- Red pepper—a hot seasoning prepared from ground dried red chili peppers.

One sweet green pepper (raw, 74 g) provides 18 calories; protein, 3.9 g; carbohydrate, 1.3 g; fat, 0.3 g; iron, 0.94 mg; potassium, 144 mg; vitamin C, 95 mg; thiamin, 0.06 mg; riboflavin, 0.04 mg; niacin, 0.41 mg. Sweet red peppers contain more vitamin A (570 retinol equivalents) and more vitamin C (141 mg).

peppermint (*Mentha piperita*)   A perennial HERB with a refreshing flavor. Peppermint is a popular choice of herb tea. Peppermint leaves are used as a flavoring in sauces, fruit salads, drinks and punches. Peppermint oil is extracted from dried plants and is used to flavor CHEWING GUM, CANDY and other consumer goods like toothpaste. Peppermint has a long history in folk medicine for treating digestive problems. Peppermint oil possesses anti-inflammatory and anti-ulcer activity and relieves symptoms associated with severe indigestion, gastritis and enteritis (inflammation of the stomach and intestine, respectively). Peppermint oil stimulates bile secretion and normalizes gastrointestinal functions. It also possesses antimicrobial activity. (See also SPICE.)

pepsin   A digestive ENZYME produced in the STOMACH that, together with STOMACH ACID, initiates protein DIGESTION. Pepsin originates in CHIEF CELLS of pyloric glands (gastric glands). Pepsin requires an acidic environment for full activity. It is manufactured as an inactive form called pepsinogen to prevent destruction of the glands. After secretion into the stomach, stomach acid rapidly activates pepsinogen to pepsin, where it breaks down food proteins into fragments, setting the stage for the powerful, pancreatic enzymes to complete the digestion of proteins to amino acids. Hydrochloric acid supplements, such as glutamic acid hydrochloride, usually contain pepsin. (See also PROTEASE.)

peptic ulcer   A sore or erosion in the lining of the stomach or upper portion of the intestine. Stress, cigarette smoking, food allergy, low-fiber diets and overdosing with ASPIRIN are linked to an increased risk of ulcers. Most peptic ulcers are associated with recurrent pain in the abdominal area after a meal, which may be called HEARTBURN. Consumption of ANTACIDS to neutralize stomach acid usually relieves the pain. Drugs that block stomach acid secretion and antacids are used in treatment. However, they have side effects and disrupt DIGESTION. Relapse rate is high with the drug cimetidine because it alters the lining of the stomach and the intestine. Raw cabbage juice and a component of LICORICE have been used in healing ulcers. Chronic infection by the bacterium HELICOBACTER PYLORI has been shown to cause a form of stomach inflammation called atrophic gastritis, and the bacterium is probably a cause of stomach ulcers as well. (See also DUODENAL ULCER; GASTRIC ULCER.)

peptide A molecule composed of a chain (polymer) of amino acids. Amino acids form chains by linking up in a "head to toe" fashion so that the amino group (nitrogen-bearing group) of one amino acid binds to an acid group (a carboxyl group) of another amino acid. The antioxidant glutathione, manufactured in cells from the amino acids glutamic acid, cysteine and glycine, is classified as a tripeptide because it contains three linked amino acids. Certain HORMONES, like OXYTOCIN and ANTIDIURETIC HORMONE, which contain nine amino acids, are classified as nonapeptides. Other peptides are biologically important. Enkephalins are brain peptides composed of five amino acids that decrease sensitivity to pain. Peptides are produced during DIGESTION, and are in turn degraded to amino acids and absorbed.

Proteins are polypeptides, long chains assembled from 20 different amino acids and ranging in size from 50 or 60 amino acids to a thousand or more. The characteristic properties of each type of polypeptide reside in the unique sequence of its amino acids. When peptides are digested by peptidases and proteolytic ENZYMES, they yield their constituent amino acids.

perch (*Perca*) A large family of freshwater game and food fish. Perch are characterized by spiny fins; they are widely distributed in lakes and streams, and even in brackish water. *P. flavescens*, the North American perch (yellow perch), is found in the United States and Canada; *P. fluviatilis* lives in central Europe. The walleye pike and yellow perch, important game fish, belong to a closely related genus. Saltwater fish such as sea bass and rockfish families are not true perch. Perch is a lean fish with a firm white meat and mild flavor. Perch is sold as fillets or whole, dressed, and can be poached, broiled or sauteed. With less than a gram of fat per serving, perch is classified as a lean fish. Nutrient content of 3 oz (85 g) is: 80 calories; protein, 15.8 g; fat, 1.4 g; calcium, 91 mg; cholesterol, 36 mg; thiamin, 0.08 mg; riboflavin, 0.094 mg; and niacin, 1.7 mg (See also SALMON.)

periodontal disease A progressive disease of gums supporting the bone of TEETH. Several stages have been identified: GINGIVITIS refers to swollen, inflamed gums that bleed easily—with flossing, for example. There may be bad breath (halitosis). Periodontitis is a more serious condition, in which gums recede and deep pockets form, harboring pathogenic (disease-producing) bacteria, and inflammation erodes the ligament binding the tooth to the jaw bone. As the infection progresses, deep tissue is damaged and teeth become loose.

The culprit of gum disease is plaque, a sticky film produced by bacteria that provides a haven for further bacterial growth. If not removed by daily brushing, plaque accumulates at the gum line and can cause gum inflammation. Plaque can become calcified or harden into tartar. Plaque deposits beneath the gum line favor the growth of pathogenic bacteria. The IMMUNE SYSTEM attacks the infection by causing INFLAMMATION. This process releases tissue-destroying enzymes to enable defensive cells to attack the site of infection. Thus inflammation leads to further tissue destruction.

The most important tactic in preventing periodontal disease is to keep teeth clean, especially along the gum line. This means careful brushing, flossing and regular prophylactic cleaning by professionals. Most often periodontitis can be controlled with personal and professional cleaning together with procedures that remove deep pockets of plaque and tartar and remove tooth layers with toxic bacteria. The risk of gum disease increases with pregnancy and with the use of oral contraceptives (which raises hormones that increase gum sensitivity); cigarette smoking (which slows healing); alcohol consumption (which reduces the flow of saliva); a depressed immune system; and medications that dry the mouth (antidepressants, antihistamines, antihypertensives, decongestants and muscle relaxants, among others). Children whose family history includes periodontal disease are at greater risk for this condition. (See DENTAL PLAQUE; TEETH.)

peristalsis The sequential wave-like contraction and relaxation of smooth muscles that moves food through the digestive tract. Once chewed, food enters the ESOPHAGUS, the passageway leading to the stomach. Powerful, involuntary muscular contractions propel food in its various stages of disintegration and DIGESTION. Circular muscular contractions constrict the walls of the esophagus, stomach and INTESTINE and squeeze the food forward. Passage of food into the stomach generally requires four to eight seconds. After food enters the stomach, slower peristaltic waves mix food with GASTRIC JUICES to produce a liquefied food (CHYME). Food may remain in the stomach an hour or so. Peristalsis then propels the chyme through the intestine, where the contractions are weaker than in the stomach and esophagus. Food remains in the small intestine for three to five hours. In the colon slow peristalsis (three to twelve contractions per minute) moves the chyme downward. Finally strong peristaltic waves drive the contents of the colon toward the rectum. Food ALLERGY and FOOD SENSITIVITY can contract smooth muscles, slowing transit through the digestive tract (a situation called hypomotility), leading to CONSTIPATION, or they may cause rapid peristalsis (hypermotility) leading to DIARRHEA. Hypermotility may interfere with digestion and absorption of nutrients. (See also DIGESTIVE TRACT.)

pernicious anemia A deficiency of normal RED BLOOD CELLS due to inadequate uptake of VITAMIN B_{12}. In this disorder, vitamin B_{12} cannot be absorbed because the stomach fails to secrete adequate amounts of vitamin B_{12} binding protein, INTRINSIC FACTOR, required for absorption of vitamin B_{12}. Chronic vitamin B_{12} deficiency limits the ability of BONE MARROW to produce red blood cells, causing anemia, characterized by a progressive decrease in the number of red BLOOD cells and the appearance of giant red blood cells, together with gastrointestinal disturbance, weakness and nerve damage. Pernicious anemia can be treated by vitamin B_{12} injections. (See also MALABSORPTION; MALNUTRITION.)

peroxidase Antioxidant ENZYMES that form part of the body's defense against highly reactive and damaging forms of oxygen (peroxides). Peroxidases readily destroy HYDROGEN PEROXIDE, an oxidizing agent produced by metabolism, and lipid peroxides. Peroxides are potentially hazardous to cells because they generate FREE RADICALS. These chemical fragments can rapidly damage cellular proteins, membranes and genetic material. Peroxidases belong to a large family of iron-containing enzymes that carry out oxidation. (See also CATALASE.)

peroxides Highly reactive oxidation products, especially of lipids and fat. Fats, oils and cholesterol react with oxygen in the presence of metal ions when heated to form peroxides. POLYUNSATURATED OILS like safflower oil are particularly sensitive to peroxidation because of their chemical structure, with multiple bonds. The resulting lipid peroxides are dangerous because they spontaneously decompose into FREE RADICALS and other unstable chemical species that may attack DNA, producing mutations and causing cancer; or they may kill cells outright. Lipid peroxides also trigger inflammation.

The body's defense system can destroy free radicals before they can attack cells and peroxidases (GLUTATHIONE PEROXIDASE) can disarm lipid peroxides to prevent further damage. The required nutrients include SELENIUM, GLUTATHIONE and VITAMIN C. Other antioxidants, including VITAMIN E and BETA CAROTENE, can quench free radicals produced by lipid peroxide breakdown. However, the reserve capacity to destroy peroxides can be overwhelmed with continuous exposure to free radicals, especially when the nutritional status is compromised by a diet based on highly processed food. Lipid peroxides occur in fatty foods that have been highly processed, as when the fat is heated and exposed to air, such as in deep fat-fried foods and in polyunsaturated vegetable oils exposed to heat, light and traces of iron or other metal ions. Whole or minimally processed foods contain ANTIOXIDANTS like vitamin E and carotenoids which protect these foods.

To minimize peroxide formation in fats and oils, use lower cooking temperatures and use OLIVE OIL instead of polyunsaturated oils like CORN OIL or SAFFLOWER oil (monounsaturated fat is less easily oxidized). Refrigerate cooking oils in sealed containers to reduce their oxidation. Consume an adequate intake of antioxidants by eating foods rich in selenium, vitamin C, beta carotene and carotenoids and supplement these with extra vitamin E as needed. Buy whole, fresh foods and minimize consumption of processed high-fat foods like chips and crackers to reduce your intake of rancid oils. (See also GLUTATHIONE PEROXIDASE; RANCIDITY.)

peroxisome A small particle found in the CYTOPLASM of most cells that perform a variety of oxidations. Peroxisomes operate independently of MITOCHONDRIA, the primary oxidative powerhouse of the cell, to degrade FATTY ACIDS, including the by-products of the chemical processing of vegetable oils called TRANS-FATTY ACIDS, with the production of HYDROGEN PEROXIDE. The oxidase enzymes of peroxisomes also break down unusual amino acids (D-amino acids) derived from microbial and plant sources. They degrade the toxic agent hydrogen peroxide. (See also FAT DIGESTION.)

pesco-vegetarian A person who consumes a diet based on plant foods that includes fish and milk and egg products, but no other animal protein. (See also VEGETARIAN.)

pesticides Substances used to control or destroy undesirable organisms, especially rodents, insects, weeds and molds. Pesticides may be synthetic chemicals or they may be made of natural materials. Rodenticides are used to control mice and rats; insecticides control insects, mites, spiders and ticks. Other classes of pesticides control slugs, snails and nematodes that attack root vegetables in particular. Herbicides control weeds; these may contain agents that change plant growth or alter leaf physiology. Fungicides control the growth of MOLD and fungus on produce.

The United States alone uses over a billion pounds of pesticides yearly, and the use of pesticides provides considerable benefits in crop production throughout the world. These chemicals protect against the natural threats of blight and insect pests that in times past decimated crops. Fifty percent of the dollars spent in pest control goes to weed control, and this has been a major factor in making farming less labor intensive. The increased availability of food has lowered food costs. Prior to 1950 consumers spent on the average 24% of the family budget on food; by 1990, consumers spent 12% on food. The cogent argument is made that the use of pesticides has dramatically lowered the cost of fruits and vegetables, making them more affordable and increasing their consumption as recommended by governmental agencies to reduce the risk of chronic illness.

The first pesticides were natural products, which continue to be important agricultural materials. As an example, large-scale production of biopesticides, living organisms or their by-products, has been successful in some instances. The soil bacterium *Bacillus thuringiensis* produces a protein toxin (poison) that specifically affects certain moths and caterpillars without affecting other insects, animals or humans. Aerial spraying programs have used this procedure to destroy infestations of the Asian gypsy moth. This biopesticide is approved for about 200 crops in the United States. However, in Hawaii, Florida and New York, as well as in the Philippines, Thailand and Japan, moths have evolved a resistance to this toxin. An alternative strategy relies on baiting traps with pheromones, chemicals that act as sex attractants for the male or female moth. Genetic engineering and biotechnology continue to be applied to develop safer, more effective biopesticides.

Synthetic chemical pesticides are recent creations (post–World War II) and played a role in launching the GREEN REVOLUTION. Among the first was DDT, an extremely potent pesticide that kills insects by altering the ability of their nerve cells to conduct nerve impulses. Presently there are approximately 50,000 registered pesticides. Most were approved before the U.S. EPA required health effects testing. The EPA has established that 67 of the 300 chemicals used in food induce CANCER. Many are concentrated in processed foods. The Federal Insecticide, Fungicide and Rodenticide Act (1972) prohibits the use of cancer-causing pesticides, and the DELANEY CLAUSE prohibits the addition of cancer-causing agents to foods. This was superseded by the Food Quality Protection Act of 1996, which established a single health-based standard for pesticide residues in all foods.

The U.S. FDA monitors pesticide levels in foods and the EPA establishes upper limits for the amounts of registered pesticides in foods. For example, 92 pesticides are registered for use on tomatoes. Each registered pesticide has a specified tolerance level. Though the FDA can screen for more than 300 different pesticides, not all testing facilities do so; thus, certain pesticides found in food may not be reported because of limited testing. As examples, the pesticide EBDC, which breaks down to form a carcinogen; Amitraz, an insecticide used on pears, and a possible carcinogen; and benomyl (in BANANAS, PEACHES, SOYBEANS, rice and other foods), a pesticide suspected of causing birth defects and cancer—are not analyzed (1996).

Natural Pesticides

Natural pesticides are widespread, apparently because plants defend themselves against predators, fungi, molds and infection by producing toxins, and it seems likely that each plant species produces its own characteristic set of toxins. Humans eat an estimated 5,000 to 10,000 natural pesticides and related compounds and consume about 1.5 g of these substances daily. For example, lima beans produce 23 toxins and cabbage yield 49 toxins and related compounds. Twenty-seven natural pesticides found to be rodent carcinogens are present in foods ranging from APPLE, basil and BRUSSELS SPROUTS to CELERY, EGGPLANT, fennel, horseradish and potato.

At the same time vegetables like ONIONS, CRUCIFEROUS VEGETABLES, including BROCCOLI and CAULIFLOWER, and most fresh FRUITS contain many nutrients and substances that counterbalance these natural pesticides and offer protection against cancer. The following is a brief listing.

1. Garlic and onions contain allylic sulfides and other organosulfur compounds that may stimulate a DETOXICATION enzyme in the liver.
2. Parsley, CARROTS, squash, sweet POTATOES, CANTALOUPE, kale and turnip greens contain beta carotene and related carotenoids that can act as antioxidants to prevent cellular damage.
3. Green TEA and berries contain TANNINS that also act as antioxidants.
4. Most fruits and vegetables contain FLAVONOIDS that act as antioxidants and some may also block the target sites of estrogen that can promote certain cancers.
5. Cabbage and related vegetables, including broccoli, as well as squash, yams, tomatoes, PEPPERS and SOY provide plant sterols that help maintain normal differentiation. The cabbage family contains indoles that increase the production of protective enzymes.
6. Mustard, horseradish and cabbage-family vegetables like broccoli contain ISOTHIOCYANATES, which also induce protective enzymes.
7. Citrus fruits contain limonoids that stimulate the production of protective enzymes in the liver.
8. TOMATOES and red grapefruit contain the red pigment LYCOPENE, which acts as an antioxidant to protect cells against damage.
9. Parsley, carrots, cruciferous vegetables in addition to squash, yams, tomatoes, peppers, mint, basil and cucumber, among others, contain monoterpenes that inhibit the metabolism of tumors, act as antioxidants and stimulate the production of protective enzymes.
10. Parsley, carrots, vegetables of the cabbage family, eggplant, pepper, citrus fruit, whole grains and berries provide polyphenols (tannins) that inhibit the formation of nitrosoamines, a cancer-causing agent; act as antioxidants; and increase levels of protective enzymes.

Safety Issues Regarding Synthetic Pesticides

The long-term effects of pesticides on health are a controversial area. One position is that foods containing legal levels of pesticide residues generally pose no health risk to adults or children, provided they eat foods produced in the United States. Because they are so prevalent in plants, some investigators contend that natural toxins in foods provide a greater hazard than synthetic pesticide residues.

A number of potential problems with pesticide use have been identified in recent years.

1. Traces of potential cancer-causing pesticides are permitted in foods provided they pose a negligible RISK. A number of older, more toxic pesticides are still permitted in processed foods because they were registered before current laws went into effect. The U.S. National Academy of Sciences has estimated that 90% of pesticides used on foods have not been adequately tested for safety. Looking at only 28 of the 53 pesticides, the academy experts concluded that about half of U.S. food is contaminated. The most highly contaminated foods are tomatoes and tomato products, followed by BEEF, potatoes, ORANGES, LETTUCE, APPLES, peaches, PORK, WHEAT, soybeans, BEANS, carrots, CHICKEN, CORN and GRAPES. Crops like STRAWBERRIES, peaches and celery can be heavily contaminated also. The FDA found that 40% of domestic grains and grain products, 51% of domestic fruits and 32% of domestic vegetables were contaminated (1992). It should be noted that less than 0.5% were found to violate federally allowed limits.
2. Formerly EPA standards for pesticide contamination in food were often set with unrealistic figures for consumption of a food. For example, the pesticide levels in AVOCADOS were established assuming the average consumption is less than two per year. Tolerances for cantaloupes were based on an annual consumption of only 7.5 oz. There are similar problems with ARTICHOKES, TANGERINES, BRUSSELS SPROUTS and other produce. A panel of the U.S. National Academy of Sciences concluded in 1994 that the regulatory agencies have based pesticide risk evaluation on an adult diet; in another 1994 report the Environmental Working Group concluded that one-third of a person's lifetime exposure to some pesticides in the United States can accumulate by the age of five. In an infant's first year, the average U.S. baby's exposure to certain pesticides can exceed the accepted cancer risk exposure threshold of causing one cancer death per 1 million people. Preschool children eat more fruit and drink more fruit juice on a weight basis than adults. Children's metabolism differs from adults' and this could make children more susceptible to pesticides.
3. There is currently a four-week testing process by the FDA. Since the FDA lacks authority to control sampled food, by the time a batch of food is found to be contaminated with illegal levels of pesticides, the food often has been sold and consumed.
4. In the light of new medical research, most pesticides need to be reevaluated. An estimated 90% of fungicides cause cancer in experimental animals. Furthermore, 28 of the 53 most common pesticides probably cause cancer.

New legislation requires the EPA to review all existing tolerances for pesticide by 2006.

5. Little is known about the safety of long-term exposure to low levels of multiple pesticide residues and to related compounds like PCBs (polychlorinated biphenyls) and PBBs (polybrominated biphenyls). Studies have linked the herbicide 2,4-D to non-Hodgkins lymphoma, a cancer of the lymphatic system. A pilot study in 1992 found that the breast fat of women with breast cancer contained more PCBs and pesticides like DDT than the breast tissue of normal women.

6. When screening pesticides, the EPA does not test whether they can imitate estrogen, a human female reproductive hormone. As an example, endosulfan, a pesticide used on carrots, lettuce, spinach and tomatoes among 40 other vegetables, possesses estrogen-like properties, comparable to DDT. Exposure to such pesticides and chemicals like PCBs can disrupt the endocrine system, possibly by mimicking hormones, thus altering fertility and sexual development in animals and perhaps in humans, and increasing the risk of breast cancer.

7. Certain pesticides, environmental pollutants and antibiotics alter the integrity of MITOCHONDRIA, the energy powerhouses of the cell. The purpose of mitochondria is to produce ATP, the chemical currency of cells. Normally about three ATP are generated for each oxygen atom consumed. However, toxic chemicals can lower this ratio, significantly decreasing ATP output. This phenomenon is called uncoupling. An individual whose mitochondria are partially uncoupled has compromised health and is susceptible to other environmental insults such as viral infection or damage from oxygen.

8. More imported food is contaminated with pesticides than domestic produce. Imported fruit and vegetables may be sprayed with pesticides banned in the United States (DDT, endrin, heptachlor, aldrin and chlordane). For example, chlordane is made in the United States but isn't allowed to be used here because it is suspected of being a carcinogen. Hamburger from beef imported from Central America was recently found to be contaminated with chlordane. According to the U.S. Government Accounting Office, the FDA can sample only 1% of the U.S. food imports (1991) and 4% of those contained unapproved pesticides. Such limited screening may miss many pesticides.

9. An estimated 25% of the currently used pesticides enter both plants and animals and cannot be easily removed.

10. Pests are increasingly resistant to pesticides, so that larger amounts have to be applied. Between 1950 and 1980 pesticide use increased by 1,000%.

Recommendations to minimize consumption of pesticide-contaminated food:

- Buy certified organically grown fruit and vegetables (produce grown without chemicals, including pesticides). Note that most non-organic fruits and certain vegetables often contain higher than usual amounts of pesticides. These include tomatoes, eggplant, pepper, peach and artichoke.
- Grow your own produce. The home gardener can either choose not to use pesticides or to use the safer varieties. Some pesticides are water-soluble and easily wash off from produce and decompose.

- Thoroughly wash produce with soap and water. Peel off the outer layers of lettuce, cabbage, carrots, peaches, cucumbers and apples. Pesticides adhering to the skin or outer leaves can be removed; but neither strategy will remove the estimated 40% of pesticides that are "systemic" (contained within the fruit or vegetable). Wax that may contain fungicides cannot be washed off.
- Buy locally grown produce in season because it is less likely to be treated with fungicides. Buy domestic rather than imported produce; it is less likely to contain residues.
- Eat a wide variety of foods. Be aware that perfect-looking fruit may be a sign that chemicals have been used to improve its cosmetic appearance.
- Trim fat off meat and poultry. Use skim milk and discard fat and drippings from cooking. Pesticides such as aldrin and chlordane accumulate in animal fat.

The Most Hazardous Pesticides

According to the National Academy of Sciences, benomyl, captan, chlordimeform, chlorothalonil, folpet, linuron, mancozeb, maneb, mitiram, permethrin and zineb are among the most dangerous pesticides now in use. Chlordimeform and permethrin contaminate cottonseed oil, and chlordthalonil (Bravo) is probably a cancer-causing agent, but residues can be washed off with soap and water. Permethrin may be a carcinogen and has possible toxic effects on pregnant animals. It too washes off with soap and water. It is concentrated in processed tomatoes. The use of atrazine, which accounts for roughly 10% of all pesticides used in the United States and has been a widespread contaminant, has been restricted by the EPA (1991). Carbofuran, a widely used insecticide and nematocide (an agent that kills nematodes), is very toxic to birds. In 1992 a federal court forbade the use of four common cancer-causing pesticides, including the fungicide benomyl, used on raisin grapes and tomatoes that will be processed; mancozeb, a fungicide found in flour and raisins; phosmet, an insecticide found in cottonseed oil; and trifluralin, an insecticide used in peppermint and spearmint.

Food Quality Protection Act of 1996

The Food Quality Protection Act of 1996 reforms the FEDERAL FOOD DRUG AND COSMETIC ACT and supersedes the DELANEY CLAUSE. It also amends the Federal Insecticide, Fungicide and Rodenticide Act by establishing a single health-based standard for pesticide residues in all foods. The new safety standard to apply to pesticides is based on being reasonably certain that a given pesticide's residue will not harm the consumer. This act allows the use of additives that pose a negligible health risk, based on modern risk assessment methods, for both raw and processed foods. Other provisions prohibit states from setting tolerances stricter than federal standards, unless approved by the EPA. It also allows economic considerations to be weighed. Thus there could be continued use of some products that could exceed the negligible risk standard if they are required to assure an adequate food supply. The EPA will have the authority to require chemical manufacturers to disclose information about their pesticides. Prior existing pesiticides will be reviewed in light of the new standard and all existing tolerances for pesticides wil be reviewed within 10 years.

Provisions to ensure the safety of children, infants and pregnant women are included. When the evidence for safety is questionable, then the allowable levels will be lowered to permit up to 10-fold more protection. The act also requires distribution of health information about pesticides in foods by food stores nation-wide. (See also CERTIFIED ORGANIC VEGETABLES; GREEN REVOLUTION; RISK DUE TO CHEMICALS IN FOOD AND WATER.)

National Research Council, U.S. Committee on Pesticides in the Diets of Infants and Children, *Pesticides in the Diets of Infants and Children.* Washington, D.C.: National Academy Press, 1993.

"Risk assessment of pesticides. C&E News Forum," *Chemical and Engineering News,* (January 7, 1991), pp. 27–55.

phagocyte A defensive cell capable of engulfing bacteria, foreign materials and cellular debris. The macrophage, a type of WHITE BLOOD CELL, is an important phagocyte of the body's IMMUNE SYSTEM. Macrophage engulf bacteria and foreign materials and release powerful chemicals, including the FREE RADICAL superoxide, HYDROGEN PEROXIDE, and NITRIC ACID to kill the invader, then digest the dead bacteria. Phagocytic cells patrol blood vessel surfaces, weeding out dead and dying cells. They avidly take up oxidized LOW-DENSITY LIPOPROTEIN, the major cholesterol carrier in the blood, and become engorged with lipid. In so doing, they become "foam" cells, which congregate on arterial walls. These events are believed to participate in the build-up of lipid deposits, leading to clogged arteries. (See also ATHEROSCLEROSIS; FREE RADICALS.)

pharynx (throat) The tube connecting the nose and mouth to the ESOPHAGUS, the tube leading down to the STOMACH. The pharynx also connects the nose to airways leading to the lungs. The pharynx guides masticated food into the esophagus. Unchewed food can become lodged in this region, causing choking. The walls of the pharynx contain important lymphoid tissues such as adenoids and tonsils. (See also DIGESTIVE TRACT; LYMPHATIC SYSTEM.)

phenylalanine (Phe, L-phenylalanine) An essential AMINO ACID that serves as a general protein building block. Phenylalanine is incorporated into brain proteins and smaller amino acid chains (neuropeptides) such as GROWTH HORMONE and enkephalin. The body cannot synthesize phenylalanine; it must be supplied by dietary protein. The typical U.S. diet supplies about 5 g of phenylalanine daily. An adult typically requires about 1 g of phenylalanine plus TYROSINE per day. In foods phenylalanine occurs in both animal and plant protein. Good sources of phenylalanine include any animal protein, including meat, fish, poultry and dairy products. For comparison, a cup of GRANOLA contains 0.65 g of phenylalanine; a cup of COTTAGE CHEESE, 1.70 g; 3 oz of hamburger, 0.53 g; and 1 can of tuna, 1.91 g.

Phenylalanine is converted to the nonessential amino acid, tyrosine. In turn, tyrosine is transformed by the NERVOUS SYSTEM into a family of NEUROTRANSMITTERS (chemicals that allow nerve impulses between cells): DOPAMINE, norepinephrine and EPINEPHRINE. The adrenal glands also convert tyrosine to epinephrine, which functions as a stress hormone (adrenaline). Eating a protein meal raises blood levels of phenylalanine and tyrosine and allows large amounts of these amino acids to enter the brain, which in turn leads to higher levels of dopamine and norepinephrine. Phenylalanine and tyrosine metabolism require many supportive nutrients: IRON, COPPER, VITAMIN B₆, NIACIN and VITAMIN C.

Phenylalanine Supplements

Phenylalanine (and tyrosine) supplements are claimed to increase alertness, to diminish pain and to improve mood. Phenylalanine has been reported to help with depression from various causes in some cases. Phenylalanine helps regulate the intestinal hormone CHOLECYSTOKININ (CCK). This hormone stimulates the pancreas and gallbladder to release digestive juices and signals the brain to turn off hunger signals.

Tyrosine and phenylalanine supplements can raise high blood pressure to dangerous, even deadly levels, especially in patients taking MAO INHIBITORS as antidepressants. Do not take tyrosine or phenylalanine supplements with MAO antidepressants. People with high blood pressure should consult their doctor before using phenylalanine. Phenylalanine aggravates migraine headaches in some patients. Phenylalanine produces toxic effects in patients with PHENYLKETONURIA (PKU), a genetic disease based on the inability to break down phenylalanine. ASPARTAME, an ARTIFICIAL SWEETENER, contains phenylalanine as a major ingredient. Because phenylalanine is a major constituent of aspartame, individuals with PKU are warned of foods and beverages containing this additive, and they should avoid phenylalanine supplements. In general, amino acids are powerful agents in the body and amino acid research in humans is still considered preliminary. In many cases the long-term effects and safe doses of phenylalanine, tyrosine or other amino acids are not known.

A synthetic form of phenylalanine, D-phenylalanine is the mirror image of the naturally occurring form of phenylalanine, L-phenylalanine. D-phenylalanine is rarely found in nature. It is not used by the body for proteins or neurotransmitters, nor is it a nutrient. D-phenylalanine seems promising as a treatment of chronic pain, particularly back pain, and dental pain. It apparently works by blocking the breakdown of ENDORPHINS, the brain's own pain killers (opiates), and also has anti-inflammatory effects. Naturally occurring phenylalanine, that is, L-phenylalanine, does not behave in this fashion. (See also DEPRESSION; DRUG/NUTRIENT INTERACTION.)

phenylketonuria (PKU) A rare genetic disease caused by the inability to degrade the essential AMINO ACID, PHENYLALANINE. PKU patients lack a critical enzyme called phenylalanine hydroxylase, which converts phenylalanine to tyrosine, a non-essential amino acid. In PKU patients, surplus phenylalanine is converted instead to phenylketone, a breakdown product that is excreted in the urine. Excessive phenylalanine and phenylketones can cause severe mental retardation within one to two years after birth unless the diet is corrected to lower phenylalanine intake.

Though PKU is rare, many states require that babies be screened for it by blood tests soon after birth. Children with PKU are fed a diet that is restricted for phenylalanine. Since phenylalanine cannot be manufactured in the body and is required for growth, the diet must supply enough to support growth while avoiding excess. As the child grows, the diet is modified to meet changing needs. The restrictive diet can often be relaxed as children mature, and they usually can go on to lead healthy lives as adults. (See also BIRTH DEFECTS.)

Medical Research Council Working Party on Phenylketonuria, "Phenylketonuria Due to Phenylalanine Hydroxylase Deficiency: an Unfolding Story," *British Medical Journal*, 306 (January 9, 1993), pp. 115–19.

phenylpropanolamine   The major active ingredient in diet pills, as well as in medications for colds and allergies. As an APPETITE SUPPRESSANT phenylpropanolamine is only partially effective. Phenylpropanolamine temporarily reduces appetite, but eventually appetite returns. This drug can cause significant side effects: dizziness, DEPRESSION and elevated blood pressure. Phenylpropanolamine increases the risk of STROKE and HEART ATTACK in some people with HYPERTENSION (high blood pressure). Diabetics should avoid propanolamine because it increases BLOOD SUGAR. Do not take this drug if you're being treated for high blood pressure, depression, inflammatory disorders, diabetes or kidney or thyroid disease. Do not take phenylpropanolamine with MAO INHIBITORS, methyl-dopa and tricyclic antidepressants because the combination can cause excessive blood pressure. (See also DIETING; DRUG/NUTRIENT INTERACTION.)

phospholipid   A class of LIPIDS related to FATS. Phospholipids contain PHOSPHATE, while fats do not. In addition, phospholipids contain a nitrogen-containing compound such as SERINE or CHOLINE, or a carbohydrate-like molecule, INOSITOL. The body can manufacture its own phospholipids, and phospholipids occur in all foods.

The most common phospholipid, LECITHIN, contains choline. In practice, dietary lecithin is the major source of choline, needed for cell membrane function and the formation of NEUROTRANSMITTERS, chemicals that help transmit nerve impulses. Many nerve fibers, especially those outside the brain and spinal cord, are insulated with a white segmented covering called myelin. This lipid covering contains phospholipids and serves as insulation. Phospholipids have the ability to emulsify fat and other water-insoluble materials. As a constituent of BILE, phospholipids emulsify cholesterol and help prevent gallstone formation, and they speed up fat digestion and absorption. Phospholipids help form LOW-DENSITY LIPOPROTEIN (LDL), HIGH-DENSITY LIPOPROTEIN (HDL) and CHYLOMICRONS, lipid carriers that transport cholesterol and fat in the bloodstream.

Phospholipids also have the ability to form double lipid layers, which are the foundation of all cell membranes. As major membrane building blocks, phospholipids form protective barriers that define the cell boundary as well as the internal structures of the cell, like the nucleus, where genetic information is stored, and MITOCHONDRIA, where energy is produced.

Phospholipids incorporated into cell membranes possess polyunsaturated FATTY ACIDS. Because these fatty acids are bent molecules they do not pack together easily, and they contribute to membrane flexibility. Membrane phospholipids serve as a reserve of fatty acids for the synthesis of hormone-like fatty acid derivatives, PROSTAGLANDINS. A cascade of events leading to INFLAMMATION begins with the liberation of ARACHIDONIC ACID, a polyunsaturated fatty acid and a precursor of proinflammatory agents, from membrane phospholipids. (See also ESSENTIAL FATTY ACIDS.)

phosphorus   A major mineral nutrient found primarily in bones and teeth. Phosphorus is the most common mineral in the body after CALCIUM and accounts for nearly 1.5 pounds of an adult's weight. Phosphorus exists in the body as phosphate, an inorganic, negatively charged ion. Phosphate and calcium metabolism are linked. They are withdrawn together from bone to maintain normal blood levels; vitamin D is required for both calcium and phosphate uptake. Calcium phosphate forms hydroxyapatite, the mineral deposit of bones and teeth, which represents 80% of the total phosphorus in the body. The remainder occurs in blood and soft tissues.

In blood, phosphate acts as a BUFFER to help maintain acid/base balance. The phosphate level in blood is increased by PARATHYROID hormone from the parathyroid gland and decreased by calcitonin, a hormone from the thyroid gland. The KIDNEY also helps to regulate phosphate. If blood phosphate levels rise, kidneys excrete phosphate; when dietary phosphate is low, they excrete less.

Tissues incorporate phosphate as PHOSPHOLIPIDS. These relatives of FAT form cell membranes and form lipid protein particles to transport fat and CHOLESTEROL through the circulation. Phosphate comprises part of the backbone structure of DNA and RNA. These substances store genetic information and control protein synthesis, cell division and growth and maintenance of the body.

Phosphate forms a building block of many COENZYMES, enzyme helpers derived from VITAMINS: NIACIN, RIBOFLAVIN, PANTOTHENIC ACID, THIAMIN, VITAMIN B_{12} and VITAMIN B_6. ATP (adenosine triphosphate) contains phosphate groups in a form representing large amounts of potential energy that can be tapped to drive biosynthetic reactions. The formation and utilization of ATP present extremely important aspects of energy utilization by all life forms.

Sources of Phosphate

Major food sources of phosphate include: FISH, MEAT, MILK and milk products, POULTRY, EGGS, NUTS, BEANS and PEAS. Though meat is a good source of phosphorus, it is a poor source of calcium; cheese is rich in calcium but low in phosphorus. Soft drinks are a major dietary source of this nutrient. Juices, fruit, and vegetables such as lettuce, celery and carrots provide negligible phosphorus. Cereal grains and grain products contain phosphorus. However, much of the phosphorus in cereal grains is in the form of PHYTIC ACID, which is not readily digested. More than 20 FOOD ADDITIVES contain phosphorus, including phosphoric acid, sodium hydrogen phosphate, pyrophosphate and POLYPHOSPHATES. These additives find use as pill stabilizers, acidifiers, chelating agents to bind up unwanted metal ions, leavening agents in baked goods, and emulsifiers in CHEESE.

Requirements

The RECOMMENDED DIETARY ALLOWANCE for phosphorus is 1,000 mg for adults. The standard U.S. diet is phosphate-rich and deficiencies are unlikely. When the ratio of calcium to phosphorus is approximately equal phosphorus uptake is adequate. An excess of dietary phosphorus over calcium can decrease calcium uptake.

People who chronically ingest excessive amounts of ANTACIDS, patients with bone fractures, and strict vegetarians eating high-fiber foods grown on phosphorus-depleted soil may become deficient in this mineral. Symptoms include loss of appetite, weakness and pain. Certain bone diseases, RICKETS in children and OSTEOMALACIA in adults, are caused by chronic deficiencies of VITAMIN D, calcium and phosphorus, or by an imbalance of calcium and phosphorus. Excessive levels of phosphorus can cause low blood calcium, with tetany and convulsions. (See also MACRONUTRIENT.)

photosynthesis The process by which plants trap the energy in sunlight and use it to convert atmospheric CARBON DIOXIDE into CARBOHYDRATE. Photosynthesis represents a non-polluting and renewable resource. Because all foods come directly or indirectly from plants, plants form the foundation of the FOOD CHAIN. Animals and fish eat plants, which in turn serve as human food sources.

About 2% of the energy in sunlight actually reaches the ground and 1% of this is transformed into plant products by photosynthesis. Photosynthesis relies upon the trapping of energy by the green plant pigment chlorophyll. In the first stage, or the light reaction of photosynthesis, water molecules are split into OXYGEN and hydrogen atoms. Oxygen is released to the atmosphere and energy is trapped in the form of ATP. In the second phase, or the dark reaction, carbon dioxide reacts with hydrogen atoms to form carbohydrate. The ATP generated by the light reaction drives this conversion. The overall process requires six molecules of carbon dioxide and six molecules of water plus sunlight to produce a single molecule of GLUCOSE, a simple sugar, plus six molecules of oxygen. The resulting glucose is converted to all other carbon compounds needed by the plant, including STARCH, CELLULOSE, FAT and other water-insoluble lipids, AMINO ACIDS and PROTEIN, and even DNA, the genetic material. Most materials produced by plants are indigestible; generally only 5% of a plant is suitable for human nutrition. (See also CARBOHYDRATE METABOLISM; NUTRIENT.)

pH regulators Food additives used to adjust the degree of acidity or alkalinity of a food or beverage. The pH scale refers to the acidity scale for water solutions and is based on the concentration of hydrogen ions. The scale runs from pH 0 to pH 14. The lower the pH and the more concentrated the acid, the higher the hydrogen ion concentration. A pH less than 7 is acidic; pH 7 is neutral (neither acidic nor basic); and a pH greater than 7 is alkaline (basic). The pH scale is a logarithmic scale: A pH of 3 is 10 times more acidic than a pH of 4 and 100 times more acidic than a pH of 5. Put another way, small changes in pH reflect large changes in hydrogen ion concentration.

STOMACH pH is normally about 2, due to hydrochloric acid, a very strong mineral acid produced in the stomach. Vinegar has a pH of about 5 and is somewhat acidic. Venous blood pH normally ranges between 7.36 and 7.41, slightly alkaline. A blood pH below 6.8 (severe ACIDOSIS) or above 7.8 (severe ALKALOSIS) is usually fatal. Urinary pH ranges from 5 to 8.

The final products of metabolism of fruits and vegetables, which are rich in potassium, tend to make the body more alkaline. Foods that make the body more alkaline include LEGUMES, SQUASH, members of the CABBAGE family and dark-green leafy vegetables. Meat, dairy products (high-protein foods), refined carbohydrate and sugar tend to acidify the body because they produce an acidic residue. Vegans (strict vegetarians) tend to produce more alkaline end products than meat eaters.

Because most enzymes and cellular processes operate effectively at pHs close to neutral, the body possesses many elaborate systems that regulate the pH of the body fluids. All physiologic processes, from cell division to nerve transmission, rely on enzymes, and they are exquisitely sensitive to pH for optimal activity. The KIDNEYS, lungs and RED BLOOD CELLS are especially involved in the regulating process. Together they help maintain a constant internal environment (HOMEOSTASIS).

pH considerations are also important in packaged foods and beverages. Excessively acidic or alkaline conditions can alter the appearance, taste and nutrient quality of prepared foods and beverages. Therefore food additives called pH regulating agents are used to control the degree of acidity or alkalinity of commercially prepared foods and beverages. Examples include CITRIC ACID and various forms of phosphates like sodium dihydrogen phosphate in SOFT DRINKS. (See also ACID INDIGESTION; BUFFER.)

physical activity See EXERCISE.

physical fitness See FITNESS.

phytic acid/phytate A plant compound containing phosphate bound to a carbohydrate-like compound called INOSITOL. Phytic acid occurs in unsprouted GRAINS, seeds and LEGUMES and is particularly rich in BRAN, the outer layer of grains. Although these foods often have a high phosphorus content, the phosphate in phytates is not released by digestion. Phytic acid can bind minerals very tightly, and in the intestine, phytic acid will bind IRON, MAGNESIUM and ZINC, limiting their uptake. When bread is leavened by YEAST, yeast enzymes degrade phytic acid, and yeast-leavened bread poses no threat to mineral absorption. Phytic acid is also destroyed by baking and FOOD PROCESSING. A balanced diet emphasizing minimally processed foods does not pose a problem, but wheat bran added to supplement a diet relying on high-sugar, high-fat processed food may interfere with mineral absorption. (See also MALABSORPTION.)

phytochemicals (plant chemicals) A very broad class of substances derived from plants that have a beneficial effect on health. In the broad sense, phytochemicals include vitamin C and compounds like beta carotene, which can be converted to vitamin A. However, phytochemicals include thousands of other substances; some are not well characterized and their effects are poorly understood. Many others remain to be identified. Inadequate consumption of phytochemicals may well be a major contributing factor in the chronic diseases prevalent in most Western societies. Much of what is currently known about phytochemicals is the result of recent research. Most attention has focused on the possible effects of phytochemicals in the development of cardiovascular disease and of cancer. Often conclusions are based upon studies with isolated cells or laboratory animals. How far such findings can be applied to humans is frequently not clear. Recent research has focused on several important classes that profoundly affect health. They occur in vegetables, fruits, seeds, legumes, tea, medicinal plants, spices, culinary herbs and even edible mushrooms. Phytochemicals are conveniently classified into the following groups: FLAVONOIDS, PHYTOSTEROLS, CAROTENOIDS, indoles, coumarins, organosulfur compounds, terpenes, saponins, lignans and ISOTHIOCYANATES. Refer to the accom-panying table for sources and possible actions of primary phytochemicals. The following examples are noteworthy.

Flavonoids Over 5,000 flavonoids have been identi-fied. Plants evolved this large class of compounds to protect themselves against oxidative damage. Flavonoids consist of multiple ring structures; the purple, blue and red color of fruits and berries represent flavonoids. Flavonoids act as ANTIOXIDANTS to squelch very reactive chemicals called FREE RADICALS, which are generated by pollutants as well as from oxygen by the body's own processes. Flavonoids can stabi-lize connective tissue and capillaries, and seem to work together with vitamin C in this regard. They also decrease inflammation by several mechanisms. They inhibit the infil-tration of immune cells that cause inflammation (neu-trophils). They block enzymes that generate inflammatory

Phytochemicals That May Benefit Health

Phytochemicals	Typical Source	Possible Roles
Flavonoids Polyphenols like quercetin, kaempferol anthocyanin	Fruits, berries, vegetables, kale, bark stems, wine	Antioxidant. May stimulate detoxication enzymes and protects liver. Strengthens capillaries. Blocks inflammation. May inhibit tumor formation.
Phytosterols Isoflavones like Genistein	Soybeans, lentils, peas	May inhibit estrogen-promoted cancers and lower high blood cholesterol to decrease the risk of atherosclerosis.
Carotenoids Carotenes like alpha carotene and beta carotene	Carrots, yams, cantaloupe butternut squash	Antioxidant. May protect against heart disease and stroke.
Lycopene	Tomatoes, red grapefruit	Antioxidant. May protect against cancers of the cervix, stomach, bladder, colon and prostate.
Xanthophylls	Dark green leafy vegetables	Antioxidant. May protect against heart disease and stroke.
Indoles	Cruciferous vegetables, such as broccoli, cabbage and brussels sprouts	May protect against breast cancer.
Coumarins	Citrus fruit, tomatoes	May prevent blood clotting and may stimulate detoxication enzymes in the liver.
Organosulfur Compounds Diallyl disulfide, S-allylcysteine, others	Garlic, onions, leeks, shallots, chives	May block carcinogens and suppress carcinogenic changes in cells. May stimulate detoxication enzymes.
Terpenes Monoterpenes Triterpenes	Citrus fruit, caraway seeds Licorice root, citrus fruit	May block action of carcinogens. May inhibit hormone related cancers.
Saponins	Soybeans, many vegetables, herbs	May have anticancer activity. May lower high blood cholesterol.
Lignans	Flaxseed, wheat, barley	An antioxidant. May protect against cancers.
Isothiocyanates Sulforaphane, and others	Cruciferous vegetables, including broccoli, watercress, cabbage, mustard, horseradish	May protect against breast cancer, stimulate detoxication enzymes and protect against cigarette smoke.

prostaglandins and leukotrienes, fatty acid derivatives with hormone-like qualities, and they desensitize mast cells, a type of immune cell embedded in tissues that release inflammatory agents like histamine when they encounter a foreign invader. Various flavonoids decrease the ability of platelets to form dangerous blood clots. Flavonoids can either activate or inhibit detoxication enzymes of the liver that help dispose of wastes and toxic materials. Such phytochemicals in wine, onions, apples and tea are believed to reduce the risk of CORONARY ARTERY DISEASE.

Isothiocyanates The cabbage family (Brassica vegetables) possesses sulfur compounds that protect against some forms of cancer. SULFORAPHANE is an example. Isothiocyanates seem to act on detoxication mechanisms, thus speeding up the inactivation and disposal of potentiallly harmful compounds like pollutants from the body.

Phytoestrogens A group of compounds found in soybean and other legumes. Saponins and isoflavones possess very weak estrogen activity. Estrogen is a female sex hormone, and by mimicking estrogen, phytoestrogens may lower the risk of certain cancers, including breast cancer.

Carotenoids Yellow-orange pigments that occur in dark green leafy vegetables and orange vegetables and fruits. Carotenoids act as antioxidants and they bolster the immune system. Beta carotene is the most famous example.

Organosulfur Compounds Onions, leeks and garlic supply a host of sulfur-containing compounds, such as dialyl sulfide and allicin, that serve the body in many ways. They strengthen the immune system, serve as antimicrobial agents, and help the body's abiltity to process potentially harmful substances.

A well balanced diet will provide ample amounts of phytochemicals. However, in the United States only 10% to 20% of the population consume the minimum recommended five servings of fruits and vegetables daily. A serving is considered only half a cup. If this trend continues, it seems likely that the inadequate consumption of phytochemicals will have a profound negative impact on health in future decades.

Huang, Mou-Tuan, "Phytochemicals and Cancer Prevention," *Nutrition Report*, 12:9 (1994), pp. 66–72.

phytoestrogens Plant products related to cholesterol that to a limited extent mimic ESTROGENS, female sex hormones. Phytoestrogens are found in a variety of medicinal HERBS, and many herbs have a long history in folk medicine. Such herbs include dong quai (angelica), LICORICE, black cohosh and FENNEL. The estrogen-like activity of phytosterols is low, perhaps only 0.25% of the activity of estrogen. They can counteract high estrogen levels or they can cause an increase in estrogenic activity, depending on the circumstances. Phytoestrogens may compete with estrogen, thus minimizing the effects of excessive estrogen. Phytoestrogens may help relieve some of the symptoms of menopause and lower the risk of OSTEOPOROSIS, a bone-thinning disease. Two broad classes of compounds describe photoestrogens: ISOFLAVONES and saponins. Isoflavones are a type of FLAVONOID found in high levels in soybeans, genestein is a primary example. Saponins are cholesterol-like molecules that can mimic steroid hormones because they possess a similar molecular shape. Saponins are widely distributed in legumes, including soybeans; chickpeas, mung beans and kidney beans. Saponins have the ability to lower blood cholesterol, to serve as antioxidants, to inhibit viruses and to inhibit certain forms of cancer. (See also, ENDOCRINE SYSTEM.)

pica An abnormal CRAVING for non-food materials. These may be STARCH, clay, dirt, wood or chalk. Clay eating among tribal peoples could have its origins in the ability of clay to bind toxic materials. Iron deficiency may be the cause of pica in some cases. Animals and livestock eat dirt when they become mineral deficient. (See also PAGOPHAGIA.)

pineapple (*Ananas comosus*) A tropical plant with stiff, spiny leaves that yields a single large FRUIT. The fruit of the pineapple is derived from the fusion of many fruitlets. The pineapple originated in Brazil and then spread to the Caribbean. Europeans spread the pineapple to Australia, South Africa and Hawaii. China, Hawaii, the Philippines, India, Brazil and Mexico are the leading producers. Most fresh pineapple marketed in the United States comes from Puerto Rico, Hawaii and Mexico. Pineapples weigh from 1 to 20 pounds depending upon the variety. A typical Hawaiian pineapple, the Smooth Cayenne variety, can weigh several pounds. This cone-shaped pineapple is the most popular fresh pineapple in the United States. Pineapple contains about 15% sugar. Unlike many fruits, pineapple does not ripen at home.

The fruit can be eaten fresh or can be cooked. Pineapple juice is canned or frozen as a concentrate. Pineapple is also used in ice cream, baked goods and salads, and is served with meat. Fresh pineapple cannot be used with gelatin-based desserts and salads because it contains BROMELAIN, a protein-degrading enzyme that breaks down jelled protein. Canning destroys the activity. Bromelain is used in meat tenderizers, in certain plant-based digestive aids, and as a beer clarifier. Pineapple is an excellent source of vitamin C. Nutrient content of 1 cup (155 g), raw, is: 76 calories; protein, 0.6 g; carbohydrate, 19.2 g; fiber, 2.95 g; fat, 0.7 g; potassium, 175 mg; vitamin C, 124 mg; thiamin, 0.14 mg; riboflavin, 0.06 mg; niacin, 0.65 mg.

pinocytosis The process by which a cell feeds itself by enveloping fluid and substances in its environment. Pinocytosis allows molecules that would normally be excluded by the outer membrane to enter the cell; most cells carry out pinocytosis. In receptor-mediated endocytosis, docking sites (receptors) on the cell surface bind external molecules or particles. As an example, large particles such as LOW-DENSITY LIPOPROTEIN (LDL), which transfers CHOLESTEROL to tissues, attach to the outer cell surface at specific receptor sites. The membrane at the point of attachment forms a pit; the pit deepens and eventually pinches off. The adhered material is engulfed, forming a membrane-bound sac, or vesicle, as the cell membrane reseals itself. The pinched-off vesicles migrate to LYSOSOMES, particles distributed throughout the cytoplasm that digest cellular debris and engulfed particles. Lysosomes then release AMINO ACIDS and cholesterol from degraded LDL to be recycled. Intestinal cells can absorb food proteins, peptides and bacterial products that have escaped digestion. The uptake of such foreign materials contributes to the burden confronting the body's immune system.

Pinocytosis differs from phagocytosis (cell eating), in which the cell sends out projections that envelope large particles like bacteria and form a sac enclosing the particle. Solid material inside the vesicle is digested by lysosomes. Few cells carry out phagocytosis. (See also ALLERGY; DIGESTION; FOOD SENSITIVITY.)

pistachio (*Pistacia vera*)   The edible seed of a small, tropical evergreen tree of the cashew family. The pistachio is native to the Mediterranean area and the Orient. Major nut-producing areas are Iran, Syria, Turkey and the United States (California). The seed occurs within a small fruit. The pale green meat is used as coloring and flavoring for candy, ice cream and baked goods. Salted nuts are eaten as snack food. Imported pistachios are often died red. To avoid this food coloring, choose tan (the natural shell color). The nutrient contents of 1 oz (28 g, dried, shelled nuts) provide 164 calories; protein, 5.9 g; carbohydrate, 7 g; fiber, 1.3 g; fat, 13.7 g; sodium, 221 mg; thiamin, 0.22 mg; riboflavin, 0.05 mg; niacin, 0.31 mg.

pituitary gland (hypophysis)   The "master gland" that regulates many other hormone-secreting (endocrine) glands. This gland is located deep in the skull beneath the region of the brain called the HYPOTHALAMUS and is about the size of a pea. It possesses two lobes, each of which produces hormones. The anterior lobe (adenohypophysis) produces GROWTH HORMONE, which regulates the METABOLISM and growth of muscle and bone. It also produces a range of stimulating factors: thyroid-stimulating hormone, which stimulates the THYROID GLAND to release thyroxine to regulate the rate of metabolism in all tissues; follicle-stimulating hormone and luteinizing hormone to regulate ovulation; PROLACTIN, which stimulates milk production; adrenocorticotropic hormone (ACTH), which activates the outer region of the ADRENAL GLAND (adrenal cortex) to secrete glucocorticoids to raise BLOOD SUGAR and mineralocorticoids to regulate sodium and water balance.

The posterior lobe (neurohypophysis) secretes OXYTOCIN, which regulates milk production and uterine contractions, and ANTIDIURETIC HORMONE (vasopressin), which conserves WATER and SODIUM in the kidney. Oxytocin and vasopressin are first synthesized in the hypothalamus and travel to the pituitary to be secreted. The pituitary and hypothalamus represent a direct link between the NERVOUS SYSTEM and the ENDOCRINE SYSTEM. The hypothalamus is that region of the brain that controls involuntary responses that regulate the internal environment: body temperature, blood pressure and water balance, among others. The pituitary gland receives signals from the hypothalamus in the form of trophic hormones. (See also HOMEOSTASIS.)

pizza   A flat, circular bread baked with a variety of toppings. The word pizza is Italian for "pie." Popularized in the United States, it now represents about half of "ethnic" food orders. The average American eats about 23 pounds yearly. Pizza dough is rolled or pressed flat, traditionally topped

with TOMATOES, tomato paste and herbs, and baked. The American variety of pizza is topped with mozzarella or Parmesan CHEESE, various types of SAUSAGE, MUSHROOMS, OLIVES, VEGETABLES, spices and anchovies, among other toppings. Pizza is often high in FAT, CALORIES and SODIUM. Cheese and MEAT toppings like pepperoni contribute the fat. Avoid the meat and cheese toppings to decrease calories.

Frozen pizza is usually highly processed; it contains imitation cheese as well as FOOD ADDITIVES. It may be labeled as containing imitation cheese or cheese substitute. Nutrient content of one slice (120 g) of a typical cheese pizza made with vegetable shortening is: 290 calories; protein, 15 g; carbohydrate, 39 g; fiber, 2.2 g; fat, 9 g; cholesterol, 56 mg; calcium, 220 mg; sodium, 700 mg; thiamin, 0.34 mg; riboflavin, 0.29 mg; niacin, 4.2 mg. (See also CONVENIENCE FOOD; PASTA; PROCESSED FOOD.)

PKU   See PHENYLKETONURIA.

placebo   In general, a blank pill or treatment that does not contain an active substance or effective material associated with a cure. Placebos may also be therapeutic procedures that lack specific effects. Placebos have a wide range of effects on human physiology and can decrease pulse rate; decrease serum cholesterol and fat levels; lower BLOOD SUGAR in diabetic patients; heal DUODENAL ULCERS; decrease stomach acid production; lower elevated blood pressure; reduce pain associated with ARTHRITIS, ACID INDIGESTION, ulcers, labor pain and PREMENSTRUAL SYNDROME, among other conditions. Placebo effects have been observed in surgery and drug therapy.

Placebo Effect

The placebo effect refers to positive changes produced by placebos that may aid in recovery. (If the placebo has a deleterious effect in the healing process, the result is called a nocebo effect.) Belief, hope or faith in a cure to alleviate a disease or symptoms can mobilize the body's ability to heal itself. Thus the relationship between physician (healer) and patient has an immediate impact on the effectiveness of a therapeutic intervention. It is ancient wisdom that a large percentage of people will get better simply after talking with someone they trust, or when they are assisted in visualizing wellness, in prayer, meditation or ritual. Placebos gained prominence in the 1960s when careful medical experimentation frequently incorporated double-blind, placebo-controlled studies. In these studies, neither the doctor nor the patients knew who was getting the therapeutic dose or who was receiving a neutral control (placebo) until after the treatment or experiment had been completed.

Apparently the expectation of relief even from a blank pill stimulates the brain to release pain-killer chemicals called ENDORPHINS. The NERVOUS SYSTEM is tightly coupled with the IMMUNE SYSTEM (the body's defense system), as well as with the ENDOCRINE SYSTEM (hormone-producing system). Thus endorphins can alter antibody production, white cell production, natural killer cell function and other important aspects of immunity. In some cases, levels increase; in others, levels decline. The autonomic nervous system, regulating involuntary processes and hormones, seems to participate in the healing process as well. (See also CLINICAL TRIAL; RISK DUE TO CHEMICALS IN FOOD AND WATER.)

Goleman, Daniel, "Placebo Effect Is Shown to Be Twice as Powerful as Expected," *New York Times*, (August 17, 1993), p. B6.

plantain (*Musa paradisiaca*)   The FRUIT that resembles a large green BANANA. The plantain is native to India and today is cultivated worldwide in tropical areas. Plantains become more palatable when baked, fried or otherwise cooked like a vegetable. Plantains contain more STARCH and less SUGAR than bananas and are made into a flour in tropical regions of the world, where it is a staple food. Powdered plantains may heal PEPTIC ULCERS. Cooking may destroy the anti-ulcer components, however. Plantains can be baked like potatoes or sliced and used in stir-fries or stews and soups. Nutritionally plantains resemble bananas. Nutrient contents of 1 cup (148 g) is: 181 calories; protein, 1.9 g; carbohydrate, 47.2 g; fiber, 0.74 g; fat, 0.55 g; potassium, 739 mg; vitamin C, 27.2 mg; thiamin 0.077 mg; riboflavin, 0.08 mg; niacin, 1.0 mg.

plaque   Deposits on teeth or on the inner surface of arteries. Dental plaque consists of a sticky mass of oral bacteria, carbohydrate secreted by bacteria and minerals. Such deposits promote tooth decay by holding bacteria close to the tooth surface. They can harden over time as more mineral is deposited. Plaque contributes to tooth decay and gum disease.

Plaque in arteries   Atherosclerotic plaques are called atheromas. They contain mineral deposits, connective TISSUE, and waxy deposits enriched in cells containing LIPIDS and CHOLESTEROL. In certain cases plaque is related to the uptake of oxidized cholesterol from the blood. These deposits contribute to stiffened, obstructed arteries and restricted blood flow and play a major role in CARDIOVASCULAR DISEASE. (See also ATHEROSCLEROSIS; LOW-DENSITY LIPOPROTEIN.)

plasma   The clear, cell-free fluid of BLOOD. Plasma contains the soluble proteins of blood, including clotting proteins, HORMONES, NUTRIENTS like glucose, gamma globulin (ANTIBODIES), nutrients like glucose and soluble waste products such as UREA, but not RED BLOOD CELLS or white blood cells. Plasma represents about 50% of the volume of the blood. It is prepared by centrifuging whole blood to remove red blood cells and white blood cells. In laboratory testing, plasma is used to measure levels of nutrients such as AMINO ACIDS and ESSENTIAL FATTY ACIDS. (See also HEMATOCRIT; SERUM.)

platelets (thrombocytes)   Small cell fragments in the blood that help initiate blood clot formation. They are oval or round discs and lack a nucleus. Platelets are produced by the fragmentation of a large precursor cell called mega-karyocyte produced on BONE marrow. Platelets are normally maintained at a concentration of 250,000 to 750,000 per milliliter of blood. Platelets plug damaged blood vessels in the following way. When they come into contact with damaged vessel walls, they attach to COLLAGEN exposed by injury and form clumps. Platelets develop irregular projections to increase cell-cell contact and then release thromboxane, a hormone-like lipid, and other factors that make platelets more sticky to help form a blood clot and seal the wound. Platelets release

SEROTONIN, which causes blood vessels to contract, to further reduce bleeding. Platelet aggregation is limited by polyunsaturated FATTY ACIDS in FISH and FISH OIL. These dietary components may decrease the rate of BLOOD CLOTTING and lower the risk of STROKE. (See also CARDIOVASCULAR DISEASE; EICOSAPENTAENOIC ACID.)

plum (*Prunus spp.*)   An oval or round FRUIT related to APRICOTS, CHERRIES and PEACHES. The Japanese plum originated in China, and plums have been grown in Europe for thousands of years. There are more than 140 varieties of plum. *P. americana* is native to North America; *P. domestica*, *P. mexicana* and *P. salicina* are common species that originated in Europe and China. The smooth skin ranges in color from yellow or green to shades of red and purple and are quite juicy. Ripe plums have a higher sugar content than most other fruits, and the flesh is usually yellow or red.

Top plum producers worldwide include Romania, the United States, China and Germany. California leads other states in domestic plum production. Plum varieties include Bearly, Burbank, Burmosa, Casselman, Duarte, Empress, French, Friar, Italian, Kelsey, Queen Rosa, President, Red Beaut, Santa Rosa, Simka and Wickson. To ripen hard plums, place them in a closed paper bag for several days at room temperature. The nutrient contents of one raw plum without its pit (66 g) are: 36 calories; protein, 0.5 g; carbohydrate, 8.6 g; fiber, 1.45 g; fat, 0.4 g; vitamin C, 6 mg; thiamin, 0.03 mg; riboflavin, 0.06 mg; niacin, 0.33 mg.

Prunes

Most plums are dried as prunes or are canned; only 20 to 30% of plums are marketed fresh. The most common variety used for prunes is the California French. California supplies almost all domestic prunes. The tree-ripened fruit is carefully dried. Prunes are a high-fiber food, containing more fiber than most other fruits and vegetables. Prune juice is rich in potassium. One cup contains 3 mg of iron, 473 mg of potassium and 182 calories. Because of its high sugar content it can be substituted for sugar in beverages, sauces or salads. Prune juice is a by-product of prune dehydration in prune production.

PMS   See PREMENSTRUAL SYNDROME.

pollock (*Pollachius virens*)   A saltwater bottom fish similar to cod in size, shape and quality of flesh. Pollock is classified as a lean fish rather than a fatty fish such as SALMON. The North Pacific pollock fishery is a $1-billion-a-year industry and represents the world's single most profitable fishing industry. Most pollock is converted to fish sticks and to SURIMI, a bland fish protein mixture. Surimi forms the basis of imitation crab meat and other imitation seafoods. Pollock can be baked, broiled, poached or used in chowders. The nutrient content of 3.5 oz (100 g) of steamed pollack is; 99 calories; protein, 23.3 g; fat, 0.9 g; cholesterol, 75 mg; potassium, 350 mg; thiamin, 0.12 mg; riboflavin, 0.26 mg; niacin, 4 mg.

polybrominated biphenyls (PBBs)   A synthetic flame-retardant that has been banned for many years in the United States. PBBs were once used to coat roofs and to treat fabric. PBBs are related to POLYCHLORINATED BIPHENYLS (PCBs); both are long-lasting environmental pollutants. PBBs are compounds containing two benzene rings, with bromine atoms attached to various positions on the rings. PBB is a generic term referring to a family of closely-related compounds. Attention was drawn to the toxicity of PBBs when a Michigan chemical company packed PBBs in bags labeled as a mineral supplement that were used as a feed additive for livestock. It was inadvertently shipped to farms, and by 1973 it had caused widespread damage to dairy herds. PBBs contaminated wildlife, Great Lakes fish, poultry and cattle, and gradually spread so that most Michigan residents were contaminated.

PBBs resist degradation in the environment by light, heat and oxygen and are only slowly broken down by microbes. As fat-soluble substances, PBBs accumulate in the fatty tissues of organisms that consume them because they are relatively resistant to cellular processes. Animals at the top of the FOOD CHAIN, like predatory fish and birds and omnivores like humans, tend to collect the highest levels of PBBs and other stable, fat-soluble pollutants. Most Americans now carry trace amounts of PBBs in their tissues.

PBBs belong to the class of halogenated hydrocarbons that are generally toxic and potentially cancer-causing agents. The long-term effect of chronic, low-level exposure to PBBs is unknown. Symptoms of severe exposure include memory loss, poor hand coordination, swollen joints, abdominal pain, diarrhea and acne. PBBs cause CANCER, in addition to impaired immunity and liver malfunction in experimental animals. In humans, acute exposure to PBBs is related to headaches and nervous disorders. PBBs accumulate in human fat and are released through breast milk. In spite of widespread contamination of breast milk by traces of pollutants, authorities agree that the advantages of BREASTFEEDING outweigh the disadvantages. (See also PESTICIDES; RISK DUE TO CHEMICALS, IN FOOD AND WATER.)

polychlorinated biphenyls (PCBs)

A widely distributed industrial pollutant. PCBs were formerly manufactured for use as insulators in electrical transformers, paints, adhesives and caulking compounds. PCBs are one of the first examples presented of environmental chemical hazards from non-PESTICIDE industrial chemicals. PCBs were first detected as environmental pollutants in Sweden in 1966. In 1968 more than a thousand Japanese were affected with Yusho (rice-oil) disease, due to PCB contamination of cooking oil. Since that time PCBs have been detected in foods such as MILK, EGGS, MEAT and FISH in many regions of the world. In 1977 polar bears from the Arctic were shown to contain significant levels of PCBs, indicating this pollutant had spread through the global FOOD CHAIN. Production of PCBs in the United States was halted in 1977.

PCBs belong to the class of CHLORINATED HYDROCARBONS, carbon compounds that generally are toxic and are potentially cancer-causing agents. PCBs are double-ring structures with chlorine atoms attached to various positions on both rings. There are over 40 different forms (isomers) in this family. They resist environmental degradation by sunlight, heat and exposure to air. Gradual microbial degradation occurs; bacteria have been isolated that remove chlorine atoms permitting PCB oxidation. Nonetheless, the rates of degradation in the environment are slow, and PCBs persist a long time. Being fat-soluble, PCBs accumulate in the cell membranes and fatty tissues of all organisms that digest them because they are relatively resistant to metabolic conversions.

By 1980, the EPA estimated that more than 90% of Americans carried PCB residues in their fatty tissues. PCB residues remain widespread. Exposure has come via many accidental routes. The most important food sources of PCBs are freshwater fish, notably from the Great Lakes, and bottom-feeding fish from waters near industrial areas, such as striped bass in the Hudson River. For example, for 30 years PCBs were discharged into the Hudson River (New York State) as waste from capacitor plants, contaminating fish. Widespread PCB pollution of Great Lakes fish was detected only after mink fed fish from Lake Michigan developed severe reproductive abnormalities or died. In 1979 contamination by PCBs in Billings, Montana, led to the destruction of hundreds of thousands of CHICKENS, eggs, and thousands of pounds of PORK. In other instances, fodder stored in silos painted with PCB-containing paint led to contaminated dairy herds and thus contaminated milk and milk products.

Symptoms of severe exposure include a form of severe acne (chloracne), visual disturbances, spasms, headaches, FATIGUE, nausea and numbness. The long-term effects of chronic low-level exposures are unknown. Chronic exposure may be linked to an increased risk of CANCER because PCBs are linked to liver tumors and reproductive problems in experimental animals. Environmental contaminants, including PCBs and by-products of the pesticide DDT, were found in higher levels in the breast fat of women who had breast cancer than in the breast tissue of women without cancer. The U.S. National Cancer Institute and the Canadian Center for Disease Control plan to study the effects on breast cancer of PCB contamination in the Great Lakes area. Dioxin, PCBs and other industrial chemicals can change fertility and sexual behavior in animals, fish and perhaps humans. These substances may alter the endocrine system by mimicking the action of the feminizing HORMONE estrogen.

Do pregnant women who consume fish contaminated with low levels of PCBs give birth to low birth weight babies with developmental abnormalities? Studies have yielded mixed results. In 1979 cooking oil contaminated with PCBs caused mass poisoning in Taiwan. Children born to Taiwanese women exposed to PCBs were more likely to have delayed development, abnormal lungs and skin and more neurological complaints than normal children. Traces of PCBs are routinely detected in the BREAST MILK of American women. Nonetheless, the World Health Organization (WHO) and the La Leche League recommend breastfeeding, agreeing that the advantages of breastfeeding outweigh the disadvantages. (See also RISK DUE TO CHEMICALS IN FOOD AND WATER.)

Pijnenburg, A.M., et al., "Polybrominated biphenyl and diphenylether flame retardants: analysis, toxicity, and environmental occurrence," *Reviews of Environmental Contamination and Toxicology*, 141(1995), pp 1–26.

polydipsia

Excessive thirst that occurs after extensive loss of body fluids. (See also DEHYDRATION; DIABETES MELLITUS.)

polyglycerol esters

Synthetic compounds resembling fat that are used to emulsify oils in foods. A key ingredient of these lipids is glycerol, a small triple alcohol that is the backbone of fat molecules. Polyglycerol esters contain several linked glycerol units, to which are attached various fatty acids. The fatty acids can be short- or long-chain, unsaturated or saturated, to create oils or solid fats. The polyglycerol esters may be either water-soluble or water-insoluble, depending on the ingredients used in their fabrication. As "hybrid" fats, they provide about 80% of the calories of true fats and oils. (See also FAT SUBSTITUTE; FOOD ADDITIVE.)

polyneuropathy A disease affecting groups of peripheral nerves. These nerves exclude the brain (cranial nerves) and the spinal column (spinal nerves). Polyneuropathy is caused by toxic exposure, nutritional deficiency or metabolic abnormality. Both sides of the body are affected; symptoms involve leg pain, muscle weakness, numbness and even partial paralysis. Both motor reactions (movement) and sensory responses (touch, response to pain) may be affected. Chronic, severe deficiencies of the B vitamins, THIAMIN, PANTOTHENIC ACID and VITAMIN B6, cause polyneuropathy. Such deficiencies can occur in alcoholics and are associated with MALNUTRITION as well as maldigestion. Uncontrolled DIABETES MELLITUS in older patients causes peripheral nerve damage due to damaged capillaries feeding peripheral tissue. Lead poisoning also causes a progressive neuropathy. (See also ALCOHOLISM; BERIBERI.)

polypeptide See PEPTIDE.

polyphosphates FOOD ADDITIVES used to bind unwanted metal ions. Polyphosphates aid in curing (preserving) meats and in enhancing meat flavors. Polyphosphates are chains of three or more phosphates, the nutrient form of PHOSPHORUS. The combined forms contain potassium, sodium or other minerals. They are readily broken down to phosphate and are considered safe food additives. (See also CHELATE.)

polysaccharides A large family of CARBOHYDRATES that possess long chains made up of many building blocks of simple sugar (monosaccharides) or sugar derivatives. Polysaccharides can be branched or unbranched. They may contain a single type of carbohydrate building block, or they may contain several types, including sugar amines such as glucosamine (nitrogen-containing sugars) or sugar acids like galacturonic acid or glucuronic acid. Polysaccharides are classified as complex carbohydrates because they are complex molecules compared to simple sugars.

The physical and chemical properties and biological function of polysaccharides depend upon the number, the kind and the sequence of sugars within the complex carbohydrates. Most polysaccharides found in food are either plant FIBER or STARCH. Fiber represents a mixture of different kinds of polysaccharides, each composed of different sets of sugars. They strengthen plant cell walls and plant tissue. Common examples are CELLULOSE, PECTIN, GUMS and HEMICELLULOSE made from modified glucose and other sugars. The primary structural polysaccharide of plants is cellulose, an insoluble fiber. Pectin represents a water-soluble form of fiber. Fiber is not digested in the small intestine, but is more or less broken down by colonic bacteria to provide important fuels for cells lining the colon.

Starch is the principal plant storage of carbohydrate and contains only GLUCOSE. It is common in grains like WHEAT, CORN and RICE, and in starchy vegetables like potatoes.

Animals make several polysaccharides. The liver and skeletal muscles store glucose in the form of long, branched chains called GLYCOGEN. Muscles release glucose from glycogen for quick energy, while the liver releases glucose from its stored glycogen into the blood-stream to help maintain steady BLOOD SUGAR levels between meals. Mucopolysaccharides (GLYCOSAMINOGLYCANS) create slippery surfaces in joints, structural materials that hold together cells (connective tissue) and the protective linings of the stomach and intestines. (See also CARBOHYDRATE DIGESTION; CARBOHYDRATE METABOLISM.)

polysorbates Synthetic polymers added to emulsify (suspend) oils and flavors in frozen desserts, bread dough, artificial whipped cream and non-dairy creamer, beverages, CANDY and ICE CREAM. Polysorbates are prepared by combining FATTY ACIDS with SORBITOL, a sugar alcohol, then linking many sorbate molecules together in long chains. The most prevalent form is polysorbate 60. The fatty acids are released by digestion and absorbed, and the remaining polymer is eliminated. Polysorbates have been used with patients to increase fat assimilation. Levels up to 5% have been fed to experimental animals and do not appear harmful. They have been in use since the 1940s and are apparently safe additives. (See also EMULSIFIERS; FOOD ADDITIVES.)

polyunsaturated fatty acids See FATTY ACIDS.

polyunsaturated oils Liquid FATS that contain a relatively high percentage of polyunsaturated FATTY ACIDS as building blocks. These bent molecules contain multiple double bonds. Because they are bent, they do not stick together tightly and thus do not solidify as easily as do SATURATED FATS, which possess straight chains. Fats containing more than 45% of their fatty acids as polyunsaturated fatty acids are oils at room temperature and are classified as polyunsaturates. Vegetable oils like COTTONSEED OIL, CORN OIL, SAFFLOWER oil and SOYBEAN oil contain LINOLEIC ACID, the omega-6 ESSENTIAL FATTY ACID with two unsaturated bonds; safflower oil is one of the richest sources of linoleic acid. A second essential fatty acid, ALPHA LINOLENIC ACID, contains three unsaturated bonds and represents the omega-3 family of fatty acids. FLAXSEED OIL is an important plant source. Neither linoleic acid nor alpha linolenic acid can be synthesized by the body; they must be supplied by the diet. It is important to note that not all vegetable oils are polyunsaturates: PALM OIL and COCONUT OIL are classified as saturated fats; OLIVE OIL and canola oil are monounsaturates because they contain monounsaturated fatty acids. Fish oils are another source of polyunsaturated oils. These oils contain high levels of EICOSAPENTAENOIC ACID, a polyunsaturated fatty acid with five unsaturated bonds, and docosahexaeonic acid, with four unsaturated bonds. Flaxseed oil and fish oil supply polyunsaturated fatty acids belonging to the omega-3 family that can help reduce inflammation, reduce levels of blood triglycerides (fats) and help lower the risk of stroke and heart attack by reducing the tendency to form blood clots.

A large body of evidence indicates that replacing dietary saturated fatty acids with polyunsaturated or monounsaturated oils decreases LDL (LOW-DENSITY LIPOPROTEIN), the less desirable form of blood CHOLESTEROL, in healthy people and in those with inherited cardiovascular diseases. However, monounsaturates do not lower HDL (HIGH-DENSITY LIPOPROTEIN), the beneficial form of blood cholesterol, and are preferable to polyunsaturated oils, which lower HDL at levels greater than 7% of total daily calories. Health concerns relating to high intakes of polyunsaturated fatty acids include possible promotion of tumors and suppression of the immune system in animals; elevated blood fats; increased susceptibility to oxidation by free radicals; and increased risk of GALLSTONES. The typical American diet presently provides 37% of calories as fat. Nearly 14% is derived from saturated fatty acids; 16% from monounsaturates; and 7% from polyunsaturates. General recommendations are to reduce consumption of fats, especially saturated fats; to increase consumption of COMPLEX CARBOHYDRATES from FRUITS and vegetables and LEGUMES; to replace part of the saturated fat with olive oil or canola oil; and to consume fatty coldwater fish like SALMON and MACKEREL several times a week to increase intake of the omega-3 polyunsaturates.

The ratio of polyunsaturated fatty acids to saturated fatty acids (P/S ratio) has been used as an index of polyunsaturated fatty acid intake. Current dietary intakes for North Americans provide a P/S ratio of about 2/1, and a ratio of 1/1 has been recommended. The P/S ratio is too simplistic for measuring the risk of blood clot formation or atherosclerosis because the polyunsaturates represent both omega-6 and omega-3 fatty acids, each responsible for different, multiple effects. (See also FAT METABOLISM.)

polyunsaturated vegetable oils See POLYUNSATURATED OILS.

popcorn
A variety of CORN characterized by kernels with a tough coat. When heated the water content within popcorn turns to steam, and the resulting pressure causes kernels to "explode." As a snack food popcorn offers many advantages: It contains high levels of complex carbohydrate and provides six times the amount of fiber as an equivalent amount of broccoli. Air-popped popcorn is virtually oil free; one cup provides only 30 calories and 0.4 g of fat. Oil- or butter-popped corn is not low-fat fare, however. One cup, salted and with butter, provides 154 calories and 14 g of fat. MICROWAVE POPCORN usually contains saturated fat (coconut oil, palm kernel oil or shortening). Even the so-called "lite" version derives 40 to 50% of its calories from added fat. Movie theater popcorn is often buttered in addition to being cooked in shortening (hydrogenated canola shortening), which is saturated fat. Added salt can increase salt intake appreciably. (See also CONVENIENCE FOOD.)

pork
A red meat from hogs. Together with BEEF, pork represents an important component of the standard American diet. Annual U.S. pork consumption is about 46 pounds per person, less than beef. Consumption of both types of red meat has declined over the last 20 years, in part due to consumers' concerns about pork and pork products being high-fat, high-SATURATED FAT and high-CHOLESTEROL foods. In response, breeders and farmers now produce hogs that yield pork that is about 30% lower in fat content.

Fresh pork is divided into various cuts—shoulder (pork roasts), loin (toploin, sirloin, tenderloin), side (spare ribs)—

that determine the fat content. Two-thirds of pork marketed in the United States is cured and smoked to preserve flavor. Bacon refers to cured pork belly, from the side of a hog after spare ribs have been removed. Canadian bacon represents cured pork loin, a less fatty alternative to bacon. HAM describes rear leg cuts of hog meat; most are sold fully cooked.

Traditionally considered a source of high-fat meat, hogs have been bred to accumulate massive amounts of fat. A broiled pork chop is 63% fat, while a lean cut of a pork rib roast is 45.2% fat. Processed pork products include sausage and hot dogs, traditional high-fat products. Pork fat (lard) is somewhat less saturated than beef fat (tallow). Unlike beef, there is no grading system for pork. Low-fat cuts of pork are comparable to the leanest cuts of beef; only the leanest cuts of pork approach skinless turkey or chicken breast. Loin supplies the leanest cuts: Tenderloin supplies 26% of its calories from fat. For comparison, ham provides 46% of its calories as fat, and extra-lean ham supplies 33% of its calories as fat.

Bacon is cured by injecting brine into a pork belly; smoke flavor may also be injected or the bacon may be smoked after curing. Most hams are cured in brine. Pork legs are injected with a solution containing salt, sodium nitrate and sugar. Hams that are dry cured are rubbed with a mixture of salt, sodium nitrite, sodium nitrate and seasoning. These "country hams" are drier, and their color is darker than well-cured hams.

The nutrient contents of 3.1 oz (87 g) of broiled pork chops (with bone) are: 275 calories; protein, 23.9 g; fat, 19.2 g; cholesterol, 84 mg; calcium, 4 mg; thiamin 0.82 mg; riboflavin, 0.24 mg; niacin, 4.35 mg. Pork roast—roasted, lean, 3 oz (85 g)—provides 187 calories; protein, 24 g; fat, 9.4 g; cholesterol, 80 mg; calcium, 6 mg; thiamin, 0.59 mg; riboflavin, 0.3 mg; niacin, 4.2 mg. (See also PROCESSED FOOD.)

postprandial
Following a meal. Postprandial HYPOGLYCEMIA refers to low BLOOD SUGAR after eating; postprandial hypertriglyceridemia refers to increased TRIGLYCERIDES (FAT) in the BLOOD after eating fatty foods. Overnight fasting is required when measuring serum lipids such as fat and CHOLESTEROL in order to avoid interference by dietary lipids.

potassium
A MINERAL nutrient found primarily within cells. Potassium is a positively charged ELECTROLYTE (cation) and serves an important role in skeletal muscle contraction, heart muscle contraction, transmission of nerve impulses and the release of ENERGY from FOOD.

Potassium in the blood helps maintain normal BLOOD PRESSURE. A variety of population studies link high-potassium diets with a decreased risk of essential HYPERTENSION (elevated blood pressure), the most common form of which has no explanation. Certain hypertensives may be helped by increasing their potassium intake, although calcium or magnesium supplementation seem effective in other cases. Adequate potassium in the diet may reduce the risk of stroke independent of effects on hypertension.

Sources

Potassium is widespread in foods. Good sources of potassium are fruits such as BANANAS, CANTALOUPE, GRAPEFRUIT, WATERMELON, dried fruit (raisins, APRICOTS, FIGS) and fruit juices; dried PEAS and BEANS; fresh FISH; beef liver; and MILK. For vegetable sources consider AVOCADO, baked POTATOES, winter SQUASH, kidney beans and mustard greens, and BRUSSELS SPROUTS. Processed foods generally contain less potassium and more sodium than unprocessed, whole foods. Thus a slice of white enriched bread provides 28 mg of potassium and 129 mg of SODIUM, in comparison with a piece of cake (71 mg of potassium and 269 mg of sodium). A baked potato with skin contains 844 mg of potassium and 16 mg of sodium, as compared to 14 potato chips (28 g) with 369 mg of potassium and 133 mg of sodium. Low-sodium salt and SALT SUBSTITUTES contain potassium chloride together with other ingredients in order to mask the metallic taste of potassium chloride.

Requirements

The recommended intake viewed as safe and adequate is 1,875 to 5,625 mg daily. The amounts needed are fairly high, similar to the sodium requirement. Potassium is excreted in urine, and excessive renal loss can be caused by DIURETICS (water pills) used to treat high blood pressure. Patients treated with diuretics generally require an extra 1,500 mg of potassium daily, and their potassium status should be monitored regularly. Symptoms of deficiency include weakness, nausea, loss of appetite, altered mental states such as fear and sleepiness, and impaired heart function. Mild potassium deficiency due to diuretic therapy can be counterbalanced by eating potassium-rich foods. Metabolic imbalances leading to the accumulation of organic acids in the blood, such as untreated diabetes, can cause METABOLIC ACIDOSIS (the accumulation of acids in the blood) associated with the excessive excretion of potassium. Prolonged DIARRHEA, vomiting and excessive use of laxatives also promote potassium losses. Potassium deficiency may also occur in patients with liver disease or who take digitalis, a medication.

Large doses of potassium can lead to electrolyte imbalances and toxic effects, especially for people with kidney disease, diabetes or heart problems. Side effects of excessive potassium include diarrhea, vomiting and irregular heartbeat in normal people. Rarely, extended-release potassium tablets and capsules can cause ulcers, bleeding and heartburn. People with kidney failure need medical advice before eating potassium-rich foods and potassium supplements.

Jefferson James W., "Potassium Supplementation in Lithium Patients: a Timely Intervention or Premature Speculation?" *Journal of Clinical Psychiatry*, 53:10 (October 1992), pp. 370–72.

potassium bromate A food additive used to age flour. When added at levels between 5 and 75 parts per million, this potassium compound improves the texture of dough for baking. Heating converts bromate to bromide, which is excreted by the kidneys and is considered safe. (See also FOOD ADDITIVES; WHEAT.)

potato (*solanum tuberosum*) A starchy underground stem (tuber) that is a major dietary staple. Potatoes belong to the nightshade plant family, which includes TOMATO and red and green PEPPER. The most widely cultivated vegetable, there are about 2,000 varieties of potato, though only eight are cultivated worldwide. Potatoes are grown in temperate regions of North America and Europe. Potato production ranks fourth in the United States, after WHEAT, RICE and CORN. Potatoes originated in the Andes Mountains of South America between 4,000 and 7,000 years ago. The Spaniards brought potatoes to Europe, and European settlers introduced potatoes to North America in the 18th century. The four leading U.S. producers of potatoes are Idaho, Washington, Maine and Oregon. Major varieties of white potatoes include Katahdin, Cobbler, Kennebec, California Long White and White Rose. Red varieties include Russet, Burbank, Red Pontiac, Red La Soda and Red McClure. Most Idaho baking potatoes are Russet and Burbanks. Only freshly harvested potatoes can be labeled "new." Special varieties appear in farmer's markets and food cooperatives; the Finnish yellow wax variety has an appealing buttery taste.

Baked potatoes, especially with skins, are recommended as a whole, unprocessed vegetable. Potatoes are also boiled, steamed, microwaved and mashed. Contact with aluminum or iron will discolor them; stainless-steel pots and cutlery are more suitable. Potatoes are used in soups, stews and cold salads. A potato supplies 20% of the RDA (RECOMMENDED DIETARY ALLOWANCE) for VITAMIN C. In the United States potatoes represent about 37% of all fresh vegetables, about 126 pounds per person per year. Because so many potatoes are eaten, they supply a substantial amount of the vitamin C requirement for Americans. Potatoes are excellent sources of POTASSIUM as well. With skins, they supply fiber. Whole potatoes are also a low-fat fare. However, added fat can change this. A plain potato with skin (200 g) provides about 200 calories, but adding a tablespoon of butter adds 100 calories. Furthermore, this increase is due to cholesterol-promoting saturated animal fat. Typical toppings like gravy, CHEESE, MARGARINE, MAYONNAISE and bacon bits offered at fast-food establishments increase both the fat and the sodium content significantly. About 65% of potatoes consumed in the United States are in the form of convenience foods like french fries, which represent increased fat and sodium content. Avoid adding fat-containing toppings to baked potatoes; use catsup or spices instead.

The nutrient content of one whole potato (with skin, baked, 202 g) is: 220 calories; protein, 4.7 g; carbohydrate, 51 g; fiber, 4.4 g; potassium, 844 mg; vitamin C, 26 mg; thiamin, 0.22 mg.; riboflavin, 0.07 mg; niacin, 3.32 mg.

Toxins in Potatoes

Greening due to exposure to sunlight or bruising causes accumulation of a toxic, bitter substance called solanine. Small amounts are normally present and account for the characteristic potato flavor. Solanine concentrates in the eyes of the potato and in blemished, bruised and green areas or in potatoes stored at high temperature. Solanine also occurs in the green leaves and stems of the potato plant, which are not edible. Excessive solanine can cause headache, diarrhea, nausea and cramps. To minimize solanine buildup, store potatoes in a dry, cool place and discard soft potatoes or potatoes with sprouts or a greenish tinge.

Processed Potato Products

The United States consumption of processed potatoes has risen steadily in recent decades. Potato chips are a very popular snack food. They are produced by deep-fat frying. To reduce water content, processing incorporates a drying step.

Instant potatoes (dehydrated potatoes) are prepared from cooked mashed potatoes that are filtered and treated with synthetic ANTIOXIDANTS like BHA and BHT and then bleached. Powdered cellulose derivatives contribute fluffiness; EMULSIFIERS contribute mixing qualities; milk solids are sometimes added; and VITAMINS like NIACIN, THIAMIN and RIBOFLAVIN may be added for fortification. The product is cooked and granulated.

Frozen french fries are prepared from sliced, blanched potatoes that have been fried in hot oil briefly, cooled and then frozen. The partially cooked slices may be coated with cellulose gum or with modified starch to maintain color during frying.

Potato flour is also available. It resembles the flour of cereal grains but lacks GLUTEN and is not suitable for bread dough. (See also CASSAVA; CONVENIENCE FOOD; SWEET POTATO.)

poultry Birds bred and raised for human consumption. Poultry and EGGS have been basic to the diet for thousands of years, and presently there are few societies that exclude poultry from the diet. In contrast several religions exclude various types of red MEAT. CHICKEN, TURKEY, ducks and geese are the most common types of poultry. Other kinds of poultry include guinea fowl, pigeons and quail. Wild ducks, pheasants and the like are considered game birds, not poultry.

A staple throughout the world, chicken can be roasted, broiled, grilled, poached, sauteed, baked and stir-fried. In the United States chicken and turkey consumption has climbed steadily over the last two decades. Consumers have moved away from BEEF due to concerns about SATURATED FAT and CHOLESTEROL as risk factors for HEART DISEASE. Roasted chicken and turkey can be low-FAT fare. White meat chicken contains 23% calories as fat. When cooked, white meat without skin provides 30 to 80% fewer fat calories than cooked beef, depending upon the type of cut. Dark meat chicken provides 20% more calories as white, with about 14 g of fat (3.5 oz). Turkey breast contains the least fat of any meat, with less than 1 g of fat per 3.5 oz serving. As with chicken, most of the fat is attached to the skin. Dark meat contains more fat than white. White meat turkey contains 14% fat calories. By comparison, lean steak provides 37% calories as fat. Both turkey and chicken are processed for roasts, pot pies, sausage, hot dogs, and cold cuts like turkey ham, bologna, pastrami, salami and the like. Often these contain as much fat as their beef counterparts. Sugar, salt, monosodium glutamate (MSG) and nitrites (potential cancer-causing agents) represent common additives.

Ground chicken and ground turkey are recent additions to the meat department. Consumers often choose these alternatives to HAMBURGER, expecting a lower fat content. However, there are currently no government standards regulating their fat content, as there are for ground beef. Ground poultry can contain as much fat as is found in the whole bird. Thus ground poultry may range from very low fat to relatively high, depending upon the proportion of skin and dark meat added.

The United States and Canada are among the leading consumers of poultry. Many reasons account for the popularity of poultry and eggs. Because hens lay eggs regularly, poultry are a ready food source, and the poultry industry can adjust more easily to market and production factors than the cattle and other livestock industries. Furthermore, poultry and poultry products are generally less expensive than red meat.

Poultry fat is less saturated than beef fat. Chicken provides 32% saturated fatty acids and 26% polyunsaturates; turkey provides 40% saturates and 35% polyunsaturates; while beef provides 45 to 46% saturates and only 3.6% polyunsaturates.

Most turkey and chicken production is part of an integrated industry in which a relatively small number of corporations control production and marketing. Poultry farms can be considered meat factories rather than farms in which chickens are mass-produced and grown in small compartments. Advocates believe that free-ranging chickens that have ample space to grow can be healthier than their mass-produced counterparts. Organically grown chicken and turkey, raised without the use of synthetic-growth promoters, are available at some markets and health food stores.

Turkeys and chickens are bred to grow faster and to be fatter than their forebears. However, much of the fat lies close to the skin, and trimming this visible fat and removing the skin substantially lowers the fat content. Growth promoters and antibiotics also play a role in poultry production, and these residues may be present. With mass production has come an increased risk of bacterial contamination. Between 25 and 33% of chicken and turkey carcasses are contaminated with SALMONELLA, a disease-producing (pathogenic) bacteria, due to fecal contamination during processing. Other dangerous species of bacteria, including campylobacter, are also present. Thorough cooking kills such pathogenic bacteria; however, consumers must be aware of the potential hazards of raw meat. Poultry must be kept refrigerated or frozen after purchase to avoid microbial growth. Meat juice and flesh should not contact other foods like raw vegetables. To avoid cross-contamination, wash everything that comes in contact with raw turkey or chicken, including hands, utensils and cutting board. Completely cook poultry. Never partially cook, then store poultry; this promotes the growth of disease-causing bacteria. Stuffing should be cooked outside the bird or placed in the carcass just before roasting.

The nutrient content of 1 cup (140 g) of chicken (roasted, both dark and light meat) is: 266 calories; protein, 40.5 g; fat, 10.4 g; cholesterol, 125 mg; calcium, 21 mg; iron, 1.7 mg; thiamin, 0.1 mg; riboflavin, 0.25 mg; niacin, 12.8 mg.

The nutrient content of 1 cup (140 g) of turkey (roasted, both dark and light meat) is: 240 calories; protein, 41 g; fat, 7 g; cholesterol, 106 mg; calcium, 35 mg; iron, 2.5 mg; thiamin, 0.09 mg; riboflavin, 0.26 mg; and niacin, 7.62 mg. (See also BEEF TALLOW; VEGETARIAN.)

powdered cellulose See IMITATION FOOD.

powdered milk See MILK.

ppb (parts per billion) An extremely small amount of material, equivalent to one-billionth of a gram in a gram of material. One part per billion is equivalent to 0.0000001% of a gram of material, or 1 mg per kilogram. Parts per billion can be visualized as one-one-thousandth of an inch in 16 miles or one cent in $10 million. PESTICIDE and CARCINOGEN contamination in food can be measured in parts per billion.

ppm (parts per million) A very small amount of material equivalent to one-millionth of a gram (1 mcg) in a gram of material. One part per million can be interpreted as 0.0001% or as 1 inch in 16 miles. TRACE MINERALS and VITAMINS can exist in these concentrations in foods and in the body.

prawn See SHRIMP.

pregnancy and nutritional requirements (Maternal nutrients needed for childbirth) Normal conception, embryonic development and fetal development depend upon the medical history, life-style and nutritional state of the mother. While healthy babies can be born to women who are poorly fed, pregnancy and lactation often leave the mother with drained reserves and jeopardized health, and there is a greater probability of a high-risk birth.

According to the Food and Nutrition Board of the National Academy of Sciences, normal weight gain during pregnancy is now viewed as 25 to 35 lb. The American College of Obstetricians and Gynecologists currently recommends 22 to 27 lb of weight gain. In any event, the desirable weight gain should be worked out between the pregnant woman and her physician. The weight gain aids fetal growth and lowers the risks of low birth weights, infant mortality and developmental problems. A large amount of new tissue is built and major changes occur in the mother's body to accommodate growth and development of the placenta and fetus. Of the weight gained, one-third is converted to fetal tissue (6 to 8 lb; the remainder forms the placenta (1 to 5 lb), extra blood (3 to 4 lb), enlarged breasts (1 to 2 lb), enlarged uterus (2 lb) and increased maternal fat stores (about 10 lb (4.5 kg)). The weight gained during pregnancy is distributed among protein, fat, water and blood.

Protein The rate of protein synthesis remains high throughout embryonic and fetal development, though most of the fetal growth occurs in the last three months of pregnancy. Tissues like the brain, heart and liver are composed mainly of protein (excluding water). New protein represents a net gain that is a positive NITROGEN BALANCE. There is an apparent correlation between maternal low blood protein levels and the risk of TOXEMIA of pregnancy, which is associated with high blood pressure and protein loss in the urine.

Fat A gain of nearly 10 lb of body fat is equivalent to 47,500 calories. This provides an ample energy reserve for the mother and fetus and for lactation.

Water Typically about 60% of the gained weight is water. All new tissues require water because it is the principal constituent of the body and body fluids. Water is also stored as a fluid reserve to compensate for blood loss at childbirth. About 40% of pregnant women will retain excess water. The maternal blood volume increases by 30% and the number of RED BLOOD CELLS increases by 18%. Maternal blood

supplies the embryo and fetus with nutrients, including amino acids for protein synthesis and glucose and fatty acids for energy.

Nutritional Requirements

Protein Dietary protein supplies amino acids, the raw materials for new protein. An estimated 1.3 g, 6.1 g and 10.7 g of protein/day are required for the first, second and third trimesters, respectively. Therefore an additional 10 g/day above the adult requirement of 50 g/day throughout pregnancy is thought to meet the needs of most healthy pregnant women. The RDA (recommended dietary allowance) for protein during pregnancy is 60 g per day.

Calories Metabolic changes occur that favor weight gain. Hormonal balance changes to maintain high blood GLUCOSE, amino acids and FATTY ACIDS to store fat while slowing maternal utilization.

Calcium, Phosphorus and vitamin D for pregnant women The RDA for CALCIUM is 1,200 mg daily; the RDA for phosphorus is 1,200 mg and the RDA for vitamin D is 10 mcg. An infant at birth possesses nearly 30 g of calcium, mainly in bone. The rate of calcium absorption jumps in the last two months of pregnancy to accommodate skeletal growth of the fetus. Dietary calcium may be better absorbed during pregnancy. However, it is important that the mother receive enough dietary calcium from conception till the end of lactation, and a calcium intake of 1,200 mg/day is advised. Though the amounts of phosphorus required for health are unknown, the total allowance should match that of calcium, namely 1,200 mg/day. Vitamin D is required for calcium uptake and assimilation. Whether pregnancy increases the vitamin D requirement is not proven; however, the RDA for vitamin D is set at 10 mcg/day for pregnant and lactating women. Early deposition of this fat-soluble vitamin provided in a balanced diet provides a reserve for later use when growth is very rapid.

Iron Extra iron is required during pregnancy for increased production of RED BLOOD CELLS, which contain iron as hemoglobin, to supply the fetus and placenta and to cope with blood loss during delivery. In the first trimester, cessation of menstruation compensates for additional needs of iron. To assure adequate iron throughout pregnancy, the RDA is set at 30 mg/day; this represents an additional 15 mg above the normal adult level. This high amount of iron cannot be supported by the usual American diet or by stored iron, and iron supplements are required to achieve this intake. Because usual menstruation is absent during lactation, iron requirements during lactation are essentially the same as those for non-pregnant women.

Folic acid Pregnancy increases the risk of deficiency when the intake of this fragile, water-soluble vitamin is marginal. The RDA for folic acid is 400 mcg during pregnancy. To meet this requirement, vigilance is necessary in selecting foods. Evidence indicates that folic acid supplementation before conception and the first months of pregnancy significantly reduces the risk of NEURAL TUBE DEFECTS. (Federal agencies now recommend that women who are considering pregnancy as well as those who are pregnant consume 400 mcg of folic acid daily.) During the first six months of lactation, the maternal RDA is 280 mg/day.

The requirements for certain other nutrients also increase during pregnancy and for lactation (the following comparisons are made relative to the RDAs for non-pregnant adult women):

Vitamin A　　Though the RDA does not increase during pregnancy, a 1.6-fold increase in the RDA during lactation is recommended (total of 1,300 mcg of retinol).

Vitamin E　　A 20% increase in the RDA during pregnancy, to 10 mg/day, is recommended. A 1.6-fold increase during the first six months of lactation, to 12 mg/day, is recommended.

Vitamin C　　Pregnancy calls for a 17% increase in the RDA to 70 mg/day. The RDA during lactation is 95 mg/day.

Thiamin　　A 50% increase in the RDA during pregnancy has been set at 1.5 mg/day. The RDA during lactation is about the same, 1.6 mg/day.

Riboflavin　　There is a 23% increase during pregnancy to 1.6 mg/day. A 38% increase in riboflavin intake to 1.8 mg/day during lactation is recommended.

Niacin　　Pregnancy entails a 13% increase in the RDA of niacin to 17 mg/day. A 23% increase during lactation to 20 mg/day is recommended.

Vitamin B$_6$　　The RDA increases by 38% during pregnancy, to 2.2 mg per day. During lactation RDA increases to 2.6 mg per day.

Magnesium　　The RDA increases to 300 mg daily during pregnancy. During lactation the RDA is 355 mg/day.

Zinc　　The RDA increases by 25% during pregnancy to 15 mg per day. During lactation the requirement is 19 mg/day.

Iodine　　The RDA increases by 17% to 175 mcg daily. During lactation the RDA is 200 mcg.

Selenium　　The RDA increases by 18% to 65 mcg/day. During lactation, the RDA is 75 mcg.

Possible nutrition-related problems during pregnancy are:

1. Anemia. Inadequate functional red blood cells are the end product of a chronic deficiency, most frequently of iron, though deficiencies of protein, COPPER and vitamins like folic acid, vitamin B$_6$, vitamin E, vitamin C or vitamin B$_{12}$ may cause ANEMIA.
2. CONSTIPATION. A decrease in muscle tone and the pressure of the growing fetus can cause constipation. Adequate water intake and fiber, in the form of vegetables, whole grains and fresh fruit, are recommended.
3. Diabetes. Certain hormones increase during pregnancy: ESTROGEN, human chorionic gonadotrophin and human placental lactogen. They counteract INSULIN, the hormone that lowers blood glucose, promoting glucose uptake by tissues. Diabetic pregnancy can cause placental malfunction, oversized infants and stillbirth.
4. Excessive weight gain. There is no ideal body weight and weight does not indicate nutritional status. Too rapid

weight gain can be caused by high-fat, high-calorie food that is low in important nutrients. Food choices need to be nutrient dense, that is, they need to contain a high percentage of vitamins, minerals and fiber relative to calories. Major effort to lose weight during pregnancy can cause abnormal mental development in infants.
5. Preeclampsia. This disorder affects about 7% of women in the third trimester of pregnancy. Water retention (EDEMA), elevated blood pressure and passage of protein in urine are signs of the more dangerous condition, toxemia, which threatens both the mother and fetus. Salt restriction and the use of DIURETICS can be hazardous and require medical supervision. The incidence of toxemia has declined with better prenatal care. High-quality protein is essential during pregnancy.
6. Heartburn. STOMACH ACID may be forced up into the esophagus by the enlarged fetus. Small, frequent meals may help avoid this problem. Avoid foods that cause digestive problems.
7. High blood pressure. Elevated blood pressure during pregnancy requires medical supervision. Acute HYPERTENSION during the last 12 weeks of pregnancy is a sign of toxemia.
8. Inadequate weight gain during pregnancy. Mothers whose nutritional deficiencies are corrected are more likely to have normal-term pregnancy and normal births.
9. Medication drug and alcohol use; smoking. The recent studies on FETAL ALCOHOL SYNDROME suggest that there is no safe dose of ALCOHOL during pregnancy. It has been suggested that alcohol is one of the most common cause of BIRTH DEFECTS and mental retardation in the United States. The use of cocaine, heroin and addictive drugs during pregnancy gives rise to "crack" babies. Drug-addicted infants experience severe withdrawal symptoms at birth. Mental disturbances such as irritability and problems with social adjustment can continue throughout childhood and into adult life. Smoking is associated with reduced birth weight because carbon monoxide in cigarette smoke reduces the oxygen supply to the fetus. Many medications pass through the placenta and adversely affect the fetus. No medication or nutritional supplement should be taken during pregnancy without medical supervision.

(See also DIETING; EDEMA.)

Czeizel A.E., et al., "Pregnancy Outcomes in a Randomized, Controlled Trial of Preconception Multivitamin Supplementation," *Archives of Gynecology and Obstetrics*, 255 (1994), pp. 131–39.

Keen, Carl L., Bendich, Adrianne, Willhite, Calvin C. eds., "Maternal Nutrition and Pregnancy Outcome," *Annals of the New York Academy of Sciences*, 678, (1993).

premenstrual syndrome (PMS; premenstrual tension)　　An array of symptoms associated with menstruation, now regarded as a major issue in women's health based upon hormonal patterns. Between 30 and 40% of American women report premenstrual symptoms. As many as 10% may experience severe forms. Most women with PMS are over 30 years of age. Typically, signs and symptoms recur one to two weeks before menstruation. A woman with PMS may experience symptoms such as bouts of irritability, DEPRESSION, tension, altered sex drive, breast pain, abdominal bloating, swollen ankles and constipation. Symptoms often occur seven to ten days before menses and progressively worsen until the onset of menstruation, when symptoms disappear.

There is considerable debate about the causes of PMS, and why some women are affected more than others is not clear. Changes in hormone levels associated with the menstrual cycle seem to be the key. PMS is divided into four categories based upon symptoms of hormonal patterns.

PMS-A The most common form of PMS. Anxiety with nervous tension, mood swings and insomnia. Women with PMS-A have imbalanced hormones with elevated ESTROGEN, a major female hormone, and lowered PROGESTERONE, a hormone that rises sharply in the second half of the menstrual cycle. Women may consume excessive amounts of dairy products and refined CARBOHYDRATES. Ratings of symptoms correlated best with high estrogen/progesterone levels. Excess estrogen seems to alter nervous system chemistry and change the levels of important NEUROTRANSMITTERS (chemicals for nerve transmission): increased amounts of EPINEPHRINE, norepinephrine and SEROTONIN, and decreased amounts of DOPAMINE and phenylethylamine. Such changes could explain certain symptoms. Epinephrine triggers anxiety, norepinephrine induces irritability, while high levels of serotonin lead to nervous tension and inability to concentrate. Elevated estrogen may also affect mood by reducing serotonin synthesis and reducing the effectiveness of blood sugar regulation. Furthermore, estrogen stimulates the production of the pituitary hormone PROLACTIN; excessive prolactin causes symptoms similar to those of PMS-A and PMS-H. Elevated estrogen may lower ENDORPHIN activity in the brain. (Endorphins are brain opiates that improve mood.)

PMS-C Symptoms include a craving for sweets, increased APPETITE, FATIGUE, dizziness, headache and heart palpitations. Women with PMS-C have altered glucose tolerance, suggestive of overproduction of INSULIN, and their MAGNESIUM levels may be low. Magnesium is required for many metabolic steps associated with energy production and neurotransmitter synthesis, and it is essential for the transmission of nerve impulses. Symptoms of long-term deficiency relate to the NERVOUS SYSTEM: weakness apathy, depression and lower pain threshold. Decreased PROSTAGLANDIN synthesis (PGE$_1$) may be implicated in some cases. Prostaglandins are hormone-like derivatives of ESSENTIAL FATTY ACIDS that help regulate many processes of the body.

PMS-D The key symptom is depression. Crying, confusion, mood swings, forgetfulness and insomnia are also reported. This form is less prevalent. Some women show signs of toxic lead accumulation, while others produce abnormally high levels of serum progesterone and low estrogen during the last two weeks of the menstrual cycle. Excess stress can increase adrenal steroid hormone production, including progesterone and androgens, hormones that promote masculine traits. These hormones could inhibit ovarian estrogen production. Still another possibility is an increased rate of breakdown of key neurotransmitters in affected women. Progesterone is a widely used therapeutic agent for PMS; however, results of treatment have been mixed. As with other approaches, progesterone may be effective only for certain individuals.

PMS-H Symptoms include cyclic weight gain, swelling of hands and feet. Bloating can cause breast tenderness. PMS-H is one of the more prevalent subgroups. Women retain water and SODIUM due to excessive production of the hormone ALDOSTERONE, produced by the adrenal glands, which increases water and sodium retention. Stress is known to stimulate adrenal hormone production, including aldosterone. Alternatively, estrogen excess causes increased secretion of ANGIOTENSIN II. This hormone, in turn, triggers fluid retention in the kidneys.

Nutritional Considerations

PMS is a condition with many possible causes; consequently, no single treatment or supplement is likely to be a cure. Nonetheless nutritional modifications can improve mood, help correct neurotransmitter imbalances, assist in optimizing blood sugar regulation and remedy nutritional deficiencies. Comparisons of women with and without PMS symptoms reveal that PMS patients often consume more refined carbohydrate, including SUGAR, more MILK and milk products, more sodium but fewer trace minerals like ZINC, IRON and magnesium. Various supplements may be effective in some cases.

Magnesium levels in PMS patients may be significantly lower than in women without symptoms. Magnesium deficiency can lead to elevated aldosterone levels and fluid retention. Low magnesium may reduce serotonin activity. Magnesium supplementation may reduce nervousness and breast tenderness.

VITAMIN B$_6$ supplementation may be effective in treating PMS in some cases, but not all, suggesting other factors may be involved. The U. S. National Institute of Mental Health is carrying out a study testing vitamin B$_6$ on PMS patients. Vitamin B$_6$ deficiency also reduces the ability of the kidney to secrete sodium and promotes fluid retention. Vitamin B$_6$ has been recommended for anxiety and depression, and many women report relief. Serious side effects such as nerve damage can occur with high doses of vitamin B$_6$ consumed over a long time. VITAMIN A via its precursor BETA CAROTENE may reduce PMS symptoms in some cases. VITAMIN E supplementation has been used to reduce PMS symptoms, including breast tenderness, with mixed results. There are few studies in this area.

Supplemental plant seed oils can be used to balance essential fatty acids. EVENING PRIMROSE OIL, BORAGE oil and BLACKCURRANT OIL contain GAMMA LINOLENIC ACID, which may promote the formation of a prostaglandin (PGE$_1$), a hormone-like substance that can help normalize certain responses, including insulin secretion and control of blood sugar.

Reduced consumption of sugar, sweets and bakery goods with white flour helps normalize BLOOD SUGAR regulation. A balanced diet based on minimally processed foods is a powerful strategy for promoting health generally. Highly processed foods, CONVENIENCE FOODS and snack foods provide fewer trace minerals, less fiber and more salt, sugar and fat. An increased consumption of complex carbohydrates and fiber with fruit and vegetables helps normalize blood sugar levels and reduces the likelihood of constipation.

Recent studies suggest that decreasing FAT in meals to 15% of daily calories and increasing complex carbohydrates with vegetables and grains may decrease breast swelling and soreness. This represents a severe cutback in fat for most people, who average more than 30% of their calories from fat. Eating less SALT before typical onset of symptoms may reduce water retention and edema. Women who drink large amounts of COFFEE are more likely to suffer from PMS. Excess CAFFEINE increases the level of epinephrine (adrenaline), a stress hormone. ALCOHOL is a depressant and can worsen depression. Regular physical EXERCISE has a long history in helping to manage stress and improve a sense of well-being. (See also ENDOCRINE SYSTEM.)

"Premenstrual syndrome: does anything help?" *Consumer Reports on Health,* 5:6 (June 1993), pp. 61–63.

Shamberger, R.J., "Nutritional and Clinical Observations in Premenstrual Syndrome," *Journal of Advancement in Medicine,* 8:2 (1995) pp. 131–45.

preservation of food   See FOOD PRESERVATION.

preservative   A chemical added to food to minimize chemical alteration or microbial degradation. Preservatives therefore increase the shelf life, safety, palatability and sensory appeal of foods. Preservatives fall into two general categories. ANTIOXIDANTS reduce the rate of oxidation of foods by OXYGEN and FREE RADICALS, extremely reactive chemical fragments that promote RANCIDITY and discoloration. Examples of antioxidant preservatives are BHA and BHT. Antimicrobial preservatives inhibit the proliferation of bacteria, yeasts and molds but do not necessarily destroy all microbes. Sodium NITRITE, CITRIC ACID and CALCIUM PROPIONATE are typical of this group. (See also FOOD ADDITIVES; FOOD PRESERVATION; PROPYL GALLATE.)

Foulke, Judith E., "A Fresh Look at Preservatives," *FDA Consumer,* 27 (October 1993), pp. 23–27.

pressor amines   Nitrogen-containing compounds that constrict blood vessels and increase blood pressure. TYRAMINE and HISTAMINE are pressor amines that occur in certain foods. Tyramine is a degradation product of the amino acid TYROSINE, while the amino acid HISTIDINE yields histamine. Pressor amines are fermentation by-products and occur in CHEESE, CHOCOLATE, WINE and pickled herring, among others. These substances can trigger severe high blood pressure in patients taking antidepressant medications called monoamine oxidase inhibitors, like isocarboxazid and phenelzine. (See also HYPERTENSION; NERVOUS SYSTEM; VASOCONSTRICTION.)

pressure cooking   Heating foods under pressure to cook them at a high temperature. Pressure cookers are containers that generate steam under tight lids and with a safety valve. With increased pressure the boiling point of water increases. This means that foods can be cooked at higher temperatures than those attainable without a sealed utensil. Pressure cookers are used commercially to produce canned meat and canned vegetables. Pressure COOKING finds practical application in high-altitude cooking. At higher elevations water boils at a lower temperature, and pressure cooking shortens cooking times. (See also FOOD PROCESSING.)

pretzel   A type of brittle CRACKER made from twisted strands of dough used as a snack food. The name originated from the Latin *brachiatus,* meaning "with branch-like arms." Pretzels can be hard or soft. The dough contains wheat flour, salt, yeast, vegetable shortening and malt. By dipping the pretzel in very hot coconut oil, pretzels become sealed, a process that greatly increases their shelf life. Nutrient contents of a Dutch twist pretzel made with enriched flour (16 g) are: 65 calories; protein, 1.5 g; carbohydrate, 12.8 g; fiber, 0.36 g; fat, 0.6 g; sodium, 258 mg; thiamin, 0.05 mg; riboflavin, 0.04 mg; niacin, 0.7 mg. (See also CONVENIENCE FOOD.)

prickly pear cactus (*Opuntia fiscus-indica, O. tuva;* Indian fig)   The most common edible cacti, characterized by large flat fleshy stems with spines. The prickly pear supplies an edible fruit called cactus pear as well as pads that are used as a vegetable. Native to deserts of the Southwestern United States and Mexico, the prickly pear cactus has spread to many warm regions, and cactus pears are a common food in many countries. Mexico, in particular, and Sicily produce large amounts of this fruit. Cactus pears are oval fruit that are formed after blossoming. They are usually less than 3 inches in diameter, with a rigid husk that can be green to magenta in color. The coarse flesh is sweet and mild-tasting and contains small, coarse seeds. The skin of cactus pears must be peeled off before the fruit can be eaten. Cactus pads or leaves are eaten as vegetables. They are despined and the "eyes" are removed; then the pads are sliced into strips and cooked like green beans. The flavor is reminiscent of bell peppers. They are used as a side dish, or with tomatoes, chili peppers and corn.

Pritikin diet   A high complex carbohydrate, very low-fat diet coupled with regular aerobic exercise. The Pritikin diet is a low-cholesterol, low-sodium diet in which fat accounts for only 5 to 10%; protein, 10 to 15%; and complex carbohydrate, 80%. Sugar, animal fat, salt, alcohol and coffee are omitted. The diet emphasizes whole grains, beans and legumes, fresh vegetables, fruits, non-fat dairy products, and small amounts of lean meat, fowl and fish in six to eight small meals throughout the day. The diet was a part of a supervised program to decrease the risk of cardiovascular disease. The unmodified diet revealed a number of defects. It did not provide adequate levels of essential fatty acids from fish and from seed oils. Ultra-low-fat diets are more difficult than other diets to follow because fats and oils satisfy hunger and provide flavor and "mouth feel" that make food satisfying. People generally have more success with reducing their fat to 20 to 25% of their calories. (See also DIET; DIETING; HIGH COMPLEX CARBOHYDRATE.)

processed food   Food that has been treated by physical and chemical procedures to increase its edibility, safety, nutrient content, convenience or attractiveness. Minimally processed foods have been treated using operations found in the typical home kitchen. Chopping, grinding, sieving, mixing, juicing and blending are examples of physical changes that produce minimally processed foods. Baking, boiling, steaming, broiling, BRAISING and FERMENTATION bring about chemical changes in food, but nutrient content is not usually drastically altered by these steps. The USDA defines "minimally processed" to mean that meat or poultry has been handled only during slaughter, cleaning and cutting. No grinding, breading or curing is involved in minimally processed meat.

Commercial processing of foods employs more drastic changes to prevent spoilage, increase ease of storage and increase consumer appeal through increased convenience or visual appeal. Highly processed foods differ significantly from their sources in terms of appearance, nutritional value, structure, texture and taste. Grinding, milling, extruding, bleaching, extracting, exposure to acids and bases, and curing are common procedures. Highly processed foods contain fewer nutrients in smaller amounts than the foods from which they were derived and are said to have a low nutrient density. Commercial processing tends to concentrate STARCH, PROTEIN, FAT, and OILS at the expense of MINERALS, VITAMINS, FIBER and ESSENTIAL FATTY ACIDS. Often extensive chemical treatment destroys fragile nutrients like water-soluble vitamins, particularly VITAMIN C, FOLIC ACID and THIAMIN. This means that the ratio of nutrients like vitamins and minerals to calories is usually lower than in the original food.

The following examples illustrate this point. Canned vegetables lose 57 to 77% of vitamin B_6. Losses of this vitamin in curing meats is about 40%. Losses of VITAMIN B_6 in CORN and RICE products, breads and flour is extensive: 86% for corn flakes; puffed rice, 66%; bran flakes, 25%. The loss of nutrients in refining whole WHEAT to white flour is also significant: thiamin, 77%; RIBOFLAVIN, 80%; NIACIN, 81%; vitamin B_6, 72%; PANTOTHENIC ACID, 50%; folacin, 67%; and VITAMIN E, 86%. Similarly, 40 to 89% of trace minerals are removed in preparing white flour. For example, white bread is lower in chromium by 71%, zinc by 77% and copper by 70% than whole wheat bread.

ENRICHMENT of white flour replaces a few of the more than 20 nutrients, such as CALCIUM, riboflavin and thiamin, depleted during extensive food processing. Fortification adds nutrients that may not originally be present, such as VITAMIN A and VITAMIN D. This is only a partial solution because foods are not enriched or fortified with vitamin B_6, folic acid, zinc, chromium, manganese, magnesium, among others.

Examples of Processed Foods

Cereals   Cold BREAKFAST CEREALS are processed grain products. Refined flour from corn, oats and wheat is molded into a huge variety of shapes and flavors for breakfast cereals, yet the basic ingredients remain essentially unchanged since they were first introduced about a hundred years ago. Many cereal products and baked goods contain extra fat, salt and sugar far beyond the levels found in the original unprocessed food.

Dairy product substitutes   Many traditional egg and milk products have been substituted for by extensively modified or synthetic foods. Ice cream substitutes, imitation cheese, imitation eggs, MARGARINE and NON-DAIRY CREAMER are a few of the many processed foods in this category. In these foods, traditional animal FAT may be replaced with VEGETABLE OIL and a wide range of thickeners, EMULSIFIERS, GUMS, binders and fillers are used to create textures analogous to the foods they replace or to create new foods.

Meat, fish, poultry and seafood substitutes   TEXTURIZED VEGETABLE PROTEIN is soy protein that has been treated chemically, extruded and colored to resemble meat or seafood. SURIMI is fish protein that has been mashed and pulverized, extruded and blended with small amounts of shellfish to create a wide range of imitation seafoods that taste like authentic shellfish.

Baked goods   Wheat, corn and rice, as well as POTATOES, are the basis for a growing variety of highly processed foods. Examples include potato chips, corn chips and frozen pizza. These foods contain high-fat, high-SODIUM and SUGAR, and an extensive array of FOOD ADDITIVES, including ARTIFICIAL FOOD COLORS, ARTIFICIAL FLAVORS, ANTIOXIDANTS like BHA and BHT to prevent rancidity; preservatives; partially hydrogenated vegetable oil, coconut or palm kernel oil; SWEETENERS like dextrose, maltodextrins and corn syrup solids.

Meal replacements   Beverage powders and sweetened bars are designed to be eaten with water or milk, rather than the mixture of foods that typify a complete meal. The nutrients of these preparations often represent combinations of sugars, soy derivatives, peanut butter, white flour, vegetable oil like coconut oil or palm kernel oil, and salt. Federal regulations specify that certain key nutrients must be present at levels equivalent to 25% of the USRDA.

Potential Problems with Processed Foods

A major concern regarding highly processed foods is that they are an increasingly large part of the typical U.S. diet, already characterized by too much sodium, too many calories, too much saturated fat, too much sugar and too much phosphate. Highly processed foods may lack as yet unrecognized, nutritionally important factors that occur in whole or minimally processed foods. Ingredients of dark-green leafy vegetables, of vegetables of the cabbage family and in fruits that seem to protect against CANCER are only partially understood or identified. Furthermore, several nutrients may work together to create a greater effect than when simply added together as whole or minimally processed foods are eaten (synergistic effect). (See also CONVENIENCE FOOD; DIETARY GUIDELINES FOR AMERICANS; FOOD GUIDE PYRAMID; JUNK FOOD.)

Friedman, M., "Dietary Impact of Food Processing," *Annual Review of Nutrition*, 12 (1992), pp. 119–37.

produce   Fruits and vegetables and other agricultural products. These are usually perishable items with a limited shelf life.

produce freshener   Chemicals added to fruits and vegetables to prevent browning and wilting. After the governmental ban of SULFITES from use as a preservative on fresh fruit and vegetables, several products have been developed for use by restaurants and fast food franchises to keep precut fruit and salads from browning. These products are odorless, tasteless, safe and "fully natural," with ingredients like VITAMIN C and SUGAR. For an inexpensive alternative, sprinkle lime or lemon juice over cut fruit. (See also FOOD ADDITIVES.)

product placement   The highlighted placement of consumer goods in TV or movie scenes to market the products. Manufacturers usually pay a retainer to the PACKAGING firm, which will work with film producers directly. Specific brands of BEER, liquor, SOFT DRINKS, CANDY, cigarettes, doughnuts, olive oil and raisins, as well as non-food items, are used as props. There are several potential problems with this practice. Children who go to the movies are impressionable, they don't see props as ADVERTISING. It is more usual for them to accept advertising as a model of behavior; hence their buying habits may be shaped.

proenzyme (zymogen)   An inactive form of a digestive enzyme. Digestive enzymes that break down PROTEINS and membrane constituents, PHOSPHOLIPIDS, are first synthesized in massive amounts as inert precursors by several tissues, especially the pancreas and the stomach lining. Premature activation of digestive enzymes can lead to cellular damage and, ultimately, tissue destruction.

During the normal course of events the proenzyme is secreted into the digestive tract, where it is specifically activated either by acid-induced changes (pepsinogen to PEPSIN in the stomach); by a specific activator enzyme (trypsinogen to TRYPSIN by intestinal ENTEROPEPTIDASE); or by self activation (autoactivation). The new enzyme is able to carry out its digestive function safely outside the tissue or organ. Other examples include the pancreatic products chymotrypsinogen, which is converted to CHYMOTRYPSIN (protein digestion); prophospholipase which is converted to phospholipase (phospholipid digestion). (See also DIGESTION; PROTEASE.)

progesterone   A steroid HORMONE from the ovaries and ADRENAL GLANDS that prepares the lining of the uterus for implantation of the fertilized egg during the latter half of the menstrual cycle. Progesterone also promotes the development and maintenance of the placenta during pregnancy. Progesterone also is a developmental hormone, regulating the maturation of mammary glands.

The ovaries synthesize estrogen, a female sex hormone, and progesterone in a cyclic pattern. At menstruation, levels of both hormones plummet, then progesterone levels again rise after ovulation. Imbalances of progesterone production are implicated in the occurrence of PREMENSTRUAL SYNDROME. Like all steroid hormones, progesterone is synthesized from CHOLESTEROL. The adrenal glands synthesize the progesterone needed to make ALDOSTERONE, a hormone regulating sodium excretion and water balance. Progesterone is also secreted by the corpus luteum and the placenta. (See also ENDOCRINE SYSTEM.)

prolactin (lactogenic hormone)   A HORMONE produced by the anterior portion of the PITUITARY GLAND that stimulates breast development. Alone, prolactin has little effect on mammary glands. After childbirth, prolactin stimulates lactation, together with the hormone OXYTOCIN, produced by the posterior pituitary gland. Lactation requires concerted actions by: ESTROGENS, female hormones; steroid hormones of the ADRENAL GLAND; GROWTH HORMONE, also from the anterior pituitary; thyroxine from the THYROID GLAND; and INSULIN from the PANCREAS.

Prolactin functions in the menstrual cycle as well. Prolactin inhibiting factor from the hypothalamus (brain) blocks prolactin release at the beginning of the cycle. When estrogen and progesterone levels fall in the late phase of the cycle, production of the inhibiting factor diminishes; the pituitary releases more prolactin and the blood level of prolactin increases. This increase may temporarily cause breast tenderness before menstruation. When the cycle begins again, the blood level of estrogen rises and prolactin again drops. In males prolactin supports luteinizing hormone to stimulate TESTOSTERONE production. Testosterone is the primary masculinizing hormone. (See also PREMENSTRUAL SYNDROME.)

prolamines   Major plant proteins that occur in cereal GRAINS. Prolamines contain a large amount of the AMINO ACID, PROLINE. Prolamines of WHEAT include GLUTEN. It is this fraction of wheat to which patients with CELIAC DISEASE are sensitive. Gliaden is the subfraction of wheat that contains very high levels of GLUTAMINE as well as proline. Wheat contains approximately 40 to 50% prolamine; RYE, 30 to 50%; OATS, 10 to 15%; maize (CORN), 50 to 55%; and MILLET, 50 to 60%. Millet contains prolamines with antigenic activity similar to the gluten of wheat. (See also FOOD SENSITIVITY.)

proline (Pro, L-proline)   One of the 20 amino acids that function as a protein building block. Proline is not a dietary essential amino acid because it can be readily synthesized by the body from another amino acid, GLUTAMIC ACID. Of 20 amino acids that serve as protein building blocks, only proline possesses a nitrogen atom bound in a ring. Its unique structure confers a distinctive structure to proteins in which it occurs in appreciable amounts. As a predominant constituent of COLLAGEN, it confers a unique helix to this very important connective tissue protein structure, allowing a characteristic rigidity. (See also AMINO ACID METABOLISM; HYDROXYPROLINE.)

proof   Refers to the alcohol (ethanol) content in alcoholic beverages. The value assigned to proof corresponds to double the actual alcohol content. Thus 100 proof vodka contains 50% grain alcohol. (See also BEER; WINE.)

propionic acid   A low molecule weight organic acid formed by the microbial FERMENTATION of CARBOHYDRATE. Propionic acid is a SHORT-CHAIN FATTY ACID containing three carbon atoms. The short-chain FATTY ACIDS, acetic acid, propionic acid and BUTYRIC ACID, are normal products of fermentation of fiber by intestinal bacteria, and they are important fuels for the colon. Propionic acid is a natural preservative in Swiss cheese; it also occurs in milk. Propionic acid is also a normal breakdown product of AMINO ACIDS and fatty acids in the body and is readily oxidized for energy production.

Sodium and calcium propionate are common preservatives that retard the growth of mold and bacteria and are considered safe FOOD ADDITIVES. (See also INTESTINAL FLORA.)

propyl gallate   A synthetic FOOD ADDITIVE used as a PRESERVATIVE to increase shelf life. Propyl gallate acts as an ANTIOXIDANT to reduce unwanted oxidations that cause fat decomposition (RANCIDITY), leading to altered color and texture in foods. It is used with BHA and BHT to preserve FAT,

LARD, VEGETABLE OIL, meat products, soup bases, chewing gum and cold breakfast cereals. Propyl gallate is often used in food packaging; it can migrate from the packaging lining into foods like cereals and potato flakes. The safety of propyl gallate has been questioned because it is linked to tumors in experimental animals. (See also CANCER.)

prostaglandins (PG) Derivatives of ESSENTIAL FATTY ACIDS, that serve as local, short-lived hormones. Prostaglandins (and related compounds—thromboxanes and LEUKOTRIENES) regulate most physiologic processes in the body, including INFLAMMATION, especially in joints, skin and eyes; pain and fever; blood pressure; production of blood clots; female reproductive cycle functions like inducing labor; stomach acid secretion; pituitary responses to brain signals; contraction of bronchial tubes and other smooth muscles; and fat degradation for energy production. Rather than circulating in the bloodstream to alter the function of a distant organ, prostaglandins affect cells and tissue in the immediate vicinity of origin. They are apparently synthesized by all mammalian cells, except red blood cells. In contrast, hormones originate only from specialized ENDOCRINE GLANDS. Prostaglandins are rapidly inactivated by oxidation and by structural modification.

Three families of prostaglandins designated by letters of the alphabet (PGA, PGE, PGI) play prominent roles. More than 30 different prostaglandins have been isolated, each with a specific function or functions. All possess 20 carbon atoms, a ring and two side chains. They differ in the number and position of double bonds. A numerical subscript designates the number of double bonds in their side chains, thus PG_1, PG_2 and PG_3 have one, two or three double bonds, respectively. This distinction is important because each type comes from a different FATTY ACID precursor. PG_1 and PG_2 are derived from the omega-6 family of essential fatty acids, based on LINOLEIC ACID. The PG_3 series is derived from alpha linolenic acid, of the omega-3 family of essential fatty acids.

Prostaglandins of the PG_1 Series

The PG_1 series, with a single double bond in a side chain, is synthesized from the essential fatty acid, linoleic acid, and its product, GAMMA LINOLENIC ACID. These prostaglandins tend to return body systems toward normal functioning (HOMEOSTASIS). As an example, PGE_1 decreases the stickiness of blood platelets, small particles in blood necessary for blood clotting, thus decreasing the tendency of clots to form. Series 1 prostaglandins thus help minimize the risk of heart attack and stroke. They also stimulate water excretion by the kidneys to counteract edema and they activate various types of T lymphocytes, the generals and foot soldiers that comprise cellular immunity. PGE_1 dilates (opens up) blood vessels, thus improving circulation and reducing blood pressure. It reduces tissue inflammation as found in ARTHRITIS. Nutrients that support the conversion of gamma linolenic acid to PGE_1 include VITAMIN B_6, ZINC, NIACIN and VITAMIN C.

Prostaglandins of the PG_2 Series

PG_2 prostaglandins are derived from ARACHIDONIC ACID, a highly unsaturated fatty acid supplied by the diet in animal fat and also produced from linoleic acid. PGE_2, a well-characterized member of this series, promotes BLOOD CLOTTING through increased platelet aggregation and induces sodium and water retention by the kidneys, leading to edema, and stimulates inflammation and associated pain.

Understanding how PG_2 prostaglandins are synthesized has shed light on the ways antiinflammatory drugs operate in the body. To begin PG_2 synthesis, arachidonic acid must first be liberated from membrane lipids by a specific lipase (fat splitting enzyme). Next, the "cyclic" pathway of arachidonic acid metabolism forms ring structures, characteristic of prostaglandins. ASPIRIN blocks pain and inflammation by inhibiting the enzyme (cyclo-oxygenase) that forms the prostaglandin ring, thus preventing PGE_2 formation. Steroid medications like hydrocortisone are effective antiinflammatory agents because they reduce inflammation by reducing the rate of arachidonic acid production.

Prostaglandins of the PG_3 Series

The PG_3 prostaglandins are derived from EICOSAPENTAENOIC ACID, (EPA), a major ingredient of fish and FISH OILS. The PG_3 prostaglandins counterbalance the PG_2 prostaglandins and return the body to normal functioning. Thus PGE_3 decreases platelet stickiness and decreases the risk of clot formation. EPA also blocks the conversion of arachidonic acid to thromboxane (TXA_2), a compound that promotes blood clotting. A diet high in fish and fish oil provides EPA and favors the production of PGI_3, another potent inhibitor of blood clotting. PGE_3 causes blood vessel dilation (vasodilation), while PGE_2 causes vessel constriction (vasoconstriction). The ultimate precursor of EPA is alpha linolenic acid, the second essential fatty acid. This is found in high levels in certain seed oils such as FLAXSEED OIL and walnut oil, and in dark-green leafy vegetables.

Several health conditions and nutrients affect the transformation of fatty acids to prostaglandins. The following factors reduce the body's ability to form the counterbalancing PG_1 series of prostaglandins: excessive CHOLESTEROL and dietary saturated fatty acids, excessive TRANS-FATTY ACIDS from processed vegetable oil, high alcohol consumption, zinc deficiency, uncontrolled DIABETES, high sugar consumption and aging.

During normal conditions the formation of prostaglandins and related substances appears to draw upon dietary polyunsaturated fatty acids. The synthesis of arachidonic acid from linoleic acid is normally quite slow, and the PG_1 prostaglandins would predominate. However, during injury, prostaglandins are derived from stored fatty acids in membranes. The principal fatty acid released in response to injury is arachidonic acid, leading to excessive PG_2 prostaglandins and inflammatory conditions. It has been suggested that diets high in saturated fatty acids, or diets with a high omega-6/omega-3 polyunsaturates ratio, facilitate PGE_2 and thromboxane (TX_2) production and promote blood clotting and inflammation. (See also IMMUNE SYTEM.)

El Attar, T.M.A. and Lin, H.S., "Effect of Vitamin C and Vitamin E on Prostaglandin Synthesis in Squamous Carcinoma Cells," *Prostaglandins, Leukotrienes and Essential Fatty Acids*, 47 (1992), pp. 253–57.

prostatic hyperplasia (benign prostatic hyperplasia, BPH) Prostate enlargement. The prostate gland is a walnut-sized gland surrounded by a portion of the urethra (tube draining the bladder through the penis). The only apparent function of the gland is to secrete fluid that both nourishes sperm and carries it through the penis. Prostate enlargement begins in many men by the age of 40. At least 50% of men up to the age of 50 have this condition, and it affects 75% of men over 70. Symptoms include a frequent, urgent need to urinate; urination at night can interrupt sleep. Urination is intermittent or delayed and has a weakened stream. Urine retained in the bladder through incomplete urination can cause urinary tract infections.

Aging processes in men favor the development of prostate problems. In the first place prostatic enlargement represents abnormal male hormone metabolism. After the age of 50, levels of dihydrotestosterone, a potent derivative of TESTOSTERONE, increase in the prostate and stimulate tissue growth. Increased levels of PROLACTIN increase the uptake of testosterone by the prostate and elevated estrogen levels block enzymes that would normally dispose of testosterone and dihydrotestosterone.

The Role of Nutrition

Prolactin levels in men increase with stress and with alcohol consumption. ZINC supplements have been reported to reduce the size of the prostate and reduce symptoms. This trace mineral nutrient inhibits the enzyme that converts testosterone to dihydrotestosterone, and it also inhibits testosterone uptake, conditions favoring increased excretion of these hormones. Furthermore, zinc inhibits prolactin secretion. Extracts of saw palmetto berries can inhibit the buildup of dihydrotestosterone and can help men with enlarged prostate.

In some patients prostatic hyperplasia reflects an imbalance in ESSENTIAL FATTY ACIDS. FLAXSEED OIL, SOYBEAN oil and EVENING PRIMROSE OIL may help correct essential fatty acid deficiencies. Extra vitamin E is needed when consumption of unsaturated fatty acids in significantly increased. Environmental pollutants like PCBs, PBBs, DIOXIN, hexachlorobenzene and pesticides can stimulate dihydrotestosterone formation and act as weak estrogens. This suggests that reduced exposure to such agents may be beneficial. A BALANCED DIET with minimally processed foods can also support the liver's ability to dispose of surplus testosterone and estrogen hormones.

Men should have regular physical exams after the age of 50. A digital exam, a blood test for prostate specific antigen, and ultrasound can help determine whether a tumor is involved. If examination rules out prostate CANCER, a problem with urination may be managed by cutting down on fluid intake in the evening. Alcoholic beverages and CAFFEINE stimulate urination, and these should be avoided. Certain medications can aggravate urinary problems. These include diuretics, tranquilizers, antidepressants and certain anticonvulsive agents. Antihistamines and decongestants promote urine retention and should be avoided. Take time to empty the bladder as completely as possible and urinate frequently to avoid stressing the bladder. (See also ENDOCRINE SYSTEM; KIDNEYS.)

Rose, David P. and Connolly, Jeanne M., "Dietary Fat, Fatty Acids and Prostate Cancer," *Lipids*, 27:10 (1992), pp. 798–803.

protease (proteolytic enzyme) An enzyme capable of digesting proteins. Proteases play important roles in digestion by breaking down food proteins to small fragments (PEPTIDES) and free AMINO ACIDS that can be absorbed by the small intestine.

PEPSIN is a protease produced in the STOMACH that initiates protein digestion and requires stomach acid for maximal activity. The PANCREAS produces a battery of powerful proteases to finish protein digestion in the small intestine. These include TRYPSIN, CHYMOTRYPSIN and carboxypeptidase. MEAT TENDERIZERS contain mixtures of plant proteases from pineapple (BROMELAIN) and papaya (PAPAIN) and from microorganisms (subtilism).

A deficiency of digestive proteases can cause MALNUTRITION because protein digestion is faulty. Inadequate digestive ENZYMES can be caused by an unhealthy stomach lining, by low stomach acid production, by pancreatic disease, by a damaged intestinal lining and by blockage of the common duct that carries juices of the pancreas and bile from the gallbladder to the intestine. (See also PANCREATITIS.)

protein A complex polymer of amino acids; the most common material in the body. The word protein is derived from the Greek word *proteios*, meaning "foremost" or "of primary importance." Perhaps as many as 100,000 different types of proteins make up 50% of the dry matter of the body. All life forms—bacteria, fungi viruses, plants and animals—rely on proteins for structure and the function of processes essential for growth and reproduction, for converting fuel to energy and using the released energy for maintenance, and for disposal of waste. Integration of organs and tissues ultimately relies on proteins.

Each type of protein contains a unique sequence of amino acids, similar to multicolored beads on a chain. By varying the numbers of different amino acids and their sequences, the body creates proteins of SKIN, BLOOD, MUSCLE, hair, BONE and nails, as well as ENZYMES, the catalysts that speed up chemical reactions of cells.

Despite this immense diversity, only 20 different amino acids are generally recognized as building blocks. It also seems likely that a SELENIUM derivative of the sulfur-containing amino acid CYSTEINE, called selenocysteine, is used occasionally as a protein precursor, making the total 21. All amino acid building blocks contain NITROGEN; therefore proteins are a dietary source of nitrogen and amino acids. The nitrogen content of protein is about 16%; crude protein content can be estimated from the nitrogen content of a food. To form proteins, amino acids are bound together by a special linkage called a peptide bond; a general name for proteins is "polypeptide." Breaking peptide bonds by acids, by alkali or by enzymes yields the constituent amino acid. It is worth pointing out that certain amino acids do not survive harsh conditions such as exposure to strong acids or alkalis or heat. GLUTAMINE and ASPARAGINE are broken down to GLUTAMIC ACID and ASPARTIC ACID, respectively.

Although 20 amino acid building blocks are incorporated into proteins, proteins may contain more than 20 different amino acids. This is explained by the fact that certain amino acids are modified after they have been linked up in mature proteins. Examples of modified amino acids formed in proteins include: PROLINE, converted to HYDROXYPROLINE, and

LYSINE, converted to hydroxylysine (in connective tissue); glutamic acid, to gama carboxyglutamic acid (in blood clotting proteins); SERINE and THREONINE, to phosphoserine and phosphothreonine (in regulatory proteins). Cysteine is oxidized to cystine to stabilize many proteins, such as KERATIN in hair.

Protein Structure

Protein chains fold up to form either condensed (globular) structures analogous to a ball of string; or they align themselves to form chains and fibers or sheet-like structures. Generally proteins that serve a dynamic role are globular structures. Enzymes, HORMONES, ANTIBODIES, HEMOGLOBIN and serum proteins like ALBUMIN are globular. The blood-clotting protein, fibrinogen, is transformed from a globular to a fibrous structure, FIBRIN, when blood-clotting is activated. Other fibrous proteins serve structural functions: COLLAGEN, elastin and keratin are fibrous proteins of skin, connective tissue and hair. Altering the unique three-dimensional structure of a protein usually causes a loss in biological function. This process is called denaturation. Denaturing agents include acidic and alkaline conditions, heat, and heavy metals like MERCURY and LEAD.

Protein Digestion

Digesting dietary proteins supplies essential amino acids that cannot be made in adequate amounts by the body. The dietary amino acids are used to assemble the body's own proteins. Any surplus is burned for ENERGY or converted to FAT. Most Americans eat more than enough protein to meet their amino acid needs.

Protein denaturation plays an important role in DIGESTION. Cooking foods denatures and partially breaks down proteins, making them more accessible to DIGESTIVE ENZYMES. Highly crosslinked proteins of hair, feathers and skin do not break down in the digestive tract because the protein chains cannot be attached to digestive enzymes.

Protein digestion normally begins in the stomach where the strong acid (hydrochloric acid) unfolds protein in food, rendering it more accessible to attack by the digestive enzymes of the stomach. The initial phase of protein digestion yields fragments called PEPTIDES, rather than individual amino acids. Digestive enzymes of the pancreas further break down protein fragments to free amino acids. Final stages of protein digestion require intestinal enzymes called peptidases that convert small fragments to free amino acids. Ultimately, individual amino acids are absorbed through the intestine and then distributed via the bloodstream to all cells of the body.

Protein Synthesis

A key question in understanding metabolism is how the cell achieves the precision required to assemble structures as complex as proteins without error. Much of the cell's exquisite machinery is devoted to this process. Life has evolved a template process for ordering amino acids in the proper sequence. The sequence is locked away in the nucleus of the cell in the form of a nucleic acid called DNA, the most complex molecules made by the cell. This genetic material stores information about protein structure as a sequence in code words. Prior to protein synthesis, copies of the genetic messages must be transported to the cytoplasm, where protein synthesis occurs. The vehicle for this transfer is a second type of NUCLEIC ACID called messenger RNA. This molecule bears the code words defining the amino acid sequence of a single protein. The messenger combines with cytoplasmic particles called ribosomes, protein synthesizing factories of cells. A third kind of RNA, called transfer RNA, transports each type of amino acid to the ribosome, matches up with appropriate code words in messenger RNA, and aligns amino acids in their proper sequence. The amino acids are then "zipped" together to construct the new protein. Energy for protein synthesis is generated by the oxidation of fuels.

Classification of Proteins

Proteins can be classified according to their functions:

- Carrier proteins, such as hemoglobin of red blood cells, serum lipoproteins LDL (LOW-DENSITY LIPOPROTEIN) and HDL (HIGH-DENSITY LIPOPROTEIN), which transport CHOLESTEROL in the blood.
- Structural proteins like collagen, found in skin, cartilage and scar tissue.
- Regulators, such as hormones (INSULIN, GLUCAGON, GROWTH HORMONE and ENDORPHINS), the brain's own painkillers).
- Contractile proteins, such as actin and MYOSIN of muscle.
- Defensive proteins, such as antibodies (gamma globulins) and blood clotting proteins.
- Enzymes, catalysts of the chemical changes that occur in the body. Examples are PEPSIN and TRYPSIN (digests proteins), LIPASE (digests fat) and AMYLASE (digests STARCH). Other enzymes synthesize many materials, including DNA and RNA; GLYCOGEN to store glucose; fat to store energy and even BLOOD SUGAR. Still other enzymes oxidize fat and carbohydrate to produce energy.

Simple proteins are also classified according to their solubilities.

- Albumins are water-soluble. They occur in serum, milk and eggs.
- Globulins are poorly soluble in water, but their solubility increases in salt solutions. They occur in serum, the fluid from clotted blood. Gamma globulin, the fraction of blood containing antibodies, is representative.
- Albuminoids are highly insoluble proteins found in hair, collagen and connective tissue.
- Glutelins are soluble in dilute acid or alkaline. These proteins occur in cereal grains. The GLUTEN of wheat contains glutelins.
- PROLAMINES are soluble in organic solvents such as alcohols. ZEIN in corn and GLIADEN in wheat are prolamines. They are rich in the amino acid proline.

Certain proteins are coupled with non-protein components.

- LIPOPROTEINS are complexes of phospholipids and fat and cholesterol. LDL (the less desirable form of cholesterol) and HDL (the more desirable form of cholesterol) are examples.

- Metalloproteins are complex metal ions. As an example, the serum protein transferrin binds COPPER, IRON and ZINC in blood.
- FERRITIN is an iron storage complex. It is measured to assess iron nutritional status.
- Mucoproteins and GLYCOPROTEINS contain carbohydrate chains of differing length and composition. They are produced by moist membranes that line the body cavities, such as the gastric intestinal tract. Mucins serve as lubricants.
- Nucleoprotein are protein complexes with RNA and DNA. Chromatin of the cell nucleus is an example of these complexes.
- Phosphoproteins, such as the milk protein CASEIN, contain phosphate.
- Flavoproteins contain COENZYMES (enzyme helpers) derived from the B vitamin RIBOFLAVIN. Flavoproteins occur in fat oxidation in energy-yielding pathways like the KREB'S CYCLE.

Dietary Protein Requirements

Worn-out proteins are degraded and replaced by new ones. A steady input of essential amino acids is therefore required even when the body is at a stable weight. The RECOMMENDED DIETARY ALLOWANCE (RDA) of 0.75 g protein per kilogram of body weight for adults was established based on long-term and short-term studies of humans. Thus an adult male weighing 174 lb requires 63 g of protein daily; and an adult female weighing 138 lb requires 50 g daily. Protein requirements were determined for individuals with a routinely high protein intake. Over time, people can adapt to low protein intake and achieve nitrogen balance without necessarily depleting their protein stores.

Children require relatively more protein than adults to support their rapid growth. The protein in an infant's body increases up to 15% during the first year. An intake of 2.2 g/kg of body weight is required per day up to the first five months of age; 1.2 g/kg from one to three years; 1.1 g/kg from four to six years; and about 1 g/kg from 7 to 14 years. During pregnancy, protein needs increase dramatically to meet the needs of the placenta, fetus and maternal tissues. Consequently the RDA is 60 g of protein throughout pregnancy—an increase of 10 g/day over the adult RDA. Breast milk is a protein-rich food that requires extra dietary protein to sustain its production. The protein RDA during lactation is between 62 and 65 g/day. These allowances are based upon the requirements of healthy people consuming high-quality protein. The DAILY REFERENCE VALUE used by the FDA for food labels is 50 g except for children: one to four years, 16 g; infants under one year, 14 g; pregnant women, 60 g; lactating mothers, 65 g. The typical U.S. diet supplies much more protein than is required. Thus the average protein intake for U.S. men is 75% above the RDA, and for women it is 35% more. Consequently, few people need protein supplements.

Nonetheless, certain groups of Americans may be at risk for protein deficiency: chronic dieters, elderly persons, persons with low incomes and low-income pregnant women. People with intestinal malabsorption disorders such as CROHN'S DISEASE and CELIAC DISEASE may need special protein or amino acid mixtures. Athletes who participate in high endurance training, such as cyclists, cross-country skiers and long distance runners, need more protein than sedentary people. Weight lifters and body builders also need somewhat more protein than sedentary people as they increase muscle mass. Weight-conscious women athletes who diet may not obtain enough protein from the food they eat.

Protein Malnutrition

Protein deficiency in its extreme form in children is called KWASHIORKOR. In developing nations children after weaning may be fed an unbalanced diet of starchy foods that are low in essential amino acids, such as BANANAS, YAMS and CASSAVAS. Mental development and functioning may be severely altered in infants following severe protein deficiency.

With inadequate dietary protein, yet with adequate calories, less muscle wasting occurs than with malnutrition due to a lack of both protein and energy sources because protein is not broken down so extensively. One reason is that less glucocorticoid is released by the adrenal glands. This hormone family switches the body into a degradative mode (CATABOLIC STATE) and causes muscle wasting to supply energy. Glucocorticoids tend to maintain blood sugar levels and increase blood amino acid levels at the expense of muscle protein.

Protein synthesis in glands and tissues is dramatically affected by a lack of essential amino acids. Digestive enzyme secretion by the PANCREAS and the intestine declines. Atrophy of all intestinal lining can lead to malabsorption, which in turn increases the risk of DIARRHEA, mineral loss and ELECTROLYTE imbalance, and dehydration. Protein deficiency reduces liver function; inadequate processing of fatty acids leads to the accumulation of fat in the liver due to the inability to transport fat out of the liver. Depleted serum protein synthesis by the liver adversely affects fluid balance. With less protein and electrolytes in the circulation, more water resides in tissue, causing EDEMA. ANEMIA can result from chronic protein deficiency because of inadequate supply of amino acids to manufacture red blood cells. With decreased dietary protein, antibody production is limited, leaving the individual prone to infection. Protein malnutrition causes apathy and irritability.

Problems with Excessive Protein Consumption

Excessive consumption of red meat correlates with a high saturated fat intake, and excessive saturated fat is linked to cardiovascular disease and to problems of overweight. Red meat contains 35 to 50% saturated fat. In contrast chicken is 25% saturated and fish is 20% saturated. In contrast, vegetables and fruit contain almost no saturated fat.

The surplus waste products from burning excess protein place an extra burden on the kidneys. This can be a problem for diabetics and for those with kidney problems. Surplus protein drains CALCIUM from the body, perhaps contributing to OSTEOPOROSIS. Excess animal protein may increase the risk of liver cancer in lab animals. Consumption of milk, egg and meat protein raises blood cholesterol in rabbits, while soy bean protein does not have this effect.

Dietary Recommendations

To lower your intake of animal fat and hence the risk of heart disease, move away from the belief that meat should be eaten every day. Instead, use meat as a condiment. A 2-oz serving of lean meat a day alone provides the RDA for most healthy adults. Replace red meat with fish or poultry. Reduce consumption of fatty meat like sausage, hot dogs and luncheon meat. Eat a variety of vegetables to obtain low-fat, balanced protein in place of red meat. Grains and vegetables provide important fiber and complex carbohydrates along with their protein.

Assessment of Protein Quality

Protein quality refers to the degree to which a food protein supplies needed amino acids. It is evaluated by several different procedures.

1. BIOLOGICAL VALUE (BV) measures the efficiency of utilization of absorbed nitrogen made under carefully standardized conditions and provides a comparison with a protein-free diet. However, few animals besides rats will consume protein-free diets long enough for such a study, limiting its usefulness. For less digestible protein, or high-fiber foods, BV is inadequate.
2. NET PROTEIN UTILIZATION (NPU) measures the efficiency of overall utilization of ingested nitrogen (from amino acids of digested protein). For completely digested proteins, NPU equals BV.
3. PROTEIN EFFICIENCY RATIO (PER) evaluates protein quality while allowing for the body's needs for maintenance. It is based upon the weight gained by lab animals fed a test diet compared to the amount of protein consumed by those animals.
4. Nitrogen balance index is used to estimate human protein needs. When proteins supply adequate amino acids, nitrogen balance is positive, that is, the amount of nitrogen provided by food is greater than the amount lost in urine and feces.
5. CHEMICAL SCORES are derived by comparing the amino acid composition of a test protein is compared with the amino acid composition of a reference protein that provides essential amino acid to meet the requirements of children. Egg protein and human milk are typically used. The content of an amino acid in the reference protein is assigned a value of 100%. Typically, chemical scores of 70 or higher are considered adequate protein sources.

(See also AMINO ACID METABOLISM; HUNGER; STARVATION.)

Houck, Jane and Slavin, Joanne, "Protein nutrition for the athlete," in *Sports Nutrition for the 90s*, Berning, J.R. and Steen, S.N., eds. Gaithersburg, Md.: Aspen Publishers, 1991.

protein complementation
Combining different types of protein in order to make up for any AMINO ACID deficiencies when each is eaten separately. Vegetable proteins often contain less than optimal amounts of certain essential AMINO ACIDS such as lysine or methionine. Making the appropriate match creates a complete protein mixture that more nearly matches a high-quality protein providing ample amounts of the essential amino acids. Eating such a mixture with each meal does not seem necessary. Eating a variety of selected, whole, minimally processed plant protein foods throughout the day can supply the body with adequate essential amino acids.

Traditional meals throughout the world often incorporate complementary proteins, in examples of folk wisdom that have evolved in different societies. Grains complement BEANS, PEAS and LENTILS; examples are rice and bean casseroles, lentil curry and rice, wheat bread and baked beans, corn tortillas and beans. Seeds like SESAME and SUNFLOWER complement peas, beans and lentils: roasted nuts with soybeans; sesame seeds in bean soup; hummus (garbanzo beans plus sesame seeds). Milk products complement grains: pasta and cheese, cheese sandwich. (See also PROTEIN QUALITY.)

protein efficiency ratio (PER)
A measure of PROTEIN quality. PER is one of the most commonly used procedures to assess the adequacy of a food protein in providing ample amounts of all dietary essential amino acids to meet the needs for maintenance and growth. In the United States PER is a basis for regulations governing protein content in food labeling and RECOMMENDED DIETARY ALLOWANCES (RDA). PER is defined as the weight (in grams) gained by growing animals divided by the protein intake (in grams) over a period of time. Studies usually use young rats over a 10-day feeding period. This procedure has important drawbacks. It assumes that all dietary protein is used for growth; no allowance is made for maintenance. Furthermore, the amino acid requirements for rats are not the same as for humans.

The PER for CASEIN (milk protein) is taken as a reference point for the protein RDA. For food labels, 50 g of a protein with a PER value comparable to casein is considered to meet 100% of the DAILY REFERENCE VALUE for non-pregnant nonlactating adults. When the PER is less than casein, at least 65 g of food protein is required to meet 100% of the USRDA. When consumption of FAT or CARBOHYDRATE is inadequate to meet energy requirements, dietary protein will not support growth regardless of its ability to supply essential AMINO ACIDS as a high-quality protein, because a minimum amount of carbohydrate is required in the diet to fuel the nervous system and maintain health.

protein quality
The degree to which a food protein supplies all dietary essential AMINO ACIDS. A high-quality food protein provides ample amounts of all amino acids the body cannot make in sufficient amounts to support growth and maintenance. Such a protein source is designated as "complete." Partially complete proteins can maintain life but cannot support growth. Low-quality protein is deficient in one or more essential amino acids and by itself cannot support growth and maintenance. Incomplete proteins neither maintain growth nor sustain life and lead to wasting of tissue protein.

Animal protein is generally high-quality protein because ample amounts of all dietary essential amino acids are represented. GELATIN is an exception. This degraded form of COLLAGEN lacks essential amino acids TRYPTOPHAN and METHIONINE.

Good sources of complete protein are MEAT, FISH, POULTRY and dairy products like EGGS. Red meat is the favored source of high-quality protein in the United States. However, these same sources provide excess cholesterol and saturated fat and lack fiber. On the other hand, meat is an exceptional source of zinc, iron and VITAMIN B_{12}.

Vegetable protein, with some exceptions, is lower in quality than animal protein because most plant proteins are generally low in at least one essential amino acid. Grains are usually low in lysine (corn, wheat, rye) while legumes are equally low in sulfur-containing amino acids methionine and cysteine. The proteins of SOYBEANS, dried BEANS, AMARANTH and QUINOA contain relatively large amounts of all essential amino acids and are of higher quality than other plant protein sources. Because flesh in all forms—red meat, poultry and fish—is so common in the Western diet, obtaining adequate protein is generally not a problem in these countries except for strict vegetarians. By eating a variety of minimally processed vegetables, grains, nuts and legumes each day, an individual can readily obtain vegetable protein to supply ample amino acids to meet daily needs. (See also PROTEIN COMPLEMENTATION; VEGETARIAN.)

protein-sparing fast　See DIET, VERY LOW CALORIE.

proteolytic enzyme　See PROTEASE.

provitamin A　See BETA CAROTENE.

prudent diet　See CHOLESTEROL.

psoralen　A chemical found in FIGS, CELERY leaves and PARSLEY that can increase sensitivity to sunlight. Psoralen is a potential MUTAGEN (an agent that causes mutations) and CARCINOGEN (cancer-causing agent). It can be activated by exposure to ultraviolet light in sunlight to attack cell membranes and the genetic material (DNA). Because of its ability to kill cells (cytotoxicity), it has been isolated and used therapeutically to treat psoriasis and certain types of cancer.

psychoneuroimmunology　The study of the relationship between emotions, the NERVOUS SYSTEM and the IMMUNE SYSTEM. Recent research reflects the renewed interest in examining a key assumption of ancient medicinal traditions, that mental states can affect the body's ability to fight illness. Modern research has demonstrated that the linkage between the brain and the immune system exists at the cellular and biochemical level. Excessive physical and emotional STRESS have been shown to decrease immune function as well as imbalance the endocrine (HORMONE) system. Proponents believe this sets the stage for DEGENERATIVE DISEASE.

The immune system is strongly affected by signals sent from the brain via at least two pathways. In the first, the HYPOTHALAMUS, the region of the brain that integrates fundamental processes, including heartbeat, digestion, body temperature, blood pressure, appetite and emotions, regulates hormone release. Neurotransmitters, brain chemicals that help carry nerve impulses, regulate the hypothalamus, so the brain can either activate or retard the immune system. In the second pathway, the autonomic nervous system, the branch of the nervous system that acts as the "autopilot" of the body, also regulates immunity. In the first pathway, the hypothalamus sends chemical signals to the PITUITARY GLAND, the "master gland." Under stressful conditions, the hypothalamus releases a chemical called corticotropin-releasing factor that signals the pituitary to secrete ACTH (ADRENOCORTI-

COTROPIC HORMONE), the hormone that activates the adrenal glands. In turn the adrenal glands release steroid hormones, glucocorticoids, into the bloodstream. High levels of glucocorticoids tend to shut down the immune response, especially the T cells, the foot-soldiers of the immune system. On the other hand, low levels of glucocorticoids can stimulate immune cells.

In a second pathway linking brain and immunity, the nerves of the autonomic nervous system are closely linked to the lymphatic tissues—the spleen, lymph nodes, bone marrow, thymus gland—where many types of immune cells reside. Thus nerves send signals via neurotransmitters directly to tissues responsible for immune activity. In turn, lymphatic tissues act as an endocrine (hormone-secreting) gland. They produce many proteins—including ENDORPHINS, ACTH, LYMPHOKINES and thymosins from the thymus—that are secreted into the bloodstream and facilitate two-way communication with the brain. These developments emphasize that research into causes of disease needs to evaluate contributions of both the brain and the immune system. (See also PLACEBO.)

Nee, L.E., "Effects of Psychosocial Interactions at a Cellular Level" Social Work, 40 (March 20, 1995). pp. 259-62.
Ballieux, R.E., "The mind and the immune system." *Theoretical Medicine*, volume 15 (Dec. 1994), pp. 387–395.

psyllium　A natural FIBER used to relieve CONSTIPATION. Psyllium is an annual herb grown in India and southern Europe. Its seeds contain high levels of a water-soluble fiber (gum), a non-digested plant carbohydrate. Psyllium fiber has long been marketed as a BULKING AGENT and LAXATIVE. Recent research suggests psyllium fiber may help lower blood CHOLESTEROL levels significantly when a typical dose is taken over several weeks. Other sources of soluble fiber, including GUAR GUM, OAT bran and PECTIN, also lower blood cholesterol levels. Foods rich in soluble fiber might lower blood cholesterol an additional 5% if the level is already below 200, or if the person is already on a low-fat diet. Diet and exercise are the first strategies to lower blood cholesterol. Psyllium fiber can cause gas and intestinal upset in some people due to its fermentation by gut bacteria. Excessive amounts can block the absorption of fat-soluble VITAMINS and of MINERALS. In addition, some individuals may be allergic to psyllium gum. Chronic constipation can indicate a serious underlying problem, and a qualified health care provider should be consulted.

pulses　Edible seeds of LEGUMES. Pulses commonly used as food include LENTILS, BEANS, CHICKPEAS, cowpeas, field peas, PEANUTS and SOYBEANS. These seeds and nuts possess a higher protein content than grains; their protein contains adequate lysine, an essential amino acid often found in low amounts in other plant protein. However, pulses generally are deficient in sulfur-containing amino acids CYSTEINE and METHIONINE. Soybeans are an exception. (See PROTEIN COMPLEMENTATION.)

pumpkin (*Cucurbita spp.*)　A member of the gourd and squash family. Pumpkins are large orange fruit with a coarse, sweet, strongly flavored flesh. The flesh, seeds and flowers are eaten. Pumpkins originated in Central

America and Mexico; ancient Aztec and Inca gardeners cultivated varieties that had sweet flesh. By the time Europeans arrived in the New World, pumpkins had spread throughout Mexico, North America, southeastern Canada and the Caribbean. Pumpkins are canned and frozen and are baked in pies, cakes and custards. Pumpkin is a rich source of vitamin A (beta carotene). The nutrient contents of 1 cup (canned, 245 g) are: 83 calories; protein 2.7 g; carbohydrate, 19.8 g; fiber, 5.6 g; fat, 0.7 g; iron, 3.4 mg; potassium, 504 mg; vitamin A, 5,400 retinol equivalents; vitamin C, 12 mg; thiamin, 0.08 mg; riboflavin, 0.19 mg; niacin, 1.0 mg.

purified cellulose   See FLOUR SUBSTITUTE.

purine   A nitrogen-containing compound that is a building block of DNA and RNA, substances that store information and guide protein synthesis in the cell. The most common purines are ADENINE and GUANINE, and they have a double ring structure. Together with THYMINE cytidine and uracil, they are the building blocks that define the genetic code. Purines are synthesized in the body and are not essential nutrients. Adenine is also linked up with the simple sugar ribose and phosphate to form ATP, the energy currency of the cell and the basis for most energy-requiring processes in cells. Degradation of purines ultimately yields URIC ACID, which is excreted in the urine. People who are susceptible to GOUT or who have abnormal purine metabolism may need to limit their intake of purine-rich foods; these include fish like ANCHOVIES, HERRING and SARDINES; organ meat like brains, kidney and liver; yeast and mushrooms. (See also DNA; RNA.)

pyramid   See FOOD GUIDE PYRAMID.

pyridoxamine   See VITAMIN B₆.

pyridoxine   See VITAMIN B₆.

pyrimidine   A widely distributed family of nitrogen-containing compounds. Three of the most common pyrimidines are THYMINE, its analog uracil, and cytidine. Together with the PURINES, ADENINE and GUANINE, they constitute the alphabet of the genetic code. The pyrimidines and purines of DNA and RNA are synthesized by the body and are not required nutrients. Unlike purines, which are degraded and excreted as URIC ACID, pyrimidines are readily broken down to easily disposed waste products, AMMONIA and simple acids. Mutagens (agents that cause MUTATIONS) often chemically alter pyrimidines and purines in DNA. (See also GENE.)

pyruvic acid   A simple organic acid that is an end product of GLUCOSE degradation. Glucose is the widely used simple sugar of the cell that serves as fuel, and is particularly necessary to the brain and nervous system. The breakdown of glucose to pyruvic acid initiates energy production from major dietary carbohydrates by a sequence of enzymes collectively called GLYCOLYSIS. With plentiful oxygen, pyruvic acid migrates from the cytoplasm into the cell's powerhouses, the MITOCHONDRIA, where the elaborate enzyme system of the KREB'S CYCLE completely oxidizes pyruvic acid to CARBON DIOXIDE and WATER. Energy released in this oxidation is trapped as ATP, the energy currency of the cell that drives biosynthetic reactions, muscle contractions, transport of materials into cells and nerve conduction.

When the access to oxygen is limited in skeletal muscle during strenuous exertion, pyruvic acid is converted to LACTIC ACID rather than being oxidized by mitochondria. Lactic acid must be shipped to the liver for disposal. Pyruvic acid readily acquires nitrogen to form the simple amino acid ALANINE; therefore, alanine is a non-essential amino acid. (See also CARBOHYDRATE METABOLISM; GLYCOGEN; OXYGEN DEBT; TRANSAMINATION.)

quercetin A widely distributed plant pigment. Quercetin, classified as a FLAVONOID, occurs in fruits like *apples*, vegetables like *onions*, and in *tea*. A typical Western diet supplies about 25 mg of quercetin daily. Onions, apples, kale, sweet cherries, grapes, red cabbage and green beans are good sources. Quercetin produces a broad range of effects in the body. It can function as an ANTIOXIDANT to quench highly reactive chemicals called FREE RADICALS. Together with vitamin C quercetin helps strengthen fragile capillaries and connective tissue. It can inhibit tumor formation and modulate enzymes in the liver that degrade drugs, pollutants and cancer-causing agents. Quercetin can reduce inflammation by blocking the formation and the release of inflammatory agents, and it possesses antimicrobial activity as well. (See also PHYTOCHEMICALS.)

Stavric, B. "Quercetin in our diet: from potent mutagen to probable anticarcinogen," *Clinical Biochemistry*, 27 (August 1994), pp. 245–48.

quince (*Cydonia cydonia*) A yellow, pear-shaped FRUIT. Quince is harvested from the cydonia tree, native to Iran and the Caucasus. The flesh is hard and extremely tart, preventing it from being eaten raw. Quince contains high levels of pectin, a gel-forming fiber. It is used in marmalades, jellies, jams, fruit preserves and syrup as a thickening agent. One quince (151 g) provides 53 calories; protein, 0.37 g; carbohydrate, 14 g; fiber, 1.6 g; potassium, 181 mg; vitamin C, 14 mg; thiamin, 0.018 mg; riboflavin, 0.028 mg; niacin, 0.18 mg. (See also CITRUS FRUIT.)

quinoa (chenopodium) A grain-like product unrelated to true grains. A cousin to spinach and swiss chard, quinoa produces edible greens in addition to its seeds. The seeds form large clusters at the end of the stalk. Domesticated and grown in South America for 5,000 years, quinoa was cultivated by the Incas. This hardy plant grows well at high elevations that experience little rainfall. Quinoa is imported from South America. Domestic supplies come from the Rocky Mountain region (Colorado). The seeds are protected by a resin-like layer (saponin), which must be removed by treatment with alkali to be edible. The cleansed grain resembles millet. Quinoa has a high protein content. Quinoa protein is well balanced in essential amino acids and has substantial amounts of lysine, unlike cereal grains. Quinoa also contains more iron than other grains and contains substantial amounts of other trace minerals and calcium, as well as B complex vitamins. The cooking time for quinoa is shorter than for rice or millet. Its delicate taste combines well with other grains in pilaf or baked grain casseroles.

The nutrient content of 3.5 oz (100 g) of dry grain is 374 calories; protein, 13 g; carbohydrate, 69 g; fat, 6 g; potassium, 740 mg; iron, 9 mg; thiamin, 0.2 mg; riboflavin, 0.4 mg; niacin, 3.0 mg.

quinone A family of lipids that readily undergo oxidation-reduction reactions. Two important quinone derivatives occur in the body: VITAMIN K and COENZYME Q. Vitamin K serves as a cofactor in the synthesis of several proteins required for BLOOD CLOTTING, while coenzyme Q functions as an electron carrier in MITOCHONDRIA, the cell's powerhouses. Coenzyme Q participates in the transfer of electrons to convert OXYGEN to water. At the same time ENERGY is trapped as ATP, a chemical form used by the cell. (See also ELECTRON TRANSPORT CHAIN; OXIDATIVE PHOSPHORYLATION.)

radiation preservation of food　See FOOD IRRADIATION.

radioactivity　See CARCINOGEN.

radish (*Raphanus sativus*)　A root vegetable with a distinctive sharp flavor; related to broccoli, kale and cabbage. These cruciferous vegetables possess anticancer properties. The radish probably originated in western Asia and was used by Babylonians and ancient Egyptians. It was introduced to China around 500 B.C., where new varieties were developed with a tangy flavor. According to the variety, radishes may be round, tapered or oblong, and the color can be white, red, yellow, purple or black. The Oriental radish, daikon, can weigh up to 5 lb. (2.3 kg). The common radish (red globe) is usually eaten raw as a condiment and as a salad vegetable. Black radishes are the size of turnips; their flesh is white and very pungent. Radishes can be cooked as a vegetable, added to soups or pickled. The nutrient contents of 10 radishes (raw, 45 g) is 7 calories; protein, 0.27 g; carbohydrate, 1.6 g; fiber, 0.24 g; vitamin C, 10 mg; riboflavin, 0.02 mg; niacin, 0.135 mg.

radon　See CARCINOGEN.

raisin　A dried form of several varieties of grapes. Half of the world's supply of raisins comes from the San Joaquin Valley of California. Muscat and Sultana, Thompson Seedless and Zante Currant represent the principal varieties of grapes suitable for raisins. Ripe grapes are dehy-drated either mechanically or are sun-dried so that raisins contain 17% water, compared to about 80% for grapes. Nutrients like sugar are much more concentrated in raisins than in the fresh fruit, and raisins are a good source of iron, potassium, B vitamins, dietary fiber, and carbohydrate (calories). Golden raisins are dried Thompson Seedless grapes that have been treated with sulfur dioxide then dehydrated in forced dry air. Other varieties include currants (from Black Corinth grapes); Sultanas (from a large green grape), popular in Europe; Muscat raisins (from green Muscat grapes), which are fruity flavored and often used in fruit cakes. Unopened packages of raisins can be stored a year when refrigerated, longer when frozen. The nutrient content of 1 cup (seedless, 145 g) is: 435 calories; protein, 4.7 g; carbohydrate, 115 g; fiber, 9.6 g; fat, 0.7 g; iron, 3.0 mg; potassium, 1,089 mg; vitamin C, 5 mg; thiamin, 0.23 mg; riboflavin, 0.13 mg; niacin, 1.29 mg.

rancidity　The process by which fats and oils become oxidized through exposure to air. Rancid fat has an off-flavor and a disagreeable odor. In meat, iron-containing protein react with oxygen to produce free radicals that cause loss of flavor accompanying fat decomposition. The oxidation of fats usually occurs spontaneously, though slowly, at room temperature. Exposure to heat, light and trace metals like IRON greatly speeds the reaction of oxygen. Rancidity lowers the content of other lipids, including VITAMIN A and VITAMIN E. Thus the rancid foods are less wholesome and less nutritious than fresh foods.

At a molecular level, oxygen and a reactive chemical species called FREE RADICALS, molecules that are electron deficient, can attack unsaturated FATTY ACIDS in fats and oils. Unsaturated fatty acids contain double bonds that lack pairs of hydrogen atoms. These bonds are fragile and susceptible to chemical modification, leading to the formation of PEROXIDES, which are potent intermediates in fat oxidation. Lipid peroxides can trigger INFLAMMATION and spontaneously decompose into more free radicals plus fragments that are both cytoxic (cell killing) and mutagenic (causing mutations).

Most cells contain an antioxidant enzyme system called GLUTATHIONE PEROXIDASE that converts unstable oxidized lipids (lipid peroxides) to harmless fatty acids that can be used for energy.

A growing family of FOOD ADDITIVES called ANTIOXIDANTS is used to control or prevent oxidation of processed vegetable oils and processed foods containing fats and oils in order to increase their stability during storage. Ascorbic acid (VITAMIN C) and vitamin E prevent oxidative damage, and additives like CITRIC ACID can bind metal ions that could otherwise catalyze a reaction with oxygen. Synthetic antioxidants, including BHA, BHT and PROPYL GALLATE, are designed to disarm free radicals before they can cause damage. Because of the safety concerns raised about synthetic antioxidants, the food industry has studied naturally occurring antioxidants that can be added to foods and fats and oils to stabilize them. As an example, rosemary extracts have proven effective in stabilizing vegetable oils. (See also FOOD PRESERVATION.)

rapeseed (*Brassica napus; B. campestris*) One of the five most important oil-producing seed crops and the only oil seed successfully grown worldwide. The origins of rapeseed are obscure, although reference to it is made in 3,000-year-old Sanskrit writings. The seed contains 40 to 50% oil. Rapeseed oil typically contains erucic acid, a fatty acid analog that interferes with FAT METABOLISM in experimental animals when consumed in large amounts. New strains of rapeseed that contain little of this acid or another antinutrient, glucosinolate, were developed in Canada and Europe. The oil derived from the new strains of rapeseed, CANOLA OIL, contains significantly more OLEIC ACID, the monounsaturate of OLIVE OIL. The fatty acid composition of canola oil resembles olive oil and it too is classified as a monounsaturate. Canola oil is used in SHORTENING, MARGARINE, salad oil, MAYONNAISE and as a cooking oil. It contains 6.9% saturated fatty acids; 34.6% polyunsaturated fatty acids; and 58.5% monounsaturated fatty acids. (See also VEGETABLE OIL.)

raspberry (*Rubus spp.*) The FRUIT of a family of brambles (Rosaceae) that includes BLACKBERRY and loganberry. Raspberries resemble blackberries, except the berry core remains on the vine when raspberries are picked. Each fruit is composed of tiny drupes, each of which can be considered a fruit. Raspberries apparently originated in eastern Asia. They now grow wild from the Arctic Circle to northern South America. Cultivation was probably initiated in Europe in the 16th century. Red raspberries are the most common variety in America, but they may be yellow, black or purple as well. Oregon and Washington are major raspberry producers. Ninety percent of the U.S. crop is processed, and most is quick frozen because it has a short shelf life. Most red or dark

blue-purple berries contain pigments (ANTHOCYANINS) that have beneficial effects on connective tissue and inflammation. These and related berries contain ellagic acid, a substance that may help prevent some forms of cancer. Raspberries are good sources of FIBER, POTASSIUM and VITAMIN C. The nutrient contents of 1 cup (raw, 123 g) are: 60 calories; protein, 1.1 g; carbohydrate, 14.2 g; fiber, 9.1 g; fat, 0.7 g; potassium, 187 mg; vitamin C, 31 mg; thiamin, 0.04 mg; riboflavin, 0.11 mg; niacin, 1.11 mg. (See also FLAVONOIDS.)

raw fish See SEAFOOD.

raw meat disease See TOXOPLASMOSIS.

raw milk See MILK.

raw shellfish See SHELLFISH.

raw sugar See SUCROSE.

RD See DIETITIAN.

RDA See USRDA.

recommended daily allowances See USRDA.

Recommended Dietary Allowances (RDA) The Food and Nutrition Board of the U.S. National Academy of Sciences has periodically published recommended average daily intakes for several nutrients selected as adequate to meet the dietary needs of most healthy Americans. Generally, the RDAs are reviewed every five years or so, the most recent edition being 1989. RDAs were established for the following categories:

- ENERGY;
- fat-soluble VITAMINS: VITAMINS A, VITAMIN D, VITAMIN E, VITAMIN K (added in 1989);
- water-soluble VITAMINS: VITAMIN C, FOLIC ACID, NIACIN, RIBOFLAVIN, THIAMIN, VITAMIN B_6, VITAMIN B_{12};
- macrominerals: CALCIUM, MAGNESIUM, PHOSPHORUS;
- trace minerals: IODINE, IRON, ZINC, MAGNESIUM, SELENIUM (added in 1989).

It should be noted that not all nutrients are included because the FNB considers the data inadequate to make recommendations. Consequently there is no recommendation for fat or for types of fat (ESSENTIAL FATTY ACIDS) or for COPPER, an essential nutrient (refer to the appendix for the 1989 version of the RDAs).

The RDAs are based upon population needs. Groups referred to in the RDA tables include: infants; children between the ages of one and three; between four and six; and between seven and ten; males or females between the ages of 11 and 14; between 15 and 18, 19 and 22, 23 and 50; men and women over 50; pregnant women; and lactating women.

All recommendations except for energy intend that nutrient intake will exceed the requirements of most healthy people. This decision was made in order to address the problem of variability in individual nutrient needs. Mathematically, RDAs have been chosen to cover 97.5% of a given group of people by selecting values lying between two standard deviations above the mean nutrient requirement for a population.

The determination of the RDAs for energy differs significantly from other recommendations for specific nutrients. The allowances for energy employ the average (mean) requirement for each population reported. The mean was chosen because a higher recommended energy allowance would significantly increase the odds that many people, who have average energy needs, would become overweight. OBESITY is considered an epidemic in America.

The RDAs were selected after evaluating evidence that comes from animal as well as human studies. Nutrient requirements are generally set at levels that ensure that body stores are adequate for normal functions, growth and development. In people, the nutrient turnover and rates of depletion of nutrient body pools are most usually unknown. Therefore experimental evidence for setting the RDAs generally relies on the following: intakes that maintain adequate blood levels; excretion of surplus doses in urine or feces; maintenance of a balance of intake and body losses; measurement of body function or metabolic process; knowledge of the amount of a nutrient needed to prevent or even cure disease in humans and sometimes in experimental animals; and examination of nutrient intakes of apparently healthy people.

Uses of RDAs

As originally intended, dietary recommendations serve as a guide in diet planning and as a yardstick by which diets of different groups in a population can be measured. They are also used to develop nutrition regulations and food guidelines, including the definition of food groups and serving selections to obtain the amounts of nutrients needed to meet the RDAs. They have been used as a basis in the certification of various institutions such as day-care centers and nursing homes, and they have been used by dietitians for food planning and food selection in institutions like hospitals. They provide guidelines for developing food assistance programs such as the National SCHOOL LUNCH PROGRAM and food for children's programs and food services. The RDAs are useful in interpreting food consumption patterns of populations and of individual persons for whom intakes have been averaged over several days. The RDAs are the averages, not single-day intakes, and therefore the recommendation is to design menus for groups with the goal of meeting RDAs over five- to ten-day intervals. The U.S. FDA has used RDAs to develop a standard for food fortification and labeling formerly called U.S. recommended daily allowances (US RDA), now called the REFERENCE DAILY INTAKES (RDI). The US RDAs represent a single set of values, based on the highest RDA of any age group using 1968 values.

RDA Limitations

There are a number of caveats in using the RDA tables.

There are no separate RDAs for people 70 years or older because the data were found to be inadequate; needs for people with special needs due to medical conditions are also not covered.

The RDAs are levels of essential nutrients deemed adequate to meet the needs of populations of healthy people eating a diet composed of a variety of foods from all the important food groups. Nutrients in food change dramatically with a diet relying on convenience food and highly PROCESSED FOODS. Part of the requirement for some nutrients can be met by consumption of other nutrients. As an example, the essential AMINO ACID, TRYPTOPHAN, is partially converted to the B vitamin NIACIN, and the amino acid methionine is converted to the sulfur amino acid CYSTEINE; when the dietary source of protein is lower in quality, the needs of these nutrients can increase.

The efficiency of DIGESTION and uptake (BIOAVAILABILITY) of a given nutrient is another factor. Nutrient uptake of minerals and vitamins varies immensely with the type of food and its preparation. Thus, iron from vegetables is much less readily absorbed than is iron from red meat.

The implicit assumption of the RDAs is that nutrient requirements probably follow a bell-shaped or normal distribution. This is the case for some, but not all nutrients.

The RDAs represent population averages assessed over a long period of time. They may be appropriate for evaluating individual intake, when intake can be averaged over a sufficiently long time. One or two days is not long enough.

The RDAs do not take into consideration life-style choices, including cigarette smoking, alcohol and substance abuse; exposure to chemical pollutants in the home or workplace; and exercise level.

RDAs have been established only for those nutrients for which there is a clear indication of a dietary requirement. The subcommittee of the Food and Nutrition Board defined a new category, "Safe and Adequate Intakes," for essential nutrients for which it considers adequate information lacking by which to develop RDAs. Ranges of intakes are provided. In this category are the B complex vitamins, BIOTIN and PANTOTHENIC ACID, the trace minerals copper, CHROMIUM, FLUORIDE, MANGANESE and MOLYBDENUM, and the major ions (electrolytes) CHLORIDE, SODIUM and POTASSIUM. Other nutrients exist for which less information is known, and new RDAs are likely to be developed with the accumulation of more data.

Bear in mind that the RDAs do not address optimal levels for maximizing health, productivity and longevity. The aggregate of evidence since the 1970s suggests that at least in some cases, such as vitamin C and vitamin E, optimal nutrient levels are significantly greater than RDAs. (See also FOOD GUIDE PYRAMID.)

King, J., "The need to consider functional endpoints in defining nutrient requirements," *American Journal of Clinical Nutrition*, 63 (1996), pp. 983S–4S.

Recommended Nutrient Intakes (for Canadians) (RNI)   Recommendations published by the Ministry of National Health and Welfare are designed to meet the needs of nearly all healthy Canadians consuming a mixed diet comprised of foods commonly available for usual levels of physical activity (1990). The subgroups for which RNIs are listed include the following: infants, 0 to 2, 3 to 5, 6 to 8, and 9 to 11 months; children, 1 year, 2 to 3, 4 to 6 years of age. After the age of six, RNIs are given for males and females: 7 to 9, 10 to 12, 13 to 15, 16 to 18, 19 to 24, 25 to 49, 50 to 74, and over 74 years of age. The RNIs are compared with the RDAs on page 377.

Comparison of Recommended Nutrient Intakes for Canadians with RDAs

Nutrient	Canadian RNI Ages 24 to 49		RDA Ages 25 to 50	
	(F, 130 lb./59 kg)	(M, 163 lb./74 kg)	(F, 130 lb./63 kg)	(M, 174 lb./79 kg)
Vitamin A	800 RE	1,000 RE*	800 RE	1,000 RE
Vitamin D	2.5 mcg	2.5 mcg	5 mcg	5 mcg
Vitamin E	6 mg	9 mg	8 mg	10 mg
Vitamin K	—	—	65 mcg	80 mcg
Vitamin C	30 mg	40 mg	60 mg	60 mg
Thiamin	0.8 mg	1.1 mg	1.1 mg	1.5 mg
Riboflavin	1.1 mg	1.5 mg	1.3 mg	1.7 mg
Niacin	15 mg	19 mg	15 mg	19 mg
Vitamin B_6	—	—	1.6 mg	2.0 mg
Folate (folacin)	175 mcg	220 mcg	180 mcg	200 mcg
Vitamin B_{12}	2.0 mcg	2.0 mcg	2.0 mcg	2.0 mcg
Calcium	700 mg	800 mg	800 mg	800 mg
Phosphorus	850 mg	1,000 mg	800 mg	800 mg
Magnesium	200 mg	250 mg	280 mg	350 mg
Iron	13 mg	9 mg	15 mg	10 mg
Zinc	9 mg	12 mg	12 mg	15 mg
Iodine	160 mcg	160 mcg	150 mcg	150 mcg
Selenium	—	—	55 mcg	70 mcg
Omega-6 fatty acids	7 g	9 g	—	—
Omega-3 fatty acids	1.1 g	1.5 g	—	—
Protein	44 g	61 g	64 g	70 g

*retinol equivalents

red blood cells (erythrocytes)   The major type of cells in blood. Red blood cells transport OXYGEN to all cells of the body, and their color reflects the high content of HEMOGLOBIN, the red oxygen transport protein. The importance of red blood cells is indicated by their numbers: The average person has 35 trillion red blood cells. Males have about 5 million red blood cells per milliliter of blood and females have about 4.5 million per milliliter. Each red blood cell contains about 280 million hemoglobin (protein) molecules. The blood of the average adult male contains 14 to 16.5 g of hemoglobin per 100 ml of blood; the average adult female has 12 to 14 g per 100 ml.

Inhalation brings fresh air into the lungs where hemoglobin binds oxygen, which is then carried to tissues via arteries. Oxygen binding is reversible so that hemoglobin releases oxygen in tissues where there is a low concentration of oxygen. Elevated CARBON DIOXIDE concentration and acid production from actively metabolizing tissues also promote oxygen release from red blood cells. Released oxygen diffuses into cells where it oxidizes fuels to carbon dioxide. Red blood cells pick up carbon dioxide for the return trip to the lungs via blood vessels. Red blood cells transport about 23% of carbon dioxide in this manner. In the lungs red blood cells release carbon dioxide and again bind incoming oxygen.

Red blood cells are highly specialized cells. The disk shape presents a larger surface area than a sphere, which helps the diffusion of oxygen into the cells. Red blood cells lack a nucleus and MITOCHONDRIA and therefore cannot divide, nor use oxygen to derive energy from the oxidation of fuel molecules. Instead they rely on GLYCOLYSIS, an oxygen-independent mechanism for oxidation of glucose (BLOOD SUGAR) to LACTIC ACID. The surface of the red blood cell possesses certain carbohydrate clusters (blood group substances) that are the basis for blood typing; for example, according to the ABO blood groups and Rh blood groups.

Formation

ERYTHROPOIESIS refers to the process of red blood cell formation. During embryonic development, red blood cells are produced by the yolk sac, liver, spleen, thymus gland, lymph nodes and bone marrow, while in adults, red blood cells come from the bone marrow of long bones like the femur, and from the cranium, sternum, ribs, vertebrae, pelvis and lymphoid tissues. The initial parent cells are called hemocytoblasts. These cells differentiate into proerythroblasts, an intermediate stage that eventually differentiates into reticulocytes (immature red blood cells), and finally into mature red blood cells (erythrocytes). The usual fraction of reticulocytes in blood is between 0.5 and 1.5%. The percentage increases with ANEMIA, when the number of functional red blood cells becomes inadequate; with bleeding; hemolysis (rapid breakdown of red blood cells); and in response to supplementation for IRON deficiency.

The kidney stimulates the production of the hormone, erythropoietin, which stimulates the production of red blood cells in response to lowered oxygen pressure, as experienced at high elevations. When the body suddenly needs more red blood cells, the kidneys become oxygen-deficient and release an enzyme that converts a blood protein to erythropoietin.

The levels of red blood cells represent a balance between the formation and destruction of red blood cells. Aged red blood cells are destroyed by the spleen and by the liver. The protein portion of hemoglobin is degraded to AMINO ACIDS; the red pigment, HEME, is degraded to BILE PIGMENT, bilirubin, which is excreted, and releases iron, which is reused.

A number of nutrients besides iron support cell division and protein synthesis in general, and red blood cell formation in particular: FOLIC ACID, PYRIDOXINE, VITAMIN B$_{12}$ and amino acids. ANTIOXIDANTS like VITAMIN E help maintain the red blood cell membrane and prevent fragility. Deficiencies of any of these nutrients can cause anemia, a condition resulting from an inadequate level of functional red blood cells. Several inborn errors of metabolism (mutations) cause abnormal hemoglobins to be formed. These in turn can alter the shape of red blood cells and shorten their life-span, resulting in anemia. Sickle cell anemia and glucose 6 phosphate dehydrogenase deficiency are the most common. (See also HEMATOCRIT; LEUKOCYTES.)

red dye numbers 2, 3, 40   See ARTIFICIAL FOOD COLORS.

red meat   See MEAT.

red tide (paralytic shellfish poisoning)   Refers to a plankton bloom often occurring in marine waters during the late summer and fall months. The term "red tide" comes from the red-brown color of plankton. The plankton produce a nerve poison (neurotoxin) that can accumulate to dangerous levels in shellfish such as CLAMS and mussels though it does not affect the shellfish. Eating contaminated clams, mussels and oysters causes paralytic shellfish poisoning. The adage of avoiding shellfish during months that end in the letter "r"—September, October, November and December—is no longer appropriate because red tide alerts now occur in other months. Red tide warnings by county health departments can be issued as early as April.

Symptoms of paralytic shellfish poisoning include stomach cramps, dizziness, difficulty in breathing, and tingling mouth. Symptoms can appear up to two hours after eating contaminated shellfish; in severe cases poisoning can be fatal. There is no antidote. Immediate medical attention is mandated. (See also SEAFOOD.)

Reference Daily Intake (RDI)   A replacement term for "U.S. RDA" (Recommended Daily Allowance), a set of reference values introduced in 1973 to be used for vitamins, minerals and protein to help consumers evaluate the nutritional content for food labels. For the time being, RDIs are identical to the U.S. RDAs except for protein, which is adjusted to the specific needs of different age groups. The current RDIs and RDIs approved for 1997 are as follows:

Nutrient	Amount
Vitamin A	5,000 International Units (IU)
Vitamin C	60 milligrams (mg)
Thiamin	1.5 mg
Riboflavin	1.7 mg
Niacin	20 mg
Calcium	1.0 gram (g)
Iron	18 mg
Vitamin D	400 IU
Vitamin E	30 IU
Vitamin B$_6$	2.0 mg
Folic acid	0.4 mg
Vitamin B$_{12}$	6 micrograms (mcg)
Phosphorus	1.0 g
Iodine	150 mcg
Magnesium	400 mg
Zinc	15 mg
Copper	2 mg
Biotin	0.3 mg
Pantothenic acid	10 mg

(Based on National Academy of Sciences' 1968 Recommended Dietary Allowances.)

Additions Jan 1, 1997	
Vitamin K	80 mcg
Molybdenum	75 mcg
Chloride	3,400 mg
Manganese	2.0 mg
Selenium	70 mcg
Chromium	120 mcg

Langseth, L., Vanderveen, J., and Frattali, V., "The New Reference Daily Intakes: for Better or for Worse," *Nutrition Reviews*, 50:4 (April 1992), pp. 119–24.

reference protein   A source of PROTEIN used as a basis for comparing food proteins according to their amino acid compositions. Reference proteins provide all essential amino acids in sufficient quantity to meet the needs of infants and children, who require substantially more protein than adults, based on their body weight, to support their higher growth rates. Another property of reference proteins is that they are highly digestible. High-quality protein sources often used as reference proteins include egg, human milk, meat and fish. The amino acid patterns for human milk and whole egg protein are as follows:

Amino Acid	Human Milk mg/100 g	Whole Egg mg/100g
Histidine	23	24
Isoleucine	56	63
Leucine	95	88
Lysine	68	68
Methionine and cysteine	40	56
Phenylalanine and tyrosine	99	98
Threonine	46	49
Tryptophan	17	16
Valine	63	72

The CHEMICAL SCORE attempts to measure the nutritive value of food protein in comparison with a reference protein. In this case, the amount of the least abundant limiting essential amino acid in the test protein is expressed as a percentage of that amino acid in the reference protein. Thus a good-quality protein source could have a chemical score of 70 or above. Most meat and dairy protein fall into this category. (See also BIOLOGICAL VALUE; PROTEIN COMPLEMENTATION; PROTEIN EFFICIENCY RATIO.)

refined carbohydrates   Highly purified SUGARS or STARCHES. These substances occur in sweeteners and in products that are mainly starch. Each type of refined carbohydrate supplies the same four calories per gram. Purified simple sugars and starches represent EMPTY CALORIES, that is, calories lacking in VITAMINS, FIBER, PROTEIN and MINERALS.

One of the most common refined carbohydrates is table sugar (SUCROSE), highly purified from sugar beets or sugar cane by repeated crystallization. The following sweeteners are only slightly less purified forms of sucrose: brown sugar, caramelized sugar, HONEY, syrup, MOLASSES and turbinado sugar.

Other refined sugars besides sucrose serve as common FOOD ADDITIVES:

- Dextrose (grape sugar) is another name for the pure compound of GLUCOSE, used by food manufacturers. Dextrose occurs in corn syrup.

- Maltodextrins are starch fragments containing several glucose units. They yield glucose upon digestion and provide no other nutrients.
- Fructose (fruit sugar) occurs as high FRUCTOSE CORN SYRUP. This sweetener also contains glucose, but no other nutrient.
- Sugar alcohols function as sweeteners: MANNITOL, SORBITOL and XYLITOL. None provides anything other than calories to overall nutrition.

Refined Starches

Purified starches are isolated from WHEAT, CORN and POTATOES, among other sources. Starch is used as a thickener in many foods. White flour is a staple of the American diet. Though not pure starch, white flour and products prepared from white bread—cold BREAKFAST CEREALS, muffins, pastry, pancake mix, pasta (spaghetti, noodles) and the like—contain much less of the vitamins, minerals, essential oils and fiber than are found in the whole grain from which they were derived. Milling wheat separates the starchy endosperm from the highly nutritious germ and bran (the hull of the seed or kernel).

Recent dietary guidelines have consistently emphasized minimally processed foods like FRUIT and VEGETABLES. U.S. DIETARY GUIDELINES FOR AMERICANS (1985) called for eating less refined sugar in the form of table sugar, syrup, honey, concentrated sweets like pastry, candy and soft drinks, while increasing intake of complex carbohydrates in the form of starchy foods: fruit, vegetables and legumes (dried peas, lentils and beans), and whole grain, enriched bread and other cereal grain products. The 1992 USDA guidelines from the Food and Nutrition Board ("Eat for Life") call for eating at least five servings of fruits and vegetables daily. Dark-green leafy vegetables, yellow vegetables and CITRUS FRUITS are recommended. The 1992 FOOD GUIDE PYRAMID of the USDA recommended three to five servings of vegetables, two to four servings of fruit and 9 to 11 servings of rice, bread, cereal and pasta daily, with the admonition to use sweets and added sugar sparingly. (See also CARBOHYDRATE METABOLISM; NATURAL SWEETENERS.)

renin   An enzyme produced by the KIDNEYS that helps increase blood pressure. In response to a drop in BLOOD PRESSURE, renin activates the HORMONE, ANGIOTENSIN, which in turn stimulates the ADRENAL GLANDS to produce ALDOSTERONE, the hormone that directs the kidneys to retain SODIUM and water. Elevated levels of renin correlate with increased risk of heart attack among people with moderate HYPERTENSION (high blood pressure). Possibly too much angiotensin can trigger reduced blood flow to the heart. (See also CARDIOVASCULAR DISEASE; PROTEASE.)

rennet (rennin)   An extract from the stomach of ruminants, such as calves, that contains the enzyme rennin. Milk protein coagulates because rennin degrades milk proteins, causing clotting (denaturation). Rennet is used in the manufacture of CHEESE to form curds. (See also DENATURED PROTEIN.)

respiration, cellular   The use of oxygen by cells to burn fuel nutrients for energy. OXYGEN delivered by the blood is taken up by MITOCHONDRIA, particles in the cytoplasm that function as the cell's powerhouses. Mitochondrial enzymes completely oxidize FAT, CARBOHYDRATE and AMINO ACIDS to CARBON DIOXIDE and chemical energy released by this process is trapped as ATP. ATP is the energy currency of cells; it provides the necessary energy for the synthesis of cellular components—proteins, RNA, DNA—as well as for transmission of nerve impulses, muscle contraction and the transport of nutrients across cell membranes. Carbon dioxide diffuses out of cells into the bloodstream, which transports it to the lungs to be expired. Respiration requires specialized enzyme machinery called the terminal ELECTRON TRANSPORT CHAIN. This sequence of linked oxidation-reduction enzymes receives electrons from individual oxidation reactions of the cell and passes them on to oxygen, which is converted to water. The sequential transfer of electrons to oxygen is coupled with the generation of ATP, a process called OXIDATIVE PHOSPHORYLATION.

Certain toxins and poisons like cyanide inhibit cellular respiration, limit ATP production and may ultimately cause death. Nutrients required to support respiration include B vitamins NIACIN, RIBOFLAVIN, THIAMIN, PANTOTHENIC ACID and trace minerals like COPPER and IRON. Another nutrient that may be required in the diet under certain conditions is COENZYME Q. This lipid helps funnel electrons into the system. (See also CARBOHYDRATE METABOLISM; FAT METABOLISM; RESPIRATORY QUOTIENT.)

respiratory chain   See ELECTRON TRANSPORT CHAIN.

respiratory quotient (R. Q.)   The ratio of the volume of expired CARBON DIOXIDE to the volume of OXYGEN consumed. This measurement can be used to determine whether PROTEIN, CARBOHYDRATE and FAT represent the major energy sources of the body. Carbohydrate and protein are more oxidized (contain more oxygen), and less oxygen is required to oxidize them completely to carbon dioxide. Therefore their R.Q. values are higher than that of fat: carbohydrate, 1.0; protein, 0.80; fat, 0.71; mixed diet, 0.82. Note that the R.Q. may exceed 1.0 if large amounts of carbohydrate are being converted to fat. (See also METABOLISM.)

retinal   The biologically activated form of VITAMIN A required to form visual purple (rhodopsin), the pigment in the retina responsible for night vision. The enzymatic conversion of vitamin A to retinal requires the trace mineral ZINC. (See also NIGHT BLINDNESS.)

retinoic acid (9-cis retinoic acid)   An oxidized form of VITAMIN A, believed to be a new, fat-soluble HORMONE. Cis retinoic acid may guide normal embryonic development and regulate normal cell division and may be involved in regulating blood CHOLESTEROL levels. CANCER is characterized by uncontrolled cell division; some patients with certain kinds of cancer, such as leukemia, respond to vitamin A. Furthermore, vitamin A treatment may lower the risk of recurrence of breast and lung cancer. Additional research is required to define the relationship among retinoic acidity, vitamin A and cancer. (See also ENDOCRINE SYSTEM).

retinoid   See BETA CAROTENE; VITAMIN A.

retinol   See VITAMIN A.

retinol equivalents (RE)   See VITAMIN A.

rheumatoid arthritis (RA)   A chronic inflammatory disease of the joints. Rheumatoid arthritis is characterized by overgrowth of joint tissue leading to swollen immobilized joints as a result of an overactive IMMUNE SYSTEM. Rheumatoid arthritis is classified as an AUTOIMMUNE DISEASE in which the immune system attacks the body by developing antibodies against joint tissue. An estimated 7 million people in the United States are affected by RA. The much more common ailment, OSTEOARTHRITIS, represents a joint "wear and tear" arthritis and does not involve the immune system, is not an autoimmune disease, and its cause is unrelated to rheumatoid arthritis.

Rheumatoid arthritis can begin in young or middle-aged adults. The triggering mechanisms are unproven. It seems likely there are many contributing factors. Infections, allergies, genetic susceptibility, life-style and nutritional factors may play a role. There is no cure, although some medications are used to reduce INFLAMMATION (anti-inflammatory drugs). ASPIRIN is the most common drug used to relieve pain and swelling, but high doses of aspirin can cause gastrointestinal bleeding, stomach irritation, even reduced hearing. Newer anti-inflammatory medicines and less irritating NSAIDS (nonsteroidal anti-inflammatory drugs) are now available as prescription drugs. Other NSAIDS include ibuprofen and indomethicin. However, NSAIDS in general can cause intestinal inflammation and increase gut permeability to potentially harmful substances. Cortisone-related drugs can relieve inflammation. Long-term use can lead to disabling side effects. These effects include suppression of the immune system, bone demineralization and thinning of skin.

Studies in the 1980s demonstrated that fasting often reduces symptoms of rheumatoid arthritis, but pain, swelling and stiffness return when fasting ends. Preliminary clinical trials suggest that a gluten-free, vegan diet (no animal protein, no wheat) for three to five months followed by a lactovegetarian diet (only milk and milk products plus plant-derived foods) for the rest of the year can significantly reduce pain, improve grip strength and reduce swelling among patients with rheumatoid arthritis. Therefore food sensitivities should be ruled out.

Imbalanced PROSTAGLANDINS are linked to chronic conditions. These derivatives of essential fatty acids help regulate many physiologic processes, including inflammation. A growing body of evidence suggests that diet can influence prostaglandin levels. Supplemental seed oils containing the polyunsaturated fatty acid GAMMA LINOLENIC ACID, such as BORAGE oil and EVENING PRIMROSE OIL can reduce arthritic pain. Gamma linolenic acid is obtained from the ESSENTIAL FATTY ACID, LINOLEIC ACID, and leads to the formation of a set of anti-inflammatory prostaglandins. Other anti-inflammatory prostaglandins are derived from omega-3 fatty acids that occur in flaxseed oil and coldwater fish like SALMON, HERRING, SARDINES and fish oils. These fish provide omega-3 fatty acids, such as EICOSAPENTAENOIC ACID, and diets rich in fish can decrease inflammation. Supplemental omega-3 oils (flaxseed oil and fish oil) may help decrease symptoms of arthritis.

Among the B vitamins, PANTOTHENIC ACID in large amounts has been used to relieve symptoms of rheumatoid arthritis. Vitamin K may help stabilize joint linings. Free radical and oxidative damage accompany inflammation, and the diet should provide ample ANTIOXIDANTS: SELENIUM, VITAMIN E and VITAMIN C. ZINC, MANGANESE and COPPER support the antioxidant enzyme, SUPEROXIDE DISMUTASE, which can protect tissues from free radical damage. Herbal preparations such as feverfew and LICORICE have been used in botanical medicine to treat rheumatoid arthritis. FLAVONOIDS such as QUERCETIN and catechin reduce inflammation by acting as antioxidants and by inhibiting mast cell degranulation, a major contributor to tissue injury. They also limit tissue destruction associated with inflammation. (See also OSTEO-MALACIA; OSTEOPOROSIS.)

Darlington, L.G., Ramsey, N.W. Mansfield, J.R., "Placebo-controlled, Blind Study of Dietary Manipulation Therapy in Rheumatoid Arthritis," *Lancet* (February 1, 1986), pp. 236–40.

Kjeldsen-Kragh, J., et. al, "Controlled trial of fasting and one-year vegetarian diet in rheumatoid arthritis," *Lancet*, 338:8772 (1991), pp. 899–902.

rhubarb (*Rheum rhaponticum*)   A cultivated perennial with thick, typically red stalks that is classified as a fruit. Only the leaf stalks of this plant are edible because roots and leaves contain a potentially toxic material, OXALIC ACID. Rhubarb stalks are cooked in pies, sauces, rhubarb crumble, and other baked goods, jams and preserves, and they can be fermented to produce wine. Rhubarb is extremely tart and requires the addition of sweeteners to make it appetizing. The calcium in rhubarb is mainly complexed as insoluble calcium oxalate, which is poorly absorbed. Like spinach, it is not a good dietary source of calcium. Nutrient content of cooked rhubarb with added sugar (1 cup, 240 g) is: 279 calories; protein, 0.9 g; carbohydrate, 75 g; fiber, 5.3 g; calcium, 348 mg; vitamin C, 8 mg; thiamin, 0.04 mg; riboflavin, 0.06 mg; and niacin, 0.48 mg.

riboflavin (vitamin B$_2$)   A bright-yellow, B complex VITAMIN. This widely distributed vitamin functions in oxidation-reduction reactions. Riboflavin works together with the B vitamins THIAMIN, NIACIN and PANTOTHENIC ACID to oxidize FAT and CARBOHYDRATE to carbon dioxide to produce ENERGY. The complete oxidation of these fuels occurs via the KREB'S CYCLE, a sequence of enzyme-catalyzed steps that represents the major energy-yielding pathway of most tissues. Riboflavin is the parent of FLAVIN ADENINE DINUCLEOTIDE (FAD) and flavin mononucleotide (FMN), two enzyme helpers (COENZYMES). Riboflavin participates in the body's defense system to oxidize toxins and foreign compounds. It supports glutathione reductase, an enzyme that replenishes an important cellular ANTIOXIDANT called glutathione. This system represents a major defense against oxidative damage. In addition, the production of steroid HORMONES by the ADRENAL GLANDS requires riboflavin. More generally, riboflavin is essential for successful reproduction in experimental animals, for healthy skin, eyes, and nerve function.

Possible Roles in Maintaining Health

Unlike niacin deficiency or thiamin deficiency, chronic riboflavin deficiency does not cause a distinctive human disease. ARIBOFLAVINOSIS, a riboflavin deficiency disease, occurs in association with deficiencies of other B complex vitamins. Symptoms of riboflavin deficiency include FATIGUE, delayed wound healing, sore mouth, cracks in the corners of the mouth, tongue inflammation (GLOSSITIS), blurred vision and light sensitivity, and eczema of face and genitalia.

Sources

Riboflavin is widely distributed among foods, but the levels vary greatly. Rich sources include organ meats (LIVER, kidney and heart); dairy products (MILK, CHEESE, YOGURT); and BREWER'S YEAST. BREAKFAST CEREAL, enriched flour, almonds, lean meat, raw mushrooms, wheat bran, enriched cornmeal, soybean flour and dark-green leafy VEGETABLES are good sources. Fifty percent of the riboflavin in milk can be lost within two hours upon exposure to light. Storing milk in cartons rather than in glass bottles markedly reduces the loss. Riboflavin is destroyed by light and by heat. Up to 20% of riboflavin is lost from milk by evaporation or by PASTEURIZATION. Raw fruits and vegetables generally provide little riboflavin.

The U.S. enrichment program for white flour was initiated in 1941. Since then, riboflavin, as well as thiamin, niacin and iron, have been added to flour and cereal products that together account for an estimated 0.33 mg of riboflavin per day for a typical American. Riboflavin is non-toxic; excesses are excreted and turn urine yellow.

Requirements

The RECOMMENDED DIETARY ALLOWANCE (RDA) of riboflavin is 1.7 mg per day for men and 1.3 mg per day for women between the ages of 25 and 50. The requirement increases somewhat for women who are pregnant or lactating. Anyone with a severely compromised diet is prone to B complex vitamin deficiency in general. This includes children of developing countries who consume inadequate eggs, meat, and milk or enriched foods; alcoholics; elderly persons with an imbalanced diet; people on severe weight loss programs; chronic users of fiber-based laxatives; those who use tranquilizers; and patients with HYPOTHYROIDISM. Vigorous EXERCISE can increase the requirement of riboflavin in women. (See also CARBOHYDRATE METABOLISM; FAT METABOLISM.)

Haller, J., "Vitamins for the Elderly: Reducing Disability and Improving the Quality of Life," *Aging, Clinical and Experimental Research*, 5: supp. 1 (1993), pp. 65–70.

rice (*Oryza sativa*)   An important cereal grain and a food staple in Asia and other parts of the world. Rice is a grass related to WHEAT, OATS and BARLEY. Rice originated from wild species that persist in southeast Asia. Rice culture occurred in China by 2200 B.C. and in Thailand by 5000 to 3500 B.C. Worldwide, China, India, Indonesia, Bangladesh and Thailand produce the most rice. In populations dependent on rice, it can account for 60 to 80% of total calories. In the Orient the average annual consumption is 200 to 400 lb (90 to 180 g) per person; in contrast the average American eats about 8 lbs (3.6 kg) annually. The U.S. produces about 1% of the world's crop.

There are many thousands of rice strains, including strains adapted to warm or cold climates, low or high elevations. Paddy rice is cultivated in flooded fields most of the growing season, while upland rice can grow in wet soil and doesn't require flooding. Many hardy strains of rice now used were products of the GREEN REVOLUTION, a concentrated effort of agriculture, science and industry to improve crop productivity in developing nations. Use of these strains, better irrigation, increased use of chemical fertilizers and synthetic pesticides created a dramatic increase in grain production in Asia, South America and Africa.

Rice is classified according to size: Short-grain rice is oval in shape, contains less AMYLOSE, a straight-chain form of STARCH, and is sticky when cooked. Medium-grain rice is more tender than long-grain rice and is used to make cold breakfast cereals. Long-grain rice has a high amylose content, and its kernels do not stick to each other when cooked. Long-grain rice accounts for about 75% of the U.S. domestic production. Waxy rice cooks to a sticky paste and is used for cakes and confections. Wild rice, *Zizania aquatica*, is native to eastern North America. Though it is an annual grass, it is a distant cousin of true rice.

White or polished rice is produced by milling to remove bran, husk and germ, which reduces the content of B vitamins. Polished rice is approximately 92% starch and only 2% additional nutrients. Notably, the content of THIAMIN in polished rice is only 18% of that of husked rice. Among populations subsisting primarily on white rice, the thiamin deficiency disease, BERIBERI, may occur.

In the United States white rice is enriched with thiamin, RIBOFLAVIN, NIACIN, IRON and CALCIUM. Removing hulls from dried, rough rice yields brown rice. Brown rice resembles whole wheat in nutrient content. The protein content is lower than wheat but the quality is higher. Nonetheless, rice protein is deficient in the AMINO ACID, LYSINE, typical of most grains. Rice contains more niacin than corn. Parboiled rice represents rough rice that has been soaked, steamed and dried to loosen husks, which are removed by milling. Greater amounts of nutrients are retained than in white rice. Rice is used as a breakfast food (puffed rice, flakes, crispies), rice flour, flaked rice, rice-based baby food, rice oil and rice bran. Rice bran contains fiber that can help reduce blood cholesterol levels and rice oil, which also has a cholesterol-lowering effect. Rice bran does not become sticky when cooked, unlike oat bran. Rice is commonly steamed or boiled. The more water used in cooking rice, the more nutrients are lost.

The nutrient content of 1 cup (205 g) of white, enriched rice (cooked without salt) is 223 calories; protein, 4.1 g; carbohydrate, 49.6 g; fiber, 0.82 g; fat, 0.2 g; iron, 2.9 mg; thiamin, 0.22 mg; riboflavin, 0.02 mg; niacin, 2.05 mg.

Miller, Janette, et al., "Rice: a High or Low Glycemic Index Food," *American Journal of Clinical Nutrition*, 56 (1992), pp. 1034–36.

rickets

A disorder of bone formation in growing children commonly due to VITAMIN D deficiency. Rickets is characterized by softening and deformation of long BONES, reflecting an interference with bone growth and altered mineralization. The bone disease in adults resulting from vitamin D deficiency is called OSTEOMALACIA. The mineral portion of bone consists mainly of CALCIUM and phosphate; thus a deficiency of either can cause rickets. Low calcium can be the result of a dietary deficiency of calcium or of vitamin D, or a problem with vitamin D's activation to the hormone form, calcitriol (1,25-dihydroxyvitamin D_3). Some people may be unable to convert vitamin D to calcitriol because of a rare genetic defect in the kidney enzyme performing the last step in the activation of vitamin D to calcitriol. Dietary vitamin D sources include fortified MILK and fish liver oils. Alternatively, ultraviolet light converts provitamin D in the skin to vitamin D; therefore, inadequate exposure to winter sunlight, particularly in populations living in northern latitudes and in institutionalized people, can lead to vitamin D deficiency. Still other problems can be caused by malabsorption syndromes associated with CELIAC DISEASE and INFLAMMATORY BOWEL DISEASE, which can limit uptake of fat-soluble vitamins, including vitamin D, even when dietary intake is normal.

Abnormally low phosphate and calcium in children's diets can also cause rickets. Hormone imbalances, such as an increased secretion of parathyroid hormone, can trigger calcium and phosphate release from bone. This loss of mineral softens bone.

Sometimes rickets accompanies kidney disease when the kidneys fail to synthesize calcitriol. Other types of rickets can be caused by genetic abnormalities in tissues so that the hormone, though present, cannot perform its physiologic functions. (See also OSTEOARTHRITIS; OSTEOPOROSIS; SKELETON.)

risk due to chemicals in food and water

The chance of injury or illness resulting from exposure to synthetic chemicals in FOOD. Logical and reasonable decisions can be made when risks are identified and their magnitude assessed. In reality, no substance is absolutely safe and there is no risk-free environment, though modern technology and policies based on simple, rapid solutions to public health problems have nurtured this common expectation.

Risk estimates are averages of populations and are not designed for individuals. Epidemiology, the study of populations, has identified several large risks for chronic diseases. In the United States, HEART DISEASE is the number-one killer, accounting for 35% of all deaths (death rate is 312 per 100,000 people). Risk increases with age, family history of heart disease, OBESITY, high blood pressure, smoking and excessive fat intake. CANCER is the number-two killer, with 22.5% of deaths (death rate of 199 per 100,000). It causes most deaths of men and women between the ages of 35 and 54. Smoking is linked to 30% of cancer cases; diet, to roughly 35%; and sexual behavior, to 7%. Stroke accounts for 6.9% of deaths (death rate of 61 per 100,000). Those at greatest risk are adults over 55, particularly over the age of 65. Risk increases with age, untreated high blood pressure, DIABETES, obesity and smoking.

Technology has posed questions about the definition of a safe level of exposure to potentially harmful agents. Sensitive analytical techniques can now readily detect traces of contaminants in foods at levels unattainable in the 1970s. Contaminant levels at parts per billion and even parts per trillion can be detected in air, water, foods and even human milk. The long-term effects on health of chronic exposure to such low levels of multiple contaminants remain unknown.

Under the Federal Insecticide, Fungicide and Rodenticide Act, the EPA is required to consider risks and benefits of agricultural chemicals. The current policy of the EPA regarding risk of pesticide exposure, has defined negligible risk as an acceptable risk, the use of a chemical like a pesticide that would cause one death per million people due to cancer over a lifetime (70 years). No cancer-causing agents can be added to foods. There is an additional problem inherent in assessing cancer risk: Estimating cancer risk poses a problem because the delay between exposure to a CARCINOGEN (cancer-causing agent) and development of cancer can be many years.

PESTICIDES and agricultural chemicals like ALAR, FOOD POISONING, ARTIFICIAL FOOD COLORS, SACCHARIN and BOVINE GROWTH HORMONE, a bioengineered hormone to stimulate milk production in cows, have been focuses of consumer concern in recent years regarding food risk fostered by technology. Despite these fears, an estimated two-thirds of all deaths and one-third of all hospitalizations in the United States are linked to life-style choices and to factors for which individuals are at least partially responsible: smoking, excessive ALCOHOL consumption, traffic accidents, obesity, excess blood CHOLESTEROL in balanced diet, decreased physical activity and high blood pressure (hypertension). The risk of disease also depends upon an individual's health history and genetic predisposition. Deficiencies in primary health care cannot be ignored because they tend to affect pregnant women, the fetus, infants, low-income people and the elderly, particularly.

Public perception of risk depends in part on the source of the risk, whether it is readily apparent, and the circumstances under which it appeared. Manmade hazards are less acceptable than natural (uncontrollable) causes. Perceived risk increases when there is no clear-cut benefit and when the risk is unfamiliar. For example, a government agency can estimate that a pesticide may cause between 1 and 100 deaths per million; this risk may be perceived as unacceptable by some. On the other hand, traffic accidents kill about 50,000 Americans yearly (an average of 125 per day). This is about 2 per 10,000, or 200 per million people, which is generally considered an acceptable modern-day risk.

Each approach to risk assessment presents strengths and weaknesses. A common experimental strategy in cancer risk assessment is based upon examining cancer risk for rats and mice exposed to high levels of an agent in order to detect an observable effect. Applying these data to human populations involves assumptions that humans will behave in the same way as animals and assumptions that the effects of a low dose can be calculated from a high dose administered to the animals. Even more uncertainty is involved if comparisons are made on the basis of extreme toxicity. On the other hand, risks calculated in a similar way can be compared; thus the risk of consuming different types of carcinogens can be compared from historical data. Exposure to similar compounds can also be used as a basis of comparison. Risks of cancer due to various chlorinated hydrocarbons in chlorinated drinking water can be similarly compared.

Questions to Ask Regarding a Risk

1. What is the absolute risk? Is it 1 per 1,000 or 10 per million? A tenfold increase in risk (a statement about relative risk) has different meanings in terms of the total numbers of people involved in each of these cases. Thus a tenfold increase in risk at 1 per 1,000 is 10 per thousand, or 10,000 people per million. A tenfold increase in risk at 10 per million is 100 people per million, meaning that far fewer people will be affected.

2. What is the likelihood of your personal exposure? Risk increases with amount of exposure or dosage and duration of exposure.

3. What are the tradeoffs? For example, is it acceptable to use a pesticide that lowers food costs substantially, yet could increase the number of cancer deaths by 1 in a million? This would be an application of a so-called "negligible risk" standard. (See also GENETIC ENGINEERING.)

Zeckhauser, Richard J. and Viscusi, W. Kip, "Risk Within Reason," *Science*, 248 (May 4, 1990), pp. 559–64.

RNA (ribonucleic acid)   The type of biomolecule that directs the synthesis of PROTEIN after receiving information from DNA. RNA is classified as a NUCLEIC ACID, the same chemical family as DNA. Three different types of RNA perform different functions in protein synthesis. "Messenger-RNA" represents a copy of the genetic material that carries the code words specifying the amino acid sequence characteristic of each protein. "Ribosomal RNA" occurs in ribosomes, cytoplasmic particles that combine with messenger RNA and provide the site of protein synthesis. A third family of RNA is "transfer RNA," which carries activated amino acids to assemble proteins. Transfer RNAs "read" code words in the messenger RNA, align amino acids in the proper sequence and permit amino acids to be joined together. Thus transfer RNAs help translate the language of DNA into the language of proteins in all cells.

In terms of composition, RNA consists of phosphate; the simple sugar, ribose; and four nitrogen-containing compounds (ADENINE, GUANINE, uracil and CYTOSINE). Three of these bases occur in DNA; only uracil is unique to RNA. RNA is assembled by the body from simple nutrients, and there is no dietary requirement for RNA. The enzyme that synthesizes RNA (RNA polymerase) requires the trace mineral nutrient ZINC for activity. (See also PURINE; PYRIMIDINE; URIC ACID.)

rosemary (*Rosmarinus officinalis*)   A perennial evergreen that grows as a shrub. Rosemary has long, thin leaves with a rich aromatic scent. Leaves of this pungent herb are used dried or fresh as a strong seasoning for pork, veal, lamb and chicken. It is used with tomato sauce, marinades, soups and ragouts. Rosemary extracts are used as an antioxidant by the food industry. The herb contains rosemaricine, which can stimulate the digestive tract, help with fat digestion and lessen joint pain. It has been used as an antiseptic mouthwash and gargle.

rotation diet (rotary diet)   A DIET plan in which related FOODS or foods within botanical families are not eaten more frequently than every four days. Studies of patients, especially children with food ALLERGIES, suggest that rotating foods and eating them in moderation reduces the tendency to develop new food allergies or to activate existing sensitivities. Rotation diets can help reduce the symptoms of food allergies and to identify problematic foods. Use of rotation diets also permits the patient to eliminate many foods. A variety of books are now available to assist in food selection, menu planning and meal preparation. Typically, foods are listed in four columns representing days one to four and grouped according to families. Typical categories include MEAT, GRAIN, FISH, FRUIT, VEGETABLES, beverages, NUTS and seeds, NATURAL SWEETENERS, MILK or milk substitutes, thickeners and fats and oils. Foods in one list do not appear in the other lists, in order to avoid selecting a food more frequently than every four days.

It is advisable to begin a rotation diet slowly because this type of diet represents major adjustments. One approach is to begin by rotating grains/starches by using wheat products on day one, then rice products on day two, then corn products on day three, with oats on day four. Grain alternatives such as AMARANTH, QUINOA, MILLET or BARLEY can be substituted for any of the above grain groups. After one to two weeks meats can be rotated, for example, beef (red meat) on day one, then turkey (poultry) on day two, then pork (red meat) on day three, then chicken (poultry) on day four. Note that veal, calf liver, venison and lamb fall within the beef category because these are related. Similarly, goose and turkey fall in the turkey group, and pheasant and quail are listed with chicken. To rotate fruits, the following are options: CITRUS FRUIT on day one, followed by the apple/grape family on day two, then by MELONS on day three and berries on day four. For vegetables, options can include CARROTS, BEETS, CHARD, SPINACH or CELERY on day one; then the LEGUMES with PEAS, BEANS, LENTILS or soy, or the squash family on day two; then nightshade vegetables, such as POTATO, EGGPLANT or PEPPERS on day three; and the cabbage family with CAULIFLOWER, BROCCOLI or BRUSSELS SPROUTS on day four. Symptoms may improve after several weeks of diet rotation. Often it is easier to use a rotation diet when other family members support each other in making major dietary changes.

Rapp, Doris, *Is This Your Child*. New York: William Morrow, 1991.

rutabaga (*Brassica napobrassica*; Swedish turnip)   A root vegetable that resembles a large TURNIP. It is believed to have originated in a hybrid between KALE and turnip, perhaps in Medieval Europe. Rutabaga is used both as food and as livestock fodder. In the United States it is grown mainly in the northern states. Unlike turnip greens, rutabaga leaves are not edible. The root can be baked, boiled and mashed with potatoes, served in souffles, casseroles, stews and soups.

Turnips and rutabagas contain small amounts of GOITROGENS, substances that block IODINE uptake. The effects of these materials can be worsened by an iodine-deficient diet and when large quantities are eaten, not a usual situation in the United States. Rutabagas are a rich source of vitamin C. The nutrient content of 1 cup (140 g) of rutabagas is: 64 calories; protein, 1.5 g; carbohydrate, 15.4 g; fiber, 1.4 g; fat, 0.28 g; vitamin A, 810 IU; vitamin C, 60 mg; thiamin, 0.1 mg; riboflavin, 0.1 mg; niacin, 0.14 mg.

rye (*Secale cereale*)   A common cereal grain related to wheat. Rye was domesticated in northern Europe in the 4th century B.C., and independently in Asia and the Middle East. In Medieval Europe rye became a staple bread grain. Presently rye flour is second only to wheat flour in terms of worldwide popularity for bread making, although it accounts for only 3% of the worldwide production of cereal grains and ranks eighth in the world. Northern Europe remains a major region for rye production. Popularity in the United States has declined steadily since 1920, and currently the United States produces 2% of the world rye crop. Ergot, a fungus that produces a poisonous substance that can cause convulsions, can infect rye. Limits have been established for ergot contamination.

Rye berries (groats), representing the husked whole grain, can be cooked like RICE. Whole rye flour is dark and contains most of the nutrients of rye berries. Light rye flour is a refined product, containing relatively more starch and less germ; it may be bleached. Bleached rye flour is less nutritious than dark flour. Cracked rye is crushed rye berries. It can be cooked like cracked wheat or OATS, as a BREAKFAST CEREAL. Rolled rye flakes are produced by heating rye berries until soft, and flattening them with steel rollers. Rye is used to produce crackers and rye flakes are used as a hamburger extender. Rye is also sprouted and served as a salad green. Rye is fermented to make whiskey.

Authentic rye bread is dense with a robust flavor. It is less responsive to yeast as a leavening agent, consequently wheat flour is often added to improve dough rising properties. Rye bread prepared with wheat flour may contain artificial coloring or other coloring to darken it. The nutrient value of rye is similar to wheat. Rye protein, like wheat protein, is deficient in the essential amino acid LYSINE. Rye flour (1 cup, dark) provides 419 calories; protein, 20.9 g; carbohydrate, 87.2 g; fiber, 3.1 g; fat, 3.3 g; calcium, 69 mg; sodium, 1 mg; thiamin, 0.78 mg; riboflavin, 0.28 mg; niacin, 3.5 mg.

saccharin   One of the oldest approved ARTIFICIAL SWEET-ENERS. Saccharin has been available for over 100 years. It is not metabolized in humans and it provides no calories. Although saccharin is 300 to 700 times sweeter than TABLE SUGAR, it is often perceived to have a bitter or "metallic" aftertaste at high concentrations. Saccharin is generally combined with a sugar, DEXTROSE, or with ASPARTAME, another artificial sweetener, for tabletop sweeteners, for instance to sweeten coffee. The compound is stable to baking and acidic conditions; this versatility contributes to its use in many products, including baked foods, salad dressings, reduced calorie jams, toothpaste, mouthwash and other personal care products. Saccharin can be added to chewing gum where it is used with SORBITOL, a sweet sugar analog.

Large doses of saccharin are linked to bladder cancer in experimental animals, suggesting that people who consume large amounts of saccharin may have an increased risk of bladder cancer. The U.S. FDA proposed banning saccharin in 1977 as a potential CARCINOGEN (cancer-causing agent). Congress voted to exempt saccharin from the federal law that prohibits the sale of cancer-causing substances, and this exemption continues today. Saccharin continues to be used as a sweetener, although CYCLAMATE, the first approved artificial sweetener, was banned under similar circumstances. The food industry feels that there is no RISK at the usual level of consumption. Foods and beverages containing saccharin are required to have a warning that "saccharin has been determined to cause cancer in laboratory animals." (See also DELANEY CLAUSE; FOOD ADDITIVES; NATURAL SWEETENERS.)

Clark, Nancy, "How Safe Are Artificial Sweeteners?" *The Physician and Sports Medicine*, 21 (February, 1993), pp. 45–46.

safflower (*Carthamus tinctorius*)   A thistle-like plant that produces oil-rich seeds resembling small sunflower seeds. Safflower is a late arrival in the United States, becoming an established crop only in the 1950s and 1960s as POLYUNSATURATED VEGETABLE OILS gained in popularity in response to fears about CHOLESTEROL and SATURATED FAT and their link to ATHEROSCLEROSIS. Varieties of safflower yielding 50% oil have been developed. Safflower is cultivated in California and Montana.

Safflower oil contains the highest percentage of polyunsaturated FATTY ACIDS and the lowest percentage of saturated fatty acids among commercially available oils. Typically safflower oil contains 74 to 77% LINOLEIC ACID, an essential polyunsaturated fatty acid; 16.4% OLEIC ACID, a monounsaturated fatty acid; and 6.6% saturated fatty acids. Like SOYBEAN oil, it has a high smoke point (440° to 480° F) and is often used in deep-fat frying and sauteing. Safflower oil is rich in VITAMIN E. As a polyunsaturated oil, it is susceptible to RANCIDITY (decomposition) when heated. These oils should not be reheated.

Like all commercial polyunsaturated cooking oils, safflower is partially hydrogenated to reduce its susceptibility to oxidation and decrease the rate of rancidity. Hydrogenation refers to the chemical hardening process that adds hydrogen atoms and decreases the level of saturation. Hydrogenated safflower oil yields MARGARINE, VEGETABLE SHORTENING, MAY-

ONNAISE and other products. Hydrogenation creates TRANS-FATTY ACIDS. The safety of these unusual products has been questioned.

The consumption of polyunsaturated vegetable oils like safflower oil can lower the level of LDL (LOW-DENSITY LIPOPROTEIN), the less desirable form of cholesterol, but at the same time a high intake can lower the level of HDL (HIGH-DENSITY LIPOPROTEIN), the desirable form of cholesterol. (See also ESSENTIAL FATTY ACIDS.)

saffron (*Crocus sativus*) This small crocus produces flowers with intense yellow-orange filaments. When dried, the stamens yield a pungent spice and brilliant yellow coloring agent. Saffron is used for rice dishes, soups and sauces, as well as certain meat dishes in Indian, Italian and Spanish cuisine. Saffron is best dissolved in a small amount of warm water before use for uniform mixing. (See also FOOD ADDITIVES; FOOD COLORING, NATURAL.)

sage (*Salvia officinalis*) A common perennial HERB whose fresh or dried leaves add a pungent, bitter taste to foods. There are over 500 varieties of sage, including the common garden sage. It is used to flavor poultry, fatty meat like pork, veal, ham or lamb, and in marinades, minestrone and sauces. Sage has long been used as a medicinal herb in folk medicine. Its name comes from the Latin *salvus*, which means healthy. It possesses bacterial and antifungal properties and it has been used to aid digestion. Sage tea has been used to reduce coughing associated with colds and for irregular menstruation. As with any medicinal herb the consumption of large amounts, for long periods of time, is not recommended. (See also PARSLEY.)

sago Starch from the trunk of a tropical palm. In the South Pacific sago palm flour and starch are staple foods. They are used as food thickeners. Commercially, sago starch is used as a non-corn source of glucose from which to manufacture corn-free VITAMIN C for certain individuals who are ultrasensitive to corn products. (See also OIL PALM; PALM OILS.)

saliva The fluid secreted by glands of the MOUTH. Three pairs of salivary glands produce saliva. Parotid glands, located on each side of the face, drain through ducts opening in the inner surface of the cheek. Sublingual glands drain into the floor of the mouth. Submaxillary glands (submandibular glands) are located beneath the base of the tongue and drain in the floor of the mouth. Tiny buccal glands in the mouth also contribute saliva. The combined saliva from all these sources amounts to a quart (1 liter) of fluid daily.

In composition, saliva is 99.5% water. Saliva serves important functions: It acts as a lubricant, as a moistening agent and as a dissolving agent for flavors as food is chewed and swallowed. Saliva contains mucins, slippery PROTEINS that provide the lubricating action. Without water and mucins, swallowing would be very difficult. Saliva contains the digestive enzyme AMYLASE, which initiates starch DIGESTION, and chewing food thoroughly to a uniform paste assists starch breakdown by this enzyme. Saliva also contains ions (electrolytes)—SODIUM, CHLORIDE and BICARBONATE. Chloride activates amylase. These minerals are later absorbed and recycled. For defense, saliva contains

lysozyme, an enzyme that ruptures some disease-producing bacteria, and a protective ANTIBODY, secretory IgA, that can bind to foreign materials, including viruses, bacteria and yeast, to reduce this risk of infection.

Salivation is controlled exclusively by the NERVOUS SYSTEM. Savory aromas, visual images, sounds of food preparation and memories can stimulate salivation. Salivation also occurs in response to irritating foods and with nausea. Saliva flow after eating flushes chemical remnants out of the mouth and adjusts the acidity to neutral. Dehydration can decrease salivation. A variety of medications, such as antihistamines (diphenylpyraline and azatidine), diminish mucous secretions, including saliva. Stress stimulates the sympathetic nervous system to reduce salivation. On the other hand dryness of the mouth promotes thirst sensations. (See also DEGLUTITION; TASTE.)

salmon (*Oncorhynchus*) A saltwater fish valued as a food fish and as a sport fish. The word salmon is derived from the Latin SALMO, which means "leaping." Salmon can weigh up to 65 lb (30 kg) and measure up to 3 ft (1 m) in length. Varieties include the Atlantic salmon and the five varieties of Pacific salmon: sockeye (red) salmon (*O. nerka*), both canned and sold fresh; Chinook (king) salmon (*O. tschawytscha*), the largest and fattiest variety; coho (sliver) salmon (*O. kisutch*), smaller fish, sold fresh; pink (humpback) salmon (*O. gorbuscha*), the smallest variety, bland flesh, sold canned; and chum (dog) salmon (*O. keta*), lower in fat and with pale flesh. Salmon are a migratory fish that spawn in fresh water. Young fish live in fresh water for two years before migrating to the sea. Pollution, dam construction and over-harvesting have drastically reduced the numbers of this food fish in many parts of the world. Commercial salmon comes from many countries such as Chile, Norway and Canada (Eastern Canada and British Columbia). Imported salmon are generally pen-raised rather than wild ranging fish. Domestic, pen-raised salmon are also readily available. In the United States, Maine, Alaska and Washington support most major salmon fisheries, and canned salmon comes from the northern Pacific. Most Atlantic salmon comes from Canada and Norway.

Salmon is an oily fish, rich in beneficial marine lipids. Salmon fat contains 30 to 40% omega-3 polyunsaturated FATTY ACIDS, mainly EPA (EICOSAPENTAENOIC ACID) and DHA (DOCASAHEXAENOIC ACID). These polyunsaturates are believed to decrease the risk of STROKE and CARDIOVASCULAR DISEASE. They decrease the risk of blood clots by inhibiting blood platelet aggregation. Platelets are cell fragments in the blood that initiate clotting.

Pen-raised salmon are more likely to be contaminated with industrial pollutants when grown in waters near industrial areas. Consumer advocates have criticized seafood safety in the United States. PCB contamination has been detected in fresh salmon though the levels were below tolerance limits set by the U.S. FDA. Canned salmon sold in the United States comes from the Pacific off the coast of Alaska, an area less likely to be polluted by industrial waste. Salmon is smoked, poached, grilled, marinated, baked or canned. The nutrient content of 3 oz (85 g) of broiled salmon is: 140 calories; protein, 21 g; fat, 5 g; cholesterol, 60 mg; thiamin, 0.18 mg; riboflavin, 0.14 mg; niacin, 5.5 g. (See also FISH OIL; OMEGA-3 FATTY ACIDS; SEAFOOD.)

salmonella A bacterium that frequently causes FOOD POISONING. Over 1,300 strains of salmonella have been identified. Salmonella does not form spores and is destroyed by heat (cooking and PASTEURIZATION). Its usual habitat is the intestinal tract of an animal host. Salmonella occurs in animal feed, food processing plants and food handling, and the bacteria are easily spread by fecal contamination. Flies, rodents and insects that contact infected fecal material may also contaminate food. Sewage-contaminated water is known to carry salmonella and cause disease.

Livestock and poultry are major sources of human infection. Salmonella bacteria now contaminate an estimated 37% of CHICKENS and TURKEYS, 12% of PORK and 5% of all BEEF. Salmonella grows readily in milk and milk-derived dishes like custard, egg dishes and salad dressing. MEAT and meat products like SAUSAGE, meat pies, sandwiches and chili can become contaminated when allowed to stand at room temperature for several hours if infected by a food handler.

Salmonellosis

A form of food poisoning caused by salmonella. Salmonellosis is one of the three most common food-borne diseases associated with bacteria, and it is one of the fastest growing food-borne illnesses. Salmonellosis affects 4 million Americans yearly. Some strains of salmonella resist antibiotics, and dairy cattle fed antibiotics were the likely source of a drug-resistant salmonella strain that caused a large U.S. outbreak of food poisoning, involving six states in 1985. This outbreak caused 1,000 deaths, 35,000 hospitalizations and left an estimated 125,000 people with increased risk of chronic illnesses such as ARTHRITIS, osteomyelitis, ankylosing spondylitis and COLITIS.

Salmonellosis often causes flu-like symptoms. Fever, abdominal cramping, headache, DIARRHEA and vomiting generally appear 12 to 36 hours after eating tainted food. Symptoms may last from two days to a week. Illness is most severe in those with weakened immune systems, commonly found in very young children and in elderly people. Maldigestion and MALABSORPTION can result from intestinal damage due to this disease.

Salmonellosis was almost unknown in the United States 40 years ago. Increased volume and speed of food production, increased drug resistance of bacteria and relaxed enforcement by government agencies contributed to widespread contamination of food, especially POULTRY. Raw milk, raw cheese, any raw or undercooked meat including salami and hamburger, and fresh eggs can be contaminated by feces and fecal bacteria and can thus be a potential source of contamination. Pasteurized eggs are used to prepare commercial MAYONNAISE and it is not a carrier. Salmonella is not likely to infect fruit or vegetables. Freshwater as well as marine fish caught from waters highly polluted by raw sewage may be contaminated by salmonella.

All food handlers should thoroughly wash their hands before handling food to eliminate fecal contamination. They should carefully clean all equipment used in food preparation, including cutting boards. Raw vegetables should not come into contact with utensils used to prepare raw meat and poultry. Food should be refrigerated. Salmonella is destroyed by heating at 140° F (60° C) for 20 minutes or at 149° F (60° C) for three minutes. (See also BOTULISM.)

Hedberg, Craig W., et al., "A multistate outbreak of *Salmonella javiana* and *Salmonella oranienburg* infections due to consumption of contaminated cheese," *Journal of the American Medical Association*, 268:22 (Dec. 9, 1992), pp. 3203–07.

salt See SODIUM.

salt substitutes (potassium chloride, lite salt, low-sodium salt) A combination of chemicals that taste like table salt but contains less SODIUM. Excessive dietary sodium causes HIGH BLOOD PRESSURE in hypertensive people who are sodium sensitive. Most salt substitutes are mixtures of table salt (sodium chloride) and POTASSIUM chloride. Potassium chloride is a different compound from sodium chloride. It tastes bitter, not salty. Potassium is an essential nutrient in its own right and can lower blood pressure in some people. Excessive potassium can irritate the stomach and might start an ulcer. Diseased or damaged kidneys may not be able to excrete potassium properly; a toxic excess can accumulate. Therefore patients taking certain DIURETICS (water pills), beta blockers or non-steroidal anti-inflammatory drugs; who are diabetic; or who have kidney disease are advised to avoid such salt substitutes. The safest strategy is to cut back on salt entirely and to use herbs and spices to improve the flavor in place of table salt. There are many different herbs to choose from, each with its own different, pleasing flavor. Consider CAYENNE pepper, basil, garlic powder, mace, marjoram, SAGE, savory and thyme, or blends. (See also FOOD ADDITIVES; HYPERTENSION.)

salt tablets See SODIUM.

sardine Various small saltwater fish, including alewife, Atlantic HERRING, pilchard and sprat. The name probably originated from the small Mediterranean fish in the vicinity of the island of Sardinia. Sardines are a fatty fish. Atlantic herring is a good source of OMEGA-3 FATTY ACIDS, the essential fatty acids thought to protect against heart attacks.

Sardines are rich sources of calcium because the fish is cooked bones and all. Its soft bones contribute to a high calcium content. A 4-oz serving of sardines provides 50% of the REFERENCE DAILY INTAKE (RDI) of calcium and 20% of the RDI of iron. Sardines contain significant levels of salt. The same 4-oz serving provides approximately 600 mg of sodium, one-third to one-half of the amount judged safe.

Sardines are often packed in oil, which increases their calories. Sardines packed in olive oil would be preferable to those packed in soybean oil because of olive oil's greater stability and protective effects against heart disease. Norwegian sardines are often packed in sardine oil, which has a high content of omega-3 fatty acids. Blot the fish in oil with a paper towel before eating them, to remove excess oil and to lower calories. Sardines packed in water are now available. The nutrient content of 3 oz (85 g) of sardines (canned, packed in soybean oil, drained and including bones) is: 175 calories; protein, 20 g; fat, 9.4 g; cholesterol, 85 mg; calcium, 371 mg; iron, 2.6 mg; thiamin, 0.03 mg; riboflavin, 0.17 mg; niacin, 4.6 mg.

sarsaparilla (*Smilax sarsaparilla*) A medicinal herb native to tropical regions of South America and the Caribbean. This perennial evergreen grows as a vine; its roots are used in botanical medicine. Europeans learned of its use from Native Americans. According to folk traditions, sarsaparilla has been used as a tonic (to improve body function) and in the treatment of coughs, digestive disorders, fever, gout, skin conditions and arthritis. Externally it has been used for burns and wounds. No toxicity has been reported, though the effects of long-term, high level consumption are unknown.

Sarsaparilla contains a family of saponins, steroid-like molecules that appear to bind cell wall materials released by bacteria in the intestine. Endotoxins can be absorbed by the gut and pass into the bloodstream unless removed by the liver. By rendering endotoxins unabsorbable, sarsaparilla may improve liver function and decrease the burden of foreign materials. The plant does not contain testosterone, the male hormone, and does not increase muscle mass, thus there is little evidence to support the contention that sarsaparilla acts as a sexual rejuvenator. Sarsaparilla extracts have been routinely used to flavor beverages, candy, baked goods and other foods.

satiety   The sense of being filled up and having APPETITE satisfied, as opposed to HUNGER. Appetite is a complex phenomenon involving many psychological and biochemical factors. No single event is likely to control it. Fat and oils in foods slow emptying of the stomach and contribute to the feeling of being full. Researchers are exploring the hypothesis that depleted fat cells may signal the brain to eat and cause hunger after weight loss. LEPTIN, a recently discovered protein produced by fat cells, has been shown to enter the brain and control the consumption of fatty foods. Dietary FIBER, undigestible plant material, swells when moistened, creating a feeling of fullness. As a further benefit, fiber displaces calorie-rich foods, so fewer calories are eaten.

Mechanical contact with food triggers the stomach and intestine to release gut peptides that trigger satiety. This feedback mechanism requires 10 to 20 minutes, while signals are being sent back to the brain. As an example the hormone CHOLECYSTOKININ signals the brain to stop sending hunger signals after eating. Whether cholecystokinin can be manipulated by dietary changes is not known for certain. Brain peptides are also probably involved in regulatory food consumption and satiety. Enterostatin decreases fat intake in experimental animals. The development of drugs to increase satiety is currently an area of active research. Strategies to promote a feeling of satiation and to curb appetite include eating a snack a half-hour before a meal, eating slowly and chewing each bite thoroughly and waiting 20 minutes before taking a second helping. These approaches give the hormone time to reach the brain and create a feeling of fullness. (See also APPETITE SUPPRESSANTS; CRAVING.)

saturated fat   FAT that contains a high percentage of saturated FATTY ACIDS and exists as a solid at room temperature. Saturation is a chemical concept, referring to the fact that carbon atoms in the fatty acid molecules are bonded to a maximum number of hydrogen atoms ("filled up"). Typical sources of saturated fat are animal fat, as found in BEEF, veal, LAMB, PORK, meat products, MILK, EGGS, BUTTER and products like ICE CREAM, milk and CHOCOLATE. Certain plant oils are also saturated, including COCONUT OIL, PALM and palm kernel oils. Unsaturated fat (vegetable oils) can be converted to saturated fats by a chemical process called hydrogenation, and these appear on the market as vegetable shortening.

Saturated Fatty Acids

Common building blocks of fats and oils, these organic acids contain a maximum number of hydrogen atoms and lack double bonds. Fatty acids are built of carbon chains, which may be long or short. Long-chain, saturated fatty acids include PALMITIC ACID (16 carbon atoms) and STEARIC ACID (18 carbon atoms). They are waxy solids at room temperature and can form fats that are also solids at room temperature. Typical short-chain saturated fatty acids include: acetic acid (containing two carbon atoms), propionic acid (with three carbon atoms), and BUTYRIC ACID (four carbon atoms). Medium-chain fatty acids include CAPRYLIC ACID (with eight carbons); capric acid (10 carbons); lauric acid (12 carbons); and myristic acid (14 carbons). All saturated fatty acids are readily oxidized by mitochondrial enzyme systems to produce energy with carbon dioxide and water as waste products. Fatty acids yield more than twice the amount of energy as carbohydrate and protein when they are burned. (See also ESSENTIAL FATTY ACIDS.)

McNamara, Donald and Howell, Warden H., "Epidemiologic Data Linking Diet to Hyperlipidemia and Arteriosclerosis; *Seminars in Liver Disease*, 12:4 (1992), pp. 347–55.

saturated vegetable oils   See TROPICAL OILS.

sauce   A flavorful relish or liquid dressing served with foods. Sauces are usually high-FAT foods. Stroganoff and orloff usually contain butter. Hollandaise and bearnaise contain butter and egg yolks; bearnaise contains undercooked raw egg yolk and so is a potential source of food poisoning. MAYONNAISE contains egg yolks, VINEGAR and a vegetable oil. Brown sauces (bordelaise and bourguignon) may be lower in fat if fat has been skimmed off and if butter has not been added. Tartar sauce and remoulade are flavored mayonnaise. When ordering an entree with a sauce, have it served separately so that you can add small amounts and limit the fat calories it contributes.

sauerkraut   Fermented white CABBAGE. Cabbage is pickled in salt, spices and cabbage juice by lactic acid-producing bacteria. The lactic acid gives sauerkraut its characteristic sour flavor. Canned sauerkraut also has a very high sodium level (up to 780 mg per half-cup). It can be strained and rinsed to decrease the sodium content. Dill seed and onion can be used to enhance the flavor of sauerkraut. (See also FERMENTATION; FOOD PRESERVATION.)

sausage   A seasoned, ground meat product usually containing high levels of SODIUM and FAT and packed in a casing. The term sausage is derived from the Latin *salsicius*, meaning "seasoned with salt." Most sausage contains highly seasoned, finely ground beef and pork and table salt. Any meat from a USDA-inspected carcass can be used to make sausage and animal fat can be added. Thus blood sausage is made from blood, pork fat and seasoning. The final product may be cured (smoked) and dry or semidry. Dry and semidry sausage may contain NITRITES as preservatives, which have been linked to an increased risk of stomach cancer if consumed in large amounts. Fresh sausage is made from raw meat and must be cooked. Semidry sausage has been smoked; dry sausage may or may not be smoked; and cooked sausage is ready to eat. Examples include BOLOGNA, braunschweiger, frankfurter, head cheese, knackwurst, liverwurst, salami, souse and Vienna sausage.

Sausages contain ample protein, iron and many B vitamins; however, they also contain almost 55% of their calories as fat. A few brands contain less than 40% of their calories as fat. Tofu and turkey sausage may contain less fat than pork or beef products. It is recommended that sausage be eaten as a condiment or flavoring with foods rather than as a main dish.

Pork sausage, cooked, can provide 72% of calories as fat; fat accounts for 31% of the weight. One link, 13 g, provides 50 calories; protein, 2.5 g; carbohydrate, 0.1 g; fat, 4 g; cholesterol, 11 mg; sodium, 168 mg; thiamin, 0.1 mg; riboflavin, 0.03 mg; niacin, 0.59 mg. (See also CHICKEN; MEAT, PROCESSED; MEAT SUBSTITUTES; POULTRY.)

saute Refers to pan frying small strips or slices of food quickly in a hot skillet with a small amount of butter or oil. Be sure oil is hot before adding foods to minimize the amounts of oil they soak up. Pork slices, veal scallops, chicken breast, fish fillet, tofu, onions, carrots, garlic and other vegetables and grains can be sauteed.

saw palmetto (*Serenoa repens*)   A small palm tree native to South Carolina, Georgia and Florida that produces berries with medicinal properties. Saw palmetto berries have a long history of use by Native Americans, while later European physicians used the berries to treat enlarged prostate (benign prostatic hyperplasia), genito-urinary tract imbalances and as a tonic to boost nutrient and general body functioning. Modern formulations employ a fat-soluble extract of saw palmetto berries containing large-molecular-weight alcohols and plant sterols, compounds related to cholesterol. Saw palmetto berry extracts block the conversion of the male sex hormone, testosterone, to a more potent compound, dehydrotestosterone, that promotes prostatic enlargement, and promote the breakdown of the more active compound. These effects may possibly explain the saw palmetto relief of common symptoms such as decreased urination at night, increased urinary flow rates, and decreased residual urine content in the bladder. No significant side effects of saw palmetto berry extracts or berries have been noted.

School Breakfast Program (National School Breakfast Program)   A federal program to provide funds for nutritious breakfasts for children. The National School Breakfast Program was established by the Child Nutrition Act of 1966 and authorized as a permanent appropriation in 1975. Fewer children participate in the BREAKFAST program than in the SCHOOL LUNCH PROGRAM: only 4.4 million children participated in the former in 1991, as compared to 24.2 million participating in the latter because many school districts are not required to offer it. Usually a state's Department of Education administers this program.

The school breakfast must contain one serving each of MILK, FRUIT, VEGETABLE or full-strength juice. It must provide either one serving of MEAT or meat alternative (eggs, peanut butter, cooked legumes or nuts), with a serving of BREAD or bread alternative; or two servings of meat or meat alternative; or two servings of bread or bread alternative (hamburger bun, cooked cereal grains, macaroni, spaghetti). The programs generally provide more PROTEIN, CALCIUM, PHOSPHORUS and MAGNESIUM, but less VITAMIN A, IRON and VITAMIN B$_6$ than typical non-school breakfasts for youngsters.

Factors weighed in planning school food service programs include: cultural and ethnic backgrounds of students, needs of handicapped students, as well as fitting meals to accommodate class and bus schedules. Practical nutrition education can be part of breakfast programs. Evaluation of school nutrition programs finds that most students participating in school breakfast programs are from low-income families.

Breakfast is considered the most important meal for both children and adults because of its positive impact on performance and alertness. Nonetheless many Americans skip breakfast, especially teenagers. Students who skip breakfast have higher rates of tardiness, higher absenteeism and lower performance, and more FATIGUE. Researchers found that low-income children who participated in the School Breakfast Program in 1987 had higher standardized achievement test scores than children not in the program that year. (See also: HUNGER; WIC.)

School Lunch Program (National School Lunch Program)   A federal program established under the National School Lunch Program of 1946 to protect the health of U.S. children through the consumption of nutritious foods. The act authorized state grant-in-aid program to provide cash and food. The cost is shared among the USDA, state and local governments, and children's families. Household income determines whether a child will receive a reduced rate or free meal. To qualify, household income must be below 185% of the federal poverty level; for free meals household income must fall below 130% of the poverty level.

The National School Lunch Program is open to public and private schools and to residential child care institutions. Schools that participate in the program receive financial assistance, donated surplus commodities and technical assistance in equipping and managing the program. In the 1970s the Nutrition Education and Training Program was developed to educate students about the relationship between nutrition and health, to train food service personnel in management, and to instruct teachers in nutrition education. The program was expanded due to increased need for low-cost, subsidized meals, especially among economically disadvantaged children.

In 1993 about 25 million students participated in the National School Lunch Program daily. Fifty-four percent of children in school participated in school lunch programs; more than half came from lower-income families and received meals either free or at a reduced cost. The program has continued to serve nutritious school lunches to children who would not likely receive lunch from another source. Furthermore, school lunches have provided approximately 33% of the RECOMMENDED DIETARY ALLOWANCES (RDAs) for children of various ages. Eligibility for participation in the program is contingent upon operating on a nonprofit basis, providing free or reduced price lunches to needy children, making lunches available to all children regardless of origin, providing dining and kitchen facilities, avoiding segregation of needy children and serving meals that conform to USDA guidelines.

The USDA surveyed school lunches in 1993 and concluded that lunches offered by schools exceeded the government's recommendations for fat and sodium. The study found that school lunches provided 38% of daily calories as fat and 15% of calories from saturated fat. Governmental guidelines call for no more than 30% of daily calories from fat, with saturated fat supplying no more than 10% of calories. School lunches provided 1,469 mg of sodium; and all meals combined gave an average of 4,633 mg per day. The National Research Council (NRC) advises a daily consumption of no more than 2,400 mg. School lunches typically provide 47% of their calories as carbohydrate. The NRC advises consuming more than 55% of daily calories as carbohydrate. Because the lunch program requires both milk and meat (or meat alternative) to be served daily, some children obtain 270% of their protein requirement from school lunches.

A 1994 proposal regulating school lunches requires 2 oz of meat or meat alternative such as peanut butter, eggs, cooked legumes or nuts; two servings of fruits or vegetables, totaling three-quarters of a cup; a slice and a half of bread; and 8 oz of milk. The average amount of fat served (per week) could not exceed 30% of total calories, and the average saturated fat consumption could not exceed 10%. Schools have until 1998 to implement these changes.

Research carried out by the USDA shows that students who participate in the School Lunch Program have better nutrient intake than children who do not. Furthermore, low-income children depend on this program for 30 to 50% of their total daily nutrient intake. (See also HUNGER; WIC.)

Burghardt, John A., and Devaney, Barbara L., eds., "School Lunch Dietary Assessment Study," *American Journal of Clinical Nutrition,* 61: supp. (January 1995), pp. 173S–257S.
Kennedy, Eileen and Goldberg, Jeanne. "What are American children eating? Implications for Public Policy," *Nutrition Reviews* 53:5 (1995), pp. 111–26.

scurvy   A disease caused by severe deficiency of VITAMIN C (ascorbic acid). Scurvy has been described since ancient times. Long sea voyages of the 15th through the 17th centuries frequently decimated the ranks of sailors. As early as 1593 a British admiral demonstrated that lemon juice cured the disease. A Scottish naval surgeon conducted the first controlled experiment in the treatment of scurvy in 1753, which proved that citrus fruits protected seamen and cured scurvy. Not until 40 years later were limes routinely issued to British seamen to prevent scurvy. However, scurvy continued into more recent times. It was prevalent during the American Civil War, and in 1912 half the men on Scott's expedition to the South Pole died of scurvy.

During initial stages of vitamin C deficiency, an individual may feel listless. Wounds may heal slowly and gums may bleed easily. Bruising occurs easily. Minute hemorrhages appear around hair follicles or stomach, buttocks, legs and arms. Later stages are characterized by weight loss, weakness, painful muscles and swollen joints; spongy gums and loss of teeth. Vitamin C plays several important roles that can be related to scurvy. Chief among these is the requirement for vitamin C in COLLAGEN. The formation of mature collagen, the major structural protein of connective tissue, relies upon the availability of key building blocks called hydroxyproline and hydroxylysine. The production of hydroxyproline from proline and of hydroxyl lysine from lysine requires vitamin C. As a versatile antioxidant and key support nutrient of the immune system, vitamin C exhibits wide-ranging benefits on health. Modest deficiencies (subclinical deficiencies) do not manifest themselves as scurvy, rather they increase the susceptibility to infections and oxidative damage leading to chronic diseases.

Infants relying on cow's milk may be prone to scurvy because much of the vitamin C is destroyed during pasteurization. Infants require proportionately higher levels of vitamin C because of their high rate of tissue growth. Breastmilk contains adequate vitamin C to support infant development.

Among adults, low-income elderly persons are susceptible to scurvy if they do not eat fresh fruit and vegetables. Overcooking destroys most vitamin C in vegetables. Chronic disease, injuries and surgery are more likely in this group, and these conditions deplete the body stores of this vitamin. (See also MALNUTRITION.)

Oeffinger, Kevin. "Scurvy: more than historical relevance," *American Family Physician,* 48:4 (September 15, 1993) pp. 609–13.

seafood   Edible marine fish and shellfish such as CLAMS, mussels, scallops, OYSTERS (mollusks), LOBSTERS and SHRIMP (crustaceans). Seafood represents an important, highly nutritious food source. It is low in saturated fat and calories and is a good source of PROTEIN, IRON, VITAMIN B$_{12}$, IODINE, PHOSPHORUS, ZINC and COPPER. Fish and fish oil are particularly rich in the omega-3 family of polyunsaturated FATTY ACIDS, which help reduce INFLAMMATION in conditions like ARTHRITIS and psoriasis, as well as reducing the risk of blood clot formation, thus offering protection against HEART ATTACKS. COD LIVER OIL contains high levels of VITAMIN A and VITAMIN D, which may be toxic when consumed in large amounts. Several servings per week of the following fatty fish are recommended: bluefish, butterfish, halibut, herring, mackerel, striped bass, orange roughy, smelt, salmon, sardines, trout and pompano.

The larva of parasitic worms may contaminate raw fish, including Pacific salmon, Pacific red snapper (rockfish) and herring; thus raw fish dishes (sushi, sashimi, CEVICHE, lomi-lomi) carry a risk of parasitic disease, such as anisakiasis. Inadequately smoked or salted fish can carry parasites. The severe abdominal pain of such a disease is due to acute intestinal inflammation. The parasite is killed by cooking marine fish thoroughly. Pregnant and nursing women, very young children and elderly people should avoid raw fish and shellfish to minimize this RISK.

Chemical Contamination

Chemical contaminants are another prominent issue in seafood safety. Fish and shellfish are generally more susceptible to chemical contamination than meat and poultry because they filter huge amounts of water through their bodies and feed on other organisms in which contaminants may be concentrated. Clams and oysters can filter 15 to 20 gallons of water daily. While thorough cooking destroys parasites and microorganisms, this does not eliminate chemical pollutants like LEAD, chlordane, DIOXIN, DDT, MERCURY, PBBs and PCBs.

Such industrial chemicals were once widely used in PESTI-CIDES, electrical insulation, plastics, dyes and other products. Over decades these environmental pollutants have crept into the FOOD CHAIN because they are not readily broken down and because they tend to accumulate in plants and animals.

Varying levels of pollutants have been reported in both domestic and imported fish. While levels of detected pollutants have generally fallen below FDA tolerance limits, those limits were set when fish consumption was lower and consequently people accumulated less of these pollutants. The level of pollutant can vary with the source, but in many markets it is often difficult for the consumer to determine the source of fish sold. Pollutant levels in salmon from Pacific waters may be lower than from other sources; however, the fish the consumer buys may come from Chile, Norway, Eastern Canada, Maine, as well as from Washington, Alaska or British Columbia.

Chemical pollutants may increase the risk of certain cancers, birth defects and neurological damage in unborn children. However, the potential health hazards of long-term, very-low-level exposure remain unknown. Because residue build-up occurs over years, it may be hard to trace a disease cause to a specific pollutant exposure.

Shellfish can accumulate disease-causing bacteria and viruses when exposed to untreated sewage. Harvesting is limited to waters that are certified as being clean, though enforcing the policy is limited by resources. Eating raw shellfish carries the risk of gastrointestinal disease with symptoms such as diarrhea, cramps, nausea and vomiting. Shellfish also transmit hepatitis A virus. Well-cooked shellfish are safer than raw or semi-cooked shellfish.

Recommendations

- Buy fresh seafood. Fish and shellfish spoil easily and should be handled with care. Fresh fish should have a mild "ocean" smell; they should not smell "fishy" or smell like ammonia.
- Purchase fresh seafood from reputable merchants who can identify their source.
- Refrigerate seafood at home immediately after purchase to prevent bacterial growth, minimize spoilage and reduce the risk of FOOD POISONING. Raw seafood that will not be eaten within two days should be frozen. Most shrimp have been frozen and thawed, and should be cooked as soon as possible.
- Thaw frozen seafood in the refrigerator or in cold running water and do not refreeze. Other raw shellfish, including lobster, should be alive when purchased.
- Refrigerate cooked shellfish and use on the same day.
- Keep mussels, clams and oysters moistened and refrigerated to keep them alive rather than storing them in plastic bags. They should not be stored for a long time in fresh water.
- Discard any shellfish that remain closed after steaming. Raw shellfish that remain closed are dead and may have begun to decompose.
- Follow the same rules in handling raw seafood as when handling raw poultry and raw meat to avoid contaminating cooked dishes or fresh vegetables with bacteria: Wash with soap and water all utensils, counter-tops, cutting boards and hands that have come into contact with raw seafood.
- Eat a variety of seafoods rather than a single source to minimize over-exposure to pollutants. Elderly people, young children, pregnant women, patients with AIDS or compromised immune systems, or with liver disease should avoid eating raw seafood.

Taylor, S.L. and Nordlee, J.A., "Chemical Additives in Seafood Products," *Clinical Reviews in Allergy*, 11 (1993), pp. 261–91.

seafood inspection   Fish and shellfish are among the most perishable foods, yet seafood is one of the least regulated foods; it remains the only flesh that does not undergo mandatory inspection. In contrast, meat and poultry processing facilities are inspected daily. A single-time FDA inspection of most U.S. seafood processing plants revealed a relatively low violation rate of up to 5.1% of plants, depending upon the region.

An estimated 20% of food-borne illness is caused by seafood. Seafood can be contaminated by bacteria, viruses, parasites and industrial wastes and pollutants. While the National Academy of Sciences has concluded that most seafood is safe to eat, this advisory organization has also recommended increased inspection and regulation of the industry. Fish testing in specific areas is left to state agencies, and testing for chemical contaminants remains scattered. Only very small numbers or samples of fish are monitored for chemical contaminants. The FDA established a new Office of Seafood in 1991 to address this issue. In 1994 the FDA launched a seafood safety initiative designed to keep contaminated seafood off the market shelves. Seafood processors need to maintain detailed records of safety procedures; to identify where shellfish were harvested; to catch fish only from waters the government has certified as being clean; and to store their catch at proper temperatures. Ready to eat seafood will have to be cooked and stored at safe temperatures as well.

sea salt   A less pure form of table salt (SODIUM chloride). Sea salt contains low levels of certain minerals found in sea water. Using 3.5 g of sea salt would supply 22% of the REF-ERENCE DAILY INTAKE (RDI) of MAGNESIUM; 2.2% of the RDI of IODINE; 2.7% of the RDI of CALCIUM. Magnesium carbonate is the additive used to prevent caking. This is more healthful than aluminum silicate used for the same purpose in refined salt. Sea salt is not iodized and lacks iodine. As a source of sodium, sea salt carries with it the same risks for HYPERTENSION (high blood pressure) as ordinary table salt in susceptible people. (See also TRACE MINERALS.)

seaweed (sea vegetables)   A large family of marine ALGAE. Edible seaweed is one of the richest sources of vitamins and minerals. Sea vegetables provide IODINE, SELENIUM, IRON, CALCIUM, PHOSPHORUS and MAGNESIUM, as well as BETA CAROTENE, VITAMIN E and the B COMPLEX. Sea vegetables are not an adequate source of vitamin B_{12} because they possess substances that are inactive analogs or forms of the compound that the body cannot use. Vegetarians who do not eat milk, eggs, fish or meat should consider taking a vitamin B_{12} supplement rather than relying on seaweed.

Traditionally, Oriental diets include a variety of seaweed. The edible algae can be categorized as brown algae and red algae. Brown algae are represented by arame, hijiki, kelp, kombu and wakame. Arame is a Japanese product; it is softened by prolonged cooking, sun-dried and finally sliced into strands and packaged. Arame contains B complex vitamins and minerals. The calcium content is 1,170 mg per 100 g. Hijiki is found in the Far East; 100 g (dry weight) contains calcium, 1,400 mg; iron, 29 mg; plus beta carotene and B complex vitamins. This seaweed is dried, steamed to stiffen it, again dried, then soaked in arame juice and dried for market. Kelp refers to a large family, and members are used commercially as a source of food additives, EMULSIFIERS, thickeners and STABILIZERS. Kelp is dried and sold whole, or powdered when it is used as a flavoring. Kelp can be steamed, pickled or boiled. It contains significant calcium and other minerals; 100 g contains calcium, 1,093 mg; sodium, 3,007 mg; and potassium, 5,273 mg.

Kombu is a general name for several species of brown algae. Dashi consists of broad strips and is used in soups, while tororo is shaved into slivers that can be marinated. Kombu is often used with root vegetables, rice and vegetables. It provides significant beta carotene, 430 retinol equivalents per 100 mg, as well as the B complex and vitamin C. Wakame comes from Japan. It is dried and processed for preservation. It can be added to soups, like miso soup, cooked as a vegetable, used as a garnish or soaked and then added to salads. Wakame contains calcium, iron and vitamins; 100 g provides calcium, 1,300 mg; iron, 13 mg; niacin, 10 mg; and vitamin C, 15 mg. Brown sea vegetables like kombu contain alginic acid and other ingredients that bind toxic heavy metals like strontium, cadmium and radium. Alginic acid is used to treat cadmium poisoning and help remove it from the body.

Red algae include carragheen and nori. Carragheen yields a gum called CARRAGEENAN that is used in prepared foods, primarily for its ability to form gels in puddings, jellies and the like. Carrageenan inhibits herpes simplex virus (oral and genital forms) as well as tumor-inducing RNA viruses in test tube experiments. It also provides (per 100 g): calcium, 885 mg; sodium, 2,892 mg; and potassium, 2,844 mg. Nori is a cultivated red sea vegetable. Fresh nori is washed, chopped into fragments, dried and packaged. Sheets of nori are wrapped around rice used in sushi and California rolls. Nori provides (per 100 g): calcium, 260 mg; iron, 12 mg; high levels of beta carotene, 11,000 retinol equivalents; thiamin, 25 mg; niacin, 10 mg; and vitamin C, 20 mg.

Seaweed has an ancient history of use in Eastern medicine, including Chinese and Indian medicine (Ayurvedic medicine). It has been used to treat intestinal parasites. GOITER, enlarged thyroid due to iodine deficiency, is effectively treated by seaweed because of its high iodine content. Certain species of seaweed have been used in folk medicine to treat high blood pressure, constipation, wounds and ulcers, GOUT, liver and kidney ailments, menstrual irregularities, and to improve digestion. Alginic acid is used in some antacids to treat ACID INDIGESTION and to treat wounds. Fucoidin is another type of complex carbohydrate (polysaccharide) from seaweed. In animals this material inhibits chemically-induced cancers. (See also FOOD ADDITIVES; MACROBIOTIC DIET.)

Wein, Bibi, "The World's Healthiest Diet," *Lifestyles*, 17:3 (March 1995), pp. 172–75.

secretin A HORMONE released by the small intestine that blocks the release of gastric juice and STOMACH ACID. Secretin slows the movement (PERISTALSIS) of material down the gastrointestinal tract. It stimulates the secretion of BICARBONATE by pancreatic duct cells to neutralize the acidic, partially digested food discharged by the STOMACH into the small intestine. To further prepare the intestine for DIGESTION, secretin stimulates bile production to aid fat digestion and the secretion of intestinal juice and digestive enzymes. Secretin release is triggered by food entering the small intestine, including partially digested carbohydrate and fat, as well as by fluids that contain high or very low concentrations of ions. (See also ENDOCRINE SYSTEM.)

selenium A TRACE MINERAL nutrient with anticancer and antiaging properties. Selenium helps protect cells against oxidative stress. As a part of the enzyme GLUTATHIONE PEROXIDASE, selenium serves as an ANTIOXIDANT by destroying highly reactive chemicals that can form FREE RADICALS. Glutathione peroxidase destroys HYDROGEN PEROXIDE, a naturally occurring chemical that is a powerful oxidizing agent. Hydrogen peroxide is produced for antimicrobial defense by macrophages, a type of white blood cell that engulfs foreign invaders, and it is a by-product of another antioxidant system (SUPEROXIDE DISMUTASE) that destroys a highly reactive form of oxygen called superoxide. Glutathione peroxidase neutralizes oxidative damage to lipids in cell membranes, thus limiting their damage due to free radical attack. Selenium may possess other antioxidant properties as well.

Selenium is generally recognized as an anticancer agent. In selenium-deficient experimental animals, LIVER cells become defective and more prone to become cancerous when activated. Studies show that populations with a low selenium intake are more prone to gastrointestinal, breast and rectal cancer. Deficiency of selenium leads to lowered glutathione peroxidase activity. Furthermore, extensive Chinese studies have suggested that selenium supplementation provides protection against hepatitis B and liver cancer. Selenium may inhibit the development of cancer by blocking the activation of certain cancer-promoting genes, by inhibiting viruses linked to cancer or by supporting healthy cell division and protecting cells against oxidative damage that could damage their DNA.

Selenium supports a healthy IMMUNE SYSTEM, where it stimulates antibody production and defensive cells (lymphocytes, macrophages and natural killer cells). Some AIDS patients may be selenium deficient. Selenium can block mercury, arsenic and cadmium poisoning. Damaged heart muscle (cardiomyopathy) has occurred in patients fed intravenously mixtures that lacked selenium, and populations in areas of China characterized by regional selenium deficiency are more disease prone. OSTEOARTHRITIS in Chinese children has also been linked to selenium deficiency.

RECOMMENDED DIETARY ALLOWANCES (RDA) published in 1989 proposed a selenium RDA for the first time as 70 mcg/day for men and 55 mcg for non-pregnant, non-lactating women. Obtaining adequate selenium is a growing problem in the United States. Regions like the Pacific Northwest, the Great Lakes region and some southern states (Georgia and the Carolinas) possess low soil concentrations of selenium, and vegetables and grains growing in depleted soils contain only low levels of selenium. Possibly acid rain prevents plants from taking up this mineral from soil. For insurance, some may wish to supplement with no more than 200 mcg of organic selenium per day. This doubles the average U.S. intake of about 100 mg/day.

Good dietary sources of selenium include organ meats, such as liver and kidney; BREWER'S YEAST; ocean FISH and SHELLFISH; and red MEAT. Vegetable sources (if grown in soil with enough selenium) are ONIONS, GARLIC, MUSHROOMS and BROCCOLI. Asparagus, cabbage and whole grains contain small amounts of selenium. FRUITS and most VEGETABLES and drinking water generally provide little selenium. Sup-plements containing inorganic selenium (sodium selenite or sodium selenate) should probably be taken separately from large amounts of vitamin C to avoid interference.

Chemically combined selenium represents the most prevalent form of the selenium in the typical diet. Selenium can replace sulfur in the amino acids CYSTEINE and METHION-INE to form the analogs, selenocysteine and selenomethion-ine. Selenocysteine occurs in a variety of proteins including glutathione peroxidase and is found in meat. Selenomethionine cannot be synthesized by the body and is supplied in the diet by a variety of foods. It can substitute for methionine in a variety of the body's proteins. The break-down of methionine and selenomethionine releases cysteine and selenocysteine, respectively.

Safety

Toxicity can occur with daily consumption of 5 mg. Toxic levels of selenium occur in agricultural drainwater in some states. Certain regions are characterized by high levels of selenium (North and South Dakota and the San Joaquin Valley of California). Soils with high selenium cause unusually high levels in plants such as wheat. Symptoms of selenium toxicity include skin sores, garlic breath, fingernails with ridges and bumps, hair loss and lethargy. Severe toxicity is indicated by fragile, black nails, metallic taste, dizziness, peripheral nerve damage, nausea, weight loss and jaundice. Children, elderly persons and people with chronic illnesses may tolerate less selenium in their diets, while physically active people may tolerate more. Sodium selenite, the inorganic form of selenium, can cause cancer at very high doses. Organic selenium that occurs in foods is not carcinogenic.

Suadicani, P., et al., "Serum Selenium Concentration and the Risk of Ischemic Heart Disease in a Prospective Cohort Study of 3,000 Males," *Atherosclerosis*, 96 (1992), pp. 33–44.

self-rising flour See BAKING SODA.

semolina Milled durum WHEAT used to produce PASTA like macaroni and spaghetti. The high protein (gluten) content of durum wheat lends itself to elastic, resilient dough that is suitable for the mechanical processing involved in making pasta.

senility (senile dementia) Memory loss associated with AGING. This phenomenon usually begins with loss of short-term memory and the ability to process new information quickly. Recollection of past events also slows down. The aging brain makes less of the NEUROTRANSMITTERS, brain chemicals required to relay nerve impulses, associated with short-term memory. ALZHEIMER'S DISEASE is not a common form of senility: Only about 5% of Americans over 65 acquire Alzheimer's disease or another degenerative brain disease.

Half the people who appear to be suffering from senile dementia and forgetfulness may experience nutritional deficiencies, including VITAMIN B_{12} deficiency due to inadequate absorption. The uptake of this vitamin declines with age, especially in those with stomach troubles. Injections of vitamin B_{12}, or taking large doses in tablet form, is a preventive measure.

Forgetfulness, learning difficulties and problems remembering new things can frequently be caused by overmedication. Nearly one-quarter of elderly U.S. citizens (65 or older) take prescription drugs they should not be using, some of which may cause confusion or amnesia. Similar problems may be due to adverse reactions to medication. As an example, DIURETICS (water pills) can cause excessive sodium loss, especially for those on a salt-restricted diet. This condition, called hyponatremia, is easily detected if the change is dramatic. However, if the change is slow, it is more difficult to detect and the symptoms match senile dementia. This condition is reversible if caught soon enough. Memory loss is also worsened by drugs blocking the formation of neurotransmitters. Drugs that fall into this category include sleeping pills and medications for reducing tremors, decreasing stomach acid and calming nerves. Other possible causes of forgetfulness include high fever, minor head injuries, DEPRESSION, loneliness and boredom. Consult a specialist in geriatrics for mental changes in older people. To combat senility, exercise the brain by keeping mentally active and avoid drugs that that characteristically cause a dry mouth because this class of drugs may interfere with neurotransmitters.

Prescription drugs Hydergine, the hormone vasopressin (antidiuretic hormone), and unipocetine have been used to enhance memory. Lipids like phosphatidylserine and phosphatidylethanolamine play structural roles in cell membranes, and treatment with these substances suggests some improvement in certain patients with Alzheimer's disease. CHOLINE and LECITHIN (the phospholipid derivative of choline) may improve short-term memory in susceptible patients. However, they do not appear to alter the course of Alzheimer's disease. Treatment with phosphatidylcholine and prescription drugs like physostigmine and Hydergine have yielded mixed results. Three decades of research suggest that phosphatidyl serine benefits cognitive function, including memory and learning in elderly people. Other studies indicate that a derivative of the amino acid CARNITINE, L-acetylcarnitine, shows promise in moderating age-related depression, as well as the effects of stroke and nerve degeneration related to DIABETES MELLITUS. (See also FOOD; GINKGO.)

Harman, Denham, "Free Radical Theory of Aging. Increasing the Functional Lifespan," *Annals of the New York Academy of Science* 717 (June 30, 1994), pp. 1–15.

sensitivity See FOOD SENSITIVITY.

sequestrants (chelating agents) Agents used to reduce color changes and SPOILAGE in canned foods, PROCESSED FOODS and bottled salad dressings. Sequestrants bind metal ions like iron, which catalyze the reaction of oxygen with sensitive materials in food. Examples of sequestering agents are CITRIC ACID, malic acid, tartaric acid and EDTA. Citric acid is used in ice cream, sherbet, fruit drinks, soft drinks, jellies, canned fruits and vegetables and cheese. It is considered a safe additive. EDTA is widely used in salad dressings, MARGARINE, MAYONNAISE and sandwich spreads, prepared fresh fruit, potatoes, canned shellfish, beer and soft drinks. EDTA too is considered safe. (See also FOOD ADDITIVES; MINERALS.)

serine (Ser, L-serine) A non-essential AMINO ACID required to synthesize proteins. Serine plays a role in many synthetic reactions that require FOLIC ACID, VITAMIN B$_6$ and NIACIN. It can be converted to the simplest amino acid, GLYCINE, and vice versa. Serine can assist in the synthesis of PURINES and PYRIMIDINES, the building blocks of DNA and RNA. Serine can be converted to ethanolamine and CHOLINE, two nitrogen-containing compounds required for phospholipid synthesis and cell membrane formation, and to certain NEUROTRANSMITTERS, brain chemicals required to transmit signals in nerves. Serine is classified as a "glycogenic" amino acid because during STARVATION it can be converted to BLOOD SUGAR to fuel the brain. (See also AMINO ACID METABOLISM.)

serotonin (5-hydroxytryptamine) A chemical found in the brain and defensive cells of connective tissue. Mast cells, a type of defensive cell lodged in connective tissue, produce serotonin from the essential amino acid TRYPTOPHAN to slow blood flow in damaged areas because it acts as a powerful vasoconstrictor (constricts blood vessels). In the brain serotonin functions as a neurotransmitter, a chemical required for the transmission of nerve impulses. Serotonin is involved in inducing sleep, sensory perception and temperature. It diminishes pain, reduces APPETITE and has a calming effect. Certain antidepressants like Prozac maintain elevated serotonin levels and inhibit binge eating. Diet can possibly affect mood by altering brain serotonin levels. Eating carbohydrate may reduce the level of most amino acids in the blood except tryptophan, so that this amino acid can more easily penetrate the BLOOD-BRAIN BARRIER without competing with other amino acids. According to this hypothesis, as the level of tryptophan rises in the brain, more serotonin is synthesized, leading to relaxation and decreased alertness. (See also NERVOUS SYSTEM.)

serum The clear, straw-colored fluid remaining after blood has clotted. Serum contains CHOLESTEROL (serum cholesterol) in the form of LDL (LOW-DENSITY LIPOPROTEIN, the less desirable form) and HDL (HIGH-DENSITY LIPOPROTEIN, the more desirable form); fat (TRIGLYCERIDES); proteins produced by the liver such as serum ALBUMIN; ELECTROLYTES (ionic minerals like SODIUM, POTASSIUM and CHLORIDE); waste materials like UREA and URIC ACID; and nutrients such as AMINO ACIDS and BLOOD SUGAR (GLUCOSE). Serum is often used in the clinical laboratory to measure these parameters for diagnosis, rather than whole blood, which contains cells that can alter these parameters. For example, red blood cells possess their own complement of enzymes, lipids and minerals.

serum albumin See ALBUMIN.

serum cholesterol See CHOLESTEROL.

serum lipids See CHOLESTEROL.

serum triglycerides See TRIGLYCERIDES.

sesame (*Sesamum indicum*) An annual tropical plant grown since ancient times for its edible seed oil. Sesame was cultivated in Palestine and Syria as early as 3000 B.C. It is now cultivated in China, India, Burma and Mexico; the United States is a major importer. Sesame seeds contain 50% oil by weight; the oil can be extracted from crushed, whole seeds. The seed is dehulled for human consumption because its hull contains 2 to 3% OXALIC ACID, which binds minerals and gives it a bitter flavor. The U.S. imports 70 million pounds of sesame seeds annually; most of this is used for hamburger buns. Ground sesame seeds are used in hummus and tahini (a sesame seed paste). Halvah is a confection made with ground sesame seeds. Sesame seeds are used with stir-fried vegetables and fried poultry in Asian cuisine.

Sesame oil is more saturated than VEGETABLE OILS like safflower, corn or soybean oil, which all contain more than 50% polyunsaturated fatty acids. Sesame oil contains 43.8% polyunsaturated fatty acid (LINOLEIC ACID); 14.6% saturated fatty acids (mainly PALMITIC ACID and STEARIC ACID); and 41.5% monounsaturated fatty acids (OLEIC ACID). The oil has a strong nutty flavor and is often used in stir-fry meals. The nutrient content of sesame seeds (15 g) is: 84 calories; protein, 3.6 g; carbohydrate, 0.6 g; fat, 7.1 g; calcium, 18 mg; iron, 1.1 mg; thiamin, 0.29 mg; riboflavin, 0.03 mg; niacin, 0.8 mg. (See also HYDROGENATED VEGETABLE OIL.)

set point See DIETING; WEIGHT MANAGEMENT.

shellfish Include two very large classes of aquatic animals, mollusks and crustaceans, long used as food sources. Univalve mollusks such as abalone are enclosed in a single shell; bivalve mollusks with a two-part shell include CLAMS mussels, OYSTERS and scallops. Cephalopods (creatures with tentacles, like squid) are a type of mollusk. Crustaceans, which possess a tough outer layer and segmented bodies and legs, include CRAB, LOBSTERS, crayfish, prawns and SHRIMP. Shellfish provide rich sources of protein low in saturated fat and total fat, and TRACE MINERALS such as IODINE, ZINC and COPPER. Generally shellfish contain the usual amounts of cholesterol as found in meat. Shrimp contain somewhat higher levels, though less than found in eggs. Like ocean fish, shellfish contain omega-3 oils that offer protection against heart disease. Raw shellfish are a major source of severe, foodborne disease. Disease organisms carried by shellfish include salmonella and hepatitis A virus. Bacteria can cause gastroenteritis (inflamed stomach and intestines) with diarrhea, nausea, vomiting and cramps. Shellfish are bottom feeders and filter vast amounts of water, therefore they tend to accumulate waste products and disease-producing bacteria and viruses when grown in waters contaminated by sewage. Clams and oysters can filter 15 to 20 gallons of seawater daily.

FDA and state inspections are designed to make certain that shellfish are harvested from clean waters. However, regulation of the shellfish industry is spotty because few agents are available to monitor 10 million acres of approved shellfish beds in U.S. coastal waters. To meet the increased consumer demand, the fishing industry is taking fish and shellfish closer to shore, where pollution is higher and the risk of polluted SEAFOOD is higher. Raw or undercooked shellfish are the major seafood hazards. The bacterium *Vibrio vulnificus* produces a toxin causing a shellfish poisoning associated with contaminated seafood, especially oysters from the Gulf Coast. Immune compromised people and those with liver disease (cirrhosis) are most vulnerable. The toxin can cause skin ulcers and occurs as normal marine flora in warmer temperate waters. Its production is not associated with pollution.

RED TIDE is an explosive growth of a microscopic marine algae. Poisonous dinoflagellates produce neurotoxins (nerve poisons) that are not destroyed by cooking. Paralytic shellfish poisoning is caused by *Gonyaulax catenella* and *G. acetenella* along Pacific coasts and *G. tamarensis* in the Bay of Fundy and in the St. Lawrence estuary on the North Atlantic. Symptoms begin with numbness in lips and tongue, spreading to arms and legs and respiratory distress. Red tide can cause blood poisoning and death in high-risk individuals—patients with liver disease, AIDS or alcoholics. Mussels gradually destroy or eliminate bound poisons after an algal bloom. In general do not eat raw oysters during the warmer months, April to October.

Razor clams from U.S. Pacific Northwest beaches can be contaminated with domoic acid, a naturally occurring neurotoxin that causes nausea, fever, abdominal cramps, short-term memory loss, coma, and death in severe cases. This toxin is produced by marine plankton. Internal organs of Dungeness crab harvested off the coasts of California, Oregon and Washington may be contaminated, though the crab meat itself is safe.

sherbet A frozen DESSERT prepared from fruit juice or fruit puree, sugar, milk, egg white, or gelatin or dipped marshmallows. In contrast, sorbets are fruit-based frozen desserts that do not contain dairy products. (See also ICE CREAM.)

shigellosis A severe type of FOOD POISONING caused by shigella, an intestinal bacterium. Symptoms include very severe DIARRHEA, lasting several days, with possible bloody stools and accompanied by fever and possibly DEHYDRATION. Most people recover fairly rapidly, even without treatment with antibiotics. However, shigellosis can be life-threatening to children and to the elderly. Shigella is carried by fecal matter, and the disease can be transmitted by food handlers with poor hygiene. State law requires that cases of shigellosis be reported to health departments. Contact your physician if you have severe diarrhea and bloody stools. (See also SALMONELLA.)

Hedberg, Craig W., et al., "An International Foodborne Outbreak of Shigellosis Associated with a Commercial Airline," *Journal of the American Medical Association*, 268:22 (December 1992), pp. 3208–12.

shiitake mushroom (*Lentinus edodes*; forest mushroom) An edible MUSHROOM popular in the Far East. Shiitake mushrooms are cultivated commercially and are available in United States markets. Shiitake contains a broad spectrum of amino acids, potassium and ergosterol, a substance that can be converted to vitamin D in the presence of sunlight. In addition, shiitake mushrooms have been used in Oriental medicine for thousands of years. Shiitake contains carbohydrate materials and polysaccharides, including lentinan, which stimulates the immune system and which has antitumor activity. Lentinan may boost white blood cells called T helper cells that gear up the immune system. Shiitake extracts also boost antiviral defenses by increasing interferon production. Extracts can lower blood cholesterol levels.

shock See ANAPHYLAXIS.

short-chain fatty acids Very small fatty acids that have an odor (volatile fatty acids). Short-chain fatty acids are produced by the anaerobic fermentation of carbohydrate by colonic bacteria. With normal digestion, typically the main source of fermentable carbohydrate is dietary FIBER, plant cell wall materials and undigested starch. Short-chain fatty acids include ACETIC ACID (acetate, a two-carbon acid); PROPIONIC ACID (propionate, a three-carbon acid); and BUTYRIC ACID (butyrate, a four-carbon acid).

Short-chain fatty acids are readily absorbed by the colon and can be considered a major factor in human energy metabolism. It is estimated that short-chain fatty acids produced by colonic bacteria can satisfy 5 to 10% of the body's energy needs. Acetic acid and propionic acid are used by the liver, while butyric acid is a preferred fuel by cells lining the gut. Indeed, butyrate is a primary energy source for these cells. In addition, butyrate helps guide the development and maintenance of colonic cells and may decrease susceptibility to colon CANCER and colitis.

More than usual amounts of fermentable carbohydrate enter the colon with high-fiber diets and during carbohydrate MALABSORPTION and maldigestion, leading to increased production of short-chain fatty acids. The production of short-chain fatty acids lowers intestinal ammonia levels liberated through bacterial metabolism and limits the uptake of this waste product. Ammonia can induce abnormalities in intestinal cells. Short-chain fatty acids also inhibit the growth of certain pathogenic species like salmonella, and the resulting lowered colonic pH (increased acidity) favors VITAMIN K absorption, MUCUS secretion and magnesium uptake. (See also FAT METABOLISM; INTESTINAL FLORA.)

Soergel, K.H., "Colonic Fermentation: Metabolic and Clinical Implications," *Clinical Investigator*, 72 (1994), pp. 742–48.

shortening A FAT added to a food item to keep it soft during baking. By dispersing fat droplets throughout a dough, starch and grain protein do not congeal into a compact mass when cooked. BUTTER (milk fat), LARD (pork fat) and TALLOW (beef fat) are traditional shortening agents. Vegetable shortenings contain hydrogenated vegetable oils. These are solids, unlike the original oils. They are prepared from hydrogenated oils with varying melting points, and with varying degrees of softness. Vegetable shortening is often prepared from CORN OIL, COTTONSEED OIL, OLIVE OIL, PEANUT oil, PALM OIL, SAFFLOWER oil, SESAME oil or SOYBEAN oil. Regardless of form, all fats and oils provide 9 calories per gram, more than twice as much as derived from carbohydrate and protein (4 calories per gram).

Shortening is used for biscuits, bread, cookies and pie crusts. The amount of shortening varies with the recipe. Bread and rolls contain 1 to 2% shortening; cakes, 10 to 20%, and pastries, 30%. When shortenings are used for baking mixes, whipped topping, icing and filling, various emulsifying agents are included. These include MONOGLYCERIDES (glycerol with only one fatty acid). Emulsifiers allow water to be mixed with the shortening without separation. (See also DIETARY GUIDELINES FOR AMERICANS; FAT METABOLISM; VEGETABLE OIL.)

shrimp   A type of shellfish possessing 10 legs. Shrimp range in size from 0.5 in (1.1 cm) to several inches in the Gulf of Mexico. Shrimp when cooked turn red, due to a chemical change in the shell pigment when heated. Typically, the parts of cooked shrimp sold at markets are the abdominal region and tail parts, after the heads have been removed. Shrimp is a high-protein food that is also a good source of CALCIUM. Shrimp contains somewhat higher than usual levels of cholesterol, though less than found in eggs. Shrimp can be canned, converted to shrimp paste, breaded and fried, or stir-fried. The nutrient content of 3.5 oz (100 g) is: 109 calories; protein, 23.8 g; fat, 1.5 g; cholesterol, 152 mg; calcium, 320 mg; iron, 2.2 mg; thiamin, 0.03 mg; riboflavin, 0.03 mg; niacin, 3.7 mg.

signs   Keys for a medical diagnosis that depend upon objective observations by the health care specialist. They entail measurements such as BLOOD PRESSURE and lab testing such as blood GLUCOSE and serum CHOLESTEROL. Vital signs refer to functions vital for life: blood pressure, rate of respiration and body temperature.

In contrast, symptoms refer to changes in body functions indicating a disease state that the patient can feel and the physician observes. Tense muscles, distended stomach, skin rashes, discolorations, tenderness, heartburn, breath odor, deformities, coughing, constipation, diarrhea and tinnitis (ringing of the ears) are typical symptoms. (See also DIET RECORD; MALNUTRITION; NUTRITIONAL STATUS.)

silicon   The second most common element on the surface of the Earth and widely distributed in plant food and water. Silicon occurs in the skin, BONE and connective tissue of animals. It is an essential nutrient in animals, required for normal skeletal development of rats and chicks, for example. It seems probable that silicon is essential for humans, though this remains to be established. No RECOMMENDED DIETARY ALLOWANCE has been established for silicon. Silicon participates in the formation of connective tissue where it forms complexes between protein and acidic polysaccharide complexes. Acidic polysaccharides (GLYCOSAMINOGLYCANS) contribute to the gelatinous material that holds cells together. In humans, the silicon content of the aorta, the skin and the thymus decreases with age.

Silicon is widely distributed in whole grains, organ meats like liver, and red meat. Most of the silicon of whole grains is lost when white flour is prepared, and highly processed foods contain little silicon. The typical diet supplies approximately 1 g per day. Within the confines of the typical diet, silicon is nontoxic. (See also SKELETON; TRACE MINERAL.)

simple carbohydrate   See CARBOHYDRATE.

Simplesse®   The first FAT SUBSTITUTE approved in the United States. Simplesse is a cream-textured product made from milk and egg protein. Particles have the same "mouth feel" as fatty foods and can make uncooked foods taste as though they are high in fat. Simplesse cannot be used in cooked products such as pies because heating denatures ("cooks") the protein. Simplesse provides 1.3 calories per gram as compared with the 9 calories per gram of fat.

Because some people may have allergic reactions to milk protein, the U.S. FDA requires that labels of Simplesse-containing foods list the milk protein and egg protein as ingredients. It remains to be proven whether using Simplesse will help lower fat intake. No FOOD ADDITIVE can substitute for changing to a lower fat diet, as frequently recommended by dietary guidelines. (See also FROZEN DESSERTS, FAT-FREE; OBESITY; WEIGHT MANAGEMENT.)

single-cell protein   Food PROTEIN derived from cultured bacteria, YEAST, fungi and algae. Algae (seaweed) has long been used as food. Brewer's yeast, a by-product of the brewing industry, and TORULA YEAST are widely available food supplements. The potential of cultured microorganisms serving as an edible protein source is huge. A single-cell fermenter covering 0.8 sq km (one-third of a square mile) could theoretically supply 10% of the protein requirement of the world's population. By-products of the food, paper and chemical industry can be fermented by many microorganisms as inexpensive energy sources. These include methane, ALCOHOL, STARCH, MOLASSES, cellulose and animal waste products. Even fewer requirements are needed for algae; photosynthetic organisms can be grown in illuminated ponds supplied with mineral nutrients.

Problems associated with single-cell protein have limited its development as a major food source. Most single-cell protein is not palatable unless processed to eliminate bitter or unpleasant tasting materials. Digestibility of single-cell protein varies with the sources. Cooking algae increases its digestibility, but the digestibility of yeast is little altered by processing. The high nucleic acid content of single-cell organisms leads to increased purine uptake. When purines are metabolized, uric acid output rises and increases the risk of GOUT in susceptible people. Furthermore, toxic materials and pollutants can contaminate single-cell protein. Another consideration is the fact that single-cell protein is generally deficient in the dietary essential AMINO ACIDS, LYSINE and METHIONINE. Though the amino acid profile is more balanced than in cereal grain protein it remains inferior to animal protein. Genetically engineered microorganisms may overcome this deficiency. (See also FOOD CHAIN; HUNGER; MEAT; PHOTOSYNTHESIS.)

skeleton   The collection of bones that provides the framework and protective covering for many organs of the body including the brain, heart and spinal cord. Unlike the NERVOUS SYSTEM, the IMMUNE SYSTEM or the ENDOCRINE SYSTEM, the skeletal system plays a passive role in maintaining normal body function (HOMEOSTASIS). The skeletal system protects internal organs; vertebrae protect the spinal column; the cranium, the brain; the rib cage, the heart and lungs; the pelvic bones, the reproductive organs. Bones store calcium and phosphorus, which can be released and distributed to other parts of the body via the bloodstream. Red bone marrow in certain bones yields blood cells: RED BLOOD CELLS, some white cells and blood PLATELETS required for blood clotting. Fat in bone marrow represents stored ENERGY. The human skeleton contains 206 bones and is held together by tough connective tissue and cartilage. Skeletal muscles adhere to bones via tendons to promote movement.

Bones range in size from the robust femur to the delicate, intricate bones of the wrist and ankle. Physical growth during maturation from infancy to adulthood entails a dramatic increase in bone mass and size. Nearly 67% of bone represents a mineral matrix, the compound calcium phosphate, composed of the nutrients CALCIUM and PHOSPHORUS. Many other nutrients are required in the growth and maintenance of the skeletal system. MAGNESIUM and FLUORIDE are also complexed with calcium phosphate to help harden the bone matrix. BORON may reduce calcium and magnesium losses from bone in post-menopausal women. The skeleton requires a healthy connective tissue. MANGANESE is required for the formation of mucopolysaccharides, while COPPER and VITAMIN C are required for the formation of COLLAGEN and ELASTIN, proteins of connective tissue and tendon, respectively. Bone-forming cells are maintained by VITAMIN A among other nutrients. VITAMIN D, together with ample calcium, phosphorus and magnesium, promotes normal skeletal development and prevents RICKETS in children. In adults vitamin D prevents bone thinning and softening. (See also OSTEOMALACIA; OSTEOPOROSIS.)

skim milk   See MILK.

skin
The outer covering of FRUITS, VEGETABLES and seeds; otherwise called husks, peels or rinds. With reference to the human body, the skin (integument) is the outer surface of the body and is the largest organ. The skin of an adult covers a surface area of 2 sq m (3,000 sq in) and forms the primary physical barrier to the external environment, bacteria and other microorganisms. The skin provides other important functions. It helps regulate body temperature through heat lost by the evaporation of sweat and by changes in blood flow to the skin. A limited amount of body wastes and chemical toxic load can also be eliminated through sweat. The skin supports the sense of touch via sensory nerve endings embedded there. These nerves react to temperature, pressure, pain and touch. The skin is responsible for synthesizing vitamin D_3 from a stored precursor when exposed to ultraviolet light. Finally, certain types of cells embedded in underlying layers are important components of immunity, the ability to ward off disease.

Nutrient Support of Skin

The chief constituent of the skin is COLLAGEN, a structural protein requiring vitamin C. Collagen and ELASTIN are fibers of connective tissue that keep the skin smooth and toned. VITAMIN C and COPPER are trace nutrients that support the synthesis of elastin proteins. Vitamin C and VITAMIN E together with SELENIUM are required for a healthy skin. They are powerful scavengers of free radicals, the highly reactive chemicals formed by sunlight and oxygen, smog, pollutants and other factors. Essential fatty acids, LINOLEIC ACID and ALPHA LINOLENIC ACID, which occur in seed oils, are important in maintaining a lustrous skin. Sebaceous glands secrete an oily material called sebum, which is a mixture of oils, cholesterol, protein and inorganic salts. This oily film protects hair and skin from drying out; prevents excessive evaporation from the skin; keeps the skin soft and pliable; and blocks the growth of certain bacteria. It forms a water-impermeable barrier and prevents the skin from becoming saturated with water.

AGING brings marked changes in the skin. The skin appears rougher, drier and thinner, and the cushioning layer of fat beneath the skin diminishes. There are fewer melanocytes, cells that produce pigment to protect against sunlight's ultraviolet damage, and there is less collagen and elastin and that which remains may be damaged.

All structures in the skin can be affected by chronic exposure to U.V. light, including overexposure to sunlight. U.V. light reacts with cells by initiating FREE RADICAL reactions. Free radicals are unstable molecules that attack cells and damage their DNA. This chemical change accounts for most skin damage and even skin cancer. Sunburn is an injury to the skin due to ultraviolet rays that may lead to cell death and mutations. The skin becomes leathery, with wrinkles, lines, sagging skin areas, wart-like or scaly precancerous growths (keratoses), yellow discoloration and abnormal elastic tissue.

Oxidative damage to the skin alters the complexion; the skin may become blemished. Sunlight-induced damage is cumulative. U.V. light can penetrate deep layers of the skin, damaging elastin and collagen and hindering their synthesis. Without adequate underlying support, the skin sags. The first line of IMMUNE SYSTEM defense in the skin are Langerhans cells. These sentries can detect the intrusion of foreign materials and quickly signal other components of the immune system to counterattack. U.V. light whether from tanning parlors or from sunlight suppresses these cells.

Photosensitivity can aggravate the reaction to the sun's rays. Certain foods (citrus fruits, for example), deodorant soaps, Retin-A, antibiotics, tranquilizers and DIURETICS (water pills) contain materials that can accentuate a reaction to sunlight such as burning and development of age spots. By minimizing ultraviolet exposure new connective tissue can replace the old with adequate nutrition.

Vitamin E, vitamin C and B complex vitamins promote repair and cellular growth. These antioxidants also function as anti-inflammatory agents that aid in the repair of cell damage. Flaxseed oil, borage oil and evening primrose oil provide essential fatty acids also needed for skin maintenance. Collagen has a moisturizing effect when applied in skin lotion, but it is not absorbed or used by the skin when applied topically. Whether the skin can be nourished by external vitamin application remains unclear. Manufacturers often add antioxidants to skin lotions, and there is some evidence that fat-soluble vitamins and other oily (lipophilic) derivatives of vitamins do penetrate the skin. A 2 to 10% concentration of these substances may be needed to be effective; often skin preparations contain low amounts. Some manufacturers incorporate materials in liposomes, microscopic sacs prepared from lipids, to aid the absorption of a variety of substances. Preparation of microscopic droplets (called micelles) also helps materials penetrate the upper dead layers of skin to reach cells of the dermis. (See also ACNE.)

Emerit, Ingrid, "Free Radicals and Ageing of the Skin," in *Free Radicals and Ageing*, Emerit, I. and Chance, B., eds. Boston, MA: Birkhauser Verlag, 1992.

skinfold test   See FATFOLD TEST.

skin test   See ALLERGY, FOOD.

small intestine (small bowel)   The tube extending from the stomach to the large intestine (COLON). Typically, the small intestine is 1 in (2.5 cm) in diameter and 21 ft (6.35 m) long. It is divided into three regions; the first 10 inches is called the DUODENUM; the JEJUNUM represents the next 8 feet; and the ILEUM occupies the lower reaches of the small intestine. The intestine carries out two distinct functions: It selectively absorbs nutrients and important materials from food and beverages, and at the same time, it excludes a vast amount of foreign substances, ranging from microorganisms and food particles to pollutants and bacterial by-products. To carry out its absorptive function the surface is highly convoluted and is covered with small projections about 1 mm high, called VILLI, giving it a velvet appearance. Within each villus is a capillary network and lymphatic vessel to aid the uptake and distribution of nutrients. The surfaces of villi are lined with absorptive cells; each cell possesses many microscopic projections called microvilli. The number of villi decreases in the ileum; most absorption occurs in the duodenum and jejunum. The total surface area of the intestine is huge. If the microvilli and villi were flattened out, the surface would be about the size of a tennis court.

The small intestine is the major site of DIGESTION. Pancreatic enzymes efficiently digest fat, protein and starch. The intestinal lining secretes fluid (intestinal juice) containing electrolytes (ions) and mucus to protect the wall of the intestine from digestive enzymes. The volume is substantial. The small intestine secretes 2 to 3 liters of juice per day. Most of the ions and water are reabsorbed and recycled.

Intestinal enzymes complete the final stages of digestion. They include MALTASE to digest maltose, the sugar released from starch digestion; SUCRASE to digest SUCROSE (table sugar); and LACTASE to digest LACTOSE (milk sugar). A milk intolerance often reflects LACTOSE INTOLERANCE that is an impaired ability to digest lactose due to inadequate lactase. Undigested lactose passes on to the colon where bacteria rapidly ferment it, often producing gas, bloating and diarrhea. The small intestine also produces peptidases to degrade small protein fragments to amino acids.

Partially digested food (chyme) moves down the intestine by localized muscle contraction, creating a mixing action. PERISTALSIS refers to the wave-like contractions moving down the gastrointestinal tract. Chyme moves at the rate of 1 cm/min; consequently, food remains in the small intestine three to five hours. The small intestine produces an array of hormones to regulate digestion. CHOLECYSTOKININ stimulates contraction of the gallbladder to release bile, and it stimulates pancreatic enzyme secretion. SECRETIN reduces gastric and duodenal motility and promotes bicarbonate secretion by the pancreas. Gastric inhibitory protein blocks stomach acid release, while stimulating insulin secretion. To exclude foreigners, the intestine maintains a physical barrier. The mucus coating is constantly being replaced as it is washed away, limiting penetration. Underlying cells are tightly bonded together to limit the leakage of unwanted substances into the body. The movement of food through the digestive tract and the presence of powerful digestive enzymes limit uptake of foreign materials. The major immune barrier is a secreted antibody called secretory IgA. This defensive protein is secreted by immune cells embedded within the intestinal wall and can bind to specific antigens (foreign substances) and prevent their adhering to the intestinal surface. Like all antibodies, specific types of IgA are produced against specific antigens.

Cells lining the intestine replenish themselves in one to two days, thus the nutrient needs of this rapidly dividing tissue are unusually high. Ample zinc and the B complex vitamins, especially FOLIC ACID, are essential for maintaining a healthy intestine. GLUTAMINE helps maintain enterocytes, the epithelial cells lining the small intestine, while butyrate (BUTYRIC ACID) is essential for the help of colonocytes, lining the colon.

If the intestine becomes inflamed, it can become more "leaky" and foreign substances can enter the body. The influx of foreign materials can trigger multiple food allergies, joint pain, skin conditions, and autoimmune disease in which the body's defenses attack itself. LEAKY GUT syndrome can be caused by alcoholism, overuse of pain medication (non-steroidal anti-inflammatory drugs), inadequate pancreatic output, infection, AIDS or Crohn's disease (ulcerated small intestine), among others. With chronic constipation, low stomach acid and aging, colon bacteria may creep upward into the small intestine, leading to a condition known as bacterial overgrowth of the small bowel. Symptoms include sensitivity to starchy food and refined carbohydrate—leading to bloating, gas, diarrhea and other discomfort. Bacterial overgrowth often leads to maldigestion and to malabsorption of vitamins, such as VITAMIN B$_{12}$. Eradicating the offending bacteria, while remedying the underlying cause, together with dietary modification can alleviate this condition. (See also AMINO ACID METABOLISM; CARBOHYDRATE METABOLISM; FAT METABOLISM.)

smell   The olfactory sense and one of the five basic senses. Smell is a chemical sense, providing a direct link with the environment. It evolved primarily to determine which substances are acceptable. When molecules escape into the air, they travel up the nose to a small region of moist tissue called the olfactory membrane. The sense of smell relies upon the binding of volatile (gaseous) compounds to cell membranes. Gaseous compounds penetrate the mucus covering the olfactory cells and bind to hairlike extensions (cilia) like tassels. Signals are sent along a nerve to olfactory bulbs at the base of the brain, where they radiate out to regions of the brain concerned with mood, strong emotions, memory and thought. There are about 1,000 different receptors or docking sites that are able to recognize some 10,000 different odors. Flavors of foods are often based on odors rather than mouth (taste) sensations. Unique flavors usually reflect a combination of smell and TASTE. When foods are placed in the mouth, odor molecules travel to the olfactory neurons up the passage linking the inside of the nose and throat. A serious loss of smell affects about 2 million Americans (a condition known as anosmia). Most commonly this is a result of allergies, certain medications and head injury.

Stoll, Andrew L. and Oepen, Godehard, "Zinc Salts for the Treatment of Olfactory and Gustatory Symptoms in Psychiatric Patients: a Case Series," *Journal of Clinical Psychiatry*, 55:7 (July 1994), pp. 309–11.

sodium   The major positively charged ion in body fluids. Due to their chemical nature, metallic elements such as sodium exist in solutions and in compounds as cations, positively charged ions, where they counterbalance negatively charged ions, such as CHLORIDE. Sodium therefore functions in maintaining ELECTROLYTE balance, that is, the balance between negatively and positively charged ions and among complex ions such as proteins in the blood. Sodium predominates in the extracellular fluid, while POTASSIUM, another cation, concentrates within cells. Normally chloride and sodium tends to leak into cells, while potassium tends to leak out. Sodium is pumped out of cells, while potassium is pumped inward by means of an energy-dependent process called "active transport." Maintaining normal cell volume (and shape) depends upon sodium and potassium pumping. The active transport of sodium and potassium is a predominant energy-consuming process of the cells, accounting for a large percentage of the total energy expenditure of the body.

Sodium plays a vital role in controlling osmotic pressure, the pressure that develops between the blood and cells due to ionic concentration differences. The total volume of extracellular fluid is determined by its sodium level, which the body maintains under tight control by means of the endocrine and nervous systems. By balancing charges of negatively charged ions like chloride, BICARBONATE and phosphate, sodium assists in maintaining the proper balance between acidic and alkaline substances (acid-base balance).

Sodium works with potassium in nerve function. To transmit a nerve impulse, the nerve cell membrane is temporarily "depolarized"; potassium temporarily leaks outside and sodium and chloride leak in. This generates a decrease in electrical potential, which triggers a voltage-dependent increase in sodium penetration. Restoration of the potential differences to the resting state allows the impulse to be transmitted as a self-propagating wave down a nerve cell. Muscles, especially heart muscles, require an interplay of sodium and potassium by similar mechanisms.

The kidney normally reabsorbs sodium that was filtered out into the urine to maintain electrolyte balance. Water follows sodium back into the blood, thus hormones that increase sodium retention by the kidney also increase water retention. Sodium concentration and water balance are controlled by an interplay of the kidney and several hormones: When the level of sodium drops, the enzyme RENIN is released by the kidney. Renin catalyzes the conversion of a blood protein to ANGIOTENSIN. In turn this hormone stimulates the adrenal gland to release ALDOSTERONE, a hormone that causes the kidney to increase the rate of sodium reabsorption from filtered fluid to correct the original sodium depletion. On the other hand, when dietary sodium intake is high, the kidney rapidly excretes sodium. Through the operation of these homeostatic (body balancing) mechanisms, the amount of sodium excreted is adjusted to equal the amount consumed. Ninety percent of ingested sodium is excreted; some is lost through sweat and feces. Excessive sodium intake and retention can lead to EDEMA.

Sources of Sodium

Most vegetables, fruits and legumes contain only low levels of sodium, unless pickled. Although the U.S. FDA estimates that processed food contributes 25 to 50% of the sodium in the typical U.S. diet, other studies of sample diets indicate that an estimate of 60 to 75% is more realistic. Ninety percent of dietary sodium comes from sodium chloride (table salt); only 15% of dietary sodium comes from the salt shaker. There are several explanations for the prevalence of sodium in foods. Salt is a very inexpensive way to flavor PROCESSED FOOD, in place of more expensive herbs and spices. Sometimes companies are not aware of the sodium content in their products. The amount of sodium in the same type of food, produced by different manufacturers, can differ by 50 to 300%. Salt is also used in recipes dating to a time when salt was not known to be potentially harmful.

The only way to detect salty food is by taste, yet this is an unreliable indicator of sodium content. For example, FRENCH FRIES may have only one-quarter the amount of sodium in an equal serving (weight) of cherry pie because sugar masks the taste of salt. Hidden salt occurs in gelatin desserts, milk shakes, cheese, canned soups, packaged and frozen dinners, and foods at fast-food restaurants; in cured ham and bacon, cured fish, corned beef, smoked herring and soy sauce. Processed meat like BOLOGNA and HOT DOGS, tomato KETCHUP, many cold BREAKFAST CEREALS, pickled foods and salad dressings provide high levels of sodium. Sodium occurs in other food additives such as baking soda and sodium aluminum sulfate (in baked goods), sodium caseinate (a milk product), sodium phosphate (the major contributor of sodium in cheese), sodium nitrite and sodium benzoate (preservatives) and MONOSODIUM GLUTAMATE (flavor enhancer). LAXATIVES and ANTACIDS can account for a large percentage of sodium for some people, especially elderly persons. Human milk contains 161 mg of sodium per liter, while cow's milk provides 483 mg per liter; therefore, cow's milk provides considerably more sodium.

Soft water contains high levels of sodium. The amount depends upon the hardness of natural water. A glass of tap water usually contains less than 3 mg of sodium. However, salt from the de-icing of roads and ion exchange resins can raise sodium levels in inland areas. Sodium from seawater can leach into the water supplies of coastal areas.

Sodium Requirements

There is no RECOMMENDED DIETARY ALLOWANCE (RDA) for sodium. A safe and adequate level was proposed by the Food and Nutrition Board as 1,100 to 3,300 mg per day in 1980. The 1989 RDA recommendations list the minimum requirements for healthy persons (adults 18 or older) as 500 mg of sodium daily. The sodium requirements of infants and small children are estimated to be about 58 mg daily. The amount of sodium required to maintain sodium equilibrium for most adults may be less than 200 mg under normal circumstances, equivalent to one-tenth a teaspoon of salt per day. The overall consensus is that Americans generally consume too much salt. The typical adult intake is 6 to 25 g of salt, with a mean of 10 g/day, equivalent to 4 g of sodium, 20 times as much as the listed minimum. The maximum recommended daily intake of sodium choloride is 6 g (2.4 g).

Few people in the United States are sodium deficient. Relatively heavy sweating is now associated with a need for extra salt, and the primary concern should be fluid replacement. Athletes undergoing strenuous physical exercise do not need salt until they have lost approximately 3 quarts of water by sweating. The kidney adapts to sodium losses in hot weather, so that less sodium, hence less water, is excreted. One typical meal will more than make up for sodium lost in sweat through moderate exercise. Note that chronic diarrhea, kidney disease or other medical conditions can limit the body's ability to retain sodium and thus increase sodium requirements. Excessive sodium can be toxic to infants because their kidneys are not fully developed; it may also be toxic to those with kidney disease or those who have adjusted to a chronically low-sodium diet.

Sodium and High Blood Pressure

Sodium has been linked to high blood pressure (HYPERTEN-SION) in extensive studies spanning decades. Perhaps 10 to 20% of Americans experience increased blood pressure when they eat excess sodium. High blood pressure increases the risk of STROKE, HEART ATTACK and kidney disease. Worldwide, a low sodium intake matches a lowered risk of hypertension. Certainly OBESTIY, genetic makeup, lack of exercise and excessive alcohol are risk factor for developing hypertension. Salt sensitivity increases with age. As people grow older, their kidneys excrete less sodium, and an increased sodium intake is more likely to raise blood pressure in susceptible people. Cutting back on salt intake may lower blood pressure by a small amount; however, even relatively small decreases in blood pressure readings could mean a significant decrease in the risk of death due to coronary heart disease. Excessive sodium increases urinary losses of calcium and can contribute to the risk of osteoporosis. Additionally, a high-salt diet is a dominant risk factor for stomach cancer. Governmental dietary guidelines recommend moderate sodium consumption, and individuals with hypertension or who have a family history of hypertension may be advised to curtail sodium consumption.

Sodium on Food Labels

Sodium must be listed on the label of any foods that list nutritional content, and on those that make nutritional claims as being "low fat" or "enriched." (Exempt foods are those made with meat or poultry.)

- "Sodium free" means less than 5 mg of sodium per serving.
- "Very low sodium" foods contain at most 140 mg per serving.
- "Low sodium" foods contain at most 140 mg per serving.
- "Reduced sodium" means the food has been processed to reduce normal sodium levels by at least 75%.
- "No sodium" and "no salt" alternatives: Several cold breakfast cereals, canned vegetables and herbal salt substitutes have been introduced to meet consumer demands. Read the label to be certain that products actually live up to their claims.

To cut back on salt, do not add salt to foods. Season with herbs or sauces instead. Cut back on processed, convenience foods. Read food labels to determine the sodium content and avoid foods with high sodium. Do not take salt tablets without consulting a doctor. Reducing high blood pressure can mean, in addition to cutting back on sodium, limiting alcohol consumption to one or two drinks per day; engaging in reg-

ular aerobic exercise; getting enough calcium, potassium and magnesium; and losing weight.

Sodium Content of Common Foods

Food	Sodium (mg) per 100 g (3 oz)
Canadian bacon	2,555
Green olives	2,400
Corned beef	1,740
Cheese	1,430
Bologna	1,300
Cold cereal (oats)	1,267
Cured ham	1,100
Wheatflake cereal	1,032
Potato chips	1,000
Sausage	958

(See also FOOD ADDITIVES; MINERALS.)

World Hypertension League. "Can Non-pharmacological Interventions Reduce Doses of Drugs Needed for the Treatment of Hypertension?" *Bulletin of the World Health Organization*, 70:6 (1992), pp. 685–90.

sodium alginate   See ALGINATE.

sodium ascorbate   See VITAMIN C.

sodium benzoate   A food preservative that retards growth of microorganisms under acidic conditions. Foods and beverages can contain up to 0.1% sodium benzoate. Soft drinks, salad dressing and fruit juices often contain this preservative. Sodium benzoate also occurs naturally in vegetables and fruit, for example, in prunes and cranberries. Sodium benzoate is a product of metabolism as well. Extensive studies indicate it is a safe additive.

sodium chloride   See SODIUM.

sodium erythroborate   See ERYTHROBORIC ACID.

sodium nitrate   See NITRATE.

sodium nitrite   See NITRITE.

soft drinks (soda pop)   Carbonated, non-alcoholic beverages. Typically soft drinks contain dissolved CARBON DIOXIDE (carbonation), sweeteners, flavoring agents, edible acids and food coloring. Between 1968 and 1991, U.S. soft drink consumption rose from 20 gallons per person per year to nearly 43 gallons. By 1990 soft drinks had become the most popular beverage in the United States. Increased soft drink consumption means increased consumption of PHOSPHORUS, ARTIFICIAL FOOD COLORS and ARTIFICIAL SWEETENERS, and sugar. In contrast, water contains none of these additives.

STANDARDS OF IDENTITY define certain aspects of the composition of foods and beverages. Soft drinks are classified as soda water and must contain more carbon dioxide than can be absorbed at normal air pressure. Alcohol content, if contributed by a flavoring agent, cannot exceed 0.5% of the weight. CAFFEINE can be added to any soda water to a final concentration of 0.02% by weight. Optional ingredients include sweeteners (synthetic and non-synthetic), edible acids, flavors, colors, preservatives, emulsifying agents to prevent ingredients from separating, thickening agents to create cloudiness and "mouth feel," and foaming agents.

SUCROSE (table sugar) is among the most common NATURAL SWEETENERS used in soft drinks. Also approved are dextrose (GLUCOSE), INVERT SUGAR, FRUCTOSE, CORN SYRUP, high FRUCTOSE CORN SYRUP (now a general soft drink sweetener) and glucose syrup. The artificial sweetener ASPARTAME is used extensively in diet soft drinks. SACCHARIN, another non-caloric sweetener, is used in soft drinks as well. Phosphoric acid is added to acidify soft drinks. Other acids used in soft drinks include ACETIC ACID, fumaric acid, LACTIC ACID and gluconic acid, an acid of glucose. The phosphate in soft drinks increases the overall phosphate consumption. This can be detrimental because a high phosphate intake is linked to an overactive thyroid gland and bone loss (OSTEOPOROSIS). Furthermore, drinking large amounts of diet soda (8 to 10 cans a day) is a cause of tooth erosion.

Types of Soft Drinks

Colas These contain extract of the cola nut and caffeine. The coloring agent is typically caramel (brown sugar) and the sugar content can be 11 to 13%.

Orange soft drinks Artificial colors, orange oil or orange juice may be added. The sugar content resembles colas and the edible acid is usually CITRIC ACID. These are not substitutes for orange juice.

Ginger ale Ginger root extract, ginger and lime oil may be the flavoring agents in these soft drinks. Caramel may be used as a coloring and citric acid is the edible acid. The sugar content ranges from 7 to 11%.

Grape-flavor soft drinks Synthetic grape flavor or grape juice may be used in flavoring and artificial coloring is used. The sugar content is generally between 11 and 13%, and the edible acid is TARTARIC ACID. (See also CONVENIENCE FOOD; EMPTY CALORIES; JUNK FOOD.)

Shuster, J., et al., "Soft Drink Consumption and Urinary Stone Recurrence: A Randomized Prevention Trial," *Journal of Clinical Epidemiology*, 45:8 (August 1992), pp. 911–16.

solanine An ALKALOID that acts as a plant's defensive agent against insects. Solanine occurs in very low levels in apples, tomatoes, eggplant and sugar beets. POTATOES contain the highest concentration of solanine, which contributes the characteristic flavor of potatoes. Solanine acts as a nerve poison by blocking the action of NEUROTRANSMITTERS, brain chemicals required for transmitting nerve impulses. Most American-grown varieties of potatoes contain low levels of solanine, so that a person would have to consume 4.5 lb (2 kg) of unbruised, non-sprouted potatoes to ingest 200 mg of solanine, a dose that could cause drowsiness, cramps, neck itchiness and DIARRHEA. However, the content of solanine in potatoes increases dramatically with bruising or sprouting, or when the skin turns green due to exposure to too much sunlight after harvest. Damaged or green-skinned potatoes should be discarded for this reason.

somatotropin See MEAT CONTAMINANTS.

sorbic acid (potassium sorbate) A food PRESERVATIVE used to inhibit the growth of molds, yeast and fungi, but not bacteria. Sorbic acid is used in CHEESE manufacture, allowing bacteria to ferment milk products while inhibiting yeast and mold growth. Because sorbic acid is effective over a wide range of pH, it is used in a variety of foods, including MAYONNAISE, cake, MARGARINE, dried fruit, SOFT DRINKS and syrup at concentrations up to 0.3%. It breaks down at high temperature and cannot be pasteurized. The body metabolizes sorbic acid like a fatty acid; consequently it is an energy source. It is considered a safe FOOD ADDITIVE.

sorbitol (hexitol) A naturally occurring sugar ALCOHOL. Sorbitol is 60% as sweet as SUCROSE (table sugar) though it is not a carbohydrate. It is used in chewing gum, confections, icing, food toppings, meat products, milk products and beverages. It reduces the rate of sugar crystal formation, maintains moisture and sequesters (binds) food ingredients.

Sorbitol occurs in many fruits, including berries, CHERRIES, PEARS, PLUMS and APPLES and in SEAWEED. Both apple juice and pear juice contain a high concentration. Sorbitol in apple juice is not absorbed well by infants and small children; it can ferment in the large intestine, producing gas, cramps and DIARRHEA. Large doses of sorbitol (50 g) can cause diarrhea in adults.

Sorbitol is synthesized by hydrogenation of the simple sugar GLUCOSE (dextrose). Sorbitol contains the same number of 4 calories per gram as carbohydrate and is burned completely to carbon dioxide. However, it does not form glucose in the body, thus it does not raise BLOOD SUGAR. Therefore, sorbitol is used as a sweetener in certain dietetic foods. Sorbitol-containing foods and chewing gums are not calorie-free, though they carry a "sugarless" or "sugar free" label. Sorbitol formation in cells occurs as a side effect of DIABETES MELLITUS. Since it cannot leak out of cells, sorbitol can gradually accumulate, leading eventually to osmotic imbalances and tissue damage. (See also ARTIFICIAL SWEETENERS; FOOD ADDITIVES; NATURAL SWEETENERS.)

sorghum (*Sorghum vulgare*; Guinea corn, kaffir corn) A major cereal GRAIN that is a staple in Africa and Asia. Sorghum ranks in the top five most important cereal grains worldwide. Well adapted to climates too hot and dry for CORN and WHEAT, sorgum has been grown in regions of Africa and Asia since 2000 B.C. The People's Republic of China, the United States, India and Argentina represent much of the world's production. In the United States sorghum is used primarily as animal fodder. Only 1 to 2% of U.S. sorghum is used for food or alcoholic fermentation.

Though related to MILLET, nutritionally sorghum resembles corn. Both grains are deficient in the essential AMINO ACID, LYSINE. In Africa and Asia sorghum is used as a flour or a porridge. Sweet sorghum is used to make an unrefined syrup, more sour than molasses. As with all refined sweeteners, the amounts are too low to be reliable sources of minerals or B complex vitamins. The nutrient content of 1 cup (3 oz, 100 g) of sorghum is: 366 calories; protein, 11.0 g; carbohydrate, 73 g; fat, 3.3 g; thiamin, 0.38 mg; riboflavin, 0.15 mg; niacin, 3.9 mg.

soul food A cuisine originating in the southern United States, where, in the antebellum era, slaves developed eating practices from their West African roots. Soul food has been modified by later generations. Typical entrees include collard greens, mustard greens, turnip greens, Dixie fried chicken, sweet potato pie and corn bread. Traditionally these are high-salt, high-fat foods. Such foods pose a potential health problem, especially among blacks who are experiencing an epidemic of high blood pressure in the United States. As with other ethnic dishes, the use of spices and herbs for seasoning is recommended to cut down on salt. Recipes can be adapted to use less FAT in cooking, such as the substitution of VEGETABLE OIL for LARD to reduce consumption of SATURATED FAT. Modifications can help make soul food dishes nutritious and heart healthy, while still tasty and appetizing. (See also DIETARY GUIDELINES FOR AMERICANS; FOOD PYRAMID; HYPERTENSION.)

soybean (*Glycine max*; soya, soy pea) The oil-rich seed of a bushy LEGUME; a food staple in the Far East. The soybean originated in eastern Asia and was cultivated in ancient China. American and Canadian cooperative agricultural projects in the 1930s yielded soybean varieties with increased yield and oil content, making soybeans more appealing as a crop. Today soybeans are the leading U.S. cash crop, ahead of WHEAT and CORN, and the United States is the world's major supplier of soybeans. Illinois, Iowa, Missouri, Minnesota and Ohio are among the top producers of soybeans, which represent the largest domestic source of VEGETABLE OIL. Dried soybeans can be cooked like dried beans and served in salads or casseroles. Roasted soybeans are a high-fat snack food.

Soybeans contain about 20 to 25% oil, 30 to 50% protein and 14 to 21% carbohydrate, but little STARCH. Processing soybeans has traditionally separated oil and protein. Soybean oil is one of the most widely used vegetable oils. Over 90% of the oil is used for food processing, cooking oil and MARGARINE. Solvents are generally used to extract oil from cracked seeds after heating. The oil must first be degummed, then bleached, partially hydrogenated to increase stability and extend its shelf life, and finally deodorized. Because of its high content of polyunsaturated FATTY ACIDS (with multiple hydrogen-deficient linkages), soybean oil is classified as a polyunsaturated oil. Soybean oil contains LINOLEIC ACID, an essential fatty acid, up to 55%; OLEIC ACID, a monounsaturate and fatty acid, up to 25%. The saturated fatty acids represent about 15%. Soybean oil is often used in cooking and in processed foods.

Soybean protein is used as a meat substitute because its protein is unusually well balanced for a plant protein. The NET PROTEIN UTILIZATION (NPU) is 65, comparable to animal protein in quality. Soy protein contains substantial amounts of LYSINE, an essential amino acid, and sulfur-containing

amino acids, especially METHIONINE, often deficient in legumes and grains. Soy-based infant formulas may be appropriate for babies who are allergic to cow's milk protein, and soy protein can increase the nutritive value of baby cereals and canned baby foods. Soy protein is used to fortify pasta products, hot cereals and various breakfast or granola bars. Because of its low cost, soy protein is often used in institutional settings. The National SCHOOL LUNCH PROGRAM is permitted to incorporate up to 30% hydrated soy protein in meat products.

Soy Products

Processed soy protein, TEXTURIZED VEGETABLE PROTEIN, soybean flour and soybean grits contain 40 to 50% protein. They are used in baked goods like bread, rolls, cakes, pancake and waffle mixes, crackers and cookies; in meat products like SAUSAGE, hot dogs, soy burgers, MEAT LOAF, meat patties, canned meats; in breakfast cereals and confections; in infant and children's foods; and in dietetic foods.

Soy protein hydrolyzate (hydrolyzed vegetable protein) is a mixture produced by degrading soy protein by any of a variety of agents: enzymes, yeast, molds, bacteria, acids or alkali. It is used in soy sauce, and as a flavoring, foaming or whipping agent.

Soy milk is prepared by first soaking beans in water, grinding the moistened beans and then filtering to remove the particles. The milk is used in soy-based infant formulas. Commercial products contain water, homogenized soybeans, vegetables, oils and sometimes kelp. Unless specified otherwise, soy milk is not fortified with vitamins A or D or minerals. Nutritionally fortified soy milk can be a good source of vitamin B_{12}.

TOFU (soybean curd) can be coagulated from soy protein by boiling or by adding lime water. The precipitating protein is pressed into blocks to prepare tofu. Tofu can be seasoned or converted to foods ranging from eggless egg salad to tofu burgers and stir-fries.

Soy sauce (shoyu, chiang-yu) is a salty sauce prepared by fermenting a mixture of wheat and soybeans and water. It contains relatively high levels of free amino acids and protein fermentation products. It is generally a high-salt seasoning. Reduced salt and varieties without wheat are available.

A variety of population studies link the consumption of soy protein with reduced risk of heart disease. As soy protein replaces animal protein in the diet, elevated blood cholesterol levels decline. Individuals with blood cholesterol levels greater than 250 and who substitute soy for animal protein may be able to lower their cholesterol by up to 25% by consuming about 40 g of soy protein daily. The reasons behind this reduction are not known; several possibilities are being examined. Soy contains complex substances called ISOFLAVONES, such as GENISTEIN which may prevent the formation of fatty deposits in arteries (plaque) by blocking the formation of oxidized LDL, believed to be the promoter of plaque formation. Isoflavones block the formation of blood clots in plaque in partially blocked arteries and to increase the flexibility of hardened (atherosclerotic) arteries. Also in experiments on animals, genistein inhibits the regrowth of plaque after balloon angioplasty. On the other hand, soy contains fiber that may bind bile salts, derived from cholesterol, and help excrete them, thus helping to flush cholesterol out of the blood. Soy may alter hormone levels: Thyroxine, a thyroid hormone, is higher in the blood of people on soy-based diets. Thyroxine may lower cholesterol levels.

A growing number of laboratory studies indicate that genistein and cholesterol analogs called saponins can block cancer development in experimental animals. Soy isoflavones and saponins may mimic the female hormone estrogen (PHYTOESTROGENS), which promotes breast and cervical cancer. By inhibiting estrogen production, isoflavones may convince the body to make less estrogen, thus lowering the cancer risk. Population studies support the protective role of soy. Asian women, who traditionally consume eight times more soy than American women have half the rate of breast cancer. How much genistein is required to offer a protective effect is not known. The estrogen-like effects of genistein and similar isoflavones may help prevent bone loss associated with osteoporosis and they may lessen the symptoms of menopause. (See also PROTEIN QUALITY; RANCIDITY.)

Anderson, J.W., Johnstone, B.M., Cook-Newell, M.E., "Meta-analysis of the Effects of Soy Protein Intake on Serum Lipids," *New England Journal of Medicine*, 333 (August 3, 1995), pp. 276–82.

Messina, M.J., et al., "Soy Intake and Cancer Risk: a Review of the In Vitro and In Vivo Data," *Nutrition and Cancer*, 21 (1994), pp. 113–31.

soy milk   See SOYBEAN.

soy sauce   See SOYBEAN.

spastic colon   See IRRITABLE BOWEL SYNDROME.

specific dynamic effect (SDE; specific dynamic activity, SDA)   The ENERGY used by the body to digest and process foods. The secretion of ENZYMES and HORMONES and the uptake of nutrients by the INTESTINE are energy-requiring processes. Smooth muscles are activated to move food through the digestive system (PERISTALSIS), and the rate of degradation of enzymes increases. The SDE amounts to an increase of 6 to 10% in energy expenditure above the fasting or basal level. This stimulation of cell processes is also called diet-induced thermogenesis because increased metabolism inevitably produces more heat. (See also CALORIES.)

spelt (*Triticum spelta*)   A GRAIN closely related to WHEAT (*Triticum sativum*). Spelt has been cultivated in Europe and the Middle East since ancient times. The protein content ranges from 13.1 to 14.3%, comparable to durum wheat (hard wheat) but significantly greater than soft wheat. Spelt protein contains somewhat more of the essential amino acid METHIONINE than wheat. This amino acid is deficient in most grains. The whole grain contains higher levels of B complex vitamins than most other grains. The nutrient content of 100 g of spelt flour is: 382 calories; protein, 14.3 g carbohydrate, 74.5 g; fat, 2.94 g; iron, 4.2 mg; thiamin, 0.649 mg; riboflavin, 0.227 mg; niacin, 8.46 mg. For comparison, white bleached flour (100 g), enriched, provides: thiamin, 0.64 mg; riboflavin, 0.40 mg; niacin, 5.22 mg; and corn, 4.35 mg. Whole wheat flour provides: thiamin, 0.57 mg; riboflavin, 0.12 mg; niacin, 0.44 mg; and iron, 4.44 mg.

spice   Seasonings prepared mainly from tropical plants. Spices are generally more pungent than herbs and have a strong flavor. They may represent seeds, roots, stems or bark, depending on which part of the plant is the most aromatic (spicey). In contrast, herbs generally utilize most of the plant. The following are representative: Allspice and red PEPPER come from the dried fruits; CLOVES from dried flower buds; cinnamon from bark; MUSTARD from seeds; black pepper from dried berries; PAPRIKA from dried pods; GINGER and horseradish from roots; SAFFRON from dried flower stigmas. Spices are among the oldest FOOD ADDITIVES; the amounts used to flavor food are too small to contribute significant nutrients, although they stimulate digestion. Certain oils possess preservative or antioxidant effects. (See also APPETITE.)

Charalambous, George. *Spices, Herbs and Edible Fungi*. New York: Elsevier, 1994.

spina bifida   A severe BIRTH DEFECT in which the spinal cord is exposed. Approximately 2,500 infants are born each year in the United States with this condition. A related defect is anencephaly, an absence of part of the brain. Much of the damage may occur in the first month of pregnancy, before women realize they are pregnant. Genetic as well as environmental factors affect the probability of this condition. Prenatal nutrition is important. VITAMIN B$_{12}$, VITAMIN C, VITAMIN D and ZINC deficiencies seem to play a role.

Current studies link a deficiency of the B vitamin, FOLIC ACID, to this defect. Women at risk for NEURAL TUBE DEFECTS who take multivitamin pills containing folic acid in around the time of conception have fewer babies with neurological birth defects, and folic acid supplements prior to and during the early stages of pregnancy have been recommended. In 1992 for the first time the U.S. government advocated a VITAMIN supplement for the general population. Extra folic acid either from supplements or from vegetables is recommended for women of childbearing age at least one month before conception. The U.S. Public Health Service contends that folic acid intake should not exceed 1 mg daily because it could mask or aggravate ANEMIA. Folic acid occurs in dark-green leafy vegetables, citrus fruit, whole grain bread and beans, and women who eat at least five servings daily can meet the guidelines. (See also HOMOCYSTEINE.)

spinach (*Spinacia oleracea*)   A dark-green leafy VEGETABLE related to chard and beets. Spinach is believed to have originated in south-western Asia. Though Moors brought spinach to Europe about 1000 A.D., it was not cultivated in northern Europe until the 1700s. The United States is a major producer of spinach, and much of the domestic crop is grown in California and Texas. As much as 75% is processed by canning or freezing.

There are three basic types of spinach: Savoy spinach with curly leaves; flat or smooth-leaf spinach, usually frozen or canned; and semi-Savoy, with slightly crinkled leaves. Spinach is an excellent source of BETA CAROTENE (provitamin A) and VITAMIN K (required for normal blood clotting) and the B vitamin folacin. Spinach is used in fillings or stuffings, souffles, casseroles and soups and it is used now in salads. Spinach contains oxalates, salts of OXALIC ACID. Oxalates bind CALCIUM and IRON, two minerals that are high in spinach, so that these minerals cannot be completely used. Consequently spinach is not the wonder food popularized by cartoons. Other vegetarian sources such as kale and turnip greens provide more of these minerals. Various studies indicate that the oxalate content of spinach does not appreciably decrease calcium uptake from other foods. Only massive amounts of spinach can create a nutritional problem. The nutrient content of 1 cup (cooked, drained, 180 g) is: 41 calories; protein, 5.3 g; carbohydrate, 6.8 g; fiber, 5.8 g; fat, 0.5 g; calcium, 244 mg; iron, 6.4 mg; potassium, 838 mg; vitamin A, 1,474 retinol equivalents; thiamin, 0.17 mg; riboflavin, 0.42 mg; niacin, 0.88 mg. (See also BIOAVAILABILITY; TRACE MINERALS.)

spirulina   A form of microscopic blue-green algae used as a food supplement. Spirulina is a rich source of BETA CAROTENE (pro-vitamin A), a blue pigment called phycocyanin, and CHLOROPHYLL, the green plant pigment. Spirulina contains 65% protein, 18% carbohydrate, 5% fat and 7% minerals. Spirulina contains appreciable iron and B complex vitamins. Although claimed to be a good source of VITAMIN B_{12}, spirulina contains vitamin B_{12} analogs or other substances that prevent its use in the body. Spirulina provides GAMMA LINOLENIC ACID, a polyunsaturated FATTY ACID. This lipid is a parent compound of a hormone-like family of lipids called PROSTAGLANDINS, which possess anti-inflammatory activity.

Spirulina has been added to soups, salads, pasta, fruit dishes and vegetable juices. The nutrient content of a 10 g (1/3 oz) serving is: protein, 6.5 g; carbohydrate, 1.8 g; fat, 0.5 g; calcium, 100 mg; iron, 15 mg; vitamin A, 2,300 retinol equivalents; thiamin, 0.31 mg; riboflavin, 0.35 mg; niacin, 1.46 mg.

spoilage   A change in food that makes it unsuitable for human consumption. Spoilage can alter the texture, odor, color, taste and nutrient content of a food, changes that are usually readily detected. Microbial spoilage is caused by growth of YEAST, MOLDS and bacteria and is favored by warm, moist conditions. Bacteria can degrade MEAT, dairy products and canned foods, while mold and yeast can grow on BREAD, CHEESE, FRUIT, VEGETABLES and sugary foods like jelly and jam.

Enzymes in foods can also lead to spoilage. Alternatively, insect pests can infest foods, making them unfit. Softening and ripening of fruit and vegetables are caused by enzymatic changes. Enzymes may survive processing and create off-flavors.

Spontaneous chemical reactions due to oxygen, light and metal ion contaminants can lead to rancidity (breakdown) of fat and oil-containing foods. Heat can increase the rate of chemical reactions leading to degradation, whether affected by enzymes or not. Alternatively, extreme cold can crack fresh foods or alter their texture. Modern food processing and preservation aims to minimize food spoilage. Canning, drying, freezing or chilling, and the use of FOOD PRESERVATIVES, as well as sanitation, play a role in preventing spoilage up to the time of purchase. As an example, food manufacturers can limit oxidation by minimizing exposure to air (vacuum-sealed containers); by adding preservatives like CITRIC ACID to bind metal ion contaminants; or by adding synthetic ANTIOXIDANTS like BHA and BHT. (See also FOOD POISONING.)

sport drinks   Electrolyte replacement beverages. It is important to drink plenty of fluids during strenuous EXER-

CISE, especially during hot weather because the body requires water for efficient cooling and for efficient operation of the kidneys in moving wastes from the blood. GLUCOSE-sodium sport drinks provide extra sugar and sodium, which also promote rapid fluid uptake by the small intestine. Some beverages contain glucose polymers (maltodextrins), small fragments of STARCH. Glucose polymer beverages may be more effective than glucose drinks in replacing carbohydrates and in increasing BLOOD SUGAR during endurance events (more than two hours in duration). They do not slow the passage of liquid through the stomach as a high-glucose concentration does.

Simple carbohydrates seem to provide their greatest benefit when exercise exceeds 60 minutes. A potential benefit of consuming glucose replacements during exercise is that fluid intake may increase if the taste is more appealing than plain water. The carbohydrate-electrolyte sport drink should be mixed so that the carbohydrate concentration is less than 10% to minimize retention by the stomach. On the other hand, the carbohydrate concentration should be at least 6% to improve endurance. When fluid loss is reduced by a cold environment such as in cross-country skiing, fluids with a carbohydrate concentration greater than 10% are appropriate.

Sport drinks often contain more sugar (glucose) and salt (SODIUM) than are needed for optimal absorption of fluids, and they often contain less POTASSIUM than a glass of ORANGE juice. Plain water, which is both easily absorbed and palatable, effectively replaces water lost with strenuous exercise. In general, there does not seem to be any need to replace electrolytes lost through sweating by consuming expensive beverages. Sport drinks appear likely to improve performance only in endurance exercise or day-long events.

Diluted fruit juices are usually adequate electrolyte replacements. Fruit juices should be diluted at least twofold from standard preparations to prevent delayed gastric emptying. Electrolytes and carbohydrates are readily replenished by eating a banana, fruit or crackers with water. Many commercial soft drinks contain CAFFEINE, which acts as a diuretic. Therefore athletes are advised to limit their intake of such beverages. (See also DEHYDRATION.)

Burke, Louise M. and Read, Richard S.D., "Dietary Supplements in Sport," *Sports Medicine*, 15:1 (1993), pp. 43–65.

sprue (non-tropical sprue, idiopathic sprue)   A digestive disorder typically characterized by weight loss, weakness, bloating and gas, loss of appetite, greasy, frothy stools, DIARRHEA and malabsorption. Poor absorption of SUGAR, fat-soluble vitamins (A, D, E and K) and MINERALS by the small intestine is responsible for the weight loss. Malabsorption of vitamin D and calcium promotes bone thinning. The intestinal surface becomes damaged, leading to nutrient malabsorption. Sprue occurs sporadically without any known cause, although FOOD SENSITIVITIES have been implicated in some individuals. Inadequate uptake of VITAMIN B_{12}, FOLIC ACID and IRON can lead to anemia. Vitamin B_{12} and folic acid shots can be given to overcome deficiencies because they cannot be taken up efficiently if given orally to these patients. Fiber supplements should not be used with any acute gastrointestinal disease (DIVERTICULITIS, CELIAC DISEASE or ulcerative COLITIS). Foods that provoke symptoms should be avoided.

Celiac Sprue

Celiac disease refers to damaged intestine due to an inherited immunologic sensitivity to wheat protein and GLUTEN. This is one of the most common malabsorption syndromes in the United States. This disease is characterized by a marked loss in flattening of the villi—the small, hairlike projections that increase the absorptive surface of the small intestine. Celiac sprue is usually diagnosed in childhood and can be cured by placing the patient on a gluten-free diet. Celiac disease increases the risk of gastric intestinal cancer, especially of the small intestine.

Tropical Sprue

Like celiac sprue, this malabsorption syndrome is also characterized by atrophy of the villi, drastically reducing the surface area. Intestinal enzyme deficiencies lead to carbohydrate and fat maldigestion and malabsorption. Anemia often develops as a consequence of vitamin B$_{12}$ and folic acid deficiencies. Tropical sprue affects populations living in Asia, Central America and the West Indies or people who have visited the tropics. Administration of vitamin B$_{12}$ and folic acid may successfully treat macrocytic anemia (anemia characterized by large, pale red blood cells). Substitutions of fat and oils by MEDIUM-CHAIN TRIGLYCERIDES (fats with smaller fatty acids) can increase fat absorption, correct fatty stools and assist with weight gain. The cause of this disease is unknown, although there are hints that specific disease-producing strains of the bacterium ESCHERICHIA COLI are involved. Response to a wheat-free (gluten free) diet is minimal but administration of broad-spectrum antibiotics may be effective. (See also IRRITABLE BOWEL SYNDROME.)

squash (Cucurbita genus) A gourd native to North and South America. Squash is related to MELONS, PUMPKINS and CUCUMBERS and was used as food in Mexico and Guatemala about 8000 B.C. Aztec, Inca and Mayan civilizations cultivated squash, corn and beans, which spread throughout Native American populations. Hundreds of varieties of squash now exist. Summer squash is a quick-growing bushy squash that produces many fruit, which are usually harvested in the summer months while still immature. They have soft shells and tender flesh. Summer squashes are about 95% water, and so are very low in calories. Examples include Patty pan, Scallop, Chayote, Cocozelle, zucchini, yellow crookneck, yellow straightneck and Caserta.

Winter squashes are harvested in the fall when fully mature. They have a tough, coarse rind that is dark-green or orange, and their flesh is darker than that of summer varieties. Winter squash is easily stored. Acorn or Danish, butternut, spaghetti, Warren turban, Hubbard and Sugar squash are common winter squashes. Squash blossom can be eaten, as well as the dried seeds. Summer squash is usually cooked unpeeled. It can be stuffed or grated and cooked as patties; or fried or baked in casseroles. Winter squash is cut in half and the seeds removed. It is then microwaved, baked, broiled or steamed. All winter squashes are excellent sources of BETA CAROTENE (provitamin A). The nutrient content of 1 cup (cooked, 180 g) of crookneck squash is: 36 calories; protein, 1.6 g; carbohydrate, 7.8 g; fiber, 3.2 g; fat, 0.6 g; iron, 0.63 mg; potassium, 455 mg; vitamin A, 43 retinol equivalents; thiamin, 0.07 mg; riboflavin, 0.07 mg; niacin, 0.77 mg.

One cup (205 g) of baked and mashed butternut winter squash provides: 83 calories; protein, 1.8 g; carbohydrate, 21.5 g; fiber, 4.9 g; iron, 1.23 mg; potassium, 583 mg; vitamin A, 1,435 retinol equivalents; thiamin, 0.15 mg; riboflavin, 0.04 mg; niacin, 2.0 mg (See also VEGETABLES.)

stabilizers   Food additives used as thickening agents in processing to avoid watery or lumpy products. Examples are CARRAGEENAN, DEXTRIN, KARAYA GUM, LECITHIN, LOCUST BEAN GUM, TRAGACANTH GUM and XANTHAN GUM.

Carrageenan comes from a SEAWEED, Irish moss. It is used to keep cocoa butter suspended in chocolate milk and fat suspended in evaporated milk, canned milk, instant breakfasts and infant formulas. It thickens SOFT DRINKS, ICE CREAM, frozen whipped topping and YOGURT. Carrageenan appears to be safe, except for premature infants.

Dextrin is partially hydrolyzed STARCH. It finds use in candy, powdered mixes of various kinds, and in soups and gravy and other foods. Dextrin is considered a safe food additive.

Karaya gum comes from India. Food manufacturers use this complex carbohydrate to stabilize whipped products, salad dressing, processed meat products like SAUSAGE and ice cream. Long-term studies on its safety have not been carried out.

Lecithin is a nutrient and a constituent of all plant and animal food. As a FOOD ADDITIVE it stabilizes MARGARINE, CHOCOLATE, baked goods like rolls and bread, and ice cream. It is classified as a safe additive.

Locust bean gum (carob seed gum) comes from the bean of the carob tree. It is used to stabilize ice cream, salad dressing, pie filling, cakes and biscuits. It often is used together with carrageenan to improve the qualities and thickening properties of that additive. Locust bean gum is considered safe.

Tragacanth gum is a product of the Middle East. It is especially useful in acidic foods, such as salad dressing, because it does not break down under acidic conditions. The safety of this additive has not been studied.

Xanthan gum is produced by a bacterium. It is widely used because it is stable in acidic media and because it thickens even at high temperatures. Xanthan gum stabilizes salad dressing, syrup, pie fillings, pudding and processed foods. It is a safe additive. (See also EMULSIFIERS.)

standards of identity   The Federal Food, Drug and Cosmetic Act defined the standard formulations or commercial "recipes" now available for about 400 common foods and condiments, like ketchup, HAMBURGER, ICE CREAM, jelly, MAYONNAISE, PEANUT BUTTER, SAUSAGE, cheese, frankfurters and bread. Manufacturers of these items do not have to list the ingredients on labels. These standards were established to ensure consistent quality and composition and to prevent fraud. The standards of identity for foods specify required levels of ingredients. As an example, ice cream must contain at least 10% milkfat, otherwise it must be renamed as frozen dessert or labeled as imitation. The U.S. FDA has been petitioned to change several standards to help market foods that could contribute to improving the American diet. Thus "ice milk" could be changed to "reduced fat ice cream." There may be new standards of identity, such as "low fat ice cream." Low fat and reduced fat now have specific meanings on food labels. The use of artificial sweeteners in standard formulations is also being explored. (See also FOOD ADDITIVES; FOOD LABELING; PROCESSED FOOD.)

staphylococcal food poisoning   An infectious type of FOOD POISONING induced by toxins released from bacteria (Staphylococcus). The bacteria form poisons (toxins) in improperly stored or cooked food, which are not easily destroyed by cooking. Staphylococci are common in the environment and are present in secretions from the nose and throat, as well as from skin infections. Therefore food exposed to air and to infected food handlers can become contaminated. Staphylococcus can rapidly multiply in certain foods stored at room temperature. They can hibernate in the food when refrigerated, and then begin reproduction when warmed to room temperature. A variety of foods are implicated, including HAM and other meats, POULTRY and chicken salad, cream-filled desserts, custards and custard-filled baked desserts, pasta salad and cheese products.

Staph-infected food does not taste different from normal food, thus there is no change in flavor to serve as a warning. Staphylococcus is destroyed by boiling, but toxins developed before heating may resist this treatment. Prevention of staph food poisoning requires cleanliness in food preparation, elimination of flies from the kitchen area, education of food handlers in personal hygiene, and refrigeration of all perishable foods. (See also BOTULISM; SALMONELLA.)

staple   A food that is consumed in large amounts and provides a large percentage of total daily calories. Staples anchor traditional diets; POTATOES, BREAD, RICE and MILK fall into this category. Staples can significantly impact health because they provide much more than calories. As whole foods—that is, foods that have been minimally processed—they provide MINERALS, VITAMINS, ESSENTIAL FATTY ACIDS, FIBER and certain non-nutrient materials that have less well-defined functions in the body. Thus, consuming ample amounts of whole GRAINS and VEGETABLES can lower the risk of CARDIOVASCULAR DISEASE, CANCER and GASTROINTESTINAL disease in populations throughout the world.

starch   The storage carbohydrate that occurs in granules in seeds, stems and roots of higher plants. Starch consists of long chains of GLUCOSE, a simple sugar, formed during PHOTOSYNTHESIS. Starch accounts for 50 to 75% of the weight of cereal GRAIN and 75% of the weight of POTATOES. Unripened apples and bananas contain starch; as these fruits ripen, much of the starch is converted to glucose. With moist heat, starch granules absorb water and rupture, releasing starch to an easily digested, water-soluble form.

Starch is classified as a COMPLEX CARBOHYDRATE because of its complex structure, which requires DIGESTION to be assimilated. Starch occurs either as long, unbranched chains (AMYLOSE) or as highly branched chains (AMYLOPECTIN). The ratio of these two types varies with the source; an average composition is 27% amylose and 73% amylopectin.

As a carbohydrate, starch produces 4 calories per gram when burned for ENERGY. Starchy foods are dietary staples throughout the world. These foods are economical and contribute a large percentage of daily calories. Examples include

RICE in Asian countries, CORN in Mexico, roots, tubers and SORGHUM in Africa. Contrary to old ideas, starch is not fattening nor is starch the major villain in the standard American diet. Fat contains more than twice the number of calories per gram as carbohydrate, and because a high-fat intake is common, fat calories are more critical in controlling weight and maintaining long-term health. Excessive dietary fat, particularly saturated fat, not starch, increases the risk of heart disease and some forms of cancer.

Starch represents the most important source of carbohydrate in the American diet where it occurs as the main ingredient of rice, WHEAT, RYE, MILLET, corn, BARLEY and OATS. Pasta and baked goods are common sources of starch from wheat. Cornstarch and potato starch are used as thickening agents in prepared foods. Starch occurs in high amounts also in LEGUMES, dried BEANS, kidney beans, black-eyed peas, CHICKPEAS and SOYBEANS. Cornstarch is converted to high FRUCTOSE CORN SYRUP, which is extensively used as a sweetener in SOFT DRINKS.

Starch Digestion

Starch digestion produces glucose. Digestion begins in the mouth with an enzyme (AMYLASE) in SALIVA; it is completed in the intestine by the combined action of pancreatic amylase, and yields fragments containing a pair of glucose units (maltose) and dextrins, composed of several glucose units. Intestinal enzymes (MALTASE, dextrinase) degrade these fragments to glucose, which is then rapidly absorbed by the small intestine. Depending upon the form of starch and other ingredients of the meal, starch can be more or less completely converted to blood glucose from one to four hours after a meal.

The rate at which food liberates glucose and increases blood sugar can be compared to the rate from eating the sugar alone. Processed starches such as white bread, white rice and instant mashed potatoes send blood glucose soaring almost as fast as sugar does. On the other hand, starch in whole foods like legumes is more slowly digested and does not cause a surge of blood sugar. Consequently, the pancreas does not need to release such a large amount of the hormone INSULIN to stimulate glucose utilization. Chronic high insulin levels can increase blood lipids.

Starch as an Additive

Corn is the primary source for commercial starch, followed by sorghum, wheat and rice, potato and ARROWROOT, among others. Waxy hybrid strains of corn and sorghum yield starches that range from almost completely amylose to those that are almost completely amylopectin, which have different uses. The tendency to gel upon cooking is caused by the presence of amylose. Some starches form gels that are more translucent than usual; others make puddings stiffer and give baked goods a velvety texture that stays fresh longer.

Starches can be modified chemically to create useful FOOD ADDITIVES. Treatment with alkali or acid yields GUMS and DEXTRINS, which are partially degraded starch. Cross-linked starches, chemically stabilized against acid and mechanical agitation, were discontinued voluntarily as food additives by the food industry when questions arose about their safety. "Derivatized" starches contain acidic groups such as ACETIC ACID, SUCCINIC ACID or phosphate, which prevent starch molecules from clumping or crystallizing. Solutions of these starches are clearer and more viscous then untreated starch and are used in frozen foods as thickening agents. Most derivatized starches have not been exhaustively studied by lifetime feeding experiments. Previously, manufacturers of baby foods used modified starches extensively to improve consistency of product and to increase the nutrient value, but they have gradually moved away from adding starches. (See also CARBOHYDRATE METABOLISM; DIETARY GUIDELINES FOR AMERICANS; GLYCEMIC INDEX; STAPLE.)

Hudnall, Marsha, "Pasta Makes You Fat Furor Raises the Question of Insulin Resistance," *Environmental Nutrition*, 18:5 (May 1995), pp. 1, 6.

starch blockers   Kidney bean proteins believed to curtail STARCH digestion in the INTESTINE. Starch blockers were marketed according to the belief that by eating them with meals, dieters could eat starchy foods without adding calories. In 1982 the U.S. FDA classified starch blockers as drugs; tests indicated that starch blockers are not effective and cause gas, bloating and DIARRHEA, and their sale was banned by the FDA in 1987. (See also CARBOHYDRATE METABOLISM; DIETING.)

starvation   A condition due to chronic food deprivation characterized by tissue wasting. Starvation can occur due to unavailability of food; self-denial of food (FASTING); institutional restriction of food intake; or anorexia. Protein-calorie malnutrition ranges from MARASMUS, in which people do not get adequate calories, to KWASHIORKOR, in which they lack adequate protein although their diet supplies adequate calories. Anorexia may be caused by severe thiamin deficiency; KETOSIS (excessive KETONE BODIES in the blood); kidney failure; or an emotional aversion to food (ANOREXIA NERVOSA). Ketone bodies are water-soluble acid derivatives of fat, produced when massive fat breakdown occurs. Disorders of the digestive tract that can lead to starvation include: severe DIARRHEA, MALABSORPTION (such as CROHN'S DISEASE), vomiting or surgical removal of part of the digestive tract. Severe malnutrition may accompany metabolic disorders such as DIABETES, wasting diseases like CANCER or severe physical trauma.

Vulnerability to famine rests upon the degree of civil tranquility, adequacy of trained personnel, institutions and infrastructure for the production, distribution and storage of food, as well as the state of general economic development. When starvation affect entire populations, the result is a famine. Historically, war or crop failure due to poor weather or both have caused most famines. The unavailability of food due to natural catastrophes such as drought, flood and earthquake, as well as to human causes such as war, civil disruption and governmental mismanagement, reduces the food supply and leads to a decline in an entitlement to food. High food prices, unemployment and loss of assets are symptoms of underlying problems. In a typical scenario experienced in regions of Africa, sequential years of crop failure produce increased agricultural prices, less farming activity and a decline in employment of workers and farm laborers. The financially privileged class may hoard food from the poor, who are then forced to sell assets. HUNGER follows poverty with the ultimate outcome of increased mortality.

Effects of Starvation

Children, infants and the elderly are the most susceptible to the effects of starvation because of their high rates of growth and/or small reserves of energy and tissue. Impaired mental development is particularly pronounced for children starved during the first years of life, and their growth may be permanently retarded. Many nutrients are required to support the normal function of the IMMUNE SYSTEM, and adults and children who have starved are more susceptible to infectious disease due to reduced immunity.

Signs and symptoms of starvation include weight loss and muscle wasting, ketosis, ketone body excretion in the urine, low blood pressure, edema, diarrhea, irritability, smaller than normal growth and body weight.

Metabolic adaptations to starvation include an increased utilization of fat stores to spare muscle, and decreased BASAL METABOLIC RATE (metabolism required to maintain the body at rest) as the body adapts to lowered nutrient intake. Body temperature may be abnormally low. Muscle protein degradation continues at a slow rate to provide amino acids that are converted to BLOOD SUGAR. The brain and nervous system cannot use FAT as a fuel and rely upon this glucose for energy. Accumulated fatty acids in the liver are converted to ketone bodies, acids that are released into the bloodstream. As levels rise, ketone bodies can enter the brain, which then uses them to meet some of its energy needs. High blood levels of ketone bodies acidify the blood; when they are excreted in the urine this causes dehydration and loss of critical minerals (ELECTROLYTES). (See also ACIDOSIS; GLUCONEOGENESIS.)

stearic acid   A common saturated FATTY ACID in animal fat. Stearic acid is classified as "saturated" because its carbon atoms cannot take up more hydrogen and it lacks double bonds. Stearic acid with 18 carbon atoms is a solid at room temperature and contributes to the hardness of animal fat. Unlike palmitic acid, stearic acid alone does not appear to raise blood CHOLESTEROL. However, stearic acid may promote blood clots more than other saturated fats; consequently its relative safety has not been determined. In addition, food occurs as fatty acid mixtures, not isolated nutrients. Thus saturated fats like BUTTER, SHORTENING and even chocolate tend to raise cholesterol levels due to their content of saturated fatty acids. Additionally, fat is a calorie-rich nutrient, and excessive calories in processed foods contribute to problems of WEIGHT MANAGEMENT and OBESITY, said to be an American epidemic. Dietary recommendations generally call for decreasing fat consumption, especially saturated fat. (See also DIETARY GUIDELINES FOR AMERICANS; FAT METABOLISM; FOOD GUIDE PYRAMID; HEART DISEASE; VEGETABLE OIL.)

steatorrhea   Smelly, fatty stools that may be tan or light colored. Steatorrhea indicates severe fat MALABSORPTION and/or fat maldigestion. Inadequate digestive enzymes from the pancreas or a blocked bile duct can lead to fatty stools because both pancreatic lipase and bile are needed for fat breakdown and absorption. Alternatively, fat malabsorption can be produced by conditions affecting the health of the small intestine, like CELIAC DISEASE and CROHN'S DISEASE. Deficiencies of fat-soluble vitamins may develop with fat malabsorption. Further weight loss and malnutrition can develop, leading to worsening malabsorption and malnutrition. (See also FAT DIGESTION.)

steroids A family of hormones related to CHOLESTEROL. Steroid HORMONES are produced by the ADRENAL GLANDS. Steroids are LIPIDS and, such as cholesterol, have an affinity for fatty materials. Steroid hormones include sex hormones, TESTOSTERONE and ESTROGEN; GLUCOCORTICOIDS, which regulate carbohydrate metabolism; and mineralocorticoids, like ALDOSTERONE, which regulate sodium and water excretion. Calcitriol, activated vitamin D$_3$, is another type of steroid hormone. (See also BILE; ENDOCRINE SYSTEM; FAT METABOLISM.)

sterol A family of fat-soluble materials (LIPIDS), of which CHOLESTEROL is the most prominent member. Cholesterol is a primary component of all membranes and is therefore essential for cell function and metabolism. Its metabolites (metabolic products) also serve important functions. BILE salts are made by the LIVER from cholesterol to aid FAT DIGESTION. In terms of chemical structure, sterols consist of interlocking rings and possess a hydroxyl group, making them ALCOHOLS. Ergosterol is a plant sterol that forms vitamin D$_2$, ERGOCALCIFEROL, when exposed to ultraviolet light. (See FORTIFICATION; MILK.)

stock Extracts of foods that form the basis of soups, gravies and sauces. Traditionally, MEAT from older animals and mature vegetables like CARROTS, CABBAGE, TURNIPS or BEANS are heated to extract juices and flavors. Meat is trimmed of excess fat, vegetables are cleaned and even blended. Bones with marrow are used for gravies and sauces. Appropriate spices include allspice, peppercorn, coriander, celery seed and bay leaf.

stomach A long J-shaped pouch that receives swallowed, masticated food from the MOUTH via the ESOPHAGUS. The stomach lies in the upper part of the abdominal cavity under the diaphragm. Muscles encircle the stomach and run lengthwise and obliquely to make the stomach one of the strongest internal organs. The muscles squeeze and churn the pulverized food and mix it thoroughly with digestive juices. Stomach muscle contraction produces PERISTALSIS, a movement that propels food down the DIGESTIVE TRACT. Without food the stomach compresses to the size of a large sausage with large folds called rugae, which allow the stomach to expand after a large meal.

Glands in the stomach wall secrete a mixture of stomach acid, a strong mineral acid called hydrochloric acid, and a DIGESTIVE ENZYME called PEPSIN to begin protein DIGESTION. Stomach acid creates a low pH required for optimal activity of this enzyme. Chief cells produce an inactive form of pepsin, which is activated by stomach acid. Acid-producing cells are called parietal cells. Stomach acid softens and denatures proteins, easing their digestion, and it sterilizes food, killing many potentially dangerous microorganisms. The stomach's thick mucus forms a layer that protects the lining against stomach acid, which maintains a strongly acidic environment. The stomach wall is impermeable to most nutrients, and usually they do not reach the blood until they reach the intestine. The stomach can absorb water, alcohol, electrolytes, aspirin and certain drugs. An alcohol oxidizing system in men's stomachs is more prevalent than in women's, which partially explains why men are more often able to imbibe more alcohol than women. Parietal cells also produce INTRINSIC FACTOR, a vitamin B$_{12}$-binding protein that is required for intestinal absorption of this vitamin.

The lower part of the stomach is called the pylorus. Here hormone-producing (enteroendocrine) cells secrete GASTRIN, a hormone that stimulates and increases gastrointestinal tract peristalsis. A pyloric sphincter (valve) retains food long enough for partial digestion to occur in the stomach, then waves of contraction squeeze small amounts of liquefied food (CHYME) into the upper region of the small intestine (DUODENUM).

Secretion of gastric juice is regulated by gastrin and by nerve stimulation. In the "reflex phase" (cephalic phase) of nerve stimulation, the sight, taste, smell or thought of food can initiate a nerve impulse via the feeding center of the brain (HYPOTHALAMUS); this in turn activates the PARASYMPATHETIC NERVOUS SYSTEM to prepare the body for feeding. In the "gastric phase," foods that fill the stomach will activate regions in the stomach wall, which relay nerve signals back to the brain that, in turn, activate gastric secretion. Partially digested protein and CAFFEINE also stimulate gastrin production. Secretion of gastrin stops when the pH drops to 2 (more acidic). This "feedback" system normally maintains the acidic pH in the stomach without over-producing acid.

The net effect of food in the small intestine is inhibition of gastrin secretion. Certain intestinal hormones can block gastrin secretion. The stomach empties its contents into the duodenum in one to four hours. Carbohydrate-rich foods leave more quickly than fat-containing foods. The rate is limited by the amount of chyme the small intestine can process. A high sugar content in beverages (greater than 10% glucose) slows gastric emptying. This is a consideration when attempting to consume fluids to rehydrate the body. (See also EXERCISE; HELICOBACTER PYLORI; SPORT DRINKS.)

stomach acid (hydrochloric acid) The very strong mineral acid, hydrochloric acid, produced by the stomach. Stomach acid is secreted by parietal cells of the gastric glands lining the wall of the stomach. Hydrochloric acid normally maintains stomach pH between 1.5 and 2.5, an acidic environment that can sterilize food and activate pepsinogen, the inactive form of PEPSIN. This enzyme initiates protein digestion in the stomach. Stomach acid also maintains an acidic environment required for pepsin activity. The mixture of food particles, digestive enzymes and acid forms an acidic mixture called CHYME, which is released into the upper small intestine (DUODENUM). Chyme stimulates secretion of alkaline BICARBONATE to neutralize the acid. Enzymes produced further down the gastrointestinal tract do not break down food (to release bound minerals like CALCIUM and IRON) efficiently when there is inadequate stomach acid. Chewing food stimulates stomach acid production via the nervous system. The process requires 15 to 30 minutes to be fully activated. Gulping down a meal does not provide adequate time to digest food completely.

Low stomach acid production is called HYPOCHLORHYDRIA. Stomach acid production declines with age; low stomach acidity is associated with diabetes mellitus, thyroid imbalance, ECZEMA, gallbladder disease, OSTEOPOROSIS,

RHEUMATOID ARTHRITIS, food allergy and FOOD SENSITIVITY. Without adequate stomach acid, intestinal flora can become imbalanced, which increases susceptibility to disease-producing microorganisms like yeast (candida) or parasites. The stomach possesses a protective mucous layer to prevent damage to the lining. Rarely, acid can break through the barrier and cause sores (ULCERS). The precise mechanisms are not known. (See also ACHLORHYDRIA; AGING; DIGESTION.)

stone age diet (paleolithic diet)   Studies of hunter-gatherer societies as well as studies of paleolithic sites have yielded information regarding the diet of our ancestors long before the domestication of plants and animals. These studies are prompted by the observation that modern hunter-gatherers are apparently free of HYPERTENSION, HEART DISEASE, DIABETES MELLITUS and certain CANCERS, diseases all too common in industrialized nations.

Evidence suggests that paleolithic peoples foraged and hunted, and ate nuts, fruits, berries and roots that are available by season. GRAINS and dairy products like MILK and CHEESE were unavailable. These became a major part of the diet only when agriculture and animal husbandry began, between 5,000 to 10,000 years ago. The stone age diet probably consisted of about 35% MEAT and 65% VEGETABLES. This diet was rich in PROTEIN, but the meat was lean and contained essential fatty acids. The FAT of game animals contains two to five times more polyunsaturated fat per gram than livestock. The opposite is true for the typical U.S. diet. The fat of game animals contains a higher percentage of the essential fatty acids of the omega-3 family, which help protect against clogged arteries and the formation of blood clots. The omega-3 fatty acids therefore lower the risk of cardiovascular disease; long-chain omega-3 fatty acids like EICOSAPENTAENOIC ACID are especially low in domestic animals.

Paleolithic people probably ate a greater variety of vegetables and plant products than obtainable in industrialized societies until the development of post-World War II supermarkets and modern food production distribution networks. The stone age diet contributed many nutrients and a high percentage of FIBER. Consequently prehistoric people are believed to have consumed more VITAMINS, especially VITAMIN C, more CALCIUM and other minerals, more high-quality protein and more polyunsaturated fats and oils than are in the diets of industrialized societies. The diet provided adequate IRON, FOLIC ACID and VITAMIN B$_{12}$, and the amount of CHOLESTEROL was about the same as in present day Western diets. (See also FOOD GUIDE PYRAMID; WHEAT.)

Haenel H., "Phylogenesis and Nutrition," *Nahrung*, 33:9 (1989), pp. 867–87.

strawberry (*Fragaria spp.*)   The juicy fruit of a herbaceous plant and a member of the rose family. Strawberries are native to both the Old World and the New World. Strawberries lead the world production of berries and berry-like fruit. The United States remains a leading producer of strawberries, and nearly 80% of the U.S. crop comes from California. Strawberries are grown in all states and are the most popular berries, containing more VITAMIN C than most other berries. About one-third of the crop is frozen. Strawberries are also processed as jam, fruit-flavored bever-

ages and other products. They are added fresh to cereals, cheesecake, fruit salads, custards, crepes, puddings, ice cream and milkshakes. Strawberries are a rich source of vitamin C. The nutrient content of 1 cup (149 g) of fresh strawberries is: 45 calories; protein, 0.9 g; carbohydrate, 10.5 g; fiber, 3.3 g; fat, 0.6 g; vitamin C, 85 mg; thiamin, 0.03 mg; riboflavin, 0.1 mg; niacin, 0.34 mg.

stress   The adjustment of the body's mechanisms to adverse conditions or changes in the environment. Stimuli ("stressors") run the gamut of disturbances from heat, cold, injury and environmental pollutants, to glare from video screens and bacterial toxins. Psychological stress relates to coping with demands of work, relationships and the demands of life in general. Coping with stress relies on the NERVOUS SYSTEM and the closely-linked ENDOCRINE SYSTEM (hormone secreting system).

Alarm Reaction

The alarm reaction or FIGHT OR FLIGHT RESPONSE is the first reaction to a stressor. Stimuli rapidly mobilize the body to defend against danger. The brain and nervous system regulate fast responses of the body to changes in the environment within seconds; the endocrine system regulates longer responses (minutes to hours) by releasing hormones. The region of the brain called the HYPOTHALAMUS activates the sympathetic nervous system, the portion of the nervous system that controls involuntary response to stress, to adapt the body to meet a challenge. The brain also stimulates the adrenal glands to release hormones like EPINEPHRINE (adrenaline) that support adaptation by increasing ENERGY and by decreasing non-essential functions such as DIGESTION and urine production.

The heart rate increases to supply oxygen and GLUCOSE (blood sugar) to the muscles and the brain, which must be very alert. Epinephrine and norepinephrine, hormones from the adrenal medulla, stimulate the breakdown of carbohydrate reserves (GLYCOGEN) in the liver to increase BLOOD SUGAR. Sympathetic nerve impulses, supplemented by hormones, prolong typical responses of the sympathetic nervous system-constricted blood vessels in skin and viscera; dilated blood vessels of the heart and skeletal muscle; increased sweating; expanded bronchial tubes; decreased production of digestive enzymes; and increased rate of breathing to bring additional oxygen to muscle.

Resistance Reaction

The second stage of the stress response is called the resistance reaction. The resistance reaction represents a long-term adjustment to stress, after the flight or fight response has worn off, in order to meet emotional crises and perform tasks. It is initiated by hormones secreted by the hypothalamus. Chronic stress causes higher than normal levels of stress hormones. Energy stockpiles are broken down to provide blood glucose, and long-term building and maintenance are slowed. The hypothalamus secretes corticotropin-releasing hormone (CRH), growth hormone-releasing hormone and thyrotropin-releasing hormone (TRH).

CRH stimulates the pituitary to increase the secretion of ADRENOCORTICOTROPIC HORMONE (ACTH), the hormone that stimulates the adrenal cortex to secrete steroid hormones. MINERALOCORTICOIDS increase sodium conservation by the kidneys, leading to water retention and elevated blood pressure. GLUCOCORTICOIDS increase protein degradation and amino acid conversion to blood glucose; reduce INFLAMMATION; and inhibit the immune response, especially production of antibodies like secretory IgA. This antibody, when released by the small intestine, protects against the onslaught of foreign materials presented in foods daily. Chronic overexposure to glucocorticoids leads to fatigue and muscle wasting, fragile bones, ulcers, impotence, infertility and lowered resistance to disease. It may worsen neurological disorders. Growth hormone stimulates the liver to increase the concentration of blood sugar and to increase fat degradation. TRH stimulates the thyroid gland to secrete thyroxine, which increases the basal metabolic rate and energy production.

The excessive activity of adrenal glands over time can lead to fatigue, susceptibility to food allergies, high blood pressure, elevated blood cholesterol and blood sugar. If the resistance stage fails to combat a stressor, the adrenal glands may become "exhausted" due to constant demands. Prolonged, excessive stress places a high demand on the endocrine system, the circulatory system and the immune system. In this situation there may be little reserve capacity to meet additional challenges. When glucocorticoids are depleted, blood glucose levels fall and the body cannot receive enough energy. Loss of potassium also contributes to exhaustion. CHRONIC FATIGUE can result, as well as DEPRESSION and anxiety.

Health Consequences of Chronic Stress

Stress is linked to a number of diseases, among them are angina (heart pain due to limited oxygen supply), GASTRITIS (inflamed stomach), ulcerative COLITIS (ulcerated and inflamed colon); irritable bowel syndrome; PEPTIC ULCERS; ASTHMA; autoimmune disease (such as RHEUMATOID ARTHRITIS); migraine headaches; CARDIOVASCULAR DISEASE; adult onset diabetes; depression; and PREMENSTRUAL SYNDROME. The inability to predict life's events and the loss of control in an unstable work environment create stress which can increase the risk of cardiovascular disease among employees. Stress hormones may damage arterial linings and may also temporarily increase blood cholesterol and blood pressure. Psychological stress is a risk factor for developing viral respiratory infections and for developing symptoms of the common cold. Hypotheses explaining these phenomena hinge upon the interaction of the central nervous system and the immune system.

Stress Management and Recovery from Stress

In the recovery stage, the body readjusts to normal functioning. Hormonal and metabolic equilibrium is reestablished. Life-style changes incorporating sound nutrition can significantly speed this stage by lowering the effects of stress on the body. Relaxation methods such as meditation, biofeedback, guided imagery, prayer, yoga and self-hypnosis can be important components of a stress management program. Such strategies favor the dominance of the parasympathetic nervous system, which counterbalances the sympathetic ner-

vous system. Expressing feelings and pent up emotions can help maintain health. Writing in a notebook or recording thoughts/feelings on a tape can improve immune function. Relaxation methods tend to normalize digestion, breathing, blood pressure, heart rate and nervous respiration, and return blood sugar levels to a normal physiologic range. Acknowledgment of emotions seems important in improving the lives of some cancer patients. Psychological intervention may help cancer patients deal with stress, enhance their immune system and thus improve long-term survival.

EXERCISE is a physical stressor, though regular exercise reduces the risk of chronic stress-related disease and inability to cope with stress. Exercise improves cardiovascular function and oxygen delivery to tissues and reduces epinephrine secretion in response to stress; it improves nutrient utilization by tissues and increases endocrine function; it also elevates mood.

There is agreement that physical stress—injury, surgery or extreme temperatures—increases nutrient needs. Whether psychological stress increases nutrient needs is controversial. Stress creates a greater turnover of water-soluble vitamins. The level of vitamin C can fluctuate depending upon the degree of physical and emotional stress. A variety of nutrients support adrenal gland function. Vitamin C, VITAMIN B$_6$, ZINC, MAGNESIUM and PANTOTHENIC ACID and the amino acid TYROSINE are required to synthesize adrenal hormones. A deficiency of pantothenic acid causes adrenal atrophy. This vitamin occurs in whole grains, legumes like lentils, vegetables like sweet potatoes, tomatoes, broccoli, salmon and liver. Adequate POTASSIUM is important in maintaining normal adrenal function. Bovine glandular extracts have been used therapeutically to control the physiologic imbalances of chronic stress. Chinese GINSENG seems to help balance the body in the face of challenges by stressors. (See also HOMEOSTATIS; PLACEBO; TOLERANCE TO TOXIC MATERIALS.)

Herbert, T.B. and Cohen, Sheldon, "Stress and Immunity in Humans: a Meta-analytic Review," *Psychosomatic Medicine*, 55 (1993), pp. 364–79.
Morse, D.R., et al., "Stress-induced Sudden Cardiac Death: Can It Be Prevented?" *Stress Medicine*, 8:1 (1992), pp. 35–46.

stroke   Damage to the brain due to interrupted blood flow. Loss of consciousness is often followed by more or less severe paralysis, depending upon the severity of oxygen deprivation to brain tissue. Strokes can usually be traced to preexisting conditions such as HYPERTENSION (high blood pressure) and diseases of the arterial walls. In cerebral thrombosis, normal blood circulation in the brain is blocked by a blood clot. ATHEROSCLEROSIS leads to clogged arteries where blood clots can form. Cerebral embolism refers to arterial blockage due to a traveling blood clot or a trapped air bubble. A leaking or burst artery can cause cerebral hemorrhage. An aneurysm or bulge in an arterial wall can burst with overexertion, overeating, extreme stress or violent coughing. A complete physical checkup may detect underlying conditions, including hypertension.

The risk for stroke increases with advanced age, heavy cigarette smoking, diabetes, present angina or history of HEART ATTACK, use of oral contraceptives in susceptible women, in addition to high blood pressure. Warning episodes of stroke include sudden dizziness, unsteadiness, numbness and difficulty in speaking. Typically these symptoms come and go quickly, indicative of temporary insufficient blood flow to the brain. The following symptoms may indicate an impending stroke: sudden temporary weakness of face, arm or leg; temporary loss of speech, or the understanding of speech; bouts of double vision; loss of vision or dimness in one eye; momentary blackout; confusion; personality changes. There are many variations. A person may experience many transient episodes (ischemia) without ever getting a stroke, while another may have a single episode followed by a permanent, serious attack. A person who has experienced transient ischemia needs a complete medical checkup.

Reducing overall fat intake and increasing unsaturated fats is recommended, especially for people with elevated blood CHOLESTEROL, high blood pressure or a family history of CARDIOVASCULAR DISEASE, especially stroke. Fatty fish like SALMON provide OMEGA-3 FATTY ACIDS, EICOSAPENTAENOIC ACID (EPA) and docosahex aenoic acid (DHA), which can reduce BLOOD CLOTTING and reduce the risk of heart attack and cerebral thrombosis. Inuits who consume large amounts of marine lipids have a low incidence of heart attack, though they experience a higher incidence of cerebral hemorrhage, likely due to decreased blood clotting ability. Adequate POTASSIUM can lessen the tendency for SODIUM to raise blood pressure in susceptible people. The addition of potassium-rich foods such as fruit and vegetables can reduce the risk of fatal stroke. MAGNESIUM deficiency is linked to sudden heart attack, angina, arrhythmia (irregular heartbeat), high blood pressure and stroke. Fruits and vegetables, as well as whole grains, supply ANTIOXIDANTS, such as VITAMIN C, VITAMIN E, and FLAVONOIDS, which reduce damage to the nervous system caused by temporary interruption of blood flow to the brain (STROKE). In general, population studies indicate that people who eat more fruits and vegetables suffer fewer coronary problems and strokes. (See also AGING; CARDIOVASCULAR DISEASE; CORONARY ARTERY DISEASE.)

Clark, Wayne M., "Need for Treatment of Elevated Plasma Fibrinogen Levels in Cardiovascular Disease," *Heart Disease and Stroke*, 2 (1993), pp. 503–06.

Laino, Charlene, "Exercise from 25 on Guards Against Stroke," *Family Practice News*, (August 24, 1993), p. 20.

strontium   A metallic element, in the same chemical family as CALCIUM and MAGNESIUM. The biological behavior of strontium resembles that of calcium. Strontium occurs in high-calcium foods like MILK and milk products. It is stored in BONES and TEETH. Notoriety surrounding strontium focuses on the radioactive isotope, strontium-90, a product of nuclear fallout. This radioactive element is stored in the bones of all vertebrates.

Presently strontium is considered a nonessential nutrient for humans. Omission of strontium from a purified diet for experimental animals led to slowed growth. The incidence of dental caries has been found to be lower in areas with high strontium levels in drinking water. Chronic consumption of highly refined foods, deficient in strontium and other nutrients, correlates with decreased bone strength. Ingesting pharmacologic doses (gram amounts) of strontium for periods up to three years has been reported to reduce bone pain and increase bone density in a group of osteoporotic patients. Typical U.S. consumption is several milligrams daily. (See also OSTEOPOROSIS.)

subclinical nutrient deficiency   A mild form of a nutrient deficiency that is not readily detected by usual clinical means because of the lack of well-defined signs and symptoms. Suboptimal nutrition contributes to decreased organ reserve. With less reserves, nutrient supply may be inadequate to mount a defense. The IMMUNE SYSTEM, the NERVOUS SYSTEM and the ENDOCRINE SYSTEM (hormone-producing system) rely upon many vitamins and minerals for maintenance and optimal functioning. The table on page 412 lists *possible* subclinical nutrient deficiencies and chronic conditions and diseases.

The recognition of subclinical nutrient deficiencies forms a basis for preventative intervention through dietary modification and life-style changes. Long before the appearance of a full-blown nutritional disease or conditions related to severe nutrient deficiency like SCURVY, RICKETS, PELLAGRA ANEMIA or EMACIATION, a variety of subtle indicators warn of impending problems. Anemia is the last stage of iron deficiency. Certain lab tests can detect these early signs of iron deficiency: elevated serum TRANSFERRIN, low serum iron (total iron binding capacity) and low iron saturation. An early symptom of a nutrient deficiency could be fatigue.

The development of accurate methods of measuring nutrient status (nutritional adequacy) has become a major focus of nutritional medicine. Serum folic acid, vitamin B_{12} and vitamin E can be measured. Functional tests for red blood cell enzymes can be used to assess thiamin, and selenium status. Measurement of minerals such as magnesium, ZINC and MANGANESE in white blood cells and potassium and COPPER in red blood cells are often useful parameters. (See also MALNUTRITION; NUTRITIONAL STATUS; SIGNS.)

subcutaneous fat   The layer of fatty tissue lying directly under the SKIN. A subcutaneous FAT layer is present in all well-nourished people where it serves as an insulation to protect individuals from heat loss in cold environments. The degree of fat deposition varies with gender, dietary choices, metabolic efficiency in converting nutrients to fat, as well as in overall body build. (See also ADIPOSE TISSUE.)

substrate   A substance that is converted by an ENZYME to its product. Substrates can be simple molecules or as complex as POLYSACCHARIDES, PROTEINS, LIPIDS and DNA, the genetic material of the cell. (See also METABOLITE.)

succinic acid   A food additive and common intermediate in the KREB'S CYCLE, major energy-producing pathway of the body. Succinic acid is present in vegetables like beets and broccoli, fruit like rhubarb, and in meat and cheese. It is sometimes added to foods to impart a distinctive flavor. When ingested, succinic acid is readily used as fuel and is considered a safe additive. There is no evidence that supplemental forms of succinic acid (succinates) increase energy production or boost athletic performance as sometimes claimed. (See also FOOD ADDITIVES.)

succistearin   A synthetic FOOD ADDITIVE used as an EMULSIFIER in VEGETABLE SHORTENING. Succistearin contains

SUCCINIC ACID and the fatty acid STEARIC ACID. Succistearin is broken down to its components, which are burned for ENERGY. It is considered a safe additive.

sucrase   An enzyme of the small intestine that digests SUCROSE (table sugar) to its simple sugar components, GLUCOSE and FRUCTOSE. This enzyme is necessary because sucrose cannot be absorbed by the intestine, while each of these simple sugars is readily assimilated. (See CARBOHYDRATE METABOLISM; DIGESTION.)

sucrose (table sugar)   The most common dietary SUGAR and SWEETENER. Chemically, sucrose is classified as a disaccharide, a chemical combination of the simple sugars GLUCOSE and FRUCTOSE, and represents the broad family of sugars, the simple CARBOHYDRATE. Sucrose is widely distributed among higher plants, but it is obtained commercially from sugar beets and sugar cane. More than 60% of refined sucrose comes from sugar cane (*Saccharum officinarum*), a jointed grass cultivated in tropical and semitropical regions of the world. Sugar cane may have originated in New Guinea. Currently, India, Brazil, Cuba, China and Mexico are major producers of cane sugar. At harvest sugar cane contains about 15% sucrose. The sugar beet (*Beta vulgaris*) is a biennial that produces a root containing 13 to 22% sugar. Regions of the former Soviet Union, the United States, France, Germany and Poland are major producers of sugar beets.

Types of Sugar Products

Raw sugar contains about 96% sucrose. It is produced by juice obtained from either sugar cane or sugar beets. The remaining syrup after sugar crystallization is called MOLASSES. A crude molasses can be recrystallized to remove more sugar. The remaining syrup is called BLACKSTRAP MOLASSES, a by-product of sugar manufacture. Repeated crystallization and decolorization ultimately yields highly purified sucrose as table sugar.

Granulated table sugar is the final product of sugar refining and contains 99.9% pure sucrose. Powdered sugar represents finely ground crystals such as confectioner's sugar. Powdered sugar is usually packaged with cornstarch to prevent caking.

Brown sugar represents the sugar that can be crystallized from syrup once the white sugar has been removed. Some brown sugar is made by adding molasses to white sugar. Brown sugar is not usually made from sugar beet molasses because it has a strong flavor.

TURBINADO SUGAR is partially refined sugar resembling raw sugar with large and coarse granules. It is about 95% pure sucrose and is no more natural than table sugar because it has gone through all but the last steps in refining.

CARAMELIZED SUGAR is used as a coloring agent. It is prepared by heating sucrose without water until it turns brown, then water is added to create a syrup.

INVERT SUGAR is the product of hydrolysis of sucrose. It contains equal amounts of fructose (levulose) and glucose (dextrose). It resists crystallization and prolongs freshness of baked goods and confectionery items.

Consumption

Although U.S. table sugar consumption has declined from about 100 lb per person per year in 1970 to about 65 lb (1991), sugar still represents a substantial portion of the daily caloric input at 20 to 25% of daily calories. Sugar represents about 300 calories per day for the average person. While sucrose consumption has declined, the use of other sweeteners such as high FRUCTOSE CORN SYRUP has more than made up for any decline, and the total annual consumption of caloric sweeteners amounts to about 140 lb (1991).

Current dietary guidelines recommend eating sugars only in moderation. The FOOD GUIDE PYRAMID recommends eating sugar and sugary foods sparingly. The U.S. Dietary Goals for Healthy Americans (1972) called for reducing by one-half the amount of sugar consumed in the typical American diet and substituting complex carbohydrate as found in whole grains, vegetables, bread and pasta. The more recent Dietary Guidelines for Americans recommended avoiding too much sugar, including sweets and soft drinks.

Possible Subclinical Nutrient Deficiencies Associated with Chronic Conditions

Condition	Possible Deficiency
Cardiovascular Disease	Magnesium, vitamin E, selenium, essential fatty acids, carnitine, folic acid, taurine
Hypertension	Magnesium, coenzyme Q_{10}
Osteoporosis	Copper, magnesium, manganese, folic acid, boron, calcium, zinc, vitamin B_6, vitamin C, vitamin K, vitamin D
Cancer (various forms)	Vitamin E, selenium, vitamin C, carotenoids, folic acid, thiamin, vitamin A, vitamin B_6, vitamin E, calcium, copper
Diabetes	Chromium, niacin, thiamin, vitamin B_6, vitamin E, calcium, magnesium, manganese, zinc, coenzyme Q_{10}, essential fatty acids
Hypertension	Magnesium, coenzyme Q_{10}, potassium, vitamin C, calcium, essential fatty acids
Chronic Infection	B complex, vitamin C, vitamin A, Vitamin E, zinc, copper, iron
Depression	Folic acid, vitamin B_6, riboflavin, thiamin, vitamin C, vitamin B_{12}, calcium, copper, iron, magnesium, potassium
Cataract (macular degeneration)	Vitamin E, vitamin C, carotenoids, zinc
Neuropathy	Vitamin B_{12}, folic acid, thiamin, niacin, vitamin B_6, vitamin E, zinc
Birth Defects	Folic acid
Chronic Fatigue	Vitamin B_{12} and other B vitamins, magnesium, zinc, copper, chromium, manganese, iron, essential fatty acids

Effects on Health

As with any nutrient, whether sugar is desirable or not depends upon the amount eaten, the types of other foods eaten and the general state of health of the individual. On one hand many people can tolerate sugar, and moderate amounts of sugar are safe for people in good health. Although diabetics have shunned sugar, recent research suggests that a little sugar eaten with high complex carbohydrates as part of a low-fat meal can be tolerated if it replaces other calories.

On the other hand, table sugar is highly purified and contributes only calories to the diet; other nutrients like FIBER, VITAMINS or MINERALS are not present. Because table sugar is one of the most common FOOD ADDITIVES, it is partially responsible for the low nutrient density of convenience and fast foods, processed foods and soft drinks. Sucrose is hidden in spaghetti, frozen dinners, BREAKFAST CEREALS, bread, KETCHUP, canned goods. It pushes out nutrient-rich food from the diet and therefore can contribute to overnutrition and excess weight. There is general agreement that sugar consumption increases tooth decay. Bacteria in the mouth live on carbohydrate and produce acids that erode tooth enamel.

Sugar can increase blood fat. Perhaps 20% of Americans are sensitive to sugar, that is, sugar will increase their risk of heart disease because of elevated serum TRIGLYCERIDES (fat). Diabetics often have a weight problem, and eating table sugar will not help dealing with this issue. In addition, blood fat tends to increase in some patients with non-insulin dependent diabetes with increased carbohydrate intake. Such patients should avoid table sugar.

Sugar is not a leading cause of obesity. Studies have found that lean people tend to eat more sugar but less fat than obese people. Fat contains more calories per teaspoon (36 vs. 16 for sucrose), and dietary fat is more efficiently converted to body fat than carbohydrate. Surplus calories, regardless of source, increase body weight. Cakes, pies, ice cream, chocolate and other sweets derive most of their calories from fat, not sugar, and surplus calories, not sugar per se, cause weight gain.

Craving of sweet foods is a common phenomena, perhaps genetically determined. Craving sweet, high-fat foods could involve a similar mechanism as addictive drugs. Baby rats tolerate pain better after eating fatty, sweet foods. While some individuals crave sugar and carbohydrate, more frequently people crave sweet-fat foods like ice cream, chocolate or cookies. The most uncontrollable food cravings affect bulimics. When some people eat sugar and carbohydrate, they often feel calm and become sleepy. Ingestion of sugar may raise the level of a brain chemical called SEROTONIN, which diminishes pain and has a calming effect. Thus sugar could theoretically operate as an antidepressant. According to this hypothesis, overeating sweets can be a method of coping with stressful situations and emotional issues. The relationship between sugar and hyperactivity is a controversial area. A substantial body of incidental reports points to a relationship between consumption of sugary foods and hyperactivity or disruptive behavior in susceptible children. Few clearcut, uncomplicated studies have been carried out to test this hypothesis. A 1986 report by a USDA task force on sugar concluded that consumption of sugar is not linked to disease or dependency, a conclusion recently confirmed by a large clinical study. Nevertheless, a child's diet that emphasizes sugar, fat, soft drinks and refined carbohydrates like chips and snack foods is likely to alter hormone balance, body chemistry and thus behavior.

Food Labels

The terms "sugar free" and "no sugar added" on food labels may not mean "low calorie." These terms mean that table sugar (sucrose) has not been used in making the product. Other calorie-containing sweeteners have been used: SORBITOL, fructose, HONEY and CORN SYRUP are possibilities. Sorbitol can affect blood sugar, though at a slower rate than sucrose. Diabetics should obtain professional advice before switching to sorbitol-sweetened foods. Sugar-free products may be sweetened with artificial sweeteners such as ACESULFAME-K, SACCHARIN and ASPARTAME to lower the calorie content. Only diabetics have a justifiable medical need for artificial sweeteners.

Sucrose in Typical Sugar-rich Foods

12-oz. sugar-containing cola drink	8 tsp
12-oz. chocolate malt shake	18 tsp
8 oz. eggnog	6 tsp
average cinnamon roll	8 tsp
brownie	4 tsp
chocolate cupcake with fudge icing	14 tsp
small serving sugar-containing fruit gelatin dessert	4.5 tsp
cup vanilla ice cream	7.5 tsp
piece apple pie	15 tsp
2 oz. candy bar	9 tsp
2 oz. milk chocolate	8 tsp
cup sugar-coated cereal	8 tsp
baking-powder biscuit, small	4 tsp
white flour pancake, plain	2.5 tsp
hard roll	4.5 tsp

(See also BULEMIA NERVOSA; CARBOHYDRATE METABOLISM; DIABETES MELLITUS; DIGESTION; OBESITY; PROCESSED FOOD; TEETH).

sucralose An ARTIFICIAL SWEETENER not yet approved by the U.S. FDA. Sucralose is a chemically modified chlorinated sugar (sucrose) that cannot be digested. Sucralose is about 600 times sweeter than table sugar. The manufacturer sought approval in 1987 to market this sweetener in SOFT DRINKS, frozen desserts and baked goods. Sucralose seems to impair the thymus gland and immune system of experimental animals. Its long-term health effects, particularly in diabetics, are being studied. (See also NATURAL SWEETENERS; SACCHARIN.)

sucrose polyester   See OLESTRA.

sugar   See NATURAL SWEETENERS; SUCROSE.

sugar beet   See SUCROSE.

sugar cane   See SUCROSE.

sugar-free foods   See SUCROSE.

sugarless gum   See CHEWING GUM.

sulfites (sulfiting agents, sodium sulfite, potassium and sodium metabisulfite, potassium-sodium bisulfite, sulfur dioxide)   Sulfur based FOOD ADDITIVES used as PRESERVATIVES. Sulfites and related compounds are added to prevent discoloration and spoilage of FRUIT and vegetables as well as PROCESSED FOODS. Restaurant foods and salad bars previously treated raw vegetables and fruits with sulfites, but this is now forbidden by federal regulations. Because sulfites can still be added to canned products, salad bars may still serve canned foods containing sulfites. Sulfites also occur in many medications.

Foods that may legally contain sulfites include POTATOES (raw, frozen or as potato chips); MUSHROOMS (canned or raw); salad mixes (unless specifically noted otherwise); vegetables and fruits (canned, frozen or dried); canned, frozen or dried shrimp, fish, clams, crabs, lobster and oysters; and vinegar and cider. Grapes are gassed with sulfur dioxide approximately once a week after they are picked, so they may contain significant sulfites. Wash this fruit before eating it.

Condiments may contain sulfites (relishes, salad dressing, pickled pepper, sauerkraut and avocado dips). Sulfites may also be present in beverages (wine, wine coolers, beer, cordials, cocktail mixes, lemon and grape juices) and baked goods (pizzas, cookies, crackers, pie crusts, tortillas).

Some individuals react to sulfite-treated foods. Perhaps a million Americans are sensitive to sulfites; most of these have asthma and allergies. Symptoms of sulfite sensitivity include nausea, headache, skin rush, swelling, flushing and diarrhea. Severe reaction can lead to asthmatic attacks and unconsciousness. Sulfites are risky additives; they have killed highly sensitive individuals by anaphylactic shock. Read food labels to determine whether your brand contains sulfites. Patients should notify their dentists if they have experienced problems with sulfites because they are often used to preserve local anesthetics. Some sulfite sensitive people find relief of their symptoms with the supplemented trace mineral molybdenum.

Lester, M.R., "Sulfite Sensitivity: Significance in Human Health," *Journal of the American College of Nutrition*, 14:3 (1995), pp. 229–32.

sulforaphane   A sulfur-containing compound found in the cabbage family and in other vegetables that helps protect against cancer-causing agents. Sulforaphane is classified as an ISOTHIOCYANATE. These compounds occur in BROCCOLI, CAULIFLOWER, mustard greens, green ONIONS and BRUSSELS SPROUTS as well as in horseradish. Population studies have shown that vegetables of the cabbage family afford protection against some forms of cancer. In general the mechanisms are not known. Isothiocyanates and sulforaphane in particular guard against cancer. Recent research suggests that sulforaphane increases the production of enzyme systems (called phase 2 enzymes) in the liver that detoxify reactive, potentially damaging molecules so that they can be flushed out of the body, thus blocking cancer induction and tumor formation. Sulforaphane is classified as a monofunctional inducer of liver enzymes, meaning that this substance increases the levels of the second stage of enzymatic detoxication (phase 2) and not those of the first stage (phase 1). Bifunctional inducers increase both phase 1 and phase 1 enzymes. Monofunctional inducers are safer than bifunctional inducers because activating phase 1 enzymes can produce reactive chemicals that can be mutagens and carcinogens (cancer-causing agents). Identification of other non-nutrients and the roles they play are actively being investigated. Current dietary guidelines recommend daily consumption of five or more servings of fruit and vegetables every day. Green and yellow vegetables are particularly important. (See also BETA CAROTENE; CRUCIFEROUS VEGETABLES; FOOD PYRAMID.)

sulfur   A non-metal element essential for life. The body contains 140 g of sulfur, primarily in the form of the sulfur-containing amino acids, METHIONINE and CYSTEINE, which function as essential protein building blocks. Proteins that require large amounts of these amino acids occur in hair, nails and skin, whose toughness is largely due to strands of KERATIN, a protein that contains 6% sulfur. In proteins cysteine often links up with an adjacent cysteine unit to yield CYSTINE, an important structural crosslink in many proteins.

The oxidized (inorganic) form of sulfur is sulfate. Dietary sulfate is poorly absorbed. Instead sulfate is produced in the body primarily by oxidation of the sulfur-containing amino acids. There is no RECOMMENDED DIETARY ALLOWANCE for sulfur or its derivatives. Methionine is an essential amino acid which is converted to cysteine by the body. Thus cysteine is not a dietary essential amino acid when the diet supplies adequate methionine. The sulfur content of most animal proteins varies from 0.4 to 1.6%. Good sources of sulfur-containing amino acids include EGGS, CHEESE, MEAT, POULTRY, nuts and legumes.

The liver uses sulfate to process waste materials. It adds sulfate to a variety of foreign compounds and metabolic end products to inactivate them and to increase their water solubility to help flush them out of the body. For example, the industrial chemical phenol is excreted as phenol sulfate, and the hormone PROGESTERONE is excreted as progesterone sulfate.

Sulfate is a component of GLYCOSAMINOGLYCANS (mucopolysaccharides). These polysaccharide molecules are long chains of sulfated carbohydrate derivatives that provide slippery surfaces, a resilient framework in the connective TISSUE, and a lubricant for joints and other surfaces of the body. Sulfur occurs in COENZYME A, the enzyme helper derived from the B vitamin PANTOTHENIC ACID and cysteine, which assists in the burning of fat and carbohydrate in energy metabolism. Cysteine is a constituent of GLU-

TATHIONE, a predominant cellular ANTIOXIDANT that protects cell membranes against oxidative damage. Cysteine is metabolized to TAURINE, an important sulfur compound that helps regulate nerves and muscles. Sulfur also appears in the B vitamins, THIAMIN and BIOTIN.

Another form of sulfur occurs frequently in the diet. SULFITE, a common food PRESERVATIVE, is not a nutrient. It is believed to be broken down by an enzyme called sulfite oxidase, which requires the trace mineral nutrient MOLYBDENUM for activity. Sulfite can trigger ASTHMA and food and chemical sensitivities. (See also GLUTATHIONE PEROXIDASE; MINERALS.)

sulfur dioxide   See SULFITES.

sunflower (*Helianthus annus*)   An annual that produces an oily seed. The sunflower is native to North America and it was cultivated first in the United States, Mexico and Peru. High-oil varieties of sunflower were developed in the Soviet Union; oilseed varieties produce seeds containing about 40% oil. Sunflower oil is presently second among vegetable oils worldwide. Today, the United States is a major producer of sunflowers, together with regions of the former Soviet Union, Argentina, Romania, Turkey and Spain, among others. Non-oil varieties of North American origin produce large seeds used in salads and baked goods.

Sunflower oil typically contains 47.3% monounsaturates, 42% polyunsaturates and 10.7% saturated FATTY ACIDS. Most of the polyunsaturated fatty acid is the essential fatty acid, LINOLEIC ACID. Sunflower seeds contain more iron than raisins, a popular source of this nutrient. Sunflower seeds are used as a snack food. The nutrient contents of a quarter-cup (34 g) of oil-roasted seeds (edible portion) is: 208 calories; protein, 7.2 g; carbohydrate, 5 g; fiber, 1.8 g; fat, 19.4 g; iron, 2.3 mg; sodium, 205 mg; thiamin, 0.11 mg; riboflavin, 0.1 mg; niacin, 1.4 mg.

supermarkets   Large, self-service retail stores offering a wide variety of foods, beverages and household items. Grocery stores expanded in the 1950s to meet divergent consumer needs in addition to the staples like BREAD, EGGS, MILK, flour and meat products. Modern supermarkets offer exotic fruit, snack foods, fish markets, take-out foods, salad bars, bakery, deli and even pizza booths. Of all retail stores, Americans visit supermarkets most often: The average U.S. consumer visits a supermarket more than twice weekly, and shopping times range between 35 and 45 minutes per trip. The majority of trips to the supermarket occur on weekends. Though traditionally women have done the most shopping at supermarkets, men now visit grocery stores more often than women.

The number of items carried by the average supermarket is now about 16,000, and a large supermarket stocks an average of 53,000 items. Nearly half of the U.S. supermarkets are open 24 hours in order to compete with convenience stores. Many supermarkets now provide hot and cold prepared foods to go. Produce can be provided almost all year round; bananas remain the largest volume item. Though the produce department accounts for only 10% of typical supermarket sales, surveys indicate that it is often a deciding factor in selecting a store and that most produce purchases are made on impulse.

Most supermarkets offer store brands or private-label products, such as canned vegetables, canned fruit and dairy products. They may be sold at prices ranging from 5 to 70% lower than comparable name-brand products. Because much of the cost of national brands goes to advertising, stores often make a higher profit on store brands. The arrangement of food items is carefully planned to increase sales. Bulk staples are often placed lower on shelves and they are placed at the back of stores. Cross merchandising increase sales. This practice entails placing high-priced items that complement one another—cocktail sauce and seafood; wine and cheese; and so on. The dairy case is usually at the farthest point from the entrance to pull customers through non-foods or health supplies that have higher profit margins. (See also ADVERTISING; PRODUCT PLACEMENT.)

Wagner, Jana L., et al., "Influences of a Supermarket Intervention on the Food Choices of Parents and Their Children," *Journal of Nutrition Education*, 24:6 (Nov–Dec 1992), pp. 306–11.

superoxide dismutase   (SOD)   An antioxidant enzyme that destroys a reactive form of OXYGEN called superoxide. Superoxide (O_2^-) is a type of FREE RADICAL. As such it is very reactive chemically. Stimulated neutrophils and macrophages, two types of immune cells responsible for eliminating foreign materials, release superoxide to kill bacteria. A mechanism that enhances the destruction of virus-infected cells also operates through superoxide. Superoxide can also occur in MITOCHONDRIA, the powerhouses of cells. They consume most of the oxygen used by cells in order to burn fuels for energy; they can produce superoxide as a by-product. Superoxide can react with cellular metal ions to produce hydroxyl radicals, an extremely reactive free radical that can attack DNA and cause mutations. Oxidative damage is believed to underlie degenerative conditions including cardiovascular disease, premature aging, cancer and even senility.

Three variants of superoxide dismutase require COPPER, and ZINC or MANGANESE. Consequently these trace mineral nutrients are classified as ANTIOXIDANTS. Copper and zinc SOD are the major forms in the body and they are essential in protecting cells against damage due to inflammation. Injected SOD has been used to treat ARTHRITIS, CROHN'S DISEASE, LUPUS ERYTHEMATOSUS and other conditions related to an imbalanced immune system and severe inflammation.

Superoxide dismutase is sold as a supplement in health food stores. The idea behind these pills is to bolster the body's enzymes. Generally the levels of superoxide dismutase in the blood have not been shown to increase after SOD supplementation. Plant-based SOD seems to resist the rigors of the digestive tract, increasing the possibility of its absorption. (See also CATALASE.)

Asada, Kozi, and Yoshikawa, Toshikazu, eds. "Frontiers of Reactive Oxygen Species in Biology and Medicine." Proceedings of the Sixth International Conference on Superoxide and Superoxide Dismutase, Kyoto, Japan. October 11–15, 1993. *Exerpta Medica*, Amsterdam (1994).

supplements   See VITAMIN.

surfactant   A food additive that acts as an antifoaming agent. Surfactants decrease the surface tension of water solutions, thus decreasing foaming. In PROCESSED FOODS, surfactants act as stabilizers to avoid watery mixtures, lumpy preparations and oil-water separation as in chocolate milk and salad dressings. There are three categories of surfactant: detergents, wetting agents and EMULSIFIERS. Emulsifiers are used to form stable mixtures of normally incompatible materials—the polar (water attracting or HYDROPHILIC) and the non-polar (lipid, water repelling or HYDROPHOBIC). Examples include BILE acids in bile to emulsify FAT for DIGESTION; and the FOOD ADDITIVES, LECITHIN, DIGLYCERIDES, POLYSORBATES, SUCCISTEARIN and XANTHAN GUM. (See also MICELLE.)

surimi   Imitation shellfish prepared from fish paste. The Japanese developed a process for preparing fish paste from inexpensive bottom fish such as POLLOCK. Whitefish is soaked extensively, mashed into a paste that looks like mashed potatoes, and then molded into the desired shape and flavored. Surimi appears as artificial crabmeat, scallops, shrimp and lobster tails. The usual imitation shellfish contains 50 to 60% surimi and only 5 to 10% of the authentic shellfish, and restaurants can profit by substituting surimi for shellfish. Surimi is popular because it provides shellfish flavor at low cost.

Surimi contains high amount of SODIUM, MONOSODIUM GLUTAMATE and ARTIFICIAL FOOD COLORS and is blended with phosphates, sugar and sorbitol. The product is low in VITAMINS and MINERALS due to extensive processing. Although the U.S. FDA requires that surimi be labeled as "artificial seafood," the packaging may mislead consumers by saying "sealegs" or the word "imitation" may be in small print. (See also FOOD ADDITIVES; IMITATION FOOD; PROCESSED FOOD.)

sushi   See SEAFOOD.

sweeteners   See NATURAL SWEETENERS.

sweetness   Refers to sweet tasting foods. The brain has taste centers that receive input from taste receptors on the tongue. Theoretically all materials that taste sweet have a common molecular shape that can make contact with a receptor docking site. This brief contact may activate a chemical or electrical signal that is relayed to the brain. Individual taste sensitivity varies immensely. A person's tongue can have as few as 500 taste buds to as many as 10,000. Quite likely, as food is homogenized and mixed with SALIVA, flavor components interact with different receptors and together convey the identity of a food. (See also NATURAL SWEETENERS; SMELL; TASTE.)

sweet potato (*Ipomoea batatas*)   A tropical plant that forms edible tubers. Sweet potatoes originated in Mexico or northern regions of South America. Europeans spread sweet potatoes to the Philippines, Africa, India and Southeast Asia. The sweet potato ranks third among leading crop vegetables worldwide; only POTATOES and CASSAVA are more popular. China and Indonesia are among the major producers. Sweet potatoes have a reddish or gray skin and their flesh may be pink, orange or purple. There are several varieties, including the Virginia (yellow flesh) and Malaga (pink flesh). Moist, orange-fleshed sweet potatoes are frequently called YAMS in the United States. However, true yams belong to a different plant family and are very large, starchy root vegetables grown in Asia and Africa. Though sweet potatoes taste sweeter than white potatoes, they don't contain more calories. Sweet potatoes are canned, dehydrated, frozen or processed for starch, sugar and syrup. Sweet potatoes may be baked, cooked in their skins, pureed or candied. Sweet potatoes are excellent sources of pro-vitamin A (BETA CAROTENE) and other carotenoids. The nutrient contents of one potato (baked with skin, 11 g) is: 118 calories; protein, 2 g; carbohydrate, 27.7 g; fiber, 3 g; vitamin A, 2,575 retinol equivalents; thiamin, 0.08 mg; riboflavin, 0.21 mg; niacin, 1 mg.

sweets   Foods that contain a high level of SUGAR. CANDY, CHOCOLATE, cake, cookies, ICE CREAM, jam, jelly, marshmallows, pastries, pie, tarts, sweetened gelatin desserts and SOFT DRINKS sweetened with sugar are sugary foods. The sweetener may be TABLE SUGAR, HONEY or another NATURAL SWEETENER. Often sweets contain a high percentage of FAT. The fat content may account for more calories than the sugar in such foods. The FOOD PYRAMID for consumers recommends using sweets sparingly because such foods contain fewer nutrients than vegetables, whole grains and fresh fruits, lentils and beans. (See also DIETARY GUIDELINES FOR AMERICANS; TEETH.)

symptom   The effects of disease that the patient observes: fever, indigestion, hives, bloating, joint pain and fatigue, to name a few. (See also SIGNS.)

syndrome   A collection of symptoms and signs (measured by diagnostic medical personnel) that indicate a disease or abnormal state. Toxic shock syndrome, malabsorption syndromes and PREMENSTRUAL SYNDROME, are examples. (See also FATIGUE.)

Syndrome X   A complex, diverse collection of signs and symptoms associated with increased blood sugar, blood lipids and blood pressure during aging. Aging Americans often experience a chain of events. Sedentary life-styles lead to weight gain, specifically around the waist (android or apple-shaped adiposity). This in turn leads to insulin resistance, in which high levels of insulin must be secreted to lower blood sugar levels. High insulin signals the body to make more fat, increasing the levels of blood triglycerides and LDL-cholesterol, the so-called "bad" form. Hypertension (elevated blood pressure) is a final feature of Syndrome X. To decrease Syndrome X, diabetes and associated risk of cardiovascular disease, middle-aged people should exercise regularly and reduce calories to avoid becoming overweight. (See also: DIET; OBESITY).

systemic   Pertaining to most or all organ systems of the body. A systemic disease can affect the NERVOUS SYSTEM, the IMMUNE SYSTEM, musculature, gastrointestinal tract or CIRCULATORY SYSTEM or a combination of these systems. (See also ALLERGY, FOOD; LUPUS ERYTHEMATOSUS.)

table salt See SODIUM.

table sugar See SUCROSE.

tahini A butter prepared from ground, hulled SESAME seeds. Tahini prepared from untoasted seeds has a mild flavor and is easily spreadable. Toasting sesame seeds yields a more oily mixture and adds a stronger flavor. Most commercial production of sesame seeds occurs in Mexico and Guatemala. Like sesame seed, tahini is a vegetarian source of iron. One tablespoon (15 g) provides 91 calories; protein, 2.7 g; carbohydrate, 2.7 g; fiber, 2.2 g; fat, 8.5 g; iron, 0.95 mg; thiamin, 0.24 mg; riboflavin, 0.02; mg niacin, 0.85 mg.

tallow FAT extracted from fatty tissue of sheep and cattle. Tallow hardens at room temperature, reflecting its relatively high content of saturated FATTY ACIDS; it contains about 46% saturated fatty acids and only 4% polyunsaturated fatty acids. Beef tallow is used in prepared foods such as chili and refried beans and french fries. It is also used industrially in soap and candle manufacture. Fat regardless of its source yields 9 calories per gram, more than double the amount of calories in carbohydrate. (See also FAT METABOLISM; LARD.)

tamari (natural shoyu, Japanese soy sauce) A soy sauce prepared from the formation of SOYBEANS and cracked, roasted WHEAT. Tamari is fermented slowly and no preservatives are added. Tamari is a salty food containing 16% salt. Although vegetarians may use seaweed, tempeh, miso and tamari from the belief that these foods are good sources of VITAMIN B$_{12}$, tamari contains little vitamin B$_{12}$ activity.

tangerine A smallish, tart CITRUS FRUIT. Tangerine is a descendent of the mandarin ORANGE and originated in China. The fruit has a thin, easily peeled skin and segments separate readily. Unlike oranges, which can be stored at room temperature for several weeks, tangerines need to be refrigerated if kept longer than a couple of days. They are eaten raw or used in fruit or gelatin-based salads. Tangerines provide less vitamin C than oranges. The edible portion of one raw tangerine (84 g) provides 37 calories; protein, 0.5 g; carbohydrate, 9.4 g; fiber, 1.6 g; fat, 0.2 g; potassium, 132 mg; vitamin C, 26 mg; thiamin, 0.09 mg; riboflavin, 0.02 mg; niacin, 0.13 mg.

tannins A family of complex compounds that occur in the bark or leaves of certain plants and trees. Tannins are classified chemically as flavonoids they are composed of two or more aromatic ring structures that act as antioxidants to quench oxidative damage due to free radicals. Polyphenols block the ability of certain compounds to cause mutations in test tube experiments and inhibit lung and skin tumors in experimental animals. Tannins are classified as hydrolyzable or condensed. Hydrolyzable tannins such as ellagic acid, gallic acid and related compounds, are often complexed with glucose. Hydrolyzable tannins could serve as anticancer agents through increasing the liver's ability to "detoxify" potential cancer-causing agents by increasing their water-solubility, thus speeding up their removal (excretion). A second type, condensed tannins (flavolans), are chains of polyphenol units that do not break down readily and combine with iron and other metals.

Individuals consuming COFFEE, TEA, COCOA and CHOCOLATE may ingest on the order of 1,000 mg of tannins daily. Tannins occur in all coffees, even decaffeinated coffee. A child consuming chocolate milk together with chocolate candy could consume 160 mg of cocoa tannin per kilogram of body weight per day. Brewed teas supply tannins. Some population studies suggest that tea drinkers have a reduced risk of dying from coronary heart disease. High levels of tannic acid can bind protein and limit digestion; limit the uptake of GLUCOSE and METHIONINE; and bind iron from vegetable sources. Acute toxicity tests with adult animals did not indicate toxicity.

tapioca A form of starch derived from the CASSAVA, a tropical root vegetable. Tapioca is prepared by drying pulped roots after fibers have been removed. Special grinding and sieving is required to produce the type of tapioca used in popular puddings. Like most starches, tapioca swells and thickens when cooked in water. It is often used to thicken soups, pies and puddings. High-grade tapioca forms milky beads with a brilliant white luster. The nutrient content of 1 cup (165 g) of tapioca cream pudding is: 221 calories; protein, 8.3 g; carbohydrate, 28.2 g; fat, 8.4 g; sodium, 257 mg; calcium, 173 mg; thiamin, 0.07 mg; riboflavin, 0.30 mg; niacin, 0.2 mg. (See also FLOUR.)

tardive dyskinesia A disabling disorder sometimes produced by the long-term use of anti-psychotic drugs and neuroleptic drugs (tranquilizers). Tardive dyskinesia occurs in 10 to 20% of patients treated with these drugs. Symptoms include involuntary twitching of mouth and face, hand trembling, spasms and speech disturbances. Sometimes these drug-induced effects are irreversible.

Supplements of the nitrogen-containing nutrient CHOLINE and of LECITHIN, the PHOSPHOLIPID from which choline is derived, reduce the abnormal movements of tardive dyskinesia, and lecithin remains an important treatment option. TRYPTOPHAN, together with NIACINAMIDE and VITAMIN B$_6$, may relieve symptoms of tardive dyskinesia. Large-scale studies have suggested that patients who supplement with NIACIN, MANGANESE and ZINC concomitantly with drug treatment experience decreased symptoms of tardive dyskinesia. The American Psychiatric Association concluded (1991) that the general clinical value of such nutrients should be confirmed with long-term, large-scale studies before acceptance. Preliminary clinical studies suggest that VITAMIN E may also decrease the severity of symptoms. (See also NERVOUS SYSTEM; PARKINSON'S DISEASE.)

Cadet, Jean Lud, "Movement Disorders: Therapeutic Role of Vitamin E," *Toxicology and Industrial Health*, 9:1–2 (1993), pp. 337–47.

target heart rate See EXERCISE.

taro (*Colocasia esculenta*) A tropical, tuber-bearing plant native to Southeast Asia. Taro cultivation gradually spread to Japan, China, the eastern Mediterranean region, Polynesia,

New Zealand, West Africa, South America and Hawaii. Taro root is a high-carbohydrate food. Poi, a staple food of Hawaii and Polynesia, is made from the taro root. A common variety of taro produces a brown-skinned root with a pale purple or white flesh. Taro root is sold in Asian markets and specialty shops. Taro leaves should not be consumed raw because some varieties contain high levels of OXALIC ACID (calcium oxalate) that can be toxic when large amounts are consumed. Taro root can be used like potatoes; it is boiled, baked or steamed. The vegetable becomes very sticky upon cooling. The tuber has a nutrient value similar to the Irish POTATO.

tarragon (*Artemesia dracunculus*) A small perennial shrub with a dark-green, narrow leaf that is used as a culinary HERB. The name comes from the French *estragon*, meaning "little dragon," because the twisted roots resemble dragons. Tarragon is used fresh or dried to create a somewhat anise-like flavor in chicken, veal and turkey dishes; in broiled fish and shellfish; omelet and egg dishes; MUSTARD; and MAYONNAISE. Tarragon is used in bearnaise sauce. Tarragon can overwhelm other seasonings, and it is not recommended in recipes calling for a blend of herbs. (See also ANISE; SPICE.)

tartaric acid An acidic FOOD ADDITIVE used to create a tart taste. Tartaric ACID occurs widely in plants, especially in fruits and ripe grapes. Commercially, tartaric acid is a byproduct of wine production. Tartaric acid is used with grape flavors and other flavoring agents in SOFT DRINKS, CANDY, gelatin-based desserts and YOGURT.

The potassium salt of tartaric acid (potassium tartrate) is called "cream of tartar." This compound is used as a leavening agent and as an anticaking agent in baking. A mixture of sodium tartrate and sodium-potassium tartrate, "Rochelle salt," is used to control acidity and to emulsify ingredients of processed foods (CHEESE and jam, among others). Intestinal bacteria produce most of the tartaric acid people ingest, and it is considered a safe food additive. (See also CITRIC ACID.)

tartrazine (FD&C yellow no. 5) One of the most widely used artificial colorings in the United States. Low levels of tartrazine are used in beverages like SOFT DRINKS; higher levels are used in BREAKFAST CEREALS, baked goods and snack foods. Health concerns have been raised because tartrazine causes allergic reactions in certain people, particularly if they are sensitive to ASPIRIN. Asthma, hives and typical "hay fever" symptoms can occur, though more severe symptoms have been reported. Tartrazine sensitivity was estimated to be prevalent in less than 100,000 Americans in the late 1970s. In 1981 the U.S. FDA required that ingredient labels on foods disclose the presence of tartrazine rather than simply noting "artificial coloring." Several European countries have banned this dye from food use. Coloring from TURMERIC and ANNATTO can be used in place of this yellow food coloring. (See also ALLERGY, FOOD; FOOD ADDITIVES; FOOD SENSITIVITY.)

taste (gustatory sensation) The flavor sensation of substances placed in the mouth. The sensation of taste relies on the stimulation of receptors (taste buds) by substances dissolved in SALIVA. An adult possesses about 2,000 taste buds located chiefly on the tongue. They occur also on the soft palate and in the throat. Typically, taste buds occur in small protuberances called papillae, which give the upper surface of the tongue a rough appearance. Taste buds possess external cells with hair-like extensions that project through a central taste pore. When a dissolved substance enters a taste pore and contacts the hair-like projections, it can generate a nerve impulse that is relayed to the brain.

Of all the seemingly endless different flavors and subtle tastes, there are only four basic taste sensations: sweet, sour, salt and bitter. Most other tastes are combinations of these modified by odors. When a person has a cold, the olfactory sensations (SMELL) do not operate normally, though the taste sensations may be normal. The olfactory system (sense of smell) is much more sensitive to stimulation than the gustatory system for a given concentration of a substance.

Taste buds located in different areas possess different sensitivities to taste sensations. Thus, the tip of the tongue reacts with all primary taste sensations, but it is highly sensitive to salty and sweet materials. The edges of the tongue respond more readily to sour substances, while the back of the tongue responds most to bitter substances.

Foods that taste bitter are generally rejected. This may be part of a protective mechanism in human evolution, because many poisonous plants contain toxic substances that produce a bitter taste. A degree of saltiness is often considered pleasant but very salty foods will be rejected. The preference for salty foods in most people is acquired. Gradually reducing the amount of salt in foods will uncover the subtle, rich flavors of minimally processed foods. Sweet tasting foods create pleasurable feelings. ARTIFICIAL SWEETENERS have been developed that will trigger the sweet receptors without contributing calories. A sour taste may be either objectionable or desirable. Dilute acid solutions such as VINEGAR can create tangy, zestful foods and beverages, while excessive acidity is not palatable. The taste threshold varies for each primary taste. Bitter substances possess the lowest taste threshold, that is, they can be distinguished at low concentrations; the threshold for sour substances is higher; and the thresholds for salt and sweet materials are higher than for sour or bitter foods. Adding sugar to highly seasoned dishes increases the ability to sense hot spices.

Children up to the age of five have more taste buds than adults, so foods taste richer to them. Babies explore their environment by tasting everything they can reach. Possible reasons for a decrease in the sense of taste include: cigarette smoking, eating excessively salty foods or drinking alcoholic beverages, and a ZINC deficiency. Elderly persons gradually lose some of their sense of taste; food tends to taste bland to them.

Cowart, Beverly J., "Relationships Between Taste and Smell Across the Adult Lifespan," *Annals of the New York Academy of Sciences*, 561 (June 30, 1989), pp. 39–55.

Frank, Marion E. and Hettinger, Thomas P., "The Sense of Taste: Neurobiology, Aging and Medication Effects," *Critical Reviews in Oral Biology and Medicine*, 3 (1992), pp. 371–93.

taurine A sulfur-containing compound produced by the liver. Taurine serves multiple functions. The liver uses taurine to convert CHOLESTEROL to BILE salts, required to digest FAT and to modify toxic chemicals to help flush them out of the body. Taurine helps regulate nerves and muscles and supports SODIUM and POTASSIUM transport across cell membranes. It is required for normal function of the heart, brain, eyes and vascular system. Taurine is the most prevalent free amino acid in the heart, where it contributes to muscle contraction. With chronic stress and when the oxygen supply to the heart drops (ischemia), taurine levels in the heart decrease. In Japan taurine is used in treating HEART DISEASE and congestive heart failure. Taurine administered to experimental animals can prevent induced heart muscle damage. In the brain taurine acts as a NEUROTRANSMITTER, a chemical released by a nerve cell (neuron) to help carry a nerve impulse to an adjacent cell. Taurine seems to be inhibitory, that is, it depresses the brain. Therefore, it is being studied as an anticonvulsant in the treatment of epilepsy. Taurine is also involved in calcium metabolism of the brain.

The body possesses a limited capacity to produce taurine, and certain individuals may require dietary taurine, depending upon their nutritional status. Pre-term and full-term infants do not synthesize appreciable taurine, which is the most abundant amino acid in breast milk. With time the taurine content of breast milk declines as the infant grows and begins to manufacture taurine. Until recently taurine was omitted from infant formulas; now it is added routinely. Taurine is concentrated in animal protein, especially organ meats, fish and milk, but is absent from plant foods.

Taurine is a nerve depressant and when used as a supplement it may affect short-term memory. Its use is considered experimental. (See also METHIONINE; NERVOUS SYSTEM.)

Chapman, R.A., et al., "Taurine and the Heart," *Cardiovascular Research* 27 (1993), pp. 358–63.

tea (*Camellia sinensis*) The dried leaves of a tropical evergreen that grows as a small tree or shrub. Brewed tea is the most popular beverage worldwide. The origin of tea is obscure, though it probably originated in regions of Tibet, western China and northern India. India, Sri Lanka and China are the leading tea growing countries. Flower, leaf, bark, roots and seeds of various plants are used in herbal teas but these are not derived from *Camellia sinensis*.

Differences in color and aroma among various types of tea reflect primarily differences in tea processing. Nearly 75% of tea ends up as black tea, in which leaves are crushed to release enzymes that oxidize substances in leaves (polyphenols) that create the rich flavor. The leaves are then dried in hot air to develop a brown/black color. For green tea, fresh leaves are steamed to destroy the oxidizing enzymes, then rolled and dried. Instant tea was developed in the United States in 1948. It is prepared by brewing a strong tea and removing water to leave a dried concentrate, which can be added to water. Oolong tea is partially fermented to create a green-brown leaf.

Brewed tea is prepared by pouring boiling water over dried tea leaves. Generally, the best flavor is obtained when tea has steeped (soaked) in boiled water for up to five minutes for black tea, one to two minutes for green tea. Longer steeping creates tea with more TANNIN and increased bitterness. Black tea, and to a lesser extent, green tea bind iron because of the tannin content. Tannins contribute to the pungency of tea. Tea is a mild stimulant because it contains CAFFEINE. A cup of black tea provides about 40 mg, about half the amount in COFFEE. Caffeine increases urination and is responsible for the diuretic effect of tea.

Brewed tea contains other substances as well. Tea is a source of FLUORIDE; a cup of tea provides about 0.3 mg. Green tea yields more fluoride and less caffeine than black tea. Green tea provides vitamin C; on the average, one cup of green tea provides as much vitamin C as half a cup of orange juice. Cancer of the esophagus, stomach and intestine are rare in regions of Japan and China where large amounts of green tea are consumed. Tea contains tannin and catechin (classified as FLAVONOIDS), widely distributed among plants. They possess ANTIOXIDANT properties. Antioxidants have been proposed as anti-cancer agents, and animal studies suggest that green tea inhibits the development of certain types of cancer, but more human study is required. Other studies link tea consumption with a lowered risk of dying from heart disease. Tea flavonoids may limit the oxidation of LDL cholesterol, believed to be an early event in atherosclerosis. However, the mechanism of action of tea flavonoids is still being investigated.

Yang, S. and Wang, Zhi-Yuan, "Tea and Cancer," *Journal of the National Cancer Institute*, 85:13 (July 7, 1993), pp. 1038–49.

teeth Boney projections from the upper and lower jaws used for chewing food. Each tooth possesses an exposed crown and one or more roots that anchor the tooth in the jaw bone. The 32 adult or permanent teeth are divided 16 per jaw. A child may develop up to 20 teeth that are replaced with permanent teeth. Incisors and cuspids (canines) are for biting off pieces of food. Bicuspids (premolars) and molars provide grinding surfaces to pulverize food.

The outer coating of the tooth is called the enamel, the hardest part of the tooth. This protective layer resists the wear of chewing and the action of bacteria. A hardened type of bone covers the roots. Dentine, a hard, mineralized layer, lies beneath the enamel. Dentine surrounds a central cavity of the tooth, filled with nerves and blood vessels. The gums (gingivae) bridge the gap between the tooth and bone. Tooth sockets are lined with a periodontal ligament and elastic connective tissue, which both anchor the tooth and act as a shock absorber.

FLUORIDE is incorporated into teeth during their formation in the first years of life. Fluoride enters the mineral structure, increasing its resistance to microbial degradation. Fluoride has its greatest effect before and during the emergence of teeth, and it is recommended in the diet until all teeth are in place. Fluoride has been recommended in drinking water up to a concentration of 1 mg per milliliter as a supplement during tooth formation.

Most adults over 50 exhibit symptoms of GINGIVITIS (inflamed gums) due to dental plaque accumulation. Plaque is the sticky mass of bacterial deposit, which can harden and become tartar. In certain cases bacterial infection spreads to deep tissues (periodontitis) and can cause tooth and bone loss. Flossing, brushing and professional cleaning are the foundation for oral health and best defense against plaque formation. Topical application of fluoride as toothpaste or oral antiseptic rinse further reduces tooth decay. (See also PERIODONTAL DISEASE.)

tempeh A type of fermented soybean cake and a meat substitute. Tempeh is a food staple in Indonesia, New Guinea and, to a lesser degree, in Malaysia. Soaked soybeans are boiled, usually with grains, then fermented (aged) with a mold, *Rhizopus oligosporus*. Mold growth forms a mat around the cooked beans that binds the mixture into a firm cake, which can be fried, baked, roasted or diced and served in soups. Tempeh contains somewhat more protein than soybean curd (TOFU).

teratogen An agent that causes BIRTH DEFECTS. The placenta acts as a barrier to many potentially damaging substances in maternal blood. However, a number of fat-soluble compounds and drugs can penetrate the placenta and can damage the embryo or fetus. In the United States alone nearly 100,000 infants are born with malformations and developmental defects that require medical treatment. This figure represents about 2.6% of live births. Additional birth defects are found in the first year of life, raising the incidence to 6 to 7%. The rate of birth defects has not declined despite huge advances in medicine and health sciences over the last decade. An estimated 14 to 16% of birth defects are genetic; 6 to 10% are due to toxic exposure; and about 70% represent unknown causes.

The catalog of teratogenic agents lists all chemicals that have been reported to be teratogenic in humans or in animals. Americans are exposed to approximately 5 million chemicals; 1,600 of these have been tested in lab animals and about 50% are known teratogens. A number of these are related to nutrients. Retinoids, a family of lipids related to VITAMIN A, affect the development of body shape, and overdoses can lead to severe malformation. Retinoic acid (C_{13} cis—retinoic acid), a vitamin A derivative used in skin treatment for severe ACNE, is a human teratogen. Some investigators believe that ETHANOL, the alcohol in alcoholic beverages, could be responsible for as much as 20% of cases of mental retardation in the United States. About one-third of all children born to alcoholic mothers are affected by FETAL ALCOHOL SYNDROME, a condition characterized by long-term growth retardation, nervous system irregularities, small head size and facial anomalies. Maternal alcohol consumption during pregnancy is also associated with cleft palate and congenital head defects. Excessive consumption of selenium can cause a condition called selenosis in which very high levels of selenium accumulate in maternal tissues. Animal studies indicate that selenium under these extreme conditions can be a teratogen. A variety of drugs are teratogens. The general recommendation is to avoid alcohol and drugs during pregnancy. Consult a physician before taking any medication during pregnancy.

terpenoid (terpene) A large family of compounds produced by plants and animals that are classified as LIPIDS. Lipids are fat-soluble (hydrophobic) compounds that dissolve oils and organic solvents. Terpenoids are ring structures assembled from acetyl COENZYME A, the activated form of ACETIC ACID derived from the degradation of CARBOHYDRATE and FAT. Terpenoids include a large number of plant and animal materials such as VITAMIN A, VITAMIN D, VITAMIN E, VITAMIN K, CHOLESTEROL, steroid hormones, BILE salts; plant oils like limonene from oil of LEMON and ORANGE; pinene from turpentine; geraniol from flowers; menthol from PEPPERMINT; zingiberene from oil of GINGER; B-selinene from oil of CELERY; and squalene from fish liver oil. (See also CARBOHYDRATE METABOLISM; FAT METABOLISM; HORMONE; STEROIDS.)

testosterone The predominant male sex HORMONE. Testosterone is the major androgenic hormone (hormones that guide the development and maintenance of male organs and secondary male characteristics, including facial hair, male musculature, with widened shoulders and narrowed hips, among others). Testosterone stimulates the accumulation of muscle and the maturation of sperm and stimulates bone growth. Testosterone, like other STEROID hormones, is synthesized from CHOLESTEROL and is secreted by the testicles. Illicit use of synthetic androgens by athletes and body builders has led to increased muscle mass above the level induced by workouts, with often disastrous side effects.

In females testosterone is synthesized by the ovaries and adrenal glands; the blood levels of testosterone in women are about 10% of a typical male. The role of androgens in female development is unclear. The effects of excessive male hormones are better documented with increased risk of diabetes, high blood pressure, heart disease, breast cancer, irregular periods and endometrial cancer. (See also ANABOLIC STEROIDS.)

tetracycline See ANTIBIOTIC-RESISTANT BACTERIA IN FOOD.

tetrahydrofolic acid (THF) The biologically active form of the B vitamin, FOLIC ACID. THF functions as a coenzyme, that is, an enzyme helper. It differs from folic acid because it possesses extra hydrogen atoms and GLUTAMIC ACID units. THF figures predominantly in the transfer of single carbon units. It helps catalyze the synthesis of the amino acid SERINE from the simplest amino acid, GLYCINE; helps catalyze the nitrogen-containing bases, PURINE and THYMINE, which are used as building blocks of genetic material, DNA; and helps catalyze EPINEPHRINE, a stress hormone released by the adrenal gland, among others. (See also COENZYME.)

texture The sensation produced in the mouth by a food or beverage, often referred to as "mouth feel." Adjectives such as chewy, sticky, creamy, hard, lumpy, soft, rough, smooth, gritty, crisp and the like describe food textures. The physical and chemical properties of a food form the basis for acceptance or rejection. Experience teaches associations between certain foods and textures. If food has a texture that differs from expectations it is judged as of lower quality. A rejected food may be stringy, slimy, gritty, greasy or contain hard to chew pieces or fragments. (See also FOOD PROCESSING; TASTE.)

texturized vegetable protein (TVP) SOYBEAN protein that has been processed to resemble meat. Protein is isolated from soybean, chemically treated, combined with additives and further processed to create colored granules, chunks or strips. TVP is made by cooking soybean flour with other ingredients and extruding the mixture to form hamburger extenders, bacon bits and the like. Spun forms are made by spinning fibers and adding flavor and color. TVP can be formed to resemble meat, fish or poultry. Imitation meat products contain many additives to create a desired texture and flavor, including MONOSODIUM GLUTAMATE, salt, ARTIFICIAL FOOD COLORS, flavors, flavor enhancers, EMULSIFIERS and various types of VEGETABLE OIL. Though low in cholesterol, imitation meat can be a high-fat option because of the added hydrogenated vegetable oil.

TVP is an inexpensive, versatile imitation meat used in a large number of manufactured foods, including simulated CHICKEN, simulated HAMBURGER, simulated HAM and BACON, simulated pepperoni and even imitation nuts. Soybean protein finds its way into casseroles, pizza toppings, stews, snacks, other CONVENIENCE FOODS and institutionalized cooking. The amount used in soy products is up to the discretion of the manufacturer. TVP is considered a safe food additive. (See also IMITATION FOOD; PROCESSED FOOD.)

thermogenesis (nonshivering thermogenesis) The generation of heat by the body in response to cold. Brown fat tissue (adipose tissue) is geared to product heat. Brown adipose is most predominant in newborn infants and decreases with age. It is much less abundant in the body than white fat, and occurs in only a few regions, especially the back of the neck and the upper back in adults. The amount of brown fat can increase with exposure to low temperatures. Fat cells in brown adipose tissue can switch over to burn fat and produce heat in response to thyroid hormone. Released heat can then warm the body. This response is more prominent in babies than in adults. (See also FAT METABOLISM; SPECIFIC DYNAMIC EFFECT.)

thiamin (vitamin B_1) A water-soluble vitamin and a member of the B complex. Thiamin is essential for the energy production from carbohydrate and fat. The active form (coenzyme), thiamin pyrophosphate, serves as an enzyme helper in the breakdown of glucose (blood sugar) and in the Kreb's cycle, the central energy-yielding pathway of the body. Thiamin is also required in the PENTOSE phosphate pathway, a sequence of enzymes that converts glucose to the smaller sugars and energy and liberates hydrogen atoms for biosynthesis. These energy-yielding pathways are critical for normal function of peripheral nerves, skeletal muscle and heart muscle, among others.

Severe thiamin deficiency causes BERIBERI. Though rare in the United States, this disease occurs all too frequently in malnourished populations in developing nations who rely on white flour and white rice that are not enriched with thiamin. When beriberi affects primarily the nervous system, it is called "dry" beriberi. Degeneration of insulation (myelin sheath) around nerves of the central nervous system occurs, leading to nerve irritation, pain, numbness and, in extreme cases, paralysis and muscle wasting. Beriberi produces a staggering gait, numbness of legs and retarded growth. Mental symptoms such as disorientation, hallucinations and depression occur as well. These symptoms usually respond to thiamin supplementation, and thiamin is also important in treating polyneuritis (nerve inflammation) associated with pregnancy and ALCOHOLISM. Thiamin deficiency can masquerade as SENILITY. Alcoholics may exhibit the mental confusion typical of beriberi. Thiamin supplementation alone does not seem to affect mental processes and memory if thiamin deficiency is not involved.

An alternate course results in "wet" beriberi, seen as problems with the heart and circulation (abnormal heart rhythm, low blood pressure, elevated levels of blood lactic acid, edema [water retention] of the legs, heart muscle weakness and, ultimately, heart failure). This form of beriberi usually responds quickly and dramatically to thiamin supplementation.

Requirements

The RECOMMENDED DIETARY ALLOWANCE (RDA) for thiamin for men is 1.5 mg and for non-pregnant women 1.1 mg, and based upon an allowance of 0.5 mg per 1,000 calories consumed daily. The requirement increases with pregnancy and lactation. Because of the prevalence of alcoholism in the United States, thiamin deficiency is not uncommon. Symptoms of moderate deficiency include FATIGUE, apathy, nausea, irritability, depression, slowed wound healing, loss of appetite, indigestion and constipation. Moderate deficiency symptoms can be caused by crash dieting, alcohol abuse or liver disease. People relying on highly processed foods are at risk, for example, elderly people; low-income persons; teenagers relying on sweets, soft drinks and low-nutrient foods; and pregnant women. Consuming large amounts of sugar as found in sweets and soft drinks increases the need for thiamin. Also at risk are patients on kidney dialysis or who are sustained for long periods by intravenous nutrients.

Factors That Increase Thiamin Requirements

- Alcohol. Thiamin assimilation is blocked by alcohol consumption. Alcohol use also injures the small intestine and reduces its ability to absorb thiamin. Alcohol decreases thiamin conversion to thiamin pyrophosphate and depletes tissues of this coenzyme.
- Thiamin antagonists. Raw SEAFOOD, such as shrimp, carp, herring, mussels and clams, and YEAST contain thiaminase, an enzyme that degrades thiamin. Eating a large amount of live yeast can reduce thiamin ABSORPTION. Cooking seafood destroys this enzyme.
- Heat-stable anti-thiamin factors have been isolated from several sources. Fermented fish contain factors that limit thiamin uptake. Tea, coffee and even decaffeinated coffee reduce thiamin absorption.
- Baking soda. Cooking with baking soda destroys thiamin.
- Cigarette smoking. Smoking adversely affects thiamin uptake and use by tissues.
- Medications. Antacids and barbiturates may interfere with thiamin uptake.

Foods that contain ample thiamin are wheat germ; meats (pork, beef, ham, organ meats); nuts (pecans, peanuts, walnuts); brewer's yeast; fortified cereals and grain products. Thiamin is used to enrich flour, breads and cereals, a practice that has eliminated the widespread thiamin deficiency that existed prior to enrichment programs. Heating food and processing destroys this fragile vitamin. The higher the cooking temperature, the greater the loss. However, microwave cooking does not seem to increase thiamin loss. Thiamin is relatively non-toxic. Very high doses rarely lead to headaches, mental instability, irritability or weakness. Some people are allergic to thiamin injections. (See also CARBOHYDRATE METABOLISM.)

Seear, Michael, et al., "Thiamine, Riboflavin and Pyridoxine Deficiencies in a Population of Critically Ill Children," *Journal of Pediatrics*, 121:4 (1992), pp. 533–38.

thickening agents (thickeners)   Food additives used to modify the consistency of ice cream, yogurt, pudding, soft drinks, soups, salad dressing and baby food, among other products. They stabilize complex mixtures in manufactured foods to prevent a lumpy or watery consistency or crystallization or to prevent oils, coloring agents and nutrients from separating. Many thickeners are naturally occurring polysaccharides (AGAR, CARRAGEENAN, PECTIN and the like). Chemically modified starches, called "derivatized starches," cellulose gums and other chemically modified materials are frequently used for this purpose. (See also GUAR GUM; GUM; SEAWEED.)

thiourea   A small sulfur compound analog that occurs in vegetables like TURNIPS and CABBAGE and other cruciferous vegetables. Thiourea inhibits the synthesis of thyroxine (thyroid hormone) and can cause goiter formation in lab animals. These vegetables nonetheless add considerable nutritional value and variety to the diet. Vegetables high in thiourea theoretically could cause a potential health problem for people with iodine-deficient diets who rely on turnips—not a likely circumstance in the United States.

thirst   A craving for WATER. Thirst sensation is caused by cells in the HYPOTHALAMUS, a small region of the brain that controls both drinking and excreting water and processes information about the external environment in order to maintain an optimal internal environment (HOMEOSTASIS). Certain cells detect the concentration of SODIUM in the blood. When the concentration increases above 310 to 340 mg per 100 ml (136 to 145 milli-equivalents per liter), cells of the thirst center begin to shrink, triggering nerve impulses that evoke the sensation of being thirsty. A 1% increase in effective ion concentration (osmolarity) can trigger this response. Intracellular DEHYDRATION can also stimulate thirst. Another nerve center of the hypothalamus triggers the release of ANTIDIURETIC HORMONE from the PITUITARY GLAND. This hormone causes the KIDNEYS to decrease urine output, effectively conserving water. (See also ELECTROLYTES.)

threonine (Thr, L-threonine)   A dietary essential AMINO ACID that serves as a building block of PROTEIN. Threonine resembles SERINE, which is a simple amino acid that can be synthesized by tissues. Severe threonine deficiency in experimental animals causes neurologic dysfunction and lameness. In addition to being a raw material for protein synthesis, animal studies suggest that threonine stimulates the THYMUS GLAND and supports the IMMUNE SYSTEM. Adults need an estimated 7 mg/kg of body weight per day. Animal protein like meat, fish, poultry and dairy products are good dietary sources of this amino acid. (See also AMINO ACID METABOLISM.)

thrombin   The enzyme derived from the serum protein prothrombin that catalyzes the final step in the BLOOD CLOTTING cascade. VITAMIN K is required in the maturation of prothrombin, and hence is indirectly responsible for thrombin formation. Hemorrhagic (bleeding) disease in newborn infants due to inadequate blood clotting may respond to vitamin K supplementation because vitamin K stores are low at birth, and the sterile gut lacks the beneficial bacteria that normally produce vitamin K in adults. Breast milk contains little vitamin K, and the American Academy of Pediatrics recommends administration of vitamin K at birth to promote normal thrombin formation and clotting.

thrombosis   The obstruction of a blood vessel by a blood clot. Detachment of a fixed blood clot (thrombus) produces a traveling blood clot (embolus) that can block a vessel at a distant site. Blockages of arteries feeding the brain lead to STROKES, while blockage of arteries feeding the heart contribute to HEART ATTACKS. (See also ATHEROSCLEROSIS; CARDIOVASCULAR DISEASE.)

thyme (*Thymus vulgaris*)   A fragrant culinary HERB. Thyme was known to Egyptians, Greeks and Romans and traditionally was used to instill courage. There are many varieties of this plant. Garden thyme is a small bushy perennial. Thyme is a powerful herb with a distinctive aroma. It can be mixed with PARSLEY and bay leaves as a seasoning, and is used in marinades and sauces. It is used sparingly with veal, pork, poultry and poultry stuffing, vegetable soups, chowders, summer squash and gumbo dishes. Thyme is also used in custards and jellies. Thyme tea has been used in folk medicine for coughs, colds, and sore throats. It has antibacterial properties and can boost the immune system. Thyme possesses powerful antifungal properties. (See also SAGE.)

thymine   A nitrogen-containing base that functions as raw material for DNA. Thymine is easily made by the body and is not a dietary necessity. However, synthesis of thymine requires FOLIC ACID, a B vitamin. Thymine consists of a six-membered ring containing four nitrogen atoms and two carbon atoms. Thymine and other bases of DNA contribute to the unique properties of DNA. DNA exists as two parallel chains linked side by side as a helix. This association relies upon a linkage of bases between the two strands; thus thymine in one DNA chain binds to a base called ADENINE on the adjacent chain. It is this specificity of base-pairing that underlies the genetic code and DNA replication during cell division. Thymine is readily broken down by the body and does not yield URIC ACID, a general waste product of DNA and RNA degradation. (See also PURINE; PYRIMIDINE.)

thymus gland   A component of the IMMUNE SYSTEM that produces HORMONES to support the development of the immune cells. The thymic hormones include thymosin, thymic humoral factor, thymic factor and thymopoietin. Together they promote the proliferation and maturation of various types of T cells, lymphocytes (white blood cells) that help defend the body against foreign invaders. Helper T cells (which activate other lymphocytes), cytotoxic T cells (which attack cells) and suppressor T cells (which limit lymphocyte activity) represent the major class of T cells.

The thymus shrinks as people age. At birth thymic tissue represents 0.4% of body weight. At the age of 70, the thymus accounts for only 0.0007%. This atrophy correlates with a gradual weakening of the immune system. Orally administered extracts of beef thymus have been used to support the function of the thymus gland. Antioxidants like VITAMIN C, VITAMIN E, BETA CAROTENE and SELENIUM are nutrients that enhance T-cell function and may retard thymic shrinkage because the gland is susceptible to oxidative damage. The amino acids ORNITHINE and ARGININE can also stimulate the thymus gland. ZINC, VITAMIN B₆ and vitamin C seem crucial to support thymic hormone production and cell-dependent immune function. *Echinacea angustifolia* and licorice enhance immune function performed by the thymus gland. Thymic factors are being studied as therapeutic agents for AIDS patients and cancer patients. (See also AGING; ENDOCRINE SYSTEM.)

thyroid gland   The gland responsible for the formation of thyroid HORMONES and calcitonin. The most plentiful thyroid hormone is thyroxine (T4), which is converted to tri-iodothyronine (T3), which is more potent but is present in smaller amounts in the blood. This conversion takes place in the liver and lungs. Thyroxine consists of the amino acid TYROSINE, to which iodine is bound. Tyrosine is a building block of the protein thyroglobulin, to which IODINE is added during its processing. Thyroxine is released from thyroglobulin when the thyroid gland is stimulated, for instance, by other hormone signals.

T3 and T4 increase the rate of oxygen uptake, the rate of oxidation of fat and carbohydrate for ENERGY, and the BASAL METABOLIC RATE, the rate at which energy maintains body function. Thyroid hormones also increase carbohydrate uptake by the intestine; regulate lipid metabolism; help regulate normal growth, brain development and skeletal maturation in children; and help regulate the central nervous system as well as the function of peripheral nerves. In children thyroid hormones help regulate growth and development by working together with GROWTH HORMONE. Furthermore, thyroid hormones regulate the activity of the nervous system, which in turn increases blood flow, increases heartbeat and blood pressure, and increases movement of the gastrointestinal tract (PERISTALSIS).

Calcitonin operates differently. This hormone lowers the level of CALCIUM and phosphate in the blood by inhibiting BONE breakdown (demineralization) and by increasing calcium and phosphate incorporation into bones. This appears to take place by inhibiting bone-destroying cells called osteoclasts.

The HYPOTHALAMUS regulates the activity of the thyroid gland. This portion of the brain regulates responses to changes in blood chemistry such as lowered blood sugar and decreased body temperature. It releases a hormone called thyrotropin releasing hormone which stimulates the pituitary to secrete thyroid stimulating hormone (TSH) into the bloodstream. In turn, TSH then stimulates the thyroid gland to release its hormones to speed up metabolism.

In decreased thyroid gland function (HYPOTHYROIDISM), body temperature decreases, reaction time is decreased and thought processes are slowed. Low basal temperature, depression, FATIGUE, dry skin, dry hair, low blood pressure and difficulty in losing weight also characterize hypothyroidism. In extreme cases a GOITER develops (enlarged thyroid gland). Iodine, ZINC, VITAMINᵉ and VITAMIN A, RIBOFLAVIN, NIACIN, VITAMIN B₆ and vitamin C are required for the formation of thyroid hormone. Exercise stimulates the thyroid gland. On the other hand an overactive thyroid gland (hyperthyroidism) is characterized by a high metabolic rate, nervousness, weight loss, heat intolerance, excessive sweating and increased heart rate. This metabolic disorder can mimic IRRITABLE BOWEL SYNDROME. (See also CATABOLISM; ENDOCRINE SYSTEM.)

McDougall, I. Ross. *Thyroid Disease in Clinical Practice.* New York: Oxford University Press, 1992.

tin A heavy metal. There is weak evidence that it is a required nutrient in animals, although it has no known metabolic function at the present time. Rigorous exclusion of tin from diets of laboratory animals impaired reproduction and caused other abnormal growth. If it functions as a nutrient in humans, typical daily ingestion of 1.5 to 5 mg per day more than meets requirements. Tin is still used to line certain cans, and acidic foods like canned PINEAPPLE and canned TOMATOES can leach out tin from the inside of a can. However, there is little evidence to indicate that tin can be toxic. (See also HEAVY METALS.)

tissue A level of cellular organization in which groups of similar cells perform similar functions. Cells of tissues adhere to each other through intercellular materials (connective tissue) and tight bonding (tight junctions). The epithelial tissue of the intestine is representative of this layer of cells and contains mucus-secreting cells and enzyme-secreting cells. Other tissues include nervous tissue, muscle tissue, connective tissue and ADIPOSE TISSUE. Nerve tissue is composed of nerve cells (neurons) and their supporting cell types (neuroglial cells). Muscle tissue contains muscle fibers assembled from muscle cells (myoblasts). Connective tissue contains fibroblasts, cells that secrete materials from an extracellular matrix, including the structural protein, COLLAGEN, together with GLYCOSAMINOGLYCANS (MUCOPOLYSACCHARIDES), consisting of long chains of modified sugars. Mucopolysaccharides absorb water and are slippery. They form a gel-like environment for connective tissue cells called ground substance. Adipose tissue is fatty connective tissue that contains fat cells (ADIPOCYTES). Reticular tissue is a fibrous connective tissue that forms the support for internal organs like the liver, spleen, lymph glands and lungs. (See also BONE; SKIN.)

tocopherol See VITAMIN E.

tofu A SOYBEAN curd prepared by coagulations of the PROTEIN in soybean milk with calcium or magnesium salts. Tofu is a white semi-solid containing 88% water, 6% protein and 3% fat. It is shaped into blocks and kept moistened and refrigerated in plastic tubs. In much of Asia, tofu is the most common soy-based food. Tofu appears as deep-fried cakes, pouches and puffs; tofu pudding; fermented tofu (beancurd cheese); tofu burgers and grilled tofu; beancurd sheets (dried yuba); Chinese-style pressed tofu; and savory pressed tofu. Tofu offers a number of advantages as a protein source. Soy protein is a high-quality protein, approaching the value of MEAT because it is rich in essential amino acids. Furthermore, soy protein is inexpensive and contains no CHOLESTEROL. Tofu supplies CALCIUM when soy milk is coagulated with lime. Such tofu contains 130 mg of calcium per 3.5-oz serving, a substantial part of the daily calcium requirement. (If tofu is prepared with magnesium, the calcium content is negligible.) Nutrient content of one piece of tofu measuring 2 in by 3 in by 1 in (120 g) is: 86 calories; protein, 9.4 g; carbohydrate, 2.9 g; fiber, 2.2 g; fat, 5 g; calcium, 108 mg; iron, 2.2 mg; thiamin, 0.18 mg; riboflavin, 0.08 mg; niacin, 0.1 mg.

tolerance to toxic materials (specific adaptive response) Refers to the body's adaptation to harmful substances. The first reactions to addictive substances or toxic materials are usually uncomfortable—gagging, choking, chest pains and/or sneezing. After repeated exposure to harmful materials the body may adapt to tolerate the material (maladaptation). In this stage, the body stops sending obvious distress signals. A CRAVING for the substance in question can develop, and when again ingested or taken up, the provoking substance can provide an emotional "high" or euphoria and decreased awareness of pain. Tolerance to the addictive or toxic material increases the risk of lowered immunity, weakened ADRENAL GLANDS and physical exhaustion. These factors in turn set the stage for DEGENERATIVE DISEASES like CANCER and heart disease. Minimizing exposure or avoidance of active agents, preventive nutrition and EXERCISE may counteract these effects. (See also ADDICTION; STRESS.)

tomato (*Lycopersicon esculentum*) A vegetable from an annual vine. Botanically speaking, the tomato is a fruit and is related to capsicum peppers, eggplant and potatoes (members of the NIGHTSHADE FAMILY). The modern tomato apparently originated from an ancestor in the region of Peru and Ecuador and was first domesticated in Mexico. Tomatoes were long regarded by Europeans as poisonous and used only as a decorative plant. It was not until the 1800s that tomatoes were generally accepted as food. Tomatoes are now a leading vegetable crop in the United States. It ranks second to potatoes, when the consumption of processed tomatoes is included.

Currently tomato varieties offer many shapes and sizes such as ribbed, pear-shaped or cherry-shaped. Colors range from the best known red varieties to green, yellow or varicolored. They range in size from less than an inch in diameter to 5 or 6 inches in diameter. Supermarket varieties fall into three categories: Cherry tomatoes are small and less juicy; plum tomatoes are egg-shaped and less juicy and have a firmer flesh; round (slicing) tomatoes (also known as beefsteak tomatoes) are large, round varieties. A genetically engineered tomato was approved by the U.S. FDA in 1994 as the first whole food to be commercially produced using biotechnology. This variety of tomato contains an altered gene that extends its shelf life. Currently the FDA does not require special labeling for this product.

One reason for the tomato's popularity is that it combines well with so many foods. Large red tomatoes and small cherry tomatoes are used for salads and sauces, while pear-shaped tomatoes are used in tomato pastes. Tomatoes are a traditional ingredient in dishes such as Italian pasta, gazpacho soup, guacamole, shrimp (seafood) cocktail, Spanish rice, stuffed tomatoes and CHUTNEY. The United States is the major producer of tomatoes. Nearly 75% of the crop is processed as canned tomatoes, KETCHUP, chili sauce, tomato juice, tomato paste, tomato powder, salad dressings and soups. Vegetable juice cocktails are usually tomato-based.

Fresh tomatoes are a good source of VITAMIN C, although the vitamin C content varies with the time of year. Because the consumption is so high, tomatoes are a major dietary source of vitamin C in the U.S. Tomatoes also provide beta carotene, though their intense orange-red color is due to another carotenoid called LYCOPENE, which lacks vitamin A activity. Lycopene acts as an antioxidant and, like beta carotene, offers protection against the damaging effects of free radicals, highly reactive molecules that can attack cells. Free radical damage is linked to cancer and aging. Tomatoes contain courmaric acid and chlorogenic acid, compounds that block nitrosoamines. Nitrosoamines are cancer-causing agents that can form in the digestive tract from nitrites in cured meat. The nutrient content of one raw tomato (123 g) is: 29 calories; protein, 1.1 g; carbohydrate, 5.3 g; fiber, 2.2 g; fat, 0.3 g; potassium, 255 mg; vitamin A, 139 retinol equivalents; vitamin C, 22 mg; thiamin, 0.07 mg; riboflavin, 0.06 mg; niacin, 0.74 mg. One cup of tomato paste (262 g) provides 220 calories; protein, 9.9 g; carbohydrate, 49.3 g; fiber, 6.2 g; fat, 2.3 g; iron, 7.8 mg; potassium, 2,442 mg; sodium, 170 mg (if salted, sodium is 2,070 mg); vitamin A, 647 retinol equivalents; thiamin, 0.41 mg; riboflavin, 0.5 mg; niacin, 8.4 mg.

tongue   This muscular organ is located in the MOUTH and partially in the PHARYNX. The tongue assists mastication, swallowing, speech and taste functions. It pushes food into the teeth for grinding; once the food is masticated, the tongue forms a ball of food (bolus) and pushes it into the throat. The upper surface of the tongue is covered by small projections called papillae. TASTE buds are located on the papillae; they are responsible for the sense of taste. Taste receptors located at the tip of the tongue are most responsive to sweet and salty foods, but respond to sour and bitter-tasting substances as well. The taste buds along the sides of the tongue respond to sour (acidic) substances, while the back of the tongue senses bitter materials more readily. (See also DEGLUTITION; SALIVA; TEETH.)

tooth   See TEETH.

tooth decay   See TEETH.

torula yeast (*Torulopsis utilis*)   A very hardy YEAST cultured as a food for human consumption and livestock feed. Torula can be grown using molasses, carbohydrates from wood processing, fruit wastes and citrus pulp extract. The dried yeast is tasteless and contains 50 to 62% protein. It is a source of the B vitamins, including vitamin B_{12}. (See also B COMPLEX.)

toxemia (toxemia of pregnancy, pregnancy-induced hypertension)   A potentially dangerous condition that may occur after the 20th week of pregnancy. Pre-eclampsia and ECLAMPSIA represent early and late stages of toxemia. Nearly 7% of pregnant women develop a degree of toxemia, characterized by elevated blood pressure, swollen neck and ankles, nausea, anorexia, puffy face and kidney problems. Eclampsia indicates an intensification of symptoms with protein in urine, severe high blood pressure, blurred vision, and a sudden weight gain in the last trimester. If not corrected, toxemia of pregnancy can lead to circulatory failure, convulsions and coma at time of labor. Although the cause of toxemia is not known, women who are young and pregnant for the first time, who lack prenatal care and who may be nutrient deficient are at greatest risk.

Kidney disturbances, endocrine and metabolic irregularities, and compromised nutrient status have been implicated as risk factors in toxemia. PROTEIN, CALCIUM, CALORIE and VITAMIN B_6 deficiencies may have a role. Studies of pregnant women suggest that oxidative damage may be related to the development of pre-eclampsia. Clinical studies suggest that CALCIUM may be beneficial and MAGNESIUM has been used to decrease complications of pregnancy, including toxemia. While well-balanced diets afford protection against complications, sodium restriction is discouraged in managing this condition. Delivery terminates the condition. Toxemia requires prompt medical attention.

toxicity   The degree to which a substance can cause injury. In toxicology, toxicity refers to doses at which a large fraction of the exposed population would be expected to die. For example, LD50 is the dose of a substance that is lethal to 50% of a population of experimental animals. Toxicity can be distinguished from side effects. Side effects refer to the action or effect of a substance beyond that which is desired. Undesirable consequences include headache, nausea, dizziness and sleepiness.

Toxicity can be the result of nutrient excess. Trace mineral nutrients like FLUORIDE, IODINE, SELENIUM, COPPER, IRON, ZINC, VITAMIN A, VITAMIN D and VITAMIN B_6 cause a variety of symptoms of toxicity when sufficiently high levels are consumed. Even water, which is required in volumes of 1.5 to 2 liters daily, becomes toxic when large volumes are ingested because the blood becomes so diluted that it exceeds the ability of the kidneys to excrete water rapidly enough. Toxicity can occur with exposure to naturally occurring plant and microbial poisons (toxins) in foods, like aflatoxin in moldy peanuts and poisonous MUSHROOMS. Heavy metals like LEAD, CADMIUM and MERCURY have no known biological roles and are toxic when present in sufficiently high concentrations. Toxic exposure may be due to synthetic chemicals like PESTICIDES, fertilizers, FOOD ADDITIVES, fuel additives, household chemicals and industrial solvents.

A hazardous material is one that poses a health RISK. Hazardous materials can produce toxic symptoms under conditions of actual or realistic use. Thus a food additive would be considered a hazard when amounts people usually consume can cause toxic signs and symptoms. The use of oyster shell and bone meal as calcium supplements is believed to be hazardous because they can be contaminated with lead. These effects on health may be subtle, such as lowered resistance to disease, increased risk of CANCER and of emphysema (due to cigarette smoking).

Margin of Safety

Food additives are generally permitted at levels several orders of magnitude lower than those at which they are believed to have no effect in order to create a "safety cushion." More generally, the margin of safety is the range between the level usually used and that which could create a hazard. The margin of safety for vitamin D is 1/40. Thus 40 times the common usage of vitamin D could cause toxic symptoms in susceptible people. Drugs may have lower margins of safety. Toxic effects of drugs and side effects with normal usage are commonplace among medications. Risks must be balanced against benefits.

The science of toxicology is imprecise for several reasons. Most information is generated from animal studies that may not relate to human risk. Most food additives have been tested for acute toxicity, but few have been tested for carcinogenicity, for long-range toxicity on the nervous system, or for additive or cumulative effects with pollutants, drugs or pesticides. Food additives react with each other and with other ingredients, and combinations can reveal unpredictable properties. This continues to be a critical area of research because people eat mixtures of chemicals in foods, rather than isolated chemicals. (See also ANTIBIOTIC RESISTANT BACTERIA IN FOOD; PESTICIDES; DIOXIN; HEAVY METALS.)

Hearn, Wayne, "Toxic Toll," *American Medical News* (February 15, 1993), pp. 39–42.

Parke, D.V. and Ioannides, C., "The Effects of Nutrition on Chemical Toxicity," *Drug Metabolism Reviews*, 26:4 (1994), pp. 739–65.

toxic metals   See HEAVY METALS.

toxin   See AFLATOXIN; ENTEROTOXIN.

toxoplasmosis   A type of FOOD POISONING caused by a parasite called toxoplasm. This disease-producing microorganism, which can contaminate raw MEAT and POULTRY and cause toxoplasmosis, affects the eyes, lungs and brain, sometimes leading to convulsions. The parasite can be transmitted via cat feces. About 40% of Americans have been exposed to toxoplasm from the family cat but have no symptoms because their IMMUNE SYSTEM destroys the invader. However, if a woman is exposed during her pregnancy, toxoplasmosis can affect the fetus as seriously as rubella (German measles). Infants exposed to toxoplasm during their fetal development may suffer from epilepsy, mental retardation and blindness. Toxoplasmosis may affect one in 1,000 births, much more frequent than German measles, PHENYLKETONURIA or syphilis in infants. U.S. physicians rarely check for toxoplasmosis in pregnant women, though this is commonly done in Europe. Healthy women who are exposed before pregnancy have antibodies that combat the parasite. Toxoplasmosis encephalitis (brain inflammation) is the most opportunistic infection among AIDS patients, affecting 5 to 10% of them. Toxoplasmosis can also become a problem after treatment with immunosuppressant drugs (drugs that slow down the immune system).

Recommendations to prevent toxoplasmosis include the following:

1. Wear gloves when handling raw meat or poultry if you have a cut on your hands.
2. Cook meat and poultry thoroughly (at 150° F).
3. Avoid nibbling raw HAMBURGER and avoid eating steak tartare. Cook eggs well.
4. Use gloves when cleaning the litter box and when gardening to minimize exposure from cat feces.

(See also GIARDIASIS.)

trace minerals (trace elements)   Nutrients that are required in minute levels, ranging from micrograms (millionths of a gram) to milligrams (thousandths of a gram). Trace MINERALS include BORON, CHROMIUM, COPPER, FLUORIDE, IODINE, IRON, MANGANESE, MOLYBDENUM, SELENIUM, SILICON and ZINC. RECOMMENDED DIETARY ALLOWANCES (RDAs) have been established for iodine, iron, selenium and zinc. "Estimated safe and adequate" dietary intakes have been recommended for chromium, copper, fluoride, manganese and molybdenum. Cobalt functions only as a constituent of

VITAMIN B$_{12}$ and has no other known function in animals. Selenium usually is ingested in organic form (selenomethionine and selenocysteine) rather than as the inorganic (uncombined) form.

The trace minerals vary in their function. A number aid ENZYMES (biological catalysts) by functioning as COFACTORS. Thus iron and copper function in oxidation reactions and help enzymes burn FAT and CARBOHYDRATES for energy. Cell division and growth require copper, zinc, iron and other minerals. Iron serves to transport oxygen as part of the red blood cell protein (HEMOGLOBIN). Zinc assists enzymes responsible for the synthesis of genetic machinery, DNA and RNA. Chromium assists INSULIN to regulate BLOOD SUGAR. Iodine is required in the synthesis of thyroid hormones. Manganese assists enzymes, notably in the formation of GLUCOSE from non-carbohydrate precursors and in protection against chemical damage. Fluoride is a constituent of bones and teeth. Selenium as well as zinc, copper and manganese function as ANTIOXIDANTS. Molybdenum assists various oxidases such as the enzyme that destroys SULFITE, a preservative. Silicon seems to be incorporated into bone and connective tissue. ARSENIC, NICKEL and boron are essential nutrients in animals. Boron may help in bone building and may prevent calcium losses in post-menopausal women. The roles of other minerals are generally not known. Vanadium is present in tissues, although it is not known whether it is required for health. (See also NUTRIENT; VITAMIN.)

Kazuo, Nomiyama, et al., "Trace Elements in Cardio-cerebrovascular Diseases," *Annals of the New York Academy of Sciences*, 676 (Nov. 15, 1993), pp. 308–26.

tragacanth gum   A gum obtained from the bark of a tragalus, a small bush that grows in the Middle East. Among vegetable gums tragacanth gum is among the most resistant to acidic solutions, making it ideal for thickening salad dressings. There is little known regarding its chemical composition, and long-term feeding experiments to evaluate its safety are lacking. Because some people are allergic to tragacanth gum, it is no longer used in any of the leading fast-food hamburger franchises. (See also FOOD ADDITIVES.)

transamination   The ENZYME-catalyzed transfer of nitrogen from AMINO ACIDS. Transamination is the first step in the degradation of most of the 20 amino acids used as protein-building blocks. The two exceptions are LYSINE and THREONINE, dietary essential amino acids. Transamination removes an amino group and transfers it to an acceptor molecule (KETO ACID), which is then converted to a new amino acid. This process frees the donor amino acid of its carbon skeleton, a new organic acid. Thus, ALANINE yields PYRUVIC ACID; GLUTAMIC ACID, alpha ketoglutaric acid; ASPARTIC ACID, OXALOACETIC ACID. Each of these acids is readily broken down for energy. Alternatively, these acids can be converted to blood glucose during fasting or STARVATION to supply fuel for the brain.

Enzymes that carry out transamination are called transaminases or aminotransferases. This class of enzyme is unique in its requirement for VITAMIN B$_6$ as the COENZYME, pyridoxal phosphate. Coenzymes are vitamin-derived enzyme helpers. Transaminases catalyze completely reversible reactions. This has important dietary implications because many amino acids can be formed simply by adding nitrogen to a keto acid with the appropriate carbon skeleton, thus they are not dietary essentials (non-essential amino acids). As examples, nitrogen can be transferred to pyruvic acid to form alanine; alpha ketoglutaric acid reforms to glutamic acid; and oxaloacetic acid reforms to aspartic acid. In certain diseases transaminases may leak out of cells into the blood, and elevated blood levels of several transaminases are used in the clinical diagnosis of heart disease, liver disease and other conditions. (See also AMINO ACID METABOLISM; PROTEIN QUALITY.)

trans-fatty acids   By-products of the processing of polyunsaturated vegetable oils. Trans-fatty acids occur in safflower, corn, sunflower seed oils and soybean oil, as well as in hardened fats like SHORTENING and MARGARINE.

Fatty acids are long chains of carbon atoms with hydrogen atoms attached. Fatty acids with fewer hydrogen-B atoms (double bonds) are called unsaturated. Manufacturers create trans-fatty acids as a by-product of chemical process called partial hydrogenation, which fills in some of the empty spaces for hydrogen and makes the fatty acid less saturated. Hydrogenation of vegetable oils extends their shelf life, cuts costs and makes vegetable oils firmer and more spreadable. During the process some of the unsaturated fatty acids are flipped from their bent shape to a straightened form, called trans-fatty acids. The resulting trans-fat possessess many properties of saturated fats.

Trans-fatty acids possess higher melting points than unaltered unsaturates and are solids at room temperature. The trans-fatty acid content of partially hydrogenated vegetable oil ranges between 5 and 16%. By comparison, canola oil and olive oil do not contain trans-fatty acids. Butter contains about 5% trans-fatty acids naturally. Margarine contains 10 to 27%, while stick margarine and shortening contain the most trans-fats. Vegetable shortening is sometimes used by food manufacturers in place of highly saturated tropical oils (coconut and palm). Fast foods are often cooked in shortening that has a high content of trans-fatty acids. For example, french fries may contain up to 38% trans-fatty acids. Food manufacturers frequently vary the oils and fats and the degree of hydrogenation in processed foods. Restaurant foods and commercially baked goods like cookies and crackers prepared with vegetable shortening represent other major sources of trans-fatty acids in the American diet. Low levels of trans-fatty acids are a normal part of the diet. However, the U.S. diet typically provides 20 times the intake of trans-fatty acids obtained from natural sources. Estimates of trans-fat intake range from 8 g to 20 g per day, reflecting an increased consumption of vegetable fat and processed foods.

Trans-fatty fats do not substitute for ESSENTIAL FATTY ACIDS, and they may worsen symptoms of essential fatty acid deficiency. They seem to antagonize the conversion of essential fatty acids to PROSTAGLANDINS, hormone-like lipids that regulate pain, smooth muscle contraction, raise or lower blood pressure depending on the type, and perform many other functions. Diets that incorporate high levels of trans-fatty acid are associated with an increased risk of coronary artery disease (heart disease). Trans-fatty acids may raise blood CHOLESTEROL as LDL (LOW-DENSITY LIPOPROTEIN, the less desirable form) while reducing the beneficial form of cholesterol, HDL (HIGH-DENSITY LIPOPROTEIN). In contrast, untreated polyunsaturated oils lower LDL. They may alter normal cell function in the heart muscle in lab animals when consumed at high levels. Experiments with animals indicate that trans-fatty acids can interfere with the function of insulin receptors, making insulin less effective and forcing the pancreas to produce more insulin to dispose of blood sugar. Such an effect on humans would increase the risk of diabetes. Whether trans-fatty acids impair the immune system or cause tumors in humans remains to be proven. Some animal studies show no effects with high trans-fatty acid consumption. The National Academy of Sciences concluded that currently consumed levels of trans-fatty acids are safe because small amounts are consumed.

New food labels do not indicate the amount of trans-fatty acids in a food. However, when a food label lists the amount of unsaturated (monounsaturated and polyunsaturated fat), it cannot include trans-fats. When a product label claims a food is "saturated fat free," the food cannot contain more than half a gram of trans-fat.

Current dietary guidelines recommend cutting back on all fats and oils, including butter and margarine. Small amounts of butter or margarine are probably safe for most healthy people. Trans-fats in margarine do not mean that it is better to overindulge in butter. Choose tub margarine or liquid margarine over stick margarine because they are less hydrogenated and contain less trans-fat. In baking it is preferable to use liquid vegetable oil rather than margarine (which has trans-fats) or butter (which has more saturated fat plus cholesterol). Use non-hydrogenated vegetable oils like olive oil and canola oil instead of margarine for cooking; they do not contain trans-fats. Avoid deep-fried foods; eat fewer cookies, crackers and chips or choose low-fat brands. "Diet" margarine or "light" margarine contain more water and fewer calories than regular margarine. (See also FAT METABOLISM; FOOD GUIDE PYRAMID.)

Enig, Mary G., "Trans Fatty Acids—An Update," *Nutrition Quarterly*, 17:4 (1993), pp. 79–95.

transferrin   A protein that transports IRON in the bloodstream. This protein can be measured by immunologic methods. Iron deficiency, pregnancy, low oxygen supply and chronic blood losses raise serum transferrin levels. Decreased transferrin occurs in PERNICIOUS ANEMIA, long-term infections, liver disease and excessive iron load. Transferrin levels respond quickly to changes in dietary protein, and low levels can reflect MALNUTRITION. The ability of transferrin to bind iron is called total iron binding capacity of serum (the straw-colored fluid remaining after blood has clotted). Depletion of iron stores is indicated by an increased total iron-binding capacity. (See also FERRITIN.)

trichinosis   A disease caused by a parasitic worm, *Trichinela spiralis*, which can infect meat. Trichinosis remains an important disease in the United States and Latin America and results from consuming infected, raw or partially cooked pork. In addition to pigs, wild carnivorous animals such as bears may carry the parasite. Symptoms of trichinosis include fever, gastrointestinal upset, swelling of infected muscles and severe muscular pain. Unusually high white cell count, recovery of larvae from blood, and immunologic tests are used for clinical diagnosis.

Prevention is best achieved by thoroughly cooking pork (137° F, 58° C) or by freezing pork continuously for at least 20 days at or below 5° F (−15° C) or for 24 hours at 2° F (−17° C). The same precautions apply to bear meat. Smoking or salting meat does not necessarily destroy this parasite. Infection in pigs can be minimized by cooking all garbage and offal from slaughter houses used as feed. All states have laws requiring that garbage be cooked prior to feeding to pigs.

Pork Tapeworm

In Asia, Africa and Latin America, pork tapeworm infection (*Taenia solium*) is common. Microscopic tapeworm eggs follow an oral-fecal route of infection. Infection can be spread by eating food when infected food handlers do not wash their hands before meal preparation. The larvae infect the brain, which causes inflammation and seizures. In the United States infection most frequently appears in communities populated by recent immigrants, for example, from Latin America. An immunologic test can detect parasite antibodies if present. Scrupulous hygienic practice and thorough cooking to avoid consumption of contaminated food are important preventative measures. (See also FOOD POISONING.)

tricyclic antidepressants   Drugs used to treat symptoms of DEPRESSION, bed wetting and occasionally to relieve pain. They commonly cause tremors and dry mouth, insomnia, increase sugar craving and infrequently cause convulsions, hallucinations or difficult urination. When taken with alcoholic beverages or medicines containing ALCOHOL, the combination causes excessive intoxication. Avoid alcohol with these medications. (See also MEDICATIONS; TARDIVE DYSKINESIA.)

triglycerides (triacylglycerols)   Fats and oils. Triglycerides are the most energy-rich nutrients; they provide 9 calories per gram, more than twice the amount in protein and carbohydrate. Triglycerides are digested in the intestine by lipases, enzymes that specifically degrade fat. Triglyceride digestion and absorption requires bile to free fatty acids and monoglycerides (fat fragments). These digestion products are reassembled into triglycerides within intestinal cells, then are packaged as CHYLOMICRONS (sub-microscopic particles that carry triglycerides) and released into the circulatory system. An enzyme in capillaries releases fatty acids from chylomicrons, to be absorbed by fat cells and stored as fat, or to be absorbed by muscle cells and burned for energy.

Triglycerides are classified as LIPIDS, because they are insoluble in water. Chemically, they are combinations of three FATTY ACIDS with a molecule of GLYCEROL, a fragment of glucose with three attachment points. Physical properties of triglycerides differ according to the types of fatty acids attached to glycerol. Thus fats solidify at room temperature while oils remain liquid. This difference in physical properties reflects the relative amounts of saturated FATTY ACIDS and unsaturated fatty acids, which contain double bonds (bonds deficient in hydrogen atoms). Most naturally occurring triglycerides contain mixtures of fatty acids, and oils generally contain more unsaturated fatty acids. Synthetic triglycerides can contain a single type of fatty acid; in this

case, the triglyceride is named after the fatty acid, e.g., tripalmitin contains only PALMITIC ACID (a fatty acid with 16 carbon atoms) and tristearin contains only STEARIC ACID (a fatty acid with 18 carbon atoms). MEDIUM-CHAIN TRIGLYCERIDES occur in COCONUT OIL and palm kernel oil and BUTTER. They contain shorter saturated fatty acids such as lauric acid (with 8 to 12 carbon atoms). Medium-chain fatty acids are taken up directly by the intestine and processed by the liver. They are used in treating conditions with fat MALABSORPTION: SPRUE, STEATORRHEA and other conditions.

Triglycerides are measured in a lab test of serum lipids. High levels of blood triglycerides increase the likelihood of blood clots and may indirectly contribute to processes leading to clogged arteries. High serum triglyceride levels have been found to increase the risk of coronary heart disease associated with high LDL (LOW-DENSITY LIPOPROTEIN, the less desirable form of cholesterol) and low HDL (HIGH-DENSITY LIPOPROTEIN). Fasting triglyceride levels in the range of 100 mg/dl are considered normal; 200 to 400 mg/dl are considered borderline high, and levels above 400 mg/dl are high. People with triglycerides over 150 and HDL levels lower than 40 can be considered at risk for heart attack, even while LDL is normal. Serum triglyceride levels temporarily increase after a meal due to digested fat. Alcohol consumption and vigorous exercise 24 hours before testing can also affect triglyceride readings. Exercising, losing weight, lowering fat intake and limiting alcohol consumption can help lower serum triglycerides. (See also ATHEROSCLEROSIS; DIGESTION; FAT METABOLISM.)

Assmann, Gerd and Schulte, Helmut, "Role of Triglycerides in Coronary Artery Disease: Lessons from the Prospective Cardiovascular Munster Study," *American Journal of Cardiology*, 70 (December 14, 1992), pp. 10H–13H.

triiodothyronine (T3)   See THYROID GLAND.

triticale (*Triticum secale*)   A hybrid cereal GRAIN derived from WHEAT (Triticum) and RYE (Secale). Extensive Canadian research has led to the development of more satisfactory varieties for milling and baking. In general triticale has a higher PROTEIN content, a somewhat better balance of essential AMINO ACIDS and is more resistant to cold than wheat. Much of current production is used for animal feed.

tropical oils (coconut oil and palm oils)   Saturated VEGETABLE OILS and common FOOD ADDITIVES. The most common tropical oils are COCONUT OIL and PALM OIL, mainstays of PROCESSED FOODS. They provide a rich taste and pleasing flavor to granola, cold BREAKFAST CEREALS, CRACKERS, cookies and other products. Tropical oils are among the most saturated FATS, even more saturated than lard and beef tallow. Coconut oil is 92% saturated; palm kernel oil is 86% saturated; while palm oil is 52% saturated. For comparison, BUTTER is 65% saturated and LARD is 41% saturated. Unlike unsaturated vegetable oils such as OLIVE OIL, CORN OIL, SAFFLOWER oil or CANOLA OIL which lower blood CHOLESTEROL, tropical oils seem to increase blood cholesterol levels among Americans. Consumption of tropical oils may increase the risk of clogged arteries and HEART DISEASE.

Tropical oil can be disguised by food labeling. Over half the products with added vegetable oil use "multiple choice labeling." The manufacturer can use the least expensive oil available and add the following descriptions on food labels. "100 percent vegetable oil"; "partially hydrogenated vegetable oil (may contain one or more of the following: coconut, soybean, corn oils)"; "hydrogenated vegetable shortening (soybean, palm, and/or palm kernel oil)"; or "contains one or more of the following: palm, palm kernel, cottonseed, peanut, soybean and safflower oil." These phrases on food labels are too vague to allow consumers to determine the exact types of oils present. Several food producers are changing their formulations and are in the process of gradually phasing out tropical oils in fast foods such as french fries. (See also DIETARY GUIDELINES FOR AMERICANS.)

tropical sprue See SPRUE.

trout (*Salmo*) A large group of mainly freshwater fish related to salmon. Several species are marine fish and ascend rivers to breed. Trout are primarily a sport fish; trout are raised commercially in pens for food use. The most widely known species of trout include rainbow trout, *Salmo gairdneri*; brook trout, *Salvelinus fontinalis*; steelhead or salmon trout, a variety of rainbow trout; cutthroat trout, *Salmo clarki*; and Dolly Varden, *Salvelinus malma*. Steelhead trout is an ocean-going rainbow trout. Lake trout is a large deep-lake trout found in Canada, the Great Lakes and in deep lakes of the Northeast. Lake trout from the Great Lakes is likely to be contaminated with industrial pollutants such as PBBs, PCBs and PESTICIDES. Great Lakes states have set limits for weekly consumption of game fish from these lakes. It is recommended that pregnant women avoid eating contaminated fish regardless of their source. Trout is sauteed, grilled, baked or poached. It can be substituted for salmon in recipes. The nutrient content of a 3-oz (85 g) trout is: 126 calories; protein, 17.7 g; fat, 5.6 g; cholesterol, 49 mg; thiamin, 0.28 mg; riboflavin, 0.26 mg; niacin, 7.6 mg (See also POLYBROMINATED BIPHENYLS; POLYCHLORINATED BIPHENYLS; PREGNANCY AND NUTRITIONAL REQUIREMENTS.)

trypsin An important protein-digesting enzyme produced by the PANCREAS. Trypsin is initially synthesized as an inactive form called trypsinogen and is released as such into the pancreatic duct, together with other inactive precursors of other digestive enzymes. Once in the small intestine, an intestinal enzyme (ENTEROPEPTIDASE) converts trypsinogen to trypsin. Trypsin then activates other protein-digesting enzymes such as CHYMOTRYPSIN and CARBOXYPEPTIDASE. Premature activation of these enzymes in the pancreas or duct can lead to localized inflammation and tissue destruction (PANCREATITIS).

Proteins consist of long chains of amino acids. Trypsin digests proteins by breaking (hydrolyzing) amino acid linkages within the protein chain. Trypsin is highly specific: It hydrolyzes bonds adjacent only at two amino acids, ARGININE and LYSINE. Another digestive enzyme, chymotrypsin, is less specific; it hydrolyzes bonds next to PHENYLALANINE, METHIONINE, TYROSINE, TRYPTOPHAN and LEUCINE. The combined activities of these and other digestive enzymes efficiently degrades most food proteins to simple amino acids. (See also DIGESTION; PROTEASE; ZYMOGEN.)

tryptophan (Trp, L-tryptophan) A dietary essential amino acid and a building block of proteins. Tryptophan must be consumed daily because the body cannot synthesize it. In addition to serving as a raw material for proteins, tryptophan is required for the synthesis of SEROTONIN, a neurotransmitter that helps conduct nerve impulses between cells. Serotonin is also released by mast cells, defensive cells embedded in tissues, and by blood platelets. Serotonin causes smooth muscle to contract; it functions as a vasoconstrictor to constrict blood vessels. Dietary sources of tryptophan include PINEAPPLE, TURKEY, CHICKEN, YOGURT, unripened CHEESE and BANANAS. The usual diet provides 1 to 2 g daily spread out over time, rather than as a single dose.

Tryptophan supplementation has been used with the following conditions:

Depression DEPRESSION is a facet of many diseases and tryptophan, together with painkillers, may help unresponsive depression in some cases. Tryptophan supplements in combination with VITAMIN B$_6$ have been tested as antidepressants. The effects of tryptophan on mania and aggressive behavior have also been examined clinically. Its use has been criticized as being less effective than standard drugs.

Food cravings Administering a combination of tryptophan and TYROSINE has been used to help with depression and CRAVING during withdrawal from addictive substances.

Difficulty in sleeping The effectiveness of tryptophan for inducing sleep is well established. Tryptophan has been used for many years in Great Britain to treat insomnia. For certain people, it enhances relaxation and sleepiness. Tryptophan seems more effective when taken before bedtime with a carbohydrate-rich food.

Side effects from oral contraceptives Women taking oral contraceptives may metabolize tryptophan abnormally, which may be helped by taking vitamin B$_6$.

Chronic pain Research suggests that tryptophan partially reduces sensitivity to pain. Administration of small doses of tryptophan throughout the day with a high carbohydrate, low-fat, low-protein diet and appropriate medication can decrease symptoms in some people. More research in this area is needed.

Toxicity and Side Effects

Amino acids are powerful agents in the body. Amino acid research in humans is still considered preliminary, and the long-term effects and safe dosages are not known for many situations. The Centers for Disease Control linked large doses of tryptophan supplements to a rare, painful blood disorder called eosinophilia-myalgia syndrome (EMS) that became an epidemic in 1989. Subsequently, the U.S. FDA issued a nationwide recall of all tryptophan products in which this amino acid is the sole or the major constituent. The only products containing tryptophan not recalled include certain protein supplements, infant formula, and special dietary foods that contain small amounts of tryptophan for nutrient fortification. No cases of EMS have been reported from this use. EMS is marked by severe muscle pain, joint pain, difficulty in breathing, swollen limbs and fever. In severe cases there are signs of congestive heart failure and paralysis. Most cases were associated with a tryptophan from a single manufacturer; it was contaminated with a related product. Moderate doses of tryptophan (as low as 1 g/day in certain individuals) may cause liver abnormalities. When used with antidepressants, side effects may worsen.

Belongia, E.A., Mayeno, A.N., Osterholm, M.T., "The Eosinophilia-myalgia Syndrome and Tryptophan," *Annual Review of Nutrition*, 12 (1992), pp. 235–56.

tuna (thunnus)   A marine food fish that is a member of the mackerel family. Tuna inhabit temperate waters throughout the world. Some varieties of this fish can reach up to 1,500 lb. Albacore, bluefin, skipjack and yellow fin are common varieties. Tuna has a red, dense flesh that lightens when cooked. Tuna is the most popular fish in the United States based on annual consumption. Tuna serves as a source of OMEGA-3 FATTY ACIDS, a group of FATTY ACIDS that reduce serum cholesterol and decrease the risk of blood clotting and hence heart attacks. Tuna is a predatory fish at the top of its food chain. Like other such fish, tuna is more likely to be contaminated with pollutants like MERCURY. It is recommended that pregnant women limit their consumption of tuna.

Ninety-five percent of tuna that is consumed in the United States is canned. Canned tuna in oil is a high-calorie food. Oil-packed tuna contains 23 g of fat and 1,400 calories per 3-oz serving, while water-packed tuna contains 1 g of fat and a total of 135 calories. Drain the oil to make the calorie content comparable. Fresh tuna is usually sold as steaks, which can be broiled, poached, baked or sauteed. The nutrient content of 3 oz (85 g) of tuna packed in oil and drained is: 165 calories; protein, 24 g; fat, 7 g; cholesterol, 55 mg; calcium, 7 mg; iron, 1.6 mg; sodium, 303 mg; thiamin, 0.04 mg; riboflavin, 0.09 mg; niacin, 10.1 mg. The same size serving, water packed, provides fewer calories (135); more protein (30 g); less fat (1 g); more sodium, (468 mg); and comparable amounts of other nutrients. (See also FISH OIL; HEAVY METALS; SEAFOOD.)

turbinado sugar   See SUCROSE.

turkey (*Meleagris gallopavo*)   A large, native American bird related to the pheasant. The domestic turkey was derived from a Mexican variety of wild turkey. The United States remains the largest producer of turkeys and accounts for over 55% of the world turkey production. Fast growing, broad-breasted, large white turkeys are typical of new varieties raised for their flesh. Turkey produces a higher proportion of edible meat per live weight than any other POULTRY. The time needed to raise a 25-lb tom turkey is 20 weeks. Fryer-roaster turkeys are young, immature turkeys under 16 weeks of age and of either sex. Young hen or tom turkeys are usually five to seven months of age. Grading by the USDA is voluntary. Unlike the grading of red meat, poultry grading is based on appearance, not fat content. Graded birds should be free of feathers and blemishes.

Turkey meat is lower in fat than most red meat, and brown meat contains more fat than light meat. Almost all of the fat lies under the skin and can be trimmed off. White meat, without skin, is a low-fat protein and is the leanest meat. Turkey white meat contains 14% calories as fat, dark meat contains 30% fat calories, while lean steak provides 37%

fat calories. Turkey fat provides 40% saturated fatty acids and 35% polyunsaturated fatty acids; in contrast, beef fat provides 45 to 46% saturates and only 3.6 to 4.4% polyunsaturates. Self-basting turkeys contain much more fat than unbasted birds, and often the injected fat is saturated (butter or coconut oil).

Ground turkey combines both white and dark meat and may include fat and skin. The amounts of skin and fat vary because there are no official standards for fat content for ground turkey. The food label may indicate the percentage of fat content: Supermarkets may provide products listed as "not more than 15 percent fat" or "not more than 20 percent fat." Turkey is also processed into hot dogs, turkey ham, turkey pastrami and turkey sausage. Turkey has become more popular than just a Thanksgiving meal, with the availability of turkey parts and turkey products and an increased consumer awareness of health problems associated with high saturated fat.

Turkey is perishable; frozen turkey should be stored frozen, then thawed in the refrigerator or under cold running water. The sell date on fresh turkeys is one week after the bird has been processed. Perhaps a third of CHICKENS and turkeys are contaminated with salmonella due to fecal exposure during processing. To prevent food poisoning, all items that come into contact with raw meat should be washed, including the cutting board and one's hands. Cook turkey thoroughly. Do not contaminate cooked meat by contact with raw or partially cooked meat; avoid cutting raw vegetables with utensils used for preparing raw meat. Stuffing should either be cooked separately or it should be added just before roasting.

Turkey is a good source of the B vitamins niacin, vitamin B_6 and vitamin B_{12} as well as minerals—iron, zinc and magnesium. Like most meat, it is not a good source of calcium. The nutrient content of 3 oz (85 g) of dark, roasted turkey meat is: 159 calories; protein, 24.3 g; fat, 6.1 g; cholesterol, 72 mg; iron, 2.0 mg; thiamin, 0.05 mg; riboflavin, 0.11 mg; niacin, 5.8 mg. Light meat, roasted (3 oz, 85 g) provides 133 calories; protein, 25.4 g; fat, 2.7 g; cholesterol, 59 mg; iron, 1.1 mg; thiamin, 0.09 mg; riboflavin, 0.26 mg; niacin, 7.6 mg.

turmeric (*Curcuma longa*)   A natural yellow food coloring. Turmeric is obtained from the underground stem of an East Indian herb related to GINGER. When turmeric is cooked and dried, it possesses a mustard-like taste and a brilliant yellow color. Turmeric is used extensively in Indian, Spanish, Mediterranean and Middle Eastern cuisine as a flavoring and coloring agent. It is used in commercial MUSTARD and is a traditional ingredient of curry. Turmeric is used with meat, poultry, fish, deviled eggs, shell-fish, egg salad and potato salad. As with most natural coloring agents, there is little information on its long-term effects from clinical studies.

Turmeric contains materials that can decrease inflammation and it is a potent antioxidant. It contains curcumin, a substance that blocks free radicals, extremely reactive molecules that can attack all cell components. Curcumin has strong anti-inflammatory effects, equivalent to typical nonsteroidal anti-inflammatory drugs though it does not reduce pain. It seems to inhibit neutrophil response (defensive white cells) that triggers inflammation and to block the formation of leukotrienes, powerful stimulants of inflammation. In folk medicine turmeric poultices are applied to relieve pain and inflammation. (See also ARTIFICIAL FOOD COLORS; FOOD COLORING, NATURAL.)

turnip (*Brassica rapa*)   A member of the cabbage family (CRUCIFEROUS VEGETABLE) with edible leaves and root. Turnips are related to the RUTABAGA. Turnips were first cultivated about 2000 B.C. in the Near East. California, Colorado and Indiana account for most of U.S. production. Turnips may be shaped like carrots, round or flat and broad. They can weigh up to 40 pounds. Turnips planted in the fall may be left in the ground until the following spring. Most of the U.S. crop is processed (frozen). Turnip roots are served with mashed potatoes, served with sauces, and cooked in casseroles, soups and stews. Turnip greens are a rich source of calcium: 1 cup of cooked greens provides 198 mg of calcium, about 68% of a cup of milk. The nutrient content of 1 cup (156 g) of cooked turnips is: 28 calories; protein, 1.2 g; carbohydrate, 7.6 g; fiber, 2.8 g; vitamin C, 18 mg; thiamin, 0.04 mg; riboflavin, 0.04 mg; niacin, 0.46 mg.

tyramine   An AMINE present in fermented or aged foods. Tyramine is produced by the degradation of the AMINO ACID, TYROSINE, either by FERMENTATION or by chemical action. This nitrogen-containing compound is a powerful vasopressor (increases blood pressure dramatically). It can cause migraine headaches in sensitive people. Normally tyramine is destroyed in the body by monoamine oxidase (MAO), the enzyme that degrades the hormone EPINEPHRINE. However, certain antidepressant drugs like isocarboxazid and phenelzine are classified as MAO INHIBITORS. By inhibiting this enzyme, they interfere with the disposal of tyramine, which can lead to headache, nausea and high blood pressure when tyramine-containing foods are eaten. In extreme cases, a normal-sized serving of a tyramine-containing food or beverage taken with such medications causes life-threatening elevated blood pressure. The tyramine content of specific foods per 100 g is as follows: pickled herring, 303 mg; cheddar cheese, 141 mg; Gruyere cheese, 52 mg; Brie, 18 mg; chianti wine, 2.5 mg; sherry, 0.4 mg; beer, 0.3 mg; beef liver, 0.5 mg. Bananas, soft drinks, pineapples, yeast extract, yogurt, anchovies, canned figs, chicken liver, chocolate, mushrooms, pastrami, peanuts, sausage, soy sauce, coffee and tea also contain significant amounts. Cottage cheese and processed cheese contain little tyramine. (See also DRUG-NUTRIENT INTERACTION.)

tyrosine (Tyr, L-tyrosine)   A non-essential AMINO ACID required to build proteins and other important compounds. Tyrosine is readily synthesized by the body from the essential amino acid PHENYLALANINE. Tyrosine in the diet decreases the requirement of phenylalanine because less needs to be shunted to tyrosine synthesis. In addition to serving as a raw material for proteins, tyrosine is converted by the nervous system into a family of NEUROTRANSMITTERS, chemicals that help transmit nerve impulses between cells. These "catecholamines" include DOPAMINE, norepinephrine and EPINEPHRINE. They play a role in sensitivity to pain and in feeling alert. In addition, the ADRENAL GLANDS convert tyrosine to epinephrine (adrenaline) and norepinephrine, which are released as hormones to gear up the body to respond to STRESS. The THYROID GLAND combines iodine with tyrosine to form the thyroid hormone thyroxine, which regulates basal metabolism. Tyrosine also forms melanin, the pigment of SKIN. Normal transformations of tyrosine require NIACIN, COPPER and VITAMIN C.

In humans, tyrosine appears to increase performance under stress. Under stress nerve cells release norepinephrine more rapidly. Tyrosine supplements could theoretically increase norepinephrine formation and indirectly help maintain vigilance. Tyrosine may help reduce DEPRESSION and FATIGUE associated with PREMENSTRUAL SYNDROME (PMS). TRYPTOPHAN and tyrosine have been used to minimize cravings and depression during withdrawal from addictive substances. In lab animals administration of tyrosine can increase brain uptake and increase brain production of neurotransmitters. One hypothesis of schizophrenia proposes that dopamine is increased in certain individuals. Some antipsychotic medications are designed to block the conversion of tyrosine to dopamine. Tyrosine seems to be most effective for nerve cells that fire frequently, therefore supplements can affect an aspect of physiology differently depending upon the conditions. For example, certain brain cells fire rapidly in HYPERTENSION (high blood pressure); thus, giving tyrosine to hypertensive rats lowers the blood pressure. With low blood pressure, sympathetic nerves outside the brain are being triggered in order to raise blood pressure. Administration of tyrosine in this case helps raise blood pressure. Liver CIRRHOSIS can lead to a brain condition called encephalopathy (hepatic encephalopathy). Unusually high blood levels of phenylalanine and tyrosine could increase brain formation of TYRAMINE, and this could disrupt normal nerve function. In any event, cirrhosis alters tyrosine formation from phenylalanine as well as altering tyrosine degradation.

Tyrosine supplements can either raise or lower blood pressure depending upon the individual, and migraine headaches can worsen, depending upon the conditions. Do not take tyrosine or phenylalanine supplements with antidepressant drugs containing monoamine oxidase inhibitors. Taken together they can raise blood pressure to fatal levels. In general, do not take amino acid supplements without medical supervision. (See also AMINO ACID METABOLISM.)

ubiquinone   See COENZYME Q.

ulcerative colitis   See COLITIS.

ulcers   See DUODENAL ULCER; PEPTIC ULCER.

ultraviolet light (UV light)   A form of radiant energy that lies between visible light and X rays in the electromagnetic spectrum. Ultraviolet light has a shorter wavelength than visible light and therefore has more energy than visible light. In fact, UV light can induce chemical reactions in the body and in manufacturing processes. UV light from the sun converts a cholesterol product in the skin called 7-dehydrocholesterol to vitamin D_1. Commercial treatment of the plant STEROL, ERGOSTEROL, with UV light produces vitamin D_2. UV light is used to sterilize milk and foods and has other industrial uses because it can destroy viruses and bacteria.

UV light is potentially harmful to eyes and SKIN. Lifelong exposure increases the risk of CATARACTS due to damage to the lens of the eye. UV exposure is also implicated in damage to the cornea and the retina. Sunburn is an immediate symptom of the dangers of overexposure to UV light. Prolonged exposure to UV light in sunlight can cause premature aging of the skin; loss of the skin's elasticity causes wrinkles. Long-term exposure to sunlight can cause rough, brownish, scaly growth on the skin, a precancerous condition called actinic keratosis. Tanning increases the risk of skin cancer, the most common type of cancer; malignant melanoma is the most serious form. A second type of skin cancer, basal cell carcinoma, does not spread to other parts of the body and is more prevalent, affecting one in eight Americans. Those at greatest risk are fair-skinned people with light-colored eyes; those who have a high incidence of moles or who have a family history of cancer; and people who spend long periods of time out of doors.

Preventing skin cancer involves protection from direct exposure to sunlight. Specialists recommend wearing UV-absorbing sunglasses and using appropriate sunscreen lotion whenever individuals are out in the sun. Nutrition seems to play an important role in limiting the effects of long-term UV exposure. The reason for this lies in the nature of the damage induced by UV light. UV light causes the formation of free radicals, highly reactive chemical fragments that randomly attack cell components like protein. When free radicals attack DNA, they can cause mutations, which can be a prelude to cancer. Nutritional ANTIOXIDANTS are agents that counter the effects of free radicals by either squelching them or by preventing their formation. Included in the family of antioxidants are VITAMIN C, VITAMIN E and BETA CAROTENE. Certain trace minerals like selenium and zinc can also effectively protect cells against oxidative damage. (See also MACULAR DEGENERATION; CARCINOGEN)

undernutrition   See MALNUTRITION.

unsaturated fat   FAT that contains a relatively high percentage of FATTY ACIDS containing chains of carbon atoms that are deficient in hydrogen atoms and possess double bonds. Each double bond lacks two hydrogen atoms:

$$-\overset{\displaystyle H}{\underset{\displaystyle H}{\overset{|}{\underset{|}{C}}}}-\overset{\displaystyle H}{\underset{\displaystyle H}{\overset{|}{\underset{|}{C}}}}-\overset{\displaystyle H}{\underset{\displaystyle H}{\overset{|}{\underset{|}{C}}}}-\overset{\displaystyle H}{\underset{\displaystyle H}{\overset{|}{\underset{|}{C}}}}-\quad\text{becomes}\quad -\overset{\displaystyle H}{\underset{\displaystyle H}{\overset{|}{\underset{|}{C}}}}-\overset{\displaystyle H}{\overset{|}{C}}=\overset{\displaystyle H}{C}-\overset{\displaystyle H}{\underset{\displaystyle H}{\overset{|}{\underset{|}{C}}}}-$$

Saturated   Unsaturated

Fish oils and most vegetable oils are unsaturates. In contrast, animal fat and shortening are saturated fats, enriched in saturated fatty acids whose carbon atom chains are filled up with hydrogen atoms. These important chemical differences govern the physical and chemical properties of fats. Unsaturated fats are liquids at room temperature and are sensitive to attack by OXYGEN, which can lead to RANCIDITY (decomposition), while saturated fats are hard at room temperature and are more stable to heat and oxidation.

Unsaturated fats fall into two groups. MONOUNSATURATED OILS are rich in the monounsaturated fatty acid, OLEIC ACID; this building block lacks a single pair of hydrogen atoms. Such oils are called "monounsaturates" or "oleic-rich" oils; OLIVE OIL is a typical example. Monounsaturates seem to lower the risk of HEART DISEASE by lowering blood CHOLESTEROL (a desirable effect) without lowering HDL (HIGH-DENSITY LIPOPROTEIN), the beneficial form of cholesterol. Monounsaturates are not usually partially hydrogenated.

Polyunsaturates are the second type of unsaturated fats. These oils are rich in polyunsaturated fatty acids, which lack many hydrogen atoms. Because they are less saturated, polyunsaturated are more susceptible to oxidation. Vitamin E protects polyunsaturates against oxidation, and the requirement for vitamin E increases with increased consumption of polyunsaturates.

An industrial process called hydrogenation is used to harden unsaturated fats by adding hydrogen atoms and making the fatty acids more saturated. Partially hydrogenated vegetable oils maintain some of their unsaturated character and possess some double bonds; such oils are less susceptible to rancidity and have a longer shelf life than untreated oils.

Polyunsaturates provide varying amounts of ESSENTIAL FATTY ACIDS, required in the diet because they cannot be manufactured by the body. Most vegetable oils like soybean oil, corn oil and safflower oil provide the essential fatty acid, LINOLEIC ACID, a polyunsaturated fatty acid of the omega-6 family, the most prevalent in the diet. These polyunsaturated oils seem to lower blood cholesterol (a desirable effect), but in large amounts they also lower the beneficial HDL. Polyunsaturates lower the risk of HEART ATTACK and STROKE because they block the formation of dangerous blood clots. On the other hand, in excess they may increase the risk of CANCER and lower immunity, at least in lab animals.

Certain seed oils like FLAXSEED OIL and fish oils supply the second essential fatty acid, ALPHA LINOLENIC ACID, and other omega-3 polyunsaturated fatty acids. Fish oils supply large polyunsaturated fatty acids that may help prevent or decrease the symptoms of heart disease and HYPERTENSION and of inflammatory conditions like RHEUMATOID ARTHRITIS.

Unsaturated fats produce essentially the same number of calories as saturated fats when burned for energy, 9 calories per gram—more than twice the amount derived from carbohydrate or protein. Both saturated and unsaturated fats when consumed in excess can lead to weight gain. Current dietary guidelines call for selecting a diet that is lower in total fat (less than 30% of total daily calories, with saturated fat representing less than 10% of calories) in order to lower the risk of cancer and heart disease. (See also FAT METABOLISM.)

Nydahl, Margaretha C., et al., "Lipid-lowering Diets Enriched with Monounsaturated or Polyunsaturated Fatty Acids but Low in Saturated Fatty Acids Have Similar Effects on Serum Lipid Concentrations in Hyperlipidemic Patients," *American Journal of Clinical Nutrition*, 59:1 (January 1994), pp. 115–22.

urea The major nitrogen-containing waste produced by the body. Urea production is the body's way of safely disposing of ammonia, the potentially dangerous product released when AMINO ACIDS are broken down. Urea is nontoxic; it accounts for 60 to 90% of total excreted nitrogen.

Urea production occurs in the LIVER as part of the body's detoxification function; the amount produced is proportional to the amount of protein consumed. The liver uses a group of specialized enzymes (the UREA CYCLE) to produce urea. Urea is released into the bloodstream and transported to the kidney for excretion in the urine. Normally 20 to 35 g of urea are excreted each day. Blood urea nitrogen (BUN) refers to the measurement of blood urea levels and is used as a diagnostic tool to assess liver and kidney function. The amount of urea nitrogen in a 24-hour urine sample can be multiplied by 6.25 to estimate the amount of protein used per day. (See also AMINO ACID METABOLISM.)

urea cycle A collection of enzymes responsible for transforming AMMONIA to UREA. Ammonia is a toxic by-product of amino acid breakdown (AMINO ACID METABOLISM) that is released into the bloodstream. The brain is extremely sensitive to ammonia; therefore its disposal is important. To detoxify this substance and simplify its elimination from the body, ammonia is efficiently removed from the blood by the liver, where it is combined with bicarbonate to create a safe product, urea, to be excreted by the kidneys. The liver also disposes of ammonia produced by gut bacteria and absorbed by the intestine. ORNITHINE, a non-protein amino acid that accepts ammonia, is regenerated when ammonia is released. It is worth noting that the urea cycle produces the amino acid ARGININE. However, the production of this amino acid can be limited during illness and periods of rapid growth, and dietary sources are important. (See also GLUTAMINE; KREB'S CYCLE.)

Kurtin, Paul S., "Nutritional Management of Patients with Renal Disease," *Hospital Medicine* (December 1991) pp. 42–51.

urethane A cancer-causing agent in alcoholic beverages. Urethane has been found to form spontaneously in WINE, BEER and hard liquors. Bourbon whiskey, fruit brandies and some desserts and table wines sold in the United States may contain high levels, exceeding levels permitted in a number of countries, including Canada. Research is underway to lessen urethane contamination of alcoholic beverages. Because the PRESERVATIVE DEPC (diethylpyrocarbonate) spontaneously breaks down into urethane, it was banned by the FDA in 1972. (See also CANCER.)

Foulke, Judith E., "Urethane in Alcoholic Beverages Under Investigation," *FDA Consumer*, 27 (January–February 1993), pp. 19–23.

uric acid   A waste product from the degradation of RNA and DNA. Uric acid is a nitrogen-containing carbon compound derived from PURINES, which are building blocks of DNA, the genetic material of the cell, and of RNA, which directs the manufacture of proteins. Because the body cannot decompose the purine ring system, enzymes convert purines to uric acid instead. Between 0.5 and 1.0 g of uric acid is secreted in the urine daily.

A high blood level of uric acid is associated with GOUT, a form of ARTHRITIS that is characterized by deposits of uric acid in joints. The risk of gout increases with a high protein diet, a family history of gout and an acidic blood pH. Uric acid can form kidney stones, particularly in patients with gout. People with gout should minimize their consumption of foods with a high purine content: liver and organ meats, fish like anchovies, MACKEREL and SARDINES, and yeast. Excessive alcohol can raise blood uric acid levels and increase the risk of kidney stones and gout. Extra fluid, 10 to 12 glasses of nonalcoholic, non-caffeinated beverages daily, can minimize uric acid deposits.

Uric acid performs a useful function for the body: It is a powerful ANTIOXIDANT that can destroy dangerous free radicals, which are linked to degenerative diseases and AGING. Evolution may have favored humans' ability to accumulate relatively high blood levels of uric acid in order to assure the presence of an antioxidant that is unrelated to diet. (See also VITAMIN C; VITAMIN E.)

urinary tract   A system made up of two kidneys, two ureters (tubes leading to the urinary bladder) and a single urethra, the duct that conveys urine to outside the body. The primary function of the urinary tract is to assist the body in maintaining a constant internal environment (homeostasis) by controlling the composition and volume of the BLOOD. Kidneys aid in eliminating toxic materials, drugs, normal waste products and even excesses of essential nutrients as urine. Kidneys assume a role in red blood cell production by secreting erythropoietin, stimulatory protein. They help regulate blood pH and form RENIN, a hormone to regulate BLOOD PRESSURE. Finally, the kidneys activate VITAMIN D to its hormone form, dihydroxycalciferol (calcitriol).

The two kidneys are located in the back just above the waistline. Usually each kidney is encased in a heavy cushion of fat for protection. An extremely thin person may lack this fatty support, and the kidneys may drop, placing a kink in the ureter. The rate of blood flow through the kidney is extremely high; about 10% of the total blood pumped each minute enters the kidneys. This high volume, together with a normal blood pressure, is required to filter the blood and to form urine.

Each kidney contains more than a million microscopic functional units called NEPHRONS. A nephron resembles a tiny funnel with an extremely long, twisted stem. Nephrons filter blood: some materials, like water, pass into the tubules, small tubes that drain the kidney. Others stay in the blood. Useful nutrients like GLUCOSE and minerals (ELECTROLYTES) are reabsorbed into the blood. The sum of these activities is urine.

Filtration usually occurs at a rate of 7,500 ml per hour, equivalent to 190 quarts of fluid filtered per day. Normally between 97 and 99% of the water is reabsorbed, together with all of the glucose because this nutrient, the primary brain fuel, is too precious to waste. However, in DIABETES MELLITUS the blood glucose concentration may exceed the rate at which it can be reabsorbed by kidney cells and is excreted in urine. Glucose in the urine (glucosuria) is a sign of uncontrolled diabetes.

Sodium reabsorption by the kidneys varies with blood pressure: When the sodium concentration in the blood is low, blood pressure drops and renin is released. This enzyme activates ANGIOTENSIN, a hormone that constricts minute arteries located at the nephron, increasing blood pressure. Angiotensin further stimulates the ADRENAL GLAND to release ALDOSTERONE, which increases sodium and water reabsorption by the tubules. Conditions that limit urine output are inadequate fluid consumption, stress, kidney disease and CARDIOVASCULAR DISEASE.

Usually urine is sterile; the closer it gets to the urethra, the greater the possibility of bacterial comtamination. The daily flow of urine out of the body and the immune defenses are usually adequate to assure a sterile urinary tract. However, bladder infections are common among women. Because over half of these infections involve the kidneys, they can be serious. Partial blockage of the urinary tract, for example by stone formation or scarring, can reduce urine flow and favor infection. Cranberry juice contains materials that prevent bacteria from sticking to the walls of the bladder or urethra, thus inhibiting bacterial infection. Garlic and onions also contain substances that limit bacterial growth. Sugar and sweetened juice can help promote bacterial growth, however. Drinking plenty of water (5 pints daily) is recommended.

Stone formation is a second frequent problem of the urinary tract; 10% of men and 5% of women in the United States will experience stone formation. Calcium as calcium carbonate or calcium oxalate can become insoluble and form crystalline deposits when water consumption is inadequate. Alternatively, uric acid can form stones when certain anticancer drugs are taken, or when excessive purines (yeast sardines, organ meats like liver, caviar) are part of the diet. Stone formation correlates with inadequate water intake and fiber consumption; high intake of foods like cocoa, spinach, parsley, rhubarb and certain nuts containing oxalate, can favor stone formation in the urinary tract. (See also AMINO ACID METABOLISM; ERYTHROPOIESIS; KIDNEY STONES; UREA CYCLE.)

urticaria   The medical term for hives, welts that form in response to irritation or allergy. Urticaria is typical of an immediate allergy reaction (immediate hypersensitivity) and is often accompanied by ASTHMA, itchy eyes and runny nose. Animal dander, pollen, house dust and certain foods can cause urticaria in susceptible people. (See also ALLERGY, IMMEDIATE.)

USDA (U.S. Department of Agriculture)   A federal agency responsible for regulating food quality and safety. The USDA operates under the authority of the Federal Meat Inspection Act and the Poultry Products Act, which assign the USDA the responsibility for assuring the safety of MEAT and POULTRY. The USDA inspects meat and meat products, as well as poultry and poultry products destined for human consumption. It inspects slaughtering and processing practices. State laws for meat and poultry inspection must equal USDA standards.

The USDA sets guidelines for meat labeling and grades beef according to eating quality for food companies that pay for this service. Programs for health and nutrition, nutrition education and research are carried out by the eight divisions of the USDA. These divisions are the Agricultural Research Service; Consumer and Marketing Service; Cooperative State Research Service; Annual and Plant Health Inspection Service; Federal Extension Service; Cooperative State Research Service; Food and Nutrition Service; Veterinary Services; Labeling and Registration Section. (See also PROCESSED FOOD.)

USRDA (U.S. recommended daily allowances)   A standard for nutrient intake for healthy people, designed by the USDA for use on food labels through 1994. The USRDAs represent the highest RECOMMENDED DIETARY ALLOWANCES (RDAs), which were developed by the Food and Nutrition Board of the National Academy of Sciences for several nutrients in 1968. The USRDAs are not to be confused with the RDAs, which are not used on food labels. The list of RDAs is much more extensive now, and several values differ from those specified in 1968.

The USRDA was replaced in 1994 by the RDI or REFERENCE DAILY INTAKE (RDI) on food labels. For the time being, the RDI is identical to the USRDA. Individual USRDAs were condensed into just four population groupings: adults and children over four years; infants up to one year; children under four years; and pregnant or lactating women. Generally the highest values for a given age group were used. Thus the USRDAs for adults and children over four years generally were the dietary allowances recommended for a teenage male.

When nutritional claims about a food were made on a food label, or if the food was labeled "enriched," or if extra nutrients were added, the manufacturer was required to list the content of several nutrients as percentages of the USRDAs. The values food manufacturers used for the most common category, adults and children over four, are shown in the accompanying table.

Nutrient	USRDA
Vitamin A	1,000 mcg
Vitamin C	60 mg
Calcium	1,000 mg
Iron	18 mg
Vitamin D	10 mcg
Vitamin E	30 IU
Thiamin	1.5 mg
Riboflavin	1.7 mg
Niacin	20 mg
Vitamin B_6	2.0 mg
Folate	400 mcg
Vitamin B_{12}	6 mcg
Biotin	300 mcg
Pantothenic Acid	10 mg
Phosphorus	1,000 mg
Magnesium	400 mg
Zinc	15 mg
Iodine	150 mcg
Selenium	N/A
Copper	2 mg

For this category the protein value is 45 g of high-quality protein (equivalent to milk protein, CASEIN), or 65 g of lower quality protein (less than casein). (See also FOOD LABELING.)

National Research Council. *Recommended Dietary Allowances*, 10th ed. Washington, D.C.: 1989.

valine (Val, L-valine) A dietary essential AMINO ACID that serves as an important protein building block. Valine is classified as a BRANCHED CHAIN AMINO ACID, along with ISOLEUCINE and LEUCINE. The daily requirement for valine is estimated to be 10 mg per kilograms of body weight, similar to the other branched chain amino acids. Infused branched chain amino acids are selectively used for energy by skeletal muscle rather than by the LIVER. Branched chain amino acids may help restore muscles in patients with liver disease or in patients who have undergone physical trauma such as surgery. However, it is not established that these amino acids have an anabolic (muscle enhancing) effect when used as supplements for healthy people.

Valine and other branched chain amino acids are useful in treating liver damage associated with ALCOHOLISM (hepatic encephalopathy). They seem to limit muscle wasting and reduce some of the neurologic effects related to this disease. Valine and branched chain amino acids may be useful in treating amyotrophic lateral sclerosis (Lou Gehrig's disease). Levels of these amino acids are low in these patients. On the other hand, animal studies indicate that an excess of one branched chain amino acid antagonizes the other two. (See also AMINO ACID METABOLISM.)

vanadium A TRACE MINERAL required by animals for normal growth and development. Deprivation of this element causes slowed growth, reproductive problems and blood abnormalities in rats and chicks. Vanadium in the form of vanadate and vanadyl sulfate improves the effect of insulin in diabetic animals; and artificially induced diabetes in rats can be reversed by vanadate. Large doses also affect serum FAT and CHOLESTEROL levels, though more research in this area is needed.

There is no RECOMMENDED DIETARY ALLOWANCE for vanadium, and the amounts required for optimal health are unknown. Nutritional requirements would likely be met by levels present in food. Black pepper and dill seeds are the richest sources. Whole grains, seafood, milk products and meat are fair sources, while beverages, vegetables and fruits contain the lowest amounts. The average daily intake in the United State is about 20 mcg, quite low in comparison to known essential trace elements. Elevated vanadium is associated with manic-depression, and high levels of vanadium may be toxic.

vanilla (*vanilla planifolia*) A tropical plant that produces pods containing vanilla, an aromatic ingredient used as a food flavoring. Vanilla is a member of a group of tropical orchids, native to Central America and Mexico. The active ingredient, ethyl vanillin, is chemically synthesized and marketed as "vanillin." Ethyl vanillin has 3.5 times the flavor intensity of vanilla bean extract. Because it lacks minor ingredients found in the extract, the taste is not identical. Vanilla is used to flavor ice cream, beverages, chocolate, candy and gelatin. Vanilla is considered a safe additive. (See also FLAVORS; FOOD ADDITIVES.)

varicose veins Bulging, sinuous veins that are close to the surface of the skin. Usually the term varicose veins refers to distended leg veins in which blood vessels become weakened, permitting blood to flow backward instead of forward to the heart. This condition affects an estimated 25% of American women, 10% of men and 50% of people over the age of 50. Often varicose veins are only a cosmetic issue with no symptoms. However, symptoms like aching legs can develop after a person has been standing for a long time. Leg cramps, swollen ankles, intense pain or tenderness along the vein at the end of the day can occur.

Occupations that require extended periods of standing increase the risk of varicose leg veins. Pregnancy also increases venous pressure in the legs and may lead to the development of varicose veins. Standing places heavy pressure against leg veins, and the extra weight of the blood stretches the walls of the vessels, which pulls apart vessel valves, causing blood to pool in the veins. This pressure can cause surface vein walls to bulge out into varicose veins.

Varicose veins can occur anywhere in the body. Hemorrhoids are a common example; they can be aggravated in straining during bowel movements because intense abdominal pressure is transmitted to all veins, even leg veins. Defective, deeper veins can become inflamed (phlebitis) and create a blood clot, resulting in a more serious condition. If the clot dislodges, it can cause blockage in vessels of the lung, the heart (HEART ATTACK or myocardial infarction) or the brain (STROKE).

In addition to inheritance, life-style and diet are believed to be predominant factors in the development of varicose veins. They seldom occur in populations relying on a diet high in unrefined, fiber-rich foods. EXERCISE such as walking and bike riding contract leg muscles that push blood along the venous system. Increasing the strength of vessel walls may minimize the risk of varicose veins. Blue-red berry pigments called anthocyanidins and proanthocyanins can strengthen vessel walls, reduce capillary fragility and help protect the venous connective tissue. BLACKBERRIES, CHERRIES and BLUEBERRIES are rich sources. People who have varicose veins may also be less able to break down FIBRIN, a clotting protein that is often deposited near varicose veins and increases the risk of clot formation. CAPSICUM (cayenne pepper), GINGER, GARLIC and ONIONS increase fibrin breakdown. (See also CIRCULATORY SYSTEM; DIET, HIGH COMPLEX CARBOHYDRATE; FIBER.)

vasoconstriction Reducing the diameter of blood vessels. Both environmental and physiologic factors can constrict vessels. For example, a drop in temperature causes vasoconstriction, an adaptation that helps conserve body heat. All blood vessels except capillaries and venules are regulated by the NERVOUS SYSTEM. Thus fear and other emotions can reduce blood flow. At wound sites, SEROTONIN and other products are liberated by blood PLATELETS, cells that stick to the walls of damaged vessels to form clots. Serotonin helps reduce blood loss by acting as a vasoconstrictor. Certain hormones act as vasoconstrictors: EPINEPHRINE and norepinephrine (released by the ADRENAL GLANDS in response to stress) and ANGIOTENSIN II (formed in the KIDNEYS in response to a drop in blood pressure).

vasodilation Increasing the diameter of blood vessels. Vasodilation increases blood flow and removes waste products while replenishing oxygen and nutrients. Decreased oxygen concentration and the accumulation of metabolic waste products help expand blood vessel walls. The accumulation of LACTIC ACID, decreased pH (more acidic blood), the build-up of carbon dioxide, and increased blood ion concentration (osmolarity) dilate blood vessels. Increased body temperature exerts a vasodilator effect to help cool the body. During inflammation, HISTAMINE is released from damaged cells and from immune cells called mast cells. Histamine is known to increase capillary leakiness, and fluid leakage out of capillaries accounts for swelling in areas of inflammation.

An important family of vasodilators is the kinins, which represent peptides, whose parents occur in the blood and in tissues. Kinins resemble histamine: They relax the smooth muscles around vessels and increase capillary leakiness and blood flow through the kidneys. Kinins occur in sweat glands, salivary glands and the PANCREAS. Kinin release is inhibited by GLUCOCORTICOIDS, hormones produced by the adrenal glands. A high protein diet also increases blood flow in the kidneys. PROSTAGLANDINS, hormone-like substances made from essential fatty acids, can have similar effects. (See also EDEMA, NITRIC OXIDE.)

vasopressin See ANTIDIURETIC HORMONE.

veal BEEF from male dairy calves, ranging in age from four to eighteen weeks. Sub-therapeutic doses of animal drugs may be used when veal calves are very young; this treatment is discontinued as the animal's immune system matures. Veal, like most red MEAT, is a good source of ZINC and other trace minerals. The nutrient content of a 3-oz (85 g) braised veal outlet is: 185 calories; protein, 23 g; fat, 9.4 g; cholesterol, 109 mg; calcium, 9 mg; iron, 0.8 mg; thiamin, 0.06 mg; riboflavin, 0.21 mg; niacin, 4.6 mg.

vegan See VEGETARIAN.

vegetable oil Edible oil extracted from seeds or nuts. Plant oils provide ENERGY, VITAMIN E and polyunsaturated FATTY ACIDS. No vegetable oil contains CHOLESTEROL because plants do not synthesize it. Vegetable oils are classified as TRIGLYCERIDES; like animal FAT, they contain three fatty acids and GLYCEROL (glycerin) and contain just as many calories as animal fat (9 calories per gram).

Vegetable oils fall into three classes: saturated, monounsaturated and polyunsaturated:

1. Saturated vegetable oils are solid at room temperature. The so-called TROPICAL OILS, palm kernel oil and COCONUT OIL, and VEGETABLE SHORTENING, a chemically hardened vegetable fat, are saturated and are solids at room temperatures. These saturated fats resemble saturated animal fat, as in LARD, BUTTERFAT and beef TALLOW. The excessive consumption of SATURATED FAT regardless of its source is believed to increase the risk of CARDIOVASCULAR DISEASE.

2. Monounsaturated oils including OLIVE OIL are rich in a fatty acid called OLEIC ACID, which lacks two hydrogen atoms and contains a single double bond. Olive oil apparently lowers blood LDL (LOW-DENSITY LIPOPROTEIN) cholesterol, the less desirable form, without lowering the "good" kind of cholesterol (HDL, HIGH-DENSITY LIPOPROTEIN), and probably lowers the risk of cardiovascular disease.

3. Polyunsaturated oils such as CORN OIL, SAFFLOWER oil, SUNFLOWER oil and SOYBEAN oil contain a preponderance of polyunsaturated fatty acids. These fat building blocks lack many hydrogen atoms and contain two or more double bonds. High consumption of polyunsaturated vegetable oils apparently lowers LDL cholesterol levels, a desirable result, but also lowers HDL levels, which is undesirable. High consumption of polyunsaturated oils increases the need for the antioxidant vitamin E.

Extraction of Oils

The first step in oil extraction involves crushing or grinding oil-bearing tissue to release oil from cells. The second step involves pressing to squeeze oil from crushed tissue. Residues from pressing are usually extracted with solvents such as hexane to remove the remaining oil. The solvent is then removed. To purify these oils, they are further extracted with alkali and heated, degummed, deodorized by steam treatment, and decolorized by treatment with charcoal or clay. Since these procedures remove or destroy vitamin E, synthetic antioxidants like BHT, BHA and PROPYL GALLATE are often added to retard RANCIDITY. Oils may be "winterized" by removing particulate matter that form upon chilling.

The assumption that cold-pressed oils have been extracted from seeds under mild conditions and contain more vitamin E and polyunsaturated fatty acids may not be valid. Cold-pressed oils are often heated between 120° F and 150° F, then refined, bleached and deodorized, processes that can involve further heating, possibly at temperatures as high as 450° F.

Certain "unrefined oils" are available. In the preparation of these oils, processors do nothing to the oils after heating ground seeds and pressing them to extract the oils. Because such oils are less pure, they have distinctive flavors and colors.

Hydrogenation

Unsaturated vegetable oils can be hardened and stabilized by chemically adding hydrogen atoms to reduce the degree of polyunsaturation. Hydrogenation increases the shelf-life of an oil by making it more resistant to rancidity. Heating vegetable oils at high temperatures does not hydrogenate oils, nor does it convert them to saturated fat. "Partially hydrogenated" vegetable oils retain some of their polyunsaturated fatty acids and remain oils at room temperature, while completely hydrogenated (saturated) oils are solid at room temperature (vegetable shortening). Hydrogenated vegetable oils as well as partially hydrogenated oils contain chemically altered fatty acids called TRANS-FATTY ACIDS; their long-term safety has been questioned.

Americans generally consume too much fat and oil, which increases the risk of HEART ATTACK, STROKE, OBESITY and certain forms of CANCER. A person with high blood cholesterol may be advised to reduce saturated fat intake. Total fat should account for less than 30% of daily calories, perhaps as low as 20% of calories according to some authorities. To reduce the decomposition and rancidity of vegetable oils, store oils in the refrigerator in sealed dark containers. Do not heat oils any more than is necessary and limit cooking with oils at high temperatures. Discard cooking oils after use.

vegetables Cultivated plants that generally provide leaves, stems, roots and flowers used as foods. Leafy vegetables include SPINACH, CHARD, CABBAGE and LETTUCE. Stem vegetables are CELERY and ASPARAGUS; BEETS, TURNIPS, YAMS, POTATOES and CARROTS are roots and tubers as opposed to stems. Vegetables like pumpkin, squash, BROCCOLI and CAULIFLOWER are flowers. GARLIC and ONIONS are bulbs. Corn is a seed vegetable. Vegetables include several botanical classes, including TOMATOES (fruit); PEAS and BEANS (legumes); and MUSHROOMS (FUNGI).

Most regions of the world have contributed vegetables, as indicated by the following examples:

- Europe, the origin of beets, broccoli, BRUSSELS SPROUTS, cabbage, CHIVE, MUSTARD GREEN, pea and turnip; the Mediterranean region: ARTICHOKE, asparagus, celery, chard, CHICKPEA, ENDIVE, KALE, KOHLRABI, OLIVE, PARSLEY, PARSNIP
- Africa: the BROAD BEAN, CRESS, OKRA, yam; the Middle East: broad bean, cabbage, carrot, cauliflower, CUCUMBER, LENTIL, lettuce, mustard green, RADISH, SPINACH
- India: EGGPLANT, MUNG BEAN; China: Chinese cabbage, SOYBEAN, water chestnut
- Central Asia: beet, chive, carrot, DANDELION, garlic, LEEK, onion, pea, shallot, turnip
- Central America: bean, corn, jicima, green PEPPER, PUMPKIN, SQUASH, SWEET POTATO, tomato
- South America: cassava, corn, lima bean, pepper potato, sweet potato, tomato

Root vegetables and tubers like yams, sweet potatoes, carrots and potatoes are by far the leading vegetable crops. They provide starch, fiber, minerals and some vitamins. Orange-colored vegetables like sweet potato and carrot provide BETA CAROTENE. Several of the most popular vegetables in the United States provide minimal nutrient content: celery, lettuce, cucumbers. The greener the vegetable, the more the beta carotene (provitamin A) and CAROTENOIDS it contains. Spinach, collard greens, dandelion greens, kale and Swiss chard are excellent sources and they provide vitamin C, iron and calcium.

The consumption of fresh vegetables in the United States has steadily increased since 1980 from about 115 lbs per person per year to over 190 lbs per year (1990). Nonetheless, fewer than 10% to 20% of U.S. citizens report eating the minimum recommended five daily servings of vegetables and fruits. Potatoes represent nearly 37% of all fresh vegetables, and their popularity accounts in part for this increased vegetable consumption. Much of this increase represents french fries and baked potatoes eaten away from home; french fries and baked potatoes with fatty sauces are high-fat foods, in comparison with baked potatoes without toppings. Lettuce, broccoli, tomatoes, carrots and cauliflower show increased popularity, probably a reflection of the increased availability of salad bars in fast-food restaurants.

There is a growing awareness that vegetables provide materials besides vitamins and minerals that are important for long-term health. Some plant substances (PHYTOCHEMICALS) are not considered essential nutrients, yet their consumption can have long-term effects on reducing the risk of CARDIOVASCULAR DISEASES, CANCER, CATARACTS, AUTOIMMUNE

DISEASES like rheumatoid arthritis, premature senility and other chronic problems associated with AGING. Plants of the cabbage family, including broccoli, cabbage and brussels sprouts, produce materials called ISOTHIOCYNATES and indoles, which seem to lower the risk of cancer. Sulfur compounds of onions, garlic, leeks and chives seem to boost the immune system and inhibit tumors. Many plants including vegetables produce FLAVONOIDS, a broad family of substances that can function as antioxidants to block the oxidative damage to cells due to free radicals. Free radical-induced damage is now believed to be a factor in some degenerative diseases, like heart disease, associated with aging. For example, dark green leafy and orange vegetables and some fruits are a rich source of CAROTENOIDS, including beta carotene. These phytochemicals function as antioxidants and they enhance the immune system. As a group they reduce the risk of some forms of cancer.

Rather than a simple ingredient, vegetables provide a wide array of known phytochemicals; undoubtedly, many more remain to be discovered. Phytochemicals appear to be most effective when supplied in combinations with a range of substances as found in minimally processed foods, including vegetables. Their effects are often synergistic, that is, the overall effect of a combination is more beneficial than any one isolated ingredient.

Vegetable Processing

Although fresh vegetables are available year round due to large refrigerated warehouses and fast transportation systems, processed vegetables remain an important part of the American diet. A variety of methods are used to prepare or to preserve vegetables. Several of the more common methods include:

Canning Developed in the 19th century in France, canning remains a major food preservation strategy. This process involves heating vegetables in metal or glass containers to a sufficiently high temperature to destroy microorganisms that cause spoilage or disease. Heat-treated contents are sealed against air to prevent oxidation.

Drying Drying food in the sun for preservation has been carried out for thousands of years. Drying must be carried out rapidly to avoid changes in nutrients, flavor or texture. The action of plant enzymes that darken produce, destroy nutrients and alter flavor can be limited by blanching (a brief heat treatment) or by treatment with preservatives like sulfites or antioxidants such as VITAMIN C.

Freezing Commercial techniques for rapid cooling and freezing allow many vegetables to retain most qualities of fresh vegetables for periods lasting up to 8 to 12 months. Blanching slows alterations in flavor, color and texture of frozen vegetables.

Pickling Vegetables can be preserved in a salt solution (brine) or in VINEGAR, or a combination of the two. Pickled cucumber and relishes are common food items. Commercially pickled products require heating to destroy microorganisms and to inactivate plant enzymes that alter vegetable properties.

Raw or Cooked Vegetables?

There are certain advantages to eating cooked vegetables. Cooking a vegetable can increase the availability of beta carotene because it is released from storage sites in plant cells. Cooking starchy vegetables breaks down starch granules so they can be digested. On the other hand there are advantages to eating vegetables raw. Raw vegetables may contain higher levels of heat-sensitive nutrients because cooking decreases the content of water-soluble vitamins. For example, baked potatoes and sweet potatoes lose about 20% of the B vitamins and vitamin C. Boiling causes lower losses. Boiling leaches B vitamins and minerals out of vegetables. Losses may be as high as 80%. Steaming and microwave cooking of vegetables greatly reduces this loss. Boiling also removes vitamins and minerals. Note that keeping foods warm on a steam table increases the loss of vitamins such as vitamin C, thiamin and riboflavin.

On the other hand, vegetables that have not been stored properly, or have been handled carelessly, can suffer similar nutrient losses. Slicing, mashing, dicing, mincing and grating break vegetable cells and expose vitamins to oxygen and degradative enzymes. Vitamin C is especially sensitive to oxygen exposure. The longer the storage period for sliced vegetables, the greater the loss of vitamin C. (See also BALANCED DIET; DIETARY GUIDELINES FOR AMERICANS; FOOD PRESERVATION; FOOD PROCESSING; FOOD GUIDE PYRAMID; ORGANIC FOODS.)

Graziano, J. M. et al., "A Prospective Study of Consumption of Carotenoids in Fruits and Vegetables and Decreased Cardiovascular Mortality in the Elderly." *Ann. Epidemiol.*, 5(1995), pp. 255–260.

vegetable shortening A form of saturated fat, prepared from vegetable oil, that resembles animal fat. A major advantage of vegetable shortening is that, unlike lard, butter or beef fat, it does not contain CHOLESTEROL. Vegetable shortening does contain the same high calories as butter or lard, however. Vegetable shortening is a product of the chemical processing called hydrogenation. This process adds hydrogen atoms to unsaturated FATTY ACIDS, thereby converting naturally liquid fat (oils) to materials with varying degrees of stiffness. Usually several different fats are blended to achieve the desired consistency of a shortening. CORN OIL, COTTONSEED OIL, SOYBEAN oil, OLIVE OIL, PALM OIL, PEANUT oil, SAFFLOWER oil and SESAME oil may be combined. Shortening, like other hydrogenated vegetable oils, contains TRANS-FATTY ACIDS as a by-product of manufacture. The long-term safety of trans-fatty acids has been questioned. A diet high in saturated fat is linked to an increased risk of HEART DISEASE and CANCER. (See also HYDROGENATED VEGETABLE OIL; VEGETABLE OIL.)

vegetarian One who eats predominantly VEGETABLES, FRUITS, GRAINS and NUTS and either limits or excludes animal products, including MEAT, FISH, SEAFOOD and dairy products, from the diet. With a thoughtful selection of a variety of foods, vegetarians can easily meet all their nutrient needs. People choose vegetarianism for a variety of reasons. Vegetarianism may be related to religious or philosophical beliefs. Ecologically, vegetarianism represents a more efficient use of energy than relying on meat and meat products. From a health perspective, plant products do not contain the growth promoters and antibiotics used in poultry and meat production nor do they contain cholesterol. Plants are excellent sources of FIBER and ESSENTIAL FATTY ACIDS.

There are varying degrees of vegetarianism:

- Vegans rely on foods of plant origin and omit all meat, poultry, fish and eggs, as well as milk and meat products.
- Fruitarians rely on dry or raw fruits, together with nuts, honey, grains, LEGUMES and OLIVE OIL while excluding animal products.
- Semi-vegetarians, occasionally eat some meat, fish or poultry, eggs and milk or cheese while relying on cereals, grains, fruit and vegetables. Most "heart healthy" diets are semi-vegetarian diets. There are a variety of such diets.
- Ovo-vegetarians include eggs with foods of plant origin in the diet.
- Lactovegetarians include milk and milk products, together with foods of plant origin.
- Lacto-ovo-vegetarians include both milk products and eggs with grains, fruits and vegetables. Vegetarians who eat dairy products tend to have higher blood cholesterol levels than those who do not.
- Pescovegetarians include fish and seafood, together with foods derived from plants.

Vegetarians may have a reduced risk of obesity, type II (adult onset) diabetes, GALLSTONES and CORONARY ARTERY DISEASE. There is evidence that vegetarian diets reduce the risk of breast CANCER, DIVERTICULOSIS, colonic cancer, hemorrhoids, OSTEOPOROSIS and dental caries.

Nutrient Needs

Vegans who are pregnant or lactating, children of vegans, and people who are ill run the greatest risk for certain nutrient deficiencies because these individuals have high nutrient needs that may not be readily met by eating a limited variety of plant foods.

Minerals   The amounts of many TRACE MINERALS are low in plant products, and the body's ability to absorb them from plant sources is often low. Milk and milk products provide most of the calcium and meat provides the most iron and zinc in the usual diet. Vegans may have difficulties in obtaining minerals such as:

- CALCIUM. Major plant sources are: BROCCOLI, KALE, COLLARD greens, kelp. PARSLEY, prunes, SESAME seeds, fortified TOFU and fortified soymilk.
- ZINC. Sources are: whole grains, BREWER'S YEAST, LIMA BEANS, SOYBEANS, sunflower seeds, PEAS, LENTILS and wheat germ.
- IRON. This nutrient occurs in dried beans and peas, dried fruit, fortified cereals and bread. Iron uptake can be significantly increased by eating iron-rich vegetable foods with vitamin C-rich foods (citrus fruit, berries, dark-green, leafy vegetables.
- COPPER. Copper occurs in AVOCADOS, BARLEY, BEANS, broccoli, BEETS, PECANS, RAISINS and soybeans.
- MANGANESE. This nutrient occurs in avocados, NUTS, seeds, whole grains, legumes, dried peas and dark-green leafy vegetables.

Energy   The energy demands of infants and growing children are quite high relative to their body size. Fat is a calorie-dense food that is an important part of a child's diet. Often vegetarian foods offer high fiber but low energy (fat) content. When the diet provides inadequate calories, a muscle protein is degraded for energy, not a desirable situation in a young, growing body.

Protein   Dietary protein must supply adequate essential AMINO ACIDS (the amino acids that cannot be fabricated in amounts to meet the body's requirements). Plant proteins may be less easily digested depending on the meal preparation. Their amino acid compositions are usually not as well balanced as animal protein. Consequently, vegetarian diets based on a single grain like corn can contribute to MALNUTRITION. Plant proteins from different sources can complement each other, so that the net amino acid intake of a mixture of plant protein can adequately meet the daily requirement for essential amino acids. For example, combining whole grain foods with legumes is a traditional practice (rice and beans, corn and beans, wheat and lentils, for example).

Vitamin D   The best sources of this vitamin are fatty fish, egg yolk, liver, and milk, and milk products—all of which are eliminated from a strictly vegetarian diet. Exposure to sunlight may meet individual needs; however, supplementation may be necessary for people living in northern regions of the United States during the winter months, as well as for institutionalized people.

B vitamins   A number of cereal grain products are enriched with RIBOFLAVIN, THIAMIN and NIACIN. Legumes and whole grains can provide significant riboflavin. VITAMIN B_{12} deficiency is a major concern for strict vegetarians. There is probably no very good plant source, other than nutritional YEAST. The amounts provided in sea vegetables, fermented soy and algae may be inadequate. The best sources are animal products such as meat; thus a strict vegetarian may need a supplement, fortified soy milk or fortified meat analog. Once vitamin B_{12} deficiency has occurred, the resulting nerve degeneration may not be reversible.

Strict vegetarian diets are not recommended for infants or children. Pregnant women should plan their diet very carefully to maximize nutrient-dense foods and:

1. emphasize unrefined, whole foods;
2. use protein-rich sources like legumes, seeds and nuts;
3. eat a variety of fruits, vegetables, legumes and whole grains to assure adequate protein complementation;
4. eat fruit and vitamin C-rich foods with each meal to enhance iron uptake;
5. consider supplemental sources of vitamin B_{12}, vitamin D, calcium and trace minerals or properly fortified sources;
6. eat enough food to provide adequate protein and energy.

(See also CHOLESTEROL-LOWERING DRUGS; COMPLETE PROTEIN.)

Dwyer, J.T., "Nutritional Consequences of Vegetarianism," *Annual Review of Nutrition*, 11 (1991), pp. 61–91.
Lawrence, Valerie, "Is Vegetarianism a Diet or an Ideology?" *Canadian Medical Association Journal*, 148:6 (1993), pp. 998–1002.

very-low-density lipoprotein (VLDL)   A lipid-protein particle that transports FAT from the LIVER to other tissues via the bloodstream. After a carbohydrate meal, the liver absorbs glucose from the blood and converts it to fat (TRIGLYCERIDES). The liver packages fat to export it to other parts of the body via the bloodstream in the form of VLDL. In composition, VLDL resembles chylomicrons, the fat transport vesicles from the intestine. VLDL contains triglycerides, a low amount of CHOLESTEROL and two types of protein designated B-100 and C-II.

When VLDL reaches the capillaries, its triglycerides are broken down by an enzyme in the walls of the capillaries called lipoprotein lipase. Tissues then absorb the released fatty acids. After releasing their fat, VLDL remnants follow an unusual pathway: They become enriched in cholesterol as they are transformed in the blood to LOW-DENSITY LIPOPROTEIN (LDL)—the particle that carries cholesterol to tissues.

The blood levels of both chylomicrons and VLDL increase for several hours after eating. Therefore lab tests that measure triglycerides in serum, the clear cell-free fluid remaining after blood clots, are usually performed after an overnight fast when levels have stabilized. Middle-aged white males with high levels of serum triglycerides (essentially VLDL) and high LDL appear to be more likely to have heart attacks than men with normal levels, even in people with somewhat elevated serum cholesterol levels. The risk of heart attack may decrease by lowering serum triglycerides and raising HDL (HIGH-DENSITY LIPOPROTEIN), the "desirable cholesterol." (See also CARDIOVASCULAR DISEASE; FAT METABOLISM.)

villi Microscopic, fuzzy layer coating the inner side of the wall of the SMALL INTESTINE like a shag carpet. Cells that line the surface of villi possess numerous, tiny projections called MICROVILLI. If all of the intestinal folds, villi and microvilli were flattened out, the total surface area would represent approximately a tennis court. Thus villi dramaticlly increase the absorptive area of the intestinal surface and facilitate efficient nutrient uptake. CELIAC DISEASE, CROHN'S DISEASE and intestinal parasitic diseases (like GIARDIASIS) can lead to a loss of the villi and subsequent MALABSORPTION and maldigestion syndromes. With appropriate treatment and dietary modification, the villi can grow back and digestion can improve. (See also DIGESTION; DIGESTIVE TRACT.)

villikinin A hormone produced by the SMALL INTESTINE that stimulates the movement of VILLI, microscopic hair-like projections that coat the inner surface of the small intestine. This action serves to mix chewed food and digestive juice (CHYME) and to increase nutrient absorption by the intestine. (See also DIGESTION; ENDOCRINE SYSTEM.)

vinegar A dilute solution of ACETIC ACID. The term is derived from the French *vinaigre*, which means sour wine. Vinegar has been used in food preservation and medicine for thousands of years. Typically vinegar contains 4 to 12% acetic ACID, which is produced by the bacterial oxidation of alcohol formed by the fermentation of sugars and fruits. Apples yield cider vinegar; grapes, wine vinegar; and sugar and hydrolyzed starches from corn and wheat, white vinegar. Depending upon the nature of the fruit fermented, the resulting vinegar will have a unique flavor without adding signficant calories. Vinegar provides only 2 calories per teaspoon. Because it is so acidic, vinegar is used to preserve foods in pickling. In salad dressing, MAYONNAISE, MUSTARD and tomato sauce, vinegar helps retard spoilage. Vinegar contains traces of minerals but it is not a significant food source. (See also FOOD PROCESSING.)

vitamin An essential organic nutrient. Minute amounts of vitamins participate in three general functions of the body: growth, protection and energy regulation. There are a total of 13 vitamins. Four are fat-soluble: vitamins A, D, E and K. The rest are water-soluble. Eight vitamins are in the B complex: RIBOFLAVIN (B_1), THIAMIN (B_2), NIACIN (B_3), VITAMIN B_6, vitamin B_{12}, FOLIC ACID, PANTOTHENIC ACID and biotin. VITAMIN C is also water-soluble but is not considered a B vitamin, which function as enzyme helpers (coenzymes).

Vitamins either cannot be synthesized by the body or they cannot be made in adequate amounts, so they must be supplied by the diet. As examples of the latter, vitamin D can be made in the skin when exposed to sunlight, while some niacin can be made from the amino acid tryptophan. The intestine is a source of BIOTIN, pantothenic acid and VITAMIN K; these are supplied by "friendly" intestinal bacteria, though the exact amounts supplied are difficult to assess.

The term "vitamin" dates from 1912, and the first vitamin to be isolated was vitamin A in 1913. Thiamin was discovered in 1926, vitamin K in 1929, and vitamin C in 1932. Vitamin B_{12} was the most recent vitamin to be discovered (1948). Before a compound can be classified as a vitamin, it must be proven that animals must obtain the compound from their diet. Typically, scientists test lab animals such as mice with a diet free of the test substance, together with a dose of antibiotics to eliminate intestinal bacteria.

Vitamins originate chiefly from plant sources. Except for vitamin D and vitamin C, vitamins are present in animal tissue only if the animal consumes foods containing them or harbors microorganisms capable of synthesizing them. B vitamins are universally distributed; fat-soluble vitamins may be absent from some types of organisms. Each of the vitamins plays a specific role in the body; a deficiency of one vitamin cannot be eliminated by consuming an excess of another.

Fat-Soluble Vitamins

VITAMIN A, VITAMIN D, VITAMIN E and vitamin K are oily materials and dissolve in fats and oils, not in water. Unlike the B complex, these vitamins generally do not serve as enzyme helpers, nor are they involved in energy production; each has an entirely different function, ranging from acting as an ANTIOXIDANT (E), to producing a visual pigment for night vision (A), to blood clotting (K) and to bone formation (D).

Fat-soluble vitamins are absorbed best when they are eaten with fats and oils. These vitamins are stored in the body, so they do not need to be consumed daily. Because they are stored, excessive consumption can lead to high tissue levels resulting in toxic side effects, especially for vitamins A and D. For example, 50,000 international units of vitamin A over several months can cause toxic symptoms in adults. Symptoms of toxicity, such as achy joints, fatigue, headaches and nausea, disappear when the high intake stops. What represents an excessive intake depends on many factors, including the type of vitamin, individual tolerance, which varies with age, and the length of time for which the supplement is taken.

Water-Soluble Vitamins

B complex vitamins help convert food into energy; they include THIAMIN (B_1), RIBOFLAVIN (B_2), NIACIN (B_3), VITAMIN B_6, pantothenic acid and biotin. FOLIC ACID AND vitamin B_{12} are involved in building new cells, while vitamin C serves as an antioxidant and helps build healthy capillaries, gums and joints. Except for vitamin B_{12}, water-soluble vitamins are not stored well in the body and must be replenished daily. Excesses are generally excreted in the urine.

Vitamin Deficiencies

Long-term vitamin deficiencies often lead to serious illness. Deficiencies can be due to an inadequate diet (MALNUTRITION); inability to digest food (maldigestion); inability to absorb vitamins due to damage to the intestine or to competition with another material such as a drug (MALABSORPTION); increased physiological need as during pregnancy; growth, injury, choice of life-style or other environmental factors.

Physicians may use lab tests to diagnose vitamin deficiencies. Most tests involve blood analyses, even though these are not always reliable. For example, a common antibody test for serum vitamin B_{12} detects both vitamin B_{12} together with inactive derivatives. Measurement of enzyme levels or levels of metabolic products can provide useful information. Dietary analysis can reveal levels of nutrients in the diet and guide a nutritional evaluation and assessment of individual needs complementing the physical examination and health history.

Natural vs. Synthetic Vitamins

Natural vitamins are those occurring in food. All substances classified as vitamins have been isolated from animal or plant sources, and most have been chemically synthesized in the lab to establish their structures. In other words, synthetic vitamins are usually identical to the product in cells. As an example, vitamin C in cells is defined chemically as L-ascorbic acid, identical to synthetic L-ascorbic acid. Most vitamins found in supplements are chemically synthesized, because there simply is not enough of most vitamins extracted from plant materials to meet world demand. Most vitamin C comes from a few major commercial sources worldwide.

A few synthetic vitamins differ from the natural forms. Synthetic vitamin E, called d, l-alpha-tocopherol, is a mixture of both left- and right-handed molecules, while the natural alpha tocopherol is a single form called d-tocopherol. The synthetic product is adjusted to provide the same biological activity as the natural form. Certain vitamins like vitamin B_{12} possess structures that are too complex for a convenient lab synthesis. Microbial sources have been selected to produce large amounts.

Vitamin Supplements

Nutritionists often recommend obtaining vitamins from foods for several reasons.

Foods supply mixtures of vitamins, minerals and other materials that may have beneficial effects. Mixtures are what the body uses. Foods supply materials that are not vitamins, yet are important. In this class are FLAVONOIDS, which work together with vitamin C to build strong capillaries and serve as antioxidants and as anti-inflammatory agents. Substances with anti-cancer properties have recently been isolated from vegetables of the cabbage family; they include isothiocyanates and indoles, in addition to the flavonoids.

Fifty to sixty percent of the U.S. adult population take supplements and spend about $3 billion yearly on vitamins, minerals and other supplements. An estimated 60% of surgeons and a similar number of dietitians take supplements. One explanation for this widespread practice is that many people have subclinical deficiencies. They are not sick, but they are not well, either. They may want to feel more energetic and to have more stable moods. Others want to take supplements as insurance in preventing certain diseases if they live in a polluted environment or if their genetic make up, medical history and life-style choices warrant it. A growing number of consumers want to promote optimal health. Although there is a natural tendency to search for an easy solution to health problems, there are limits regarding what vitamins can do for health. No single supplement can compensate for overindulgence, physical inactivity or genetic predisposition.

Deciding who needs vitamin supplements and how much should be taken is a controversial area. Conventional wisdom says that by following DIETARY GUIDELINES FOR AMERICANS and using a recommended plan such as the FOOD PYRAMID, an individual should be assured of an adequate supply of nutrients. Thus if an individual is healthy and is eating a BALANCED DIET, vitamin supplements would not be needed. There is general agreement that individuals with well recognized needs may require supplements. These people include:

- women with heavy menstrual bleeding (extra IRON)
- women taking oral contraceptives (may need extra vitamin B_6)
- pregnant women (extra iron, folic acid and CALCIUM)
- malnourished individuals, including dieters, elderly people with a low caloric intake, chronic alcoholics and those with other chemical dependencies
- strict vegetarians (many need extra iron, zinc, calcium and vitamin B_{12})
- newborn infants (may be deficient in vitamin E and vitamin K)
- individuals with chronic disorders, such as patients with OSTEOPOROSIS (may need extra vitamin D, calcium, magnesium and trace minerals)
- hospitalized patients. Patients in hospitals and institutionalized people may become deficient in one or more vitamin.
- people who smoke (extra vitamin C)

Another viewpoint is that many people who live in modern, industrial societies and are exposed to environmental stressors and rely on refined foods, often can benefit from supplements for optimal health and maximal longevity. However, the optimal amounts for any vitamin are merely estimates. Other individuals may benefit from supplements when their nutrient consumption is below normal though they lack symptoms of serious deficiency diseases. It has been proposed that nutrient needs increase with:

- exposure to pollution
- physical and mental stress
- frequent skipping of meals

- increased reliance on highly processed foods
- inadequate exercise and rest
- use of recreational drugs and alcohol
- widespread chemical and food sensitivities
- increased prevalence of conditions characterized by suppressed immunity, including AIDS
- dieting

There are numerous advantages in obtaining nutrients from food: It is practically impossible to get an overdose. Food supplies mixtures of nutrients and mixtures are what the body needs; food supplies other substances that may have beneficial effects and are not found in a pill or capsule. But supplements can be used as part of a wellness program to prevent illness and promote well-being. Such a program should include physical exercise, eating wholesome meals, maintaining psychological fitness and emotional stability.

The following recommendations can help define a personal strategy for using nutritional supplements.

1. Do not self-medicate. Before beginning a dietary supplement program, get feedback from a knowledgeable professional to determine whether your plan will interfere with treatment for a condition or illness. The RDAs (RECOMMENDED DIETARY ALLOWANCES) were designed to avoid deficiency-induced diseases, not to treat chronic conditions or subclinical deficiencies. The RDAs assume a healthful diet and healthy populations.

2. If you are pregnant, do not take any supplement or medication without a physician's supervision.

3. Focus on individual needs as determined with a nutrition counselor; depending upon the circumstances, additional vitamin C, calcium and magnesium may be prudent. "More" does not necessarily equal "better." It is generally advised not to exceed five times the RDA for vitamins and minerals without medical supervision. Certain vitamins, particularly A and D, are stored in the body and levels can build up over time with high daily doses. Too much of vitamin B_6 can injure nerves, for example. The incidence of vitamin toxicity nationwide is very low, however.

4. Certain supplements interfere with diagnostic blood tests. When a doctor orders a test to measure a red blood cell count (hematocrit), inform him or her whether you are taking folic acid either by itself or as part of a multivitamin supplement. For diabetics monitoring their urinary glucose, vitamin C can alter results. (There is a urine testing kit that is not affected by vitamin C.) Vitamin C can also prevent the detection of blood in the test for colorectal cancer (occult blood).

5. Those who are sensitive to wheat, soy, yeast, corn, milk products, artificial coloring or starch, may react to these products in supplements.

6. Select supplements that contain multiple nutrients, with a full range of vitamins and minerals. Many nutrients work best when they are balanced, that is, the proportions should be close to those given in the RDA tables without any one being extremely high.

7. Supplements should dissolve to be effective. Place a tablet in a cup of warm water with a tablespoon of vinegar. Stir occasionally without touching the tablet. It should disintegrate within 30 to 45 minutes to be effective. Emulsified vitamins A, D, E and K are homogenized into tiny droplets and become water-soluble to help speed their uptake.

8. Keep vitamins and mineral supplements out of children's reach. Store them in a cool, dry place out of direct sunlight.

9. Take personal responsibility for your health. Monitor how you feel when you take any supplement or medication.

(See also ORTHOMOLECULAR MEDICINE; SUBCLINICAL NUTRIENT DEFICIENCY.)

Frei, Balz, "Reactive, Oxygen Species and Antioxidant Vitamins: Mechanisms of Action," *American Journal of Medicine*, 97: supp. 3A (1994), pp. 3A–5S.

Sauberlich, Howerde E., Machlin, Lawrence J., eds. "Beyond Deficiency, New Views on the Function and Health Effects of Vitamins," *Annals of the New York Academy of Sciences*, 669 (1992).

Skerrett, P.J., "Mighty Vitamins: The One-a-day Wonders Bidding to Outstrip Their Role as Supplements," *Medical World News*, January 1993, 34:1 pp. 24–32.

vitamin A (retinol) A fat-soluble vitamin and one of the first vitamins to be discovered. Vitamin A is required for a healthy immune system, vision, growth and reproduction. Vitamin A supports normal tissue development, which accounts for its influence on taste and hearing. The liver stores 90% or more of this vitamin. Many plants produce a parent compound of vitamin A called BETA CAROTENE, also called "provitamin A." This orange-yellow pigment is stored in fat tissue and other tissues, but comparatively little is stored in the liver, unlike vitamin A. Beta carotene is cleaved to form retinol and an inactive molecule called retinoic acid, which lacks vitamin A activity.

Vitamin A and vision Perhaps the best known role for vitamin A is its effect on vision. Vitamin A forms a pigment in the eye called visual purple, required for night vision, and outright deficiency causes NIGHT BLINDNESS. Large amounts of vitamin A taken daily can delay blindness caused by retinitis pigmentosa, an inherited disease that leads to degeneration of the retina. It is worth noting that vitamin A has no effect on defective vision from other causes, and most vision problems do not involve vitamin A.

Wound healing Both vitamin A and beta carotene speed wound healing in lab animals. The effect is quite pronounced when the animals are vitamin-A deficient.

Resistance to infection Population studies in developing nations have demonstrated that vitamin A reduces death by increasing resistance to infections, such as measles. This is not surprising because vitamin A supports a healthy IMMUNE SYSTEM, including increased production of antibodies and various lymphocytes (disease-fighting cells). Beta carotene, which is non-toxic, increases T-helper cells even in normal people. Lowered immunity due to surgery has been blocked in patients given large amounts of vitamin A, and it increases the resistance of the digestive system and the respiratory tract to infection. Vitamin A can minimize decreased immunity due to radiation and chemotherapy.

Cancer Vitamin A and beta carotene possess anticancer properties. Vitamin A can block cancer cells in cultures, and even block malignancy in animals exposed to cancer-causing agents (CARCINOGENS). A diet rich in beta carotene and other carotenoids may lower the risk of lung, bladder, larynx, esophagus, stomach, prostate and colon cancer.

Vitamin A, a product of vitamin A called retinoic acid, and beta carotene may be able to prevent or eliminate pre-cancerous sores (leukoplakia) in the mouths of smokers. Retinoic acid may also prevent recurring tumors of the head and neck. Another derivative of vitamin A, tretinoin (retin A), may be able to combat precancerous cervical conditions.

Skin conditions Vitamin A can clear up ACNE but extremely large doses are required to do so, increasing the risk of toxicity. Derivatives are more effective; for example, tretinoin clears up the most common form of acne, acne vulgaris, and another derivative (etretinate) may be useful for psoriasis. Tretinoin helps with sun-damaged skin, though long-term effects on aging skin are not clear.

Other conditions Vitamin A supports the maintenance and healing of lung tissue and the intestine, and it has been used to treat peptic ulcers and inflammatory bowel disease. Vitamin A deficiency associated with AIDS is linked to decreased T-helper lymphocytes and a higher rate of mortality due to HIV. Because retinoic acid may increase HIV replication, beta carotene could be the preferred form for supplementation.

Sources

Vitamin A is either supplied as such in food, or it is formed from beta carotene in the body. Fish liver oil and liver are rich in vitamin A. Milk is fortified with vitamin A. Vitamin A palmitate is often the form of the vitamin found in supplements. Its advantage is that it is easily suspended in water, therefore it is easily absorbed by the body. Beta carotene occurs in yams, winter SQUASH, carrots and CANTALOUPE, as well as in dark-green leafy vegetables like KALE and SPINACH.

Requirements

The amount of vitamin A in a food can be given in terms of retinol equivalents (RE). One RE is defined as 1 mcg of retinol or 6 mcg of beta carotene. The uptake of beta carotene is less than retinol and its conversion to retinol is incomplete. Vitamin A activity may also be expressed in international units (IU). One IU of vitamin A activity equals 0.3 mcg of retinol or 0.6 mcg of beta carotene. Put another way, 1 retinol equivalent equals 3.33 IU of retinol (preformed vitamin A from animal sources) or 10 IU of beta carotene (plant sources).

The RECOMMENDED DIETARY ALLOWANCE (RDA) for vitamin A for men (25 to 50 years) is 1,000 mcg of retinol or retinol equivalents and 800 mcg (RE) for non-pregnant women. In pregnancy the requirement increases to 1,300 mcg. Vitamin A deficiency is common in non-industrialized societies, but a significant number of Americans might also be deficient in vitamin A, particularly young children and others consuming highly processed foods. Factors that increase the need for vitamin A include a high-fiber diet, chronic fat MALABSORPTION, stress and high alcohol consumption. Symptoms of deficiency include coarse dry skin, slow growth, night blindness, frequent infections and anemia.

Safety

Women who are pregnant should not take vitamin A supplements. Amounts greater than 10,000 IU (3,000 RE) increase the risk of birth defects. On the other hand, there is no evidence that beta carotene produces birth defects. Vitamin A is stored by the body and it is possible to accumulate too much, leading to toxicity (HYPERVITAMINOSIS). The response to high doses of vitamin A is quite variable. A high intake of 50,000 IU daily (15,000 RE) may be tolerated by some; others may have a reaction with 20,000 IU (6,000 RE). Symptoms of vitamin A overdose include headache, fatigue, dry skin, weakness, nausea, hair loss, blurred vision, bone aches and loss of appetite. Jaundice and liver damage are possible. These symptoms usually disappear rapidly when vitamin A supplementation is stopped. In contrast, beta carotene is relatively safe because it is converted to vitamin A only as needed.

Tretinoin, accutane and etretinate should not be taken by pregnant women or by women who do not use birth control because of the high risk of BIRTH DEFECTS. Vitamin A may cause bone disease in individuals with chronic kidney problems.

Bates, C.J., "Vitamin A," *Lancet*, 345 (January 7, 1995), pp. 31–35.

vitamin B₁   See THIAMIN.

vitamin B₂   See RIBOFLAVIN.

vitamin B₃   See NIACIN.

vitamin B₆   An essential water-soluble nutrient and a member of the B COMPLEX. The term "vitamin B₆" pertains to two forms, pyridoxine and pyridoxamine, which can be converted back and forth. Vitamin B₆ is required by the body to produce non-essential AMINO ACIDS, to break down most amino acids, and to support healthy immune systems, normal immunity and nerve function. However, before it can help enzymes, vitamin B₆ like other B complex vitamins must be activated. The enzyme helper (COENZYME) in this case is pyridoxal phosphate, employed by a family of enzymes called transaminases required in the first stage of amino acid utilization by the body.

Chemicals known as hydrazides and hydrazines interfere with the functions of vitamin B₆. These chemicals are widely used in industry and contaminate the food supply. Derivatives of hydrazines appear in cigarette smoke and food additives, thus the environmental burden could deplete this nutrient.

Possible Roles in Maintaining Health

Red blood cells Vitamin B₆ is essential for the production of RED BLOOD CELLS. Vitamin B₆ plays a role in protein synthesis as well as in the synthesis of DNA and RNA, and it is required to make HEME, the red pigment of the oxygen transport protein of blood (HEMOGLOBIN). A deficiency can cause anemia.

Nervous system The formation of certain brain chemicals (NEUROTRANSMITTERS) from amino acids requires this vitamin, hence it affects the NERVOUS SYSTEM. Certain inherited metabolic disorders lead to convulsions in infants, and B$_6$ supplementation usually abolishes their seizures.

Immune system   Vitamin B$_6$ is one of the most important B vitamins in maintaining a robust IMMUNE SYSTEM. Vitamin B$_6$ supplements can boost immunity in older people who may not consume enough of this important vitamin. Vitamin B$_6$ deficiency decreases immune function in humans and lab animals, and low vitamin B$_6$ levels are common in people with weakened immunity, including people with CANCER and AIDS. Vitamin B$_6$ also protects against certain types of cancer in lab animals.

Premenstrual syndrome (PMS)   Vitamin B$_6$ has long been claimed to relieve an array of symptoms occurring in the week to 10 days prior to menstruation. PMS affects the synthesis of several hormones believed to be involved in the cycle. Vitamin B$_6$ has been used to correct for some of the imbalances caused by estrogen-type birth control pills.

Carpal tunnel syndrome   Vitamin B$_6$ supplementation is often an effective treatment of carpal tunnel syndrome, in which there is compression of a nerve in the wrist. Large doses are used for several months.

High blood sugar   Vitamin B$_6$ has been used to help treat diabetic patients whose condition can be attributed in part to a deficiency of this vitamin. B$_6$ supplementation has increased GLUCOSE TOLERANCE, the body's ability to remove glucose from the blood, and decreased insulin requirements in certain patients with gestational diabetes. INSULIN is the pancreatic hormone that stimulates tissue uptake of glucose.

Cardiovascular disease   Vitamin B$_6$ may decrease the stickiness of platelets, cell fragments in the blood needed for clot formation, and thus the tendency to form blood clots. A deficiency of this vitamin has been linked to ATHEROSCLEROSIS in some instances, due to an accumulation of excessive amounts of an amino acid breakdown product.

Senility   Vitamin B$_6$ deficiency is linked to long-term memory loss in some elderly patients.

Other Conditions   Some forms of arthritis and joint pain respond to extra vitamin B$_6$. In combination with magnesium this vitamin can lower the risk of calcium oxalate kidney stones, the most common kind. Vitamin B$_6$ deficiency is common among patients with asthma.

Sources

Vitamin B$_6$ occurs in FISH; MEAT, including liver and kidneys; BLACKSTRAP MOLASSES; NUTS and whole GRAINS; BREWER'S YEAST; and many VEGETABLES.

Requirements

The Recommended Dietary Allowances (RDA) for adults (25 to 50 years) is 2.0 mg for men and 1.6 mg for women. Many people do not obtain adequate amounts of this vitamin and it is one of the most common deficiencies. Those most at risk are older persons; it has been found that 61- to 71-year-olds need more vitamin B$_6$ than the RDA. Others who may not consume enough vitamin B$_6$ include adolescent women and pregnant and lactating women, alcoholics, and those with other chemical dependencies.

Factors that may increase the need for vitamin B$_6$ include alcohol, several medications (L-dopa, penicillamine, hydralazine, isoniazid), smoking, a high protein diet, deficiencies of magnesium, ZINC and RIBOFLAVIN. A mild deficiency is sometimes associated with lowered immunity and nervous disorders. Severe deficiency causes depression, confusion, convulsions, inflamed mouth, and tongue, and skin disorders. The optimal amount for maximal health and longevity is not known.

Safety

There is general agreement that amounts up to 50 mg per day are relatively safe. Higher levels should be taken only with professional advice. Excessive consumption of vitamin B$_6$ can damage the nervous system and lead to numbness of hands and feet (peripheral neuropathy). Insomnia and anxiety are possible symptoms of excessive intake. Vitamin B$_6$ reduces the effectiveness of levodopa, a drug used to treat PARKINSON'S DISEASE. (See also AMINO ACID METABOLISM; DIABETES MELLITUS; TRANSAMINATION.)

Dakshinamurti, Krishnamurti, ed., "Vitamin B6," *Annals of the New York Academy of Sciences*, 585 (1990).

vitamin B$_{12}$ (cyanocobalamin)   An essential water-soluble nutrient belonging to the B COMPLEX that is required in extremely minute amounts for cell division and growth. Vitamin B$_{12}$ is unique in several respects: It is the only B vitamin stored in the body and the only known nutrient to contain the trace mineral COBALT. Like all B vitamins, vitamin B$_{12}$ must be chemically modified to form a coenzyme (enzyme helper) before it can participate in metabolism. Vitamin B$_{12}$ has important, though very limited, roles in metabolism. It assists in the utilization of single carbon (methyl) groups transfer from the amino acid, methionine, to donors, including thymin, a building block for DNA. Vitamin B$_{12}$ also helps to oxidize certain fatty acids and it supports the maintenance of healthy nerves. With deficiencies possible irreversible brain damage and nervous disorders can occur.

The body has evolved an efficient mechanism to absorb this vitamin. To begin the process, the stomach normally secretes INTRINSIC FACTOR, a protein that binds vitamin B$_{12}$ and carries it to the INTESTINE where it aids B$_{12}$ absorption. An estimated 20% of people in their 60s and 40% of people in their 80s develop atrophic gastritis, in which the stomach does not produce enough acid and intrinsic factor. With inadequate stomach acid to sterilize the stomach, certain bacteria can grow, consuming the vitamin that otherwise would be absorbed by the intestine. Vitamin B$_{12}$, together with another B vitamin, FOLIC ACID, functions in DNA synthesis and cell division, and supports red blood cell production. A large dose of folic acid to treat anemia can mask a vitamin B$_{12}$ deficiency; folic acid often is administered with B$_{12}$.

Possible Roles in Maintaining Health

Anemia   A deficiency of intrinsic factor causes PERNICIOUS ANEMIA, a disease caused by inadequate B$_{12}$ absorption despite adequate dietary supplies.

Nervous disorders   Mental deterioration, SENILITY and neuropsychiatric disorders—including dementia, DEPRESSION and loss of balance—may respond to extra vitamin B_{12}. An estimated 10% of elderly persons have marked vitamin B_{12} deficiencies, and many patients with senile dementia are B_{12}-deficient. Vitamin B_{12} may help in the treatment of chronic fatigue and age-related decline in energy level and well-being.

Cigarette smoking   Smokers have low vitamin B_{12} and folic acid levels. Preliminary clinical studies suggest that supplementation with both vitamins reduces the amount of precancerous bronchial tissue.

Chronic pain   Vitamin B_{12} has been used to treat bronchial spasm (ASTHMA), bursitis and bone spur pain. Neurolgia pain radiating along nerves may respond to intramuscular infections of vitamin B_{12}.

Wound healing   Anecdotal evidence from both patients and physicians suggests that certain individuals are helped by supplemental vitamin B_{12} to recover more rapidly from illness and surgical procedures.

Sources

Vitamin B_{12} occurs mainly in animal products—MEAT, POULTRY, FISH, EGGS and SHELLFISH. Some fortified foods like nutritional yeast contain vitamin B_{12}. Tamari, tempeh and miso were found to be essentially lacking in this vitamin, although sometimes these foods are claimed to be rich sources of the vitamin. SPIRULINA contains much less usable vitamins than formerly believed; the amount in seaweed is variable. Part of the problem seems to be that seaweed contains B_{12} analogs that do not form coenzymes in the body. Therefore strict vegetarians (those who eat no animal products) may need to support their diet with vitamin B_{12} supplements.

Requirements

The RECOMMENDED DIETARY ALLOWANCE (RDA) for vitamin B_{12} for normal adults is 2 mcg daily. Severe vitamin B_{12} deficiency is rare. Newer, more sensitive laboratory blood tests and metabolic indicators have turned up low-level B_{12} deficiencies with surprising frequency. Those who are most likely to be deficient include strict vegetarians; elderly persons; alcoholics; patients with CROHN'S DISEASE, severe food allergies or chemical sensitivities; and people who have undergone stomach surgery or who have a family history of anemia. About 5% of adults over the age of 50 have low vitamin B_{12} levels. Half of these may have difficulty in absorbing the vitamin from food. Low folic acid intake and some antibiotics interfere with vitamin B_{12} uptake. People suffering from anxiety or depression who take antidepressants (tricyclics and chloromazine) may block vitamin B_{12} uptake.

Signs of vitamin B_{12} deficiency include weakness in the arms and legs, difficulty in walking, and even paralysis. Irreversible nerve damage is possible. Prolonged vitamin B_{12} deficiency causes neurological symptoms and anemia. Injections of this vitamin clear up pernicious anemia. Vitamin B_{12} is not toxic when taken orally. Nasal or sublingual (under the tongue) vitamin B_{12} gels or vitamin injections are effective for vegetarians and for those with malabsorption problems. There is no known toxicity associated with

this vitamin when taken orally. Often, elevated vitamin B_{12} in the blood is most readily obtained through B_{12} injections. Occasionally some people are allergic to injections. (See also ACHLORHYDRIA; AGING; DIGESTION; MALABSORPTION.)

Lindenbaum, J., et al., "Neuropsychiatric Disorders Caused by Cobalamin Deficiency in the Absence of Anemia or Macrocytosis," *New England Journal of Medicine*, 318:26 (1988), pp. 1720–28.
Naurath, Hans J., et al., "Effects of Vitamin B_{12}, Folate and Vitamin B_6 Supplements in Elderly People with Normal Serum Vitamin Concentrations," *Lancet*, 346 (July 8, 1995), pp. 85–89.

vitamin C (ascorbic acid, sodium ascorbate, calcium ascorbate)   A water-soluble vitamin that promotes wound healing and healthy blood vessels, joints, gums and connective tissue. Vitamin C helps in the synthesis of COLLAGEN, a structural protein that provides strength to bones and tissues. Most animals make ample vitamin C; exceptions include guinea pigs, humans and other primates, and certain bats.

Vitamin C occurs in high levels in endocrine (hormone-secreting) glands. It is needed by the ADRENAL GLANDS to make hormones: EPINEPHRINE (adrenaline), a stress hormone, plus the steroids regulating BLOOD SUGAR and the hormones regulating blood minerals, and assists in the activation of other hormones. Vitamin C also occurs in high levels in the brain, and it plays a role in nerve transmission through the production of SEROTONIN and norepinephrine, brain chemicals called NEUROTRANSMITTERS. Neurotransmitters are chemicals synthesized by nerve cells to conduct impulses between cells. Vitamin C is involved in the metabolism of folic acid.

Vitamin C serves as a powerful antioxidant and helps to prevent oxidative damage in the body. It can block many types of highly reactive chemical species called FREE RADICALS, including superoxide and hydroxyl radicals in blood and body fluids, as well as regenerating VITAMIN E, the free radical scavenger of cell membranes and lipids. As a versatile antioxidant, vitamin C offers protection against airborne pollutants and supports drug detoxication by the liver. Dietary vitamin C can increase the absorption of heme iron (the form in meat) two- to fourfold. Vitamin C suppresses the formation of NITROSOAMINES and quinones, known to cause cancer (carcinogens). On the other hand, it is possible that vitamin C can participate in the BHA-induced tissue growth in the stomach of rats, thus enhancing carcinogenesis. However, a higher consumption of vitamin C contributes to higher plasma levels of other antioxidants, including vitamin E.

Possible Role of Vitamin C in Disease

The functions of vitamin C in the body and the amounts required for optimal health remain one of the most controversial areas in nutrition. The following topics have been the focus of recent research.

Scurvy   This full-blown vitamin C deficiency disease is characterized by swollen joints, poor wound healing, muscle wasting, bleeding gums and susceptibility to infection. In scurvy, defective COLLAGEN is formed, leading to diseased connective tissue. Vitamin C is required to synthesize collagen building blocks, hydroxylysine and hydroxyproline, for normal collagen formation. Scurvy has largely been eradicated from industrialized nations, though it continues to affect certain populations: the elderly, alcoholics and chronically ill people. When large amounts of vitamin C are consumed, the body adapts by accelerating excretion and metabolism. When consumption suddenly drops, a person may experience a short-term vitamin C deficiency until the body readapts ("rebound scurvy"). Infants born to mothers who have taken large amounts of vitamin C may experience rebound scurvy after birth unless they are supplemented.

Infection and colds   Whether vitamin C can cure the common cold has remained a controversial issue since Dr. Linus Pauling first suggested it in 1970. The research that has been conducted since that time has yielded mixed results, possibly reflecting flaws in experiment design. There is general agreement that vitamin C can decrease the duration and severity of colds. The vitamin can affect the outcome by blocking viruses, as well as by helping the IMMUNE SYSTEM. White cells that devour bacteria and abnormal cells require vitamin C for normal functioning; vitamin C levels decline in these cells during infection and exposure to drugs, medications, alcohol and cigarette smoking.

Cancer   A variety of population studies suggest that a low vitamin C intake correlates with a higher rate of CANCER and that vitamin C has a protective effect for cancer of the oral cavity, larynx, esophagus and stomach. Data supporting a beneficial relationship between vitamin C and bladder, cervix, endometrium and breast cancer are not as convincing, though suggestive. Vitamin C supplementation reduces the rate of precancerous changes in the stomach. It protects against cervical dysplasia, a predisposing condition to cervical cancer, and it inhibits human leukemia cells in culture. Vitamin C can block the formation of cancer-causing agents like NITROSOAMINES, and it is a powerful blocker of free radicals, which can be carcinogenic. Whether vitamin C does more than prevent certain cancers, and whether it can extend the lives of terminally ill cancer patients, remains controversial. More research is needed to resolve these issues.

Cardiovascular disease   A popular hypothesis for the origin of atherosclerosis (cholesterol clogged arteries) states that the oxidation of LDL promotes the disease process. Vitamin C may help prevent oxidative damage to LDL (LOW-DENSITY LIPOPROTEINS), lipid-transport particles implicated in clogging arteries. Vitamin C can increase HDL, the beneficial form of cholesterol, and it may lower total cholesterol values. However, epidemiologic studies did not detect a correlation between vitamin C intake and the risk of cardiovascular disease, and there as yet have not been randomized clinical studies of vitamin C in reducing cardiovascular risk. Population studies have found an increased risk of elevated blood pressure with low vitamin C intake or low vitamin C plasma levels; however, studies of treatment of hypertension with vitamin C have not been conclusive. Mortality from all causes of death was strongly inversely related to vitamin C intake, but other studies of vitamin C in preventing cardiovascular disease have yielded negative results. Additional research is justified.

Aging   Free radical damage is implicated in aging, which can be viewed as the result of accumulated damaged protein and DNA and of damaged repair mechanisms.

Population studies suggest that the consumption of ample fruits and vegetables, including those that are rich sources of vitamin C, decrease the risks of degenerative diseases associated with aging. Of the multitude of beneficial substances in these foods with antioxidant activity, vitamin C appears likely to play a central role.

Allergies   Vitamin C can help reduce asthma in certain asthmatics, and it may reduce the severity of allergy symptoms by alleviating stuffy sinuses, achy joints and puffy eyes. Vitamin C helps detoxify HISTAMINE, which promotes these inflammation symptoms.

Cataracts   Free radicals probably promote cataracts and macular degeneration with aging. Thus animals fed vitamin E–deficient diets develop macular degeneration and people with low-levels of antioxidants in their blood have a higher risk of cataracts. Adequate vitamin C, carotenoids and vitamin E consumption are related to a decreased risk of cataracts associated with aging. Several studies have suggested that antioxidant supplements, including vitamin C, decrease the risk of cataract formation. Vitamin C supplementation may halt or retard cataract development.

Other conditions   A variety of studies suggest that supplements of vitamin C can: decrease the risk of PERIODONTAL DISEASE, help diabetics maintain healthy gums; help overcome infertility in male smokers; and ease muscle soreness in athletes.

Sources

Fresh vegetables and fresh food are the best sources of vitamin C, including CITRUS FRUIT, CANTALOUPE, green PEPPERS, BROCCOLI, PAPAYA, berries and green leafy vegetables. Grains lack vitamin C. Vitamin C is the most unstable vitamin: In food it is destroyed by heat and by exposure to air, and cooking and processing of foods leads to extensive destruction. Microwave cooking minimizes losses. Destruction in fruit and vegetables is faster at room temperature than in the refrigerator, and is fastest if the vegetable is chopped or peeled. Ascorbic acid powder is stable indefinitely if kept dry.

Requirements

Currently, the RECOMMENDED DIETARY ALLOWANCE (RDA) for vitamin C is 60 mg for non-smokers and 100 mg for smokers. Many nutritional scientists believe this is too little for optimal health, though fewer advocate consuming as much as 2 to 10 g daily. Nonetheless there is substantial agreement that from 200 to 1,000 mg daily can provide insurance for a diet compromised by processed food. The level actually needed to saturate tissues has recently been studied. Data published in 1996 indicate that RDA for adults should be 200 mg. Steady state plasma and tissue concentrations of vitamin C were measured at varying doses in healthy volunteers, after first being depleted with a vitamin C–deficient diet. Bioavailability was maximal at 200 mg of vitamin C per day, higher levels of vitamin C did not appreciably change tissue saturation. Vitamin C needs are highly individualistic and exposure to pollutants, drugs, medications, smoking, infections, recovery from injury or surgery, high stress levels and heavy drinking often increases the need for vitamin C above the usual intake. The elderly or people who rely on medications like aspirin, barbiturates, L-dopa, phenacetin and cortisone need more vitamin C.

Safety

Vitamin C may have a dark side. Vitamin C increases iron uptake and hypothetically this could lead to iron accumulation in those with an inherited tendency to store iron. Iron and vitamin C spontaneously form free radicals (prooxidant effect). Excessive vitamin C supplementation together with excessive iron storage may be detrimental. However, under usual physiologic conditions, the amount of free iron would likely be very small; it would be stored in the iron binding protein FERRITIN. With injury or inflammation some iron could be released and could react with hydrogen peroxide to produce damaging free radicals. In susceptible people large amounts of vitamin C could promote the appearance of oxalate in the urine, thus increasing the risk of kidney stones. Supplementing with magnesium and extra vitamin B_6 can diminish this risk.

Side effects of excessive vitamin C supplements include diarrhea and cramps, and over time this could promote MALABSORPTION. If diarrhea and upset stomach occur, cut back on the dose. Chewable vitamin C can erode tooth enamel, and taking aspirin with vitamin C can aggravate gastric bleeding caused by aspirin. Extremely high intakes of vitamin C may increase the need for COPPER, and may increase the risk of GOUT in individuals who are genetically susceptible to those conditions. If you are prone to gout or kidney stones, or if you are pregnant, do not supplement with vitamin C without first consulting your physician.

Vitamin C interferes with the effectiveness of amphetamines, blood thinning drugs, and tricyclic antidepressants like ritalin, and it can alter lab tests like urinary glucose and occult blood for bowel cancer. Inform your physician if you are taking vitamin C or any other supplements before having diagnostic laboratory tests. Taper off gradually when you stop supplementation of 500 mg or more to avoid possible short-term scurvy-like symptoms and temporary lowered resistance to infections. (See also DETOXICATION; MEGADOSE.)

Bendich, Adrianne and Langseth, L., "The Health Effects of Vitamin C Supplementation: a Review," *Journal of the American College of Nutrition*, 14:2 (1995), pp. 124–36.

Block, Gladys, "Vitamin C and Cancer Prevention: the Epidemiologic Evidence," *American Journal of Clinical Nutrition*, 53:1 Suppl. (1991), pp. 270S–82S.

Levine, Mark, et al. "Vitamin C Pharmacokinetics in Healthy Volunteers: Evidence for a Recommended Dietary Allowance," *Proceedings of the National Academy of Science*, 93 (April 1996), pp. 3704–09.

vitamin D   A fat-soluble trace nutrient required for healthy BONES and teeth. Vitamin D_2 (ERGOCALCIFEROL) occurs in plants, yeast and fungi. Commercially, vitamin D_2 is produced by exposing a plant sterol, ergosterol, to UV light. Vitamin D_3, cholecalciferol (25-hydroxy cholecalciferol), is the form found in animal tissue and in the oil of fatty fish, and it is also synthesized in the skin from a cholesterol derivative when exposed to sunlight (UV light). Vitamin D is the only VITAMIN to be formed in this manner. This fat-soluble vitamin is stored in fatty tissue as well as in the LIVER, bones, skin and muscle. Vitamin D is required for calcium uptake, and so is linked to the formation of bones and teeth.

Vitamin D is the only vitamin that is converted to a HORMONE. Vitamin D is transported to the KIDNEYS, where it is again oxidized, yielding calcitriol (1,25 dihydroxy cholecalciferol), which is a hormone. Calcitriol in the bloodstream travels to the intestine where it stimulates the formation of calcium transport proteins. In addition calcitriol can increase bone rebuilding by working together with parathyroid hormone. It also stimulates calcium reabsorption by the kidney.

Vitamin D as calcitriol influences many glands and tissues. This hormone affects the PANCREAS (insulin secretion), the PARATHYROID GLANDS, PITUITARY GLAND, ovaries, testes, COLON, placenta, uterus, heart, THYMUS, mammary tissue and brain (cerebellum). In a very real sense calcitriol is an immune enhancer. Calcitriol stimulates WHITE BLOOD CELLS, especially macrophages, and influences B and T lymphocytes—major classes of cells responsible for antibody production and the surveillance mechanism of the IMMUNE SYSTEM.

Possible Roles in Maintaining Health

Chronic vitamin D deficiency in children leads to RICKETS, characterized by abnormal calcification of bones. As a result, bones are soft and become deformed. Teeth do not develop normally and are subject to decay. Rickets is rare in Western societies owing to the prevalent practice of food FORTIFICATION with forms of vitamin D.

The adult equivalent of rickets is OSTEOMALACIA. In this disease bones become depleted of calcium and phosphorus. Osteomalacia is more common during pregnancy and lactation, as well as during old age. Supplementation with vitamin D can reduce the risk of osteomalacia. Though vitamin D is necessary for normal calcium metabolism, it does not seem to protect against OSTEOPOROSIS in postmenopausal women. Osteoporosis is mitigated by MAGNESIUM, CALCIUM, and possibly FLUORIDE, BORON, MANGANESE and VITAMIN K.

Population studies suggest that vitamin D and calcium deficiencies account in part for the high rate of colorectal cancer and breast cancer worldwide. CALCIFEROL inhibits cancer cells in the test tube and inhibits chemically induced cancer in mice. Vitamin D applied to the skin or taken orally may clear up psoriasis, a condition characterized by scaly, itchy red patches of skin.

Sources

There are few good food sources of vitamin D, which is the least prevalent vitamin in the food supply. Vitamin D occurs in fatty fish, fish liver oils, egg yolk and liver. Vitamin D is used to fortify MILK, and either vitamin D_3 or vitamin D_2 are used. Whole milk, low-fat milk, non-fat milk and non-fat dry milk are fortified with 400 IUs, equivalent to 10 mcg of vitamin D per quart, though spotchecks have revealed variations in this level. Other foods may be fortified with vitamin D: breakfast cereal, infant cereal, bread, chocolate beverages and margarine.

Requirements

Human requirements are difficult to establish because varying levels of this vitamin are synthesized by the skin. The RECOMMENDED DIETARY ALLOWANCE (RDA) for people over 25 is 5 mcg daily, which is equivalent to 200 IU. Factors that increase the risk of vitamin D deficiency include: gallbladder removal, severe food allergies, poor fat absorption (for instance, due to CELIAC DISEASE) and liver disease. Several medications can interfere with vitamin D uptake: certain anticonvulsant agents, barbiturates and cortisone. Mineral oil blocks the uptake of this and other fat-soluble vitamins. People with kidney disease or diabetes may not be able to activate vitamin D. Institutionalized people who get little exposure to sunlight, strict vegetarians and elderly persons are more at risk for vitamin D deficiency. The efficiency of the skin's production of this vitamin declines with age.

Safety

Vitamin D can be toxic, due to high blood calcium levels (hypercalcemia) and the calcification of soft tissue. Symptoms include constipation, vomiting, fatigue, drowsiness, lack of appetite and, in severe cases, high blood pressure, kidney stones, and even kidney failure and coma. Doses at two or three times the RDA seem unlikely to cause toxicity. Young children are more susceptible, and as little as 1,800 IU of vitamin D per day may cause toxicity. Moderately high consumption over a long period of time may increase the risk of atherosclerosis. Those with elevated blood calcium levels should not supplement with vitamin D without medical supervision. (See also ENRICHMENT; HYPERVITAMINOSIS.)

Fraser, D.R., "Vitamin D," *Lancet*, 345 (January 14, 1995), pp. 104–07.

vitamin E (tocopherol)　A fat-soluble essential nutrient that stabilizes cell membranes. Naturally occurring tocopherols are a mixture of closely related compounds (isomers) designated alpha-tocopherol, beta-tocopherol, gamma-tocopherol and delta tocopherol. Alpha tocopherol has the greatest vitamin E activity in the body. Synthetic vitamin E, designated as dl-tocopherol or rac-tocopherol, is less active. Supplements usually incorporate vitamin E bound to simple acids to prevent its oxidation. Alpha tocopheryl acetate and succinate are common forms; the acetate and succinate are forms broken down by intestinal enzymes to release vitamin E.

Free radicals　Vitamin E is the major lipid antioxidant in the body, the property for which it is best known. It squelches free radicals, highly reactive molecules that can attack neighboring molecules and damage polyunsaturated fatty acids in membrane lipids, proteins and DNA, damaging cells and leading to disease. Free radical damage is linked to CANCER, HEART DISEASE, CATARACTS and aging. This vitamin plays important roles in the immune system, the nervous system and the endocine (hormonal) system.

Possible Roles in Maintaining Health

Cancer　Population studies suggest that low blood levels of vitamin E and BETA CAROTENE correlate with an increased risk of lung cancer. Mammary dysplasia, a precancerous condition of breast tissue, has been treated with vitamin E.

Cardiovascular disease　Supplementation with vitamin E has been effective in treating pain in the lower leg due to narrowed leg arteries (intermittent claudication). In research

with experimental animals vitamin E was found to slow plaque build-up in arteries and seems to inhibit blood clot formation. Men with higher levels of vitamin E were found to have a decreased risk of angina, a type of chest pain that often occurs before a heart attack. The World Health Organization found that a low blood level of vitamin E was the highest risk factor in predicting heart disease and death. Healthy men and women who supplemented with at least 100 IU of vitamin E daily had less heart disease. They may have experienced less oxidative damage to LDL (LOW-DENSITY LIPOPROTEIN, the undesirable form of blood cholesterol). In the test tube vitamin E is a potent inhibitor of LDL oxidation. Oxidation of LDL by free radicals and its uptake by cells in arterial walls may initiate the development of ATHEROSCLEROSIS. Patients with severe heart disease enrolled in the Cambridge Heart Antioxidant Study were treated with either 400 or 800 IU of vitamin E daily. After 17 months they had a significantly lower risk of developing heart attacks than those who received a placebo (blank) pill. A longer study may be needed to reveal an overall decline in death rate with supplementation. Other research suggests that the accumulation of plaque in arteries slows down with supplementation of 100 IU of vitamin E or more daily.

Neurologic disorders　Vitamin E plays an important role in maintaining normal nerve function. Vitamin E deficiency is usually associated with symptoms of peripheral NEUROPATHY. Recent results suggest that low vitamin E content in nerves precedes nerve degeneration. Vitamin E has been found to be beneficial in reducing the severity of symptoms of TARDIVE DYSKINESIA, a side effect of long-term use of tranquilizers (phenothiazines) that produces involuntary movements.

Eye diseases　Population studies indicate that cataract-free people consume more vitamin E and vitamin C than those with cataracts. Premature infants can develop vitamin E deficiencies because they possess almost no FAT, hence fat-soluble vitamin stores are marginal. Premature infants receive vitamin E to prevent anemia and retinopathy.

Immune system　Moderate amounts of vitamin E seem to increase the ability of macrophages to destroy bacteria and to boost activity of T lymphocytes, the foot-soldiers and generals of the IMMUNE SYSTEM. Vitamin E may alter production of certain PROSTAGLANDINS, hormone-like substances derived from essential fatty acids that promote INFLAMMATION. It has been used to manage autoimmune conditions like LUPUS ERYTHEMATOSUS. Healthy elderly men and women supplemented with moderate amounts of vitamin E can show greater immune responsiveness than those who do not supplement with this vitamin. On the other hand, very high levels of vitamin E may inhibit immune function.

Other conditions　Case studies support claims that vitamin E promotes wound healing and minimizes scar tissue formation. Vitamin E supplementation has been suggested to reduce symptoms of PREMENSTRUAL SYNDROME. Most careful studies on the effects of vitamin E supplementation on muscular strength, maximum oxygen consumption or endurance have failed to demonstrate benefits. It is possible vitamin E can reduce oxygen debt and increase maximum oxygen consumption in adapting to high elevations.

Diabetes Sometimes supplementation with vitamins can improve glucose tolerance and insulin sensitivity in diabetic patients, and reduce the level of secondary damage due to the buildup of glucose-bound proteins.

Osteoarthritis Vitamin E possesses mild and inflammatory activity, which may explain why it can help lessen pain associated with osteoarthritis.

Skin conditions A variety of skin conditions such as Raynaud's phenomenon and polymitosis have been treated with vitamin E.

Eye conditions Oxidative damage probably promotes CATARACTS and macular degeneration associated with aging. Animals fed vitamin E-deficient diets develop macular degeneration. People with low-levels of antioxidants in blood have a higher risk of cataracts.

Sources

The highest levels of vitamin E occur in VEGETABLE OILS (safflower, soybean and sunflower oils), BUTTER and MARGARINE, NUTS, wheat germ, whole-grain CEREALS, EGGS and green leafy vegetables. Most fruits and white bread contain negligible vitamin E. To obtain 100 IU of vitamin E, a level found to reduce the risk of heart disease, a person would have to eat six cups of kale, or 4.5 cups of sweet potatoes. Vitamin E supplements should not be taken together with iron because they interfere with each other.

Requirements

The RECOMMENDED DIETARY ALLOWANCE (RDA) for vitamin E is 10 mg (14.9 IU) of alpha tocopherol equivalents per day for men and 8 mg (11.9 IU) per day for women over 25 years of age. Typical intakes in the United States range from 5 to 10 mg daily. It is generally believed that few individuals are frankly vitamin E deficient. However, surveys have revealed that 45% of affluent, elderly Americans may consume less than the RDA, and even susceptible but healthy persons eating a BALANCED DIET may benefit from vitamin E supplements, with less free radical damage and less risk of cancer and heart disease. Premature infants, individuals on very-low-calorie/low-fat diets or who do not absorb fat very well (including some elderly people) may be deficient. Chronic malabsorption of fat and fat-soluble vitamins, including vitamin E, can accompany cystic fibrosis, SPRUE and non-tropical sprue, chronic PANCREATITIS, CELIAC DISEASE and bile duct inflammation or blockage, among other conditions.

Symptoms of severe vitamin E deficiency include ANEMIA and neurologic disorders. Newborn infants, especially premature infants with vitamin E deficiency, experience EDEMA and blood abnormalities. The requirement for vitamin E increases with increased consumption of polyunsaturated oils due to the increased susceptibility to peroxidation. However, the optimal ratio is unclear. In extreme situations the requirement may exceed the RDA.

Safety

Vitamin E is one of the least toxic fat-soluble vitamins when administered orally, and most healthy adults can tolerate 100 to 800 mg daily. Excessive vitamin E may cause fatigue, muscle weakness, stomach upset, headache, nausea and skin disorders. In certain patients with high blood pressure, vitamin E may elevate blood pressure. Those with HYPERTENSION, rheumatic heart disease or diabetes should seek medical advice before supplementing with vitamin E. People taking anticoagulant medications or who are deficient in VITAMIN K, or who have blood clots, should follow their physician's advice regarding vitamin E supplements to avoid the potential problem with increased bleeding. Iron and oral contraceptives can interfere with absorbing vitamin E. (See also AGING; DEGENERATIVE DISEASES.)

Meydani, Mohsen, "Vitamin E," *Lancet*, 345 (January 21, 1995), pp. 170–75.

vitamin F See ESSENTIAL FATTY ACIDS.

vitamin H See BIOTIN.

vitamin K A fat-soluble vitamin required for normal BLOOD CLOTTING. As with VITAMIN E and VITAMIN B_6, the term vitamin K represents several closely related forms: the most prevalent, naturally occurring forms are vitamin K_1 (philloquinone or hytonadione) and vitamin K_2 (menaquinone). Vitamin K_3 is MENADIONE, a synthetic form that can be activated in the LIVER.

Vitamin K serves as a cofactor for the processing of six proteins required in the complex chain of reactions that regulates blood clotting. One of these proteins is prothrombin, the inactive precursor of the enzyme that creates fibrin clots from fibrinogen, and vitamin K has been used to treat clotting disorders due to vitamin K deficiency. Vitamin K also assists in the synthesis of osteocalcin, a bone protein that forms the matrix for mineralization and bone building.

Possible Roles in Maintaining Health

Vitamin K is required for healing fractured bone and in the maintenance of normal bone. Elderly patients with osteoporosis (thin bone disease) may be low in vitamin K. Vitamin K supplementation may decrease calcium excretion and help protect against osteoporosis. A deficiency of vitamin K causes hemorrhaging. Pediatricians administer vitamin K to newborn infants to reduce their risk of spontaneous bleeding. Infants also run the risk of being permanently brain damaged by vitamin K deficiency in the first six months of life. There may be other important functions of this vitamin; vitamin K-dependent modified proteins occur in kidneys and other tissues as well, though their function is unclear.

Sources

Vitamin K occurs in highest levels in green, leafy vegetables. Dairy products are good sources, and small amounts occur in cereals, meats and other vegetables. Vitamin K occurs in low levels in breastmilk. Newborn infants are often given vitamin K to help their clotting mechanism. Bacteria colonizing the mature small intestine produce vitamin K; LACTOBACILLUS ACIDOPHILUS is an example of such a beneficial gut bacteria. Vitamin K_3 is prescribed to treat vitamin K deficiencies.

Requirements

The RECOMMENDED DIETARY ALLOWANCE for normal adults is 80 mcg/day for men and 65 mcg/day for women. There are hints that optimal bone metabolism is more sensitive to inadequate vitamin K and the needs may be higher. Because vitamin K is widely distributed in food and is formed by normal gut flora, vitamin K deficiency is not believed to be common. Deficiency could occur in people who consume few vegetables, in people with lipid MALABSORPTION and in those with CELIAC DISEASE or bile duct obstruction. The prolonged use of oral antibiotics; certain medications like cholesterol lowering drugs, mineral oil, anticonvulsants (Dilantin) and some antibiotics (aphalosporins); and PARENTERAL NUTRITION (venous feeding) increase the risk. Vitamin K status needs to be monitored in patients being treated with anticoagulants (like coumadin). Symptoms of severe deficiency include a tendency to bleed and disturbed bone formation.

Safety

Naturally occurring forms of vitamin K are relatively nontoxic. The synthetic form may rarely cause liver problems. An allergic-type reaction can occur with high doses. A high intake of vitamin E may cause bleeding similar to vitamin K deficiency. Those who have a vitamin K deficiency need medical supervision. Patients taking anticoagulants should take vitamin K only with the advice of a physician. (See also VITAMIN A; VITAMIN D.)

vitamin P   See FLAVONOIDS.

VLDL   See VERY LOW-DENSITY LIPOPROTEIN.

walnut (*Juglans spp.*)   A popular commercial nut with a hard, deeply furrowed shell surrounding the meat. The English walnut (*J. regia*) is the most important commercial walnut. It is native to southeastern Europe and western Asia and probably originated in Persia. The black walnut (*J. nigra*) is native to the Mississippi Valley and Appalachians of the United States; there is limited commercial production of black walnuts, however. The United States produces over half the world crop; most of it comes from California. About 40% of the walnut crop is marketed in shells, the remainder is processed. Machine-shelled nuts may be blanched to remove the inner skins, which give walnuts their somewhat bitter aftertaste. They may be blanched to even out the color.

Walnuts contain a large percentage of oil, with 66% of it as polyunsaturated fatty acids. It is a good source of alpha linolenic acid, an omega-3 fatty acid essential to the diet. Cholesterol-lowering diets in which meat and dairy products are substituted by walnuts may lower blood cholesterol levels because of their polyunsaturated fat. Shelled nuts are subject to rancidity; they should be vacuum-packed or stored in sealed plastic bags in the freezer. On the other hand, whole walnuts can be stored for months in a cool environment. If antioxidants are added to extend shelflife, they are listed on the food label. Walnuts are used in baking and confections. The nutrient content of 1 cup (120 g) of chopped English walnuts is: 770 calories; protein, 17.2 g; carbohydrate, 22 g; fiber, 8.4 g; fat, 74.2 g; iron, 2.8 mg; potassium, 602 mg; thiamine, 0.46 mg; riboflavin, 0.18 mg; niacin, 1.256 mg.

water   A clear, colorless, odorless liquid that is essential for all life forms. Water is the most abundant nutrient in the body. More water is needed daily than any other nutrient because cells contain mainly water. A human embryo represents about 98% water; an infant's weight is about 75% water; and water accounts for 50 to 65% of an adult's weight. EXTRACELLULAR FLUID including blood and lymph accounts for 20% of body weight; INTRACELLULAR FLUID, the water within cells, accounts for 45%. Water represents 75% of muscle tissue and 92% of the cell-free fluid of blood (plasma). Excessive water can accumulate in tissues, a condition called EDEMA. Edema is caused by heart failure, low blood pressure due to low blood protein resulting from STARVATION, or to increased capillary leakiness due to INFLAMMATION.

Water serves many roles for the body. Water functions as a lubricant and is a major constituent of joint fluid. It helps internal organs slide by each other, for example, during PERISTALSIS, the muscular contraction that moves food down the digestive tract. Water comprises the major constituent of fluids important in digestion: SALIVA, MUCUS, gastric juice, BILE, pancreatic juices and intestinal secretions. Because water is so prevalent in cells, most cellular macromolecules of the body like DNA, RNA, proteins and polysaccharides function in a water environment. Water participates in many chemical reactions of the body. Thus DIGESTION refers to the hydrolysis of nutrients, that is, the breaking of chemical bonds by means of water molecules.

Because water is an excellent solvent, it readily transports nutrients and waste products in the bloodstream. Water also absorbs and releases heat slowly so that it can slow changes in body temperature as environmental temperatures fluctuate. Water possesses a high heat of vaporization; that is, a lot of heat is used up in evaporation. Thus when water evaporates as sweat, it provides an effective means of cooling the body. Gases dissolve readily in water, and moist tissue surfaces promote the absorption of gases like OXYGEN and the release of CARBON DIOXIDE in the lungs.

Water Balance

Water balance refers to the ability of the body to adjust water output to water intake. When a large volume of water is consumed, urine excretion increases; with limited water intake, urine production declines. Water is lost daily from the skin (450 ml), urine (1,400 ml), expired air from the lungs (350 ml) and in stools (200 ml). To make up for these losses, a typical adult uses 2 to 2.9 quarts (2 to 2.7 liters) of water daily. Beverages provide about 1.5 l; foods contribute about 0.70 l, and water from metabolism yields 0.20 l. RESPIRATION, the oxidation of nutrients to carbon dioxide, produces on the average 13 g of water per 100 calories with a typical diet. Thus oxidation of 100 g of carbohydrate yields 60 g of water; the oxidation of 100 g of protein, 42 g of water; and 100 g of fat, 110 g of water.

Water is also recycled. Each day the intestine receives 8 to 10 liters of secretions, including saliva, gastric juices and glandular products. Most water is reabsorbed; only 100 to 200 ml of water is lost through feces. Exceptions are DIARRHEA and vomiting. The kidneys play a major role in water conservation while removing waste materials in urine. Each day the kidneys filter nearly 2,000 liters of blood. Only 0.1% of this volume is released as urine.

Water balance is regulated by an elegant feedback system involving the brain and hormones. Nerve centers in the region of the brain called the HYPOTHALAMUS regulate hunger, thirst and urine output. A loss of about 1% of body water creates the sensation of THIRST. Decreased water and elevated sodium in the blood are detected by osmoreceptor cells, regulatory cells located in the hypothalamus. As the effective ion concentration of blood increases, water leaves these cells and they shrink, generating nerve impulses that trigger thirst and stimulate the release of ANTIDIURETIC HORMONE (ADH) from the PITUITARY GLAND. ADH in turn increases the ability of NEPHRONS (the kidneys' filtration device) to absorb water that would otherwise be lost as urine. As a result, the sodium concentration of the blood decreases, cells of the hypothalamus regain water, and the thirst sensation diminishes.

Dehydration

DEHYDRATION can be caused by evaporation, diarrhea, blood losses, burns or excessive urine production, as in uncontrolled diabetes. Physical activity increases water loss through perspiration and breathing. Water depletion can become a serious problem with prolonged EXERCISE. With elevated temperatures, strenuous exercise can increase water losses three- to tenfold above normal. DIURETICS (water pills) increase urine output by increasing water and sodium excretion, as do CAFFEINE and related compounds like theophylline. ALCOHOL increases urination because it inhibits the release of ADH. Dehydration can cause discomfort, flushed skin, tingling in hands and feet, then increased heart rate, increased body temperature, weakness, confusion, spastic muscles and decreased blood volume.

Overhydration

With excessive water intake, brain cells become swollen. This can cause drowsiness, lowered blood pressure, weakened heart, weakness and even convulsions and coma. Patients administered excessive IV solutions too rapidly or who have impaired ADH production may develop symptoms of water intoxication.

Minerals in Drinking Water

All water except distilled water contains minerals, and domestic water supplies vary in their mineral content.

Hard water contains calcium and magnesium salts of bicarbonate and sulfate. The mineral content can be sufficiently high to contribute to daily requirements of these minerals. Boiling hard water converts bicarbonate to carbonate, and insoluble magnesium and calcium carbonate deposits form in tea kettles, hot water and steam pipes. Calcium and magnesium in hard water also form solids with typical soaps.

Soft water contains sodium sulfate and sodium bicarbonate, which are soluble and do not form solids as water is boiled, nor do they react with soap. Soft water is associated with an increased risk of CARDIOVASCULAR DISEASE, possibly because low dietary calcium and magnesium increase the risk of heart disease. When drinking water contains more than 20 mg of sodium per liter, it represents a significant source of sodium for people on sodium-restricted diets. Soft water is more corrosive to plumbing and can dissolve CADMIUM and LEAD from galvanized pipes and soldered joints.

Water hardness is expressed in parts per million (ppm) equivalent to calcium carbonate, though magnesium or other minerals may be present. Water with a hardness less than 100 ppm of calcium carbonate is considered soft, while water with a hardness greater than 300 ppm is considered hard.

Over half of the municipal water supplies in the United States add FLUORIDE to reduce tooth decay. This has become a controversial issue because too much fluoride can cause health problems.

Demineralized water that is free of mineral ions, like calcium, magnesium and carbonate, is prepared by ion exchange columns that replace calcium and magnesium with sodium and hydrogen ions, and replace carbonate with sulfate. Non-ionic materials such as pesticides are not removed.

Distillation, in which water is converted to steam and then condensed and collected, removes most organic residues as well as minerals. Volatile materials (those that readily vaporize) such as solvents may not be removed by distillation.

Disinfecting Drinking Water

Chlorination has long been used as a chemical treatment to disinfect water. In most industrialized countries, water treatment by chlorination has removed the threat of water-borne diseases like cholera, typhoid, dysentery and gastroenteritis. However, inadequate treatment of sewage leads to periodic outbreaks of hepatitis A and other diseases. There are hints that chlorination by-products slightly increase the risk of cancer. Most public health officials agree that the health risks of not disinfecting water are very much greater than those posed by chlorination.

An alternative treatment to kill disease-causing microbes, chloramination, incorporates chlorine and ammonia to treat water supplies. It is as effective as chlorine, and this method is used by about 20% of the largest municipal water supplies. Ozonation disinfects water with ozone, with a follow-up chlorination or chloramination treatment to destroy microbes that may multiply after ozone wears off. Less than 1% of water systems use this method.

Parasites can contaminate water supplies in the United States. In 1993 an estimated 370,000 people in Milwaukee experienced diarrhea and flu-like symptoms due to water contamination by a parasite called Cryptosporidium. Elevated levels of particulate matter in drinking water in Washington, D.C., the same year caused the EPA to issue an alert to boil drinking water as a defense against Cryptosporidium, which resists chlorination. Though most people experience only mild discomfort with infection, Cryptosporidium can cause life threatening illness in newborn infants and in people with impaired immune systems.

Presently there are no standards for acceptable levels of this parasite in drinking water. Giardia, another intestinal parasite that can also cause intestinal distress, is larger than Cryptosporidium and is more easily removed by filtration in municipal water treatments. The presence of this parasite in water is essentially unacceptable to the EPA.

Suggestions for Water Purification When Camping

Boiling water up to 20 minutes is a tried and true method of disinfecting drinking water, and it is probably the safest. Using iodine to disinfect water may pose a hazard because excessive amounts of iodine can be toxic. Another form of iodine, hypoperiodide, is safer. To remove the unpleasant taste from the sterilized water, add a couple of tablets of activated charcoal per quart and shake. Avoid drinking tap water and iced drinks when traveling in countries where water quality is questionable. If water used to make ice cubes is contaminated, the iced beverage will be too.

Chemical Water Pollutants

Industrialization has introduced thousands of new chemicals into the environment, and about 700 chemical contaminants have been detected in drinking water in the United States including PESTICIDES; industrial solvents; toxic heavy metals like lead and MERCURY; NITRATES from fertilizer use; and radioactive contaminants like radon. Under the Safe Drinking Water Act of 1974, the Environmental Protection Agency is charged with setting standards of water quality for all local water systems and to make certain that states enforce the standards. In 1991 the EPA reported that 10% of community water supply wells were contaminated with pesticides, but that fewer than 1% were estimated to be above levels that could be harmful.

Over 80 compounds and toxic substances are regulated in terms of maximum upper limits for concentrations in drinking water. The legal limits, called maximum contaminant levels (MCLs), are administered by individual states. Included are minerals like ARSENIC; nitrates; heavy metals like cadmium; lead; mercury; solvents like benzene and phenol; pesticides like Endrin, Diquat, Dalapon, and Simazine; products of incomplete combustion like BENZOPYRENE and DIOXIN. Antimony, NICKEL, pesticides like dinoseb (a pesticide used on soybeans and other crops), atrazine (a herbicide used on corn) and halogenated hydrocarbons are among the most commonly found compounds in water supplies.

Halogenated hydrocarbons are quite stable in the environment and can contaminate the environment for decades. One class is called CHLORINATED HYDROCARBONS. As an example, trichloroethylene (TCE) and its degradation products are important contaminants of ground water. TCE was used as a degreasing agent. Since TCE is volatile, drinking water can be treated by air evaporation process (air stripping). Other regulated volatile chlorinated hydrocarbons include dichloromethane and trihalomethane, by-products of the reaction of chlorine with organic materials in drinking water. Because they evaporate easily, they may pose a hazard when taking a shower.

Home Water Treatment

No single device removes all contaminants. Water purifiers remove bacteria while water filters remove non-bacterial contaminants but not bacteria. The best systems can remove up to 99% of the chlorine and over 70% of other contaminants. Units should be certified by the nonprofit National Sanitation Foundation in Ann Arbor, Michigan. Water softeners or water treatment units to improve the taste or smell of drinking water may be certified by the Water Quality Association.

Activated carbon filtration units with high-quality carbon can absorb chlorine and organic compounds but are not very effective in removing minerals like IRON, lead or fluoride. Carbon filters must be replaced about once a month. Some filters can become breeding grounds for harmful bacteria unless properly maintained. The best filters are solid blocks of activated charcoal with a diversion valve, so that unfiltered water can be used for dishes. Filters need to be changed regularly.

Reverse osmosis filtration forces water through a porous membrane at high pressures. Reverse osmosis effectively removes inorganic ions like fluoride and a few organic contaminants, but reverse osmosis also wastes about 75% of the water and the membranes need to be replaced periodically.

Water softener units incorporate ion exchangers, which will remove iron, calcium and other minerals of hard water and replace them with sodium. Cooking with or drinking softened water is not advised due to the high sodium content.

Home distillation removes minerals and non-volatile organic compounds (those that do not evaporate), but the process is slow and costly because of heating costs.

BOTTLED WATER is another alternative to tap water. Bottled water is classified as a food product by the U.S. FDA, but this is no guarantee that it will be safe or wholesome. Producers are not required to list the source of the water. Most bottled water comes from wells or springs, but it may be municipal water. Bottled water is less well regulated than tap water, and spot-checks have turned up traces of organic solvents, nitrates and toxic heavy metals—and the sodium content can be high. Tests of domestic bottled water have seldom turned up harmful levels of chemical contaminants, though sampled bottled water may only meet, not exceed, health department standards. Bottled water is disinfected by ozone, not chlorine treatment, and it is not fluoridated.

Recommendations

To minimize chemical contaminants, use cold tap water for drinking because hot water tends to dissolve metals from pipes. Let the cold tap run until the water gets cold. This water contains the least amount of contaminants leached from metal pipes.

Water suppliers will provide the results of water tests for regulated contaminants upon request. Contact the EPA safe water hotline (1-800-476-4791) to find out whether the contaminants exceed federal standards. The EPA also can supply the name of your state's certifying officer, for referrals to qualified local water testing labs.

Though bottled water generally appears to be good quality it may be prudent to request the latest chemical analysis from the bottler, or have a sample tested independently. To minimize the RISK of exposure to contaminants, vary your water supply from time to time.

Akhter, M.E. et al., *Mortality and Weekly Report*, 43 (1994), Atlanta: Centers for Disease Control, pp. 661–63..

"Assessment of Inadequately Filtered Public Drinking Water— Washington, D.C., December, 1993," *Journal of the American Medical Association*, 272:18 (1994), pp. 1401–02.

"Over 50 Million Drink Water Failing Health Standards," *Nutrition Week*, 25:22 (June 9, 1995), p. 6.

watermelon (*Citrullus vulgaris*)   The fruit of an annual vine belonging to the squash and melon family. This round or cylindrical fruit can weigh from 5 lb to 85 lb (2.3 to 38.3 kg). There are more than 50 varieties, including seedless watermelons. The juicy flesh may be red, pink, orange, yellow or white. Watermelons originated in Africa and have been cultivated since ancient times in the Mediterranean region, Egypt and India. Watermelons are now cultivated throughout the world from tropical to temperate regions. Florida, Texas and California lead domestic production. The fruit is eaten fresh. Watermelon is a good source of vitamin C; it contains about 90% water and 8% sugar. The nutrient content of a slice of raw watermelon that is 1 in thick and 10 in in diameter, without refuse (480 g), is: 152 calories; protein, 3 g; carbohydrate, 34.6 g; fiber, 2.4 g; fat, 2.1 g; iron, 0.82 g; potassium, 560 mg; vitamin A, 176 retinol equivalents; vitamin C, 47 mg; thiamin, 0.3 mg; riboflavin, 0.1 mg; niacin, 0.96 mg.

water pills   See DIURETICS.

water-soluble vitamins   See VITAMIN.

wax   A family of water resistant compounds that are solids or thick (viscous) liquids. Waxes consist of long chains of carbon atoms, and are obtained from petroleum products (paraffin), fat, beeswax, synthetic resins and palm oil derivatives. Only insect-based waxes and vegetable waxes are applied on domestic produce, though imported produce may contain animal-based waxes. Commercially, waxes are generally sprayed as a thin film on produce to prevent loss of moisture and to enhance consumer appeal after polishing. Naturally occurring protective waxes on fruits and vegetables are generally washed off when the produce is harvested. Producers commonly wax APPLES, AVOCADOS, BEETS, green PEPPERS, CUCUMBERS, EGGPLANT, MELONS, certain nuts, PAPAYAS, PEACHES, PINEAPPLES, POTATOES, SQUASH, TANGERINES, TOMATOES, SWEET POTATOES and WATERMELONS.

Waxes are classified as PRESERVATIVES, and the U.S. FDA regulations specify that waxes must be identified where the consumer purchases the produce. The type of wax applied is not specified, a concern for those following dietary laws or making dietary choices such as KOSHER, Muslim, Seventh Day Adventist or vegetarian diets.

FUNGICIDES are generally applied before waxing or are mixed with waxes before application, and waxed produce cannot be washed free of fungicides. Benomyl, thiabendazole, phenol, captan, folpet, dicloran and others are permitted to be used with waxes. The U.S. National Academy of Sciences estimates that 90% of fungicides are potential cancer-causing agents (carcinogens). Specifically, benomyl, captan and folpet increase the risk of cancer. (See also DELANEY CLAUSE; FOOD ADDITIVES; ORGANIC FOODS; PESTICIDES.)

weight management   Generally, programs designed to assist individuals to lose weight or to maintain a desired body weight. Americans who diet to lose weight frequently participate in weight management programs for many reasons. Statistics show that meeting external expectations motivates most dieters. Current American images of attractiveness and success place a premium on being slender, especially for women. Theoretically a normal, healthy man's body weight should be between 15 and 18% FAT. Women normally possess more body fat then men, and a healthy woman's body should be between 18 and 22% fat.

A second motivation to manage weight is an awareness of the ramifications of being excessively overweight. OBESITY, defined as being 30% over a desirable body weight, carries increased risks for diabetes, HYPERTENSION and CARDIOVASCULAR DISEASE. Certain people tend to gain excess fat on their upper body, and upper body fat increases the waist to hip ratio, which correlates with a greater risk of heart disease.

Strategies for Weight Loss

Short-term weight loss readily can be attained by extreme measures: a drastic reduction in caloric intake (semi-starvation); CRASH DIETING; unbalanced diets emphasizing high fat and high protein with little or no CARBOHYDRATE. However, most of this lost weight represents WATER and muscle protein loss rather than fat loss. Without a commitment to changing long-term behavior, pounds lost will be rapidly regained; frequently lost muscle is replaced by fat at the termination of the weight loss program. Several popular, doctor-supervised, very-low-calorie programs are available. There is little published data on the success rates of most weight management programs. The limited information available suggests that only 2 to 10% of people who have enrolled in such programs successfully keep off lost pounds for a year or more. These strategies can lead to weight losses of several pounds per week and often employ liquid protein meal replacements. Current liquid formula diets are much improved over 1970s versions. Regular food allotments plus three meal replacements can bring the total calories up to 1,200 per day, and with supervision they are often safe for several weeks. A major disadvantage: They often reinforce the unhealthy pattern of eating lightly at breakfast and lunch, and eating heavily at dinner or later.

Under starvation or semi-starvation conditions, usually less than 1,200 calories per day, the body's metabolism compensates for decreased caloric intake by gearing down the rate at which calories are burned. In other words the BASAL METABOLIC RATE declines as a protective adaptation. Furthermore the body preferentially breaks down protein in the early stages of semi-starvation to meet energy requirements; paradoxically, the body can therefore become proportionately fatter during this period. Programs that incorporate medications to curb CRAVING as well as increased exercise and restricted caloric intake have been recommended for obese people.

Recommendations for Weight Management

People who have lost weight permanently and have maintained a desired weight for a number of years share certain characteristics that permit several generalizations for managing weight successfully.

Committing to exercising for life   Daily exercises can temporarily increase the basal metabolic rate and thus increase the efficiency of burning calories, even when calories are restricted. Even a daily half-hour of vigorous walking will help maintain weight. Regular exercise is often sufficient to lose a small amount of weight and to become leaner. Moderate exercise is more effective for weight management because it preferentially burns fat, and intense exercise burns carbohydrate (glycogen), which is easily replenished.

Committing to changing eating habits   Eat fewer fatty, high-calorie foods, typically the CONVENIENCE FOODS that make up a large percentage of the American diet. Fat provides more than twice as many calories per gram as carbohydrate or protein, and fat calories are more readily converted to body fat. Eating less fat will help bring about weight loss. High dietary fat correlates with increased risk of disease; generally, dietary guidelines call for consuming less saturated fat while increasing fresh fruits and vegetables, whole grains and legumes. Foods containing high levels of refined carbohydrate, like sugar, white flour and fat, provide few other nutrients. People relying on such foods need to select extra nutrient-rich foods to make up for this deficiency, not a usual pattern in the United States. A combination of exercise and improved food selection is often adequate to lose 10 to 20 pounds a year without dieting.

Dieting and exercising combined   To lose up to 50 pounds, dieting combined with exercise is recommended:

1. Lose weight gradually, no more than a pound per week. Conditions that promote rapid weight loss cause the body's METABOLISM to switch to favor loss of muscle protein and water and, less rapidly, fat. Severe caloric restriction reduces thyroid gland activity, slowing the metabolism and slowing fat loss.

2. Consume at least 1,200 calories daily with adequate intake of high-quality protein, vitamins and minerals to meet daily needs in order to accomplish gradual weight loss. Generally 45 to 60 g of FISH, POULTRY, lean MEAT, soy protein or other complete protein will meet daily requirements of all essential amino acids. This step will assure an adequate supply of all essential amino acids and will help prevent loss of muscle. Diets supplying less than 1,500 calories per day require supplementation—for example, with calcium—to achieve adequate intake. VITAMIN C, the B COMPLEX and TRACE MINERALS are known to help metabolize fat, and adequate intakes are important.

3. Meals should supply adequate FIBER: Both soluble fiber, as found in fresh FRUITS, VEGETABLES, LEGUMES and certain grains, and insoluble fiber, as found in whole grains and bran. Fiber contributes to normal digestion, maintenance of the digestive tract and a feeling of satiety.

4. Drink plenty of water. The kidneys require water to excrete metabolic wastes and fat breakdown products.

Seeking out emotional support   Overeating usually is symptomatic of deeper emotional issues. Until these are dealt with, long-term changes in eating behavior are difficult to achieve. When people substitute eating for self-acceptance or for avoiding emotional pain, weight management becomes increasingly difficult. Overeaters Anonymous and other support groups can help nurture self-esteem and self-forgiveness. (See also ANOREXIA NERVOSA; BULIMIA NERVOSA; DIETARY GUIDELINES FOR AMERICANS; DIETING; EATING DISORDERS.)

Gibbs, W.W., "Gaining on Fat," *Scientific American*, 275:2 (1996), pp. 88–94.

Goldstein, D.J. and Potvin, J.H., "Long-term Weight Loss: the Effects of Pharmacologic Agents, *American Journal of Clinical Nutrition*, 60 (1994), pp. 647–57.

weights and measures   See MEASURES.

Wernicke's disease (Wernicke-Korsakoff syndrome) A disorder of the NERVOUS SYSTEM usually associated with a deficiency of the B vitamin, THIAMIN. Typical symptoms include: poor balance and uncoordinated walk, double vision, confusion, delusion and psychosis. It can occur in chronic ALCOHOLISM, BERIBERI and STARVATION. Some alcoholics apparently possess enzymes that require higher than normal levels of thiamin for energy production from carbohydrate. When the diet is depleted in B vitamins and the need for B vitamins increases, these individuals are more prone to thiamin deficiency symptoms. Wernicke's disease represents a medical emergency. Massive doses of thiamin are used therapeutically. (See also MALNUTRITION; NEUROPATHY; PERIPHERAL.)

wheat   A cereal GRAIN that serves as a staple for one-third of the world's population. Wheat accounts for 40 to 60% of the calorie and protein intake in many developing countries. Wheat is related to other true grains including RICE, CORN, BARLEY and RYE. Wheat apparently developed from a wild grass in southwestern Asia, and it was cultivated as early as 6000 B.C. in the regions of China, Egypt and Iraq. The United States, southeastern European nations, India, Canada and Australia rank among the leading wheat producing countries. In the United States, wheat ranks second to corn in terms of total grain production and is still the most important cereal grain for human consumption. The general trend in grain consumption since the early 1900s has been a gradual decline as processed sugar and fat have become more prominent carbohydrates.

During the 1960s new high-yield strains of wheat and rice were developed and cultivated in the Philippines, Mexico, India and Pakistan. These advances, together with increased use of pesticides and irrigation, ushered in the GREEN REVOLUTION, which dramatically increased grain production. Despite the Green Revolution, domestic food production remains critical in many regions of the world.

Efforts continue to develop new strains of wheat. In the past, development of new wheat strains required up to 10 years. Now biotechnology offers new techniques for screening different strains and for breeding wheat. A new wheat strain is likely to be profitable for only an estimated 10 years before it is improved upon or becomes susceptible to pests and disease. Efforts are being directed toward breeding pesticide-resistant strains. Nonetheless, food production alone cannot eradicate hunger in countries disrupted by civil strife, breakdown of governmental services, drought, poverty, illiteracy and high birth rates.

Types of Wheat

Thousands of varieties of wheat exist today; currently about 100 varieties are cultivated in the United States. Wheat varieties fall into two broad categories: winter wheat and spring wheat. Winter wheat is planted in the fall and harvested the following summer in the midwestern United States. Spring wheat is planted in the spring in regions where winters are severe and harvested later in the summer. Most bread is made from hard, red winter wheat grown in the United States. As an example, durum wheat is grown mainly for PASTA, like spaghetti and noodles. Hard wheats contain a higher protein content than spring wheat. Soft, white winter wheat is best suited for pastries and Asian noodles.

Wheat Products

Wheat berries are kernels after the chaff (husk) has been removed by threshing. The wheat kernel has a tough outer layer with FIBER (BRAN); a soft, oily, nutrient-rich section (germ); and a starchy endosperm or inner core that represents about 80% of the kernel. The endosperm is the source of wheat flour.

Wheat germ represents 2.5% of the kernel. It contains many nutrients, including essential fatty acids and high-quality protein. Wheat germ can be used to supplement cereals, breads, cookies and hot dishes. Because wheat germ can become rancid, it should be refrigerated after opening the container or frozen for long-term storage.

The kernel is surrounded with a tough outer coating called bran. Milling or grinding wheat kernels separates the starchy endosperm from the germ and bran to produce flour. Stone ground flour is thought to be more nutritious because the flour is not heated as much as it is in conventional milling. Different types of wheat yield flour with different properties. For example, bakery flour with a higher protein concentra-

tion creates doughs strong enough to permit extensive mechanical kneading.

Wheat flour contains a protein fraction called GLUTEN, consisting of GLIADEN and glutenin. When mixed with water they form an elastic dough that traps the carbon dioxide released by LEAVENING AGENTS. This accounts for the unique leavening properties of wheat doughs. The use of leavening agents is credited to the Egyptians who introduced yeast.

Representative Nutrient Contents of Wheat

Nutrient	Whole Wheat	White Flour*
Energy, calories	330	355
Crude fiber	2.3 g	0.3 g
Linoleic acid	1.5 g	0.75 g
Protein	13 g	11 g
Biotin	0.010 mg	0.002 mg
Vitamin B$_6$	0.30 mg	0.05 mg
Calcium	35 mg	17 mg
Choline	170 mg	80 mg
Chromium	0.06 mg	0.02 mg
Copper	0.5 mg	0.1 mg
Vitamin E	1.5 IU	0.03 IU
Fluoride	0.1 mg	0.06 mg
Folic acid	0.04 mg	0.01 mg
Vitamin K	0.017 mg	0.004 mg
Iron	3.0 mg	0.6 (3.0) mg
Magnesium	140 mg	25 mg
Manganese	3 mg	0.3 mg
Molybdenum	0.05 mg	0.025 mg
Niacin	5 mg	1.0 (5.3) mg
Pantothenic acid	1.0 mg	0.5 mg
Phosphorus	350 mg	90 mg
Potassium	400 mg	90 mg
Riboflavin	0.12 mg	0.04 (0.4) mg
Selenium	0.04 mg	0.03 mg
Thiamin	0.5 mg	0.09 (0.64) mg
Zinc	3 mg	0.6 mg

*Based on 60% to 72% extraction white flour, per 100 g (13% moisture basis). Values in parentheses are after U.S. enrichment and are valid only for iron, niacin, riboflavin and thiamin. Amounts are representative of U.S. samples, which may vary widely in composition especially for minerals.

Beating or kneading dough traps air bubbles in the mixture to give baked goods a lighter texture. Starch yields glucose, which is broken down by the yeast enzymes to carbon dioxide. Bubbles of carbon dioxide are trapped in elastic doughs. Alternatively, BAKING POWDER can be used as a leavening agent; it contains chemicals that yield carbon dioxide upon mixing and heating the dough.

White bleached flour accounts for more than 95% of the wheat flour used in the United States. In terms of nutrients, the annual consumption of 120 lb of refined wheat products per year is comparable to consuming 30 lb of whole wheat plus 90 lb of pure starch. White flour is aged to increase its elasticity as a dough, using several oxidizing agents to modify gluten. It may contain phosphate and other additives to shorten kneading time. All-purpose flour was developed in the 1960s for greater convenience in home cooking. The flour does not form clumps readily, it is dust free, and it disperses in cold water. Special flours have also been developed for cakes, pastries, Italian and French breads and rolls. The food label will indicate whether the flour has been bleached.

Whole wheat flour represents 95% of the whole kernel contents. It provides all common nutrients except VITAMIN A, VITAMIN B$_{12}$, VITAMIN C and IODINE. Whole wheat also contains trace minerals like tin and nickel for which there is no established role in the body. The amounts of nutrients vary according to the variety of wheat and the soil conditions where it was grown. Whole wheat flour is less stable than bleached white flour because it contains wheat germ oils and can become rancid upon storage. Whole wheat flour should be used soon after purchase and refrigerated to preserve freshness.

White flour represents a refined or purified carbohydrate with lesser amounts of key nutrients than whole wheat flour. The production of white flour requires about two dozen different steps that remove or destroy substantial amounts of nutrients found in whole wheat. White flour retains starch and about 70% of the protein, but losses of other nutrients average 70 to 80%. In order to partially remedy this deficiency, an enrichment program increases the levels of IRON, THIAMIN and NIACIN to those approximating whole wheat. RIBOFLAVIN is increased threefold; CALCIUM is often added. Canada and Britain have similar enrichment programs. Other nutrients—including FOLIC ACID, VITAMIN B$_6$, VITAMIN E, BIOTIN, CHROMIUM, COPPER, MAGNESIUM, MANGANESE ZINC and fiber—are not added back. All white flour produced in the United States is enriched, as are about 90% of commercial baked goods prepared from white flour. The accompanying table compares the nutrient contents of whole wheat, non-enriched white flour and enriched flour.

(See also BREAKFAST CEREAL.)

white blood cells   See LEUKOCYTES.

WIC (Supplemental Food Program for Women, Infants, Children)

A federal program initiated in 1972 to improve pregnant women's health and the health of their children by providing them with a good diet. Since 1972 WIC has assisted state agencies in giving food to impoverished women and children. Due to sharp increases in food prices, and a scarcity of funding, thousands of recipients in many states were dropped from assistance programs in 1990, when a House Select Committee on Hunger found at least 50,000 people were dropped in 27 states. In 1992 the program had 5.0 million enrolled women and cost $2.6 billion yearly.

The original philosophy was preventative, rather than therapeutic. Full disclosure of a comprehensive study of its efficacy revealed that between 1972 and 1980 WIC reduced infant mortality. There is a possibility that WIC food supplements might have increased skull growth and mental development in poor children. Other studies since 1980 have shown that adequate prenatal nutrition helps prevent low birth weight babies and reduces long-term medical expenses that would otherwise be publicly financed. The U.S. General Accounting Office reported that the WIC funding of $2.6 billion for 1992 paid for itself in a year due to reduced health costs.

Each state WIC program authorizes food that will be redeemable with WIC checks. WIC clients are provided with coupons to obtain fresh fruit and vegetables, in addition to milk, eggs, cheese, cereal, juice and infant formula. WIC actively promotes breastfeeding, but the program supplies formula for infants up to one year of age. For any new food to be authorized, in general the food manufacturer must submit a request for authorization, the product must meet state requirements in packaging, the food must be available statewide, and the product must be consistent with the WIC program promotion of healthy, economic food purchasing practices. (See also PREGNANCY AND NUTRITIONAL REQUIREMENTS; SCHOOL LUNCH PROGRAM.)

Auruch, S. Cackley, A.P., "Savings Achieved by Giving WIC Benefits to Women Prenatally," *Public Health Report*, 110:7 (Jan–Feb 1995), pp. 27–34.

Buescher, P.A., Larson, L.C., Nelson, M.D. Jr, Lenihan, A.J., "Prenatal WIC participation can reduce low birth weight and newborn medical costs: a cost benefit analysis of WIC participation in North Carolina," *Journal of the American, Dietetic Association,* 93 (February 1993), pp. 163–66.

wild rice (*Zizania aquatica*; Indian rice)

The only native cereal GRAIN domesticated in North America. Wild RICE grows in Minnesota and Wisconsin in the United States, and in Manitoba, Canada. Harvesting has traditionally been performed by hand because kernels of wild rice fall off the stalks as they ripen. Improved varieties can be harvested mechanically like wheat and barley, and 90% of the annual wild rice crop in Minnesota is grown in paddies and harvested by combines.

Wild rice is cooked like regular rice: The larger the kernel and the darker its color, the longer the required cooking time. Its protein content is higher than typical grains. The nutrient content of a half-cup (100 g) of cooked wild rice is: 92 calories; protein, 3.6 g; carbohydrate, 11 g; fiber, 2.6 g; fat, 0.2 g; iron, 1.1 mg; thiamin, 0.11 mg; riboflavin, 0.16 mg; niacin, 1.6 mg.

wine

The fermented juice of grapes. When other fruit juices are fermented, the name of the fruit is given, as in blackberry wine or plum wine. Archaeological evidence indicates that wine was prepared between 6000 and 5000 B.C. in the Middle East. Wine making was described in Egypt by 2500 B.C. American grapes, *Vitus labrusca*, are pest-resistant, and European varieties, *V. vinifera*, are grafted onto American root stocks. The Concord grape, developed in 1852 in Massachusetts, yields a full-bodied wine. Grapes grown in cooler regions of California, Oregon and Washington yield grapes with the higher acid content and the low to medium alcohol content of typical table wines. Dessert wines require grapes with a high sugar content.

To prepare wine, grapes are crushed and treated with sulfur dioxide to kill wild yeasts on the grapes. Additional dextrose (glucose) may be added if the sugar content is inadequate and the mixture is inoculated with a culture of a pure yeast strain. Fermentation is then carried out in temperature-controlled vats. Red wines are produced by fermenting grape pulp with skins; white wines are fermented with only minimal contact with skin. After fermentation the wine is clarified by adding gelatin or egg white protein to coagulate suspended materials. After settling, the mixture is filtered. Most wine is mellowed by aging from several months to several years to remove bitter or harsh flavors. Among the many chemical changes that occur, acidic substances slowly form fragrant compounds called esters. Wooden barrels have traditionally been used for aging because they absorb astringent substances and contribute their own subtle flavors. Wine is filtered and usually treated with sulfur dioxide to prevent spoilage. Aging continues after the wine is bottled.

Drinking red wine may lower LDL (LOW-DENSITY LIPOPROTEINS), the less desirable form of blood cholesterol. During fermentation of grape skins, a compound called resveratrol leaches out of the skin. Resveratrol is responsible in part for the cholesterol-lowering effect of red wine in experimental animals. It occurs naturally in grapes and offers natural protection against fungus. Heat treatment of Concord grapes, used to prepare red grape juice, releases resveratrol also. The cholesterol lowering effect of alcoholic beverages declines rapidly after more than one or two drinks are consumed daily. Alcohol is inappropriate for people with a history of ALCOHOLISM, HYPERTENSION, liver disease, smoking, DIABETES, OBESITY or PEPTIC ULCERS.

Red wine contains substantial amounts of IRON. However, the amounts of most nutrients found in grapes are quite low. Red wine also contains a mixture of FLAVONOIDS, complex plant substances that can function as ANTIOXIDANTS. Test-tube experiments demonstrated that red wine flavonoids can protect LDL-cholesterol, the most prevalent form of cholesterol in blood, from oxidation. Whether this occurs in the body remains unclear. The so-called "French Paradox" describes the phenomenon of those who consume wine, together with substantial animal fat and meat, yet have lower rates of heart disease than those who do not consume wine. Moderate consumption of alcoholic beverages, regardless of the source, raise HDL-cholesterol, the beneficial form. In addition, the MEDITERRANEAN DIET entails a higher consumption of fruits, legumes and vegetables than in the typical U.S. diet. These factors also decrease the risk of heart disease. Wine like all alcoholic beverages has a low nutrient density and displaces more nutrient-rich sources of calories when consumed in excess. An estimated 4% of domestic and imported wines contain 0.3 parts per million of LEAD. The lead cap can leach a lead residue that dissolves as the wine is poured. The nutrient contents of 3.5 fl oz of wine is: 74 calories; protein, 0.2 g; carbohydrate, 1.8 g; iron, 0.44 mg; potassium, 115 mg; riboflavin, 0.03 mg; niacin, 0.08 mg; and about 10 ml of pure ethanol. (See also BEER; CARDIOVASCULAR DISEASE.)

Vinson, Joe L. and Hontz Barbara, A. "Phenol Antioxidant Index: Comparative Antioxidant Effectiveness of Red and White Wines, *Journal of Agriculture and Food Chemistry*, 43 (1995), pp. 401–03..

World Health Organization (WHO)   A specialized agency of the United Nations founded in 1948 to promote international cooperation to improve health. Member governments finance WHO with annual contributions on the basis of their relative ability to pay. WHO works in conjunction with the FOOD AND AGRICULTURAL ORGANIZATION and it focuses on three areas:

1. International sanitary regulations. WHO provides current information regarding such matters as control of drug addicts, vaccination practices, advances in nutrition, cancer research and hazards of nuclear radiation. It standardizes quarantine measures.
2. Support of member health programs. Upon request, WHO provides technical advice, assists in setting up health centers and aids in training of medical personnel.
3. Control of epidemics. WHO promotes nationwide vaccination programs, clinics for disease prevention, clean water supplies and modern sanitation systems, health education, antibiotic use and insecticide application. It has helped wage campaigns against tuberculosis, smallpox, malaria and, more recently, the AIDS epidemic.

(See also GREEN REVOLUTION.)

xanthan gum   A food additive used as an emulsifier in salad dressing, syrup and pie fillings where viscous mixtures are desired. Xanthan gum is stable to heat and acidic conditions, making it a versatile stabilizer. A water-soluble POLYSACCHARIDE, xanthan gum is produced by bacteria and is considered a safe additive.

As a supplement, xanthan gum is a source of water-soluble FIBER, and it improves the body's ability to use glucose (BLOOD SUGAR), decreasing the need for INSULIN, the hormone responsible for lowering blood sugar. Xanthan gum improves GLUCOSE TOLERANCE in diabetics, apparently by slowing starch digestion and preventing glucose from being dumped into the bloodstream. Xanthan gum may also help lower blood CHOLESTEROL. (See also DIABETES MELLITUS; FOOD ADDITIVES.)

xanthophyll   A yellow pigment related to BETA CAROTENE that cannot be converted to vitamin A. XANTHOPYLL belongs to the family of CAROTENOIDS, widely distributed yellow-orange pigments found in many plants. It is often added to poultry feed to color poultry skin yellow and to deepen the color of egg yolks. Consumers often associate these color changes with quality.

xenobiotic   Any compound found in the body that originated from the external environment. Xenobiotics represent a diverse group of chemicals, ranging from PESTICIDES to drugs, industrial solvents and cigarette tar. Xenobiotics are either stored in fatty tissues, such as adipose (fat) tissue and nerves, or they are processed by enzymes and eliminated through the bile, urine and, to a certain extent, in sweat. However, long-term exposure to environmental chemicals in the home or the workplace can lead to their build-up in the body, ultimately leading to illness.

Chemical modification of xenobiotics occurs chiefly in the LIVER; lungs, kidneys and intestines also play a role. Enzymes of these organs convert foreign compounds to more water-soluble forms, so that they can be excreted. To accomplish this feat, the body employs a battery of oxidizing enzymes, called Phase 1 enzymes. These enzymes require IRON, NIACIN and RIBOFLAVIN for their activity. A second battery of enzymes, called Phase 2 enzymes, then attaches compounds—including amino acids, sulfate and sugar acids—to the modified xenobiotic. The "conjugated" product is generally much more soluble in body fluids, is more easily excreted and is less harmful that the unprocessed *xenobiotic*. Key nutrients support Phase 2 processes: the sulfur-containing amino acid CYSTEINE, VITAMIN C, PANTOTHENIC ACID and niacin. (See also CANCER; DETOXICATION; GLUTATHIONE.)

Crotty, Brendan, "Ulcerative Colitis and Xenobiotic Metabolism," *Lancet*, 343:8888 (January 1, 1994), pp. 35–38.

xylitol   A sugar alcohol used as a sweetener. Xylitol is a derivative of a common pentose (small sugar) that is as sweet as SUCROSE (table sugar). Small amounts occur naturally in PLUMS, RASPBERRIES, STRAWBERRIES and vegetables like CAULIFLOWER and EGGPLANT. The commercial source is birch bark. Xylitol is used in sugar-free gum and diet foods like jams and jellies. It has little effect on BLOOD SUGAR.

Like other sugar alcohols, such as MANNITOL and SOR-BITOL, xylitol resists fermentation by oral bacteria. Early studies indicated that chewing sugarless gum sweetened with xylitol after eating sugar-rich foods reduced the rate of dental cavities. More recently, children given xylitol daily seemed to develop less tooth decay. Xylitol may interfere with decay-causing bacteria by blocking their utilization of other sugars. However, the safety of this additive is questionable. Bladder and adrenal gland tumors can form and organs can be damaged when animals consume xylitol for long periods. (See also ARTIFICIAL SWEETENERS; NATURAL SWEETENERS; TEETH.)

yam (*Dioscorea spp.*)   A starchy tuber of a tropical plant. Yams are unrelated to the rich SWEET POTATOES sold in the United States, which they resemble. Yams were cultivated in Africa and Asia as early as 8000 B.C. and are now a staple among people living in tropical regions. They are produced in West Africa, Southeast Asia and the Polynesian islands. The cush cush yam (*D. trifida*), the Asiatic yam (*D. alata*) and the white yam (*D. rotunda*) are important food yams. Yams can be baked, broiled, roasted or fried. Unlike sweet potatoes, true yams contain little BETA CAROTENE. Compared to POTATOES, yams contain the same amount of protein, but 50% more starch. They contain half as much vitamin C as potatoes.

Several varieties of yams contain ALKALOIDS, plant substances that possess powerful physiologic effects. The Asiatic bitter yam, *D. hispida*, contains diosorine, a toxin that can be removed by soaking or boiling it in water. Chinese yams, *D. opposita* and *D. batatas*, are used in Oriental medicine. Certain wild types of yams yield STEROIDS, hormone-like substances that have been used to prepare oral contraceptives and arthritis medications.

yeast   See BAKER'S YEAST; BREWER'S YEAST; CANDIDA ALBICANS.

yellow no. 5 and no. 6   See ARTIFICIAL FOOD COLORS.

yogurt   A fermented milk product. Yogurt is one of the oldest cultured dairy foods. Commercially, a mixture of fresh, skimmed and non-fat dry MILKS are inoculated with bacteria that ferment milk sugar to LACTIC ACID, which both curdles the milk and acts as a PRESERVATIVE.

In terms of nutrients, yogurt resembles the milk from which it was prepared, including the calcium content. The nutritional quality varies with the type of milk, type of lactic acid cultures, fermentation conditions, storage conditions and additives. Producers may add thickeners (CARRAGEENAN, modified starch, PECTIN or AGAR), non-fat dry milk solids and SUGAR, as well as fruit flavor, to yogurt. Acid-producing bacteria such as LACTOBACILLUS ACIDOPHILUS, *L. bulgaricus*, and *Streptococcus thermophilus* are sometimes added as well.

Various claims have been made regarding the possible health benefits of yogurt. Studies have shown that yogurt with live cultures of lactic acid-producing bacteria is tolerated by lactose-sensitive people, presumably due to the presence of bacterial enzymes capable of degrading LACTOSE (milk sugar) to simple sugars. The conjecture that yogurt offers protection against coronary heart disease by lowering blood CHOLESTEROL arose from observations of Masai tribesmen of East Africa who consume large amounts of yogurt-like foods, yet maintain low blood cholesterol levels. Subsequent studies have failed to support this hypothesis. Data on the effects of yogurt on gastrointestinal infections are conflicting. Yogurt's role in increasing longevity remains unproven.

Yogurt has become popular in the United States since the 1960s due to its convenience, the variety of flavors and its image as a health food. Many varieties of yogurt are available: fat and non-fat, plain and flavored, frozen yogurts and yogurt drinks. Yogurt may be pasteurized, so the live bacteria are destroyed. Manufacturers may add back acid-producing bacteria. Non-fat yogurt contains 6% of its calories as fat; low-fat yogurt, 24%; and whole milk yogurt, 48%. The nutrient content of 1 cup (227 g) of non-fat yogurt is: 127 calories; protein, 13 g; carbohydrate, 17.4 g; fat, 0.41 g; cholesterol, 4 mg; calcium, 452 mg; potassium, 579 mg; thiamin, 0.11 mg; riboflavin, 0.53 mg; niacin, 0.28 mg. One cup of yogurt made from whole milk (227 g) provides 138 calories; protein, 7.9 g; carbohydrate, 10.6 g; fat, 7.6 g; cholesterol, 29 mg; calcium, 275 mg; potassium, 216 mg; thiamin, 0.07 mg; riboflavin, 0.32 mg; niacin, 0.17 mg.

Hilton, Eileen, et al., "Ingestion of Yogurt Containing Lactobacillus Acidophilus as Prophylaxis for Candidal Vaginitis," *Annals of Internal Medicine*, 116:5 (March 1, 1992), pp. 353–57.

yo-yo dieting (diet-induced obesity)   A pattern of repeated losing and regaining of weight. This pattern of weight fluctuation may carry added health risks for overweight people. People whose weight fluctuates repeatedly suffer increased mortality from heart disease as well as other causes. With on-again off-again DIETING, some people may gradually adapt to using food more efficiently, possibly making weight loss more difficult with repeated dieting cycles, although there is no consensus on the long-term consequences.

There are other possibilities: Yo-yo dieting may increase a dieter's desire for fatty foods and it may lower self-esteem, leading to other ineffective weight-loss strategies. Fat regained after drastic weight loss tends to cluster in the upper body and the abdominal cavity. The so-called android pattern, with a waist to hip ratio greater than 1.0, increases the risk of CARDIOVASCULAR DISEASE. The National Task Force on the Prevention and Treatment of Obesity concluded that yo-yo dieting may not pose serious health risks (1994). OBESITY is a complex phenomenon due to many factors, including inheritance and environmental influences. More study is needed to define long-term health effects of repeated dieting. (See also WEIGHT MANAGEMENT.)

National Task Force on the Prevention and Treatment of Obesity, "Weight Cycling," *Journal of the American Medical Association*, 272 (1994), pp. 1196–1202.

zein   A protein from CORN. Zein is deficient in two dietary essential AMINO ACIDS, LYSINE and TRYPTOPHAN. High lysine varieties of corn have been developed to partially remedy this deficiency. Zein is commercially produced by treating cornmeal with alcohol. It is used as an edible coating for CANDY and shelled nuts and finds many industrial uses, ranging from paper coating to microencapsulation. (See also GLUTEN.)

zen macrobiotic diet   See MACROBIOTIC DIET.

zinc   An essential trace mineral nutrient required for a wide array of metabolic processes. The body contains about 2.2 g of zinc, more than any trace mineral except iron. The highest concentrations occur in the skin, prostate gland, eyes, nails and hair, though it is widely distributed among tissues. Over 100 different ENZYMES (biological catalysts) require zinc. For example, zinc is required by DNA polymerase, an enzyme required for the synthesis of DNA (responsible for inheritance), and by RNA polymerase, an enzyme required for the synthesis of RNA. RNA guides the synthesis of proteins using the genetic information stored in DNA. Gene activators that regulate the expression of genetic information often utilize proteins containing zinc to bind to specific regions on the DNA molecule.

Possible Roles in Maintaining Health

Other roles range from protection against oxidation to digestion and BLOOD SUGAR regulation. Thus zinc is classified as an ANTIOXIDANT when it functions as a cofactor for SUPEROXIDE DISMUTASE, the enzyme that disarms a particularly reactive form of oxygen. In digestion, the pancreatic PROTEASE, CARBOXYPEPTIDASE, requires zinc for its protein-degrading action. Furthermore, the hormone INSULIN is processed and packaged as a zinc complex. Zinc also aids the interaction of insulin with its target tissues to facilitate the uptake of blood sugar.

Zinc supports normal cell division and growth, the function of cell membranes, the IMMUNE SYSTEM, BONE calcification and the development and function of male reproductive organs. Many trace minerals and vitamins, including zinc, are required for normal growth and development. Zinc deficiency can cause birth defects, complicated deliveries and low birth weight, as well as impaired learning and delayed sexual development.

Immune system   It is well established that zinc stimulates the IMMUNE SYSTEM. Zinc activates T-lymphocytes, the soldiers and generals of the immune system. Furthermore, zinc deficiency in the womb can lead to a weakened immune system at birth and enhanced risk of infection in newborn infants. Furthermore, zinc deficiency may be partially responsible for the weakened immunity that so frequently accompanies AGING. Zinc supplementation can improve white cell counts and antibody production in healthy, elderly people. There are intriguing hints that the zinc status of some AIDS patients is marginal; these patients have a severely imbalanced immune system. Zinc may help lessen symptoms of such autoimmune diseases as

RHEUMATOID ARTHRITIS, when the body begins to attack its own tissues.

Cancer   A healthy immune system helps prevent cancer, and zinc-deficient animals are more sensitive to carcinogens (cancer-causing agents). Patients with prostate cancer have significantly lower zinc levels, as do those with esophageal cancer. Whether zinc supplementation alone corrects prostate enlargement or slows prostate cancer is unproven.

Male fertility   Zinc is implicated in normal prostate functions and male infertility. The male sex hormone, TESTOS-TERONE, may regulate zinc metabolism in the prostate, and zinc, in turn, may affect testosterone metabolism in the prostate. Zinc deficiency leads to a lowered sperm count as well as impotence, and initial studies suggest that zinc can be used therapeutically in these cases.

Vision   Zinc plays a role in vision. Conversion of VITA-MIN A to its biologically active form, retinal, requires zinc. Zinc-deficient alcoholics may suffer from night blindness, and zinc has been used in this situation. Aging frequently brings blindness. In certain cases zinc supplementation may slow the progress of vision loss due to this condition.

Tissue repair   Zinc seems to promote wound healing, particularly in zinc-deficient individuals. Zinc is necessary for tissue repair and growth. Zinc ointments have been used to treat ACNE.

Taste   Zinc deficiency leads to altered taste and smell sensitivity; diminished taste acuity may respond to zinc.

Requirements   The RECOMMENDED DIETARY ALLOWANCE for adults (25 to 50 years of age) has been set at 12 mg for women and 15 mg for men. Pregnancy and lactation increase a woman's requirements.

Sources   The best sources of zinc are animal products. SEAFOODS, MEAT and POULTRY provide readily absorbed forms of zinc. BREWER'S YEAST, whole GRAINS and BRAN contain zinc. Zinc in vegetables and grains is tightly bound, limiting its BIOAVAILABILITY. Recently zinc has been added to parenteral (IV) nutrient formulations and to breakfast cereals.

Marginal (subclinical) zinc deficiency can be a problem for many Americans. Early symptoms of a subclinical deficiency include loss of appetite, altered taste and smell, decreased appetite, as well as slow growth in children. Lethargy, white spots on fingernails, slow wound healing, impotence and delayed sexual development may follow. Chronic dieters, alcoholics, strict vegetarians, and young children with diets compromised by junk food often consume inadequate zinc and other trace nutrients. Some patients with EATING DISOR-DERS may be zinc deficient. Zinc may help patients recovering from injury or infection. Pregnant and lactating women require zinc and other trace minerals. Elderly people may rely on zinc-deficient foods, a situation that is compounded by their reduced ability to absorb trace minerals like zinc. Strenuous exercise increases zinc loss through sweating and increased excretion, consequently an athlete's need for zinc increases.

Factors that increase the need for zinc include kidney disease, diabetes, cystic fibrosis, INFLAMMATORY BOWEL DIS-EASE, inherited zinc deficiency, and the use of diuretics and laxatives. A high-fiber diet and foods containing PHYTIC ACID can bind trace minerals and limit zinc uptake when large amounts are eaten. Likewise, excessive COPPER, IRON or CALCIUM displace zinc and limit its uptake.

Safety   Zinc is relatively non-toxic, and modest zinc supplementation for insurance may be appropriate particularly when the diet is compromised or there is maldigestion or malabsorption. The ratio of zinc to copper should be about seven to one, the ratio of the RDAs. Symptoms of zinc excess include nausea, bloating, abdominal cramps, diarrhea and fever. A high zinc intake (100 to 300 mg daily) may suppress the immune system, lower HDL (HIGH-DENSITY LIPOPROTEIN, believed to protect against heart disease) and block the absorption of copper, creating a copper deficiency. Copper deficiency in turn can increase blood CHOLESTEROL (LDL, LOW-DENSITY LIPOPROTEIN, the undesirable form) and lower HDL, thus increasing the risk of CARDIOVASCULAR DISEASE. (See also ATHEROSCLEROSIS.)

Mares-Perlman, J.A., et al., "Zinc Intake and Sources in the U.S. Adult Population 1976–1980," *Journal of the American College of Nutrition*, 14:4 (1995), pp. 349–57.

Odeh, M., "The Role of Zinc in Acquired Immunodeficiency Syndrome," *Journal of Internal Medicine*, 231 (1992), pp. 463–69.

zymogen (proenzyme)   An inactive form of an enzyme that is converted in the body to an active enzyme. Examples include pepsinogen, secreted by the STOMACH to form PEPSIN for protein digestion in the stomach; chymotrypsinogen and trypsinogen secreted by the PANCREAS to form CHYMOTRYPSIN and TRYPSIN for protein DIGESTION in the intestine. Secretion of these DIGESTIVE ENZYMES as zymogens normally assures their safe transit through the cell before activation so they do not attack the tissue that is their source.

Index

Page numbers in **boldface** indicate article titles.

hyperacidity *see*
  hyperchlorhydria
hyperactivity (attention
  deficit-hyperactivity
  disorder, ADHD) 173–174,
  198, **234**, 413
hyperalimentation 234
hyperblastic/hypertrophic
  obesity 319
hypercalcemia 234
hyperchlorhydria
  (hyperacidity) 234–235
hypercholesterolemia 235
  atherosclerosis 36–37
  DNA mutations 141
  familial 164–165, 245
  low-density lipoprotein 276
  saturated fat 334
  tropical oils 428
  see also cardiovascular
    disease; coronary artery
    disease
hyperglycemia 55, 127, 213, 235
hyperinsulinism 235
hyperkalemia 235
hyperlipemia 235
hyperlipoproteinemia 235–236
hyperplasia 7, 236
hypertension (high blood
  pressure) **236–237**
  alcoholism link 12, 13
  angiotensin 22
  beta blocker therapy 47
  biochemical individuality
    51
  as cardiovascular risk 79,
    111, 112, 199
  diastolic pressure indicator
    55, 129
  diuretics for 140
  eclampsia 147
  free radicals 200
  MAO inhibitors treatment
    284
  nutrient deficiencies 411
  obesity link 319, 405
  potassium benefits 356
  pregnancy-related 146, 360,
    425
  pressor amines 362
  renin 379
  senility link 124
  sodium 139, 387, 400
  stress link 410
  stroke 410
  Syndrome X 80, 416
hyperthyroidism 237, 423
hypertriglyceridemia **237–238**,
  356
hyperuricemia 218, 238
hypervitaminosis 104, 238, 292,
  441, 444, 445, 448, 449
hypoalbuminemia 238
hypocalcemia 238
hypochlorhydria 137, 238
  achlorhydria vs. 3
  alkalemia 14
  causes 408–409
  gastrointestinal disorders 3,
    207
  intestinal flora effects
    249–250
  intrinsic factor 250–251, 445
  lupus erythematosus 277
  malabsorption 282
  parietal cells 338
  stomach acid booster 48
hypoglycemia, fasting 55, 99,
  213, 235, 238
hypoglycemia, postprandial
  238–239, 356
  cortisol 7, 113
  mood effects 194–195
  triggers 88, 161, 235, 248
hypokalemia 239
hypophysis *see* pituitary gland
hypothalamic-pituitary-adrenal
  axis (HPA axis) 26, **239**, 308,
  320, 352, 370, 422, 423

hypothalamus **239–240**
  ACTH regulation 7
  ADH release 26
  depression/imbalance link
    125
  enkephalins 152
  functions 151, 220, 229, 230,
    239–240, 260, 308, 319,
    332, 370, 409–410, 423
  hunger/thirst regulation
    29, 94, 213, 231, 239, 320,
    422, 453
  thyroid gland 423
  see also
    hypothalamic-pituitary-ad
    renal axis
hypothyroidism 124, 171, **240**,
  251, 305, 423

I

iatrogenic malnutrition *see*
  hospital-induced malnutrition
IBD *see* inflammatory bowel
  disease
IBS *see* irritable bowel syndrome
ibuprofen 21
ice cream 241
  carob bean gum 81
  consumption 145
  emulsifiers 150
  standard of identity
    405–406
  substitutes 119–120
  sucrose content 413
ICF *see* intracellular fluid
IDDM *see* diabetes mellitus
ideal body weight 224, **241–242**,
  319, 330
idiopathic **242**
IgA *see* antibodies; mucous
  membrane
IgE *see* antibodies; histamine
IgG *see* antibodies; gamma
  globulin
ileitis *see* Crohn's disease
ileum 1, 106, 138, **242**, 251, 398
illness (sickness) 242–243, 294
  epidemiology 156
  etiology 160
  nutraceutical foods 315–316
  signs 396
  stress linkage 410
  symptom 416
  syndrome 416
  see also deficiency disease;
    degenerative diseases; fat
    and chronic disease;
    immune system; *specific
    conditions*
imitation fat *see* fat substitute;
  Olestra; Simplesse(R)
imitation flour *see* flour
  substitute
imitation food 197, **243**, 286
  cheese 87
  fat 170–171, 318, 323, 396
  flour 183
  meat 288–289, 290, 421
  non-dairy 119–120, 241, 314
  nutritional equivalency
    definition 316–317
  processed 363
  shellfish 113, 202, 353, 416
immediate hypersensitivity *see*
  allergy, immediate
immune system **243–245**
  aging 8, 9
  AIDS 10–11
  allergen effects 15, 16
  anaphylactic reaction 16, 21
  antibodies 25, 243
  antigen 26, 243
  antioxidant boosters 9, 47
  chronic fatigue 99
  circulatory system 100
  DHEA 126–127
  digestive tract 398
  endorphin effects 352

food intolerance 190, 196
gamma globulins 25, 54,
  205, 244
garlic/onion benefits 11,
  205, 439
HPA axis 239, 309
illness 242, 243
interferon 248–249
iron 252, 253
leaky gut 267
leukocytes 54, 269–270
lymphatic system 278
lymphokines 243, 278
malabsorption 282
mast cell 286
nitric oxide production 312
nutrient deficiencies 411
phagocyte 347
psychoneuroimmunology
  245, 309, 370
selenium benefits 392
stimulants 217, 336
stress effects on 113, 245,
  370, 409–410
thymus gland 230, 423
vitamin A benefits 443
vitamin B6 benefits 445
vitamin C benefits 447
vitamin D hormone
  (calcitriol) 448
vitamin E benefits 449
zinc activation of 464–465
see also autoimmune
  diseases
immunity 244
immunoglobulins *see* gamma
  globulins
IMP *see* disodium inosinate
inborn errors of metabolism 245
  see also specific diseases
indigestion *see* acid indigestion;
  dyspepsia; gastritis
individuality *see* biochemical
  individuality
Indocin 12
indoles 64, 65, 73, 115
induction (enzyme) **245**
infant formula 245–246, 274
  aluminum compounds in 17
  chloride in 93
  corn oil as base 110
  in developing countries 232
  fortification 68, 297
  labeling rules 191
  nitrate in 312
  soy as base 402
taurine in 419
inflammation (inflammatory
  response) **246**
  analgesics for 21
  antineuritic 26
  cortisol reduction 113
  flavonoid benefits 24, 181,
    328
  histamine trigger 229
  leukotriene trigger 246, 270,
    271, 348
  mast cell 286
  prostaglandins 365
  tumeric as countering
    agent 430–431
  see also arthritis; asthma;
    colitis; dermatitis;
    diverticulitis;
    gallbladder; lupus
    erythematosus;
    pancreatitis
inflammatory bowel disease
  (IBD) 38, **246–247**, 250
  colitis 105–106
  Crohn's disease 115
  elemental diet 149
  leaky gut 266
inhibition 155, 173, **247**
inositol (myoinositol) 247, 274,
  349
Insecticide, Fungicide and
  Rodenticide Act of 1972 123,
  344, 346, 382

insecticides *see* pesticides
insect infestation of food
  247–248, 262
insoluble fiber *see* fiber
insulin 151, **248**, 334
  as anabolic stimulant 294
  blood sugar 55, 126, 173,
    213, 235
  cysteine 116
  diabetes 127, 248
  digestion 137
  fat metabolism 6, 294
  glucose tolerance factor 213
  hyperinsulinism 235
  obesity 320
  pregnancy 127
  resistance 248
  resistance/cardiovascular
    disease link 79, 80
  trans-fatty acid interference
    427
  zinc 464
insulin-dependent diabetes *see*
  diabetes mellitus
intercellular fluid *see* interstitial
  fluid
interferon 243, **248–249**
international unit (IU) 249, 444
interstitial fluid (intercellular)
  249
intestinal flora (bacteria)
  182–183, **249–250**, 266
  see also acidophilus;
    bacteria, intestinal;
    bifidobacteria; *Candida
    albicans*; *Escherichia coli*;
    Lactobacillus acidophilus
intestine 250
  digestive enzymes 138, 154
  lamina propria 265
  mucus secretion 136, 398
  vitamin synthesis 441
  see also gastrointestinal
    disorders
intestine, large *see* colon
intestine, small *see* small
  intestine
intoxication *see* alcohol
intracellular fluid (ICF) 56, 163,
  250, 452
intravenous feeding *see*
  parenteral nutrition
intrinsic factor **250–251**
  parietal cells 92, 338, 408
  pernicious anemia 22, 251,
    445
  vitamin B12 138, 251, 445
inulin 251
invert sugar 251, 412
iodine (iodide) **251**
  deficiency effects 122, 217,
    240
  pregnancy/lacation
    requirements 360
  RDA 376, 377
  RDI/USRDA 251, 378, 435
  RNI (Canadian) 377
iodized salt 189, 217, 251
iron 251–253
  aging deficiencies 9
  apoferritin 28, 174
  chelating agents 88
  deficiency, subclinical 121,
    252, 310, 412
  deficiency anemia 21–22,
    122, 252–253
  deficiency effects 252
  enriched/fortified products
    86, 187, 459
  as enzyme catalyst 295
  excessive deposits 225, 226,
    253
  ferritin 26, 28, 174, 252, 253,
    368, 427
  function 426
  heme as 225, 378
  immune system benefits 244
  malabsorption 282

pregnancy/lactation
  requirements 359
RDA 252–253, 376, 377
RDI/USRDA 378, 435
RNI (Canadian) 377
sources 120, 252, 340, 440,
  457
storage protein 174
supplement safety 253
transferrin 427
vitamin C effects on 448
irradiated food *see* food
  irradiation
irritable bowel syndrome (IBS;
  spastic colon) 197, 247, 250,
  253, 410
ischemia 253, 419
islets of Langerhans 151, 230,
  248
isoflavone 10, 27, 73, 181, **253**,
  268, 316, 351, 402
isoleucine 19, 54, 60, 158,
  253–254, 379
isoniazid 28
isothiocyanate 10, 254
  sources/health benefits 64,
    65, 115, 254, 316, 345, 350,
    351, 414, 439
isotretinoin 1
IU *see* international unit

J

jam 255
jaundice 50, 82, 225, 226, 255
jejunum 138, **255**, 398
jelly 255–256
Jewish dietary laws 261
joint inflammation *see* arthritis
joule 256, 261
juice 256
  citrus 101, 219, 325
  cranberry 53, 114, 203, 434
  fortified 187, 189, 197, 199
  fruit 203, 219, 404
  grape 219, 259
  orange 69, 153, 325
junk food 256–257
  advertising 7
  B complex inadequacy 44
  empty calories 150
  fast food as 165
  obesity 322
juvenile diabetes *see* diabetes
  mellitus

K

kabob 258
kaempferol 181
kale 106, **258**, 345
karaya gum 258, 405
kasha 220, **258**
kefir 258–259
kelp 14
keratin 116, **259**
ketchup (catsup) 259
keto acid 259
ketogenic 259, 269
ketone bodies **259**
  acetoacetic acid 2, 3
  acetone 2, 3
  acidosis 4
  beta hydroxybutyric acid 48
  blood-brain barrier passage
    by 54
  fasting 166
  starvation diets 130, 135,
    164, 407
  urine production 161, 211,
    260
ketosis 2, 23, 48, 54, 164, **259**
kidneys 259–260
  fluid balance 182, 453
  function 434
  mineralocorticoids 6, 13
  nephron 257–258, 307–308,
    434
  phosphate regulation 348
  renin 379